TYPE 1 DIABETES – PATHOGENESIS, GENETICS AND IMMUNOTHERAPY

Edited by **David Wagner**

INTECHOPEN.COM

Type 1 Diabetes – Pathogenesis, Genetics and Immunotherapy
Edited by David Wagner

CBS, Edition **2017**

Published by InTech

Janeza Trdine 9, 51000 Rijeka, Croatia

Notice
Statements and opinions expressed in the chapters are these of the individual contributors and not necessarily those of the editors or publisher. No responsibility is accepted for the accuracy of information contained in the published chapters. The publisher assumes no responsibility for any damage or injury to persons or property arising out of the use of any materials, instructions, methods or ideas contained in the book.

Publishing Process Manager Sandra Bakic

Technical Editor Teodora Smiljanic

Cover Designer InTech Design Team

Image Copyright Roxana Bashyrova, 2011. Used under license from Shutterstock.com

Additional hard copies can be obtained from orders@intechopen.com

Type 1 Diabetes – Pathogenesis, Genetics and Immunotherapy, Edited by David Wagner
p. cm.
ISBN 978-953-307-362-0

INTECH

open science | open minds

Contents

Contents

Contents

Preface

This book is a compilation that includes mechanisms of type 1 diabetes pathogenesis, genetics, beta cell replacement therapy and immunotherapies. Authors have reviewed current literature on each of these topics to provide an excellent compendium on current understanding of how type 1 diabetes evolves and progresses and on the current status of treatment strategies.

The etiology of diabetes remains a mystery. There are suggestions that viral or other environmental agents are causal. The autoimmune nature of the disease including CD4+ and CD8+ T cells have been extensively explored; yet why these cells become pathogenic and the underlying causes of pathogenesis are not fully understood. The section includes description of recently defined biomarkers for pathogenic T cells. There are many ventures in to immunotherapy, attempting to control auto-aggressive T and B cells and some of these approaches and rationales are discussed.

The section on genetics covers what is known from genome – wide associated studies (GWAS) and other studies. A section on imaging includes the current status of examining beta cells during diabetogenesis and a section on beta cell replacement describes the current status of that treatment option. This book is an excellent review of the most current understanding on development of disease, imaging of disease pathogenesis and treatment opportunities.

David Wagner,
Webb-Waring Center and Department of Medicine,
University of Colorado,
USA

Part 1

Pathogenesis

1

Autoimmunity and Immunotherapy of Type 1 Diabetes

Mourad Aribi
Tlemcen Abou-Bekr Belkaïd University
Algeria

1. Introduction

Type 1 diabetes, formerly termed insulin-dependent diabetes mellitus (IDDM), is a chronic organ-specific autoimmune disorder thought to be caused by proinflammatory autoreactive CD4+ and CD8+ T cells, which mediate progressive and selective damage of insulin-producing pancreatic beta-cells (Atkinson & Eisenbarth, 2001). The reduction of beta-cell mass leads to a lack of insulin and thereby loss of blood glucose control (Boettler & von Herrath, 2010).

The worldwide prevalence of T1D was estimated to be 171 million cases among the adult population (Wild et al., 2004). Its annual incidence varies widely from one country to another (from less than 1 per 100,000 inhabitants in Asia to approximately up to 25/100,000 population/year in North America, more than 30 per 100,000 in Scandinavia and up to 41/100,000 population/year in Europe). It is in steady increase across the globe, especially among children aged less than five years (Kajander et al., 2000; Vija et al., 2009).

According to the European Diabetes (EURODIAB) study group, the prevalence of T1D in Europe will increase significantly in children younger than 15 years of age to reach 160,000 cases in 2020 (Patterson et al., 2009). These data will result in an increasing number of patients with longstanding diabetes and with a risk of serious complications (Kessler, 2010). These include heart diseases and strokes, high blood pressure, renal failure and ketoacidosis (DKA) (Boettler & von Herrath, 2010).

To date, it has not been possible to prevent the autoimmune response to beta-cells in human, due probably to its unknown aetiology, although it is known that development of T1D is genetically controlled and thought to be initiated in susceptible individuals by environmental factors such as virus infections (Luo et al., 2010; Mukherjee & DiLorenzo, 2010; von Herrath, 2009).

It is now evident that targeted destruction may go undetected for many years, but antibodies to various beta-cell antigens can be easily demonstrable in the sera of patients at risk before clinical onset (Achenbach et al., 2005). Additionally, some endogenous insulin secretion is generally present at the onset of clinical diabetes (Scheen, 2004), during which time, immunotherapeutic intervention may be effective (Staeva-Vieira et al., 2007).

This chapter emphasizes the principal immunological risk markers of T1D and especially the role of cell-mediated immune response leading to pancreatic beta-cells destruction, as well as the most promising immunotherapeutic approaches for prevention and treatment of the disease.

2. Autoimmunity of the type 1 diabetes

The autoimmune nature of T1D is initially affirmed by several arguments that are primarily indirect, including the association with other autoimmune diseases (Barker, 2006), such as the autoimmune thyroid disease (Hashimoto thyroiditis or Graves disease) (Criswell et al., 2005; Levin et al., 2004), Addison disease (Barker et al., 2005), myasthenia or Biermer's anemia, and the detection of various autoantibodies (Seyfert-Margolis et al., 2006) and islet lymphocytes infiltrates (Bach, 1979).

2.1 Humoral markers of type 1 diabetes

Although T1D is primarily mediated by mononuclear cells (Carel et al., 1999), diagnosis means of the preclinical period are primarily markers of humoral immune response that are represented, for instance, by antibodies to beta-cell antigens, including glutamic acid decarboxylase 65, insulin, insulinoma-associated protein 2 islet tyrosine phosphatase, islet cell cytoplasm and more recently zinc transporter 8 (Luo et al., 2010) (Fig. 1). Studies of twins or in subjects with a family history of autoimmune diabetes have shown that these markers, when associated in the same subject, confer very high risk of developing diabetes within 5 years (Verge et al., 1996). The predictive value increases from less than 5% in the absence of antibodies to more than 90% when antibodies to GAD, tyrosine phosphatase IA-2 and insulin are present (Bingley et al., 1999; Verge et al., 1996). Additionally, taken in aggregate, the use of the level of autoantibody can provide additional predictive information for the persistence of autoantibodies and development of T1D (Barker et al., 2004). Moreover, among metabolic risk markers, the loss of first phase insulin response to intravenous glucose has the same prediction value with multiple positive antibodies when it is associated with one of these autoantibodies (Krischer et al., 2003). Furthermore, the predictive value of having multiple autoantibodies can increase significantly by the presence of a high-risk genotype, with a positive predictive value of 67% in multiple antibody-positive DR3/4 individuals, versus 20% in those without DR3/4 (Yamamoto et al., 1998). While, high sensitivity and specificity are required for detection of prediabetes in the general population where the prevalence is of the order of 0.3% even when genetic susceptibility markers are also included (Hermann et al., 2004).

2.1.1 Islet cell autoantibodies

These are markers with best predictive value (Bonifacio & Christie, 1997), because of their high sensitivity to the pancreatic insulite (Kulmala et al., 1998) and their high specificity for T1D (Gorsuch et al., 1981).

Islet cell autoantibodies (ICAs) have been the first disease-specific autoantibodies to be described in patients with T1D (Bottazzo et al., 1974). They appear until ten years before the clinical onset of diabetes (Riley et al., 1990). ICA corresponds to a compounding of different specificities antibodies, because they can be fixed on all cellular types of antigenic structures present in the islet cell cytoplasm (Atkinson & Maclaren, 1993).

High ICA levels could be a marker of strong autoimmune reaction and accelerated depletion of beta-cell function (Zamaklar et al., 2002). In prediabetic subjects, a higher ICA titer is associated with a higher risk for T1D development (Mire-Sluis et al., 2000). In newly diagnosed type 1 diabetic patients, ICAs are present in 80%, and ICA reactivity often waned after diagnosis, with no more than 5% to 10% of patients remaining ICA positive after 10

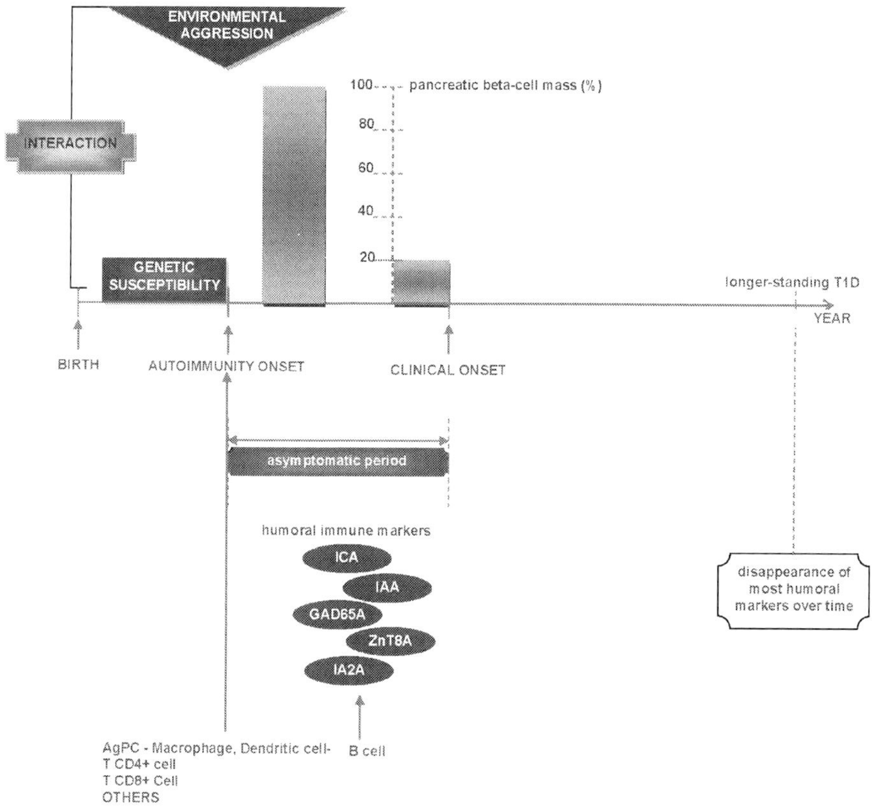

Fig. 1. Natural history of type 1 diabetes. *AgPC: antigen-presenting cell; GAD65A: glutamic acid decarboxylase 65 autoantibody; IAA: insulin autoantibody; ICA: islet cell autoantibody; ZnT8A: zinc transporter 8 autoantibody.*

years (Gilliam et al., 2004). The frequency of the positive ICA is 80% to 100% (Schatz et al., 1994) of revelation for a 25 years old T1D or less (Elfving et al., 2003). It decreases remotely by the primo-decompensation, reaching approximately 3% in related subjects aged of less than 20 years (Schatz et al., 1994).

ICAs are highlighted by indirect immunofluorescence (Borg et al., 2002a; Elfving et al., 2003; Perez-Bravo et al., 2001) on sera incubated with human blood group O pancreas (Takahashi et al., 1995; Thivolet & Carel, 1996). They can be also detected by complementary-fixing antibody (Knip et al., 1994; Montana et al., 1991), since they mainly belong to the IgG1 subclass antibodies (Bottazzo et al., 1980). The increase in ICAs may indicate the presence of other autoantibodies, corresponding to more IgG1subclasses (Dozio et al., 1994). Association with other autoantibodies increases the test specificity, with a decrease in sensitivity however (Thivolet & Carel, 1996). ICA levels that exceed 80 JDF (Juvenile Diabetes Foundation) units at the time of diagnosis despite better beta-cell function are associated with short clinical remission (Zamaklar et al., 2002), and include 53% of disease development risk in five years following their revelation (Dozio et al., 1994). Nevertheless, the high levels of ICA found in the family relatives do not necessarily lead to T1D development (Bingley, 1996). Likewise, the low rates of these antibodies lessen the disease risk (Bonifacio et al., 1990).

2.1.2 Insulin autoantibodies

It would be important to recall that protective alleles of insulin gene *INS VNTR* (variable number of tandem repeats) are associated with higher levels of *INS* messenger RNA expression in the thymus (Aribi, 2008; Pugliese et al., 1997; Vafiadis et al., 1997). Insulin would then be the main antigens engaged in thymic T cell education and immune tolerance induction. Therefore, it has been the first diabetes-related autoantigen to be identified (Gilliam et al., 2004).

Insulin autoantibodies (IAAs) are of weak prevalence at the time of diagnosis (Breidert et al., 1998). Their levels are increased especially in prediabetics (Palmer et al., 1983), but also in newly diagnosed type 1 diabetic subjects. Additionally, IAAs could be confused with insulin antibodies (IAs) produced following injection of exogenous insulin; therefore, we cannot assess the real level of IAAs in treated patients (Gilliam et al., 2004).

On the other hand, various studies have shown that the elevated IAA frequency and levels are observed mainly in young children (Landin-Olsson et al., 1992) and HLA DR4 subjects (Achenbach et al., 2004; Savola et al., 1998; Ziegler et al., 1991). Moreover, IAAs could be detected in all children who develop diabetes when they are associated with multiple autoantibodies. Furthermore, these antibodies confer high risk in T1D relatives (Ziegler et al., 1989), essentially in combination with other autoimmune markers (Bingley et al. 1999; Thivolet et al., 2002; Winnock et al., 2001). However, the actual frequency of positivity varies considerably from one study to another, according to the IAA assay, age at diagnosis, as well as the populations studied (Gilliam et al., 2004).

Interestingly, IAAs do not necessarily reflect beta-cell destruction. Indeed, they have been reported to occur in other autoimmune diseases, such as Hashimoto thyroiditis, Addison disease, chronic hepatitis, pernicious anemia, systemic lupus erythematosis, and rheumatoid arthritis (Di Mario et al., 1990).

IAAs can be detected by two assay methods, a fluid-phase radioimmunoassay (RIA) and a solid-phase enzyme-linked immunosorbent assay (ELISA); however, it has been shown that IAAs measured by RIA were more closely linked to T1D development than those measured by ELISA (Murayama et al., 2006; Schlosser et al., 2004; Schneider et al., 1976; Wilkin et al., 1988).

2.1.3 Glutamic acid decarboxylase autoantibodies

Of note, a 64kDa islet cell protein was initially isolated by precipitation with autoantibodies present in sera of patients with T1D (Baekkeskov et al., 1982). After laborious searches, this protein was identified as glutamic acid decarboxylase (GAD) (Baekkeskov et al., 1990); the enzyme that synthesizes the gamma-aminobutyric acid neurotransmitter in neurons and pancreatic beta-cells (Dirkx et al., 1995). At that time, GAD autoantibodies had been demonstrated to have a common identity in patients with stiff-man syndrome (SMS) and T1D (Baekkeskov et al., 1990; Solimena et al., 1988). During the same period, GAD complementary deoxyribonucleic acid (GAD cDNA) cloning demonstrate that there are two different genes of GAD, designated GAD1 and GAD2 (Bu et al., 1992; Erlander et al., 1991; Karlsen et al., 1991), located on chromosome 2q31.1 and chromosome 10p11.23, respectively (Bennett et al., 2005). GAD1 mRNA has been reported to be translated into GAD67, which is not detected in human islets (Karlsen et al., 1991), but is predominantly found in mouse islets (Petersen et al., 1993; Velloso et al., 1994). The mRNA for GAD2 gene encodes the GAD65kDa isoform that is expressed in human pancreatic islets and brain (Gilliam et al., 2004).

GAD65 autoantibodies (GAD65A) are revealed in 70% to 80% of cases among prediabetic subjects and newly diagnosed patients (Kulmala et al., 1998). They are considered as a good retrospective marker of the autoimmune progression, because of their persistence in the sera of patients with T1D for many years following diagnosis (Borg et al., 2002b). Whereas, these antibodies have a low positive predictive value for beta-cell failure (47%) compared to ICAs (74%) (Borg et al., 2001) and can be revealed in patients with neurological disorders, including those with gamma-aminobutyric acid (GABA)-ergic alterations (Piquer et al., 2005; Solimena et al., 1990). Similarly, they can be present in patients who have other autoimmune diseases (Davenport et al., 1998; Nemni et al., 1994; Tree et al., 2000) as well as in patients with type 2 diabetes (Hagopian et al., 1993; Tuomi et al., 1993). Consequently, they don't seem to be specific to pancreatic beta-cells destruction (Wie et al., 2004; Costa et al., 2002).

GADAs are usually detected by radioligand-binding assay, which is reported to have higher sensitivity, specificity, and reproducibility than other methods using ELISA, enzymatic immunoprecipitation, and immunofluorescence assays (Damanhouri et al., 2005; Knowles et al., 2002; Kobayashi et al., 2003).

2.1.4 Anti-tyrosin phosphatase autoantibodies

These antibodies are directed against two digestion fragments (Jun & Yoon, 1994; Maugendre et al., 1997) resulting from trypsin hydrolysis of transmembrane protein expressed in islets and the brain, and are present in two related forms with distinct molecular weights, 40kDa and 37kDa (Bonifacio et al., 1995a; Li et al., 1997; Yamada et al., 1997).

Of note, the 40kDa antigen is the receptor tyrosine phosphatase-like protein IA-2 associated with the insulin secretory granules of pancreatic beta-cells (Trajkovski et al., 2004), also called islet cell autoantigen 512 (ICA512)/IA-2 (Bonifacio et al., 1995b; Payton et al., 1995). The 37kDa antigen is a tryptic fragment related protein tyrosine phosphatase, designated IA-2β/phogrin (Kawasaki & Eisenbarth, 2002), or islet cell autoantigen-related protein tyrosine phosphatase (IAR) (Lu et al., 1996).

It has been shown that antibodies to the two antigens have similar sensitivity; however, epitope mapping studies have suggested that antibodies to IA-2 (IA-2A, insulinoma-associated protein 2 islet tyrosine phosphatase) appear to be more important for the pathogenesis of T1D than those to IA-2β (Savola, 2000; Schmidli et al., 1998). In fact, the binding of phogrin autoantibodies could be totally blocked if adding ICA512 to sera positive for both ICA512 and phogrin, while the binding of ICA512 antibodies cannot be fully blocked with phogrin (Savola, 2000).

IA-2As can be evaluated by radioligand-binding assay and ELISA (Bonifacio et al., 2001; Chen et al., 2005a; Kotani et al., 2002); whereas, RIAs performed much better than ELISAs, as was found for GAD65A assays (Verge et al., 1998).

2.1.5 Zinc transporter 8 autoantibodies

The human beta-cell-specific zinc transporter Slc30A8 (ZnT8) is a member of the large cation efflux family of which at least seven are expressed in islets (Chimienti et al., 2004). It has been recently defined as a major target of humoral autoimmunity in human T1D based on a bioinformatics analysis (Dang et al., 2011; Wenzlau et al., 2009). Autoantibodies to ZnT8 (ZnT8A) have been therefore detected in high prevalence in newly diagnosed type 1 diabetic patients (Yang et al., 2010) and obviously overlap with GADA, IA2A, and IAA (Wenzlau et al., 2007).

Of note, ZnT8 autoimmunity could be an independent marker of T1D, given that ZnT8As can be present in antibody-negative individuals and in type 2 diabetes, and in patients with other autoimmune disorders (Wenzlau et al., 2008).

Antibodies to ZnT8 can be measured by radioimmunoprecipitation assay using 35^S labelled methionine *in vitro* translation products of different fragments of human ZnT8 (Lampasona et al., 2010).

2.2 Immunological anomalies of type 1 diabetes and cellular autoimmunity

In reality, our understanding of the exact cellular immune mechanisms that lead to the development of T1D is limited, and it is possible that the potential target autoantigens may be less well defined and more diverse, probably because of the epitopes diversification.

The immune reaction against beta-cells is due primarily to a deficit in the establishment of central thymic tolerance and the activation of potentially dangerous autoreactive T cells and B cells that recognize islet antigens. Additionally, aggression of the beta-cells may be initiated by other cells and components of the innate immune system. In fact, it has been observed that the immune cells peripheral infiltration of the Langerhans islets, a process termed perished-insulitis, begins initially with the monocytes/macrophages and dendritic cells (DCs) (Rothe et al., 2001; Yoon et al., 2005; Yoon et al., 2001). Upon exposure to antigens, islet-resident antigen presenting cells, likely DCs, undergo maturation, leading to the expression of cell surface markers that are subsequently required for T cell activation in the pancreatic lymph nodes (panLN). CD4+ T cells and macrophages home to islets and release pro-inflammatory cytokines and other death signals that acutely trigger necrotic and pro-apoptotic pathways (Fig. 2).

2.2.1 T cells and B cells

Although both humoral and cell-mediated immune mechanisms are active during T1D, CD4+ and CD8+ T cells recognizing islet autoantigens are the main actors of beta-cells death (DiLorenzo et al., 2007; Gianani & Eisenbarth, 2005; Toma et al., 2005). B cells may play a role in inducing inflammation and presentation of self-antigen to diabetogenic CD4+ T cells (Silveira et al., 2007).

It has been repeatedly observed that the pancreatic islets of diabetic patients prior to and at diagnosis are infiltrated by T lymphocytes of both CD4 and CD8 subsets (Hanninen et al., 1992; Imagawa et al., 2001; Kent et al., 2005). Additionally, their circulating number among type 1 diabetic patients is higher than those of B cells (Martin et al., 2001). Moreover, the disease can be transferred to NOD-*scid* mice that are genetically deficient in lymphocytes (Christianson et al., 1993; Sainio-Pollanen et al., 1999; Yamada et al., 2003), or to newborn NOD mice exposed to atomic radiation (Miller et al., 1988; Yagui et al., 1992) by injection of T CD4+ and CD8+ spleenocytes from prediabetics. However, injection of anti-islets antibodies does not induce autoimmunity (Timist, 1996) and beta-cell damage may develop in individuals with severe B cells deficiency (Martin et al., 2001).

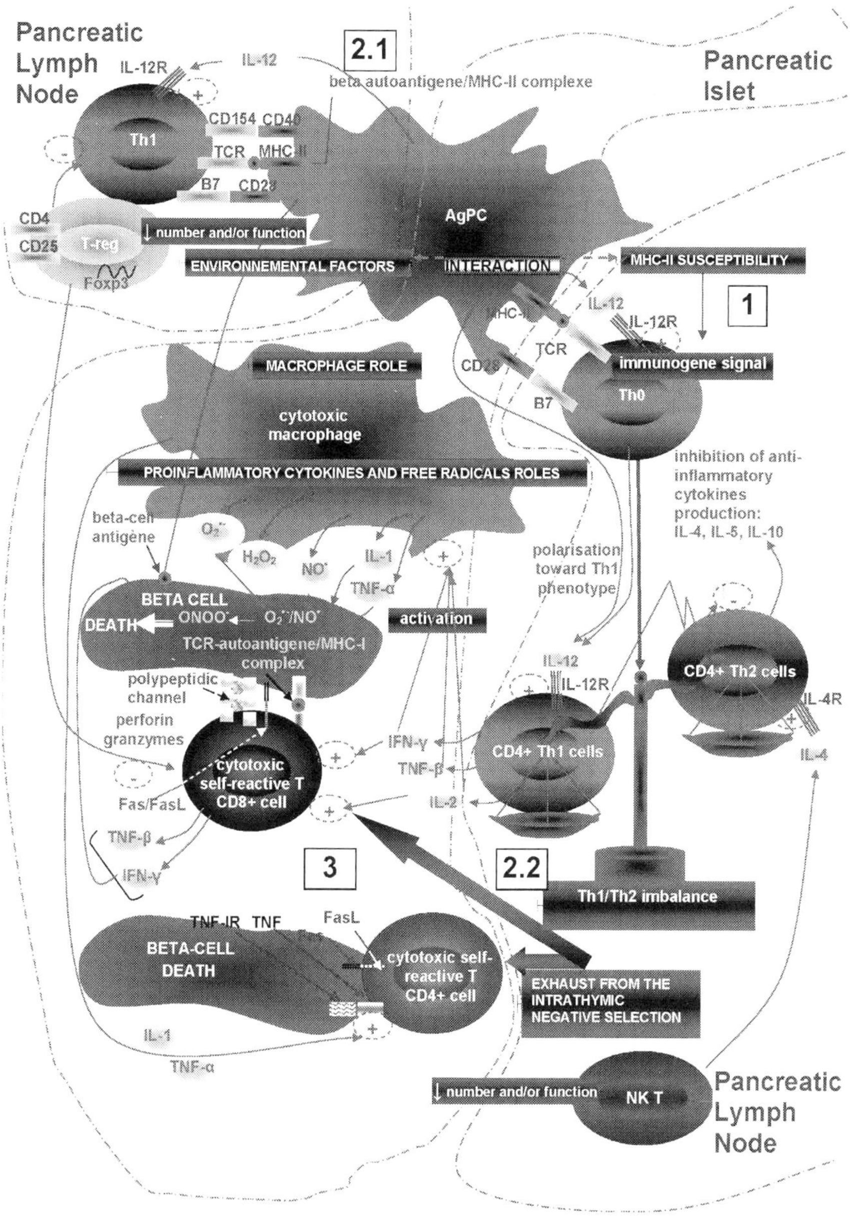

Fig. 2. Hypothetical scheme of the autoimmune response of type 1 diabetes: cellular interaction and molecules that can be involved within the destruction of pancreatic islets beta-cells. *(1) Antigen exposure and TCR signalling pathway: AgPC exposes epithopes derived from*

beta-cells on its membrane surface by some class II MHC molecules that are involved in the susceptibility of T1D. The autoantigens/class II MHC complex, adhesion molecules, particularly B7, IL-12 derived from AgPC, and possibly other immunogenic signals, could join and cause the activation of CD4+ Th0 cells. Many factors (physical, psychological, and chemical stress) are able to guide the Th0 differentiation towards Th1 cell. (2.1 and 2.2) Activation of Th1 cells: immunogenic signals resulting from class II MHC/peptide-TCR, CD40-CD154 and CD28-B7 interactions induce the activation of Th1 cells. (3) Beta-cells destruction: activated Th1 cells produce IL-2, TNF-β and IFN-γ cytokines, increasing the activation of islet-infiltrated macrophage and autoreactive cytotoxic CD8+ cells. These cells can destroy pancreatic beta cells by proinflammatory cytokines, granzymes and perforin, FasL-Fas interaction, and oxygen/nitrogen free radicals. Anomalies of autoreactive T cells suppression could be due to the decreased number and/or function of peripheral regulatory cells affecting both NK T cells and natural CD4+CD25+/CD25highFoxp3+ T-reg cells. AgPC: antigen-presenting cell, CD: cluster of differentiation, DC: dendritic cell, Fas/FasL: CD95/CD95 Ligand, Foxp3: transcription factor forkhead box P3, IFN: interferon, IL: interleukin, MHC: major histocompatibility complex, NK T: natural killer T cell, T1D: type 1 diabetes, TCR: T cell receptor, Th: T helper, TNF: tumor necrosis factor.TNF-RI: tumor necrosis factor receptor type I.

2.2.2 CD4+ and CD8+ T cells and ways of beta-cells destruction

The precise role of each of these cells in pancreatic islets destruction remains unclear and controversial. Therefore, two main pathways may be involved in triggering the disease, both of which are activated following recognition of beta-cell autoantigens.

According to the indirect way, the critical role in T1D development could be attributed to autoreactive CD4 T cells, as exemplified by the observation that the major histocompatibility complex class II (MHC II) genes are the main candidate genes to which a key role can be assigned in the autoimmune process according to their strong association with the disease (Aribi, 2008; Concannon et al., 2009). These cells can initiate beta-cells destruction and lead to tissue cell damage (Peterson & Haskins, 1996), through the secretion of cytokines with toxic effects (Amrani et al., 2000), then recruit T CD8+ lymphocytes (McGregor et al., 2004).

According to the direct way, autoreactive T CD8+ lymphocytes (Anderson et al., 1999) could initiate beta-cells destruction, as shown in transgenic TCR (NOD/ AI4αβ Tg) NOD mice, that T1D autoimmunity beginning can be achieved in total absence of CD4+ T cells and requires only CD8+ T cells (Graser et al., 2000). Additionally, disease development is reduced only when adult NOD mice are injected with anti-class I MHC molecules or anti-CD8 mAb molecules (Wang et al., 1996). Moreover, β2-microglobulin-deficient ($\beta 2m^{-/-}$) and anti-CD8 mAb-treated NOD mice, yet deficient in CD8+ T cells develop neither insulitis nor T1D (Yang et al., 2004).

However, direct evidence for these observations is compelling only in animal models in which adoptive transfer experiments are feasible ethically (Di Lorenzo et al., 2007). Additionally, several differences can be revealed between men and animal models of T1D. For example, in men, immunohistological studies of type 1 diabetic pancreatic-biopsy showed a strong number of islet-infiltrated CD8+ cytotoxic T cells compared to that of islet-infiltrated CD4+ T helper cells (Itoh et al., 1993). In contrast, in NOD mice, pancreatic islets are infiltrated predominantly by CD4 + T cells compared to CD8+ T cells (Kida et al., 1998).

2.2.3 Regulatory T cells/effectors T cells imbalance

The primary function of Treg cells is the maintenance of self-tolerance in order to prevent the development of autoimmune diseases (Sakaguchi et al., 1995). They also have the ability to control a runaway immune response by different feedback mechanisms, involving the production of anti-inflammatory cytokines, direct cell-cell contact or modulating the activation state of antigen-presenting cells (AgPCs) (Corvaisier-Chiron & Beauvillaina, 2010). Normal tolerance to self-antigens is an active process that has a central component and a peripheral component. Central tolerance implies induction of tolerance in developing lymphocyte when they encounter self-antigens that are present in high concentration in the thymus or bone marrow; while peripheral tolerance is maintained by mechanisms of self-reactive T cells elimination by clonal deletion, anergy or ignorance (Wallace et al., 2007). Among these three mechanisms only the deletion is induced by Treg cells (Corvaisier-Chiron & Beauvillaina, 2010).

Different subpopulations of Treg cells have been identified: natural Treg (nTreg) cells that drived from the thymus and migrate to peripheral tissues, and peripherally induced Treg (iTreg) (Corvaisier-Chiron & Beauvillaina, 2010). nTreg cells represent 2-4% of circulating lymphocytes in humans (Wahlberg et al., 2005) and are characterized by the expression of CD4, $CD25^{high}$, $CD127^{low}$ molecules and high levels of the transcription factor FoxP3 (forkhead box P3) (Corvaisier-Chiron & Beauvillaina, 2010; Wahlberg et al., 2005). They also express surface CTLA-4 (cytotoxic T lymphocyte-associated antigen 4) and GITR (TNF receptor family glucocorticoidinduced-related gene) involved in membrane mechanisms of Treg suppression (Corvaisier-Chiron & Beauvillaina, 2010).

Except pathological conditions, there is a balance between regulatory T cells and effector T cells. Some genetic and environmental factors might cause deregulation of this balance in favor of self-reactive lymphocytes that may induce or predispose to the development of autoimmune diseases, including T1D (Brusko et al., 2008).

In NOD mice and diabetic patients and in several organ-specific animal models of autoimmunity as well as in humans (Furtado et al., 2001; Kriegel et al., 2004; Kukreja et al., 2002), it has been demonstrated that number and/or function of peripheral regulatory cells affecting both nTreg cells (CD4+CD25+Foxp3+) (Fontenot et al., 2003; Hori et al., 2003; Khattri al., 2003) and natural killer (NK) T cells (Duarte et al., 2004; Hong et al., 2001) are decreased; while self-reactive peripheral T cells number is increased (Berzins et al., 2003). Additionally, decreased contacts between effectors and nT-reg cells seem to belong to additional events leading to autoreactive T cells activation and proliferation (Lindley et al., 2005; Maloy & Powrie, 2001; Piccirillo et al., 2005).

On the other hand, various studies showed that T1D in both humans and NOD mice could be due to the weak secretion of IL-4 resulting from a deficiency in NK T cells (Lehuen et al., 1998; Wilson et al., 1999) and that diabetes can be prevented in mice by transfer of NK T cell-enriched $CD4^{-}CD8^{-}$ double negative cells (Baxter et al., 1997; Falcone et al., 1999; Lehuen et al., 1998) or of thymic-derived nT-reg cells (Chen et al., 2005b; Lindley et al., 2005; Luo et al., 2007).

2.2.4 Regulatory T cells/Th17 cells imbalance

Th17 cells represent a subtype of T cells that can be generated in the presence of IL-23 even from cells deficient in transcription factors required for Th1 (T-bet) or Th2 (GATA-3) cells development (Harrington et al., 2005; Park et al., 2005). However, IL-23 would not be a factor for Th17 cells differentiation but rather intervene in their survival and proliferation. In fact, naive T cells do not express receptors for IL-23 and do not differentiate into Th17 cells only in the presence of IL-23 (Mangan et al., 2006). Additionally, Th17 cells express a specific transcription factor, RORC2 (retinoic acid receptor-related orphan receptor C2, known as RORγt in mice), which is crucial for the generation of Th17 cells, especially *via* the transcriptional induction of the gene encoding IL-17 and the expression of IL-23 receptor (Ivanov et al., 2006). To acquire a full differentiation of such cells, RORC2 acts in cooperation with other transcription factors, including RORα, STAT3, IRF-4 and Runx1 (Miossec et al., 2009).

The discovery of factors involved in the differentiation of Th17 and Treg cells suggests the existence of Treg/Th17 balance, controlled by IL-6 (Kimura et al., 2011). More recently, increased Th17 immune responses or imbalance of nTreg cells and IL-17 producing Th17 have been found to be associated to the onset of the disease in both humans and NOD mice or Diabetes-prone BioBreeding (DP-BB) rats (Honkanen et al., 2010; Shi et al., 2009; van den Brandt et al., 2010). While, these observations should be confirmed further.

2.2.5 Th1/Th2 imbalance

Different factors, including physical, psychological, and chemical stress (Ernerudh et al., 2004) can produce imbalance in the proportions of CD4+ Th1 cell and CD4+ Th2 cell subsets (Eizirik et al., 2001; Rabinovitch et al., 1994; Thorvaldson et al., 2005). Several studies have shown that the autoimmune aggression leading to T1D involves Th1 cells (Kida et al., 1999; Sharif et al., 2002; Yoon & Jun, 2005). However, Th2 cells seem to be associated with protection against beta-cells destruction (Cameron et al., 1997; Ko et al., 2001; Suarez-Pinzon & Rabinovitch, 2001).

In NOD mouse model, T1D can be transferred among animals through the injection of Th1 cells (Kukreja et al., 2002). T1D-sex relationship has been linked to the type of produced cytokines. Lymphocytes infiltrating female mice pancreatic islets produce high levels of Th1 cytokine mRNA and low levels of Th2 cytokine mRNA. On the other hand, male mice are more resistant to T1D because they produce more Th2 cytokine mRNA and less cytokine Th1 mRNA (Azar et al., 1999; Fox & Danska, 1997). Likewise, young NOD mice spleenocytes expressing CD62L and CD25, *i.e.* CD4+CD45RB^{low} (memory/activated cells) which are involved in dominant protection against T1D development, show an overproduction of Th2 cytokines, yet tend towards an overproduction of Th1 cytokines right before diabetes onset (Shimada et al., 1996). Besides, female NOD mice have more spleenocytes CD45RB^{low} CD4+ and more spleenocytes CD4+CD25+ activated helper cells than do male NOD mice have (Azar et al., 1999). Moreover, it is possible to prevent T1D in NOD mice with a single injection of insulin or GAD peptide (Han et al., 2005), because it causes a reduction in levels of Th1 cytokines and an increase in the ones of Th2 cytokines (Muir et al., 1995; Sai et al., 1996).

2.2.6 Innate immunity

It has been recently observed that innate immunity may play a critical role in the development of T1D. This observation has been supported by works showing that infusions of alpha-1 antitrypsin, a serine protease inhibitor that protects tissues from enzymes produced from inflammatory cells, were found to reverse new-onset diabetes in NOD mice (Koulmanda et al., 2008). Many effects have been described, including reduced insulitis, enhanced beta-cell regeneration, and improvement in peripheral insulin sensitivity (Luo et al., 2010).

Thanks to many experiments conducted in animal models, it has been shown that toll-like receptors (TLRs), as part of the innate immune system, may have an important role in T1D development (Filippi & von Herrath, 2010). For example, injection of low dose of TLR-3 stimulus poly I:C has been shown to prevent diabetes in the disease-prone Biobreeding rat model (Sobel et al., 1998). In addition, TLR deficiency has been associated with decreased number of some Treg. Indeed, T cells with a regulatory phenotype can express TLR-2, TLR-4, TLR-5, TLR-7 and TLR-8 (Caramalho et al., 2003; Sutmuller et al., 2006), and the proliferation of Treg cells has been observed especially following the administration of TLR-2 ligands to TLR-2-deficient mice (Sutmuller et al., 2006). Moreover, it has been suggested that protection against T1D in NOD mice through infection with Lymphocytic Choriomeningitis Virus (LCMV) is dependent on the emergence of Tregs and TLR-2 (Boettler & von Herrath, 2011).

2.2.7 Macrophages

Macrophages play a significant role in the oxidative stress (Ishii et al., 1999; Rozenberg et al., 2003), innate immunity (Bedoui et al., 2005; Lawrence et al., 2005) and inflammation (Ishii et al., 1999; Lawrence et al., 2005). Macrophages and other AgPCs in the panLN (Pearl-Yafe et al., 2007) initiate T cell sensitization, and concomitantly activate regulatory mechanisms (Kaminitz et al., 2007). The central role of macrophages in the cellular immune response (Durum et al., 1985) and in the development and activation of beta-cell-cytotoxic T cells during T1D (Yoon & Jun, 2001) has been previously proven in BioBreeding (BB) rats where a macrophage insulitis preceding lymphocyte insulitis could be prevented by a silica intraperitoneal injection (Albina et al., 1991). However, macrophages are also able to exert a suppressor effect on lymphocyte proliferation (Albina et al., 1991; Taylor et al., 1998; Zhang & McMurray, 1998). This effect is exerted on T and B cells alike and is mediated by several ways involving especially prostaglandins and nitric oxide as metabolic mediators (Albina et al., 1991; Ding et al., 1988; Jiang et al., 1992).

A mechanism by which macrophages intervene preferentially in Th1 and Th2 clones differentiation has been suggested. Hence, macrophages can interact with Th cells and induce polarization toward the Th1 or Th2 cell subset depending on the oxidation level of their glutathione content. With low levels of oxidized glutathione, they induce a polarization toward Th1 phenotype, whereas high levels of oxidized glutathione lead to Th2 differentiation (Murata et al., 2002). Additionally, some IL-12 antigenic stimulations induce Th1 cells activation (Hsieh et al., 1993). Th2 cells activation goes through the action of IL-4 and IL-10, which can also be produced by activated macrophages in the presence of immune complexes (Fiorentino et al., 1991).

2.2.8 Dendritic cells

DCs play an important role in initiating the immune response and antigen presentation, as well as in maintaining peripheral self-tolerance (Steinman et al., 2003). There are mostly immature DCs (iDCs), which have poor antigen presentation functions (de Vries et al., 2003), may be involved in immunoregulatory functions in autoimmune processes (Dorman et al., 1997). These functions depend largely on co-stimulation during the maturation process. Thus, tolerogenic DCs are iDCs with reduced allostimulatory capacities and low expression levels of costimulatory molecules, like CD40, CD80 and CD86 molecules. However, the transition to the mature state, following exposure to pathogens, leads to increased antigen presentation and expression of T cell co-stimulatory molecules and T cell responses (Steinman & Banchereau, 2007).

Nevertheless, the acquisition of a high degree of maturity and expression of adhesion molecules, especially CD86 molecule, allows the DCs to provoke the activation of $CD4^{+}CD25^{+}$ regulatory T cells capable of inhibiting autoimmune disease (Yamazaki et al., 2003). It is therefore quite possible that the DCs involved in triggering the autoimmune process leading to T1D (Clare-Salzler et al., 1992; Feutren et al., 1986; Mathis et al., 2001), are mature cells with a large capacity for antigen presentation, but without effect on regulatory T cells.

Additionally, it has been shown that DCs are the initiators of the islet infiltration in NOD mice (DiLorenzo et al., 2007). Such cells isolated from the panLN could prevent diabetes development when transferred adoptively to young recipients (Bekris et al., 2005), while those from other sites could not, suggesting that the activation of autoreactive T cells occurs at this site and that their suppression would be due to deletion or regulation mechanisms (Belz et al., 2002; Hugues et al., 2002).

2.2.9 Adhesion and costimulation molecules and cell signaling

T-cell-receptor (TCR)-mediated recognition of pancreatic autoantigens is a central step in the diabetes pathogenesis (Bach, 2002). Interaction between TCR and pancreatic peptides aberrantly complexed with class II MHC molecules on pancreatic beta-cells (Foulis, 1996) or expressed on the AgPCs in panLN is required for the activation of Th1 lymphocytes. Similarly, TCR interaction with autoantigen peptides presented by class I MHC molecules on pancreatic beta-cells is essential for the activation of cytotoxic CD8+ autoreactive T lymphocytes in pancreatic islet. Activated Th1 cells induce positive signals involving IL-2, TNF-β and IFN-γ cytokines to increase the activation of islet-infiltrated macrophage and cytotoxic CD8+ cells.

Beta-cells aggression can be mediated by proinflammatory cytokine-mediated cell killing (IL-1 (Aribi et al., 2007; Sparre et al., 2005), TNF-α (Christen et al., 2001; Lee et al., 2005), TNF-β, IFN-γ, IL-18 (Nakanishi et al., 2001; Szeszko et al., 2006), IL-12 (Giulietti et al., 2004; Holtz et al., 2001), IL-6 (Kristiansen & Mandrup-Poulsen, 2005; Targher et al., 2001), and IL-8 (Erbağci et al., 2001; Lo et al., 2004), etc.), granzymes (GRZ) and perforin (PRF1), FasL-Fas (CD95L-CD95) interactions, hydrogen peroxide and free radicals (Mukherjee & DiLorenzo, 2010).

Numerous adhesion molecules and signalling proteins, can amplify activation of the CD3/TCR complex leading to self-reactive T cells proliferation within panLN. Experimental NOD mice studies highlighted three principal costimulation pathways for such activation: CD28-B7, CD40-CD40L (CD 154) (Bour-Jordan et al., 2004) and NKG2D-RAE-1 (von Boehmer, 2004). Therefore, it has been previously shown that the T1D occurrence is decreased by injection of anti-B7.2 mAb's (Lenschow et al., 1995). Meanwhile, invalidation of B7.2 (CD86) (NOD/B7.2$^{-/-}$) confers protection against the disease (Salomon et al., 2001). Additionally, ablation of CD40-CD40L pathway with neutralizing antibodies (anti-CD40L mAb's) or with invalidation of CD40L (NOD/B7.2$^{-/-}$) prevents the early stages of T cell activation in the panLN (Green et al., 2000). Moreover, it has been demonstrated that the activated islet-infiltrated CD8+ T cells express NKG2D molecules and that the treatment of NOD mice with anti-NKG2D mAb's can prevent T1D development (Ogasawara et al., 2004).

2.2.10 Vitamin D status

The gradual increase in the frequency of T1D from the Equator to the Poles, especially among children born in spring or early summer and in the winter months has been

interpreted as the consequence of limited exposure to sun and low vitamin D status. Additionally, case-control studies have consistently demonstrated an association between the incidence of T1D and vitamin D status in children and pregnant women, and an inverse relationship between vitamin D intake from diet and supplements and seasonal variations in the incidence of T1D (Pittas & Dawson-Hughes, 2010).
Experimental data could also confront the observation about the relationship between vitamin D and T1D. Indeed, the insulin-producing beta-cells, as well as other cell types of the immune system (Stoffels et al., 2006), express the vitamin D receptor (VDR) and 1-alpha-hydroxylase enzyme (Nikalji & Bargman, 2011). By regulating the extracellular calcium concentration and transmembrane calcium fluxes, vitamin D may extend to preservation of insulin secretion and insulin sensitivity. Besides, vitamin D has immunomodulatory properties and is able to affect the autoimmune process leading to T1D (Bobryshev, 2010).

3. Immunotherapy of type 1 diabetes

Intervention and prevention strategies currently under consideration for T1D aim to reverse immune autoreactivity and restore beta-cell mass (Boettler & von Herrath, 2010; Bougneres et al., 1988). Immunotherapy can be used to induce immunological tolerance to beta-cell antigens using various protocols (Haase et al., 2010), involving both islets antigen-non-specific and antigen-specific approaches, but so far success has been limited.
Immunomodulation strategies have been generally achieved in two stages of the disease: prior to clinical onset but after the appearance of islet autoantibodies (secondary prevention) and immediately after diagnosis (intervention) (Staeva-Vieira et al., 2007) (Fig. 3). Based on the preclinical and clinical outcomes of studies using these therapies, combination with islet

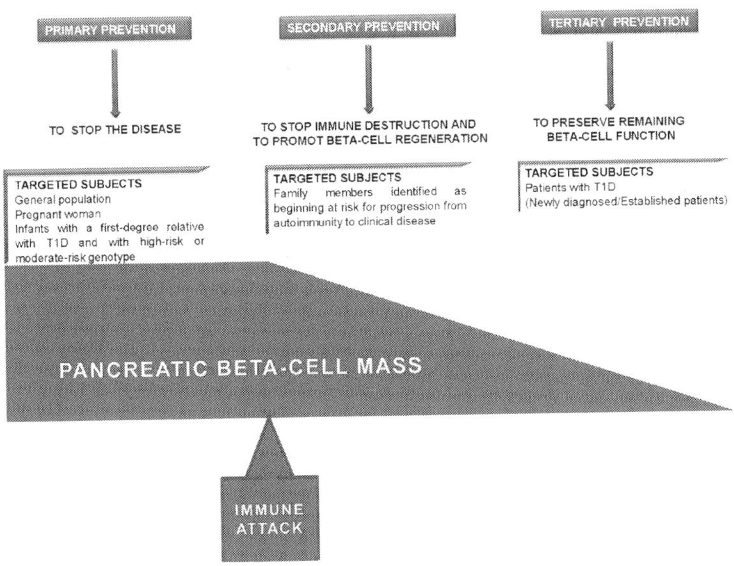

Fig. 3. Stages of type 1 diabetes prevention: objectives and selective targeting.

transplantation or stem cells for beta-cell regeneration are required in order to re-establish peripheral tolerance and to achieve a lasting remission (Marin-Gallen et al., 2010). Nevertheless, it is important to select eligible patients for such therapy, both to avoid toxicity and improve the chances of successful treatment (June & Blazar, 2006).

3.1 Non-antigen-specific immunotherapeutic approach for type 1 diabetes

For non-antigen-specific immunomodulation approch, many protocols using chemical- and antibody-mediated therapies have shown promise to the effects of various immunosuppressive drugs, including cyclosporine A (CsA), corticoïdes, azathioprine, T cell modulators (anti-CD3, anti-thymocyte globulin (ATG)), B cell-depleting agents (Rituximab: anti-CD20), anti-inflammatory molecules (anti-interleukin (IL)-1, anti-tumour necrosis factor (TNF)-α and anti-TNF-γ), cytokine-receptor-directed therapies and small-molecule protease inhibitors (Boettler & von Herrath, 2011; Luo et al., 2010; Sia, 2005; Silverstein et al., 1988) (Table 1). However, we have to acknowledge that these drugs increase the risk of developing infections and malignancies, favor the occurrence of metabolic complications such as dyslipidemia and hypertension and that some of them have been shown to inhibit beta-cell regeneration (Nir et al., 2007; Vantyghem et al., 2009). In addition to the immunosuppressant toxicity, recurrence or persistence of the autoimmune process has been observed after withdrawal of the immunosuppressive agents.

Immunomodulation therapies with nicotinamide and Bacillus Calmette-Guérin (BCG) have been tested in many clinical T1D prevention trials, but they showed no advantageous effects (Huppmann et al., 2005). Despite these negative results, large placebo-controlled clinical trials continue to illustrate the efficacy of these drugs in preventing T1D in newly diagnosed patients or in first-degree relatives of subjects with the disease.

Other immunomodulatory drugs that directly target immune cells have also been tested with success, especially in animal models of T1D, but some of them have run into major difficulties. They include DCs-based therapy, mainly the endocytic receptor involved in antigen processing and presentation DCs (DEC-205 (Ly75/CD205)), drugs targeting T cells (CTLA4-Ig: anti-CD4, anti-CD45) (Staeva-Vieira et al., 2007; Gregori et al., 2005), AgPCs (antibodies to CD40L or CD40) and NK T cells (alpha-galactosyl-ceramide (α-Gal-Cer), etc. (Chen et al., 2005c; Hong et al., 2001; Rewers & Gottlieb, 2009).

Although most of the immunomodulator treatments induce Treg cells activation, the direct infusion of ex vivo-expanded regulatory T cells has been considered to be a potential to prevent T1D (Lundsgaard et al., 2005; Tang et al., 2004; Tarbell et al., 2004) as well as other diseases, such as systemic lupus erythematosus (SLE) (Zheng et al., 2004), multiple sclerosis (MS) (Kohm et al., 2002) and inflammatory bowel disease (IBD) (Mottet et al., 2003). Treg-based cell therapy must meet at least four important therapeutic criteria: to (1) avoid the induction of immunogenicity of the infused cells; (2) prevent or delay cellular immunosenescence; (3) maximize help; and (4) be cognizant of the known differences between mouse and human T-cell biology (June & Blazar, 2006).

Moreover, drugs targeting adhesion molecules, such as Alefacept (antibody to leucocyte function-associated antigen-3 (LFA-3)), Efalizumab (antibody to LFA-1), FTY720 (immunosuppressive drug inhibiting activated T cell extravasation and trafficking to sites of inflammation), show promise in a significant proportion of patients with other diseases and are therefore of high potential interest for testing in T1D (Staeva-Vieira et al., 2007).

Therapeutic agent	Methodof delivery	Phase	Population targeted	ClinicalTrials.gov identifier
Otelixizumab	SC	III	ND	NCT00946257 NCT00451321 NCT00678886 NCT01123083
Teplizumab	IV, SC	I/II	ND	NCT01030861 NCT00378508 NCT00870818 NCT00806572
INGAP peptide	SC	II	EP	NCT00995540 NCT00071409
Peptide-MHC class II dimmers	PRT	//	//	*No trials on humans*
CsA	O	PS	ND	*NCT/URL links no longer available*
Nicotinamide	O	ES	SR	*NCT/URL links no longer available*
Atorvastatin	O	I	ND	NCT00974740
BCG	ID	I	ND	NCT00607230
Gluten-free diet	O	OG	NR	NCT01115621 NCT00279318
DHA	O	II	CR	NCT00333554
BP/Hyd. casein	O	II	CR	NCT01055080 NCT00607230
Vitamin D3	O	I	NR	NCT00141986
Diazoxide	O	IV	ND	NCT00131755
hrIFN-α	O	II	ND	NCT00024518
hrIL-1Ra	SC	III	ND	NCT00711503 NCT00645840
Canakinumab	SC	II	ND	NCT00947427
AAT	O	I	ND	NCT01319331
Rituximab	IV	III	ND	NCT00279305
Alemtuzumab	IV	I	ND	NCT00214214
ATG	IV	II	ND	NCT00515099
CTLA4-Ig	IV	II	ND	NCT00505375
Auto UCB	INF	II	EP	NCT00305344
Auto ODN DC	INF	I	EP	NCT00445913
Prochymal	IV	II	ND	NCT00690066

Table 1. Non-antigen-specific tolerance-based clinical trials for type 1 diabetes. *AAT: alpha 1-antitrypsin (Aralast NP); Alemtuzumab: anti-CD52 monoclonal antibody (Campath 1H®); ATG: anti-thymocyte globulin; Auto ODN DC: autologous dendritic cells treated ex vivo with the mixture of the antisense oligodeoxynucleotides; Auto UCB: autologous umbilical cord blood; BCG: Bacillus Calmette-Guérin; BP/Hyd. casein: bovine protein (cow's milk) or hydrolyzed casein formula; Canakinumab: human anti-interleukin-1β monoclonal antibody; CR: children at risk of T1D; CTLA4-Ig: cytotoxic T lymphocyte antigen-4 immunoglobulin (Abatacept); DHA: docosahexaenoic acid (omega-3 fatty acid supplementation diet); EP: established patients; ES: efficacy studies; hrIFN-α: human recombinant interferon-α (Roferon, Roche); hrIL-1Ra: human recombinant interleukin-1 receptor antagonist (Anakinra [Kineret®]); ID: intradermal; INF: infusion; INGAP: islet neogenesis associated protein (15 amino-acid sequence in INGAP peptide, Exsulin); CsA: cyclosporin A; IV: intravenously; ND: newly diagnosed; NR: newborns at risk of T1D; O: oral; OG: ongoing; Otelixizumab: ChAglyCD3 (aglycosylated human anti-CD3 monoclonal antibody, TRX4); Prochymal: mesenchymal stem cells; PRT: parenteral vaccination; PS: pilot studies; Rituximab: anti-CD20 monoclonal antibody; SC: subcutaneously; SR: subjects at risk of T1D; Teplizumab: hOKT3γ 1 (ala-ala) (mutated human anti-CD3 monoclonal antibody).*

3.2 Antigen-specific tolerance strategies for type 1 diabetes

The interest in induction of antigen-specific tolerance to beta-cell antigens for immune prevention of T1D development increased due to the lack of mild non-antigen-specific immunosuppressive agents. This therapeutic approach improves remarkable longevity and long term health in T1D patients and allows most of them to escape the major degenerative complications (Bach, 2003). It can occur as a result of clonal anergy and deletion of antigen-specific autoreactive T cells or induction of regulatory cells and immune deviation (Peakman & Dayan, 2001).

Paradoxically, the induction of tolerance may not be limited to the immune response against the injected antigen, but could be extended to responses against other antigens by a close proximity mechanism involving immunosuppressive cytokines (Bach, 2003). Therefore, the administration of the antigenic epitope specifically recognized by receptors on autoreactive T cells as part of the beta-cells would be more attractive than the whole antigen administration, given the higher levels of its specificity, but also the relatively modest costs of its synthesis (Atassi & Casali, 2008) (Fig. 4).

Different antigen-specific therapeutic approaches have shown efficacy in mouse models of T1D and have been studied most intensively in terms of inducing tolerance in humans (Boettler & von Herrath, 2010). They mainly include administration of immunogenic epitope peptide or whole protein from islet autoantigen, through parenteral, oral and nasal routes. Most of these approaches have been translated into clinic, but none of them have shown convincing promise in recent-onset T1D so far.

The most important clinical trials that have been reported with particular interest have focused on oral administration of parenteral and oral insulin clinical trials, efficacy and safety study on subcutaneous administration of heat-shock protein peptide (hsp60), DiaPep277, in C-peptide positive type 1 diabetes patients and safety experience on subcutaneous injection with the 65kDa isoform of glutamic acid decarboxylase in alum (GAD-alum) and an altered peptide ligand based on putative major autoantigenic sites in the insulin B9-23 chain, which had induced strong Th2 responses in animal models (Alleva et al., 2006; Alleva et al., 2002; Thrower & Bingley, 2009) (Table 2).

It has been observed in the Diabetes Prevention trial - Type1 (DPT-1) that oral administration of insulin in a group of patients with high IAA titers might allow an important delay in T1D onset (Skyler et al., 2005). TrialNet is now testing the efficacy of oral insulin in decreasing the chances of high-risk individuals converting to T1D (Haller et al., 2007). The immunomodulation with hsp60 has shown to provide some preservation of C-peptide in newly diagnosed adult type 1 diabetics and a significant reduction in inflammation of the pancreas with continued insulin production, suggesting that the progression of the disease may be prevented (Elias et al., 2006; Lazar et al., 2007; Raz et al., 2001). Additionally, the safety experience with subcutaneous GAD65 (Diamyd's GAD65) has been demonstrated in latent autoimmune diabetes of adulthood (LADA) patients (Agardh et al., 2005). The results indicate that this treatment increases fasting p-C-peptide concentrations after 24 weeks in subjects treated with a moderate dose (20 μg) but not in subjects treated with higher doses (100 or 500 μg) or lower doses (4 μg) (Stenström et al., 2005).

Other trials using a DNA vaccine-based approaches include BHT-3021 (Bayhill Therapeutics) (Burn, 2010), a plasmid encoding proinsulin, designed to target specific pathogenic immune cells. BHT-3021 has shown considerable effectiveness in the new-onset

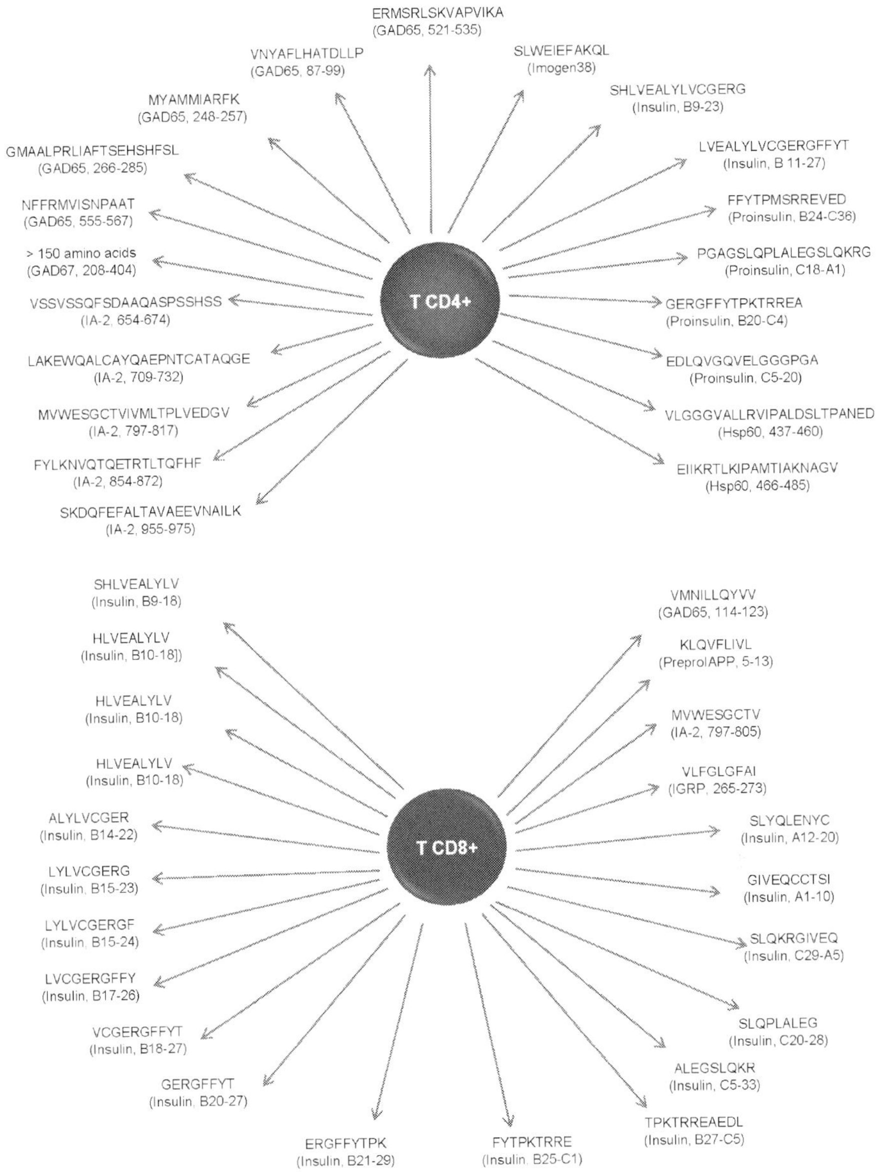

Fig. 4. CD4 and CD8 T cell epitopes for human pancreatic beta-cell antigens. *(Amino acid positions are indicated in brackets.)*

diabetes in the NOD mice. In the current phase I/II clinical trial, BHT-3021, administered by intra-muscular route, demonstrated preservation of C-peptide and an acceptable safety and tolerance in patients with T1D (Sanjeevi, 2009).

Therapeutic agent	Methodof delivery	Phase	Population targeted	ClinicalTrials.gov identifier
Insulin	O	III	RR	NCT00004984
	IN	III	CR	NCT00223613 NCT00336674
	PRT	II	RR	NCT00654121
IBC-VS01	IM	I	ND	NCT00057499
NBI-6024	SC	I	ND	NCT00873561
BHT-3021	IM	I	EP	NCT00453375
rhGAD-alum	SC	II	ND	NCT00529399 NCT01129232
DiaPep277	SC	III	ND	NCT01103284 NCT00615264 NCT00644501

Table 2. Antigen-specific tolerance-based clinical trials for type 1 diabetes. *CR: children at risk of T1D; EP: established patients; DiaPep277: Hsp60 immunodominant peptide p277; IBC-VS01: human insulin B chain in incomplete Freund's adjuvant (IFA) vaccine; IM: intramuscular; IN: intranasal; NBI-6024: altered peptide ligand (APL) insulin B9-23; ND: newly diagnosed; PRT: parenteral; rhGAD-alum: recombinant human glutamic acid decarboxylase (rhGAD65) formulated in alum; RR: relatives at risk of T1D; SC: subcutaneously; SR: subjects at risk of T1D.*

3.3 Combination immunotherapy approaches

Failure to induce a lasting complete remission in patients with T1D using any single agent suggests that combination therapies may be needed for effective prevention of the disease or reversal of new-onset T1D (Luo et al., 2010). Among these approaches that are currently being tried, combinations between immunosuppressive or anti-inflammatory and antigen-specific vaccines are of particular interest, because of their quite promising early preclinical trial results. The most potent and promising ones were schemes based on a combination of anti-CD3 treatment with GAD-alum, intranasal proinsulin peptide (Bresson et al., 2006), proinsulin DNA (BHT-3021), oral insulin or anti-inflammatory drugs (Matthews et al., 2010) (Fig. 5).

4. Conclusions

T1D results from selective autoimmune destruction of insulin-producing pancreatic islet beta-cells.

Although the cause of the disease is still not fully understood, multiple immune abnormalities, involving dysfunctional regulation of the immune system that leads to the activation of self-reactive CD4+ and CD8+ T cells as well as DCs and macrophages, are believed to be a major component behind beta-cells destruction.

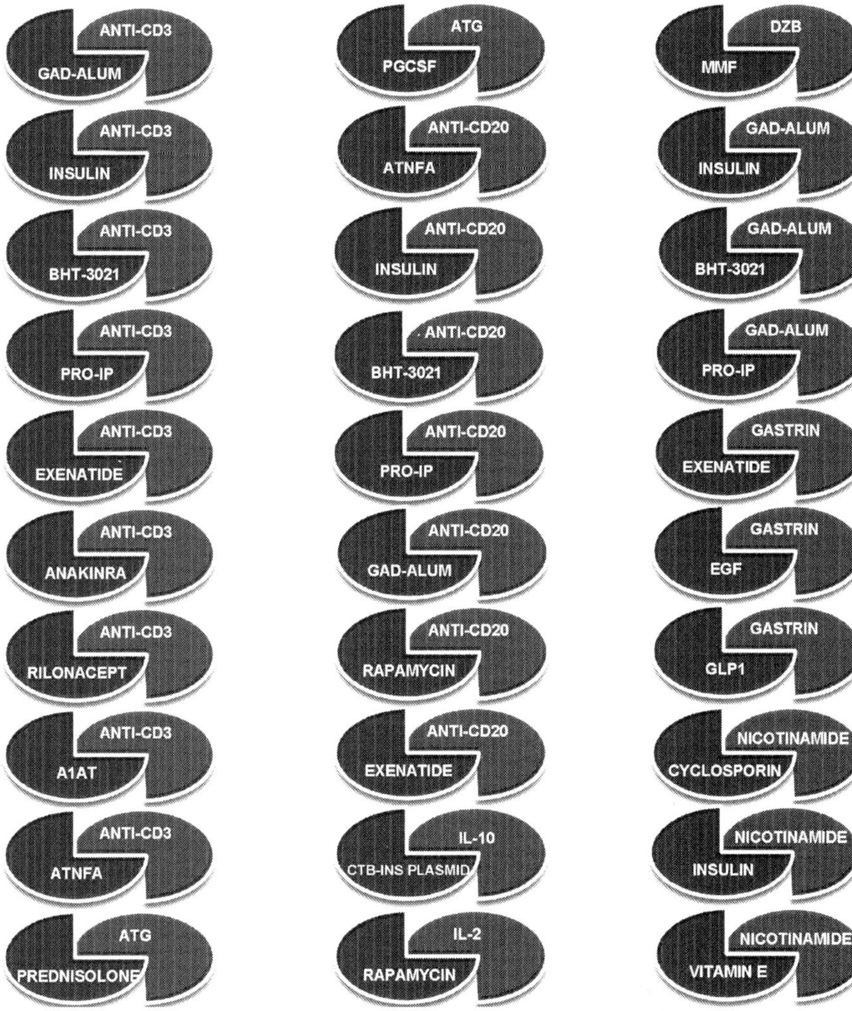

Fig. 5. Main combination immunotherapies for type 1 diabetes. *A1AT: alpha 1-antitrypsin; Anakinra: IL-1RA (Amgen); ATG: anti-thymocyte globulin; ATNFA: anti-tumor necrosis factor alpha; BHT-3021: proinsulin deoxyribonucleic acid; CTB-INS plasmid: cholera toxin B chain insulin; DZB: daclizumab (anti-CD25 monoclonal antibody); GAD-ALUM: glutamic acid decarboxylase formulated in Alum (Diamyd); GLP1: glucagon-like peptide-1; MMF: mycophenolate mofetil; PGCSF: pegylated granulocyte colony stimulating factor; PRO-IP: proinsulin peptide ; Rilonacept: IL-1 Trap.*

Given that there is evidence that the inflammatory phase preceding the destruction of beta-cells may be reversible and that humoral markers of the autoimmunity are usually present many years prior to and at the time of diagnosis, various approaches are being explored in order to slow down the progression of diabetes using antigen-specific and non-antigen-specific immunotherapies. The most promising results could be based on the induction of specific immunotolerance, because of the harmful health effects that could be observed when non-antigen-specific drugs are used.
Finally, it is possible that the etiological factors may be different from one patient to another and humoral immune response would be a relatively late marker for the disease progression. Most clinical trials have therefore been hampered by the lack of cellular markers of the immune processes that cause the disease.

5. Acknowledgment

I would like to thank most sincerely Maliha Meziane for proofreading of this chapter.

6. References

Achenbach, P., Koczwara, K., Knopff, A., Naserke, H., Ziegler, A.G. & Bonifacio, E. (2004). Mature high-affinity immune responses to (pro)insulin anticipate the autoimmune cascade that leads to type 1 diabetes. *The Journal of Clinical Investigation,* Vol.114, No.4, (August 2004), pp. 589-97, ISSN 0021-9738

Achenbach, P., Bonifacio,E. & Ziegler, A.G. (2005). Predicting type 1 diabetes. *Current Diabetes Reports,* Vol.5, No.2, (April 2005), pp. 98-103, ISSN 1534-4827

Agardh, C.D., Cilio, C.M., Lethagen, A., Lynch, K., Leslie, R.D.G., Palmer, M., Harris, R.A., Robertson, J.A. & Lernmark, Å. (2005). Clinical evidence for the safety of GAD65 immunomodulation in adult-onset autoimmune diabetes. *Journal of Diabetes and its Complications,* Vol.19, No.4, (July-August 2005), pp. 238-246, ISSN 1056-8727

Albina, J.E., Abate J.A. & Henry, Jr.W.L. (1991). Nitric oxide production is required for murine resident peritoneal macrophages to suppress mitogen-stimulated T cell proliferation. Role of IFN-g in the induction of the nitric oxide-synthesizing pathway. *Journal of Immunology (Baltimore, Md.: 1950),* (July 1991), Vol.147, No.1, pp. 144-148, ISSN 0022-1767

Alleva, D.G., Gaur, A., Jin, L., Wegmann, D., Gottlieb, P.A., Pahuja, A., Johnson, E.B., Motheral, T., Putnam, A., Crowe, P.D., Ling, N., Boehme, S.A. & Conlon, P.J. (2002). Immunological characterization and therapeutic activity of an altered-peptide ligand, NBI-6024, based on the immunodominant type 1 diabetes autoantigen insulin B-chain (9–23) peptide. *Diabetes,* (July 2002), Vol.51, No.7, pp. 2126-2134, ISSN 0012-1797

Alleva, D.G., Maki, R.A., Putnam, A.L., Robinson, J.M., Kipnes, M.S., Dandona, P., Marks, J.B., Simmons, D.L., Greenbaum, C.J., Jimenez, R.G., Conlon, P.J. & Gottlieb, P.A. (2006). Immunomodulation in type 1 diabetes by NBI-6024, an altered peptide ligand of the insulin B epitope. *Scand Journal of Immunology,* (January 2006), Vol.63, No.1, pp. 59-69, ISSN 0300-9475

Amrani, A., Verdaguer, J., Thiessen, S., Bou, S. & Santamaria, P. (2000). IL-1alpha, IL-1beta, and IFN-gamma mark beta cells for Fas-dependent destruction by diabetogenic

CD4(+) T lymphocytes. *The Journal of Clinical Investigation,* (February 2000), Vol.105, No.4, pp. 459-468, ISSN 0021-9738

Anderson, B., Park, B.J., Verdaguer, J., Amrani, A. & Santamaria, P. (1999). Prevalent CD8(+) T cell response against one peptide/MHC complex in autoimmune diabetes. *Proceedings of the National Academy of Sciences of the United States of America,* (August 1999), Vol.96, No.16, pp. 9311-9316, ISSN 0027-8424

Aribi, M. (2008). Candidate genes implicated in type 1 diabetes susceptibility. *Current Diabetes Reviews,* (May 2008), Vol.4, No.2, pp. 110-121, ISSN: 1573-3998

Aribi, M., Moulessehoul, S., Kendouci-Tani, M., Benabadji, A.B., Hichami, A. & Khan, N.A. (2007). Relationship between interleukin-1beta and lipids in type 1 diabetic patients. *Medical Science Monitor: International Medical Journal of Experimental and Clinical Research,* (August 2007), Vol.13, No.8, pp. CR372-378, ISSN 1234-1010

Atassi, M.Z., Casali, P. (2008). Molecular mechanisms of autoimmunity. *Autoimmunity,* (March 2008), Vol.41, No.2, pp. 123-132, ISSN 0891-6934

Atkinson, M.A. & Eisenbarth, G.S. (2001). Type 1 diabetes: New perspectives on disease pathogenesis and treatment. *Lancet,* (July 2001), Vol.358, No.9277, pp. 221-229, ISSN 0140-6736

Atkinson, M.A. & Maclaren, N.K. (1993). Islet cell autoantigens in insulin-dependent diabetes. *The Journal of Clinical Investigation,* (October 1993), Vol.92, No.4, pp. 1608-1616, ISSN 0021-9738

Azar, S.T., Tamim, H., Beyhum, H.N., Habbal, M.Z. & Almawi, W.Y. (1999). Type I (insulin-dependent) diabetes is a Th1- and Th2-mediated autoimmune disease. Clinical *and Diagnostic Laboratory Immunology,* (May 1999), Vol.6, No.3, pp. 306-310, ISSN 1071-412X

Bach, J.F. (2002). Immunotherapy of type 1 diabetes: lessons for other autoimmune diseases. *Arthritis Research* (May 2002), Vol.4, No.Suppl 3, pp. S3-S15, ISSN 1465-9905

Bach, J.F. (2003). Prevent and cure insulin-dependent diabetes. *Pathologie-Biologie,* (April 2003), Vol.51, No.3, pp. 151-155, ISSN 0369-8114

Baekkeskov, S., Aanstoot, H.J., Christgau, S., Reetz, A., Solimena, M., Cascalho, M., Folli, F., Richter-Olesen, H. & De Camilli, P. (1990). Identification of the 64K autoantigen in insulin-dependent diabetes as the GABA-synthesizing enzyme glutamic acid decarboxylase. *Nature,* (September 1990), Vol.347, No.6289, pp. 151, ISSN 0028-0836

Baekkeskov, S., Nielsen, J.H., Marner, B., Bilde, T., Ludvigsson, J. & Lernmark, A. (1982). Autoantibodies in newly diagnosed diabetic children immunoprecipitate human pancreatic islet cell proteins. *Nature,* (July 1982), Vol.298, No.5870, pp. 167, ISSN 0028-0836

Barker, J.M. (2006). Clinical review: Type 1 diabetes associated autoimmunity: Natural History, Genetic Associations and Screening. *The Journal of Clinical Endocrinology and Metabolism,* (April 2006), Vol.91, No4., pp. 1210-1217, ISSN 0021-972X

Barker, J.M., Barriga, K.J., Yu, L., Miao, D., Erlich., H.A., Norris, J.M., Eisenbarth, G.S. & Rewers, M. (2004). Diabetes Autoimmunity Study in the Young. Prediction of autoantibody positivity and progression to type 1 diabetes: Diabetes Autoimmunity Study in the Young (DAISY). *The Journal of Clinical Endocrinology and Metabolism,* (August 2004), Vol.89, No.8, pp. 3896-3902, ISSN 0021-972X

Barker, J.M., Ide, A., Hostetler, C., Yu, L., Miao, D., Fain, P.R., Eisenbarth, G.S. & Gottlieb, P.A. (2005). Endocrine and immunogenetic testing in individuals with type 1 diabetes and 21-hydroxylase autoantibodies: Addison's disease in a high-risk population. *The Journal of Clinical Endocrinology and Metabolism,* (January 2005), Vol.90, No.1, pp. 128-134, ISSN 0021-972X

Baxter, A.G., Kinder, S.J., Hammond, K.J., Scollay, R. & Godfrey, D.I. (1997). Association between alphabetaTCR+CD4-CD8- T-cell deficiency and IDDM in NOD/Lt mice. *Diabetes* (April 1997), Vol.46, No.4, pp. 572-582, ISSN 0012-1797

Bedoui, S., Velkoska, E., Bozinovski, S., Jones, J.E., Anderson, G.P. & Morris, M.J. (2005). Unaltered TNF-alpha production by macrophages and monocytes in diet-induced obesity in the rat. *Journal of Inflammation (London, England),* (March 2005), Vol.2, No.1, pp. 2, ESSN 1476-9255

Bekris, L.M., Shephard, C., Peterson, M., Hoehna, J., Van Yserloo, B., Rutledge, E., Farin, F., Kavanagh, T.J. & Lernmark, A. (2005). Glutathione-s-transferase M1 and T1 polymorphisms and associations with type 1 diabetes age-at-onset. *Autoimmunity,* (December 2005), Vol.38, No.8, pp. 567-575, ISSN 0891-6934

Belz, G.T., Behrens, G.M., Smith, C.M., Miller, J.F., Jones, C., Lejon, K., Fathman, C.G., Mueller, S.N., Shortman, K., Carbone, F.R. & Heath, W.R. (2002). The CD8alpha(+) dendritic cell is responsible for inducing peripheral self-tolerance to tissue-associated antigens. *The Journal of Experimental Medicine,* (October 2002), Vol.196, No.8, pp. 1099-1104, ISSN 0022-1007

Bennett, C.L., Huynh, H.M., Chance, P.F., Glass, I.A. & Gospe, S.M.Jr. (2005). Genetic heterogeneity for autosomal recessive pyridoxine-dependent seizures. *Neurogenetics,* (September 2005), Vol.6, No.3, pp. 143-149, ISSN 1364-6745

Berzins, S.P., Venanzi, E.S., Benoist, C. & Mathis, D. (2003). T-cell compartments of prediabetic NOD mice. *Diabetes,* (February 2003), Vol.52, No.2, pp. 327-334, ISSN 0012-1797

Bingley, P.J. (1996). Interactions of age, islet cell antibodies, insulin autoantibodies, and first-phase insulin response in predicting risk of progression to IDDM in ICA+ relatives: the ICARUS data set. Islet Cell Antibody Register Users Study. *Diabetes,* (December 1996), Vol.45, No.12, pp. 1720-1728, ISSN 0012-1797

Bingley, P.J., Williams, A.J. & Gale, E.A. (1999). Optimized autoantibody-based risk assessment in family members. Implications for future intervention trials. *Diabetes Care,* (November 1999), Vol.22, No.11, pp. 1796-1801, ISSN 0149-5992

Bobryshev, Y.V. (2010). Vitamin D3 suppresses immune reactions in atherosclerosis, affecting regulatory T cells and dendritic cell function. *Arteriosclerosis, Thrombosis, and Vascular Biology,* (December 2010), Vol.30, No.12, pp. 2317-2319, ISSN 1079-5642

Boettler, T. & von Herrath M. (2010). Immunotherapy of type 1 diabetes--how to rationally prioritize combination therapies in T1D. *International Immunopharmacology,* (December 2010) Vol.10, No.12, pp. 1491-1495, ISSN 1567-5769

Boettler, T. & von Herrath, M. (2011). Protection against or triggering of Type 1 diabetes? Different roles for viral infections. *Expert Review of Clinical Immunology,* (January 2011), Vol.7, No.1, pp. 45-53, ISSN 1744-666X

Bonifacio, E. & Christie, M.R. (1997). Islet cell antigens in the prediction and prevention in insulin-dependent diabetes mellitus. *Annals of Medicine,* (October 1997), Vol.29, No.5, pp. 405-412, ISSN 0785-3890

Bonifacio, E., Atkinson, M., Eisenbarth, G., Serreze, D., Kay, T.W., Lee-Chan, E. & Singh, B. (2001). International Workshop on Lessons From Animal Models for Human Type 1 Diabetes: identification of insulin but not glutamic acid decarboxylase or IA-2 as specific autoantigens of humoral autoimmunity in nonobese diabetic mice. *Diabetes,* (November 2001), Vol.50, No.11, pp. 2451-2458, ISSN 0012-1797

Bonifacio, E., Bingley, P.J., Shattock, M., Dean, B.M., Dunger, D., Gale, E.A. & Bottazzo, G.F. (1990). Quantification of islet-cell antibodies and prediction of insulin-dependent diabetes. *Lancet,* (January 1990), Vol.335, No.8682, pp. 147-149, ISSN 0140-6736

Bonifacio, E., Genovese, S., Braghi, S., Bazzigaluppi, E., Lampasona, V., Bingley, P.J., Rogge, L., Pastore, M.R., Bognetti, E. & Bottazzo, G.F., et al. (1995a). Islet autoantibody markers in IDDM: risk assessment strategies yielding high sensitivity. *Diabetologia,* (July 1995), Vol.38, No.7, pp. 816-822, ISSN 0012-186X

Bonifacio, E., Lampasona, V., Genovese, S., Ferrari, M. & Bosi, E. (1995b). Identification of protein tyrosine phosphatase-like IA-2 (islet cell antigen 512) as the insulin-dependent diabetes-related 37/40K autoantigen and a target of islet-cell antibodies. *Journal of Immunology (Baltimore, Md.: 1950),* (December 1995), Vol.155, No.11, pp. 5419-5426, ISSN 0022-1767

Borg, H., Gottsater, A., Fernlund, P. & Sundkvist, G. (2002a). A 12-year prospective study of the relationship between islet antibodies and beta-cell function at and after the diagnosis in patients with adult-onset diabetes. *Diabetes,* (June 2002), Vol.51, No.6, pp. 1754-1762, ISSN 0012-1797

Borg, H., Gottsater, A., Landin-Olsson, M., Fernlund, P. & Sundkvist G. (2001). High levels of antigen-specific islet antibodies predict future beta-cell failure in patients with onset of diabetes in adult age. *The Journal of Clinical Endocrinology and Metabolism,* (July 2001), Vol.86, No.7, pp. 3032-3038, ISSN 0021-972X

Borg, H., Marcus, C., Sjoblad, S., Fernlund, P. & Sundkvist, G. (2002b). Insulin autoantibodies are of less value compared with islet antibodies in the clinical diagnosis of autoimmune type 1 diabetes in children older than 3 yr of age. *Pediatric Diabetes,* (September 2002), Vol.3, No.3, pp. 149-154, ISSN 1399-543X

Bottazzo, G.F., Dean, B.M., Gorsuch, A.N., Cudworth, A.G. & Doniach, D. (1980). Complement-fixing islet-cell antibodies in type-I diabetes: possible monitors of active beta-cell damage. *Lancet,* (March 1980), Vol.1, No.8170, pp. 668-672, ISSN 0140-6736

Bottazzo, G.F., Florin-Christensen, A. & Doniach, D. (1974). Islet cell antibodies in diabetes mellitus with autoimmune polyendocrine deficiencies. *Lancet,* (November 1974), Vol.2, No.7892, pp. 1279-1283, ISSN 0140-6736

Bougneres, P.F., Carel, J.C., Castano, L., Boitard, C., Gardin, J.P., Landais, P., Hors, J., Mihatsch, M.J., Paillard, M. & Chaussain, J.L., et al. (1988). Factors associated with early remission of type I diabetes in children treated with cyclosporine. *The New England Journal of Medicine,* (March 1988), Vol.318, No.11, pp. 663–670, ISSN 0028-4793

Bour-Jordan, H., Salomon, B.L., Thompson, H.L., Szot, G.L., Bernhard, M.R. & Bluestone, J.A. (2004). Costimulation controls diabetes by altering the balance of pathogenic and regulatory T cells. *The Journal of Clinical Investigation,* (October 2004), Vol.114, No.7, pp. 979-987, ISSN 0021-9738

Breidert, M., Temelkova-Kurktschiev, T., Hanefeld, M., Leonhardt, W., Schmoeckel, A. & Seissler, J. (1998). Prevalence of diabetes-specific autoantibodies in patients at risk for adult onset diabetes mellitus. *Experimental and Clinical Endocrinology & Diabetes: Official Journal, German Society of Endocrinology [and] German Diabetes Association,* (1998), Vol.106, No.2, pp. 113-116, ISSN 0947-7349

Bresson, D., Togher, L., Rodrigo, E., Chen, Y., Bluestone, J.A., Herold, K.C. & von Herrath, M. (2006). Anti-CD3 and nasal proinsulin combination therapy enhances remission from recent-onset autoimmune diabetes by inducing Tregs. *The Journal of Clinical Investigation,* (May 2006), Vol.116, No.5, pp. 1371-1381, ISSN 0021-9738

Brusko, T.M., Putnam, A.L. & Bluestone, JA. (2008). Human regulatory T cells: role in autoimmune disease and therapeutic opportunities. *Immunological Reviews,* (June 2008), Vol.223, No.1, pp. 371-390, ISSN 0105-2896

Bu, D.F., Erlander, M.G., Hitz, B.C., Tillakaratne, N.J., Kaufman, D.L., Wagner-McPherson, C.B., Evans, G.A. & Tobin, A.J. (1992). Two human glutamate decarboxylases, 65-kDa GAD and 67-kDa GAD, are each encoded by a single gene. *Proceedings of the National Academy of Sciences of the United States of America,* (March 1992), Vol.89, No.6, pp. 2115, ISSN 0027-8424

Burn, P. (2010). Type 1 diabetes. *Nature Reviews. Drug Discovery,* (March 2010), Vol.9, No.3, pp. 187-188, ISSN 1474-1776

Cameron MJ, Arreaza GA, Zucker P, Chensue SW, Strieter RM, Chakrabarti S, Delovitch TL. (1997). IL-4 prevents insulitis and insulin-dependent diabetes mellitus in nonobese diabetic mice by potentiation of regulatory T helper-2 cell function. *Journal of Immunology (Baltimore, Md.: 1950),* (November 1997), Vol.159, No.10, pp. 4686-4692, ISSN 0022-1767

Caramalho, I., Lopes-Carvalho, T., Ostler, D., Zelenay, S,. Haury, M. & Demengeot, J. (2003). Regulatory T cells selectively express Toll-like receptors and are activated by lipopolysaccharide. *The Journal of Experimental Medicine,* (2003), Vol.197, No.4, pp. 403-411, ISSN 0022-1007

Carel, J.C., Lotton, C., Timisit, J., Bougnères, P. & Boitard, C. (1999). Auto-anticorps dans le diabète auto-immun. Signification et utilisation pratique. *Médecine thérapeutique Endocrinologie & Reproduction,* (May-June 1999), Vol.1, No.1, pp. 47-54, ISSN 1295-9359

Chen, S., Willis, J., Maclean, C., Ananieva-Jordanova, R., Amoroso, M.A., Brooking, H., Powell, M., Collins, A., Bennett, S., Mitchell, S., Burne, P., Furmaniak, J. & Smith, B.R. (2005a). Sensitive non-isotopic assays for autoantibodies to IA-2 and to a combination of both IA-2 and GAD65. *Clinica Chimica Acta; International Journal of Clinical Chemistry,* (July 2005), Vol.357, No.1, pp. 74-83, ISSN 0009-8981

Chen, Y.G., Choisy-Rossi, C.M., Holl, T.M., Chapman, H.D., Besra, G.S., Porcelli, S.A., Shaffer, D.J., Roopenian, D., Wilson, S.B. & Serreze, D.V. (2005b). Activated NKT cells inhibit autoimmune diabetes through tolerogenic recruitment of dendritic cells to pancreatic lymph nodes. *Journal of Immunology (Baltimore, Md.: 1950)*, (February 2005), Vol.174, No.3, pp. 1196-1204, ISSN 0022-1767

Chen, Z., Herman, A.E., Matos, M., Mathis, D. & Benoist, C. (2005c). Where CD4+CD25+ T reg cells impinge on autoimmune diabetes. *The Journal of Experimental Medicine*, (November 2005), Vol.202, No.10, pp. 1387-1397, ISSN 0022-1007

Chimienti, F., Devergnas, S., Favier, A. & Seve, M. (Identification and cloning of a beta-cell-specific zinc transporter, ZnT-8, localized into insulin secretory granules. *Diabetes*, (September 2004), Vol.53, No9, pp. 2330-2337, ISSN 0012-1797

Christen, U., Wolfe, T., Möhrle, U., Hughes, A.C., Rodrigo, E., Green, E.A., Flavell, R.A. & von Herrath, M.G. (2001). A dual role for TNF-alpha in type 1 diabetes: islet-specific expression abrogates the ongoing autoimmune process when induced late but not early during pathogenesis. *Journal of Immunology (Baltimore, Md.: 1950)*, (June 2001), Vol.166, No.12, pp. 7023-7032, ISSN 0022-1767

Christianson, S.W., Shultz, L.D. & Leiter, E.H. (1993). Adoptive transfer of diabetes into immunodeficient NOD-scid/scid mice. Relative contributions of CD4+ and CD8+ T-cells from diabetic versus prediabetic NOD. NON-Thy-1a donors. *Diabetes*, (January 1993), Vol.42, No.1, pp. 44-55, ISSN 0012-1797

Clare-Salzler, M.J., Brooks, J., Chai, A., Van Herle, K. & Anderson, C. (1992). Prevention of diabetes in nonobese diabetic mice by dendritic cell transfer. *The Journal of Clinical Investigation*, (September 1992), Vol.90, No.3, pp. 741-748, ISSN 0021-9738

Concannon, P., Rich, S.S. & Nepom, G.T. (2009). Genetics of type 1A diabetes. *The New England Journal of Medicine*, (April 2009), Vol.360, No.16, pp. 1646-1654, ISSN 0028-4793

Corvaisier-Chiron, M. & Beauvillaina, C. (2010). T regulator and Th17 lymphocytes: physiological and pathological functions. *Revue Francophone des Laboratoires*, (July-August 2010), Vol.40, No.424, pp. 31-40 ISSN 1773-035X

Costa, M., Saiz, A., Casamitjana, R., Castañer, M.F., Sanmartí, A., Graus, F. & Jaraquemada, D. (2002). T-cell reactivity to glutamic acid decarboxylase in stiff-man syndrome and cerebellar ataxia associated with polyendocrine autoimmunity. *Clinical and Experimental Immunology*, (September 2002), Vol.129, No.3, pp. 471-478, ISSN 0009-9104

Criswell, L.A., Pfeiffer, K.A., Lum, R.F., Gonzales, B., Novitzke, J., Kern, M., Moser, K.L., Begovich, A.B., Carlton, V.E., Li, W., Lee, A.T., Ortmann, W., Behrens, T.W. & Gregersen, P.K. (2005). Analysis of families in the multiple autoimmune disease genetics consortium (MADGC) collection: the PTPN22 620W allele associates with multiple autoimmune phenotypes. *American Journal of Human Genetics*, (April 2005), Vol.76, No.4, pp. 561-571, ISSN 0002-9297

Damanhouri, L.H., Dromey, J.A., Christie, M.R., Nasrat, H.A., Ardawi, M.S., Robins, R.A. & Todd, I. (2005). Autoantibodies to GAD and IA-2 in Saudi Arabian diabetic patients. *Diabetic Medicine: a Journal of the British Diabetic Association*, (April 2005), Vol.22, No.4, pp. 448-452, ISSN 0742-3071

Dang, M., Rockell, J., Wagner, R., Wenzlau, J.M., Yu, L., Hutton, J.C., Gottlieb, P.A. & Davidson, H.W. (2011). Human Type 1 Diabetes Is Associated with T Cell Autoimmunity to Zinc Transporter 8. *Journal of Immunology (Baltimore, Md.: 1950)*, (April 2011) [Epub ahead of print], ISSN 0022-1767

Davenport, C., Radford, P.M., Al-Bukhari, T.A., Lai, M., Bottazzo, G.F. & Todd, I. (1998). Heterogeneity in the occurrence of a subset of autoantibodies to glutamic acid decarboxylase in autoimmune polyendocrine patients with islet cell antibodies. *Clinical and Experimental Immunology,* (March 1998), Vol.111, No.3, pp. 497-505, ISSN 0009-9104

de Vries, I.J., Lesterhuis, W.J., Scharenborg, N.M., Engelen, L.P., Ruiter, D.J., Gerritsen, M.J., Croockewit, S., Britten, C.M., Torensma, R., Adema, G.J., Figdor, C.G. & Punt, CJ. (2003). Maturation of dendritic cells is a prerequisite for inducing immune responses in advanced melanoma patients. *Clinical Cancer Research: an Official Journal of the American Association for Cancer Research,* (November 2003), Vol.9, No.14, pp. 5091-5100, ISSN 1078-0432

Di Mario U, Perfetti R, Anastasi E, Contreas G, Crisà L, Tiberti C, Amendolea MA, Masala C. (1990). Autoantibodies to insulin do appear in non-diabetic patients with autoimmune disorders: comparison with anti-immunoglobulin antibodies and other autoimmune phenomena. *Acta Endocrinologica,* (March 1990), Vol.122, No.3, pp. 303, ISSN 0001-5598

DiLorenzo, T.P., Peakman, M. & Roep, B.O. (2007). Translational mini-review series on type 1 diabetes: systematic analysis of T cell epitopes in autoimmune diabetes. *Clinical and Experimental Immunology,* (April 2007) Vol.148, No.1, pp. 1-16, ISSN 0009-9104

Ding, A.H., Nathan, C.F., & Stuehr, D.J. (1988). Release of reactive nitrogen intermediates and reactive oxygen intermediates from mouse peritoneal macrophages. Comparison of activating cytokines and evidence for independent production. *Journal of Immunology (Baltimore, Md.: 1950),* (October 1988), Vol.141, No.7, pp. 2407-2412, ISSN 0022-1767

Dirkx, R. Jr., Thomas, A., Li, L., Lernmark, A., Sherwin, R.S., De Camilli, P. & Solimena, M. (1995). Targeting of the 67-kDa isoform of glutamic acid decarboxylase to intracellular organelles is mediated by its interaction with the NH2-terminal region of the 65-kDa isoform of glutamic acid decarboxylase. *The Journal of Biological Chemistry,* (February 1995), Vol.270, No.5, pp. 2241-2246, ISSN 0021-9258

Dorman, J. (1997). Molecular epidemiology of insulin-dependent diabetes mellitus: WHO DiaMond Project. WHO DiaMond Molecular Epidemiology Sub-Project Group. *Gaceta Medica de Mexico,* pp. 151-154. Vol.133, No.Suppl 1, ISSN 0016-3813

Dozio, N., Belloni, C., Girardi, A.M., Genovese, S., Sodoyez, J.C., Bottazzo, G.F., Pozza, G. & Bosi, E. (1994). Heterogeneous IgG subclass distribution of islet cell antibodies. *Journal of Autoimmunity,* (February 1994), Vol.7, No.1, pp. 45-53, ISSN 0896-8411

Duarte, N., Stenström, M., Campino, S., Bergman, M.L., Lundholm, M., Holmberg, D. & Cardell, S.L. (2004). Prevention of diabetes in nonobese diabetic mice mediated by CD1d-restricted nonclassical NKT cells. *Journal of Immunology (Baltimore, Md.: 1950),* (September 2004), pp. 3112-3118. Vol.173, No.5, ISSN 0022-1767

Durum, S.K., Schmidt, J.A. & Oppenheim, J.J. (1985). Interleukin 1: an immunological perspective. *Annual Review of Immunology,* (April 1985), Vol.3, No.1, pp. 263-287, ISSN 0732-0582

Eizirik, D.L. & Darville, M.I. (2001). Beta-cell apoptosis and defense mechanisms: lessons from type 1 diabetes. *Diabetes,* Vol.50, No. Suppl 1, pp. S64-S69, ISSN 0012-1797

Elfving, A.M., Lindberg, B.A., Nystrom, L., Sundkvist, G., Lernmark, A., Ivarsson, S.A. & DISS Study Group. (2003). Islet autoantibodies in cord blood from patients who developed type 1 diabetes mellitus at 15-30 years of age. *Autoimmunity,* (June 2003), Vol.36, No.4, pp. 227-231, ISSN 0891-6934

Elias, D., Avron, A., Tamir, M. & Raz, I. (2006). DiaPep277 preserves endogenous insulin production by immunomodulation in type 1 diabetes. *Annals of the New York Academy of Sciences,* (October 2006), Vol.1079, No.1, pp. 340-344, ISSN 0077-8923

Erbağci, A.B, Tarakçioğlu, M., Coşkun, Y., Sivasli, E. & Namiduru, E.S. (2001). Mediators of inflammation in children with type 1 diabetes mellitus: cytokines in type 1 diabetic children. *Clinical Biochemistry,* (November 2001), pp. 645-650. Vol.34, No.4, ISSN 0009-9120

Erlander MG, Tillakaratne NJ, Feldblum S, Patel N, Tobin AJ. (1991). Two genes encode distinct glutamate decarboxylases. *Neuron,* (July 1991), Vol.7, No.1, pp. 91, ISSN 0896-6273

Ernerudh, J., Ludvigsson, J., Berlin, G. & Samuelsson, U. (2004). Effect of photopheresis on lymphocyte population in children with newly diagnosed type 1 diabetes. *Clinical and Diagnostic Laboratory Immunology,* (September 2004), Vol.11, No.5, pp. 856-861, ISSN 1071-412X

Falcone, M., Yeung, B., Tucker, L., Rodriguez, E. & Sarvetnick, N. (1999). A defect in interleukin 12-induced activation and interferon gamma secretion of peripheral natural killer T cells in nonobese diabetic mice suggests new pathogenic mechanisms for insulin-dependent diabetes mellitus. *The Journal of Experimental Medicine,* (October 1999), pp. 963-972. Vol.190, No.7, ISSN 0022-1007

Feutren, G., Papoz, L., Assan, R., Vialettes, B., Karsenty, G., Vexiau, P., Du Rostu, H., Rodier, M., Sirmai, J. & Lallemand A., et al. (1986). Cyclosporin increases the rate and length of remissions in insulin-dependent diabetes of recent onset. Results of a multicentre double-blind trial. *Lancet,* (July 1986), Vol.2, No.8499, pp. 119-124, ISSN 0140-6736

Filippi, C.M. & von Herrath, M.G. (2010). 99th Dahlem conference on infection, inflammation and chronic inflammatory disorders: viruses, autoimmunity and immunoregulation. *Clinical and Experimental Immunology,* (2010), Vol.160, No.1, pp. 113-119, ISSN 0009-9104

Fiorentino, D.F., Zlotnik, A., Mosmann, T.R., Howard, M. & O'Garra, A. (1991). IL-10 inhibits cytokine production par activated macrophages. *Journal of Immunology (Baltimore, Md.: 1950),* (December 1991), pp. 3815-3822. Vol.147, No.11, ISSN 0022-1767

Fontenot, J.D., Gavin, M.A. & Rudensky, A.Y. (2003). Foxp3 programs the development and function of CD4+CD25+ regulatory T cells. *Nature Immunology,* (April 2003), Vol.4, No.4, pp. 330-336, ISSN 1529-2908

Foulis, A.K. (1996). The pathology of the endocrine pancreas in type 1 (insulin-dependent) diabetes mellitus. *APMIS : Acta Pathologica, Microbiologica, et Immunologica Scandinavica,* (March 1996), Vol.104, No.3, pp. 161-167, ISSN 0903-4641

Fox, C.J. & Danska, J.S. (1997). IL-4 expression at the onset of islet inflammation predicts nondestructive insulinitis in nonobese dibetic mice. *Journal of Immunology (Baltimore, Md.: 1950),* (March 1997), Vol.158, No.5, pp. 2414-2424, ISSN 0022-1767

Furtado, G.C., Olivares-Villagomez, D., Curotto de Lafaille, M.A., Wensky, A.K., Latkowski, J.A. & Lafaille, J.J. (2001). Regulatory T cells in spontaneous autoimmune encephalomyelitis. *Immunological Reviews,* (August 2001), Vol.182, No.1, pp. 122-134, ISSN 0105-2896

Gianani, R. & Eisenbarth, G.S. (2005). The stages of type 1A diabetes: 2005. *Immunological Reviews,* (April 2005), Vol.204, No.1, pp. 232-249, ISSN 0105-2896

Gilliam, L.K., Palmer, J.P. & Lernmark, Å. (2004). Autoantibodies and the disease process of type 1 diabetes mellitus, In: *Diabetes Mellitus: A Fundamental and Clinical Text,* D. LeRoith, S.I. Taylor & J.M., Olefsky, (Eds), 499-518, Lippincott, ISBN 0-7817-4097-5 (hc), Philadelphia PA 19106, USA

Giulietti, A., Stoffels, K., Decallonne, B., Overbergh, L. & Mathieu, C. (2004). Monocytic expression behavior of cytokines in diabetic patients upon inflammatory stimulation. *Annals of the New York Academy of Sciences,* (December 2004), Vol.1037, No.1, pp. 74-78, ISSN 0077-8923

Gorsuch, A.N., Spencer, K.M., Lister, J., McNally, J.M., Dean, B.M., Bottazzo, G.F. & Cudworth, A.G. (1981). Evidence for a long prediabetic period in type I (insulin-dependent) diabetes mellitus. *Lancet,* (December 1981), Vol.2, No8260-61., pp. 1363-1365, ISSN 0140-6736

Graser, R.T., DiLorenzo, T.P., Wang, F., Christianson, G.J., Chapman, H.D., Roopenian, D.C., Nathenson, S.G. & Serreze, D.V. (2000). Identification of a CD8 T cell that can independently mediate autoimmune diabetes development in the complete absence of CD4 T cell helper functions. *Journal of Immunology (Baltimore, Md.: 1950),* (April 2000), Vol.164, No.7, pp. 3913-3918, ISSN 0022-1767

Green, E.A., Wong, F.S., Eshima, K., Mora, C. & Flavell, R.A. (2000). Neonatal tumor necrosis factor alpha promotes diabetes in nonobese diabetic mice by CD154-independent antigen presentation to CD8(+) T cells. *The Journal of Experimental Medicine,* (January 2000), Vol.191, No.2, pp. 225-238, ISSN 0022-1007

Gregori, S., Mangia, P., Bacchetta, R., Tresoldi, E., Kolbinger, F., Traversari, C., Carballido, J.M., de Vries, J.E., Korthäuer, U. & Roncarolo, M.G. (2005). An anti-CD45RO/RB monoclonal antibody modulates T cell responses via induction of apoptosis and generation of regulatory T cells. *The Journal of Experimental Medicine,* (April 2005), Vol.201, No.8, pp. 1293-1305, ISSN 0022-1007

Haase, C., Yu, L., Eisenbarth, G. & Markholst, H. (2010). Antigen-dependent immunotherapy of non-obese diabetic mice with immature dendritic cells. *Clinical and Experimental Immunology,* (June 2010), Vol.160, No.3, pp. 331-339, ISSN 0009-9104

Hagopian, W.A., Karlsen, A.E., Gottsäter, A., Landin-Olsson, M., Grubin, C.E., Sundkvist, G., Petersen, J.S., Boel, E., Dyrberg, T. & Lernmark, A. (1993). Quantitative assay using recombinant human islet glutamic acid decarboxylase (GAD65) shows that 64k autoantibody positivity at onset predicts diabetes type. *The Journal of Clinical Investigation,* (January 1993), Vol.91, No.1, pp. 368, ISSN 0021-9738

Haller, M.J., Gottlieb, P.A. & Schatz, D.A. (2007). Type 1 diabetes intervention trials 2007: where are we and where are we going? *Current Opinion in Endocrinology, Diabetes, and Obesity,* (August 2007), Vol.14, No.4, pp. 283-7, ISSN 1752-296X

Han, G., Li, Y., Wang, J., Wang, R., Chen, G., Song, L., Xu, R., Yu, M., Wu, X., Qian, J. & Shen, B. (2005). Active tolerance induction and prevention of autoimmune diabetes by immunogene therapy using recombinant adenoassociated virus expressing glutamic acid decarboxylase 65 peptide GAD(500-585). *Journal of Immunology (Baltimore, Md.: 1950),* (April 2005), Vol.174, No.8, pp. 4516-4524, ISSN 0022-1767

Hanninen, A., Jalkanen, S., Salmi, M., Toikkanen, S., Nikolakaros, G. & Simel, O. (1992). Macrophages, T cell receptor usage, and endothelial cell activation in the pancreas at the onset of insulin-dependent diabetes mellitus. *The Journal of Clinical Investigation, ISSN 0021-9738* (November 1992), Vol.90, No.5, pp. 1901-1910, ISSN

Harrington, L.E., Hatton, R.D., Mangan, P.R., Turner, H., Murphy, T.L., Murphy, K.M. & Weaver, CT. (2005). Interleukin 17-produc- producing CD4+ effector T cells develop via a lineage distinct from the T helper type 1 and 2 lineages. *Nature Immunology,* (November 2005), pp. 1123-1132. Vol.6, No.11, ISSN 1529-2908

Hermann, R., Bartsocas, C.S., Soltész, G., Vazeou, A., Paschou, P., Bozas, E., Malamitsi-Puchner, A., Simell, O., Knip, M. & Ilonen, J. (2004). *Diabetes/Metabolism Research and Reviews,* (July-August 2004), Vol.20, No.4, pp. 322–329, ISSN 1520-7552

Holz, A., Brett, K. & Oldstone, M.B. (2001). Constitutive beta cell expression of IL-12 does not perturb self-tolerance but intensifies established autoimmune diabetes. *The Journal of Clinical Investigation,* (December 2001), Vol.108, No.12, pp.1749-1758, ISSN 0021-9738

Hong S, Wilson MT, Serizawa I, Wu L, Singh N, Naidenko OV, Miura T, Haba T, Scherer DC, Wei J, Kronenberg M, Koezuka Y, Van Kaer L. (2001). The natural killer T-cell ligand alpha-galactosylceramide prevents autoimmune diabetes in nonobese diabetic mice. *Nature Medicine,* (September 2001), Vol.7, No.9, pp. 1052-1056, ISSN 1078-8956

Honkanen, J., Nieminen, J.K., Gao, R., Luopajarvi, K., Salo, H.M., Ilonen, J,. Knip, M., Otonkoski, T. & Vaarala, O. (2010). IL-17 immunity in human type 1 diabetes. *Journal of Immunology (Baltimore, Md.: 1950),* (August 2010), Vol.185, No.3, pp. 1959-1967, ISSN 0022-1767

Hori, S., Nomura, T. & Sakaguchi, S. (2003). Control of regulatory T cell development by the transcription factor Foxp3. *Science (New York, N.Y.),* (February 2003), Vol.299, No.5609, pp. 1057-1061, ISSN 0036-8075

Hsieh, C.S., Macatonia, S.E., Tripp, C.S., Wolf, S.F., O'Garra, A. & Murphy, K.M. (1993). Development of Th1 CD4+ T cells through IL-12 produced by listeria-induced macrophages. *Science (New York, N.Y.),* (1993), pp. 547-549. Vol.260, No., ISSN 0036-8075

Hugues, S., Mougneau, E., Ferlin, W., Jeske, D., Hofman, P., Homann, D., Beaudoin, L., Schrike, C., Von Herrath, M., Lehuen, A. & Glaichenhaus, N. (2002). Tolerance to islet antigens and prevention from diabetes induced by limited apoptosis of pancreatic β cells. *Immunity,* (February 2002), Vol.16, No.2, pp. 169-181, ISSN 1074-7613

Huppmann, M., Baumgarten, A., Ziegler, A.G. & Bonifacio, E. (2005). Neonatal Bacille Calmette-Guerin vaccination and type 1 diabetes. *Diabetes Care,* (May 2005), Vol.28, No.5, pp. 1204, ISSN 0149-5992

Imagawa, A., Hanafusa, T., Tamura, S., Moriwaki, M., Itoh, N., Yamamoto, K., Iwahashi, H., Yamagata, K, Waguri, M., Nanmo, T., Uno, S., Nakajima, H., Namba, M., Kawata, S., Miyagawa, J.I. & Matsuzawa, Y. (2001). Pancreatic biopsy as a procedure for detecting in situ autoimmune phenomena in type 1 diabetes: close correlation between serological markers and histological evidence of cellular autoimmunity. *Diabetes,* (June 2001), pp. 1269-73. Vol.50, No.6, ISSN 0012-1797

Ishii, T., Itoh, K., Sato, H. & Bannai, S. (1999). Oxidative stress-inducible proteins in macrophages. *Free Radical Research,* (1999), pp. 351-355. Vol.31, No., ISSN 1071-5762

Itoh, N., Hanafusa, T., Miyazaki, A., Miyagawa, J., Yamagata, K., Yamamoto, K., Waguri, M., Imagawa, A., Tamura, S., Inada, M., Kawata, S., Tarui, S., Kono, N. & Matsuzawa, Y. (1993). Mononuclear cell infiltration and its relation to the expression of major histocompatibility complex antigens and adhesion molecules in pancreas biopsy specimens from newly diagnosed insulin-dependent diabetes mellitus patients. *The Journal of Clinical Investigation,* (November 1993), Vol.92, No.5, pp. 2313-2322, ISSN 0021-9738

Ivanov, I.I., McKenzie, B.S., Zhou, L., Tadokoro, C.E., Lepelley, A., Lafaille, J.J., Cua, D.J. & Littman, D.R. (2006). The orphan nuclear receptor RORgammat directs the differentiation program of proinflammatory IL-17+ T helper cells. *Cell,* (September 2006), pp. 1121-1133. Vol.126, No.6, ISSN 0092-8674

Jiang, H., Stewart, C.A., Fast, D.J. & Leu, R.W. (1992). Tumor target-derived soluble factor synergizes with IFN-g and IL-2 to activate macrophages for tumor necrosis factor and nitric oxide production to mediate cytotoxicity of the same target. *Journal of Immunology (Baltimore, Md.: 1950),* (September 1992), pp. 2137-2146. Vol.149, No.6, ISSN 0022-1767

Jun, H.S. & Yoon, J.W. (1994). Initiation of autoimmune type 1 diabetes and molecular cloning of a gene encoding for islet cell-specific 37kd autoantigen. *Advances in Experimental Medicine and Biology,* (January 1994), Vol.347, No.1, pp. 207-220, ISSN 0065-2598

June, C.H. & Blazar, B.R. (2006). Clinical application of expanded CD4+25+ cells. *Seminars in Immunology,* (April 2006), pp. 78-88. Vol.18, No.2, ISSN 1044-5323

Kajander, M., Moltchanova, E., Libman, I., LaPorte, R. & Tuomilehto, J. (2000). Incidence of childhood type 1 diabetes worldwide. Diabetes Mondiale (DiaMond) Project Group. *Diabetes Care,* (October 2000), Vol.23, No.10, pp. 1516-1526, ISSN 0149-5992

Kaminitz, A., Stein, J., Yaniv, I. & Askenasy, N. (2007). The vicious cycle of apoptotic β-cell death in type 1 Diabetes. *Immunol Cell Biol,* (November-December 2007), Vol.85, No.8, pp. 582-589, ISSN 0818-9641

Karlsen, A.E., Hagopian, W.A., Grubin, C.E., Dube, S., Disteche, C.M., Adler, D.A., Bärmeier, H., Mathewes, S., Grant, F.J. & Foster, D., et al. (1991). Cloning and primary structure of a human islet isoform of glutamic acid decarboxylase from chromosome 10. *Proceedings of the National Academy of Sciences of the United States of America,* (0ctober 1991), pp. 8337-8341, Vol.88, No.19, ISSN 0027-8424

Kawasaki, E. & Eisenbarth, G.S. (2000). High-throughput radioassays for autoantibodies to recombinant autoantigens. *Frontiers in Bioscience: a Journal and Virtual Library,* (November 2000), Vol.5, No.1, pp. E181-E190, ISSN 1093-9946

Kent, S.C., Chen, Y., Bregoli, L., Clemmings, S.M., Kenyon, N.S., Ricordi, C., Hering, B.J. & Hafler, D.A. (2005). Expanded T cells from pancreatic lymph nodes of type 1 diabetic subjects recognize an insulin epitope. *Nature,* (May 2005), Vol.435, No.7039, pp. 224-228, ISSN 0028-0836

Kessler, L. (2010). Human pancreatic islet transplantation in type 1 diabetes. State of this art. *Médecine Nucléaire - Imagerie Fonctionnelle et Métabolique,* (October 2010), Vol.34, No.10, pp. 589-596, ISSN 0928-1258

Khattri, R., Cox, T., Yasayko, S.A. & Ramsdell, F. (2003). An essential role for Scurfin in CD4+CD25+ T regulatory cells. *Nature Immunology,* (April 2003), Vol.4, No.4, pp. 337-342, ISSN 1529-2908

Kida, K., Kaino, Y., It,o T. & Hirai, H. (1998). Controversies on the prevention of insulin-dependent diabetes mellitus by immunomodulation: lessons from NOD mice treated with beta-1,6;1,3-D-glucan and rhIGF-I. *Journal of Pediatric Endocrinology & Metabolism: JPEM,* (April 1998), Vol.11, No.Suppl2, pp. 327-333, ISSN 0334-018X

Kida, K., Kaino, Y., Ito, T., Hirai, H. & Nakamura, K. (1999). Immunogenetics of insulin-dependent diabetes mellitus. *Acta Paediatrica,* (January 1999), Vol.82, No.Suppl427, pp. 3-7, ISSN 0001-656X

Kimura, A. & Kishimoto, T. (2011). Th17 cells in inflammation. *International Immunopharmacology,* (March 2011), pp. 319-322, Vol.11, No.3, ISSN 1567-5769

Knip, M., Vahasalo, P., Karjalainen, J., Lounamaa, R. & Akerblom, H.K. (1994). Natural history of preclinical IDDM in high risk siblings. Childhood Diabetes in Finland Study Group. *Diabetologia,* (April 1994), Vol.37, No.4, pp. 388-393, ISSN 0012-186X

Knowles, C.H., Lang, B., Clover, L., Scott, S.M., Gotti, C., Vincent, A. & Martin, J.E. (2002). A role for autoantibodies in some cases of acquired non-paraneoplastic gut dysmotility. *Scandinavian Journal of Gastroenterology,* (February 2002), Vol.37, No.2, pp. 166-170, ISSN 0036-5521

Ko, K.S., Lee, M., Koh, J.J. & Kim, S.W. (2001). Combined administration of plasmids encoding IL-4 and IL-10 prevents the developments of autoimmune diabetes in nonobese diabetic mice. *Molecular Therapy: the Journal of the American Society of Gene Therapy,* (October 2001), Vol.4, No.4, pp. 313-316, ISSN 1525-0016

Kobayashi, T., Tanaka, S., Okubo, M., Nakanishi, K., Murase, T. & Lernmark, A. (2003). Unique epitopes of glutamic acid decarboxylase autoantibodies in slowly progressive type 1 diabetes. *The Journal of Clinical Endocrinology and Metabolism,* (October 2003), Vol.88, No.10, pp. 4768-4775, ISSN 0021-972X

Kohm, A.P., Carpentier, P.A., Anger, H.A. & Miller, S.D. (2002). Cutting edge: CD4+CD25+ regulatory T cells suppress antigen-specific autoreactive immune responses and central nervous system inflammation during active experimental autoimmune encephalomyelitis. *Journal of Immunology (Baltimore, Md.: 1950)* (November 2002), Vol.169, No.9, pp. 4712-4716, ISSN 0022-1767

Kotani, R., Nagata, M., Moriyama, H., Nakayama, M., Yamada, K., Chowdhury, S.A., Chakrabarty, S., Jin, Z., Yasuda, H. & Yokono, K. (2002). Detection of GAD65-reactive T-Cells in type 1 diabetes by immunoglobulin-free ELISPOT assays. *Diabetes Care,* (August 2002), Vol.25, No.8, pp. 1390-1397, ISSN 0149-5992

Koulmanda, M., Bhasin, M., Hoffman, L., Fan, Z., Qipo, A., Shi, H., Bonner-Weir, S., Putheti, P., Degauque, N., Libermann, T.A., Auchincloss, H.Jr., Flier, J.S. & Strom, T.B.

(2008). Curative and beta cell regenerative effects of alpha1-antitrypsin treatment in autoimmune diabetic NOD mice. *Proceedings of the National Academy of Sciences of the United States of America,* (October 2008), Vol.105, No.42, pp. 16242-16247, ISSN 0027-8424

Kriegel, MA, Lohmann, T, Gabler, C, Blank, N, Kalden, JR, Lorenz, HM. (2004). Defective suppressor function of human CD4+ CD25+ regulatory T cells in autoimmune polyglandular syndrome type II. *The Journal of Experimental Medicine,* (May 2004), Vol.199, No.9, pp. 1285-1291, ISSN 0022-1007

Krischer, J.P., Cuthbertson, D.D., Yu, L., Orban, T., Maclaren, N., Jackson, R., Winter, W.E., Schatz, D.A., Palmer, J.P. & Eisenbarth, G.S. (2003). Screening strategies for the identification of multiple antibody-positive relatives of individuals with type 1 diabetes. *The Journal of Clinical Endocrinology and Metabolism,* (January 2003), Vol.88, No.1, pp. 103-108, ISSN 0021-972X

Kristiansen, O.P. & Mandrup-Poulsen, T. (2005). Interleukin-6 and diabetes: the good, the bad, or the indifferent? *Diabetes,* (December 2005), Vol.54, No.Suppl 2, pp. S114-S124, ISSN 0012-1797

Kukreja, A., Cost, G., Marker, J., Zhang, C., Sun, Z., Lin-Su, K., Ten, S., Sanz, M., Exley, M., Wilson, B., Porcelli, S. & Maclaren, N. (2002). Multiple immuno-regulatory defects in type-1 diabetes. *The Clinical Investigator,* (January 2002), Vol.109, No.1, pp. 131-140, ISSN 0941-0198

Kulmala, P., Savola, K., Petersen, J.S., Vähäsalo, P., Karjalainen, J., Löppönen, T., Dyrberg, T., Akerblom, H.K. & Knip, M. (1998). Prediction of insulin-dependent diabetes mellitus in siblings of children with diabetes. A population-based study. The Childhood Diabetes in Finland Study Group. *The Journal of Clinical Investigation,* (January 1998), Vol.101, No.2, pp. 327-336, ISSN 0021-9738

Lampasona, V., Petrone, A., Tiberti, C., Capizzi, M., Spoletini, M., di Pietro, S., Songini, M., Bonicchio, S., Giorgino, F., Bonifacio, E., Bosi E., Buzzetti, R. & Non Insulin Requiring Autoimmune Diabetes (NIRAD) Study Group. (2010). Zinc transporter 8 antibodies complement GAD and IA-2 antibodies in the identification and characterization of adult-onset autoimmune diabetes: Non Insulin Requiring Autoimmune Diabetes (NIRAD) 4. *Diabetes Care,* (January 2010), Vol.33, No.1, pp. 104-108, ISSN 0149-5992

Landin-Olsson, M., Palmer, J.P., Lernmark, A., Blom, L., Sundkvist, G., Nyström, L. & Dahlquist, G. (1992). Predictive value of islet cell and insulin autoantibodies for type 1 (insulin-dependent) diabetes mellitus in a population-based study of newly-diagnosed diabetic and matched control children. *Diabetologia,* (November 1992), Vol.35, No.11, pp. 1068-1073, ISSN 0012-186X

Lawrence, T., Bebien, M., Liu., G.Y., Nizet, V. & Karin, M. (2005). IKKalpha limits macrophage NF-kappaB activation and contributes to the resolution of inflammation. *Nature,* (April 2005), Vol.434, No.7037, pp. 1138-1143, ISSN 0028-0836

Lazar, L., Ofan, R., Weintrob, N., Avron, A., Tamir, M., Elias, D., Phillip, M. & Josefsberg, Z. (2007). Heat-shock protein peptide DiaPep277 treatment in children with newly diagnosed type 1 diabetes: a randomised, double-blind phase II study. *Diabetes/Metabolism Research and Reviews,* (May 2007), Vol.23, No.4, pp. 286-291, ISSN 1520-7552

Lee, L.F., Xu, B., Michie, S.A., Beilhack, G.F., Warganich, T., Turley, S. & McDevitt, H.O. (2005). The role of TNF-alpha in the pathogenesis of type 1 diabetes in the nonobese diabetic mouse: analysis of dendritic cell maturation. *Proceedings of the National Academy of Sciences of the United States of America,* (November 2005), Vol.102, No.44, pp. 15995-16000, ISSN 0027-8424

Lehuen, A., Lantz, O., Beaudoin, L., Laloux, V., Carnaud, C., Bendelac, A., Bach, J.F. & Monteiro, R.C. (1998). Overexpression of natural killer T cells protects Vα14- Jα281 transgenic nonobese diabetic mice against diabetes. *The Journal of Experimental Medicine,* (November 1998), Vol.188, No.10, pp. 1831-1839, ISSN 0022-1007

Lenschow, D.J., Ho, S.C., Sattar, H., Rhee, L., Gray, G., Nabavi, N., Herold, K.C. & Bluestone, J.A. (1995). Differential effects of anti-B7-1 and anti-B7-2 monoclonal antibody treatment on the development of diabetes in the nonobese diabetic mouse. *The Journal of Experimental Medicine,* (March 1995), Vol.181, No.3, pp. 1145-1155, ISSN 0022-1007

Levin, L., Ban Y., Concepcion, E., Davies, T.F., Greenberg, D.A. & Tomer, Y. (2004). Analysis of HLA genes in families with autoimmune diabetes and thyroiditis. *Human Immunology,* (June 2004), Vol.65, No.6, pp. 640-647, ISSN 0198-8859

Li, Q., Borovitskaya, A.E., DeSilva, M.G., Wasserfall, C., Maclaren, N.K., Notkins, A.L. & Lan, M.S. (1997). Autoantigens in insulin-dependent diabetes mellitus: molecular cloning and characterization of human IA-2 beta. *Proceedings of the Association of American Physicians,* (July 1995), Vol.109, No.4, pp. 429-439, ISSN 1081-650X

Lindley, S., Dayan, C.M., Bishop, A., Roep, B.O., Peakman, M. & Tree, T.I. (2005). Defective suppressor function in CD4(+)CD25(+) T-cells from patients with type 1 diabetes. *Diabetes,* (January 2005), Vol.54, No.1, pp. 92-99, ISSN 0012-1797

Lo, H.C., Lin, S.C. & Wang, Y.M. (2004). The relationship among serum cytokines, chemokine, nitric oxide, and leptin in children with type 1 diabetes mellitus. *Clinical Biochemistry,* (August 2004), Vol.37, No.8, pp. 666-672, ISSN 0009-9120

Lu, J., Li, Q., Xie, H., Chen, Z.J., Borovitskaya, A.E., Maclaren, N.K., Notkins, A.L. & Lan, M.S. (1996). Identification of a second transmembrane protein tyrosine phosphatase, IA-2beta, as an autoantigen in insulin-dependent diabetes mellitus: precursor of the 37-kDa tryptic fragment. *Proceedings of the National Academy of Sciences of the United States of America,* (March 1996), Vol.93, No.6, pp. 2307-2311, ISSN 0027-8424

Lundsgaard, D., Holm, T.L., Hornum, L. & Markholst, H. (2005). In Vivo Control of Diabetogenic T-Cells by Regulatory CD4+CD25+ T-Cells Expressing Foxp3. *Diabetes,* (April 2005), Vol.54, No.4, pp. 1040-1047, ISSN 0012-1797

Luo, X., Herold, K.C. & Miller, S.D. (2010). Immunotherapy of type 1 diabetes: where are we and where should we be going? *Immunity,* (April 2010), Vol.32, No.4, pp. 488-499, ISSN 1074-7613

Luo, X., Tarbell, K.V., Yang, H., Pothoven, K., Bailey, S.L., Ding, R., Steinman, R.M. & Suthanthiran, M. (2007). Dendritic cells with TGF-β1 differentiate naïve CD4+CD25- T cells into islet-protective Foxp3+ regulatory T cells. *Proceedings of the National Academy of Sciences of the United States of America,* (February 2007), Vol.104, No.8, pp. 2821-2826, ISSN 0027-8424

Maloy, K.J. & Powrie, F. (2001). Regulatory T cells in the control of immune pathology. *Nature Immunology,* (September 2001), Vol.2, No.9, pp. 816-822, ISSN 1529-2908

Mangan, P.R., Harrington, L.E., O'Quinn, D.B., Helms, W.S., Bullard, D.C., Elson, C.O., Hatton, R.D., Wahl, S.M., Schoeb, T.R. & Weaver, C.T. (2006). Transforming growth factor-beta induces development of the T(H)17 lineage. *Nature,* (2006), Vol.441, No.7090, pp. 231-234, ISSN 0028-0836

Marin-Gallen, S., Clemente-Casares, X., Planas, R., Pujol-Autonell, I., Carrascal, J., Carrillo, J., Ampudia, R., Verdaguer, J., Pujol-Borrell, R., Borràs, F.E. & Vives-Pi, M. (2010). Dendritic cells pulsed with antigen-specific apoptotic bodies prevent experimental type 1 diabetes. *Clinical and Experimental Immunology,* (May 2010), Vol.160, No.2, pp. 207-214, ISSN 0009-9104

Martin, S., Wolf-Eichbaum, D., Duinkerken, G., Scherbaum, W.A., Kolb, H., Noordzij, J.G. & Roep, B.O. (2001). Development of type 1 diabetes despite severe hereditary B-lymphocyte deficiency. *The New England Journal of Medicine,* (October 2001), Vol.345, No.14, pp. 1036-1040, ISSN 0028-4793

Mathis, D., Vence, L. & Benoist, C. (2001). Beta-Cell death during progression to diabetes. *Nature,* (December 2001), Vol.414, No.6865, pp. 792-798, ISSN 0028-0836

Matthews, J.B., Staeva, T.P., Bernstein, P.L., Peakman, M. & von Herrath, M. (2010). ITN-JDRF Type 1 Diabetes Combination Therapy Assessment Group. Developing combination immunotherapies for type 1 diabetes: recommendations from the ITN-JDRF Type 1 Diabetes Combination Therapy Assessment Group. *Clinical and Experimental Immunology,* (May 2010), pp. 176-84. Vol.160, No.2, ISSN 0009-9104

Maugendre, D., Chaillous, L., Rohmer, V., Lecomte, P., Marechaud, R., Sai, P., Marre, M., Charbonnel, B., Allannic, H. & Delamaire, M. (1997). Multiple antibody status in type 1 diabetic patients and subjects at various risk with islet-cell antibodies. *Diabetes & Metabolism,* (September 1997), Vol.23, No.4, pp. 320-326, ISSN 1262-3636

McGregor, C.M., Schoenberger, S.P. & Green, EA. (2004). CD154 is a negative regulator of autoaggressive CD8+ T cells in type 1 diabetes. *Proceedings of the National Academy of Sciences of the United States of America,* (June 2004), Vol.101, No.25, pp. 9345-9350, ISSN 0027-8424

Miller, B.J., Appel, M.C., O'Neil, J. & Wicker, L.S. (1988). Both the Lyt-2+ and L3T4+ T cell subsets are required for the transfer of diabetes in nonobese diabetic mice. *Journal of Immunology (Baltimore, Md.: 1950),* (January 1988), Vol.140, No.1, pp. 52-58, ISSN 0022-1767

Miossec, P., Korn, T. & Kuchroo, V.K. (2009). Interleukin-17 and type 17 helper T cells. *The New England Journal of Medicine,* (August 2009), Vol.361, No.9, pp. 888-898, ISSN 0028-4793

Mire-Sluis, A.R., Das, R.G. & Lernmark, Å. (2000). The World Health Organization International Collaborative Study for Islet Cell Antibodies. *Diabetologia,* (October 2000), Vol.43, No.10, pp. 1282, ISSN 0012-186X

Montana, E., Fernandez-Castaner, M., Rosel, P., Gomez, J. & Soler, J. (1991). Age, sex and ICA influence on beta-cell secretion during the first year after the diagnosis of type 1 diabetes mellitus. *Diabete & Metabolisme,* (September-October 1991), pp. 460-468. Vol.17, No.5, ISSN 0338-1684

Mottet, C., Uhlig, H.H. & Powrie, F. (2003). Cutting edge: cure of colitis by CD4+CD25+ regulatory T cells. *Journal of Immunology (Baltimore, Md.: 1950),* (April 2003), Vol.170, No.8, pp. 3939-3943, ISSN 0022-1767

Muir, A., Peck, A. & Clare-Salzler, M. (1995). Insulin immunization of nonobese diabetic mice induces a protective insulitis characterized by adminished intraislet interferon-r transcription. *The Journal of Clinical Investigation,* (February 1995), Vol.95, No.2, pp. 628-634, ISSN 0021-9738

Mukherjee, G. & Dilorenzo, T.P. (2010). The immunotherapeutic potential of dendritic cells in type 1 diabetes. *Clinical and Experimental Immunology,* (August 2010), Vol.161, No.2, pp. 197-207, ISSN 0009-9104

Murata, Y., Shimamura, T. & Hamuro, J. (2002). The polarization of T(h)1/T(h)2 balance is dependent on the intracellular thiol redox status of macrophages due to the distinctive cytokine production. *International Immunology,* (February 2002), Vol.14, No.2, pp. 201-212, ISSN 0953-8178

Murayama, H., Matsuura, N., Kawamura, T., Maruyama, T., Kikuchi, N., Kobayashi, T., Nishibe, F. & Nagata, A. (2006). A sensitive radioimmunoassay of insulin autoantibody: Reduction of non-specific binding of [(125)I]insulin. *Journal of Autoimmunity,* (March 2006), Vol.26, No.2, pp. 127-132, ISSN 0896-8411

Nakanishi, K., Yoshimoto, T., Tsutsui, H. & Okamura, H. (2001). Interleukin-18 is a unique cytokine that stimulates both Th1 and Th2 responses depending on its cytokine milieu. *Cytokine & Growth Factor Reviews,* (March 2001), Vol. 12, No.1, pp. 53-72, ISSN 1359-6101

Nemni, R., Braghi, S., Natali-Sora, M.G., Lampasona, V., Bonifacio, E., Comi, G. & Canal, N. (1994). Autoantibodies to glutamic acid decarboxylase in palatal myoclonus and epilepsy. *Annals of Neurology,* (October 1994), Vol.36, No.4, pp. 665-667, ISSN 0364-5134

Nikalji, R. & Bargman, J.M. (2011). Severe hypoglycemia with endogenous hyperinsulinemia in a nondiabetic hemodialysis patient following parathyroidectomy. *Nephrology, Dialysis, Transplantation: Official Publication of the European Dialysis and Transplant Association - European Renal Association,* (June 2011), Vol. 26, No.6, pp. 2050-2053 ISSN 0931-0509

Nir, T., Melton, D.A. & Dor, Y. (2007). Recovery from diabetes in mice by beta cell regeneration. *The Journal of Clinical Investigation,* (September 2007), pp. 2553-25561. Vol.117, No.9, ISSN 0021-9738

Ogasawara, K., Hamerman, J.A., Ehrlich, L.R., Bour-Jordan, H., Santamaria, P., Bluestone, J.A. & Lanier, L.L. (2004). NKG2D blockade prevents autoimmune diabetes in NOD mice. NKG2D blockade prevents autoimmune diabetes in NOD mice. *Immunity,* (June 2004), Vol.20, No.6, pp. 757-767, ISSN 1074-7613

Palmer, J.P., Asplin, C.M., Clemons, P., Lyen, K., Tatpati, O., Raghu, P.K. & Paquette, T.L. (1983). Insulin antibodies in insulin-dependent diabetics before insulin treatment. *Science (New York, N.Y.),* (December 1983), Vol.222, No.4630, pp. 1337-1339, ISSN 0036-8075

Park, H., Li Z., Yang, X.O., Chang, S.H., Nurieva, R., Wang, Y.H., Wang, Y., Hood, L., Zhu, Z., Tian, Q. & Dong, C. (2005). A distinct lineage of CD4 T cells regulates tissue inflammation by producing interleukin 17. *Nature Immunology,* (November 2005), Vol.6, No.11, pp. 1133-1141, ISSN 1529-2908

Patterson, C.C., Dahlquist, G.G., Gyürüs, E., Green, A., Soltész, G. & EURODIAB Study Group. (2009). Incidence trends for childhood type 1 diabetes in Europe during 1989-2003 and predicted new cases 2005-20: a multicentre prospective registration study. *Lancet,* (June 2009), Vol.373, No.9680, pp. 2027-2033, ISSN 0140-6736

Payton, M.A., Hawkes, C.J. & Christie, M.R. (1995). Relationship of the 37,000- and 40,000-Mr tryptic fragments of islet antigens in insulin-dependent diabetes to the protein tyrosine phosphatase-like molecule IA-2 (ICA512). *The Journal of Clinical Investigation,* (September 1995), Vol.96, No.3, pp. 1506-1511, ISSN 0021-9738

Peakman, M. & Dayan, CM. (2001). Antigen-specific immunotherapy for autoimmune disease: fighting fire with fire? *Immunology,* (December 2001), Vol.104, No.4, pp. 361-366, ISSN 0019-2805

Pearl-Yafe, M., Kaminitz, A., Yolcu, E.S., Yaniv, I., Stein, J. & Askenasy, N. (2007). Pancreatic islets under attack: cellular and molecular effectors. *Current Pharmaceutical Design,* (December 2007), pp. 749-760. Vol.13, No.7, ISSN 1381-6128

Perez-Bravo, F., Santos, J.L., Carrasco, E., Calvillan, M., Albala, C., Puig-Domingo, M., Piquer, S. & De Leiva, A. (2001). Transmission of high-risk HLA-DQB1 alleles in Chilean type 1 diabetic patients and their parents: stratification by the presence of ICA or GAD65 autoantibodies. *Autoimmunity,* (April 2001), pp. 285-291. Vol.33, No.4, ISSN 0891-6934

Petersen, J.S., Russel, S., Marshall, M.O., Kofod, H., Buschard, K., Cambon, N., Karlsen, A.E., Boel, E., Hagopian, W.A. & Hejnaes, K.R., et al. (1993). Differential expression of glutamic acid decarboxylase in rat and human islets. *Diabetes,* (March 1993), Vol.42, No.3, pp. 484-495, ISSN 0012-1797

Peterson, J. & Haskins, K. (1996). Transfer of diabetes in the NOD-scid mouse by CD4 T cell clones. Differential requirement for CD8 T cells. *Diabetes,* (March 1996), Vol.45, No.3, pp. 328-336, ISSN 0012-1797

Piccirillo, C.A., Tritt, M., Sgouroudis, E., Albanese, A., Pyzik, M. & Hay, V. (2005). Control of type 1 autoimmune diabetes by naturally occurring cd4+cd25+ regulatory T lymphocytes in neonatal NOD mice. *Annals of the New York Academy of Science,* (June 2005), Vol.1051, No.1, pp. 72-87, ISSN 0077-8923

Piquer, S., Belloni, C., Lampasona, V., Bazzigaluppi, E., Vianello, M., Giometto, B., Bosi, E., Bottazzo, G.F. & Bonifacio, E. (2005). Humoral autoimmune responses to glutamic acid decarboxylase have similar target epitopes and subclass that show titer-dependent disease association. *Clinical Immunology (Orlando, Fla.),* (October 2005), Vol.117, No.1, pp. 31-35, ISSN 1521-6616

Pittas, A.G. & Dawson-Hughes, B. (2010). Vitamin D and diabetes. *The Journal of Steroid Biochemistry and Molecular Biology,* (July 2010), Vol.121, No.1-2, pp. 425-429, ISSN 0960-0760

Pugliese, A., Zeller, M., Fernandez, A.Jr., Zalcberg, L.J., Bartlett, R.J., Ricordi, C., Pietropaolo, M., Eisenbarth, G.S., Bennett, S.T. & Patel, D.D. (1997). The insulin gene transcribed in the human thymus and transcription level correlate with allelic variation at the INS VNTR-IDDM2 susceptibility locus for type 1 diabetes. *Nature Genetics,* (March 1997), Vol.15, No.3, pp. 293-297, ISSN 1061-4036

Rabinovitch, A. (1994). Immunoregulatory and cytokine imbalance in the pathogenesis of IDDM. *Diabetes,* (May 1994), Vol.43, No.5, pp. 613-621, ISSN 0012-1797

Raz, I., Elias, D., Avron, A., Tamir, M., Metzger, M. & Cohen, I.R. (2001). Beta-cell function in new-onset type 1 diabetes and immunomodulation with a heat-shock protein peptide (DiaPep277): a randomised, double-blind, phase II trial. *Lancet,* (November 2001), Vol.358, No.9295, pp. 1749-1753, ISSN 0140-6736

Rewers, M. & Gottlieb, P. (2009). Immunotherapy for the prevention and treatment of type 1 diabetes: human trials and a look into the future. *Diabetes Care,* (October 2009), Vol.32, No.10, pp. 1769-1782, ISSN 0149-5992

Riley, W.J., Maclaren, N.K., Krischer, J., Spillar, R.P., Silverstein, J.H., Schatz, D.A., Schwartz, S., Malone, J., Shah, S. & Vadheim, C., et al. (1990). A prospective study of the development of diabetes in relatives of patients with insulin-dependent diabetes. *The New England Journal of Medicine,* (October 1990), Vol.323, No.17, pp. 1167-1172, ISSN 0028-4793

Rothe, H., Ito, Y. & Kolb, H. (2001). Disease resistant, NOD related strains reveal checkpoints of immunoregulation in the pancreas. *Journal of Molecular Medicine,* (May 2001), Vol.79, No.4, pp. 190-197, ISSN 0377-046X

Rozenberg, O., Rosenblat, M., Coleman, R., Shih, D.M. & Aviram, M. (2003). Paraoxonase (PON1) deficiency is associated with increased macrophage oxidative stress: studies in PON1-knockout mice. *Free Radical Biology & Medicine,* (March 2003), Vol.34, No.6, pp. 774-784, ISSN 0891-5849

Sai, P., Rivereau, A.S., Granier, C., Haertle, T.H. & Martignat, L. (1996). Immunization of non-obese diabetic (NOD) mice with glutamic acid decarboxylase-derived peptide 524-543 reduces cyclophosphamide-accelerated diabetes. *Clinical and Experimental Immunology,* (August 1996), Vol.105, No.2, pp. 330-337, ISSN 0009-9104

Sainio-Pollanen, S., Liukas, A., Pollanen, P. & Simell, O. (1999). The role of CD8+ cells, cell degeneration, and Fas ligand in insulitis after intraperitoneal transfer of NOD splenocytes. *Pancreas,* (April 1999), pp. 282-293. Vol.18, No.3, ISSN 0885-3177

Sakaguchi, S., Sakaguchi, N., Asano, M., Itoh, M. & Toda, M. (1995). Immunologic self-tolerance maintained by activated T cells expressing IL-2 receptor alpha-chains (CD25). Breakdown of a single mechanism of self-tolerance causes various autoimmune diseases. *Journal of Immunology (Baltimore, Md.: 1950),* (August 1995), Vol.155, No.3, pp. 1151-1164, ISSN 0022-1767

Salomon, B., Rhee, L., Bour-Jordan, H., Hsin, H., Montag, A., Soliven, B., Arcella, J., Girvin, A.M., Padilla, J., Miller, S.D. & Bluestone, J.A. (2001). Development of spontaneous autoimmune peripheral polyneuropathy in B7-2-deficient NOD mice. *The Journal of Experimental Medicine,* (September 2001), Vol.194, No.5, pp. 677-84, ISSN 0022-1007

Sanjeevi, C.B. (2009). Type 1 diabetes research: Newer approaches and exciting developments. *International Journal of Diabetes in Developing Countries,* (April 2009), pp. 49-51. Vol.29, No.2, ISSN 0973-3930

Savola, K., Bonifacio, E., Sabbah, E., Kulmala, P., Vahasalo, P., Karjalainen, J., Tuomilehto-Wolf, E., Merilainen, J., Akerblom, H.K. & Knip, M. (1998). IA-2 antibodies--a sensitive marker of IDDM with clinical onset in childhood and adolescence.

Childhood Diabetes in Finland Study Group. *Diabetologia,* (April 1998), Vol.41, No.4, pp. 424-429, ISSN 0012-186X

Savola., K. (2000). *Role of IA-2 antibodies in clinical and preclinical type 1 diabetes. Academic Dissertation to be presented with the assent of the Faculty of Medicine, University of Oulu, for public discussion in Auditorium 12 of the University Hospital of Oulu, on June 16th, 2000, at 12 noon.* Oulu University Library, ISBN 951-42-5677-8, Oulu: Finland

Schatz, D., Krischer, J., Horne, G., Riley, W., Spillar, R., Silverstein, J., Winter, W., Muir, A., Derovanesian, D. & Shah, S., et al. (1994). Islet cell antibodies predict insulin-dependent diabetes in United States school age children as powerfully as in unaffected relatives. *The Journal of Clinical Investigation,* (June 1994), Vol.93, No.6, pp. 2403-2407, ISSN 0021-9738

Scheen, J. (2004). Pathophysiology of insulin secretion. *Annales d'Endocrinologie,* (February 2004), pp. 29-36 Vol.65, No.1, ISSN 0003-4266

Schlosser, M., Strebelow, M., Rjasanowski, I., Kerner, W., Wassmuth, R. & Ziegler, M. (2004). Prevalence of diabetes-associated autoantibodies in schoolchildren: the Karlsburg Type 1 Diabetes Risk Study. *Annals of the New York Academy of Science,* (December 2004), Vol.1037, No.1, pp. 114-117, ISSN 0077-8923

Schmidli, R.S., Colman, P.G., Cui, L., Yu, W.P., Kewming, K., Jankulovski, C., Harrison, L.C., Pallen, C.J. & DeAizpurua, H.J. (1998). Antibodies to the protein tyrosine phosphatases IAR and IA-2 are associated with progression to insulin-dependent diabetes (IDDM) in first-degree relatives at-risk for IDDM. *Autoimmunity,* (January 1998), Vol.28, No.1, pp. 15-23, ISSN 0891-6934

Schneider, B., Staraus, E. & Yalow, R.S. (1976). Some considerations in the preparation of raioiodoisulin for radioimmunoassay and receptor assay. *Diabetes,* (April 1976), Vol.25, No.4, pp. 260-267, ISSN 0012-1797

Seyfert-Margolis V, Gisler TD, Asare AL, Wang RS, Dosch HM, Brooks-Worrell B, Eisenbarth GS, Palmer JP, Greenbaum CJ, Gitelman SE, Nepom GT, Bluestone JA, Herold KC. (2006). Analysis of T-cell assays to measure autoimmune responses in subjects with type 1 diabetes: results of a blinded controlled study. *Diabetes,* (September 2006), Vol.55, No.9, pp. 2588-2594, ISSN 0012-1797

Sharif, S., Arreaza, G.A., Zucker, P. & Delovitch, T.L. (2002). Regulatory natural killer T cells protect against spontaneous and recurrent type 1 diabetes. *Annals of the New York Academy of Sciences,* (April 2002), Vol.958, No.1, pp. 77-88, ISSN 0077-8923

Shi, B., Wang, Z., Jin, H., Chen, Y.W., Wang, Q. & Qian, Y. (2009). Immunoregulatory Cordyceps sinensis increases regulatory T cells to Th17 cell ratio and delays diabetes in NOD mice. *International Immunopharmacology,* (May 2009), pp. 582-586. Vol.9, No.5, ISSN 1567-5769

Shimada, A., Charlton, B., Taylor-Edwards, C. & Fathman, G. (1996). B-cell destruction may be a late consequence of the autoimmune process in nonobese diabetic mice. *Diabetes,* (August 1996), Vol.45, No.8, pp. 1063-1067, ISSN 0012-1797

Sia, C. (2005). Imbalance in Th cell polarization and its relevance in type 1 diabetes mellitus. *The Review of Diabetic Studies: RDS,* (Winter 2005), Vol.2, No.4, pp. 182-186, ISSN 1613-6071

Silveira, P.A., Serreze, D.V. & Grey, S.T. (2007). Invasion of the killer B's in type 1 diabetes. *Frontiers in Bioscience: a Journal and Virtual Library,* (January 2007), pp. 2183-2193. Vol.12, No.1, ISSN 1093-9946

Silverstein, J., Maclaren, N., Riley, W., Spillar, R., Radjenovic, D. & Johnson, S. (1988). Immunosuppression with azathioprine and prednisone in recent-onset insulin-dependent diabetes mellitus. *The New England Journal of Medicine,* (September 1988), Vol.319, No.10, pp. 599–604, ISSN 0028-4793

Skyler, J.S., Krischer, J.P., Wolfsdorf, J., Cowie, C., Palmer, J.P., Greenbaum, C., Cuthbertson, D., Rafkin-Mervis, L.E., Chase, H.P. & Leschek, E. (2005). Effects of oral insulin in relatives of patients with type 1 diabetes: The Diabetes Prevention Trial--Type 1. *Diabetes Care,* (May 2005), Vol.28, No.5, pp. 1068-76, ISSN 0149-5992

Sobel, D.O., Goyal, D., Ahvazi, B., Yoon, J.W., Chung, Y.H., Bagg, A. & Harlan, D.M. (1998). Low dose poly I:C prevents diabetes in the diabetes prone BB rat. *Journal of Autoimmunity,* (August 1998), Vol.11, No.4, pp. 343–352, ISSN 0896-8411

Solimena, M., Folli, F., Aparisi, R., Pozza, G. & De Camilli, P. (1990). Autoantibodies to GABA-ergic neurons and pancreatic beta cells in stiff-man syndrome. *The New England Journal of Medicine,* (May 1990), pp. 1555-1560. Vol.322, No.22, ISSN 0028-4793

Solimena, M., Folli, F., Denis-Donini, S., Comi, G.C., Pozza, G., De Camilli, P. & Vicari, A.M. (1988). Autoantibodies to glutamic acid decarboxylase in a patient with stiff-man syndrome, epilepsy, and type I diabetes mellitus. *The New England Journal of Medicine,* (April 1988), Vol.318, No.16, pp. 1012-1020, ISSN 0028-4793

Sparre, T., Larsen, M.R., Heding, P.E., Karlsen, A.E., Jensen, O.N. & Pociot, F. (2005). Unraveling the pathogenesis of type 1 diabetes with proteomics: present and future directions. *Molecular & Cellular Proteomics: MCP,* (April 2005), Vol.4, No.4, pp. 441-457, ISSN 1535-9476

Staeva-Vieira T, Peakman M, von Herrath M. (2007). Translational mini-review series on type 1 diabetes: Immune-based therapeutic approaches for type 1 diabetes. *Clinical and Experimental Immunology,* (April 2007), Vol.148, No.1, pp. 17-31, ISSN 0009-9104

Steinman, R.M. & Banchereau, J. (2007). Taking dendritic cells into medicine. *Nature,* (September 2007), Vol.449, No.7171, pp. 419-426, ISSN 0028-0836

Steinman, R.M., Hawiger, D. & Nussenzweig, M.C. (2003). Tolerogenic dendritic cells. *Annual Review of Immunology,* (December 2003), pp. 685–711. Vol.21, No., ISSN 0732-0582

Stenström, G., Gottsäter, A., Bakhtadze, E., Berger, B. & Sundkvist, G. (2005). Latent Autoimmune Diabetes in Adults Definition, Prevalence, β-Cell Function, and Treatment. *Diabetes,* (December 2005), Vol.54, No.Suppl2, pp. S68-S72, ISSN 0012-1797

Stoffels, K., Overbergh, L., Giulietti, A., Verlinden, L., Bouillon, R. & Mathieu, C. (2006). Immune regulation of 25-hydroxyvitamin-D3-1alpha-hydroxylase in human monocytes. *Journal of Bone and Mineral Research: the Official Journal of the American Society for Bone and Mineral Research,* (January 2006), pp. 37-47. Vol.21, No.1, ISSN 0884-0431

Suarez-Pinzon, W.L. & Rabinovitch, A. (2001). Approaches to type 1 diabetes prevention by intervention in cytokine immunoregulatory circuits. *International Journal of Experimental Diabetes Research,* (January 2001), Vol.2, No.1, pp. 3-17, ISSN 1560-4284

Sutmuller, R.P., den Brok, M.H., Kramer, M., Bennink, E.J., Toonen, L.W., Kullberg, B.J., Joosten, L.A., Akira, S., Netea, M.G. & Adema, G.J. (2006). Toll-like receptor 2 controls expansion and function of regulatory T cells. *The Journal of Clinical Investigation,* (February 2006), Vol.116, No.2, pp. 485-494, ISSN 0021-9738

Szeszko, J.S., Howson, J.M., Cooper, J.D., Walker, N.M., Twells, R.C., Stevens, H.E., Nutland, S.L. & Todd, J.A. (2006). Analysis of polymorphisms of the interleukin-18 gene in type 1 diabetes and Hardy-Weinberg equilibrium testing. *Diabetes,* (February 2006), Vol.55, No.2, pp. 559-562, ISSN 0012-1797

Takahashi, K., Tasaka, H. & Hasegawa, Y. (1995). Sensitivity and specificity for detection of islet cell cytoplasmic antibodies using rat pancreatic sections. *Japanese Journal of Clinical Immunology,* (April 1995), Vol.18, No.2, pp. 188-196, ISSN 0911-4300

Tang, Q., Henriksen, K.J., Bi, M., Finger, E.B., Szot, G., Ye, J., Masteller, E.L., McDevitt, H., Bonyhadi, M. & Bluestone, J.A. (2004). In vitro-expanded antigen-specific regulatory T cells suppress autoimmune diabetes. *The Journal of Experimental Medicine,* (June 2004), Vol.199, No.11, pp. 1455-1465, ISSN 0022-1007

Tarbell, K.V., Yamazaki, S., Olson, K., Toy, P. & Steinman, R.M. (2004). CD25+ CD4+ T cells, expanded with dendritic cells presenting a single autoantigenic peptide, suppress autoimmune diabetes. *The Journal of Experimental Medicine,* (June 2004), pp. 1467-1477. Vol.199, No.11, ISSN 0022-1007

Targher, G., Zenari, L., Bertolini, L., Muggeo, M. & Zoppini, G. (2001). Elevated levels of interleukin-6 in young adults with type 1 diabetes without clinical evidence of microvascular and macrovascular complications. *Diabetes Care,* (May 2001), Vol.24, No.5, pp. 956-957, ISSN 0149-5992

Taylor, A.W., Yee, D.G. & Streilein, J.W. (1998). Suppression of nitric oxide generated by inflammatory macrophages by calcitonin gene-related peptide in aqueous humor. *Investigative Ophthalmology & Visual Science,* (July 1998), pp. Vol.39, No.8, 1372-1378, ISSN 0146-0404

Thivolet, C. & Carel, J.C. (1996). Screening and prediction of diabetes mellitus in children. *La Revue du Praticien,* (March 1996), Vol.46, No.5, pp. 565-569, ISSN 0035-2640

Thivolet, C., Nicolino, M., Monbeig, S., Estour, B., Halimi, S., Robert, M., Orgiazzi, J., Chatelain, P. & GRADI study. (2002). Combination of autoantibody markers and risk for development of type 1 diabetes: results from a large french cohort of family members. *Diabetes & metabolism,* (September 2002), Vol.28, No. 4 Pt 1, pp. 279-285, ISSN 1262-3636

Thorvaldson, L., Johansson, S.E., Hoglund, P. & Sandler, S. (2005). Impact of plastic adhesion in vitro on analysis of Th1 and Th2 cytokines and immune cell distribution from mice with multiple low-dose streptozotocin-induced diabetes. *Journal of Immunological Methods,* (December 2005), pp. 73-81. Vol.307, No.1-2, ISSN 0022-1759

Thrower, S.L. & Bingley, P.J. (2009). Strategies to prevent type 1 diabetes. *Diabetes, obesity & metabolism,* (October 2009), pp. 931-938. Vol.11, No.10, ISSN 1462-8902

Timist, J. (1996). Etiopathogenesis of type 1 diabetes mellitus. *La Revue du Praticien,* (March 1996), pp. 560-564. Vol.46, No.5, ISSN 0035-2640

Toma, A., Haddouk, S., Briand, J.P., Camoin, L., Gahery, H., Connan, F., Dubois-Laforgue, D., Caillat-Zucman, S., Guillet, J.G., Carel, J.C., Muller, S., Choppin, J. & Boitard, C. (2005). Recognition of a subregion of human proinsulin by class I-restricted T cells in type 1 diabetic patients. *Proceedings of the National Academy of Sciences of the United States of America,* (July 2005), Vol.102, No.30, pp. 10581-10586, ISSN 0027-8424

Trajkovski, M., Mziaut, H., Altkruger, A., Ouwendijk, J., Knoch, K.P., Muller, S. & Solimena, M. (2004). Nuclear translocation of an ICA512 cytosolic fragment couples granule exocytosis and insulin expression in {beta}-cells. *The Journal of Cell Biology,* (December 2004), pp. 1063-1074. Vol.167, No.6, ISSN 0021-9525

Tree, T.I., Morgenthaler, N.G., Duhindan, N., Hicks, K.E., Madec, A.M., Scherbaum, W.A. & Banga, J.P. (2000). Two amino acids in glutamic acid decarboxylase act in concert for maintenance of conformational determinants recognised by Type I diabetic autoantibodies. *Diabetologia,* (July 2000), pp. 881-889. Vol.43, No.7, ISSN 0012-186X

Tuomi, T., Groop, L.C., Zimmet, P.Z., Rowley, M.J., Knowles, W. & Mackay, I.R. (1993). Antibodies to glutamic acid decarboxylase reveal latent autoimmune diabetes mellitus in adults with a non-insulin-dependent onset of disease. *Diabetes,* (February 1993), Vol.42, No.2, pp. 359-362, ISSN 0012-1797

Vafiadis, P., Bennett, S.T., Todd, J.A., Nadeau, J., Grabs, R., Goodyer, C.G., Wickramasinghe, S., Colle, E. & Polychronakos, C. (1997). Insulin expression in human thymus is modulated by INS VNTR alleles at the IDDM2 locus. *Nature Genetics,* (March 1997), pp. 289-292, Vol.15, No.3, ISSN 1061-4036

van den Brandt, J., Fischery, H.J., Waltery, L., Hünigy, T., Klötingy, I. & Reichardty H.M. (2010). Type 1 diabetes in BioBreeding rats is critically linked to an imbalance between Th17 and regulatory T cells and an altered TCR repertoire. *Journal of Immunology (Baltimore, Md.: 1950),* (August 2010), Vol.185, No.4, pp. 2285-2294, ISSN 0022-1767

Vantyghem, M.C, Balavoiney, A.S, Kerr-Contey, J., Pattouy, F. & Noely C. (2009). Who should benefit from diabetes cell therapy? *Annales d'Endocrinologie,* (December 2009), Vol.70, No.6, pp. 443-448, ISSN 0003-4266

Velloso, L.A., Eiziricky, D.L., Karlsson, F.A., Kämpe, O. (1994). Absence of autoantibodies against glutamate decarboxylase (GAD) in the non-obese diabetic (NOD) mouse and low expression of the enzyme in mouse islets. *Clinical and Experimental Immunology,* (April 1994), Vol.96, No.1, pp. 129-137, ISSN 0009-9104

Verge, C.F, Stenger, D., Bonifacio, E., Colman, P.G., Pilcher, C., Bingley, P.J. & Eisenbarth, G.S. (1998). Combined use of autoantibodies (IA-2 autoantibody, GAD autoantibody, insulin autoantibody, cytoplasmic islet cell antibodies) in type 1 diabetes: combinatorial islet autoantibody workshop. *Diabetes,* (December 1998), Vol.47, No.12, pp. 1857-1866, ISSN 0012-1797

Verge, C.F., Gianani, R., Kawasaki, E., Yu, L., Pietropaolo, M., Jackson, R.A., Chase, H.P. & Eisenbarth, GS. (1996). Prediction of type I diabetes in first-degree relatives using a combination of insulin, GAD, and ICA512bdc/IA-2 autoantibodies. *Diabetes,* (July 1996), Vol.45, No.7, pp. 926-933, ISSN 0012-1797

Vija, L., Farge, D., Gautier, J.F., Vexiau, P., Dumitrache, C., Bourgarit, A., Verrecchia, F. & Larghero, J. (2009). Mesenchymal stem cells: Stem cell therapy perspectives for type 1 diabetes. *Diabetes & Metabolism,* (April 2009), Vol.35, No.2, pp. 85-93, ISSN 1262-3636

von Boehmer, H. (2004). Type 1 diabetes: focus on prevention. *Nature Medicine,* (August 2004), Vol.10, No.8, pp. 783-784, ISSN 1078-8956

von Herrath, M. (2009). Diabetes: A virus-gene collaboration. *Nature,* (May 2009), Vol.459, No.7246, pp. 518-519, ISSN 0028-0836

Wahlberg, J., Fredriksson, J., Nikolic, E., Vaarala, O. & Ludvigsson, J. (2005). The ABIS-Study Group. Environmental factors related to the induction of beta-cell autoantibodies in 1-yr-old healthy children. *Pediatric Diabetes,* (December 2005), Vol.6, No.4, pp. 199-205, ISSN 1399-543X

Wallace, D.J., Hahn, B. & Dubois, E.L. (2007). *Dubois' lupus erythematosus,* Lippincott Williams & Wilkins, ISBN(13) 978-0-7817-9394-0, Philadelphia PA 19106, USA

Wang, B., Gonzalez, A., Benoist, C. & Mathis, D. (1996). The role of CD8+ T cells in the initiation of insulin-dependent diabetes mellitus. *European Journal of Immunology,* (August 1996), Vol.26, No.8, pp. 1762-1769, ISSN 0014-2980

Wenzlau, J.M., Frisch, L.M., Gardner, T.J., Sarkar, S., Hutton, J.C. & Davidson, H.W. (2009). Novel antigens in type 1 diabetes: the importance of ZnT8. *Current Diabetes Reports,* (April 2009), Vol.9, No.2, pp.105-112, ISSN 1534-4827

Wenzlau, J.M., Juhl, K., Yu, L., Moua, O., Sarkar, S.A., Gottlieb, P., Rewers, M., Eisenbarth, G.S., Jensen, J., Davidson, H.W. & Hutton, J.C. (2007). The cation efflux transporter ZnT8 (Slc30A8) is a major autoantigen in human type 1 diabetes. *Proceedings of the National Academy of Sciences of the United States of America,* (October 2007), Vol.104, No.43, pp.17040-17045, ISSN 0027-8424

Wenzlau, J.M., Moua, O., Sarkar, S.A., Yu, L., Rewers, M., Eisenbarth, G.S., Davidson, H.W. & Hutton, J.C. (2008). SlC30A8 is a major target of humoral autoimmunity in type 1 diabetes and a predictive marker in prediabetes. *Annals of the New York Academy of Sciences,* (December 2008), Vol.1150, No.12, pp. 256-259, ISSN 0077-8923

Wie, J., Davis, K.M., Wu, H. & Wu, J.Y. (2004). Protein phosphorylation of human brain glutamic acid decarboxylase (GAD)65 and GAD67 and its physiological implications. *Biochemistry,* (May 2004), Vol.43, No.20, pp. 6182-6189, ISSN 0006-2960

Wild, S., Roglic, G., Green, A., Sicree, R. & King, H. (2004). Global prevalence of diabetes: estimates for the year 2000 and projections for 2030. *Diabetes Care,* (May 2004), Vol.27, No.5, pp. 1047-1053, ISSN 0149-5992

Wilkin, T., Palmer J., Kurtz, A., Bonifacio E. & Diaz JL. (1988). The second international workshop on the standardization of insulin autoantibody (IAA) measurement. *Diabetologia,* (July 1988), Vol.31, No.7, pp. 449-450, ISSN 0012-186X

Wilson, S.B., Kent, S.C., Patton, K.T., Orban, T., Jackson, R.A., Exley, M., Porcelli, S., Schatz, D.A., Atkinson, M.A., Balk, S.P., Strominger, J.L. & Hafler, D.A. (1998). Extreme Th1 bias of invariant Valpha24JalphaQ T cells in type 1 diabetes. *Nature,* (January 1998), Vol.391, No.6663, pp. 177-181, ISSN 0028-0836

Winnock, F., Christie, M.R., Batstra, M.R., Aanstoot, H.J., Weets, I., Decochez, K., Jopart, P., Nicolaij, D., Gorus, F.K. & Belgian Diabetes Registry. (2001). Autoantibodies to a 38-kDa glycosylated islet cell membrane-associated antigen in (pre)type 1 diabetes: association with IA-2 and islet cell autoantibodies. *Diabetes Care,* (July 2001), Vol.24, No.7, pp. 1181-1186, ISSN 0149-5992

Yagui, H., Matsumoto, M., Kunimoto, K., Kawaguchi, J., Makino, S. & Harada, M. (1992). Analysis of the roles of CD4+ and CD8+ T cells in autoimmune diabetes of NOD mice using transfer to NOD athymic nude mice. *European Journal of Immunology,* (September 1992), Vol.22, No.9, pp. 2387-2393, ISSN 0014-2980

Yamada, K., Yuan, X., Inada, C., Hayashi, H., Koyama, K., Ichikawa, F., Eisenbarth, G.S. & Nonaka, K. (1997). Combined measurements of GAD65 and ICA512 antibodies in acute onset and slowly progressive IDDM. *Diabetes Research and Clinical Practice,* (March 1997), Vol.35, No.2-3, pp. 91-98, ISSN 0168-8227

Yamada, S., Irie, J., Shimada, A., Kodama, K., Morimoto, J., Suzuki, R., Oikawa, Y. & Saruta, T. (2003). Assessment of beta cell mass and oxidative peritoneal exudate cells in murine type 1 diabetes using adoptive transfer system. *Autoimmunity,* (March 2003), Vol.36, No.2, pp. 63-70, ISSN 0891-6934

Yamamoto, A.M., Deschamps, I., Garchon, H.J., Roussely, H., Moreau, N., Beaurain, G., Robert, J.J. & Bach, J.F. (1998). Young age and HLA markers enhance the risk of progression to type 1 diabetes in antibody-positive siblings of diabetic children. *Journal of Autoimmunity,* (December 1998), Vol.11, No.6, pp. 643-650, ISSN 0896-8411

Yamazaki, S., Iyoda, T., Tarbell, K., Olson, K., Velinzon, K., Inaba, K. & Steinman, R.M. (2003). Direct expansion of functional CD25+CD4+ regulatory T cells by antigen-processing dendritic cells. *The Journal of Experimental Medicine,* (July 2003), Vol.198, No.2, pp. 235-247, ISSN 0022-1007

Yang, L., Luo, S., Huang, G., Peng, J., Li, X., Yan, X., Lin, J., Wenzlau, J.M., Davidson, H.W., Hutton, J.C. & Zhou, Z. (2010). The diagnostic value of zinc transporter 8 autoantibody (ZnT8A) for type 1 diabetes in Chinese. *Diabetes/Metabolism Research and Reviews,* (October 2010), Vol.26, No.7, pp.579-584, ISSN 1520-7552

Yang, W., Hussain, S., Mi, Q.S., Santamaria, P. & Delovitch, T.L. (2004). Perturbed homeostasis of peripheral T cells elicits decreased susceptibility to anti-CD3-induced apoptosis in prediabetic nonobese diabetic mice. *Journal of Immunology (Baltimore, Md.: 1950),* (October 2004), Vol.173, No.7, pp. 4407-4416, ISSN 0022-1767

Yoon, J,W. & Jun, H.S. (2005). Autoimmune destruction of pancreatic beta cells. *American Journal of Therapeutics,* (November-December 2005), Vol.12, No.6, pp. 580-591, ISSN 1075-2765

Yoon, J.W. & Jun, H.S. (2001). Cellular and molecular pathogenic mechanisms of insulin-dependent diabetes mellitus. *Annals of the New York Academy of Sciences,* (April 2001), Vol.928, No.1, pp. 200-211, ISSN 0077-8923

Zamaklar, M., Jotic, A., Lalic, N., Lalic, K., Rajkovic, N. & Milicic, T. (2002). Relation between course of disease in type 1 diabetes and islet cell antibodies. *Annals of the New York Academy of Sciences,* (April 2002), Vol.958, No.1, pp. 251-253, ISSN 0077-8923

Zhang, X. & McMurray, D.N. (1998). Suppression of lymphoproliferation by alveolar macrophages in the guinea pig. *Tubercle and Lung Disease: the Official Journal of the International Union against Tuberculosis and Lung Disease,* (January 1998), pp. 119-126. Vol.79, No.2, ISSN 0962-8479

Zheng, S.G., Wang, J.H., Koss, M.N., Quismorio, Jr.F., Gray, J.D. & Horwitz, D.A. (2004). CD4+ and CD8+ regulatory T cells generated ex vivo with IL-2 and TGF-beta suppress a stimulatory graft-versus-host disease with a lupus-like syndrome. *Journal of Immunology (Baltimore, Md.: 1950),* (February 2004), Vol.172, No.3, pp. 1531-1539, ISSN 0022-1767

Ziegler, A.G., Standl, E., Albert, E. & Mehnert, H. (1991). HLA-associated insulin autoantibody formation in newly diagnosed type I diabetic patients. *Diabetes,* (September 1991), Vol.40, No.9, pp. 1146-1149, ISSN 0012-1797

Ziegler, A.G., Ziegler, R., Vardi, P., Jackson, R.A., Soeldner, J.S., & Eisenbarth, G.S. (1989). Life-table analysis of progression to diabetes of anti-insulin autoantibody-positive relatives of individuals with type I diabetes. *Diabetes,* (October 1989), Vol.38, No.10, pp. 1320-1325, ISSN 0012-1797

2

Use of Congenic Mouse Strains for Gene Identification in Type 1 Diabetes

Ute Christine Rogner
*Institut Pasteur & Centre National de la Recherche Scientifique
Paris,
France*

1. Introduction

Type 1 diabetes (T1D) affects about 0.25 % of the Caucasian population and is a major health problem due to early disease onset (before the age of 20 in half of the patients), the increasing disease incidence in most populations, the absence of an effective curative treatment, and the high vascular burden associated with residual hyperglycaemia in insulin-treated T1D patients. The disease results from the autoimmune destruction of the insulin secreting pancreatic beta-cells. Indirect evidence implicating auto-immunity in human diabetes relies on the detection of insulitis, islet cell antibodies, T cell responses to ß-cell antigens and association with a restricted set of class II Major Histocompatibility Complex (MHC) haplotypes.

Type 1 or insulin dependent diabetes (IDDM) is under both multifactorial and polygenic control, with the MHC class II locus and the insulin locus being two of the best studied genetic loci (Serreze & Leiter, 2001; Todd & Wicker, 2001; Maier & Wicker, 2005). Genetic studies of T1D aetiology in man have often proved difficult, reflecting the complexity of the genetic control, genetic heterogeneity, and in many cases the lack of intrinsic power of the studies. However, recent advances in human genetics, for example, the availability of the human genome sequence, the establishment of the HapMap (Zeggini et al., 2005; Taylor et al., 2006), the development of high throughput genotyping, the availability of larger sample collections (2007), and the increasing statistical power of the studies provided more promising results. The underlying genetic complexity of T1D and the difficulty of undertaking functional studies in human provide a strong argument for undertaking complementary genetic studies in a model animal system in which genetic heterogeneity and environmental factors can be more easily controlled. Only model animal studies moreover allow the functional genomic studies, which provide definitive proof of genetic causality.

The nonobese diabetes (NOD) mouse (Makino et al., 1980; Hattori et al., 1986) is a well-characterized animal model of IDDM. The NOD mouse spontaneously develops T1D, which shares most of the characteristics of the human disease. However one distinctive feature is that female mice have much higher prevalence than male mice: approximately 80% in females versus 40% in males at 8 months of age. More than forty murine insulin dependent diabetes susceptibility loci (*Idd*) have been genetically localised, although little information has been obtained about the nature of many of these non-MHC *Idd* genes. Identification and characterisation of particular *Idd* genes in the mouse will allow testing of the involvement of the human homologue in T1D and more particularly, since there is unlikely to be just a one to one correspondence between human and mouse, allow the identification of the underlying metabolic network for systematic candidate gene testing in human. An improved knowledge of the underlying genetics of T1D in both mouse and men should provide information about potential drug targets and lead to improved possibilities for earlier diagnostics.

2. Generation and analysis of NOD congenic mice

The mouse is the organism of choice as a model for human disease. Not only that many thousands of mutations are already isolated and projects to inactivate all mouse genes are underway (Grimm, 2006), but also 450 inbred strains have been described (Beck et al., 2000) with a wealth of genetic and phenotypic diversity. This collection of inbred strains provides a basis for studying phenotypes under complex genetic control. The Mouse Phenome Project has been organized to establish a collection of baseline phenotypic data on commonly used and genetically diverse inbred mouse strains and to make this information publicly available through a web-accessible database (see database links).

2.1 Definition of recombinant inbred, consomic and congenic strains

Different breeding systems have been established in the mouse (Figure 1). Recombinant inbred (RI) strains contain a unique admixture of genetic contributions in approximately equal proportions from its two original progenitor inbred strains. Recombinant inbred (RI) strains are established by crossing animals of two inbred strains, followed then by 20 or more generations of brother/sister matings (Bailey, 1971). The Complex Trait Consortium (Churchill et al., 2004) represents the largest community effort to date to generate some 1000 RIs from eight different parental strains to identify genes involved in complex disorders. Recombinant Congenic (RC) strains are also established by an initial crossing between two inbred strains, but this is followed by a few, usually two, backcrosses of the resulting F1 hybrids to one of the parental strains, called the 'recipient' strain, with subsequent brother/sister intercrossing (Demant & Hart, 1986). In both RI and RC strains the result is a mosaic genetic structure with blocks of genetic material from one parent interspersed with blocks of genetic material from the other parent. RI and RC strains differ however in the relative contribution of the two parents.

Consomics and congenics are inbred strains in which part of the genome of one mouse strain is transferred to another by backcrossing the donor strain to the recipient strain, followed by intercrossing in later generations to ensure homozygosity. In the case of the NOD congenic strains the recipient is the NOD mouse and the donor in most cases a C57BL/6 mouse. Genetic selection is systematically practised to ensure retention of the desired genetic material from the donor strain in each backcross. Most genetic markers and their alleles can be conveniently looked up in the Mouse Genome Informatics (MGI) database. The breeding method was first described by Snell who produced histo-incompatible congenic strains, that were originally called 'congenic resistant' strains (Snell, 1978). In the case of a consomic strain an entire chromosome is transferred (Nadeau et al., 2000; Santos et al., 2002). In the case of a congenic strain a chromosomal segment, also termed the differential segment, is transferred (Boyse & Bentley, 1977; Wakeland et al., 1997). Congenic strains will normally carry differential regions of 10-20 Mb in size (Peirce,

2001) unless specific efforts are made to reduce the size of the differential segment (see below). Many of the existing congenic strains, including many of the NOD congenics, can already be retrieved directly via the Jackson Laboratories. Congenic strains need to be distinguished from co-isogenic strains that differ at only a single locus from their parental strain (Roths et al., 1984). Co-isogenics can be derived by gene targeting, for example through homologous recombination, or by mutagenesis approaches. All above described strains have in common that they allow repeated phenotyping of large numbers of genetically homogenous animals under very defined environmental conditions. This would never be possible by studying human subjects.

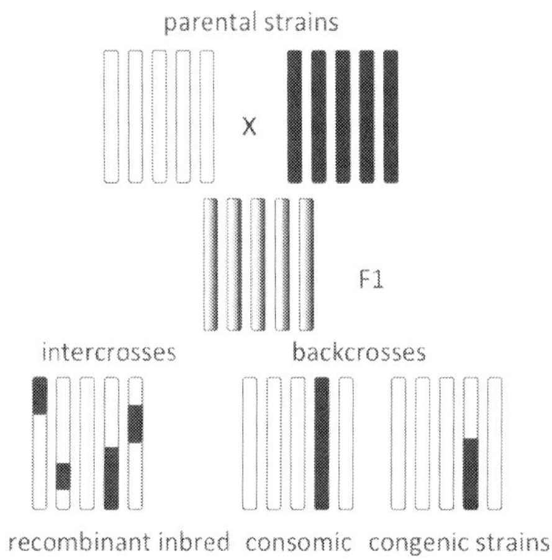

Fig. 1. Recombinant inbred strains, consomics, and congenics.

Recombinant inbred strains are generated by intercrosses of F1 mice and subsequent brother-sister interbreeding. Consomic strains are generated by repeated backcrossing to the parental receiver strain (NOD mouse), but only one chromosome is derived from the diabetes resistant donor strain. In congenic strains only the differential chromosome segment is derived from the donor strain.

2.2 Establishment of congenic strains

The starting point for the identification of a genetic locus controlling a Complex trait, or Quantitative trait locus (QTL), or in the case of T1D diabetes an *Idd* locus, is most often the generation of an F1 intercross from two parental inbred strains differing in phenotype for the trait under study and the subsequent intercrossing of F1 progeny to produce an F2 generation that can be subject to genetic analysis. Alternatives may involve the backcrossing of the F1 progeny to either one or the other parental strains, to generate first stage backcross generation animals (BC1) and/or eventually backcross 2 animals (BC2). The number of animals needed for the F2, BC1 or BC2 analysis depends on the strength of the phenotypic effect conferred by each QTL under study and also on the size of the genetic interval(s) to be identified. Generally, experimental cohort sizes are in the range of several hundred animals. Most of the easily identified QTL present rather extreme phenotypes that confer above average contributions to the overall phenotype. Consulting the Mouse Genome Informatics (MGI) database (see below) reveals for example that whilst an initial localisation has been described for some 2000 quantitative trait loci, in less than 1 % of the cases has the gene(s) been identified. Contributions of the average single QTL to the overall phenotype has been estimated to be 5% or less (Flint et al., 2005).

Alternatives to performing new crosses involve the use of existing sets of recombinant inbred lines (RI) and/or recombinant congenic (RC) strains. The analytical power of an RI set depends on the number of generated lines and the degree of genetic/phenotypic variation in the parental strains. Whilst RI sets can deliver higher mapping resolution than F2 mice (Flint et al., 2005), current RI sets will often have insufficient power to identify genes with a small effect on the QTL. In contrast to RI sets, sets of RC strains have the property of limiting the amount of the genome that has to be searched for multiple genes involved in QTLs as long as they have been selected for the phenotype of interest. The genome of a standard RC strain comprises, on average, only 12.5% from the donor strain (Stassen et al., 1996).

Consomic and especially congenic strains are key resources for the dissection of T1D QTLs. Understanding the role of an individual QTL is often hampered by the complexity of its genetic and phenotypic interactions with other participating QTLs. Considering susceptibility to type 1 diabetes and the well-known disease model for type 1 diabetes, the nondiabetes (NOD) mouse (Makino et al., 1980; Hattori et al., 1986), it turns out that diabetes sensitive strains such as NOD carry not only diabetes sensitivity loci but also QTL loci conferring diabetes resistance. Conversely, diabetes resistant strains such as C57Bl/6 and C3H/HeJ (Rogner et al., 2001) carry loci conferring diabetes susceptibility as well as resistance genes. For example, on mouse chromosome 6 we have identified three loci involved in T1D, termed *Idd6, Idd19, Idd20. Idd6* (Carnaud et al., 2001) and *Idd20* (Morin et al., 2006) are both NOD susceptibility loci and *Idd19* (Melanitou et al., 1998) is a NOD resistant locus. Furthermore, *Idd19* can mask *Idd6* phenotypes and *Idd20* can mask *Idd19* phenotypes. It is therefore the overall balance and interactions in a given congenic strain and an inbred strain, which determines the final phenotype (Yang & Santamaria, 2006). Some idea of the overall complexity is given by the forty or more murine insulin dependent diabetes loci (*Idd*), which have been genetically identified. In this complex situation, sets of congenic strains have been of critical importance for breaking down the overall genetic complexity. The second reason to generate congenic strains is to study the effects of a gene mutation, a knockout, a knockin, or a transgene on one or several different genetic backgrounds. This approach is of particular interest for studies on genetic modifiers (Montagutelli, 2000; Nadeau, 2001). The use of congenics, although often onerous, remains less time consuming than introducing the same modification in parallel onto different genetic backgrounds by gene targeting or transgenesis. Indeed in many cases the latter approach may be impossible as the appropriate ES cell lines may not be available. When congenic construction is used, it should however be born in mind that it is not a single gene that is being transferred but the gene and its surrounding genetic region. There have been examples showing that such genomic fragments can contribute to the phenotype or in even confer a new phenotype. Different breeding strategies to minimise such problems have been discussed (Wolfer et al., 2002).

Congenic strains are derived by repeated backcrossing of the donor strain to the recipient strain with selection for the differential segment. This breeding is then followed by sister/brother interbreeding of the backcrossed progeny. In practice, female F1 animals are mated with recipient strain males to establish the BC1 generation. If males are used at this stage, the final congenic strain may still carry the donor derived Y-chromosome. Males heterozygous for the selected chromosome region are then repeatedly backcrossed to recipient females (e.g. NOD females) during congenic strain derivation. Congenic strains are then rendered homozygous for the genetic intervals under study by intercrossing heterozygous males and females of the same genotype and subsequently maintained by brother and sister mating. When repeated backcrossing is used to establish a congenic strain a minimum of nine generations of backcrossing is normally recommended to remove 99.9% of the unwanted donor material (Silver, 1995), though the exact number of required backcross generations appears somewhat arbitrary (Festing, 1979). A genome scan should be carried out before fixing the congenic interval so that if further backcrossing is necessary to remove a contaminating genomic fragment this can be carried out before the congenic strain is rendered homozygous. When choosing recombinants to fix genetic intervals we recommend ensuring the highest possible density of markers within the differential fragment (at least 1-2 cM) to avoid partial heterozygosity. A good advice is also to check the interval of interest for eventual heterozygosity once the strains have been fixed because recombinations may have occurred in the parental heterozygous animals.

Alternative congenic breeding schemes have been established that involve both positive selection for the desired differential segment and negative selection against the rest of the donor genome during early backcross generations. In such breeding schemes, which are called 'speed congenics', the genetically 'best' animals, i.e. those carrying the differential segment and minimal detectable donor strain material elsewhere in the genome, are selected. Theoretically the process can lead to the creation of a congenic strain with less than 0.5% contaminating donor genome unlinked to the differential segment within a total of five generations or four backcrosses (Markel et al., 1997). Simulations suggest that screening between 16 and 20 male progeny per generation with markers spaced every 25 cM most efficiently reduces unlinked contaminating donor genome. Use of larger progeny cohorts and higher marker density seems of little advantage in reducing contaminating donor genome until later backcross generations. High-density genotyping of the differential segment in later generations is however necessary to reduce the size of the target region below 20-30 cM (Wakeland et al., 1997). Experience suggests that both 'best' and 'second best' males should routinely be kept for breeding, in particular when poor breeding performance may occur. Simulation studies have suggested that marker-assisted breeding strategies can lead to increased background heterogeneity, or 'gaps', in the recipient genetic background as compared to standard breeding procedures. This suggests that additional backcrossing may still be required in order to reduce the number and length of such gaps (Armstrong et al., 2006). On the assumption of putative remaining gaps, it may be of interest to derive a given set of congenic strains from a single breeding pair and to generate at least one congenic strain carrying no differential fragment as an internal control for phenotyping.

The benefit that can be obtained from a panel of congenic strains is critically dependent on the quality of the phenotyping available, which in turn, obviously depends on the disease under study. The availability of sub-phenotypes for characterisation is often critical to the fine dissection of the trait. Analysis often starts with the most robust and basic phenotype before proceeding to more subtle analysis of sub-phenotypes. Phenotyping employed in autoimmune disorders ranges from histology, evaluation of physiological parameters, to metabolomics and transcriptional profiling.

2.3 Methods to the analysis of type 1 diabetes in the NOD mouse model

The baseline for a systematic analysis of a given NOD congenic strain compared to the original NOD mouse or better also to a NOD control congenic strain is the follow-up of spontaneous diabetes development during a period of about 30 weeks. Overt diabetes starts around 10 to 12 weeks of age. For the monitoring of diabetes, measurement of glucose levels in the urine is usually sufficient. This simple test is in itself not much invasive to the animals, but importantly, the number of animals in the test series should be high enough to allow the detection of small changes in diabetes incidence. At this stage, generally 30 to 50 female mice and sometimes more are required. Using such a high number of animals avoids overestimation of changes occurring due to 'environmental' effects, e.g. the sometimes observed cage-specific effects. Some investigators prefer to keep their congenics together with the NOD controls in the same cage during diabetes testing. Young female animals from different NOD congenic strains usually do not aggress each other when kept in the same cage, but good attention should still be paid to the behaviour of the animals. Overcrowed cages lead to additional stress amongst the animals and this can have an influence on the diabetes incidence. Also, pregnant females should not be included in the testing because hormonal changes influence diabetes development.

Additional monitoring of diabetes incidence may involve an accelerated form of diabetes after injection of drugs such as cyclophosphamide (CY). CY is an alkylating agent that leads to the depletion of regulatory T cells, whereas IFN-gamma producing lymphocytes are CY resistant (Ablamunits et al., 1999). This method allows evaluating diabetes incidence within a much shorter period of 12 weeks only, but is not necessarily appropriate to analyse all T1D associated loci. For example, loci that reveal diabetes protection due to activity of regulatory T-cells may not be discovered because CY eliminates these cells (Rogner et al., 2001). Both methods to monitor T1D incidence can be combined with the evaluation of insulitis by rating the infiltration of the pancreatic islets with immune cells. This histological analysis is mostly performed at 12 weeks of age and usually requires about 10 animals per strain. It can be performed at earlier ages, but much less insulits and peri-insulitis should be expected, and usually no signs of insulitis are found before the age of three weeks.

The systematic evaluation of the number of immune cells (T cells, B cells and other relevant cell types) in different organs (thymus, spleen, lymph nodes, islets, etc.), of the cytokine, insulin and antigen levels can be much helpful to get further insights into the protective mechanism underlying the T1D locus under study. The number of animals used for these tests can often be limited to six, and different tests can be combined at this stage. It is also useful to perform the tests at different ages (4, 8, 12, and 16 weeks) to relate phenotypes to different stages of diabetes development. Finally, extended testing of cell activation or proliferation and adoptive transfer assays are good methods to complete the analysis. Since several examples have shown that T1D diabetes loci overlap with other autoimmune loci, NOD congenic strains may exhibit phenotypes in other organs and tissues than those directly involved in diabetes. One typical and well studied example of this is sialitis (Hjelmervik et al., 2007). In any case, the defined subphenotypes may be very helpful in following up QTLs during genetic dissection as they may vary less than the diabetes incidence.

2.4 Refining the candidate region

2.4.1 Generation of subcongenic strains

The genetic interval conferring a particular phenotype in a given congenic strain can often be reduced and refined by identification of new recombinants during further backcrossing.

It becomes increasingly difficult to obtain the necessary recombinants as the genetic distance under study is reduced and then much larger breeding populations are needed. Several studies have shown the existence of sex-specific differences in recombination frequency (Shiroishi et al., 1991; Lynn et al., 2005; Morelli & Cohen, 2005) and it can therefore, on occasions, be useful to change the direction of the cross and use heterozygous females instead of males or *vice versa*. It should be noted that recombination does not occur with random efficiency throughout the genome and is often higher at so called 'hotspots'. Some hypotheses predict that recombination will occur more often in regions where genes density is higher and less often in what has been termed 'gene deserts'. This was observed in the human genome, where recombination rates are found to be higher in regions with higher gene density (Fullerton et al., 2001). The informative polymorphic markers necessary to characterize the mouse recombinants are listed in the MGI database and only rarely additional comparative sequencing efforts will be required to identify additional polymorphisms.

When analysing congenic strains, it has been observed that the phenotypic effects often get smaller as the genetic interval is reduced and subcongenics are generated (Hung et al., 2006). This most often occurs when the original effect was due to the combination of several genes and this may reflect the relatively frequent occurrence of QTLs as haplotype blocks. In other cases, genetic interactions may lead to the suppression of phenotypes when intervals are combined (Rogner et al., 2001). In theses cases, complexity within the genetic interval can normally still be successfully addressed, although it may require larger number of animals and more strains to be phenotyped and studied.

2.4.2 Haplotype analysis

In silico mapping has been suggested to be a powerful computational based method for predicting chromosomal regions regulating phenotypic traits (Grupe et al., 2001). Single nucleotide polymorphisms (SNPs) in different inbred mouse strains are organised in an alternating mosaic pattern of relatively large, typically 1-2 Mb, genomic regions (blocks) of low or high polymorphic variation (Lindblad-Toh et al., 2000; Wade et al., 2002). Regions that are poor in polymorphic markers have been assigned as regions of common ancestry. Haplotype blocks are defined as genomic segments harbouring sets of coupled polymorphisms that reflect a common ancestral origin (Frazer et al., 2004; Yalcin et al., 2004). Genome-wide association studies involving the correlation of a phenotype, for instance disease prone and disease resistance, over a wide selection of different inbred mouse strains, to patterns of genetic variation in these same strains have been suggested to provide powerful indications of potential candidate regions (Grupe et al., 2001). QTL genes are likely to be found in regions of different ancestry among any pair of differentially affected strains, whilst a given phenotype observed in common in different strains will likely be controlled by a region that is held in common between these strains (Guo et al., 2006). The approach requires that well standardised parental phenotype data is available for many inbred strains. The PHENOME project was established in part with this type of application in mind.

Applied to congenic strain analysis, knowledge of the haplotype block structure within a congenic interval may focus interest on a particular subregion within the congenic candidate region (Figure 2). There are several examples in the literature that have demonstrated the value of this type of combined approach (Ikegami et al., 1995; Lyons et al., 2000; Hillebrandt

et al., 2005). Haplotype mapping in the NOD mouse appears however less powerful as only one sensitive strain can be compared to the panel of diabetes resistant strains.
In whatever way *in silico* mapping is applied, the success of the strategy depends on the size of the underlying haplotype blocks and the panel of relevant mouse strains. The approach also depends on rates of mutation within regions of shared haplotype being sufficiently low as to not obscure the underlying patterns of haplotype variation. Other work indicates that the definition of haplotype blocks is not that robust and that methods for QTL mapping may fail if they assume a simple block-like structure (Yalcin et al., 2004).

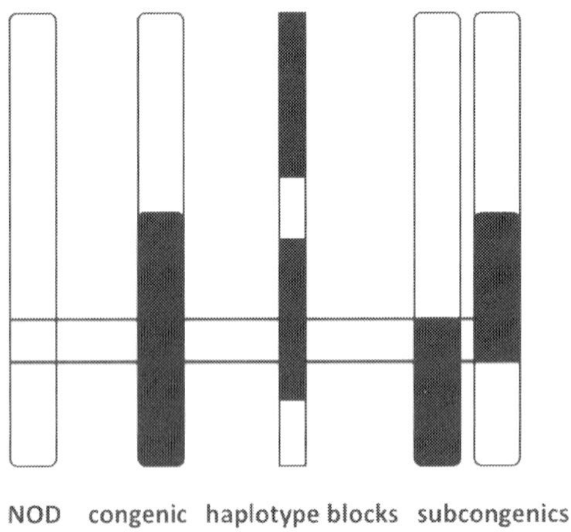

Fig. 2. Reduction of the candidate region of an *Idd* using congenics, haplotype mapping and subcongenics.

Comparison of the SNP distribution within the candidate interval between disease sensitive (NOD, chromosome represented by a white bar) and resistant (black segments) strains and generation of subcongenic strains may allow the initial candidate region to be reduced. The reduced interval is indicated by two black lines.

2.5 Transcriptional profiling

The use of expression profiling for candidate gene identification is based around the idea that in many cases the QTL will reflect also quantitative changes in the expression of the underlying gene(s). This approach has proven to be particularly successful in cases where the phenotype of the disease under study has provided clues as to the class(es) of genes or to the tissues in which the candidate gene is likely to be expressed. Annotated lists of genes for the region under study obtained from e.g. Ensembl, MGI or NCBI databases, including *in silico* expression profiling approaches based on exploiting data from sources such as Serial Analysis of Gene Expression (SAGE) libraries, microarray analysis based datasets, and cumulative data on Expressed Sequence Tags (ESTs), allow the tissue expression profiles of the genes to be established. Where necessary this data is then validated for the most promising candidates by comparative expression profiling of the discriminatory congenic strains using techniques such as quantitative real-time PCR. A complementary approach uses genome wide microarray based expression profiling to identify possible genetic pathways (Eaves et al., 2002). The efficiency of both strategies depends on the completeness of the gene annotations and the exhaustiveness of the gene representation that is being exploited and is influenced by both the cellular complexity of the target tissue and relative transcript expression levels. In the case of complex tissues sensitivity maybe increased by analysing cellular subpopulations of the tissue in question (Lock et al., 2002; Scearce et al., 2002).

A recent Genome-Wide Association Study (GWAS) has defined over 150 genomic regions containing variation predisposing to immune-mediated disease. The results provide evidence that for many of the complex diseases common genetic associations implicate regions encoding proteins that physically interact (Rossin et al., 2011). This type of analysis demonstrates how bioinformatics tools can be applied to the identification of gene networks in complex diseases.

2.6 Resequencing and search for polymorphisms

Once a candidate region has been defined and characterized, the crucial difficulty of identifying and validating the causative gene(s) arises. It is important to realise that there is rarely one single approach but rather a spectrum of complementarity approaches that can be used to identify without ambiguity the gene(s) underlying a QTL.

The identification of changes in primary nucleotide sequence, which is powerfully diagnostic in the case of mutations in monogenic disorders, is of much less certain value in the case of QTL characterisation. Nonsense or stop codons that completely abolish gene function are much less likely to underlie QTL variation than in mutations affecting monogenic traits, and it is often unknown whether to expect changes in coding sequences or in non-coding regulatory sequences. Extensive nucleotide variation may also occur outside of the exon sequences of some genes, which renders the identification of causal polymorphisms in such regions more difficult or impossible. This indeterminacy may moreover be compounded if the causal gene lies within a region, which shows a high degree of polymorphism between the parental strains. In such cases the polymorphism within the genomic sequence of the causal gene will likely be no more marked than that of the surrounding genes. Such regions of elevated polymorphism are to be found throughout the mouse genome and reflect the breeding history of the mouse inbred strains (see above). Such caveats suggest that resequencing of entire regions in the donor and recipient strains is an approach that can help to exclude a certain proportion of candidate genes rather than lead to the unambiguous identification of the responsible gene. The researcher can already benefit from the ongoing resequencing projects that include the NOD mouse.

2.7 Further validation: overlap with other autoimmune loci and interspecies comparison

The genome-scale analysis in type 1 diabetes has resulted in a number of non-major histocompatibility complex loci of varying levels of statistical significance. Comparative analysis of the position of loci for type 1 diabetes with candidate loci from other autoimmune diseases has shown considerable overlap (Becker et al., 1998). This supports a hypothesis that the underlying genetic susceptibility to type 1 diabetes may be shared with other clinically distinct autoimmune diseases such as systemic lupus erythemastosus, multiple sclerosis, and Crohn's Disease. This is less surprising when looking at the cellular and molecular levels that indicate similar mechanisms and pathways underpinning the diseases. An interesting way to further analyse T1D regions of interest is therefore to study their link to other autoimmune diseases (Jiang et al., 2009). For example, several loci involved peripheral neuropathy overlap with T1D loci in the NOD mouse. The MGI database lists phenotypes that have already been linked to genomic regions. The T1D database provides directly all known locations and genes in human and in mouse. Another approach is to analyse the syntenic regions in human and in rat. The Rat Genome database provides a tool to visualize syntenic regions for all three species. The Davis Human/Mouse Homology Map shows syntenic regions between mouse and human.

2.8 Gene manipulation in the NOD mouse

Neither the identification of sequence variation nor of altered expression profiles is of itself sufficient to establish causality. For this, techniques of gene inactivation, gene overexpression and replacement of the allele of one strain by that of the other strain, need to be undertaken. Ongoing programmes for inactivation or mutating all mouse genes will increasingly provide embryonic stem (ES) cells carrying a knockout for the candidate genes under study. Interestingly, some of the constructs used in the global knockout programmes may facilitate application of a knockin strategy, which would enable the integration of alternative functional allelic forms of the gene to be undertaken (Garcia-Otin & Guillou, 2006). Database links that provide information about existing knockouts and mutants are listed below. Exploiting such resources for QTL validation may in many cases be complicated by the need to cross the knockout onto the relevant genetic background. Direct gene targeting and deriving mouse models on the T1D background are however possible since a germline competent embryonic stem cell line from the nonobese diabetic mouse has been established (Nichols et al., 2009).

An alternative strategy to gene disabling is the use of small interfering RNA (siRNA) to inhibit/knock-down gene expression. RNA interference (RNAi) is a highly evolutionary conserved process of post-transcriptional gene silencing (PTGS) in which double stranded RNA (dsRNA), when introduced into a cell, causes sequence-specific degradation of homologous mRNA sequences (Fire et al., 1998). Double-stranded RNAs of around 21 nucleotides in length inhibit the expression of specific genes (Hasuwa et al., 2002; Xia et al., 2002; Qin et al., 2003). Whilst it has turned out that RNA silencing can be causative in disease development, it also provides a useful research tool in type 1 diabetes (Kissler et al., 2006). The RNAi WEB database provides a good summary of such studies and excellent practical advices. The long-term and stable inhibition of gene function normally necessary for assessing the effect of a QTL implies that delivery systems capable of supporting stable and persistent expression *in vivo* are necessary. Cloning of stable interfering short hairpin (sh) RNA molecules and use of several viral vectors and transposon based non-viral vectors have been reported that fulfil this requirement (Naldini, 1998; Yant et al., 2002). Interestingly, such RNAi approaches can be used with embryos circumventing the strain restriction bottleneck associated with ES cell use. Although there are problems associated with off target non-specificity of RNAi that require stringent control, RNAi can be engineered to be specific for a particular allelic forms of a given gene. Providing technical problems can be overcome, experiments aimed at targeting RNAi to one or other alleles of a candidate gene in F1 animals from two discriminatory congenic strains should prove particularly informative.

Overexpression studies provide an alternative if less stringent way of either further reducing the size of the candidate region or to validate formally candidate genes, when the trait under consideration is dominantly or co-dominantly expressed (Symula et al., 1999; Giraldo & Montoliu, 2001). Such approaches are often carried out using BAC clones, which may be one to several hundred kilobases in size and therefore allow the gene to be tested along with many of the cis-acting sequences necessary for its regulated expression. Such studies are being facilitated by the construction of BAC libraries for many mouse strains other than C57Bl/6 and 129/Sv (Osoegawa et al., 2000). The fingerprinting of these libraries, the ready availability of both mouse genomic draft and finished sequences (Waterston et al., 2002) and of strain resequencing programmes, allow the DNA hybridisation probes necessary for BAC isolation to be easily designed. Although BAC transgenesis is an efficient process, it should be noted that both copy number variation and variation in site of integration in the genome leading to position effects may lead to modification in gene expression profiles which might hamper or obscure the identification of the gene where subtle phenotypes are concerned.

It should be noted that less laborious but also less complete approaches include the transfection of particular cell types prior to adoptive transfer experiments and *ex vivo* studies.

2.9 Identification of new candidate genes using NOD congenic strains

The use of congenic strains has proven to be a successful approach to the identification of several T1D candidate genes. Amongst non-major Histocompatibility Complex (MHC) *Idd* genes that have been cloned are *Idd3* for which *Il2* has been implicated (Lyons et al., 2000), *Idd5.1* where *Ctla4* and *Icos* were suggested (Greve et al., 2004), and *Idd5.2* where *Nramp* is a likely candidate (Kissler et al., 2006).

Our own research has focused on understanding the *Idd6* locus on mouse chromosome 6 (Rogner et al., 2001; Rogner et al., 2006). We have shown that the congenic strain NOD.C3H 6.VIII (6.VIII), carrying C3H alleles at the 5.8 Mb *Idd6* genetic locus, is resistant to the spontaneous development of diabetes and that splenocytes and $CD4^+$ T cell populations from this strain suppress the development of diabetes in NOD.SCID mice more efficiently than those from NOD mice in diabetes transfer experiments. Congenic fine-mapping has further localized genetic control of the increased splenocyte suppressive activity to the 700 kb candidate *Idd6.3* interval. Transcriptional profiling studies of genes in the *Idd6.3* interval revealed *Arntl2* as a promising candidate gene for diabetes protection (Hung et al., 2006). Arntl2 belongs to the basic helix-loop-helix/Per-Arnt-Sim (bHLH/PAS) family of transcription factors that are involved in the control of circadian rhythm (Jones, 2004). Interestingly two other members of the *ARNT* family, *ARNT* (Gunton et al., 2005) and *ARNTL1* (Woon et al., 2007; Ando et al., 2008) have already been implicated in type 2 diabetes. Taken together these studies suggest a potentially important role for these circadian rhythm related genes in insulin and sugar metabolism. Other members of the bHLH/PAS family such as the Aryl-hydrocarbon receptor (AhR) have been shown to control key regulatory immune functions and to be involved in autoimmunity (Quintana et al., 2008; Veldhoen et al., 2008). We recently reported functional studies aimed at correlating *Arntl2* expression to T cell activation and diabetes transfer. Our results show that upregulation of *Arntl2* inhibits the proliferation rate of $CD4^+$ T cells *ex vivo* and suppresses the disease promoting activity of diabetogenic splenocytes *in vivo*, whilst suppression of *Arntl2* by RNAi leads to expansion of $CD4^+$ T cells *in vivo*, to decreased levels of regulatory T cells and to increased diabetes incidence (He et al., 2010a, 2010b).

Available mouse models	http://jaxmice.jax.org/index.html
Center of Rodent Genetics	http://www.niehs.nih.gov/research/resources/collab/crg
Complex Trait Consortium	http://www.complextrait.org/
Gene expression data	http://www.informatics.jax.org/menus/expression_menu.shtml http://www.ncbi.nlm.nih.gov/UniGene/clust.cgi?ORG=Mm
Human/Mouse relationships	http://www.ncbi.nlm.nih.gov/Omim/Homology
Knockout mouse project	http://www.nih.gov/science/models/mouse/knockout/index.html
Mouse Genome Informatics database (MGI)	http://www.informatics.jax.org
Mouse Phenome Database	http://www.jax.org/phenome
Mouse sequence databases	http://www.ncbi.nlm.nih.gov http://www.ensembl.org http://mrcseq.har.mrc.ac.uk http://www.genome.ucsc.edu
Online books on mouse genetics and human molecular genetics	http://www.informatics.jax.org/silver/index.shtml http://www.ncbi.nlm.nih.gov/books/bv.fcgi?rid=hmg
Online Mendelian Inheritance in Man, OMIM	http://www.ncbi.nlm.nih.gov/entrez/query.fcgi?db=OMIM
Rat Genome Database	http://rgd.mcw.edu

Table 1. Links to databases and tools

The table lists useful links to existing databases and to other tools.

3. Conclusion

Despite the past 75 million years of separate evolution, only about 300 genes, corresponding to 1 percent of the 25000 - 30,000 genes in the mouse genome, were found to be without a counterpart in the human genome. (Marshall, 2002; Okazaki et al., 2002). This leads to the idea that in the majority of cases the physiology of processes in man and mouse will be similar or identical. Most studies of mouse models of human disease are applied on this basis. Diseases under monogenic control provided often support for this assumption (Villasenor et al., 2005). When mutations in a given gene failed to produce the same phenotype in human and mouse, the differences were mainly imputable to differences in physiology, to subtle differences in gene regulation, epigenetic factors, or differences in the specific mutation itself rather than to the complete absence of the gene. The predictive value of QTLs identified in one species for the other is generally considerably weaker. This is almost certainly due to the genetic heterogeneity underlying most complex traits, to differences in penetrance, and to differences in the range of naturally occurring variation at a given locus in man and mouse. This however does not necessarily imply that the underlying genetic networks are highly divergent and indeed in type 1 diabetes this is clearly not the case. Indeed the identification of causative genes for the autoimmune disease type 1 diabetes (T1D) in humans and in the NOD mouse has shown that susceptibility or resistance to type 1 diabetes, involving genes and pathways contributing to the disease are often held in common by both species. For example, gene variants for the interacting molecules IL2 and IL-2R-α (CD25), which are members of a same pathway that is essential for immune homeostasis, are present in both mice and humans (Wicker et al., 2005). In this context identifying the mouse genes involved in T1D and consolidating our knowledge of the pathway underlying the pathogenesis will identify novel genes, which can be studied for their implication in the human disease.

4. Acknowledgment

I thank Philip Avner and Christian Boitard for scientific discussion, and the ANR, the ARD, the EFSD/JDRF/Novo Nordisk Programme, the CNRS, INSERM and the Pasteur Institute for funding of our research.

5. References

Ablamunits, V.; Quintana, F.; Reshef, T.; Elias, D.; Cohen, I. R.; Podolin, P. L.; Denny, P.; Armitage, N.; Lord, C. J.; Hill, N. J., et al. (1999). Acceleration of autoimmune diabetes by cyclophosphamide is associated with an enhanced IFN-gamma secretion pathway. *J Autoimmun*, Vol.13, No.4, (n.d.), pp. 383-392

Ando, H.; Takamura, T.; Matsuzawa-Nagata, N.; Shima, K. R.; Eto, T.; Misu, H.; Shiramoto, M.; Tsuru, T.; Irie, S.; Fujimura, A., et al. (2008). Clock gene expression in peripheral leucocytes of patients with type 2 diabetes. *Diabetologia*, (Oct 2008), pp. 201-207

Armstrong, N. J.; Brodnicki, T. C. & Speed, T. P. (2006). Mind the gap: analysis of marker-assisted breeding strategies for inbred mouse strains. *Mamm Genome*, Vol.17, No.4, (Apr 2006), pp. 273-287

Bailey, D. W. (1971). Recombinant-inbred strains. An aid to finding identity, linkage, and function of histocompatibility and other genes. *Transplantation*, Vol.11, No.3, (Mar 1971), pp. 325-327

Beck, J. A.; Lloyd, S.; Hafezparast, M.; Lennon-Pierce, M.; Eppig, J. T.; Festing, M. F. & Fisher, E. M. (2000). Genealogies of mouse inbred strains. *Nat Genet*, Vol.24, No.1, (Jan 2000), pp. 23-25

Becker, K. G.; Simon, R. M.; Bailey-Wilson, J. E.; Freidlin, B.; Biddison, W. E.; McFarland, H. F. & Trent, J. M. (1998). Clustering of non-major histocompatibility complex susceptibility candidate loci in human autoimmune diseases. *Proc Natl Acad Sci U S A*, Vol.95, No.17, (n.d.), pp. 9979-9984

Boyse, E. A. & Bentley, D. R. (1977). The increasing value of congenic mice in biomedical research. *Lab Anim Sci*, Vol.27, No.5, (n.d), pp. 771-781

Carnaud, C.; Gombert, J.; Donnars, O.; Garchon, H. & Herbelin, A. (2001). Protection against diabetes and improved NK/NKT cell performance in NOD.NK1.1 mice congenic at the NK complex. *J Immunol*, Vol.166, No.4, (n.d.), pp. 2404-2411

Churchill, G. A.; Airey, D. C.; Allayee, H.; Angel, J. M.; Attie, A. D.; Beatty, J.; Beavis, W. D.; Belknap, J. K.; Bennett, B.; Berrettini, W., et al. (2004). The Collaborative Cross, a community resource for the genetic analysis of complex traits. *Nat Genet*, Vol.36, No.11, (Nov 2004), pp. 1133-1137

Demant, P. & Hart, A. A. (1986). Recombinant congenic strains--a new tool for analyzing genetic traits determined by more than one gene. *Immunogenetics*, Vol.24, No.6, (n.d.), pp. 416-422

Eaves, I. A.; Wicker, L. S.; Ghandour, G.; Lyons, P. A.; Peterson, L. B.; Todd, J. A. & Glynne, R. J. (2002). Combining mouse congenic strains and microarray gene expression analyses to study a complex trait: the NOD model of type 1 diabetes. *Genome Res*, Vol.12, No.2, (n.d.), pp. 232-243

Festing, M. F. W. (1979). *Inbred Strains in Biomedical Research.* (1st edition) The Macmillian Press LTD, London and Basingstoke UK

Fire, A.; Xu, S.; Montgomery, M. K.; Kostas, S. A.; Driver, S. E. & Mello, C. C. (1998). Potent and specific genetic interference by double-stranded RNA in Caenorhabditis elegans. *Nature*, Vol.391, No.6669, (Feb 1998), pp. 806-811

Flint, J.; Valdar, W.; Shifman, S. & Mott, R. (2005). Strategies for mapping and cloning quantitative trait genes in rodents. *Nat Rev Genet*, Vol.6, No.4, (Apr 2005), pp. 271-286

Frazer, K. A.; Wade, C. M.; Hinds, D. A.; Patil, N.; Cox, D. R. & Daly, M. J. (2004). Segmental phylogenetic relationships of inbred mouse strains revealed by fine-scale analysis of sequence variation across 4.6 mb of mouse genome. *Genome Res*, Vol.14, No.8, (Aug 2004), pp. 1493-1500

Fullerton, S. M.; Bernardo Carvalho, A. & Clark, A. G. (2001). Local rates of recombination are positively correlated with GC content in the human genome. *Mol Biol Evol*, Vol.18, No.6, (Jun 2001), pp. 1139-1142

Garcia-Otin, A. L. & Guillou, F. (2006). Mammalian genome targeting using site-specific recombinases. *Front Biosci*, Vol.11, (n.d.), pp. 1108-1136

Giraldo, P. & Montoliu, L. (2001). Size matters: use of YACs, BACs and PACs in transgenic animals. *Transgenic Res*, Vol.10, No.2, (n.d.), pp. 83-103

Greve, B.; Vijayakrishnan, L.; Kubal, A.; Sobel, R. A.; Peterson, L. B.; Wicker, L. S. & Kuchroo, V. K. (2004). The diabetes susceptibility locus Idd5.1 on mouse chromosome 1 regulates ICOS expression and modulates murine experimental autoimmune encephalomyelitis. *J Immunol*, Vol.173, No.1, (Jul 2004), pp. 157-163

Grimm, D. (2006). Mouse genetics. A mouse for every gene. *Science*, Vol.312, No.5782, (Jun 2006), pp. 1862-1866

Grupe, A.; Germer, S.; Usuka, J.; Aud, D.; Belknap, J. K.; Klein, R. F.; Ahluwalia, M. K.; Higuchi, R. & Peltz, G. (2001). In silico mapping of complex disease-related traits in mice. *Science*, Vol.292, No.5523, (Jun 2001), pp. 1915-1918

Gunton, J. E.; Kulkarni, R. N.; Yim, S.; Okada, T.; Hawthorne, W. J.; Tseng, Y. H.; Roberson, R. S.; Ricordi, C.; O'Connell, P. J.; Gonzalez, F. J., et al. (2005). Loss of ARNT/HIF1beta mediates altered gene expression and pancreatic-islet dysfunction in human type 2 diabetes. *Cell*, Vol.122, No.3, (Aug 2005), pp. 337-349

Guo, Y.; Weller, P.; Farrell, E.; Cheung, P.; Fitch, B.; Clark, D.; Wu, S. Y.; Wang, J.; Liao, G.; Zhang, Z., et al. (2006). In silico pharmacogenetics of warfarin metabolism. *Nat Biotechnol*, Vol.24, No.5, (May 2006), pp. 531-536

Hasuwa, H.; Kaseda, K.; Einarsdottir, T. & Okabe, M. (2002). Small interfering RNA and gene silencing in transgenic mice and rats. *FEBS Letters*, Vol.532, No.1-2, (Dec 2002), pp. 227-230

Hattori, M.; Buse, J. B.; Jackson, R. A.; Glimcher, L.; Dorf, M. E.; Minami, M.; Makino, S.; Moriwaki, K.; Kuzuya, H.; Imura, H., et al. (1986). The NOD mouse: recessive diabetogenic gene in the major histocompatibility complex. *Science*, Vol.231, No.4739, (n.d.), pp. 733-735

He, C. X.; Avner, P.; Boitard, C. & Rogner, U. C. (2010a). Downregulation of the circadian rhythm related gene Arntl2 suppresses diabetes protection in Idd6 NOD.C3H congenic mice. *Clin Exp Pharmacol Physiol*, Vol.37, No.12, (Dec 2010), pp. 1154-1158

He, C. X.; Prevot, N.; Boitard, C.; Avner, P. & Rogner, U. C. (2010b). Inhibition of type 1 diabetes by upregulation of the circadian rhythm-related aryl hydrocarbon receptor nuclear translocator-like 2. *Immunogenetics*, Vol.62, No.9, (Sep 2010), pp. 585-592

Hillebrandt, S.; Wasmuth, H. E.; Weiskirchen, R.; Hellerbrand, C.; Keppeler, H.; Werth, A.; Schirin-Sokhan, R.; Wilkens, G.; Geier, A.; Lorenzen, J., et al. (2005). Complement factor 5 is a quantitative trait gene that modifies liver fibrogenesis in mice and humans. *Nat Genet*, Vol.37, No.8, (Aug 2005), pp. 835-843

Hjelmervik, T. O.; Lindqvist, A. K.; Petersen, K.; Johannesson, M.; Stavrum, A. K.; Johansson, A.; Jonsson, R.; Holmdahl, R. & Bolstad, A. I. (2007). The influence of the NOD Nss1/Idd5 loci on sialadenitis and gene expression in salivary glands of congenic mice. *Arthritis Res Ther*, Vol.9, No.5, (n.d.), pp. R99, 1478-6362 (Electronic) 1478-6354 (Linking)

Hung, M. S.; Avner, P. & Rogner, U. C. (2006). Identification of the transcription factor ARNTL2 as a candidate gene for the type 1 diabetes locus Idd6. *Hum Mol Genet*, Vol.15, No.18, (Sep 2006), pp. 2732-2742

Ikegami, H.; Makino, S.; Yamato, E.; Kawaguchi, Y.; Ueda, H.; Sakamoto, T.; Takekawa, K. & Ogihara, T. (1995). Identification of a new susceptibility locus for insulin-dependent diabetes mellitus by ancestral haplotype congenic mapping. *J Clin Invest*, Vol.96, No.4, (n.d.), pp. 1936-1942

Jiang, F.; Yoshida, T.; Nakaki, F.; Terawaki, S.; Chikuma, S.; Kato, Y.; Okazaki, I. M.; Honjo, T. & Okazaki, T. (2009). Identification of QTLs that modify peripheral neuropathy in NOD.H2b-Pdcd1-/- mice. *Int Immunol*, Vol.21, No.5, (May 2009), pp. 499-509, 1460-2377 (Electronic) 0953-8178 (Linking)

Jones, S. (2004). An overview of the basic helix-loop-helix proteins. *Genome Biol*, Vol.5, No.6, (n.d.), pp. 226, 1465-6914 (Electronic)

Kissler, S.; Stern, P.; Takahashi, K.; Hunter, K.; Peterson, L. B. & Wicker, L. S. (2006). In vivo RNA interference demonstrates a role for Nramp1 in modifying susceptibility to type 1 diabetes. *Nat Genet*, Vol.38, No.4, (Apr 2006), pp. 479-483

Lindblad-Toh, K.; Winchester, E.; Daly, M. J.; Wang, D. G.; Hirschhorn, J. N.; Laviolette, J. P.; Ardlie, K.; Reich, D. E.; Robinson, E.; Sklar, P., et al. (2000). Large-scale discovery and genotyping of single-nucleotide polymorphisms in the mouse. *Nat Genet*, Vol.24, No.4, (n.d.), pp. 381-386

Lock, C.; Hermans, G.; Pedotti, R.; Brendolan, A.; Schadt, E.; Garren, H.; Langer-Gould, A.; Strober, S.; Cannella, B.; Allard, J., et al. (2002). Gene-microarray analysis of multiple sclerosis lesions yields new targets validated in autoimmune encephalomyelitis. *Nat Med*, Vol.8, No.5, (n.d.), pp. 500-508

Lynn, A.; Schrump, S.; Cherry, J.; Hassold, T. & Hunt, P. (2005). Sex, not genotype, determines recombination levels in mice. *Am J Hum Genet*, Vol.77, No.4, (Oct 2005), pp. 670-675

Lyons, P. A.; Armitage, N.; Argentina, F.; Denny, P.; Hill, N. J.; Lord, C. J.; Wilusz, M. B.; Peterson, L. B.; Wicker, L. S. & Todd, J. A. (2000). Congenic mapping of the type 1 diabetes locus, Idd3, to a 780-kb region of mouse chromosome 3: identification of a candidate segment of ancestral DNA by haplotype mapping. *Genome Res*, Vol.10, No.4, (n.d.), pp. 446-453

Maier, L. M. & Wicker, L. S. (2005). Genetic susceptibility to type 1 diabetes. *Curr Opin Immunol*, Vol.17, No.6, (Dec 2005), pp. 601-608

Makino, S.; Kunimoto, K.; Muraoka, Y.; Mizushima, Y.; Katagiri, K. & Tochino, Y. (1980). Breeding of a non-obese, diabetic strain of mice. *Jikken Dobutsu*, Vol.29, No.1, (n.d.), pp. 1-13

Markel, P.; Shu, P.; Ebeling, C.; Carlson, G. A.; Nagle, D. L.; Smutko, J. S. & Moore, K. J. (1997). Theoretical and empirical issues for marker-assisted breeding of congenic mouse strains. *Nat Genet*, Vol.17, No.3, (n.d.), pp. 280-284

Marshall, E. (2002). Genome sequencing. Public group completes draft of the mouse. *Science*, Vol.296, No.5570, (May 2002), pp. 1005

Melanitou, E.; Joly, F.; Lathrop, M.; Boitard, C. & Avner, P. (1998). Evidence for the presence of insulin-dependent diabetes-associated alleles on the distal part of mouse chromosome 6. *Genome Res*, Vol.8, No.6, (n.d.), pp. 608-620

Montagutelli, X. (2000). Effect of the genetic background on the phenotype of mouse mutations. *J Am Soc Nephrol*, Vol.11 Suppl 16, (Nov 2000), pp. S101-105

Morelli, M. A. & Cohen, P. E. (2005). Not all germ cells are created equal: aspects of sexual dimorphism in mammalian meiosis. *Reproduction*, Vol.130, No.6, (Dec 2005), pp. 761-781

Morin, J.; Boitard, C.; Vallois, D.; Avner, P. & Rogner, U. C. (2006). Mapping of the murine type 1 diabetes locus Idd20 by genetic interaction. *Mamm Genome*, Vol.17, No.11, (Nov 2006), pp. 1105-1112

Nadeau, J. H. (2001). Modifier genes in mice and humans. *Nat Rev Genet*, Vol.2, No.3, (Mar 2001), pp. 165-174

Nadeau, J. H.; Singer, J. B.; Matin, A. & Lander, E. S. (2000). Analysing complex genetic traits with chromosome substitution strains. *Nat Genet*, Vol.24, No.3, (n.d.), pp. 221-225

Naldini, L. (1998). Lentiviruses as gene transfer agents for delivery to non-dividing cells. *Current Opinion in Biotechnology*, Vol.9, No.5, (Oct 1998), pp. 457-463

Nichols, J.; Jones, K.; Phillips, J. M.; Newland, S. A.; Roode, M.; Mansfield, W.; Smith, A. & Cooke, A. (2009). Validated germline-competent embryonic stem cell lines from nonobese diabetic mice. *Nat Med*, Vol.15, No.7, (Jul 2009), pp. 814-818

Okazaki, Y.; Furuno, M.; Kasukawa, T.; Adachi, J.; Bono, H.; Kondo, S.; Nikaido, I.; Osato, N.; Saito, R.; Suzuki, H., et al. (2002). Analysis of the mouse transcriptome based on functional annotation of 60,770 full-length cDNAs. *Nature*, Vol.420, No.69 (n.d.), pp. 563-573

Osoegawa, K.; Tateno, M.; Woon, P. Y.; Frengen, E.; Mammoser, A. G.; Catanese, J. J.; Hayashizaki, Y. & de Jong, P. J. (2000). Bacterial artificial chromosome libraries for mouse sequencing and functional analysis. *Genome Res*, Vol.10, No.1, (Jan 2000), pp. 116-128

Peirce, J. (2001). Looking at old tools in new ways: using knockouts as congenics to study QTLs. *Genome Res*, Vol.11, No.9, (n.d.), pp. 1469-1471

Qin, X. F.; An, D. S.; Chen, I. S. & Baltimore, D. (2003). Inhibiting HIV-1 infection in human T cells by lentiviral-mediated delivery of small interfering RNA against CCR5. *Proc Natl Acad Sci U S A*, Vol.100, No.1, (Jan 2003), pp. 183-188

Quintana, F. J.; Basso, A. S.; Iglesias, A. H.; Korn, T.; Farez, M. F.; Bettelli, E.; Caccamo, M.; Oukka, M. & Weiner, H. L. (2008). Control of T(reg) and T(H)17 cell differentiation by the aryl hydrocarbon receptor. *Nature*, Vol.453, No.7191, (May 2008), pp. 65-71

Rogner, U. C.; Boitard, C.; Morin, J.; Melanitou, E. & Avner, P. (2001). Three loci on mouse chromosome 6 influence onset and final incidence of type I diabetes in NOD.C3H congenic strains. *Genomics*, Vol.74, No.2, (n.d.), pp. 163-171

Rogner, U. C.; Lepault, F.; Gagnerault, M. C.; Vallois, D.; Morin, J.; Avner, P. & Boitard, C. (2006). The Diabetes Type 1 Locus Idd6 Modulates Activity of CD4+CD25+ Regulatory T-Cells. *Diabetes*, Vol.55, No.1, (Jan 2006), pp. 186-192

Rossin, E. J.; Lage, K.; Raychaudhuri, S.; Xavier, R. J.; Tatar, D.; Benita, Y.; Cotsapas, C. & Daly, M. J. (2011). Proteins encoded in genomic regions associated with immune-mediated disease physically interact and suggest underlying biology. *PLoS Genet*, Vol.7, No.1, (n.d.), pp. e1001273, 1553-7404 (Electronic) 1553-7390 (Linking)

Roths, J. B.; Murphy, E. D. & Eicher, E. M. (1984). A new mutation, gld, that produces lymphoproliferation and autoimmunity in C3H/HeJ mice. *J Exp Med*, Vol.159, No.1, (Jan 1984), pp. 1-20

Santos, J.; Montagutelli, X.; Acevedo, A.; Lopez, P.; Vaquero, C.; Fernandez, M.; Arnau, M. R.; Szatanik, M.; Salido, E.; Guenet, J. L., et al. (2002). A new locus for resistance to gamma-radiation-induced thymic lymphoma identified using inter-specific consomic and inter-specific recombinant congenic strains of mice. *Oncogene*, Vol.21, No.43, (n.d.), pp. 6680-6683

Scearce, L. M.; Brestelli, J. E.; McWeeney, S. K.; Lee, C. S.; Mazzarelli, J.; Pinney, D. F.; Pizarro, A.; Stoeckert, C. J., Jr.; Clifton, S. W.; Permutt, M. A., et al. (2002). Functional genomics of the endocrine pancreas: the pancreas clone set and PancChip, new resources for diabetes research. *Diabetes*, Vol.51, No.7, (n.d.), pp. 1997-2004

Serreze, D. V. & Leiter, E. H. (2001). Genes and cellular requirements for autoimmune diabetes susceptibility in nonobese diabetic mice. *Curr Dir Autoimmun*, Vol.4, (n.d.), pp. 31-67

Shiroishi, T.; Sagai, T.; Hanzawa, N.; Gotoh, H. & Moriwaki, K. (1991). Genetic control of sex-dependent meiotic recombination in the major histocompatibility complex of the mouse. *Embo J*, Vol.10, No.3, (Mar 1991), pp. 681-686

Silver, L. M. (1995). *Mouse Genetics Concepts and Applications.* Oxford University Press, New York, ISBN 0195075544.

Snell, G. D. (1978). Congenic resistant strains of mice. In:*Origins of Inbred Mice*, Morse, H. C., eds., pp. 1-31, Academic Press, New York

Stassen, A. P.; Groot, P. C.; Eppig, J. T. & Demant, P. (1996). Genetic composition of the recombinant congenic strains. *Mamm Genome*, Vol.7, No.1, (Jan 1996), pp. 55-58

Symula, D. J.; Frazer, K. A.; Ueda, Y.; Denefle, P.; Stevens, M. E.; Wang, Z. E.; Locksley, R. & Rubin, E. M. (1999). Functional screening of an asthma QTL in YAC transgenic mice. *Nat Genet*, Vol.23, No.2, (n.d.), pp. 241-244

Taylor, J. A.; Xu, Z. L.; Kaplan, N. L. & Morris, R. W. (2006). How well do HapMap haplotypes identify common haplotypes of genes? A comparison with haplotypes of 334 genes resequenced in the environmental genome project. *Cancer Epidemiol Biomarkers Prev*, Vol.15, No.1, (Jan 2006), pp. 133-137

Todd, J. A. & Wicker, L. S. (2001). Genetic protection from the inflammatory disease type 1 diabetes in humans and animal models. *Immunity*, Vol.15, No.3, (n.d.), pp. 387-395

Veldhoen, M.; Hirota, K.; Westendorf, A. M.; Buer, J.; Dumoutier, L.; Renauld, J. C. & Stockinger, B. (2008). The aryl hydrocarbon receptor links TH17-cell-mediated autoimmunity to environmental toxins. *Nature*, Vol.453, No.7191, (May 2008), pp. 106-109

Villasenor, J.; Benoist, C. & Mathis, D. (2005). AIRE and APECED: molecular insights into an autoimmune disease. *Immunol Rev*, Vol.204, (Apr 2005), pp. 156-164

Wade, C. M.; Kulbokas, E. J.; Kirby, A. W.; Zody, M. C.; Mullikin, J. C.; Lander, E. S.; Lindblad-Toh, K. & Daly, M. J. (2002). The mosaic structure of variation in the laboratory mouse genome. *Nature*, Vol.420, No.6915, (n.d.), pp. 574-578

Wakeland, E.; Morel, L.; Achey, K.; Yui, M. & Longmate, J. (1997). Speed congenics: a classic technique in the fast lane (relatively speaking). *Immunol Today*, Vol.18, No.10, (n.d.), pp. 472-477

Waterston, R. H.; Lindblad-Toh, K.; Birney, E.; Rogers, J.; Abril, J. F.; Agarwal, P.; Agarwala, R.; Ainscough, R.; Alexandersson, M.; An, P., et al. (2002). Initial sequencing and comparative analysis of the mouse genome. *Nature*, Vol.420, No.6915, (Dec 2002), pp. 520-562

Wellcome Trust Case Control Consortium (2007). Genome-wide association study of 14,000 cases of seven common diseases and 3,000 shared controls. *Nature*, Vol.447, No.7145, (Jun 2007), pp. 661-678

Wicker, L. S.; Clark, J.; Fraser, H. I.; Garner, V. E.; Gonzalez-Munoz, A.; Healy, B.; Howlett, S.; Hunter, K.; Rainbow, D.; Rosa, R. L., et al. (2005). Type 1 diabetes genes and pathways shared by humans and NOD mice. *J Autoimmun*, Vol.25 Suppl, (n.d.), pp. 29-33

Wolfer, D. P.; Crusio, W. E. & Lipp, H. P. (2002). Knockout mice: simple solutions to the problems of genetic background and flanking genes. *Trends Neurosci*, Vol.25, No.7, (Jul 2002), pp. 336-340

Woon, P. Y.; Kaisaki, P. J.; Braganca, J.; Bihoreau, M. T.; Levy, J. C.; Farrall, M. & Gauguier, D. (2007). Aryl hydrocarbon receptor nuclear translocator-like (BMAL1) is associated with susceptibility to hypertension and type 2 diabetes. *Proc Natl Acad Sci U S A*, Vol.104, No.36, (Sep 2007), pp. 14412-14417

Xia, H.; Mao, Q.; Paulson, H. L. & Davidson, B. L. (2002). siRNA-mediated gene silencing in vitro and in vivo. *Nat Biotechnol*, Vol.20, No.10, (Oct 2002), pp. 1006-1010

Yalcin, B.; Fullerton, J.; Miller, S.; Keays, D. A.; Brady, S.; Bhomra, A.; Jefferson, A.; Volpi, E.; Copley, R. R.; Flint, J., et al. (n.d.). Unexpected complexity in the haplotypes of commonly used inbred strains of laboratory mice. *Proc Natl Acad Sci U S A*, Vol.101, No.26, (Jun 2004), pp. 9734-9739

Yang, Y. & Santamaria, P. (2006). Lessons on autoimmune diabetes from animal models. *Clin Sci (Lond)*, Vol.110, No.6, (Jun 2006), pp. 627-639

Yant, S. R.; Ehrhardt, A.; Mikkelsen, J. G.; Meuse, L.; Pham, T. & Kay, M. A. (2002). Transposition from a gutless adeno-transposon vector stabilizes transgene expression in vivo. *Nat Biotechnol*, Vol.20, No.10, (Oct 2002), pp. 999-1005

Zeggini, E.; Rayner, W.; Morris, A. P.; Hattersley, A. T.; Walker, M.; Hitman, G. A.; Deloukas, P.; Cardon, L. R. & McCarthy, M. I. (2005). An evaluation of HapMap sample size and tagging SNP performance in large-scale empirical and simulated data sets. *Nat Genet*, Vol.37, No.12, (Dec 2005), pp. 1320-1322

3

Relationship of Type 1 Diabetes with Human Leukocyte Antigen (HLA) Class II Antigens Except for DR3 and DR4

Masahito Katahira
Department of Endocrinology and Diabetes, Ichinomiya Municipal Hospital
Japan

1. Introduction

Type 1 diabetes (T1D) is the form of the disease that occurs primarily as a result of β-cell destruction. The American Diabetes Association (ADA) and the World Health Organization (WHO) have classified T1D into 2 categories, namely, immune-mediated (autoimmune) and idiopathic (Alberti & Zimmet, 1998; Expert Committee on the Diagnosis and Classification of Diabetes Mellitus, 1997). In autoimmune T1D (type 1A diabetes), the rate of β-cell destruction is quite variable, being rapid in some individuals and slow in others (Zimmet et al., 1994). Markers of immune destruction, including islet cell autoantibodies (ICA), autoantibodies to insulin (IAA), autoantibodies to glutamic acid decarboxylase (GAD65), and autoantibodies to tyrosine phosphatases IA-2, are present in 85–90% of individuals with T1D when fasting diabetic hyperglycemia is initially detected (Verge et al., 1996). The rapid-onset ("classic") form of T1D is commonly observed in children, but also may occur in adults (Humphrey et al., 1998). The slow-onset form of T1D generally occurs in adults and is sometimes referred to as latent autoimmune diabetes in adults (LADA) (Zimmet et al., 1994). This term has been commonly used to refer to autoimmune forms of diabetes that do not initially require insulin. However, it is now clear that diabetes in these patients is not latent and is not limited to adults (Borg et al., 2003; Fourlanos et al., 2005; Landin-Olsson et al., 1992; Turner et al., 1997). On the other hand, idiopathic T1D (type 1B diabetes) lacks immunological evidence for β-cell autoimmunity (Alberti & Zimmet, 1998; Expert Committee on the Diagnosis and Classification of Diabetes Mellitus, 1997). A new subtype known as "fulminant T1D" has been described in Japan. The clinical characteristics of this form of diabetes are remarkably abrupt onset of disease, very short (< 1 week) duration of diabetic symptoms, and virtually no C-peptide secretion (< 10 µg/day in urine) (Imagawa et al., 2000a). Although more than 250 patients with fulminant T1D have been reported in Japan, only few patients with fulminant T1D have been reported outside Japan (Imagawa & Hanafusa, 2005). Therefore, in the Japanese population, in contrast to other ethnic groups, there are 3 prevalent subtypes of T1D: rapid-onset ("classic"), slow-onset, and fulminant T1D.

T1D is a multifactorial disease caused by a complex interaction of genetic and environmental factors. It is beyond doubt that the human leukocyte antigen (HLA) complex constitutes the most relevant susceptibility region. The HLA complex contributes 50% of the inherited risk for T1D (Steenkiste et al., 2007). An additional 17 genes with variable but small effects, named *IDDM2-IDDM18*, located on different chromosomes, have been described. The HLA gene (*IDDM1*) is located on 6p21.3. The remainder are found on chromosomes 2, 3, 5, 10, 11, 14, 15, and 18, and three additional regions on chromosome 6q. Worldwide studies and many other individual reports have clearly shown that HLA class II loci have the most intense susceptibility determinants for T1D. However, population studies have shown that HLA associations may vary depending on the ethnic origin. In the Caucasian population, susceptibility to T1D is strongly associated with DRB1*03:01-DQA1*05:01-DQB1*02:01 (DR3) and/or DRB1*04-DQA1*03:01-DQB1*03:02 (DR4). These haplotypes are very frequent among Caucasian patients with T1D, and only approximately 10% of Caucasian patients with T1D carry neither of these haplotypes (Rønningen et al., 1991; Sanjeevi et al., 1995). Hence, the subgroup of patients who do not carry these haplotypes is generally very small, and therefore the data have been difficult to evaluate. However, the DR3 haplotype is absent and the DR4 haplotype is rare in the Japanese population, which is probably why Japan has one of the lowest incidences of T1D in the world (Matsuura et al., 1998; Tuomilehto et al., 1995). Therefore, the Japanese population is a good model for understanding the clinical stages of T1D and for examining the susceptibility of HLA DR-DQ haplotypes, except DR3 and DR4, to T1D.

In this chapter, we suggest that T1D can be divided into six subtypes based on the mode of disease onset, markers of immune destruction, and insulin deficiency; thus we intend to classify T1D, but not other types of diabetes such as Type 2 diabetes (T2D) or gestational diabetes. An appropriate staging would improve our understanding of the pathogenesis of T1D and allow for easier discrimination between T1D and T2D. Moreover, we discuss the relationship between HLA class II genes and T1D in the Japanese population based on a comparison with other ethnic groups.

2. Criteria of staging

For the better understanding of the clinical stages of T1D, we selected 3 clinical markers: islet autoantibodies, mode of disease onset, and insulin deficiency. On the other hand, the age at disease onset was the main classification criterion in the early 1970s because the peak incidence of autoimmune and rapid-onset T1D occurs in childhood and adolescence. However, onset of T1D may occur at any age, ranging from childhood to the ninth decade of life (Mølbak et al., 1994). Fulminant T1D also occurs at any age, ranging from 1 to 80 years (Imagawa et al., 2003). Since LADA is considered to be confined to adulthood, terms such as "LADY-like" (latent autoimmune diabetes in the young) (Lohmann et al., 2000) and "LADC" (latent autoimmune diabetes in children) (Aycan et al., 2004) were recently introduced for cases of autoimmune and slow-onset T1D occurring in childhood and adolescence. Based on these findings, we did not include the age at disease onset as a staging criterion.

2.1 Islet autoantibodies

The presence of islet autoantibodies has provided the main classification criterion for T1D since the ADA and WHO proposed the current classification of diabetes. Markers of immune destruction are also useful in distinguishing T1D from T2D. We divided diabetic patients, which included both T1D and T2D, into two categories; autoimmune and idiopathic. Autoimmune diabetic patients have at least one marker of immunological β-cell destruction such as ICA, IAA, autoantibodies to GAD65 (GADAb), or autoantibodies to IA-2 (IA-2Ab). In contrast, idiopathic diabetic patients have no markers of immunological β-cell destruction.

2.2 Mode of disease onset

The mode of disease onset allows us to identify three subtypes of the condition: fulminant-onset, rapid-onset, and slow-onset such as LADA. According to the criteria for definitive diagnosis of fulminant T1D (Imagawa & Hanafusa, 2006), the duration of the disease is within 1 week in general and within 2 weeks at most. According to the definition of LADA (Stenström et al., 2005), slow-onset diabetes can be distinguished from rapid-onset diabetes as patients with slow-onset diabetes had no requirement for insulin at diagnosis and for a minimum of 6 months after diagnosis.

2.3 Insulin deficiency

For many years, insulin deficiency was thought to characterize autoimmune and rapid-onset T1D. Insulin deficiency was clinically characterized by decreased urinary and/or serum C-peptide levels. In fulminant-onset diabetes, the urinary C-peptide level is < 10 μg/day (3.3 nmol/day), fasting serum C-peptide is < 0.3 ng/ml (0.1 nmol/L), or serum C-peptide is < 0.5 ng/ml (0.17 nmol/L) after glucagon injection (or meal) load (Imagawa & Hanafusa, 2006; Imagawa et al., 2003). In rapid-onset diabetes, the urinary C-peptide level is < 20 μg/day (6.6 nmol/day), fasting serum C-peptide is < 0.4 ng/ml (0.13 nmol/L), or serum C-peptide is < 1.0 ng/ml (0.33 nmol/L) after glucagon injection (or meal) load (Stenström et al., 2005). Fulminant-onset and rapid-onset types of diabetes are insulin deficient when fasting diabetic hyperglycemia is detected, while slow-onset type of diabetes has two stages, i.e., insulin-deficient and non-insulin-deficient.

3. Clinical types of diabetes

Table 1 shows the clinical types of diabetes based on islet autoantibodies, mode of disease onset and insulin deficiency. The first marker is islet autoantibodies—(A) positive (autoimmune) or (B) negative (idiopathic). The second marker is mode of disease onset and insulin deficiency. Therefore, there are 4 clinical stages of T1D (numbered for convenience sake): fulminant-onset (0), rapid-onset (1), slow-onset with insulin deficiency (2), and slow-onset without insulin deficiency (3). Islet autoantibodies are arranged along the vertical axis, and the mode of disease onset and insulin deficiency are arranged along the horizontal axis. The combination of autoimmunity (A or B) and clinical stages (0–3) indicates the clinical types of diabetes.

<table>
<tr><td>Insulin deficiency</td><td colspan="3">Insulin-deficient</td><td>Non-insulin-deficient</td></tr>
<tr><td>Mode of disease onset</td><td>Fulminant</td><td>Rapid</td><td colspan="2">Slow</td></tr>
<tr><td>Clinical stages / Islet autoantibodies</td><td>0</td><td>1</td><td>2</td><td>3</td></tr>
<tr><td>A) positive (autoimmune)</td><td>A0</td><td>A1</td><td>A2</td><td>A3</td></tr>
<tr><td>B) negative (idiopathic)</td><td>B0</td><td>B1</td><td>B2</td><td>B3</td></tr>
</table>

Table 1. Clinical types of diabetes based on islet autoantibodies, mode of disease onset, and insulin deficiency.

In Table 1, the region of T1D is the sum of A0, A1, A2, A3, B0, and B1 areas (shaded region), whereas the areas of B2 and B3 belong to T2D. The region of fulminant T1D is the sum of A0 and B0 areas, that of classic T1D is the sum of A1 and B1 areas, and that of LADA is the sum of A2 and A3 areas, where the onset of disease is in adulthood.

3.1 Fulminant T1D (Clinical stage 0)

3.1.1 Fulminant-onset and autoimmune (A0) area

Although fulminant T1D is a subtype of idiopathic T1D, it has been shown that 4.8% of patients with fulminant T1D were positive for GADAb (Imagawa et al., 2003). The ADA and WHO criteria cannot explain this form of diabetes, which corresponds to fulminant-onset and autoimmune (A0) area in Table 1. Recently, a fulminant T1D patient with positive IA-2Ab has also been reported (K. Katsumata & K. Katsumata, 2005). Although, it has been shown that there are few patients with fulminant T1D among Caucasian populations (Maldonado et al., 2003; Pozzilli et al., 2000), the high incidence of autoimmune T1D might conceal the presence of the A0 type of diabetes amongst Caucasians (Imagawa & Hanafusa, 2005).

3.1.2 Fulminant-onset and idiopathic (B0) area

Imagawa et al. reported, for the first time, 11 patients with fulminant T1D who do not have islet autoantibodies and proposed that this form of diabetes is a "nonautoimmune fulminant" T1D (Imagawa et al., 2000a). This form of diabetes corresponds to fulminant-onset and idiopathic (B0) area in Table 1. Although more than 250 patients with B0 area have been reported in Japan, few patients have been reported outside of Japan (Imagawa & Hanafusa, 2005). Despite its classification as an idiopathic form of T1D, the B0 type of diabetes is associated with HLA (Imagawa et al., 2005).

3.2 Rapid-onset T1D (Clinical stage 1)

3.2.1 Rapid-onset and autoimmune (A1) area

Rapid-onset and autoimmune T1D is the most common form of T1D and accounts for the majority of cases of "classic" T1D. This form of diabetes corresponds to rapid-onset and autoimmune (A1) area in Table 1. The A1 type of diabetes has strong HLA associations, with linkage to the DQA and B genes, and is influenced by the DRB genes (Cantor et al., 1995; Huang et al., 1996). These HLA-DR/DQ alleles can be either predisposing or protective.

3.2.2 Rapid-onset and idiopathic (B1) area

This form of diabetes corresponds to idiopathic T1D except for fulminant T1D and has no known etiology. Imagawa et al. called the B1 type of diabetes the nonautoimmune nonfulminant (chronic) T1D in contrast to the B0 and A1 types of diabetes (Imagawa et al., 2000a, 2000b).

3.3 Slow-onset diabetes (Clinical stages 2 and 3)

Although slow-onset T1D is known as LADA throughout the world, it is referred to as slowly progressice T1D in Japan (Kobayashi et al., 1993). However, there are some differences between LADA and slowly progressive T1D (Table 2): LADA patients are typically adults at diagnosis (usually aged >30 years), do not require insulin at least during the first 6 months after diagnosis, and are not necessarily insulin deficient (Stenström et al., 2005; Tuomi et al., 1999). Patients with slowly progressive T1D, who usually are insulin deficient, have variable age at disease onset, and insulin treatment is typically initiated >12 months after diagnosis (Kobayashi et al., 1993).

	LADA	Slowly progressive T1D	Slow-onset T1D
Islet autoantibodies	Positive	Positive	Positive
Age of diabetes onset	Usually >30 years	Any age	Any age
Duration not requiring insulin after diagnosis	>6 months	>12 months	>6 months
Insulin deficiency	Not necessarily deficient	Usually deficient	Not necessarily deficient

Table 2. Clinical characteristics of LADA, slowly progressive T1D, and slow-onset T1D. LADA, latent autoimmune diabetes in adults; T1D, Type 1 diabetes.

3.3.1 Slow-onset, insulin-deficient and autoimmune (A2) area

This form of diabetes corresponds to insulin-deficient LADA, LADY (Lohmann et al., 2000), and LADC (Aycan et al., 2004) or slowly progressive T1D in Japan. LADA has strong HLA associations apart from the same contribution of HLA in LADA and classic Type 1 diabetes (Desai et al., 2007; Hosszúfalusi et al., 2003; Stenström et al., 2003; Tuomi et al., 1999). Therefore, it is possible that the A2 type of diabetes is associated with HLA. Previous studies investigating the relationship between HLA class II genes and slow-onset T1D in Japan have focused on the relationship between these genes and the A2 type of diabetes (Kobayashi et al., 1993; Maruyama et al., 1994; Murao et al., 2004; Ohtsu et al., 2005) .

3.3.2 Slow-onset, insulin-deficient and idiopathic (B2) area

This form of diabetes corresponds to insulin-deficient T2D. Individuals with extensive insulin secretory defects, and therefore no residual insulin secretion, require insulin for survival. The B2 type of diabetes is thus a form of T2D, not T1D.

3.3.3 Slow-onset, non-insulin-deficient and autoimmune (A3) area

This form of diabetes corresponds to non-insulin-deficient LADA, LADY (Lohmann et al., 2000), and LADC (Aycan et al., 2004). The A3 type of diabetes is thus a form of T1D, not T2D. The association of the A3 type of diabetes with HLA is unknown. This form of diabetes ultimately progresses to the A2 type of diabetes.

3.3.4 Slow-onset, non-insulin-deficient and idiopathic (B3) area

This form of diabetes corresponds to non-insulin-deficient T2D, where insulin is not required at all or is required for adequate glycemic control, but not for survival. The B3 type of diabetes is "typical" T2D. Progression of this form of diabetes to the B2 type of diabetes is not common.

3.4 Correspondence to previous classification methods

Table 3 shows how various classification methods correspond to each area in Table 1. As stated above, the region of fulminant T1D is the sum of A0 and B0 areas. The region of classic, rapid-onset, or acute-onset T1D is the sum of A1 and B1 areas. The region of insulin-dependent diabetes mellitus (IDDM) is the sum of A0, A1, B0, and B1 areas. The region of autoimmune T1D (type 1A diabetes) is the sum of A0, A1, A2, and A3 areas. The region of idiopathic T1D (type 1B diabetes) is the sum of B0 and B1 areas. The region of slowly progressive IDDM (SPIDDM) is the sum of A2 and B2 areas. The region of LADA is the sum of A2 and A3 areas, where the onset of disease is in adulthood. The region of mon-insulin-dependent diabetes mellitus (NIDDM) is the sum of A3 and B3 areas.

Classifications of diabetes	Area(s) of diabetes
Fulminant T1D	A0 + B0
Nonautoimmune fulminant T1D	B0
Classic (rapid-onset or acute-onset) T1D	A1 +B1
Insulin-dependent diabetes mellitus (IDDM)	A0 + A1 + B0 + B1
Autoimmune T1D (type 1A diabetes)	A0 + A1 + A2 + A3
Idiopathic T1D (type 1B diabetes)	B0 + B1
Nonautoimmune nonfulminant (chronic) T1D	B1
Slowly progressive IDDM (SPIDDM)	A2 + B2
Latent autoimmune diabetes in adults (LADA)	A2 + A3
T1D	A0 + A1 + A2 + A3 + B0 + B1
Non-insulin-dependent diabetes mellitus (NIDDM)	A3 + B3
T2D	B2 + B3

Table 3. Correspondence of various classifications of diabetes to area(s) of diabetes. T1D, Type 1 diabetes; T2D, Type 2 diabetes.

4. HLA class II genes and T1D in the Japanese population

More than 90% of patients with T1D of Caucasian origin are carriers of DR3 or DR4 (Rønningen et al., 1991; Sanjeevi et al., 1995). In the Japanese population, in contrast to Caucasians and other Asians, DRB1*04:05-DQA1*03:03-DQB1*04:01—which is different from the DR4 haplotype in Caucasians—, DRB1*08:02-DQA1*03:01-DQB1*03:02 (DR8), DRB1*09:01-DQA1*03:02-DQB1*03:03 (DR9), and DRB1*13:02-DQA1*01:02-DQB1*06:04 (DR13) haplotypes confer susceptibility to T1D. In this section, we discuss the relationship between HLA class II genes and T1D in the Japanese population based on a comparison with other ethnic groups.

4.1 DRB1*04:05-DQA1*03:03-DQB1*04:01 haplotype

The DRB1*04:05-DQA1*03:03-DQB1*04:01 haplotype is frequently observed in East Asians, including the Japanese, but is rare in other ethnic groups such as Caucasians and Blacks (Thomson et al. 2007). Among East Asians, this haplotype confers susceptibility to T1D only in the Japanese, Taiwanese (Chuang et al., 1995; Huang et al., 1995), and Filipinos (Bugawan et al., 2002), but not in Koreans (Park et al., 2000), Hong Kong Chinese (Chang et al., 1998), and Singapore Chinese (Chan et al., 1995). DRB1*04:05-DQA1*03:03-DQB1*04:01 and DR9 are the most frequently observed susceptibility haplotypes in the Japanese (Awata et al., 1992; Imagawa et al., 2005; Kawabata et al., 2002; Kobayashi et al., 1993; Maruyama et al., 1994; Murao et al., 2004; Tanaka et al., 2002; Yasunaga et al., 1996). However, studies conducted before the discovery of fulminant T1D may have included patients with fulminant T1D. Fulminant T1D accounts for approximately 20% of rapid-onset T1D in the Japanese population (Imagawa et al., 2003). A nationwide survey in Japan revealed that 41.8% of fulminant T1D patients possessed the DR4-DQ4 (encoded by DRB1*04:05-DQA1*03:03-DQB1*04:01) haplotype (Imagawa et al., 2005). Table 4 shows the phenotype frequencies of DRB1*04:05-DQA1*03:03-DQB1*04:01 and DR9 haplotypes in rapid-onset T1D with fulminant T1D (A0 + A1 + B0 + B1 areas) (Awata et al., 1992; Kawabata et al., 2002; Kobayashi et al., 1993; Maruyama et al., 1994; Yasunaga et al., 1996), rapid-onset T1D (which includes A1 area and excludes B0 area) (Imagawa et al., 2005; Murao et al., 2004; Tanaka et al., 2002), and fulminant T1D (B0 area) (Imagawa et al., 2005; Tanaka et al., 2002).

Mode of onset	Author (publication year)	Area(s) of diabetes	DRB1*04:05-DQA1*03:03-DQB1*04:01		DR9	
			PF	OR	PF	OR
Rapid-onset T1D	Imagawa et al. (2005)	A1	39.5%	2.2	56.8%	3.4
	Tanaka et al. (2002)	A0 + A1	43.6%	3.0	50.0%	4.3
	Murao et al. (2004)	A1 + B1	46.0%	3.1	65.1%	4.9
Rapid-onset T1D with fulminant T1D	Kobayashi et al. (1993)	A0 + A1 + B0 + B1	48.9%	3.1	44.3%	5.2
	Maruyama et al. (1994)		52.4%	4.3	38.1%	NS
	Awata et al. (1992)		52.5%	4.4	51.5%	2.2
	Kawabata et al. (2002)		53.8%	2.7	34.2%	2.1*
	Yasunaga et al. (1996)		56.8%	3.6	36.0%	1.3
Fulminant T1D	Imagawa et al. (2005)	B0	65.9%	6.6	36.3%	NS
	Tanaka et al. (2002)		68.2%	8.4	36.4%	NS

Table 4. Phenotype frequencies of DRB1*04:05-DQA1*03:03-DQB1*04:01 and DR9 haplotypes in Japanese T1D. DR9, DRB1*09:01-DQA1*03:02-DQB1*03:03; T1D, Type 1 diabetes; PF, Phenotype frequency; OR, Odds ratio; NS, not significant. Corrected $P < 0.05$ with haplotype frequency.

Before the existence of fulminant T1D was clarified (Imagawa et al., 2000a), the frequency and odds ratio (OR) of the DRB1*04:05-DQA1*03:03-DQB1*04:01 haplotype were higher than those of the DR9 haplotype in rapid-onset T1D with fulminant T1D (Awata et al., 1992; Kawabata et al., 2002; Kobayashi et al., 1993; Maruyama et al., 1994; Yasunaga et al., 1996). However, the frequency and OR of the DRB1*04:05-DQA1*03:03-DQB1*04:01 haplotype in rapid-onset T1D are lower than those of the DRB1*04:05-DQA1*03:03-DQB1*04:01 haplotype in rapid-onset T1D with fulminant T1D and those of the DR9 haplotype in rapid-onset T1D (Imagawa et al., 2005; Murao et al., 2004; Tanaka et al., 2002). On the other hand, the frequency and OR of the DRB1*04:05-DQA1*03:03-DQB1*04:01 haplotype in fulminant T1D are higher than those of the DRB1*04:05-DQA1*03:03-DQB1*04:01 haplotype in rapid-onset T1D. The DR9 haplotype is less frequent in fulminant T1D than in rapid-onset T1D and does not confer susceptibility to fulminant T1D (Imagawa et al., 2005; Tanaka et al., 2002).

The role of HLA class II has been emphasized in the context of the antigen-presenting process in autoimmune T1D (Eisenbarth et al., 2003), but it remains to be elucidated how a certain HLA class II can contribute toward the molecular mechanisms of β-cell destruction in fulminant T1D. One possibility is that the HLA molecule is associated with immune reaction of fulminant T1D similar to autoimmune T1D; another is that it may interact with some type of virus, as shown in mice (Wykes et al., 1993). The HLA gene, or a gene showing linkage disequilibrium to the HLA gene, contributes to the development of fulminant T1D (Imagawa et al., 2006). It is suggested that idiopathic T1D (B0 + B1 areas) accounts for approximately 40% of rapid-onset T1D with fulminant T1D (A0 + A1 + B0 + B1 areas) in the Japanese (Imagawa et al., 2000b). It is reported that 81.8% of the Japanese with idiopathic T1D (B0 + B1 areas) possess the HLA DRB1*0405 allele compared to the 58.8% with autoimmune T1D (Urakami et al., 2002). Further investigations of idiopathic T1D except fulminant T1D (B1 area) might clarify the relationship between the DRB1*04:05-DQA1*03:03-DQB1*04:01 haplotype and T1D.

4.2 DRB1*08:02-DQA1*03:01-DQB1*03:02 (DR8) haplotype

The DRB1*04:01, *04:02, or *04:05-DQA1*03:01-DQB1*03:02 (DR4) haplotype confers susceptibility to T1D in almost all ethnic groups such as Caucasians, Blacks, and East Asians (Thomson et al., 2007), but is rare in the Japanese. Conversely, the DR8 haplotype confers susceptibility to Japanese T1D (Awata et al., 1992; Kawabata et al., 2002; Kobayashi et al., 1993; Murao et al., 2004; Ohtsu et al., 2005; Yasunaga et al., 1996) and is present only in Japanese and Korean T1D (Thomson et al., 2007). However, some studies have found no evidence that the DR8 haplotype confers susceptibility to Japanese T1D (Maruyama et al., 1994; Murao et al., 2004; Tanaka et al., 2002). Table 5 shows the phenotype frequency of the DR8 haplotype and the mean onset age of T1D in previous studies.

Mode of onset	Author (publication year)	Area(s) of diabetes	DR8		Mean onset age
			PF	OR	
Rapid-onset T1D with or without fulminant T1D	Murao et al. (2004)	A1 + B1	18.8%	3.8	8
	Ohtsu et al. (2005)	A1 + B1	12.9%	4.6	8
	Kawabata et al. (2002)	A0 + A1 + B0 + B1	13.6%	6.0	16
	Kobayashi et al. (1993)	A0 + A1 + B0 + B1	30.7%	5.2	22
	Awata et al. (1992)	A0 + A1 + B0 + B1	14.1%	9.7	26
	Maruyama et al. (1994)	A0 + A1 + B0 + B1	8.3%	NS	30
	Tanaka et al. (2002)	A0 + A1	15.4%	NS	34
	Murao et al. (2004)	A1 + B1	7.9%	NS	39
Slow-onset T1D with or without rapid-onset T1D	Ohtsu et al. (2005)	A2 + B2	6.3%	NS	11
	Maruyama et al. (1994)	A2 + B2	6.3%	NS	35
	Katahira et al. (2008)	A1 + A2 + B1	14.5%	4.2	35
	Kobayashi et al. (1993)	A2 + B2	18.8%	NS	38
	Takeda et al. (2002)	A1 + A2	16.9%	3.3	41
	Murao et al. (2004)	A2	10.7%	NS	47

Table 5. Phenotype frequencies of the DR8 haplotype and the mean onset age in Japanese T1D. DR8, DRB1*08:02-DQA1*03:01-DQB1*03:02; T1D, Type 1 diabetes; PF, Phenotype frequency; OR, Odds ratio; NS, not significant.

This haplotype appears to confer susceptibility to rapid-onset T1D where the mean onset age is young (≤26 years) (Awata et al., 1992; Kawabata et al., 2002; Kobayashi et al., 1993; Murao et al., 2004; Ohtsu et al., 2005). Even if the mean onset age is older than 30 years old, this haplotype appears to confer susceptibility to rapid-onset T1D with slow-onset T1D (which includes both A1 and A2 areas) (Katahira et al., 2008; Takeda et al., 2002). However, there are no studies reporting that this haplotype confers susceptibility to slow-onset T1D (which includes A2 area and excludes A1 area) even if the mean onset age is young (Kobayashi et al., 1993; Maruyama et al., 1994; Murao et al., 2004; Ohtsu et al., 2005).
The effects of DRB1*04 subtypes on the DQA1*03:01-DQB1*03:02 haplotype vary from susceptibility to T1D (DRB1*04:01, *04:02, or *04:05) to protection against T1D (DRB1*04:03 or *04:06). The Korean population is unique in that the DR8 haplotype is present in addition to the DRB1*04-DQA1*03:01-DQB1*03:02 haplotype. Table 6 shows the frequencies of DRB1*04 and DRB1*08 subtypes linked to the DQA1*03:01-DQB1*03:02 haplotype in available Japanese (Kawabata et al., 2002; Murao et al., 2004) and Korean (Park et al., 2000) studies.

Ethnic	Japanese						Korean		
Author (publication year)	Kawabata et al. (2002)			Murao et al. (2004)			Park et al. (2000)		
DRB1 allele	n	%	OR	n	%	OR	n	%	OR
*04:01	0	0	–	0	0	–	15	27.8	13.9
*04:02	0	0	–	0	0	–	2	4.1	NS
*04:03	4	12.5	NS	1	5.3	0.16	2	3.7	NS
*04:04	0	0	–	0	0	–	5	9.3	NS
*04:05	5	15.6	13.3	0	0	–	11	20.4	10.1
*04:06	1	3.1	0.12	0	0	–	3	5.6	NS
*04:07	4	12.5	NS	2	10.5	NS	7	13.0	13.6
*08:02	18	56.3	5.67	16	84.2	4.88	9	16.7	NS
Total	32	100	–	19	100	–	54	100	–

Table 6. Frequencies of DRB1*04 and DRB1*08 subtypes linked to the DQA1*03:01-DQB1*03:02 haplotype in Japanese and Korean rapid-onset T1D. T1D, Type 1 diabetes; OR, Odds ratio; NS, not significant.

The DRB1*08:02 subtype is the most frequent in DRB1*04 and DRB1*08 subtypes linked to the DQA1*03:01-DQB1*03:02 haplotype (56.3% and 84.2%, respectively) and confers susceptibility to rapid-onset T1D in the Japanese population, whereas the DRB1*08 subtype is the third most frequent (16.7%) after DRB1*04:01 and *04:05 and does not confer susceptibility to rapid-onset T1D in the Korean population. The susceptibility of the DR8 haplotype to Japanese rapid-onset T1D might originate from the distribution of DRB1*04 and DRB1*08 subtypes linked to the DQA1*03:01-DQB1*03:02 haplotype.

4.3 DRB1*09:01-DQA1*03:02-DQB1*03:03 (DR9) haplotype

As with the DRB1*04:05-DQA1*03:03-DQB1*04:01 haplotype, the DR9 haplotype is frequently observed in East Asians, including the Japanese. However, although the DR9 haplotype is present in Caucasians, it is rare in Blacks and Mexican-Americans (Thomson et al., 2007). This haplotype confers susceptibility to T1D in East Asians such as the Japanese,

Koreans (Park et al., 2000), and Filipinos (Bugawan et al., 2002), but generally not in Caucasians (Hermann et al., 2003; Koeleman et al., 2004; Lambert et al., 2004). However, exploratory analyses revealed that the DR9 haplotype confers risk for T1D in Norwegians who do not carry the DR3 or the DR4 haplotype (Undlien et al., 1999). Moreover, Graham et al. demonstrated that the risk of T1D decreased with age for the DR9 haplotype in a Swedish population (Graham et al., 1999). In the Japanese population, it has been reported that the frequency of the DR9 haplotype with an onset age <5 years is greater than that with an onset age >5 years of age at onset (61.5% *vs.* 43.1%) in childhood-onset T1D (Ohtsu et al., 2005), whereas the ratio of the DR9/DR4 frequency increases with the onset age in childhood- or adult-onset T1D (Murao et al., 2004). Fig. 1 shows the relationship between the frequency of the DR9 phenotype and the mean onset age in previous studies where the DR9 haplotype confers susceptibility to adult-onset T1D in the Japanese (Awata et al., 1992; Imagawa et al., 2005; Kawabata et al., 2002; Kobayashi et al., 1993; Murao et al., 2004; Tanaka et al., 2002). A significant positive correlation is observed between the frequency of the DR9 phenotype and the mean onset age ($r^2 = 0.742$, $P = 0.0274$). The frequency of the DR9 phenotype increases with the mean onset age of T1D in adult-onset Japanese T1D.

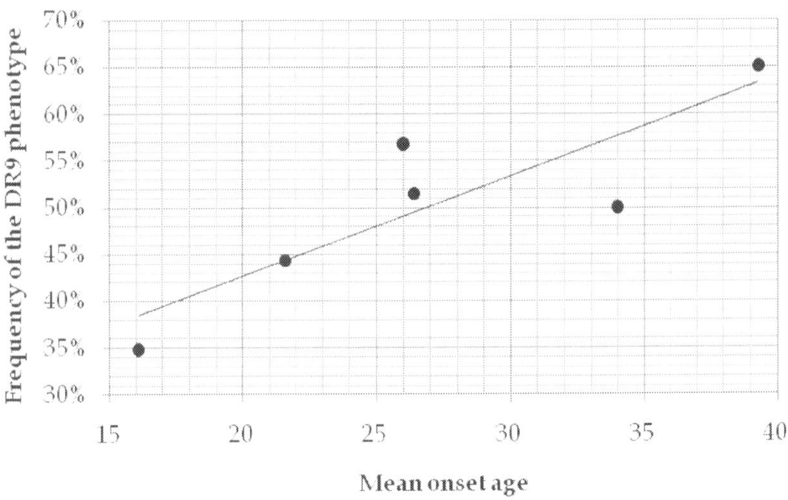

Fig. 1. Relationship between the frequency of the DR9 phenotype and the mean onset age. A significant positive correlation is observed between the frequency of the DR9 haplotype and the mean onset age ($r^2 = 0.742$, $P = 0.0274$). DR9, DRB1*09:01-DQA1*03:02-DQB1*03:03.

4.4 DRB1*13:02-DQA1*01:02-DQB1*06:04 (DR13) haplotype

Although the DR13 haplotype is observed in almost all ethnic groups (Thomson et al., 2007), a few investigators have demonstrated that this haplotype confers susceptibility to T1D in the Japanese (Katahira et al., 2008; Matsuda et al., 1988; Murao et al., 2004), Caucasians (Graham et al., 1999; Undlien et al., 1999), and Latin Americans (Cruz et al., 2004; Balducci-Silano et al., 1994). Table 7 shows the phenotype and haplotype frequencies of the DR13 haplotype in adult-onset Japanese T1D.

Author (publication year)	Mode of onset	Area(s) of diabetes	DR13			Mean onset age
			PF	HF	OR	
Kawabata et al. (2002)	fulminant + rapid	A0 + A1 + B0 + B1	13.6%	6.8%	NS	16
Kobayashi et al. (1993)	fulminant + rapid	A0 + A1 + B0 + B1	13.6%	–	NS	22
Imagawa et al. (2005)	rapid	A1	–	11.7%	NS	26
Awata et al. (1992)	fulminant + rapid	A0 + A1 + B0 + B1	22.2%	–	NS	26
Maruyama et al. (1994)	fulminant + rapid	A0 + A1 + B0 + B1	19.0%	–	NS	30
Tanaka et al. (2002)	rapid	A0 + A1	24.4%	–	NS	34
Katahira et al. (2008)	rapid + slow	A1 + A2 + B1	28.9%	15.1%	3.1	35
Murao et al. (2004)	rapid	A1 + B1	–	7.9%	4.6	39

Table 7. Phenotype and haplotype frequencies of the DR13 haplotype and the mean onset age in Japanese T1D. DR13, DRB1*13:02-DQA1*01:02-DQB1*06:04; T1D, Type 1 diabetes; PF, Phenotype frequeny; HF, Haplotype frequency; OR, Odds ratio; NS, not significant.

The average age at onset of diabetes was relatively low in previous studies (Awata et al., 1992; Imagawa et al., 2005; Kawabata et al., 2002; Kobayashi et al., 1993; Maruyama et al., 1994; Tanaka et al., 2002) which did not find a significant susceptibility to DR13 (16–34 years). In contrast, the average age at onset of diabetes was relatively high in previous studies (Katahira et al., 2008; Murao et al., 2004) which did find susceptibility to DR13 (≥35 years). Exploratory analyses revealed that the DR13 haplotype might also confer risk for T1D in subjects in Norway, Sweden (Graham et al., 1999; Undlien et al., 1999), and Venezuela (Balducci-Silano et al., 1994) who do not carry the DR3 or the DR4 haplotype. Moreover, Graham et al. demonstrated that the risk of T1D increased with age for the DR13 haplotype (Graham et al., 1999). It has been demonstrated that the DPB1*0301 allele, which exhibits linkage disequilibrium with the DR13 haplotype in Puerto Ricans, confers susceptibility to T1D in this ethnic group (Cruz et al., 2004).

The DR13 haplotype shares the same DQA1 allele with the DRB1*1501-DQA1*0102-DQB1*0602 haplotype which is strongly associated with T1D protection in almost all ethnic groups (Thomson et al., 2007). Moreover, DQB1*0604 and DQB1*0602 differ at seven amino acids, six of which are within the first external domain at β9, β30, β57, β70, β86, and β87, and one within the second external domain at β130. Some investigators have suggested that differences in peptide binding between DQB1*0604 and DQB1*0602 contribute to the mechanism of their association with T1D (Ettinger et al., 2006; Sanjeevi et al., 2002).

4.5 Haplotypes associated with T1D protection

The DRB1*1501-DQA1*0102-DQB1*0602 haplotype confers protection against T1D in almost all ethnic groups such as Caucasians and East Asians (Thomson et al., 2007), and the similar

DRB1*1503-DQA1*0102-DQB1*0602 haplotype confers protection against T1D in Blacks, suggesting that the DQA1*0102-DQB1*0602 haplotype is a primary protective molecule in all ethnic groups. On the other hand, DRB1*1502-DQA1*0103-DQB1*0601 and DRB1*0803-DQA1*0103-DQB1*0601 haplotypes are present in East Asians, but rare in Caucasians and Blacks (Thomson et al., 2007). These haplotypes confer weak protection against T1D in the Japanese (Katahira et al., 2008; Yasunaga et al., 1996) and Koreans (Park et al., 2000). As with the DQA1*0102-DQB1*0602 haplotype, the DQA1*0103-DQB1*0601 haplotype encodes "non-Arg," an amino acid other than arginine, at position 52 in DQα and aspartic acid at position 57 in DQβ. These are thought to be strongly negatively associated with the development of T1D (Khalil et al., 1990; Todd et al., 1987). Although the DRB1*11-DQA1*05-DQB1*0301 haplotype is observed in almost all ethnic groups (Thomson et al., 2007) and confers protection against T1D in Caucasians (Hermann et al., 2003; Undlien et al., 1999; Yasunaga et al., 1996) and Latin Americans (Volpini et al., 2001), this haplotype confers very weak (Huang et al., 1995; Awata et al., 1992; Katahira et al., 2008) or no protection (Bugawan et al., 2002; Park et al., 2000) against T1D in East Asians, including the Japanese.

5. Conclusions

T1D can be divided into six subtypes based on the mode of disease onset, markers of immune destruction, and insulin deficiency. The relationship between DRB1*04:05-DQA1*03:03-DQB1*04:01, DR8, DR9 and DR13 haplotypes and T1D depends on the mode of disease onset and the mean onset age of the disease. The DRB1*04:05-DQA1*03:03-DQB1*04:01 haplotype is the most frequent in fulminant T1D and solely confers susceptibility to fulminant T1D. The DR8 haplotype confers susceptibility to rapid-onset T1D with onset at a young age. The DR9 haplotype, the frequency of which increases with the mean onset age of T1D, is the most frequent in rapid-onset T1D. The DR13 haplotype confers susceptibility to rapid-onset T1D, with onset at a relatively old age. On the other hand, the DQA1*0102-DQB1*0602 haplotype is the common protective haplotype against T1D in all ethnic groups.

6. References

Alberti, K.G. & Zimmet, P.Z. (1998) Definition, diagnosis and classification of diabetes mellitus and its complications. Part 1: Diagnosis and classification of diabetes mellitus provisional report of a WHO consultation. *Diabet Med*, Vol. 15 (No. 7): 539-553.

Awata, T., Kuzuya, T., Matsuda, A., Iwamoto, Y. & Kanazawa, Y. (1992) Genetic analysis of HLA class II alleles and susceptibility to type 1 (insulin-dependent) diabetes mellitus in Japanese subjects. *Diabetologia*, Vol. 35 (No. 5): 419–424.

Aycan, Z., Berberoglu, M., Adiyaman, P., Ergür, A.T., Ensari, A., Evliyaoglu, O., Siklar, Z. & Ocal, G. (2004) Latent autoimmune diabetes mellitus in children (LADC) with autoimmune thyroiditis and Celiac disease. *J Pediatr Endocrinol Metab*, Vol. 17 (No. 11): 1565–1569.

Balducci-Silano, P.L., Layrisse, Z., Dominguez, E., Amaro, R., Gunczler, P., Lanes, R. & Zaro, R. (1994) HLA-DQA1 and DQB1 allele and genotype contribution to IDDM susceptibility in an ethnically mixed population. *Eur J Immunogenet*, Vol. 21 (No. 6): 405–414.

Borg, H., Arnqvist, H.J., Björk, E., Bolinder, J., Eriksson, J.W., Nyström, L., Jeppsson, J.O. & Sundkvist, G. (2003) Evaluation of the new ADA and WHO criteria for classification of diabetes mellitus in young adult people (15-34 yrs) in the Diabetes Incidence Study in Sweden (DISS). *Diabetologia*, Vol. 46 (No. 2): 173–181.

Bugawan, T.L., Klitz, W., Alejandrino, M., Ching, J., Panelo, A., Solfelix, C.M., Petrone, A., Buzzetti, R., Pozzilli, P. & Erlich, H.A. (2002) The association of specific HLA class I and II alleles with type 1 diabetes among Filipinos. *Tissue Antigens*, Vol. 59 (No. 6): 452–469.

Cantor, A.B., Krischer, J.P., Cuthbertson, D.D., Schatz, D.A., Riley, W.J., Malone, J., Schwartz, S., Quattrin, T. & Maclaren, N.K. (1995) Age and family relationship accentuate the risk of insulin-dependent diabetes mellitus (IDDM) in relatives of patients with IDDM. *J Clin Endocrinol Metab*, Vol. 80 (No. 12): 3739–3743.

Chan, S.H., Thai, A.C., Lin, Y.N., Liu, K.F. & Wee, G.B. (1995) Influence of gender and age at onset on the HLA associations in Chinese with insulin-dependent diabetes mellitus. *Hum Immunol*, Vol. 44 (No. 3): 175–180.

Chang, Y.W., Lam, K.S. & Hawkins, B.R. (1998) Strong association between DQA1/DQB1 genotype and early-onset IDDM in Chinese: the association is with alleles rather than specific residues. *Eur J Immunogenet*, Vol. 25 (No. 4): 273–280.

Chuang, L.M., Wu, H.P., Tsai, W.Y., Lin, B.J. & Tai TY. (1995) Transcomplementation of HLA DQA1-DQB1 in DR3/DR4 and DR3/DR9 heterozygotes and IDDM in Taiwanese families. *Diabetes Care*, Vol. 18 (No. 11): 1483–1486.

Cruz, T.D., Valdes, A.M., Santiago, A., Frazer de Llado, T., Raffel, L.J., Zeidler, A., Rotter, J.I., Erlich, H.A., Rewers, M., Bugawan, T. & Noble, J.A. (2004) DPB1 alleles are associated with type 1 diabetes susceptibility in multiple ethnic groups. *Diabetes*, Vol. 53 (No. 8) :2158–2163.

Desai, M., Zeggini, E., Horton, V.A., Owen, K.R., Hattersley, A.T., Levy, J.C., Walker, M., Gillespie, K.M., Bingley, P.J., Hitman, G.A., Holman, R.R., McCarthy, M.I. & Clark, A. (2007) An association analysis of the HLA gene region in latent autoimmune diabetes in adults. *Diabetologia*, Vol. 50 (No. 1): 68–73.

Eisenbarth, G.S., Polonsky, K.S. & Buse, J.B. (2003) Type 1 diabetes mellitus, In: *William Textbook of Endocrinology 10th ed.*, Larsen, P.R., Kronenberg, H.M., Melmed, S. & Polonsky, K.S. (Ed.), 1485–1504, Saunders, ISBN 0-7216-9184-6, Philadelphia, USA

Ettinger, R.A., Papadopoulos, G.K., Moustakas, A.K., Nepom, G.T. & Kwok, W.W. (2006) Allelic variation in key peptide-binding pockets discriminates between closely related diabetes-protective and diabetes-susceptible HLA-DQB1*06 alleles. *J Immunol*, Vol. 176 (No. 3): 1988–1998.

Expert Committee on the Diagnosis and Classification of Diabetes Mellitus. (1997) Report of the Expert Committee on the Diagnosis and Classification of Diabetes Mellitus. *Diabetes Care*, Vol. 20 (No. 7): 1183–1197.

Fourlanos, S., Dotta, F., Greenbaum, C.J. Palmer, J.P., Rolandsson, O., Colman, P.G. & Harrison, L.C. (2005) Latent autoimmune diabetes in adults (LADA) should be less latent. *Diabetologia*, Vol. 48 (No. 11): 2206–2212.

Graham, J., Kockum, I., Sanjeevi, C.B., Landin-Olsson, M., Nyström, L., Sundkvist, G., Arnqvist, H., Blohmé, G., Lithner, F., Littorin, B., Scherstén, B., Wibell, L., Ostman, J., Lernmark, Å., Breslow, N. & Dahlquist G. (1999) Negative association between type 1 diabetes and HLA DQB1*0602-DQA1*0102 is attenuated with age at onset. *Eur J Immunogenet*, Vol. 26 (No. 2-3): 117-127.

Hermann, R., Turpeinen, H., Laine, A.P., Veijola, R., Knip, M., Simell, O., Sipilä, I., Åkerblom, H.K. & Ilonen J. (2003) HLA DR-DQ-encoded genetic determinants of childhood-onset type 1 diabetes in Finland: an analysis of 622 nuclear families. *Tissue Antigens*, Vol. 62 (No. 2): 162–169.

Hosszúfalusi, N., Vatay, A., Rajczy, K., Prohászka, Z., Pozsonyi, E., Horváth, L., Grosz, A., Gerõ, L., Madácsy, L., Romics, L., Karádi, I., Füst, G. & Pánczél, P. (2003) Similar genetic features and different islet cell autoantibody pattern of latent autoimmune diabetes in adults (LADA) compared with adult-onset type 1 diabetes with rapid progression. *Diabetes Care*, Vol. 26 (No. 2): 452–457.

Huang, H.S., Peng, J.T., She, J.Y., Zhang, L.P., Chao, C.C., Liu, K.H. & She, J.X. (1995) HLA-encoded susceptibility to insulin-dependent diabetes mellitus is determined by DR and DQ genes as well as their linkage disequilibria in a Chinese population. *Hum Immunol*, Vol. 44 (No. 4): 210–219.

Huang, W., Connor, E., Rosa, T.D., Muir, A., Schatz, D., Silverstein, J., Crockett, S., She, J.X. & Maclaren, N.K. (1996) Although DR3-DQB1*0201 may be associated with multiple component diseases of the autoimmune polyglandular syndromes, the human leukocyte antigen DR4-DQB1*0302 haplotype is implicated only in beta-cell autoimmunity. *J Clin Endocrinol Metab*, Vol. 81 (No. 7): 2559–2563.

Humphrey, A.R., McCarty, D.J., Mackay, I.R., Rowley, M.J., Dwyer, T. & Zimmet, P. (1998) Autoantibodies to glutamic acid decarboxylase and phenotypic features associated with early insulin treatment in individuals with adult-onset diabetes mellitus. *Diabet Med*, Vol. 15 (No. 2): 113–119.

Imagawa, A., Hanafusa, T., Miyagawa, J. & Matsuzawa Y. (2000a) A novel subtype of type 1 diabetes mellitus characterized by a rapid onset and an absence of diabetes-related antibodies. *N Engl J Med*, Vol. 342 (No. 5): 301–307.

Imagawa, A., Hanafusa, T., Miyagawa, J. & Matsuzawa, Y. (2000b) A proposal of three distinct subtypes of type 1 diabetes mellitus based on clinical and pathological evidence. *Ann Med*, Vol. 32 (No. 8): 539–543.

Imagawa, A., Hanafusa, T., Uchigata, Y., Kanatsuka, A., Kawasaki, E., Kobayashi, T., Shimada, A., Shimizu, I., Toyoda, T., Maruyama, T. & Makino, H. (2003) Fulminant type 1 diabetes: A nationwide survey in Japan. *Diabetes Care*, Vol. 26 (No. 8) : 2345–2352.

Imagawa, A. & Hanafusa, T. (2005) Fulminant type 1 diabetes-is it an Asianoriented disease? (2005) *Intern Med*, Vol. 44 (No. 9): 913–914.

Imagawa, A., Hanafusa, T., Uchigata, Y., Kanatsuka, A., Kawasaki, E., Kobayashi, T., Shimada, A., Shimizu, I., Maruyama, T. & Makino H. (2005) Different contribution of class II HLA in fulminant and typical autoimmune type 1 diabetes mellitus. *Diabetologia*, Vol. 48 (No. 2): 294–300.

Imagawa, A. & Hanafusa, T. (2006) Fulminant type 1 diabetes mellitus. *Endocr J*, Vol. 53 (No. 5): 577–584.

Katahira, M., Ishiguro, T., Segawa, S., Kuzuya-Nagao, K., Hara, I. & Nishisaki, T. (2008) Reevaluation of human leukocyte antigen DR-DQ haplotype and genotype in type 1 diabetes in the Japanese population. *Horm Res*, Vol. 69 (No. 5): 284–289.

Katsumata, K. & Katsumata, K. (2005) A Chinese patient presenting with clinical signs of fulminant type 1 diabetes mellitus. *Intern Med*, Vol. 44 (No. 9): 967–969.

Kawabata, Y., Ikegami, H., Kawaguchi, Y., Fujisawa, T., Shintani, M., Ono, M., Nishino, M., Uchigata, Y., Lee, I. & Ogihara, T. (2002) Asian-specific HLA haplotypes reveal heterogeneity of the contribution of HLA-DR and -DQ haplotypes to susceptibility to type 1 diabetes. *Diabetes*, Vol. 51 (No. 2): 545–551.

Khalil, I., d'Auriol, L., Gobet, M., Morin, L., Lepage, V., Deschamps, I., Park, M.S., Degos, L., Galibert, F. & Hors, J. (1990) A combination of HLA-DQβ Asp57-negative and HLA DQα Arg52 confers susceptibility to insulin-dependent diabetes mellitus. *J Clin Invest*, Vol. 85 (No. 4): 1315–1319.

Kobayashi, T., Tamemoto, K., Nakanishi, K., Kato, N., Okubo, M., Kajio, H., Sugimoto, T., Murase, T. & Kosaka K. (1993) Immunogenetic and clinical characterization of slowly progressive IDDM. *Diabetes Care*, Vol. 16 (No. 5): 780–788.

Koeleman, B.P., Lie, B.A., Undlien, D.E., Dudbridge, F., Thorsby, E., de Vries, R.R., Cucca, F., Roep, B.O., Giphart, M.J. & Todd, J.A. (2004) Genotype effects and epistasis in type 1 diabetes and HLA-DQ trans dimer associations with disease. *Genes Immun*, Vol. 5 (No. 5): 381–388.

Lambert, A.P., Gillespie, K.M., Thomson, G., Cordell, H.J., Todd, J.A., Gale, E.A. & Bingley, P.J. (2004) Absolute risk of childhood-onset type 1 diabetes defined by human leukocyte antigen class II genotype: a population-based study in the United Kingdom. *J Clin Endocrinol Metab*, Vol. 89 (No. 8): 4037–4043.

Landin-Olsson, M., Karlsson, F.A., Lernmark, Å. & Sundkvist, G. (1992) Islet cell and thyrogastric antibodies in 633 consecutive 15- to 34-yr-old patients in the diabetes incidence study in Sweden. *Diabetes*, Vol. 41 (No. 8): 1022–1027.

Lohmann, T., Nietzschmann, U. & Kiess, W. (2000) "Lady-like": Is there a latent autoimmune diabetes in the young? *Diabetes Care*, Vol. 23 (No. 11): 1707–1708.

Maldonado, M., Hampe, C.S., Gaur, L.K., D'Amico, S., Iyer, D., Hammerle, L.P., Bolgiano, D., Rodriguez, L., Rajan, A., Lernmark, Å. & Balasubramanyam A. (2003) Ketosis-prone diabetes: dissection of a heterogeneous syndrome using an Immunogenetic and beta-cell functional classification, prospective analysis, and clinical outcomes. *J Clin Endocrinol Metab*, Vol. 88 (No. 11): 5090–5098.

Maruyama, T., Shimada, A., Kasuga, A., Kasatani, T., Ozawa, Y., Ishii, M., Takei, I., Suzuki, Y., Kobayashi, A., Takeda, S., Matsubara, K. & Saruta, T. (1994) Analysis of MHC class II antigens in Japanese IDDM by a novel HLA-typing method, hybridization protection assay. *Diabetes Res Clin Pract*, Vol. 23 (No. 2):77–84.

Matsuda, A., Kuzuya, T., Iwamoto, Y., Yoshioka, N., Awata, T., Kumakura, S. & Ohwada N. (1988) HLA DR antigens in adult-onset and juvenile-onset Japanese insulin-dependent diabetic patients. *Diabetes Res Clin Pract*, Vol. 13 (No. 5): 107–112.

Matsuura, N., Fukuda, K., Okuno, A., Harada, S., Fukushima, N., Koike, A., Ito, Y. & Hotsubo, T. (1998) Descriptive epidemiology of IDDM in Hokkaido, Japan: the Childhood IDDM Hokkaido Registry. *Diabetes Care*, Vol. 21 (No. 10): 1632–1636.

Mølbak, A.G., Christau, B., Marner, B., Borch-Johnsen, K. & Nerup J. (1994) Incidence of insulin-dependent diabetes mellitus in age groups over 30 years in Denmark. *Diabet Med*, Vol. 11 (No. 7): 650–655.

Murao, S., Makino, H., Kaino, Y., Konoue, E., Ohashi, J., Kida, K., Fujii, Y., Shimizu, I., Kawasaki, E., Fujiyama, M., Kondo, S., Tanaka, K., Tarumi, Y., Seto, I., Kato, K.,

Ohno, K., Kusunoki, Y., Ebisui, O., Takada, Y., Tanabe, K., Takemoto, K., Onuma, H., Nishimiya, T. & Osawa, H. (2004) Differences in the contribution of HLA-DR and -DQ haplotypes to susceptibility to adult- and childhood-onset type 1 diabetes in Japanese patients. *Diabetes*, Vol. 53 (No. 10): 2684–2690.

Ohtsu, S., Takubo, N., Kazahari, M., Nomoto, K., Yokota, F., Kikuchi, N., Koike, A. & Matsuura, N. (2005) Slowly progressing form of type 1 diabetes mellitus in children: genetic analysis compared with other forms of diabetes mellitus in Japanese children. *Pediatr Diabetes*, Vol. 6 (No. 4): 221–229.

Park, Y., She, J.X., Wang, C.Y., Lee, H., Babu, S., Erlich, H.A., Noble, J.A. & Eisenbarth G.S. (2000) Common susceptibility and transmission pattern of human leukocyte antigen DRB1-DQB1 haplotypes to Korean and Caucasian patients with type 1 diabetes. *J Clin Endocrinol Metab*, Vol. 85 (No. 12): 4538–4542.

Pozzilli, P., Visalli, N. & Leslie, D. (2000) No evidence of rapid onset (Japanese) Type I diabetes in Caucasian patients. *Diabetologia*, Vol. 43 (No. 10): 1332–1333.

Rønningen, K.S., Spurkland, A., Iwe, T., Vartdal, F. & Thorsby, E. (1991) Distribution of HLA-DRB1, -DQA1 and -DQB1 alleles and DQA1-DQB1 genotypes among Norwegian patients with insulin-dependent diabetes mellitus. *Tissue Antigens*, Vol. 37 (No. 3): 105–111.

Sanjeevi, C.B., Lybrand, T.P., DeWeese, C., Landin-Olsson, M., Kockum, I., Dahlquist, G., Sundkvist, G., Stenger, D. & Lernmark, Å. (1995) Polymorphic amino acid variations in HLA-DQ are associated with systematic physical property changes and occurrence of IDDM. *Diabetes*, Vol. 44 (No. 1): 125–131.

Sanjeevi, C.B., Lybrand, T.P., Stevanovic, S. & Rammensee, H.G. (2002) Molecular modeling of eluted peptides from DQ6 molecules (DQB1*0602 and DQB1*0604) negatively and positively associated with type 1 diabetes. *Ann N Y Acad Sci*, 2002; Vol. 958 (Apr): 317-320.

Steenkiste, A., Valdes, A.M., Feolo, M., Hoffman, D., Concannon, P., Noble, J., Schoch, G., Hansen, J., Helmberg, W., Dorman, J.S., Thomson, G., Pugliese, A. & 13th IHWS 1 Diabetes Component participating investigators. (2007) 14th International HLA and Immunogenetics Workshop: report on the HLA component of type 1 diabetes. *Tissue Antigens*, Vol. 69 (Suppl. 1): 214–225.

Stenström, G., Berger, B., Borg, H., Fernlund, P., Dorman, J.S. & Sundkvist G. (2002) HLA-DQ genotypes in classic type 1 diabetes and in latent autoimmune diabetes of the adult. *Am J Epidemiol*, Vol. 156 (No. 9): 787–796.

Stenström, G., Gottsäter, A., Bakhtadze, E., Berger, B. & Sundkvist, G. (2005) Latent autoimmune diabetes in adults: Definition, prevalence, betacell function, and treatment. *Diabetes*, Vol. 54 (Suppl. 2): S68–S72.

Takeda, H., Kawasaki, E., Shimizu, I., Konoue, E., Fujiyama, M., Murao, S., Tanaka, K., Mori, K., Tarumi, Y., Seto, I., Fujii, Y., Kato, K., Kondo, S., Takada, Y., Kitsuki, N., Kaino, Y., Kida, K., Hashimoto, N., Yamane, Y., Yamawaki, T., Onuma, H., Nishimiya, T., Osawa, H., Saito, Y. & Makino, H. (2002) Clinical, autoimmune, and genetic characteristics of adult-onset diabetic patients with GAD autoantibodies in Japan (Ehime Study). *Diabetes Care*, Vol. 25 (No. 6): 995-1001.

Tanaka, S., Kobayashi, T., Nakanishi, K., Koyama, R., Okubo, M., Murase, T., Odawara, M. & Inoko, H. (2002) Association of HLA-DQ genotype in autoantibody-negative and rapid-onset type 1 diabetes. *Diabetes Care*, Vol. 25 (No. 12): 2302–2307.

Thomson, G., Valdes, A.M., Noble, J.A., Kockum, I., Grote, M.N., Najman, J., Erlich, H.A., Cucca, F., Pugliese, A., Steenkiste, A., Dorman, J.S., Caillat-Zucman, S., Hermann, R., Ilonen, J., Lambert, A.P., Bingley, P.J., Gillespie, K.M., Lernmark, Å., Sanjeevi, C.B., Rønningen, K.S., Undlien, D.E., Thorsby, E., Petrone, A., Buzzetti, R., Koeleman, B.P., Roep, B.O., Saruhan-Direskeneli, G., Uyar, F.A., Günoz, H., Gorodezky, C., Alaez, C., Boehm, B.O., Mlynarski, W., Ikegami, H., Berrino, M., Fasano, M.E., Dametto, E., Israel, S., Brautbar, C., Santiago-Cortes, A., Frazer de Llado, T., She, J.X., Bugawan, T.L., Rotter, J.I., Raffel, L., Zeidler, A., Leyva-Cobian, F., Hawkins, B.R., Chan, S.H., Castano, L., Pociot, F. & Nerup, J. (2007) Relative predispositional effects of HLA class II DRB1-DQB1 haplotypes and genotypes on type 1 diabetes: a meta-analysis. *Tissue Antigens*, Vol. 70 (No. 2): 110-127.

Todd, J.A., Bell, J.I. & McDevitt, H.O. (1987) HLA-DQβ gene contributes to susceptibility and resistance to insulin-dependent diabetes mellitus. *Nature*, Vol. 329 (No. 6140): 599-604.

Tuomi, T., Carlsson, A., Li, H., Miettinen, A., Nilsson, A., Nissén, M., Ehrnström, B.O., Forsén, B., Snickars, B., Lahti, K., Forsblom, C., Saloranta, C., Taskinen, M.R. & Groop, L.C. (1999) Clinical and genetic characteristics of type 2 diabetes with and without GAD antibodies. *Diabetes*, Vol. 48 (No. 1): 150-157.

Tuomilehto, J., Virtala, E., Karvonen, M., Lounamaa, R., Pitkäniemi, J., Reunanen, A., Tuomilehto-Wolf, E. & Toivanen, L. (1995) Increase in incidence of insulin-dependent diabetes mellitus among children in Finland. Int J Epidemiol, Vol. 24 (No. 5): 984-992.

Turner, R., Stratton, I., Horton, V., Manley, S., Zimmet, P., Mackay, I.R., Shattock, M., Bottazzo, G.F. & Holman, R. (1997) UKPDS 25: Autoantibodies to islet-cell cytoplasm and glutamic acid decarboxylase for prediction of insulin requirement in type 2 diabetes. *Lancet*, Vol. 350 (No. 9087): 1288-1293.

Undlien, D.E., Kockum, I., Rønningen, K.S., Lowe, R., Sanjeevi, C.B., Graham, J., Lie, B.A., Akselsen, H.E., Lernmark, Å. & Thorsby, E. (1999) HLA associations in type 1 diabetes among patients not carrying high-risk DR3-DQ2 or DR4-DQ8 haplotypes. *Tissue Antigens*, Vol. 54 (No. 6): 543-551.

Urakami, T., Inami, I., Morimoto, S., Kubota, S. & Owada, M. (2002) Clinical characteristics of non-immune-mediated, idiopathic type 1 (type 1B) diabetes mellitus in Japanese children and adolescents. *J Pediatr Endocrinol Metab*, Vol. 15 (No. 3): 283-288.

Verge, C.F., Gianani, R., Kawasaki, E., Yu, L., Pietropaolo, M., Jackson, R.A., Chase, H.P. & Eisenbarth, G.S. (1996) Prediction of type I diabetes in first-degree relatives using a combination of insulin, GAD, and ICA512bdc/IA-2 autoantibodies. (1996) *Diabetes*, Vol. 45 (No. 7): 926-933.

Volpini, W.M., Testa, G.V., Marques, S.B., Alves, L.I., Silva, M.E., Dib, S.A., Guerra, G. Jr., Paulino, M.F., Marini, S.H., Persoli, L.B. & Caillat-Zucman, S. (2001) Family-based association of HLA class II alleles and haplotypes with type I diabetes in Brazilians reveals some characteristics of a highly diversified population. *Hum Immunol*, Vol. 62 (No. 11): 1226-1233.

Wykes, M.N., Shellam, G.R., McCluskey, J., Kast, W.M., Dallas, P.B. & Price, P. (1993) Murine cytomegalovirus interacts with major histocompatibility complex class I molecules to establish cellular infection. *J Virol*, Vol. 67 (No. 7): 4182-4189.

Yasunaga, S., Kimura, A., Hamaguchi, K., Rønningen, K.S. & Sasazuki, T. (1996) Different contribution of HLA-DR and -DQ genes in susceptibility and resistance to insulin-dependent diabetes mellitus (IDDM). *Tissue Antigens*, Vol. 47 (No. 1): 37–48.

Zimmet, P.Z., Tuomi, T., Mackay, I.R. Rowley, M.J., Knowles, W., Cohen, M. & Lang DA. (1994) Latent autoimmune diabetes mellitus in adults (LADA): The role of antibodies to glutamic acid decarboxylase in diagnosis and prediction of insulin dependency. *Diabet Med*, Vol. 11 (No. 3): 299–303.

4

The Role of T Cells in Type 1 Diabetes

David Wagner
Webb-Waring Center and Department of Medicine, University of Colorado, Denver, CO, USA

1. Introduction

The role of T cells as pathogenic effector cells in type 1 diabetes (T1D) is well established. Both $CD4^+$ and $CD8^+$ cells can play distinct and highly pathogenic roles mediating diabetogenesis. Other cell types including NK, B cells, macrophages and dendritic cells also play coordinate roles. Ultimately auto-aggressive T cells invade pancreatic islets focusing destructive force on the beta cells that produce insulin. The initial insult may be solely inflammation but nonetheless results in loss of insulin production. This chapter will focus on the different T cell subtypes including a newly described helper T cell subtype, Th40, which is highly pathogenic in T1D. Discussion will include how auto-aggressive T cells can arise and suggest alternative means to control auto-aggressive T cells. The ultimate goal for a successful treatment is to control pathogenic effector cells without causing immune suppression, a feat that has yet to be achieved. Considering new paradigms about diabetogenesis may provide substantive clues towards effectively curing this ravaging disease.

2. $CD4^+$ T cells and inflammation

$CD4^+$ T cells differentiate and based on immunologic functions and cytokine production are grouped into different sub types of T "helper" (Th) cells. Help is provided to CD8 cells in the form of IL-2 to drive viral protection or to B cells in the form of IL-4/IL-5 to promote the humoral immune arm. Other forms of help include IFNγ (1, 2) to create activated macrophages that aid innate immunity. Naive T cells are polarized by IL-12 to a Th1 phenotype producing IFNγ, TNFα, IL-2, IL-1β *etc.*, (Fig. 1) leading to localized inflammation (3, 4). IL-4 polarizes Th2 cells to produce IL-4, IL-5, IL-10, IL-13 etc., and is associated with an anti-inflammatory response. Of further interest is IL-6, which is categorized as a Th2 cytokine, but atypical of that family IL-6 is pro-inflammatory; suggesting that IL-6 would have better fit with Th1 cytokines.

T cell subsets impact each other's functional capabilities; IFNγ inhibits Th2 cells while promoting Th1 cells and IL-4 inhibits the Th1 response (5). These T helper subtypes provide an interesting back drop for T1D. Th1 cytokines like IFNγ and TNFα have been shown to be prominent in driving disease (6). However, $IFN\gamma^{-/-}$ mice still develop T1D and when IFNγ is blocked with a neutralizing antibody early in diabetogenesis, disease is exacerbated (7). An additional complication is that T cells isolated from $IFN\gamma^{-/-}$ mice transfer disease very effectively, suggesting that IFNγ is important for trafficking rather than islet destruction (8). When IFNγ is not available Th17 cells drastically increase in number (7), suggesting a role for Th17 cells in T1D development.

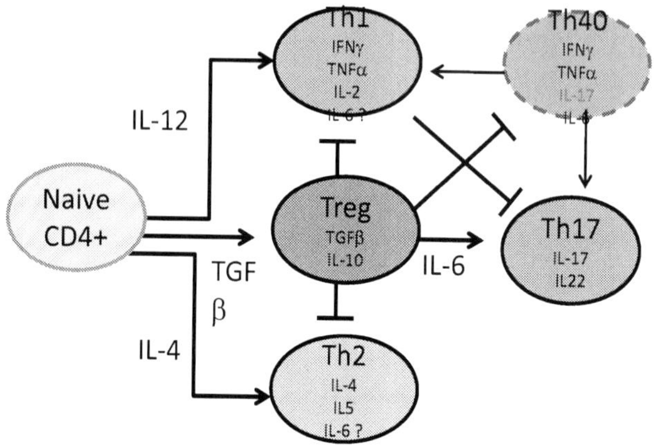

Fig. 1. Stages of helper T cells

Th17 cells have been postulated as a distinct T helper subtype that produces IL-17 and IL-22 (9). Th17 cells are linked to microbial immunity (10, 11) and to autoimmune diseases including multiple sclerosis and the experimental autoimmune encephalitis (EAE) mouse model of that disease. Studies further link Th17 cells to experimental autoimmune uveitis (EAU) (12-14), rheumatoid arthritis (15), systemic lupus erythematosus (16) and to delayed airway hypersensitivity (17). Th1 or Th17 cells are capable of becoming pathogenic effector cells, however distinguishing surface biomarkers that identify predominantly auto-aggressive T cells rarely have been forthcoming. The role of Th17 cells as pathogenic effector cells in T1D is still debated. Th17 and diabetes was further explored using a T cell receptor (TCR) transgenic model. Cells were isolated from BDC2.5.TCR transgenic mice and polarized to a Th1 or Th17 phenotype (18), then transferred to NOD.scid recipients. Th1 recipients became diabetic more quickly than Th17 recipients (18). When Th17 cells were removed and analyzed it was determined that a majority of those cells produced IFNγ. The interpretation was that Th17 cells could convert to Th1 phenotype and the Th1 phenotype alone was responsible for disease. However, given that the BDC2.5 TCR recognizes an islet antigen, recently determined to be Chromogranin-A and that antigen is always present, the T cells from BDC2.5.TCR.Tg mice could never be considered truly naïve. This therefore could impact the polarization process.

Another T helper produced cytokine with high potential in diabetogenesis is IL-6. IL-6 levels were reported generally increased in T1D subjects, including long - term diabetics (19) . However it also was reported that IL-6 levels are not predictive of outcome or disease progression (20). In another demonstration of discordance between human and mouse transitional studies, it was shown that blocking IL-6 in young NOD mice prevents disease onset (6, 21). While not examined in that study, the inhibition of IL-6 may have impeded the generation of Th17 cells. Administration of IL-12 to young NOD mice induces increases in IFNγ producing cells, but interestingly also induces diabetes in IFNγ receptor knockout mice (21). This suggests that control of IFNγ producing cells alone is inadequate for controlling diabetogenesis. These studies indicate a complicated picture with no tightly characterized cell type dominating the disease process.

3. Tregs and T1D

A critical player in the T cell dyad of the inflammatory/anti-inflammatory milieu is the regulatory T cell subset (Tregs). Tregs function to control effector cells and to diminish the inflammatory response. Tregs are generally classified by expression of CD4, $CD25^{hi}$ (the alpha chain of the IL-2 receptor) and the transcription factor FoxP3 (22). Other molecules are associated with Tregs including GITR, CTLA-4, CD103, $CD127^{lo}$, and CD62L. Tregs can arise naturally or be induced in the periphery. Naturally arising Tregs develop in the thymus and require self-antigen recognition for development. This was demonstrated using recombination activating gene, (RAG1 and RAG2) knockout mice that do not develop Tregs (23, 24). In a TCR transgenic mouse model it was shown that Tregs develop in the thymus as long as RAG1 and RAG2 are available (24). In the TCR transgenic mice that are $RAG^{-/-}$ and therefore do not express endogenous TCR molecules, Tregs do not develop (25, 26). This poses an interesting scenario that a set of self - antigen reactive T cells are able to preferentially escape negative selection. That possibility poses the central question of whether those cells ultimately become pathogenic.

The other type of Treg is induced in the periphery requiring interactions with antigen and polarizing exposure to TGFβ (Fig. 1). An interesting aspect is that Th17 effector cells can arise directly from Tregs (Fig. 1). Polarization studies show that treating Tregs with IL-6 promotes a Th17 phenotype (27). Given that Tregs from the thymus are auto-antigen reactive and that a later burst of IL-6 promotes Th17 cells, this could constitute a mechanism for central tolerance escape.

Studies in mouse autoimmune models have shown that knocking out Tregs favors autoimmunity. In T1D studies there remains disparity as to the role of Tregs in controlling disease. It has been reported in mouse (28) and in human (29) T1D subjects that the actual number and function of Tregs is normal. An interesting observation was made however that Tregs from pancreatic lymph nodes of T1D subjects are dysregulated in function (30), when compared to Tregs from peripheral blood. Another study has shown that regulatory CD8+ T cells that recognize the atypical HLA-E presenting the self - antigen Hsp60 are defective in T1D (31). This suggests that the disparity in Treg number and function in autoimmune disease may relate to the location and classification of the Tregs.

4. Th40 cells: a biomarker for pathogenic effector T cells

In numerous studies CD40 has been identified as a biomarker for auto-aggressive T cells (19, 28, 32-36). A panel of highly pathogenic, auto-aggressive T cell clones, including the well described BDC2.5 clone express CD40 (34-36). Although CD40 has been typically associated with antigen presenting cells, it was demonstrated on primary T cells in NOD mice, the type 1 diabetes model, and in the process identified a unique effector $CD4^+$ T cell population, characterized as $CD4^+CD40^+$ [Th40] (19, 28, 32-37). Importantly, Th40 cells were detected in both autoimmune and non-autoimmune mouse strains but occurring at a significantly greater percentage and cell number in autoimmunity (19, 28, 32-35). In fact, the percentage of Th40 cells increased proportionately with increasing insulitis leading to eventual diabetes in NOD mice (34). Primary Th40 cells isolated directly from the pancreata of pre-diabetic and diabetic NOD mice transferred progressive insulitis and diabetes to NOD.*scid* recipients (34, 36), demonstrating pathogenicity of these T cells. In other studies it was shown that Th40 cells are sufficient and necessary for T1D transfer (28, 36, 38, 39). CD40 depleted and

Treg depleted T cells are incapable of disease transfer, even when those cells are pre-activated (28).

Extending these studies, Th40 cells are highly significantly expanded in human T1D, but not in T2D or control subjects (19). Th40 cells from T1D subjects were responsive to diabetes associated antigens including insulin peptides, GAD peptides and whole islets. Th40 cells from T1D subjects but not from controls proliferate when exposed to self-antigens and are induced to produce and secrete cytokines. Typically Th1 cytokines are favored (19). However it was further demonstrated that Th40 cells also can produce IL-17 and furthermore that a subset of Th40 cells produce IL-17 and IFNγ at the same time (40). As such, Th40 cells can be categorized between Th1 and Th17 phenotypes having characteristics of both (Fig. 1). Another interesting feature is that Th40 cells from human T1D subjects produce a substantially elevated level of IL-6; but unlike the other cytokines produced by these T cells, IL-6 production is not dependent upon antigen recognition (19). This could align with the notion that autoimmune diabetes favors a loss of Tregs by providing a mechanism to convert Tregs to Th17 cells (Fig. 1). This process may proceed through the Th40 subset, which as mentioned are greatly expanded in number in T1D (19, 28, 32, 35-41).

Blocking CD40 interaction with its natural ligand CD154 provides a useful treatment strategy in autoimmunity and T1D in particular. CD40 - CD154 interactions have proven crucial in several autoimmune diseases including T1D (42-44). Blocking CD40 - CD154 interactions at 3-weeks of age in NOD mice prevents T1D onset (44). Taken further, blocking CD40 - CD154 interactions in NOD prevented the expansion of auto-aggressive T cells while allowing expansion of innate regulatory, $CD4^{+}CD25^{+}$ T cells (34). Thus, blocking CD40 - CD154 interaction restores T cell homeostasis. CD154 is temporally induced on activated T cells (45, 46), is found on platelets (47-49), smooth muscle, vascular endothelial cells and antigen presenting cells (50). CD154 is a member of the TNF super-family, demonstrating high protein sequence homology with TNF (51). Like TNF, CD154 occurs in a soluble form and may behave as a cytokine (52, 53). Interestingly, CD154 including the soluble form is hyper-expressed in T1D (54).

5. T cell co-stimulation and disease

A primary paradigm of immunology states that T cells require two signals to achieve effector status; an antigen specific recognition signal and a second co-stimulus (55). The classic T cell co-stimulus is CD28 on T cells interacting with B7 on APC. However $CD28^{-/-}$ mice that did not develop disease after initial injections, developed fulminant EAE after a second round of induction (56) . In that model a faster, more severe EAE occurred in the absence of the CD28 T cell co-stimulatory pathway. It has been repeatedly shown that TCR engagement alone is insufficient for effector functions. Given that T cells require a co-stimulus for activation the above study suggests a second, perhaps more pernicious T cell co-stimulatory mechanism. Interestingly in that study, blocking CD40 - CD154 through administration of an anti-CD154 resulted in significant long-term inhibition of clinical EAE relapse (56). While CD40 signaling directly impacts antigen presenting cells, in contrast to established paradigms, CD40 has been shown to function effectively as a T cell co-stimulus (57, 58). In fact, CD40 engagement of T cells proved as effective as CD28 co-stimulus (40, 58, 59).

6. Th40 cells and TCR revision

Another paradigm of immunology holds that TCR molecules are generated in the thymus without further alteration. However, it has been demonstrated that RAG1 and RAG2, the recombinase proteins that are responsible for TCR generation, are inducible in peripheral T cells (35, 60-70). Following induction of RAGs, altered expression of TCRα (34, 35) and TCRβ (64, 65, 71) molecules on peripheral T cells, (TCR revision) was demonstrated. This has serious implications for T cell function and autoimmune potential. TCR revision could directly create auto-aggressive T cells that would not be negatively selected. Regardless of whether auto-aggressive T cells are thymic escapees or generated in the periphery, they accumulate under autoimmune conditions (72). Another intriguing finding is that IL-17 producing T cells are more likely to undergo TCR revisions (60). Cumulatively, these findings have direct implications for T1D and other autoimmune diseases. Eventual TCR revision of the initial auto-aggressive T cells could promote tolerance by altering antigen specificity of pathogenic T cells; thus resulting in remission. Alternatively, TCR revision by necessity dictates that T cells with TCR that were never exposed to thymic selection conditions are found in the periphery and therefore may have initiated the autoimmune insult.

7. Conclusions

T cells play a critical role in diabetogenesis as do other cells. Different categories of T cells, Th1, Th17 and now Th40 are being identified in this disease, yet a major concern for understanding and ultimately treating the disease requires a global outlook. How is it that each of these cell types contribute to the overall disease and how do they work in concert to establish and maintain debilitating inflammation. Controlling the inflammatory process without inducing unwanted immune suppression will require surgical precision. It is likely that no one treatment option will prove completely successful, and focusing on any one cell type will diminish the ability to comprehend the overall picture of the disease process. Creating a comprehensive framework of study will be essential for successful treatment.

8. References

[1] Stout, R. D., S. K. Watkins, and J. Suttles. 2009. Functional plasticity of macrophages: in situ reprogramming of tumor-associated macrophages. *J Leukoc Biol* 86:1105-1109.

[2] Suttles, J., and R. Stout. 1997. The many roles of CD40 in cell-mediated inflammatory responses. *Immunol. Today* 17:487-492.

[3] Crane, I. J., and J. V. Forrester. 2005. Th1 and th2 lymphocytes in autoimmune disease. *Crit Rev Immunol* 25:75-102.

[4] Lafaille, J. J. 1998. The role of helper T cell subsets in autoimmune diseases. *Cytokine Growth Factor Rev* 9:139-151.

[5] Romagnani, S. 2000. T-cell subsets (Th1 versus Th2). *Ann Allergy Asthma Immunol* 85:9-18; quiz 18, 21.

[6] Campbell, I. L., T. W. Kay, L. Oxbrow, and L. C. Harrison. 1991. Essential role for interferon-gamma and interleukin-6 in autoimmune insulin-dependent diabetes in NOD/Wehi mice. *J Clin Invest* 87:739-742.

[7] Jain, R., D. M. Tartar, R. K. Gregg, R. D. Divekar, J. J. Bell, H. H. Lee, P. Yu, J. S. Ellis, C. M. Hoeman, C. L. Franklin, and H. Zaghouani. 2008. Innocuous IFNgamma induced by adjuvant-free antigen restores normoglycemia in NOD mice through inhibition of IL-17 production. *J Exp Med* 205:207-218.

[8] Savinov, A. Y., F. S. Wong, and A. V. Chervonsky. 2001. IFN-gamma affects homing of diabetogenic T cells. *J Immunol* 167:6637-6643.

[9] Korn, T., E. Bettelli, M. Oukka, and V. K. Kuchroo. 2009. IL-17 and Th17 Cells. *Annu Rev Immunol* 27:485-517.

[10] Schulz, S. M., G. Kohler, C. Holscher, Y. Iwakura, and G. Alber. 2008. IL-17A is produced by Th17, gammadelta T cells and other CD4- lymphocytes during infection with Salmonella enterica serovar Enteritidis and has a mild effect in bacterial clearance. *Int Immunol* 20:1129-1138.

[11] Steinman, L. 2008. A rush to judgment on Th17. *J Exp Med* 205:1517-1522.

[12] Weaver, C. T., L. E. Harrington, P. R. Mangan, M. Gavrieli, and K. M. Murphy. 2006. Th17: an effector CD4 T cell lineage with regulatory T cell ties. *Immunity* 24:677-688.

[13] Bettelli, E., M. Oukka, and V. K. Kuchroo. 2007. T(H)-17 cells in the circle of immunity and autoimmunity. *Nat Immunol* 8:345-350.

[14] Luger, D., P. B. Silver, J. Tang, D. Cua, Z. Chen, Y. Iwakura, E. P. Bowman, N. M. Sgambellone, C. C. Chan, and R. R. Caspi. 2008. Either a Th17 or a Th1 effector response can drive autoimmunity: conditions of disease induction affect dominant effector category. *J Exp Med* 205:799-810.

[15] Wong, P. K., J. M. Quinn, N. A. Sims, A. van Nieuwenhuijze, I. K. Campbell, and I. P. Wicks. 2006. Interleukin-6 modulates production of T lymphocyte-derived cytokines in antigen-induced arthritis and drives inflammation-induced osteoclastogenesis. *Arthritis Rheum* 54:158-168.

[16] Garrett-Sinha, L. A., S. John, and S. L. Gaffen. 2008. IL-17 and the Th17 lineage in systemic lupus erythematosus. *Curr Opin Rheumatol* 20:519-525.

[17] Komiyama, Y., S. Nakae, T. Matsuki, A. Nambu, H. Ishigame, S. Kakuta, K. Sudo, and Y. Iwakura. 2006. IL-17 plays an important role in the development of experimental autoimmune encephalomyelitis. *J Immunol* 177:566-573.

[18] Bending, D., H. De La Pena, M. Veldhoen, J. M. Phillips, C. Uyttenhove, B. Stockinger, and A. Cooke. 2009. Highly purified Th17 cells from BDC2.5NOD mice convert into Th1-like cells in NOD/SCID recipient mice. *J Clin Invest.*

[19] Waid, D. M., R. J. Wagner, A. Putnam, G. M. Vaitaitis, N. D. Pennock, D. C. Calverley, P. Gottlieb, and D. H. Wagner, Jr. 2007. A unique T cell subset described as CD4loCD40+ T cells (TCD40) in human type 1 diabetes. *Clin Immunol* 124:138-148.

[20] Kaas, A., C. Pfleger, L. Hansen, K. Buschard, N. C. Schloot, B. O. Roep, and H. B. Mortensen. Association of adiponectin, interleukin (IL)-1ra, inducible protein 10, IL-6 and number of islet autoantibodies with progression patterns of type 1 diabetes the first year after diagnosis. *Clin Exp Immunol* 161:444-452.

[21] Trembleau, S., G. Penna, S. Gregori, N. Giarratana, and L. Adorini. 2003. IL-12 administration accelerates autoimmune diabetes in both wild-type and IFN-gamma-deficient nonobese diabetic mice, revealing pathogenic and protective effects of IL-12-induced IFN-gamma. *J Immunol* 170:5491-5501.

[22] Sakaguchi, S., M. Ono, R. Setoguchi, H. Yagi, S. Hori, Z. Fehervari, J. Shimizu, T. Takahashi, and T. Nomura. 2006. Foxp3+ CD25+ CD4+ natural regulatory T cells in dominant self-tolerance and autoimmune disease. *Immunol Rev* 212:8-27.

[23] Sakaguchi, S., T. Yamaguchi, T. Nomura, and M. Ono. 2008. Regulatory T cells and immune tolerance. *Cell* 133:775-787.

[24] Yamaguchi, T., K. Hirota, K. Nagahama, K. Ohkawa, T. Takahashi, T. Nomura, and S. Sakaguchi. 2007. Control of immune responses by antigen-specific regulatory T cells expressing the folate receptor. *Immunity* 27:145-159.

[25] Kersh, G. J., D. L. Donermeyer, K. E. Frederick, J. M. White, B. L. Hsu, and P. M. Allen. 1998. TCR transgenic mice in which usage of transgenic alpha- and beta-chains is highly dependent on the level of selecting ligand. *J Immunol* 161:585-593.

[26] Koh, W. P., E. Chan, K. Scott, G. McCaughan, M. France, and B. Fazekas de St Groth. 1999. TCR-mediated involvement of CD4+ transgenic T cells in spontaneous inflammatory bowel disease in lymphopenic mice. *J Immunol* 162:7208-7216.

[27] Suto, A., D. Kashiwakuma, S. Kagami, K. Hirose, N. Watanabe, K. Yokote, Y. Saito, T. Nakayama, M. J. Grusby, I. Iwamoto, and H. Nakajima. 2008. Development and characterization of IL-21-producing CD4+ T cells. *J Exp Med* 205:1369-1379.

[28] Waid, D. M., G. M. Vaitaitis, N. D. Pennock, and D. H. Wagner, Jr. 2008. Disruption of the homeostatic balance between autoaggressive (CD4+CD40+) and regulatory (CD4+CD25+FoxP3+) T cells promotes diabetes. *J Leukoc Biol* 84:431-439.

[29] Schneider, A., M. Rieck, S. Sanda, C. Pihoker, C. Greenbaum, and J. H. Buckner. 2008. The effector T cells of diabetic subjects are resistant to regulation via CD4+ FOXP3+ regulatory T cells. *J Immunol* 181:7350-7355.

[30] Gagliani, N., A. Ferraro, M. G. Roncarolo, and M. Battaglia. 2009. Autoimmune diabetic patients undergoing allogeneic islet transplantation: are we ready for a regulatory T-cell therapy? *Immunol Lett* 127:1-7.

[31] Jiang, H., S. M. Canfield, M. P. Gallagher, H. H. Jiang, Y. Jiang, Z. Zheng, and L. Chess. HLA-E-restricted regulatory CD8(+) T cells are involved in development and control of human autoimmune type 1 diabetes. *J Clin Invest* 120:3641-3650.

[32] Vaitaitis, G. M., and D. H. Wagner, Jr. 2008. High distribution of CD40 and TRAF2 in Th40 T cell rafts leads to preferential survival of this auto-aggressive population in autoimmunity. *PLoS One* 3:e2076.

[33] Siebert, J. C., M. Inokuma, D. M. Waid, N. D. Pennock, G. M. Vaitaitis, M. L. Disis, J. F. Dunne, D. H. Wagner, Jr., and H. T. Maecker. 2008. An analytical workflow for investigating cytokine profiles. *Cytometry A* 73:289-298.

[34] Waid, D. M., G. M. Vaitaitis, and J. Wagner, D.H. 2004. Peripheral Expansion of $CD4^{lo}CD40^{+}$ Auto-Aggressive T Cells During Insulin-Dependent Diabetes Mellitus. *European Journal of Immunology* 34:1488-1497.

[35] Vaitaitis, G. M., M. Poulin, R. J. Sanderson, K. J. Haskins, and D. H. Wagner Jr. 2003. CD40-Induced Expression of Recombination Activating Gene (RAG) 1 and RAG2: A Mechanism for the Generation of Autoaggressive T Cells in the Periphery. *Cutting Edge, J. Immunol.* 170:3455-3459.

[36] Wagner, D. H., Jr., G. Vaitaitis, R. Sanderson, M. Poulin, C. Dobbs, and K. Haskins. 2002. Expression of CD40 identifies a unique pathogenic T cell population in type 1 diabetes. *Proc Natl Acad Sci U S A* 99:3782-3787.

[37] Vaitaitis, G., and D. H. Wagner Jr. 2010. CD40 Glycoforms and TNF-Receptors 1 and 2 in the Formation of CD40 Receptor(s) in Autoimmunity. *Mol. Immunol.* 47:2303-2313.

[38] Waid, D. M., G. M. Vaitaitis, and D. H. Wagner, Jr. 2004. Peripheral CD4loCD40+ auto-aggressive T cell expansion during insulin-dependent diabetes mellitus. *Eur J Immunol* 34:1488-1497.

[39] Vaitaitis, G. M., M. Poulin, R. J. Sanderson, K. Haskins, and D. H. Wagner, Jr. 2003. Cutting edge: CD40-induced expression of recombination activating gene (RAG) 1 and RAG2: a mechanism for the generation of autoaggressive T cells in the periphery. *J Immunol* 170:3455-3459.

[40] Vaitaitis, G., D. M. Waid, and D. H. Wagner Jr. 2010. The expanding role of TNF-receptor super family member CD40 (tnfrsf5) in autoimmune disease: Focus on Th40 cells. *Curr Immunol Rev* 6:130-136.

[41] Vaitaitis, G. M., and D. H. Wagner, Jr. CD40 glycoforms and TNF-receptors 1 and 2 in the formation of CD40 receptor(s) in autoimmunity. *Mol Immunol* 47:2303-2313.

[42] Durie, F. H., R. A. Fava, T. M. Foy, A. Aruffo, J. A. Ledbetter, and R. J. Noelle. 1993. Prevention of collagen-induced arthritis with an antibody to gp30 the ligand for CD40. *Science* 281:1328-1330.

[43] Lutgens, E., L. Gorelik, M. J. Daemen, E. D. de Muinck, I. S. Grewal, V. E. Koteliansky, and R. A. Flavell. 1999. Requirement for CD154 in the progression of atherosclerosis. *Nat Med* 5:1313-1316.

[44] Balasa, B., T. Krahl, G. Patstone, J. Lee, R. Tisch, H. O. McDevitt, and N. Sarvetnick. 1997. CD40 Ligand-CD40 interactions are necessary for the initiation of insulitis and diabetes in nonobese diabetic mice. *Journal of Immunology* 159:4620-4627.

[45] Yellin, M. J., J. Sinning, L. R. Covey, W. Sherman, J. J. Lee, E. Glickman-Nir, K. C. Sippel, J. Rogers, A. M. Cleary, M. Parker, L. Chess, and S. Lederman. 1994. T Lymphocytes T cell-B cell activating molecule/ CD40-L molecules induce normal B cells or Chronic Lymphocytic Leukemia B cells to express CD80(B7/BB1) and enhance their costimulatory activity. *Journal of Immunology* 153:666-674.

[46] Noelle, R. 1995. The role of gp39 (CD40L) in immunity. *Clinical Immunology and Immunopathology* 76:5203-5207.

[47] Wang, C. L., Y. T. Wu, C. A. Liu, M. W. Lin, C. J. Lee, L. T. Huang, and K. D. Yang. 2003. Expression of CD40 ligand on CD4+ T-cells and platelets correlated to the coronary artery lesion and disease progress in Kawasaki disease. *Pediatrics* 111:E140-147.

[48] Andre, P., L. Nannizzi-Alaimo, S. K. Prasad, and D. R. Phillips. 2002. Platelet-derived CD40L: the switch-hitting player of cardiovascular disease. *Circulation* 106:896-899.

[49] Hermann, A., B. H. Rauch, M. Braun, K. Schror, and A. A. Weber. 2001. Platelet CD40 ligand (CD40L)--subcellular localization, regulation of expression, and inhibition by clopidogrel. *Platelets* 12:74-82.

[50] Mach, F., U. Schonbeck, G. K. Sukhova, T. Bourcier, J. Y. Bonnefoy, J. S. Pober, and P. Libby. 1997. Functional CD40 ligand is expressed on human vascular endothelial cells, smooth muscle cells, and macrophages: implications for CD40-CD40 ligand signaling in atherosclerosis. *Proc Natl Acad Sci U S A* 94:1931-1936.

[51] Stone, G. W., S. Barzee, V. Snarsky, K. Kee, C. A. Spina, X. F. Yu, and R. S. Kornbluth. 2006. Multimeric soluble CD40 ligand and GITR ligand as adjuvants for human immunodeficiency virus DNA vaccines. *J Virol* 80:1762-1772.

[52] Stumpf, C., C. Lehner, S. Eskafi, D. Raaz, A. Yilmaz, S. Ropers, A. Schmeisser, J. Ludwig, W. G. Daniel, and C. D. Garlichs. 2003. Enhanced levels of CD154 (CD40 ligand) on platelets in patients with chronic heart failure. *Eur J Heart Fail* 5:629-637.
[53] Toubi, E., and Y. Shoenfeld. 2004. The role of CD40-CD154 interactions in autoimmunity and the benefit of disrupting this pathway. *Autoimmunity* 37:457-464.
[54] Jinchuan, Y., W. Zonggui, C. Jinming, L. Li, and K. Xiantao. 2004. Upregulation of CD40--CD40 ligand system in patients with diabetes mellitus. *Clin Chim Acta* 339:85-90.
[55] Bachmaier, K., C. Pummerer, A. Shahinian, J. Ionescu, N. Neu, T. W. Mak, and J. M. Penninger. 1996. Induction of autoimmunity in the absence of CD28 costimulation. *J Immunol* 157:1752-1757.
[56] Girvin, A. M., M. C. Dal Canto, and S. D. Miller. 2002. CD40/CD40L interaction is essential for the induction of EAE in the absence of CD28-mediated co-stimulation. *J Autoimmun* 18:83-94.
[57] Munroe, M. E., and G. A. Bishop. 2007. A costimulatory function for T cell CD40. *Journal of Immunology* 178:671-682.
[58] Baker, R. L., D. H. Wagner, Jr., and K. Haskins. 2008. CD40 on NOD CD4 T cells contributes to their activation and pathogenicity. *J Autoimmun* 31:385-392.
[59] Munroe, M. E., and G. A. Bishop. 2007. A costimulatory function for T cell CD40. *J Immunol* 178:671-682.
[60] Zehn, D., M. J. Bevan, and P. J. Fink. 2007. Cutting edge: TCR revision affects predominantly Foxp3 cells and skews them toward the Th17 lineage. *J Immunol* 179:5653-5657.
[61] Cooper, C. J., G. L. Turk, M. Sun, A. G. Farr, and P. J. Fink. 2004. Cutting edge: TCR revision occurs in germinal centers. *J Immunol* 173:6532-6536.
[62] Cooper, C. J., M. T. Orr, C. J. McMahan, and P. J. Fink. 2003. T cell receptor revision does not solely target recent thymic emigrants. *J Immunol* 171:226-233.
[63] Ali, M., M. Weinreich, S. Balcaitis, C. J. Cooper, and P. J. Fink. 2003. Differential regulation of peripheral CD4+ T cell tolerance induced by deletion and TCR revision. *J Immunol* 171:6290-6296.
[64] McMahan, C., and P. Fink. 2000. Receptor revision in peripheral T cells creates a diverse V beta repertoire. *J Immunol* 165:690206907.
[65] Fink, P. J., and C. J. McMahan. 2000. Lymphocytes rearrange, edit and revise their antigen receptors to be useful yet safe. *Immunol Today* 21:561-566.
[66] McMahan, C. J., and P. J. Fink. 1998. RAG reexpression and DNA recombination at T cell receptor loci in peripheral CD4+ T cells. *Immunity* 9:637-647.
[67] Takase, M., E. M. Kanagawa, and O. Kanagawa. 2007. Age-dependent TCR revision mediated by interaction between alphabeta TCR and self-antigens. *J Immunol* 179:2163-2169.
[68] Huang, C. Y., B. P. Sleckman, and O. Kanagawa. 2005. Revision of T cell receptor {alpha} chain genes is required for normal T lymphocyte development. *Proc Natl Acad Sci U S A* 102:14356-14361.
[69] Nagafuchi, H., H. Yoshikawa, Y. Takeba, K. Nara, K. Miura, M. S. Kurokawa, and N. Suzuki. 2004. Recombination activating genes (RAG) induce secondary Ig gene rearrangement in and subsequent apoptosis of human peripheral blood circulating B lymphocytes. *Clin Exp Immunol* 136:76-84.

[70] Huang, C. Y., R. Golub, G. E. Wu, and O. Kanagawa. 2002. Superantigen-induced TCR alpha locus secondary rearrangement: role in tolerance induction. *J Immunol* 168:3259-3265.
[71] Blish, C., B. Gallay, G. Turk, K. Kline, W. Wheat, and P. Fink. 1999. Chronic modulation of the TCR repertoire in the lymphoid periphery. *J Immunol* 162:3131-3140.
[72] Wagner, J., D.H. 2007. Reshaping the T cell repertoire: TCR editing and TCR revision for Good and for Bad. *Clin Immunol* I123:1-6.

5

Beta-Cell Function and Failure in Type 1 Diabetes

Maria-Luisa Lazo de la Vega-Monroy and Cristina Fernandez-Mejia
Unidad de Genética de la Nutrición, Instituto de Investigaciones Biomédicas, Universidad Nacional Autónoma de México/ Instituto Nacional de Pediatría, Mexico City, Mexico

1. Introduction

Glucose is an essential energy source for all cells. Therefore, maintaining glucose levels within a normal range is essential for life in vertebrates. Glucose homeostasis in the organism is tightly regulated by insulin, a hormone that acts on the major glucose metabolic tissues such as muscle, liver and adipose tissue. Insulin's main effects include promoting glucose uptake, glycogen synthesis in the liver and muscle, triglyceride formation to be stored in adipocytes, and protein synthesis. Insulin secretion is held by the pancreatic beta-cells, and it is modulated by glucose levels. Insufficient insulin secretion and consequent impairment of insulin's actions lead to Diabetes Mellitus.

Diabetes is a group of metabolic diseases characterized by hyperglycemia, caused by a defect on insulin production, insulin action or both. Type 1 diabetes in particular is due to an autoimmune destruction of the insulin producing pancreatic beta-cell, which usually leads to absolute insulin deficiency (ADA 2009). This type of diabetes accounts for 5-10% of the total cases of diabetes worldwide, and although its onset is commonly during childhood and adolescence, it can occur at any age, even during late adulthood.

As the loss of beta-cells is determinant for the development of overt type 1 diabetes, understanding beta-cell's normal physiology, namely insulin secretion, and how it may be affected during the progression of this disease is essential. Moreover, the development of new therapeutic interventions for type 1 diabetes, such as islet transplantation, beta cell maintenance and replacement, or stem cell therapy, requires a profound knowledge of how the presence of different nutrients and signals may regulate insulin secretion and beta-cell mass.

In this chapter we aim to review the mechanisms involved in normal beta-cell function and beta-cell mass regulation, and how this function may be modulated by glucose, nutrients and signals in the beta-cell milieu. We also review how these mechanisms may be affected by the onset and progression of type 1 diabetes.

2. Normal function of the beta-cell - glucose stimulated insulin secretion

The pancreas is an endocrine and exocrine gland. The exocrine portion corresponds to acinar tissue, responsible for secreting digestive enzymes into the pancreatic juice, while the endocrine portion comprises the pancreatic islets, which consist of several cell types secreting different hormones: β-cells (insulin), α-cells (glucagon), δ-cells (somatostatin), PP-cells (pancreatic polypeptide) and ε-cells (ghrelin). The endocrine pancreas represents 1% to 5% of the total pancreatic mass (Kim, S.K. & Hebrok, M. 2001). In the islet, beta-cells (β-cells) are approximately 70% to 80% of the total islet cells.

Beta-cells are responsible for secreting insulin in response to rises in blood nutrient levels during the postprandial state. Glucose is the most important nutrient for insulin secretion. The process by which glucose promotes insulin secretion requires its sensing and metabolism by the beta-cell, a process called glucose-stimulated insulin secretion.

2.1 Insulin is secreted in a pulsatile and biphasic fashion

Glucose-stimulated insulin secretion is biphasic and pulsatile (Stagner, J.I. et al. 1980). The secretory pulses of beta-cells are associated with synchronous Ca^{2+} oscillations in response to glucose stimulus (Bergsten, P. et al. 1994), and they have been suggested to be coupled to glycolysis oscillations of the beta cell (Kar, S. & Shankar Ray, D. 2005). Secretory pulses are also regulated and synchronized within the other islet cell types. Insulin and glucagon secretion show asynchronous patterns (Grapengiesser, E. et al. 2006; Stagner, J.I. et al. 1980), whereas somatostatin pulses are synchronized with insulin secretion (Stagner, J.I. et al. 1980).

Glucose-stimulated insulin secretion also shows a biphasic pattern. Shortly after glucose stimulus, a first burst of insulin secretion occurs, followed by a decrease in the rate of secretion. A second sustained phase of insulin secretion can be observed just after this decrease, which can continue for up to several hours until euglycemia is achieved (Curry, D.L. et al. 1968) (Figure 1).

Although the mechanisms involved in the first phase of insulin secretion (termed the triggering pathway) are well understood, mechanisms regulating the sustained second phase (or the amplifying pathway) are yet to be deciphered, and different players that account for it have been proposed (Henquin, J.C. 2009). Notably, most of them are related to glucose metabolism inside the beta-cell.

2.1.1 Mechanisms involved in the first phase of insulin secretion - the triggering pathway

The first phase of glucose-stimulated insulin secretion is a multistep process that requires transport and oxidation of glucose, electrophysiological changes and fusion of insulin-containing secretory granules with the beta-cell plasma membrane (Figure 1). Glucose enters the cell by facilitated diffusion mediated by glucose transporters (GLUT2 in rodents, GLUT1 in humans). Glucose is then phosphorylated to form glucose-6-phosphate by glucokinase. This enzyme plays a critical role in glucose-stimulated insulin secretion and is considered the glucosensor of the pancreatic beta cell. Due to its kinetic characteristics, glucokinase is a determining factor for glucose phosphorylation (Matschinsky, F.M. 1996) and hence for its metabolism through glycolysis and oxidation.

The generation of ATP by glycolysis, the Krebs cycle and the respiratory chain leads to closure of the ATP-sensitive K+ channel (K_{ATP}), a hetero-octamer comprised of four subunits of the sulphonylurea 1 receptor (SUR1) and four subunits of the inwardly rectifying K^+ channel Kir6.2 (Aguilar-Bryan, L. et al. 1998). The closure of K_{ATP} channels, permit the background sodium (Na^+) entry without balance. These two events depolarize the membrane to a range that allows the opening of voltage-dependent T-type calcium (Ca^{2+})

and sodium (Na^+) channels. Na^+ and Ca^{2+} entry further depolarizes the membrane and L-type and maybe other voltage-dependent calcium channels (VDCC) open. Their activation triggers action potentials that increase in intracellular Ca^{2+} ($[Ca^{2+}]i$) (Hiriart, M. & Aguilar-Bryan, L. 2008). Together with calcium mobilized from intracellular stores, this Ca^{2+} increase leads to fusion of insulin-containing secretory granules with the plasma membrane and the release of insulin into the circulation (Rorsman, P. & Renstrom, E. 2003). Following glucose metabolism, the rate-limiting-step for the first phase lies in the rate of signal transduction between sensing the rise in $[Ca^{2+}]i$ and exocytosis of the immediately releasable granules (Straub, S.G. & Sharp, G.W. 2002).

2.1.2 Mechanisms involved in the second phase insulin secretion - the amplifying pathway

The existence of a second phase of insulin secretion was first reported in the 1960s. Curry et. al.(Curry, D.L. et al. 1968) observed that, in total pancreas perfusion with glucose, insulin release showed an early and rapid increase at 2 min after glucose infusion, peaking at 4 min. A second or "slow" phase, characterized by an increasing rate of insulin secretion was sustained during the whole period of glucose infusion. On the other hand, when the pancreas was perfused with tolbutamide, a sulfonylurea that blocks the potassium channels, only the first rapid release peak was observed, suggesting this biphasic insulin secretion is only generated in glucose-stimulated insulin secretion (Curry, D.L. et al. 1968). It was until the 1990s that evidence of mechanisms for glucose-stimulated insulin secretion independent of ionic action (i.e. K_{ATP} potassium channel activation) was found (Aizawa, T. et al. 1998; Gembal, M. et al. 1992). Since then, the concept of a rapid first phase glucose-stimulated insulin secretion, caused by a triggering pathway (or K_{ATP}-dependent mechanism), followed by a sustained second phase due to an amplifying pathway (or K_{ATP}-independent mechanism) has developed (Aizawa, T. et al. 2002; Henquin, J.C. 2000).

Biphasic insulin secretion has been explained by the existence of different pools of insulin-containing granules inside the beta cell (Aizawa, T. & Komatsu, M. 2005; Straub, S.G. & Sharp, G.W. 2004). There is a reserve pool of granules located in the cytoplasm which accounts for approximately 94% of the total granules, and a releasable pool of granules which are docked to the plasma membrane. It has been suggested that the docked granules have different ability to be released and therefore constitute two subsets, the readily releasable pool, and the immediately releasable pool. The granules from the immediately releasable pool are the first to be secreted in response to intracellular Ca^{2+} increase during the triggering pathway, leading to the first phase of insulin secretion. At the lowest point of secretion in between the two phases, the granules from the readily releasable pool are converted to the immediately releasable pool, an ATP-dependent process termed "priming". This priming has been suggested to be the rate-limiting step for exocytosis, and the target process for signals involved in the amplifying pathway that leads to the sustained second phase of insulin secretion (Straub, S.G. & Sharp, G.W. 2004) (Figure 1). Given the glucose-stimulated nature of biphasic insulin secretion and the ATP-dependence of priming, most of these signals are proposed to be derived from glucose metabolism. Some of these signals are reviewed in the next section.

2.2 Transcription factors regulating beta cell function

Transcription factors in the beta-cell act in a cooperative manner, forming transcriptional networks, to induce not only insulin expression, but also the expression of other genes

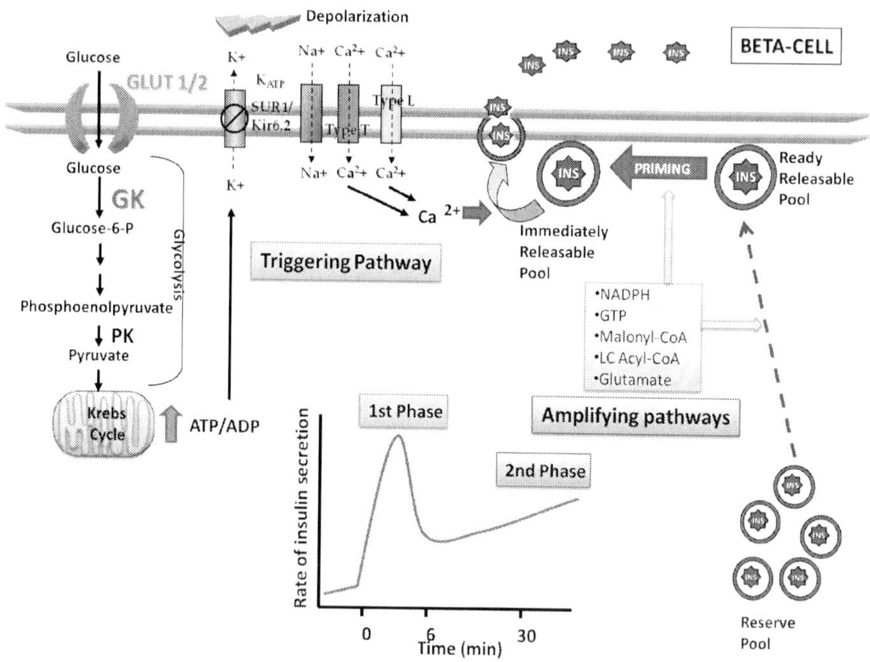

Fig. 1. Mechanism of biphasic glucose-stimulated insulin secretion.
Glucose enters the cell by glucose transporters (GLUT2 in rodents, GLUT1 in humans) and is then phosphorylated for its metabolism through glycolysis and oxidation. The generation of ATP by glycolysis, the Krebs cycle and the respiratory chain closes the ATP-sensitive K+ channel (KATP), allowing sodium (Na^+) entry without balance. These two events depolarize the membrane and open voltage-dependent T-type calcium (Ca^{2+}) and sodium (Na^+) channels. Na^+ and Ca^{2+} entry further depolarizes the membrane and L-type and maybe other voltage-dependent calcium channels (VDCC) open. This activation increases intracellular Ca^{2+} ($[Ca^{2+}]i$), which leads to fusion of insulin-containing secretory granules with the plasma membrane and the first phase insulin secretion. A sustained second phase of insulin secretion is held when the granules from the readily releasable pool are converted to the immediately releasable pool, an ATP-dependent process termed "priming". Most of the signals involved in this process also come from glucose mitochondrial metabolism, comprising the amplifying pathways.

involved in insulin gene regulation and insulin secretion, thus establishing and maintaining beta-cell's phenotype and function (Lazo-de-la-Vega-Monroy, M.L. & Fernandez-Mejia, C. 2009). Some of these factors include PDX-1, HNF4α, MAFA, FOXA2 and NeuroD1 (Lazo-de-la-Vega-Monroy, M.L. & Fernandez-Mejia, C. 2009).

PDX-1 is one of the most important transcription factors regulating the insulin gene transcription. This factor is determinant for pancreatic function. β-cell-specific knockout studies show that when *pdx1* is ablated, β-cell function is impaired and mice present diabetic phenotypes (Ahlgren, U. et al. 1998). Many of the target genes for *pdx1* are crucial for glucose-induced insulin secretion, such as glucose transporter *glut2* (Ahlgren, U. et al. 1998), the insulin gene (Chakrabarti, S.K. et al. 2002), and other transcription factors (Ahlgren, U. et al. 1998; Chakrabarti, S.K. et al. 2002; Raum, J.C. et al. 2006; Thomas, H. et al. 2001). PDX1 plays a role in the maintenance and proliferation of beta-cells as well (Holland, A.M. et al. 2005). Its overexpression in diabetic mice (*Irs2* knockouts) participates in beta-cell mass recovery and helps ameliorate glucose tolerance (Kushner, J.A. et al. 2002), whereas *pdx1* haploinsufficiency causes β-cell apoptosis (Kulkarni, R.N. et al. 2004).

PDX1 decrease has also been associated with apoptosis and reduced expression of the anti-apoptotic genes Bcl_{XL} and Bcl-2 (Johnson, J.D. et al. 2006), defects in post-translational processing of insulin, inhibition of GLP-1 receptor expression (Wang, H. et al. 2005), glucotoxicity (Olson, L.K. et al. 1993) and lipotoxicity (Gremlich, S. et al. 1997; Hagman, D.K. et al. 2005).

2.3 Metabolic coupling factors and glucose-stimulated insulin secretion

As noted earlier, an ATP/ADP ratio increase caused by glucose metabolism in the beta-cells is the mechanism by which the first phase of glucose-stimulated insulin secretion is triggered. However, glucose metabolism can also render a series of signals, or metabolic coupling factors, that may initiate and sustain the second phase of insulin secretion, presumably by favoring mobilization of the insulin granules form the reserve pool and the replenishment of the immediately releasable pool of insulin granules. Some of these metabolic coupling factors participate in mitochondrial shuttles, involving NADPH, pyruvate, malate, citrate, isocitrate, acyl-CoAs, and glutamate (Jitrapakdee, S. et.al. 2010). There are also various signaling pathways that, when activated, may contribute to maintaining or increasing glucose-stimulated insulin secretion, including the CaMKII (Calcium-Calmodulin-Dependent Protein Kinase II) , PKA (Protein Kinase A), PKC (Protein Kinase C) and PKG (Protein kinase G) pathways. Notably, most of other insulin secretagogues, namely nutrients, hormones and neurotransmitters, also modulate insulin secretion by these pathways.

2.3.1 Mitochondrial signalling

The role of mitochondria in the second phase of glucose-induced insulin secretion has been established by several studies in cell lines and humans (Jitrapakdee, S. et.al. 2010; Maechler, P. & Wollheim, C.B. 2001). There is even evidence of an uncommon subform of diabetes, mitochondrial diabetes, where mutations in mitochondrial DNA cause pancreatic beta-cell dysfunction (Maechler, P. & Wollheim, C.B. 2001).

Besides rendering the initial increase of ATP/ADP ratio, mitochondrial metabolism and anaplerotic metabolites are also involved in sustaining second phase insulin secretion. Pyruvate, the end product of glycolysis, plays an important role in this process, as it participates in several cycles whose final products constitute amplifying signals for insulin secretion. Particularly, NADPH, GTP, Malonyl-CoA, long-chain acyl-CoA, and glutamate have been suggested to sustain insulin secretion, although the exact mechanisms by which they have their effects remain to be elucidated (Jitrapakdee, S. et.al. 2010).

Once entering the mitochondria, pyruvate may be either converted to Acetyl-CoA by pyruvate dehydrogenase, or carboxylated to oxalacetate by pyruvate carboxylase, and therefore enter the Krebs cycle (Figure 2). Notably, there is a high expression of pyruvate carboxylase in the pancreatic islets comparable to that in gluconeogenic tissues, but islets lack phosphoenolpyruvate carboxykinase (PEPCK), the first enzyme in the glyconeogenic pathway (MacDonald, M.J. 1995). Moreover, several studies have correlated pyruvate carboxylation with insulin secretion (Han, J. & Liu, Y.Q.; Hasan, N.M. et al. 2008; Lu, D. et al. 2002; Xu, J. et al. 2008).

Oxalacetate from pyruvate carboxylation may be converted to malate, exit the mitochondria, and re-converted to pyruvate, producing NADPH (Pyruvate/malate cycle). Oxalacetate may also condense with acetyl-CoA to form citrate, which either continues in the TCA cycle, or exits the mitochondria, and converts again to oxalacetate and acetyl-CoA by the ATP-citrate lyase (pyruvate/citrate cycle). Oxalacetate may re-enter the pyruvate/malate cycle which will produce NADPH, while acetyl-CoA is carboxylated by Acetyl-CoA carboxylase and form malonyl-CoA, the initial step of fatty acid synthesis (Jitrapakdee, S. et.al. 2010). As the pancreatic islet is not a lipogenic tissue, the fact that acetyl-CoA activity is high in this tissue may indicate that malonyl-CoA can also act as a metabolic coupling factor for insulin secretion (Prentki, M. et al. 1992).

Metabolites from the Krebs cycle can also exit the mitochondria and enter other cycles. Isocitrate, for example, is converted to α-ketoglutarate by the NADP-dependent isocitrate dehydrogenase, rendering NADPH. α-ketoglutarate may re-enter the mitochondria to continue in the TCA cycle, or can be converted to glutamate by the glutamate dehydrogenase (GDH). Glutamate has been suggested to be another metabolic coupling factor for insulin secretion, possibly by entering insulin secretory granules and promoting exocytosis (Maechler, P. & Wollheim, C.B. 1999).

Finally, GTP may be produced by an isoform of the succinyl-CoA synthetase, which catalyzes the conversion of succinyl-CoA to succinate in the TCA cycle. It has been suggested that GTP participates in insulin secretion. In beta-cells, suppression of GTP production by this pathway reduced glucose-induced insulin secretion, independently of changes in NADPH or the ATP/ADP ratio (Kibbey, R.G. et al. 2007).

2.3.2 Calcium signaling and calcium-calmodulin-dependent protein kinase II (CaMKII)

As noted earlier, glucose-stimulated insulin secretion is a Ca^{2+}-mediated process. The increase of cytosolic calcium inside the beta-cell must be sensed and transduced in order to exert a secretory response. One of the candidate proteins involved in this transducing system is CaMK II. CaMK II activation has been correlated with glucose-stimulated insulin secretion. Besides being localized at the insulin secretory granules, CaMKII phosphorylates proteins involved in the secretory machinery, including synapsin I (Matsumoto, K. et al. 1995), MAP-2 (microtubule-associated protein 2) (Krueger, K.A. et al. 1997), VAMP/synaptobrevin (Nielander, H.B. et al. 1995) and others. Insulin release is then suggested to be modulated by CaMK II by mobilizing the secretory granules toward the cell membrane by MAP-2 phosphorylation and by potentially regulating the docking or priming mechanisms via VAMP and synapsin I protein phosphorylation. Since CaM kinase II remains active after glucose stimulation, it is suggested as a mechanism of readily releasable pool replenishment. (Easom, R.A. 1999).

2.3.3 The G-protein coupled signaling pathways: PKA and PKC

The guanyl-nucleotide-binding (GTP) protein system or G-protein coupled system plays an important role on insulin secretion. In the beta-cells, two G-protein regulated pathways, the Adenylate cyclase (AC)/PKA, and the phospholipase C (PLC)/PKC pathways, modulate

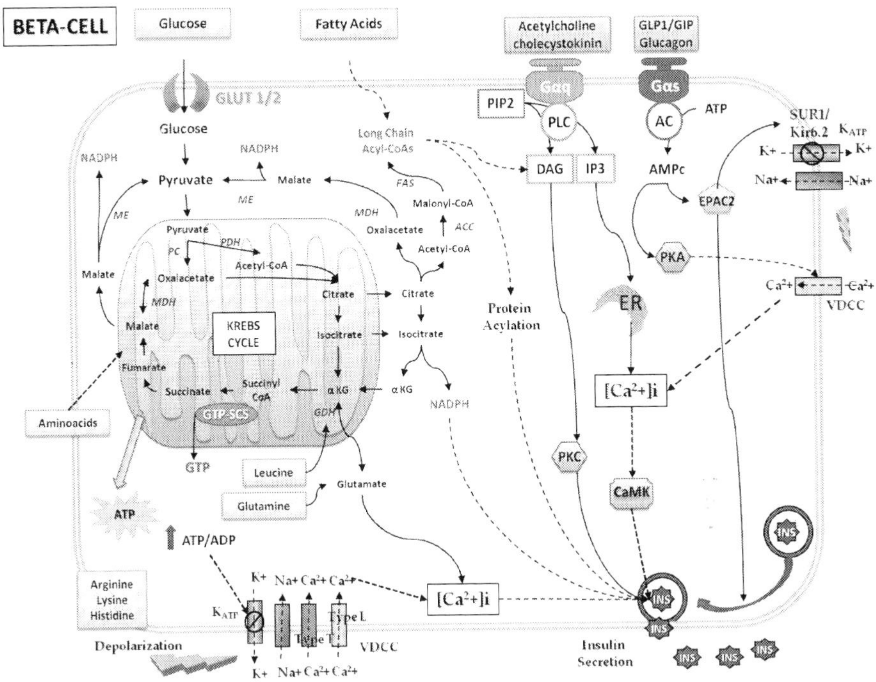

Fig. 2. Regulation of glucose-stimulated insulin secretion by nutrients, hormones and neurotransmitters.

Glucose-stimulated insulin secretion may be modulated by several mechanisms. Glucose metabolism increase ATP/ADP ratio and closes ATP-sensitive pottasium channels (K_{ATP}), depolarizing the membrane, opening voltage-dependent calcium channels (VDCC), and thus increasing intracellular calcium ([Ca2+]i). Glucose metabolism by the Krebs Cycle also renders a series of metabolic coupling factors that may initiate and sustain insulin secretion. These metabolic coupling factors participate in mitochondrial shuttles, involving NADPH, pyruvate, malate, citrate, isocitrate, acyl-CoAs, and glutamate. Signaling pathways that contribute to maintaining or increasing glucose-stimulated insulin secretion include PKA and PKC. Glucagon, glucagon-Like peptide 1 (GLP-1), and glucose-dependent insulinotropic peptide (GIP) act through PKA pathway, while acetylcholine and cholecystokinine act through the PKC pathway. Fatty acids may contribute to insulin secretion through the PKC pathway through formation of diacylglycerol (DAG) or through protein acylation. Aminoacids may stimulate insulin release by increasing ATP production from the Krebs Cycle, by membrane depolarization, or by participating in intracellular calcium increase. (αKG: alpha-ketoglutarate, ACC: Acetyl CoA Carboxylase, FAS: Fatty Acid Synthase, GDH: Glutamate Dehydrogenase, GTP-SCS: GTP-Succinyl CoA Synthetase, ER: endoplasmic Reticulum, ME: Malic enzyme, MDH: Malate Dehydrogenase, PC: Pyruvate Carboxylase, PHD: Pyruvate Dehydrogenase, PIP2: Phosphatidyl Inositol Biphosphante, IP3: inositol 1,4,5-trisphosphate).

insulin secretion in response to nutrients and other peripheral signals (Doyle, M.E. & Egan, J.M. 2003). Depending on the type of Gα subunit present, these signals will activate or inhibit Adenylate Cyclase ($G\alpha_s$ and $G\alpha_i$ subunits respectively). $G\alpha_q$ subunits are associated with the phosphatidyl inositol system (Gomperts, B.D. et al. 2003).

When the Adenylate Cyclase is activated in the beta-cell, it converts ATP in cyclic AMP (cAMP), which in turn can activate the cAMP-dependent protein kinase (PKA) and the Rap guanine nucleotide exchange factor (GEF) 4 or Epac2. PKA will phosphorylate several proteins, including L-type voltage-dependent calcium channels and proteins from the exocytotic machinery, increasing sustained insulin secretion (Ammala, C. et al. 1993) . Epac2 has been shown to favor insulin secretion by increasing the size of the reserve pool and facilitating the recruitment of the granules to the plasma membrane (Shibasaki, T. et al. 2007), mediating pulsatility of insulin secretion (Idevall-Hagren, O. et al. 2010), and binding to the SUR1 subunit of the K_{ATP} channels (Zhang, C.L. et al. 2009). The insulin gene itself has cAMP response elements in its promoter that modulate insulin transcription in response to this nucleotide (Melloul, D. et al. 2002).

Therefore, ligands that increase the activity of adenylate cyclase and cAMP have a positive effect on insulin synthesis and secretion (Sharp, G.W. 1979), while ligands that decrease adenylate cyclase activity affect insulin secretion in a negative way (Jones, P.M. & Persaud, S.J. 1998). Hormones and neurotransmitters mostly act on insulin secretion by this pathway (see below).

Phospholipase C (PLC) is the other effector protein regulated by G-protein coupled receptors in the beta-cell. PLC activation cleaves phosphoinositides into two second messengers, inositol 1,4,5-trisphosphate (IP_3), involved in Ca^{2+} release from the endoplasmic reticulum, and diacylglycerol (DAG). DAG is involved in the activation of the Protein kinase C (PKC). PKC phosphorylates the K_{ATP} channels and the voltage-dependent Ca^{2+} channels and mobilize the secretory vesicles (Doyle, M.E. & Egan, J.M. 2003), therefore promoting insulin secretion. Both nutrients and neurotransmitters may act through PKC activation, albeit by different mechanisms. It has been proposed that nutrients may activate atypical isoforms of PKC (-ζ, -ι, and -μ) by a non-identified mechanism independent of DAG, while the typical isoforms (-α, -β, -δ, and -ϵ) of PKC (Protein Kinase C) are activated by DAG (Jones, P.M. & Persaud, S.J. 1998).

2.3.4 The cGMP/PKG pathway

The cyclic GMP (cGMP) pathway is regulated basically by two factors: calcium and protein kinase G (PKG). Calcium increases the activity of calcium-dependent nitric oxide synthases, a key step in the synthesis of cGMP by soluble guanylyl cyclase (cGC). Calcium may also decrease cGMP synthesis by activating a calcium-dependent phosphodiesterase (PDE1). On the other hand, protein kinase G (PKG), an enzyme activated by cGMP, may phoshporylate different targets and modulate intracellular calcium concentration, primarily closing K_{ATP} channels (Soria, B. et al. 2004).

Although several studies have pointed to a role of sGC and cGMP on insulin secretion (Laychock, S.G. et al. 1991; Russell, M.A. & Morgan, N. 2010), a precise mechanism of action has not been yet elucidated for this pathway. As phosphorylation of PKG has been identified in rat islets (Jones, P.M. & Persaud, S.J. 1998), this is likely the enzyme mediating cGMP actions on insulin secretion. It has also been shown that PKG activity is necessary to increase ATP content in response to cGMP (Vilches-Flores, A. et al. 2009), and that glucose produces small increases in islet cGMP content (Laychock, S.G. et al. 1991; Schmidt, H.H. et al. 1992).

3. Nutrient modulation of insulin secretion

Beta-cells may be considered fuel sensors, as they are continually monitoring and responding to nutrient concentration in the circulation in order to secrete insulin and therefore, regulate glucose homeostasis. Given that meals are composed by multiple nutrients, it is important to examine the interplay between glucose-sensing in the beta-cell and other dietary nutrients, such as amino acids, fatty acids and vitamins. Cumulatively, the mixed nutrient sensing generates the metabolic coupling factors working as signals for insulin exocytosis.

3.1 Insulin secretion in response to fatty acids

While it would appear that free fatty acids do not stimulate insulin secretion in the absence of glucose, there is a substantial body of evidence that they are essential for glucose-stimulated insulin secretion (Salehi, A. et al. 2005). It has been proposed that, in the presence of glucose, fatty acid oxidation is inhibited, due to formation of malonyl-CoA by acetyl-CoA carboxylase. This permits the accumulation of long-chain acyl-CoA in the cytosol that then stimulate insulin secretion directly or through the formation of other lipid compounds such as diacylglycerol and various phospholipids (Nolan, C.J. et al. 2006). The mechanisms which could be involved in this process are (Yaney, G.C. & Corkey, B.E. 2003): a) activation of protein kinase-C enzymes; b) enhanced fusion of insulin-secretory vesicles with plasma membrane and insulin release; c) modulation of K_{ATP} channel activity directly or via complex lipid formation; d) Stimulation of Ca2+-ATPases; e) Protein acylation of GTP-binding proteins; f) Inhibition of lipase activity.

The effects of fatty acids on glucose-stimulated insulin secretion are directly correlated with chain length and the degree of unsaturation, where long-chain fatty acids (such as palmitate or linoleate) acutely improve insulin release, however, chronic increase of long-chain fatty acids reduce insulin release in response to glucose stimulation (Newsholme, P. et al. 2007b).

3.2 Insulin secretion in response to amino acids

In addition to fatty acid involvement in glucose-stimulated insulin secretion, amino acids derived from dietary proteins and those released from intestinal epithelial cells, in combination with glucose; stimulate insulin secretion, *in vivo*. Amino acids individually are poor insulin secretagogues and a relatively small number of amino acids promote or synergistically enhance glucose stimulated insulin release from pancreatic beta-cells (Newsholme, P. et al. 2010). Leucine, glutamine, alanine, arginine, lysine, and histidine induce insulin secretion. The mechanisms by which these amino acids elicit insulin release may vary.

Glutamine and alanine are quantitatively the most abundant amino acids in blood and extracellular fluids and therefore might be the most relevant to insulin secretion (Newsholme, P. et al. 2010). Alanine increase ATP production in islet beta-cells, an event that has potential to promote the K+ATP channel triggering pathway. Alanine is also one of the electrogenic amino acids, being co-transported with Na+ so that its import depolarizes the plasma membrane and promotes Ca2+ influx, events that trigger insulin secretion (McClenaghan, N.H. et al. 1998). Although glutamine is rapidly transported and metabolized by islets, it does not promote insulin secretion by itself or enhance glucose-stimulated insulin secretion, but can elicit insulin release in the presence of leucine (Newsholme, P. et al. 2007a). It is believed that this is because leucine activates glutamic

dehydrogenase, which then increases the capacity of glutamine to contribute to anaplerosis via alpha-ketoglutarate (Newsholme, P. et al. 2007a).
Similarly as glucose-stimulated insulin release, leucine acts by generating ATP thought its metabolism, thus causing closure of ATP-sensitive potassium channels, membrane depolarization via opening of the L-voltage-dependent calcium channels, leading to calcium influx and increased cytoplasmic calcium concentrations. Furthermore, leucine acutely stimulates insulin secretion by serving as both metabolic fuel and allosteric activator of glutamate dehydrogenase, resulting in conversion of glutamate to 2-ketoglutarate, a compound that has been proposed to be a common mediator of glucose, amino acid, and organic acid insulin secretion (Odegaard, M.L. et al. 2010). Additionally, transamination of leucine to α-ketoisocaproate and entry into TCA cycle via acetyl-CoA can contribute to ATP generation by increasing the oxidation rate of the amino acid and thus stimulation of insulin secretion.
Other amino acids also stimulate insulin secretion by elevating cytosolic calcium concentration, although their mechanisms are achieved independently of ATP generation. Positive charged amino acids such as arginine, lysine and histidine, elicit insulin secretion by beta-cell inward transport of positive charge, triggering depolarization of cytoplasm membrane, and influx of extracellular calcium (Newsholme, P. et al. 2010).

3.3 Insulin secretion in response to vitamins

3.3.1 Vitamin A

Vitamin A is found in the organism either as retinol, retinal or retinoic acid forms. Retinoic acid is the active form, and the majority of its effects involve the activation of ligand-dependent transcription factors from the superfamily of hormonal nuclear receptors. Two of these receptors are known: the retinoic acid receptors (RARs) and the rexinoid receptors (RXRs). These can bind as heterodimers to specific DNA sequences named Retinoic Acid Response Elements, (RAREs) in the promoters of their target genes, or interact with other receptors such as Vitamin D receptors (VDRs), thyroid hormone receptors and PPARs (Peroxisome Proliferation Activating Receptors).
Retinol is essential for insulin secretion (Chertow, B.S. et al. 1987) and retinoic acid increases insulin secretion in cultured islets (Cabrera-Valladares, G. et al. 1999), presumably by its stimulatory effect on pancreatic glucokinase expression and activity (Cabrera-Valladares, G. et al. 1999). Retinoic acid is also capable of increasing insulin (Cabrera-Valladares, G. et al. 1999) and GLUT2 mRNA (Blumentrath, J. et al. 2001).

3.3.2 Vitamin D

Vitamin D is syntethized under the skin thanks to exposure to UVB radiation. It can also be obtained from food in the form of ergocalcipherol (vitamin D2) or cholechalcipherol (vitamin D3). When UVB radiation is absorbed through the skin, 7-dehydrocholesterol reserves form the pre-vitamin D3, which is transformed into vitamin D3 ($1,25(OH_2)D_3$) in a further process, by the action of the $25(OH_2)D_3$ hydroxylase (Holick, M.F. 2003). Vitamin D acts on Vitamin D receptors (VDRs), which are either in the nucleus or in the membrane, rendering two different mechanisms of action, genomic, and non-genomic (rapid response) (Norman, A.W. et al. 2001)
Both VDRs (Johnson, J.A. et al. 1994) and $25(OH_2)D_3$ hydroxylase are expressed in the pancreatic beta-cells (Bland, R. et al. 2004), suggesting there may be vitamin D synthesis and

effects in these cells. In vitro, 1,25(OH_2)D induces the biosynthesis of insulin in rat beta-cells (Bourlon, P.M. et al. 1999). It has been suggested that increases in cytosolic Ca^{2+}, a non-genomic effect of vitamin D, can increase insulin secretion (Norman, A.W. 2006). This increase may be modulated by activation of the PKC (Billaudel, B.J. et al. 1995) and PKA (Bourlon, P.M. et al. 1997) signaling pathways (d'Emden, M.C. et al. 1989).

3.3.3 Biotin

Biotin is a water-soluble vitamin that acts as a prosthetic group of carboxylases. Unrelated to this classic role, pharmacological concentrations of biotin regulate gene expression at both the transcriptional and the translational level (Rodriguez-Melendez, R. & Zempleni, J. 2003; Zempleni, J. 2005), and have a wide repertoire of effects on systemic processes such as development (Watanabe, T. 1996), reproduction (Baez-Saldana, A. et al. 2009; Paul, P.K. & Duttagupta, P.N. 1976; Simmins, P.H. & Brooks, P.H. 1983), and metabolism (Dakshinamurti, K. 2005; Fernandez-Mejia, C. 2005).

Biotin exerts beneficial effects on endocrine pancreas physiology. We have found that biotin stimulates insulin and pancreatic glucokinase expression(Romero-Navarro, G. et al. 1999), an enzyme that plays an important role in glucose homeostasis regulating insulin secretion in response to changes in blood glucose concentrations. Our group found that biotin concentrations of 10 to 1000 nM augmented glucokinase activity and mRNA abundance in cultured rat pancreatic islets (Romero-Navarro, G. et al. 1999). A similar stimulatory effect on pancreatic glucokinase was observed in the insulinoma RIN 1046-38 cell line (Borboni, P. et al. 1996). A positive effect of biotin on insulin secretion has been reported (Romero-Navarro, G. et al. 1999; Sone, H. et al. 2000; Sone, H. et al. 1999; Vilches-Flores, A. et al. 2009). Studies by our group (Romero-Navarro, G. et al. 1999; Vilches-Flores, A. et al. 2009) and others (Sone, H. et al. 2000; Sone, H. et al. 1999) have revealed that glucose-stimulated insulin secretion increases in response to acute exposure to pharmacological doses of biotin in either primary cultured islets (Romero-Navarro, G. et al. 1999), perifused pancreas (Sone, H. et al. 1999) or perifused islets (Sone, H. et al. 2000). This effect of biotin on insulin secretion also appears to be dose-dependent (Sone, H. et al. 1999). In isolated pancreatic islets, using blockers and inhibitors of different signaling pathways, we have discovered that the induction of glucokinase mRNA and the increase on insulin secretion by biotin involves guanylate cyclase and PKG activation, which triggers ATP production (Vilches-Flores, A. et al. 2009). The increase of ATP induces insulin secretion via ATP-sensitive potassium channels. Insulin, in an autocrine manner, activates PI3K/Akt signaling, which increases pancreatic glucokinase mRNA expression (Vilches-Flores, A. et al. 2009).

Although the acute effect of biotin on *in* vitro insulin secretion has been well documented, further studies addressing the effect of this vitamin on *in vivo* models, resembling the actual doses and periods of treatment currently recommended for diabetes treatment, need to be done.

4. Other modulatory signals of insulin secretion - hormones and neurotransmitters

Insulin secretion in response to the plasmatic concentration of glucose can be increased or decreased by several hormones (including insulin itself) and neurotransmitters via activation of their membrane receptors on the beta-cells (Flat, P.R. 1996). The G protein receptors and adenylate cyclase pathway are responsible for mediating most of these effects.

The adenylate cyclase pathway may be activated by some neurotransmitters, like acetylcholine, and hormones like GLP-1. GLP-1 is also an important factor for insulin synthesis and secretion, having a trophic effect on the beta-cells as well (Baggio, L.L. & Drucker, D.J. 2007). Other modulating pathways are activated in the beta-cells in response to oxidative stress caused by high glucose levels, like the JNK pathway, which ablates insulin synthesis and interferes with its action (Kaneto, H. et al. 2006).

4.1 Insulin and the beta-cell autocrine signaling

Various studies have shown an autocrine role of insulin on beta-cell function and survival (Aikin, R. et al. 2006; Navarro-Tableros, V. et al. 2004; Xu, G.G. & Rothenberg, P.L. 1998). In this process, insulin binding to tyrosine-kinase receptors located in the beta-cell promotes the receptor's autophosphorylation, catalyzing subsequent tyrosine phosphorylation of other proteins like IRS (IRS1 and IRS2). Once phosphorylated, these proteins interact with signaling molecules, which results in a phosphorylation cascade where PI3K, PDK and Akt are sequentially activated. Akt is a serine/threonine kinase which regulates cell survival, proliferation, growth and nutrient metabolism, through phosphorylation of different proteins like GSK3, FOXO and CREB (Song, G. et al. 2005). The activated receptor may act on the Ras signaling pathway, which in turn activates MAP kinases ERK1/2, in this way regulating growth, cellular differentiation and protein synthesis (Kahn, S.E. et al. 2006). In human islets, insulin has a positive effect on insulin production at the transcriptional level, as well as on beta-cell proliferation (Persaud, S.J. et al. 2008) .

4.2 Insulin secretion in response to glucagon

Glucagon is considered the contrarregulatory hormone of insulin, as its systemic actions are contrary to the ones exerted by insulin. Glucagon stimulates glucose production, glycogen degradation, and lipolysis. Paradoxically, it has been shown that glucagon stimulates insulin secretion both in rats (Kawai, K. et al. 1995) and humans (Ahren, B. et al. 1987). Glucagon induces a transient increase in plasma insulin up to 1 mg glucagon concentrations, and this increase is seen before glucose levels rise (Ahren, B. et al. 1987). There is evidence that the positive effect of glucagon on insulin secretion is mediated by activation of glucagon receptors in the beta-cells (Kawai, K. et al. 1995), and this activation may increase cAMP levels, leading to the PKA pathway.

4.3 Effects of incretins on insulin secretion

Incretins are hormones secreted in the postprandial state by the enteroendocrine cells in the gut. Their main physiological role is to modulate insulin secretion. Two incretins have been described GIP (glucose-dependent insulinotropic peptide) and GLP-1 (glucagon-like peptide-1) (Brubaker, P.L. 2010).

GLP-1 is released rapidly into the circulation after oral nutrient ingestion, and its secretion occurs in a biphasic pattern starting with an early (within10–15 min) phase that is followed by a longer (30 -60 min) second phase (Herrmann, C. et al. 1995). Incretin-receptor activation leads to activation of adenylate cyclase and elevation of cAMP. Its actions include stimulation of glucose-dependent insulin secretion, induction of beta-cell proliferation, and enhanced resistance to islet cells apoptosis (Brubaker, P.L. 2010). GLP-1 stimulates insulin secretion via mechanisms that include the following: 1) direct inhibition of K_{ATP} channels, which leads to beta-cell membrane depolarization; 2) increases in intracellular calcium levels resulting from GLP-1-dependent influx of extracellular calcium through voltage-dependent calcium, channels, activation of nonselective cation channels, and mobilization of intracellular calcium stores; 3) increases in mitochondrial ATP synthesis, which lead to further membrane depolarization; 4) closure of voltage-dependent potassium (Kv) channels and consequent reductions in Kv currents, thereby preventing beta-cell repolarization; and 5) direct effects on beta-cell insulin storage granule exocytosis that occur distal to increases in ATP and intracellular calcium (Baggio, L.L. & Drucker, D.J. 2007).

Both GIP and GLP-1 are cleaved and inactivated by the enzyme dipeptidyl peptidase 4 (DPP4). The rapid degradation of GLP-1 by DPP4 has led to the development of degradation-resistant GLP-1-receptor agonists and dipeptidyl peptidase-4 inhibitors, in order to increase the incretin effects. These drugs are currently used for diabetes treatment (Brubaker, P.L. 2010).

4.4 Neurotransmitters in the regulation of insulin secretion

Besides nutrients, neurohormonal signals such as autonomic innervation can markedly modulate glucose-stimulated insulin secretion. Islets are thoroughly innervated by autonomic nerves, which contain an extensive variety of neuropeptide transmitters. Increased sympathetic activity affects insulin secretion in situations of stress, exercise and trauma. Activation of parasympathetic nerves before and during feeding by the smell, taste and digestive tract, along with incretin hormones derived from the gut are responsible for enhancing insulin response to meals.

Parasympathetic neurotransmitters that stimulate insulin secretion include acetylcholine, vasoactive intestinal polypeptide and gastrin-releasing polypeptide. Sympathetic neurotransmitters inhibit insulin release; these include norepinephrine, galanin and neuropeptide Y. The enteroinsular axis, mediated by incretin hormones, explains why the insulin response to an ingested nutrient load is greater than when the same load is given parenterally. Gastrointestinal hormones such as gastric inhibitory peptide, glucagon-like peptide-1 (7-36) and cholecystokinin exert physiological relevant insulinotrophic effects (Flatt, P.R. 2003). In particular glucagon-like peptide-1 (7-36) has attracted attention by its potential role in the treatment of diabetes (see above).

There are at least three potential sites were insulin can be modulated by hormones, peptides and neurotransmitters. Firstly, these may affect the ion channels that regulate membrane potential and calcium influx. Secondly, they may influence the mobilization of intracellular calcium stores, mainly the endoplasmic reticulum, and therefore cytosolic calcium concentration. Thirdly, they may modify the calcium sensibility of the contractile protein interactions that lead to the release of the insulin secretory granules (Flatt, P.R. 2003). The two better known targets of hormones, peptides and neurotransmitters within the beta-cell are related to adenylate cyclase and phospholipase C.

Activation of adenylate cyclase produces cyclic adenosine monophosphate (cAMP), which inhibits calcium sequestration within intracellular stores. Activation of cAMP-dependent protein kinase (PKA) results in phosphorylation of intracellular proteins that enhance calcium sensitization. PKA also promotes phosphorylation of voltage-dependent calcium channels thereby increasing calcium influx (Flatt, P.R. 2003).

Phospholipase C activation cleaves phosphatidylinosistol in the membrane producing inositol-1,4,5 triphosphate wich in turn inhibits calcium sequestration into the endoplasmic reticulum, while the adjacent cleavage product, diacylglycerol activates protein kinase C. Similarly to the effects of adenylate cyclase signaling pathway, activation of phospholipase

C alters insulin secretion by mechanisms related to calcium sensitivity and protein phosphorylation (Flatt, P.R. 2003).

5. Beta-cell mass

Besides a correct beta-cell function, the organism's beta-cell mass is also important for maintaining adequate insulin production and secretion. Beta-cell mass is determined by cell number as well as cell size, and it increases progressively during fetal, neonatal and growth periods in the life of an organism, reaching a plateau during adulthood and decaying gradually with age (Ackermann, A.M. & Gannon, M. 2007).

Diverse processes participate in increasing and maintaining the beta cell mass, such as neogenesis (newly forming of cells from precursors), proliferation (cell replication), beta-cell size increase (hypertrophy), and apoptosis (cell death) (Ackermann, A.M. & Gannon, M. 2007). Although beta-cell progenitors have been identified in the pancreas (Bonner-Weir, S. et al. 2008; Xu, X. et al. 2008), the participation of neogenesis during post-natal and adult beta cell mass is limited (Dor, Y. et al. 2004), being proliferation (Meier, J.J. et al. 2008) and hypertrophy (Montanya, E. et al. 2000) the mainly responsible mechanisms for post-natal beta cell expansion (Ackermann, A.M. & Gannon, M. 2007). The organism is also capable of modifying beta-cell mass depending on its insulin requirements. In insulin resistance states, such as pregnancy and obesity, beta-cell mass is increased (Rhodes, C.J. 2005) a process driven by proliferation (Ackermann, A.M. & Gannon, M. 2007).

The mechanisms by which adult beta-cell proliferation is driven remain unknown. Nevertheless, some of the factors regulating this process have been identified, such as growth factors (growth hormone, lactogens, insulin, insulin-like growth factors), incretins, cell cycle proteins, and transcription factors (PDX-1) (Ackermann, A.M. & Gannon, M. 2007). Although many of the molecular regulators of postnatal beta-cell mass and beta-cell turnover have been identified in rodent models, it has been observed that human beta-cells' ability to proliferate under the same signals is very restricted compared to rodent ones (Parnaud, G. et al. 2008). Moreover, in humans, beta-cell proliferation has suggested to occur only until early adulthood, as proliferation studies in humans have shown that there is no beta-cell replication after the first 30 years of life (Perl, S. et al. 2010).

6. Beta-cell failure and death in type 1 DM

Overt hyperglycemia and therefore, the onset of type 1 diabetes occurs when 70-80% of the beta-cell mass is gone. But the progressive loss of beta-cells is suggested to occur slowly over several years (Cnop, M. et al. 2005). This progressive damage may also account for a reduction of the first-phase insulin secretion seen in patients positive to islet cell antibodies but who had not developed hyperglycemia yet (Srikanta, S. et al. 1983). Nevertheless, the rate of beta-cell destruction in type 1 diabetes patients is variable and so can be the first manifestations of the disease. While some patients, mainly children and teenagers, may present ketoacidosis as first sign of diabetes, others (usually adults) could show modest fasting hyperglycemia, which may not evolve to severe hyperglycemia nor ketoacidosis for several years due to remaining function of the beta-cell (ADA 2009).

Regardless this variable nature, type 1 diabetes progression after the initiation of the autoimmune response may be divided in two different phases: insulitis and overt diabetes (Mathis, D. et al. 2001) (Figure 3). Apoptosis of the beta-cell is present even in the initiation and, evidently, both in insulitis and diabetes. These observations suggest that the beta-cell has a more important role in the pathophysiology of the disease than previously thought (Eizirik, D.L. et al. 2009; Mathis, D. et al. 2001).

It has been proposed that beta-cell death possibly participates in the initiation of the autoimmune response, particularly in autoantigen presentation (Filippi, C.M. & von Herrath, M.G. 2007; Kaminitz, A. et al. 2007; Mathis, D. et al. 2001). It is known that beta-cells, both in rodents (Finegood, D.T. et al. 1995) and humans (Kassem, S.A. et al. 2000), may undergo physiological periods of apoptosis, particularly during the perinatal period. Moreover, viral infections or inflammatory cytokines may induce accumulation of misfolded proteins, causing ER stress, which can also lead to beta-cell apoptosis (Eizirik, D.L. et al. 2009). Immunological

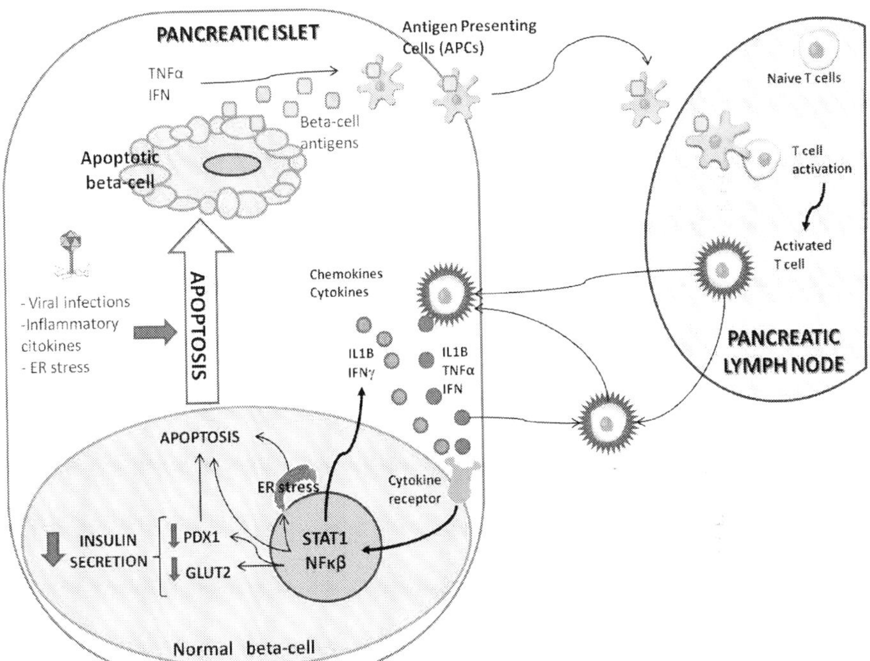

Fig. 3. Induction and progression of insulitis.
Viral infections or inflammatory processes may lead to beta-cell apoptosis. Apoptotic beta-cells undergoing secondary necrosis may release beta-cell antigens, which would activate the antigen presenting cells. These cells could activate naive T cells in the pancreatic lymph nodes. When T cells reencounter the islet-antigens, they are retained in the islet, releasing inflammatory factors and inducing insulitis. Inflammatory cytokines activate transcription factors NFκβ and STAT-1, which decrease PDX1 and GLUT1 expression, leading to insufficient insulin production and secretion. Activation of NFκβ and STAT-1 also trigger ER stress, apoptotic processes and beta-cell release of citokines, leading to a vicious cycle of inflammation/beta-cell destruction that maintains and eventually amplifies the autoimmune attack.

recognition of antigens released by apoptotic beta-cells undergoing secondary necrosis, particularly in the presence of inflammatory factors such as TNF or interferons, could be an important signal to activate antigen presenting cells, which may then reach the pancreatic lymph nodes and be recognized by T cells (Filippi, C.M. & von Herrath, M.G. 2007). When these T cells reencounter the islet-antigens, they are retained in the islet, triggering the inflammatory process or insulitis (Mathis, D. et al. 2001).

Beta-cells also participate in the progression of insulitis (Eizirik, D.L. et al. 2009; Kaminitz, A. et al. 2007). Beta-cells themselves are capable of producing chemokines and cytokines in response to inflammatory factors such as IL-1β and IFNγ (Cardozo, A.K. et al. 2003), a process mediated by activation of the transcription factors NFκβ and STAT-1 (Cardozo, A.K. et al. 2001; Cnop, M. et al. 2005). This cytokines, besides promoting beta-cell death, can contribute to the recruitment and activation immune cells (Eizirik, D.L. et al. 2009). A localized inflammatory process starts within the islet beta-cell milieu, in which immune cells produce more inflammatory cytokines (IL-1β, TNF and interferons) that would activate NFκβ and STAT-1, leading to a vicious cycle of inflammation/beta-cell destruction that maintains and eventually amplifies the autoimmune attack (Eizirik, D.L. et al. 2009; Kaminitz, A. et al. 2007).

Once insulitis is established, selective destruction of the beta-cells occur mainly by two proposed mechanisms: a recognition-linked mechanism and activation-linked mechanism. The former involves direct recognition of the beta-cell antigens by cytotoxic T-cells, while the latter is caused by exposure of soluble mediators secreted by T-cells that induce beta-cell death (Cnop, M. et al. 2005; Mathis, D. et al. 2001) such as cytokines, perforin or Fas/Fas ligand interactions, nitric oxide and reactive oxygen species (Cnop, M. et al. 2005; Mathis, D. et al. 2001).

Insulitis can be maintained in certain patients without evolving to overt diabetes. Studies in NOD mice have suggested that before the appearance of hyperglycemia, and after insulitis has been triggered, beta-cell function impairment precedes beta-cell apoptosis in response to the autoimmune attack (Strandell, E. et al. 1990). Surprisingly, beta-cell function may be recovered if the islets of these animals are either removed from their inflammatory milieu and cultured *in vitro* or if the inflammation is stopped with antibodies against the effector T cells (Strandell, E. et al. 1990), suggesting beta-cell damage in this stage is reversible. In addition, there is evidence that NFκβ activation in response to inflammatory factors also reduces PDX1 and GLUT2 expression (Cardozo, A.K. et al. 2003), two proteins which are crucial for insulin production and secretion.

Together with an initial loss of beta-cell function, the inflammatory process found in type 1 diabetes appears to stimulate beta-cell proliferation during the first stage of the disease. An increase in beta-cell mass may maintain metabolic demands for the period before the development of hyperglycemia, but it may also expose more and new epitopes, favoring and increasing the autoimmune destruction (Akirav, E. et al. 2008).

Given the important role of the beta-cell during the initiating and progression stages of insulitis that may lead to type 1 diabetes, current research is being directed toward maintenance and improvement of beta-cell function and mass before and during the inflammatory process, establishing important therapeutic targets. New therapeutic approaches suggest that using combinatory treatments comprising a first immune intervention, followed by stimulation of beta-cell proliferation and function (perhaps with GLP-1-receptor agonists), and maintenance of normal glucose levels, together with the already used immunomodulatory therapy, may help not only to stop the progression of the disease, but even to recover the remaining beta-cell mass and function (Akirav, E. et al. 2008; Weir, G.C. & Bonner-Weir, S. 2010).

7. Conclusions

Type 1 diabetes is one of the most serious chronic diseases of childhood. In spite of all the efforts in finding efficient therapeutic approaches for this disease, insulin keeps being the only effective treatment, as islet transplantation and beta-cell generation from stem cells have shown difficulties in getting donors or generating effective glucose-coupled insulin secreting cells.

As the loss of beta-cells is determinant for the development of overt type 1 diabetes, understanding beta-cell normal physiology, namely insulin secretion, and how it may be affected during the progression of this disease is essential. Moreover, the development of new therapeutic interventions for type 1 diabetes, such as islet transplantation, beta cell maintenance and replacement, or stem cell therapy, require a profound knowledge of how the presence of different nutrients and signals may regulate insulin secretion and beta-cell mass.

Recent studies on the different stages of type 1 diabetes have shed light on an important role of beta-cell in the progression of the inflammatory process, and even evidence of reversal of the beta-cell damage present in the disease. These findings may provide tools to propose new integral and combinatorial therapeutic interventions that may aid in fighting this disease.

8. Acknowledgements

This work was supported by grants from CONACyT: 99294-M, and from the Dirección General de Asuntos del Personal Académico: IN221908 Universidad Nacional Autónoma de México. Maria-Luisa Lazo de la Vega-Monroy is recipient of the CONACyT scholarship number CVU/Becario: 217876/207055.

9. References

Ackermann, A. M.& Gannon, M. (2007). Molecular regulation of pancreatic beta-cell mass development, maintenance, and expansion. *J Mol Endocrinol,* Vol. 38,No. 1-2, pp. 193-206.

ADA (2009). Diagnosis and classification of diabetes mellitus. *Diabetes Care,* Vol. 32,No. supplement 1, pp. S62-67.

Aguilar-Bryan, L., Clement, J. P. t., Gonzalez, G. et al. (1998). Toward understanding the assembly and structure of KATP channels. *Physiol Rev,* Vol. 78,No. 1, pp. 227-245.

Ahlgren, U., Jonsson, J., Jonsson, L. et al. (1998). beta-cell-specific inactivation of the mouse Ipf1/Pdx1 gene results in loss of the beta-cell phenotype and maturity onset diabetes. *Genes Dev,* Vol. 12,No. 12, pp. 1763-1768.

Ahren, B., Nobin, A.& Schersten, B. (1987). Insulin and C-peptide secretory responses to glucagon in man: studies on the dose-response relationships. *Acta Med Scand,* Vol. 221,No. 2, pp. 185-190.

Aikin, R., Hanley, S., Maysinger, D. et al. (2006). Autocrine insulin action activates Akt and increases survival of isolated human islets. *Diabetologia,* Vol. 49,No. 12, pp. 2900-2909.

Aizawa, T.& Komatsu, M. (2005). Rab27a: a new face in beta cell metabolism-secretion coupling. *J Clin Invest,* Vol. 115,No. 2, pp. 227-230.

Aizawa, T., Sato, Y.& Komatsu, M. (2002). Importance of nonionic signals for glucose-induced biphasic insulin secretion. *Diabetes,* Vol. 51 Suppl 1,No. pp. S96-98.

Aizawa, T., Komatsu, M., Asanuma, N. et al. (1998). Glucose action 'beyond ionic events' in the pancreatic beta cell. *Trends Pharmacol Sci,* Vol. 19,No. 12, pp. 496-499.

Akirav, E., Kushner, J. A.& Herold, K. C. (2008). Beta-cell mass and type 1 diabetes: going, going, gone? *Diabetes,* Vol. 57,No. 11, pp. 2883-2888.

Ammala, C., Ashcroft, F. M.& Rorsman, P. (1993). Calcium-independent potentiation of insulin release by cyclic AMP in single beta-cells. *Nature,* Vol. 363,No. 6427, pp. 356-358.

Baez-Saldana, A., Camacho-Arroyo, I., Espinosa-Aguirre, J. J. et al. (2009). Biotin deficiency and biotin excess: effects on the female reproductive system. *Steroids,* Vol. 74,No. 10-11, pp. 863-869.

Baggio, L. L.& Drucker, D. J. (2007). Biology of incretins: GLP-1 and GIP. *Gastroenterology,* Vol. 132,No. 6, pp. 2131-2157.

Bergsten, P., Grapengiesser, E., Gylfe, E. et al. (1994). Synchronous oscillations of cytoplasmic Ca2+ and insulin release in glucose-stimulated pancreatic islets. *J Biol Chem,* Vol. 269,No. 12, pp. 8749-8753.

Billaudel, B. J., Bourlon, P. M., Sutter, B. C. et al. (1995). Regulatory effect of 1,25-dihydroxyvitamin D3 on insulin release and calcium handling via the phospholipid pathway in islets from vitamin D-deficient rats. *J Endocrinol Invest,* Vol. 18,No. 9, pp. 673-682.

Bland, R., Markovic, D., Hills, C. E. et al. (2004). Expression of 25-hydroxyvitamin D3-1alpha-hydroxylase in pancreatic islets. *J Steroid Biochem Mol Biol,* Vol. 89-90,No. 1-5, pp. 121-125.

Blumentrath, J., Neye, H.& Verspohl, E. J. (2001). Effects of retinoids and thiazolidinediones on proliferation, insulin release, insulin mRNA, GLUT 2 transporter protein and mRNA of INS-1 cells. *Cell Biochem Funct,* Vol. 19,No. 3, pp. 159-169.

Bonner-Weir, S., Inada, A., Yatoh, S. et al. (2008). Transdifferentiation of pancreatic ductal cells to endocrine beta-cells. *Biochem Soc Trans,* Vol. 36,No. Pt 3, pp. 353-356.

Borboni, P., Magnaterra, R., Rabini, R. A. et al. (1996). Effect of biotin on glucokinase activity, mRNA expression and insulin release in cultured beta-cells. *Acta Diabetol,* Vol. 33,No. 2, pp. 154-158.

Bourlon, P. M., Faure-Dussert, A.& Billaudel, B. (1997). Modulatory role of 1,25 dihydroxyvitamin D3 on pancreatic islet insulin release via the cyclic AMP pathway in the rat. *Br J Pharmacol,* Vol. 121,No. 4, pp. 751-758.

Bourlon, P. M., Billaudel, B.& Faure-Dussert, A. (1999). Influence of vitamin D3 deficiency and 1,25 dihydroxyvitamin D3 on de novo insulin biosynthesis in the islets of the rat endocrine pancreas. *J Endocrinol,* Vol. 160,No. 1, pp. 87-95.

Brubaker, P. L. (2010). Minireview: update on incretin biology: focus on glucagon-like peptide-1. *Endocrinology,* Vol. 151,No. 5, pp. 1984-1989.

Cabrera-Valladares, G., German, M. S., Matschinsky, F. M. et al. (1999). Effect of retinoic acid on glucokinase activity and gene expression and on insulin secretion in primary cultures of pancreatic islets. *Endocrinology,* Vol. 140,No. 7, pp. 3091-3096.

Cardozo, A. K., Proost, P., Gysemans, C. et al. (2003). IL-1beta and IFN-gamma induce the expression of diverse chemokines and IL-15 in human and rat pancreatic islet cells, and in islets from pre-diabetic NOD mice. *Diabetologia,* Vol. 46,No. 2, pp. 255-266.

Cardozo, A. K., Heimberg, H., Heremans, Y. et al. (2001). A comprehensive analysis of cytokine-induced and nuclear factor-kappa B-dependent genes in primary rat pancreatic beta-cells. *J Biol Chem,* Vol. 276,No. 52, pp. 48879-48886.

Chakrabarti, S. K., James, J. C.& Mirmira, R. G. (2002). Quantitative assessment of gene targeting in vitro and in vivo by the pancreatic transcription factor, Pdx1. Importance of chromatin structure in directing promoter binding. *J Biol Chem,* Vol. 277,No. 15, pp. 13286-13293.

Chertow, B. S., Blaner, W. S., Baranetsky, N. G. et al. (1987). Effects of vitamin A deficiency and repletion on rat insulin secretion in vivo and in vitro from isolated islets. *J Clin Invest,* Vol. 79,No. 1, pp. 163-169.

Cnop, M., Welsh, N., Jonas, J. C. et al. (2005). Mechanisms of pancreatic beta-cell death in type 1 and type 2 diabetes: many differences, few similarities. *Diabetes,* Vol. 54 Suppl 2,No. pp. S97-107.

Curry, D. L., Bennett, L. L.& Grodsky, G. M. (1968). Dynamics of insulin secretion by the perfused rat pancreas. *Endocrinology,* Vol. 83,No. 3, pp. 572-584.

d'Emden, M. C., Dunlop, M., Larkins, R. G. et al. (1989). The in vitro effect of 1 alpha,25-dihydroxyvitamin D3 on insulin production by neonatal rat islets. *Biochem Biophys Res Commun,* Vol. 164,No. 1, pp. 413-418.

Dakshinamurti, K. (2005). Biotin--a regulator of gene expression. *J Nutr Biochem,* Vol. 16,No. 7, pp. 419-423.

Dor, Y., Brown, J., Martinez, O. I. et al. (2004). Adult pancreatic beta-cells are formed by self-duplication rather than stem-cell differentiation. *Nature,* Vol. 429,No. 6987, pp. 41-46.

Doyle, M. E.& Egan, J. M. (2003). Pharmacological agents that directly modulate insulin secretion. *Pharmacol Rev,* Vol. 55,No. 1, pp. 105-131.

Easom, R. A. (1999). CaM kinase II: a protein kinase with extraordinary talents germane to insulin exocytosis. *Diabetes,* Vol. 48,No. 4, pp. 675-684.

Eizirik, D. L., Colli, M. L.& Ortis, F. (2009). The role of inflammation in insulitis and beta-cell loss in type 1 diabetes. *Nat Rev Endocrinol,* Vol. 5,No. 4, pp. 219-226.

Fernandez-Mejia, C. (2005). Pharmacological effects of biotin. *J Nutr Biochem,* Vol. 16,No. 7, pp. 424-427.

Filippi, C. M.& von Herrath, M. G. (2007). Islet beta-cell death - fuel to sustain autoimmunity? *Immunity,* Vol. 27,No. 2, pp. 183-185.

Finegood, D. T., Scaglia, L.& Bonner-Weir, S. (1995). Dynamics of beta-cell mass in the growing rat pancreas. Estimation with a simple mathematical model. *Diabetes,* Vol. 44,No. 3, pp. 249-256.

Flat, P. R. (1996) The hormonal and neural control of endocrine pancreatic function; Pickup J, GW, editor. Oxford: Blackwell Science. 9.1-9.15 p.

Flatt, P. R. (2003) The hormonal and neural control of endocrine pancreatic function. In: Pickup, JC& Garteth, W, editors(ed.), *Textbook of Diabetes,* 3rd ed. Malden, MA, USA, Blackwell Publishing Company.

Gembal, M., Gilon, P.& Henquin, J. C. (1992). Evidence that glucose can control insulin release independently from its action on ATP-sensitive K+ channels in mouse B cells. *J Clin Invest,* Vol. 89,No. 4, pp. 1288-1295.

Gomperts, B. D., Kramer, I. M.& Tatham, P. E. R. (2003) Signal Transduction. London, UK: Elsevier Academic Press.

Grapengiesser, E., Salehi, A., Qader, S. S. et al. (2006). Glucose induces glucagon release pulses antisynchronous with insulin and sensitive to purinoceptor inhibition. *Endocrinology,* Vol. 147,No. 7, pp. 3472-3477.

Gremlich, S., Bonny, C., Waeber, G. et al. (1997). Fatty acids decrease IDX-1 expression in rat pancreatic islets and reduce GLUT2, glucokinase, insulin, and somatostatin levels. *J Biol Chem,* Vol. 272,No. 48, pp. 30261-30269.

Hagman, D. K., Hays, L. B., Parazzoli, S. D. et al. (2005). Palmitate inhibits insulin gene expression by altering PDX-1 nuclear localization and reducing MafA expression in isolated rat islets of Langerhans. *J Biol Chem,* Vol. 280,No. 37, pp. 32413-32418.

Han, J.& Liu, Y. Q. Reduction of islet pyruvate carboxylase activity might be related to the development of type 2 diabetes mellitus in Agouti-K mice. *J Endocrinol,* Vol. 204,No. 2, pp. 143-152.

Hasan, N. M., Longacre, M. J., Stoker, S. W. et al. (2008). Impaired anaplerosis and insulin secretion in insulinoma cells caused by small interfering RNA-mediated suppression of pyruvate carboxylase. *J Biol Chem,* Vol. 283,No. 42, pp. 28048-28059.

Henquin, J. C. (2000). Triggering and amplifying pathways of regulation of insulin secretion by glucose. *Diabetes,* Vol. 49,No. 11, pp. 1751-1760.

Henquin, J. C. (2009). Regulation of insulin secretion: a matter of phase control and amplitude modulation. *Diabetologia,* Vol. 52,No. 5, pp. 739-751.

Herrmann, C., Goke, R., Richter, G. et al. (1995). Glucagon-like peptide-1 and glucose-dependent insulin-releasing polypeptide plasma levels in response to nutrients. *Digestion,* Vol. 56,No. 2, pp. 117-126.

Hiriart, M.& Aguilar-Bryan, L. (2008). Channel regulation of glucose sensing in the pancreatic beta-cell. *Am J Physiol Endocrinol Metab,* Vol. 295,No. 6, pp. E1298-1306.

Holick, M. F. (2003). Vitamin D: A millenium perspective. *J Cell Biochem,* Vol. 88,No. 2, pp. 296-307.

Holland, A. M., Gonez, L. J., Naselli, G. et al. (2005). Conditional expression demonstrates the role of the homeodomain transcription factor Pdx1 in maintenance and regeneration of beta-cells in the adult pancreas. *Diabetes,* Vol. 54,No. 9, pp. 2586-2595.

Idevall-Hagren, O., Barg, S., Gylfe, E. et al. (2010). cAMP mediators of pulsatile insulin secretion from glucose-stimulated single beta-cells. *J Biol Chem,* Vol. 285,No. 30, pp. 23007-23018.

Jitrapakdee, S., Wutthisathapornchai, A., Wallace, J. C. et al. (2010). Regulation of insulin secretion: role of mitochondrial signalling. *Diabetologia,* Vol. 53,No. 6, pp. 1019-1032

Johnson, J. A., Grande, J. P., Roche, P. C. et al. (1994). Immunohistochemical localization of the 1,25(OH)2D3 receptor and calbindin D28k in human and rat pancreas. *Am J Physiol,* Vol. 267,No. 3 Pt 1, pp. E356-360.

Johnson, J. D., Bernal-Mizrachi, E., Alejandro, E. U. et al. (2006). Insulin protects islets from apoptosis via Pdx1 and specific changes in the human islet proteome. *Proc Natl Acad Sci U S A,* Vol. 103,No. 51, pp. 19575-19580.

Jones, P. M.& Persaud, S. J. (1998). Protein kinases, protein phosphorylation, and the regulation of insulin secretion from pancreatic beta-cells. *Endocr Rev,* Vol. 19,No. 4, pp. 429-461.

Kahn, S. E., Hull, R. L.& Utzschneider, K. M. (2006). Mechanisms linking obesity to insulin resistance and type 2 diabetes. *Nature,* Vol. 444,No. 7121, pp. 840-846.

Kaminitz, A., Stein, J., Yaniv, I. et al. (2007). The vicious cycle of apoptotic beta-cell death in type 1 diabetes. *Immunol Cell Biol,* Vol. 85,No. 8, pp. 582-589.

Kaneto, H., Nakatani, Y., Kawamori, D. et al. (2006). Role of oxidative stress, endoplasmic reticulum stress, and c-Jun N-terminal kinase in pancreatic beta-cell dysfunction and insulin resistance. *Int J Biochem Cell Biol,* Vol. 38,No. 5-6, pp. 782-793.

Kar, S.& Shankar Ray, D. (2005). Sustained simultaneous glycolytic and insulin oscillations in beta-cells. *J Theor Biol,* Vol. 237,No. 1, pp. 58-66.

Kassem, S. A., Ariel, I., Thornton, P. S. et al. (2000). Beta-cell proliferation and apoptosis in the developing normal human pancreas and in hyperinsulinism of infancy. *Diabetes,* Vol. 49,No. 8, pp. 1325-1333.

Kawai, K., Yokota, C., Ohashi, S. et al. (1995). Evidence that glucagon stimulates insulin secretion through its own receptor in rats. *Diabetologia,* Vol. 38,No. 3, pp. 274-276.

Kibbey, R. G., Pongratz, R. L., Romanelli, A. J. et al. (2007). Mitochondrial GTP regulates glucose-stimulated insulin secretion. *Cell Metab,* Vol. 5,No. 4, pp. 253-264.

Kim, S. K.& Hebrok, M. (2001). Intercellular signals regulating pancreas development and function. *Genes Dev,* Vol. 15,No. 2, pp. 111-127.

Krueger, K. A., Bhatt, H., Landt, M. et al. (1997). Calcium-stimulated phosphorylation of MAP-2 in pancreatic betaTC3-cells is mediated by Ca2+/calmodulin-dependent kinase II. *J Biol Chem,* Vol. 272,No. 43, pp. 27464-27469.

Kulkarni, R. N., Jhala, U. S., Winnay, J. N. et al. (2004). PDX-1 haploinsufficiency limits the compensatory islet hyperplasia that occurs in response to insulin resistance. *J Clin Invest,* Vol. 114,No. 6, pp. 828-836.

Kushner, J. A., Ye, J., Schubert, M. et al. (2002). Pdx1 restores beta cell function in Irs2 knockout mice. *J Clin Invest,* Vol. 109,No. 9, pp. 1193-1201.

Laychock, S. G., Modica, M. E.& Cavanaugh, C. T. (1991). L-arginine stimulates cyclic guanosine 3',5'-monophosphate formation in rat islets of Langerhans and RINm5F insulinoma cells: evidence for L-arginine:nitric oxide synthase. *Endocrinology,* Vol. 129,No. 6, pp. 3043-3052.

Lazo-de-la-Vega-Monroy, M. L.& Fernandez-Mejia, C. (2009). [Transcription factors in the adult beta cell]. *Rev Invest Clin,* Vol. 61,No. 5, pp. 428-446.

Lu, D., Mulder, H., Zhao, P. et al. (2002). 13C NMR isotopomer analysis reveals a connection between pyruvate cycling and glucose-stimulated insulin secretion (GSIS). *Proc Natl Acad Sci U S A,* Vol. 99,No. 5, pp. 2708-2713.

MacDonald, M. J. (1995). Influence of glucose on pyruvate carboxylase expression in pancreatic islets. *Arch Biochem Biophys,* Vol. 319,No. 1, pp. 128-132.

Maechler, P.& Wollheim, C. B. (1999). Mitochondrial glutamate acts as a messenger in glucose-induced insulin exocytosis. *Nature,* Vol. 402,No. 6762, pp. 685-689.

Maechler, P.& Wollheim, C. B. (2001). Mitochondrial function in normal and diabetic beta-cells. *Nature,* Vol. 414,No. 6865, pp. 807-812.

Mathis, D., Vence, L.& Benoist, C. (2001). beta-Cell death during progression to diabetes. *Nature,* Vol. 414,No. 6865, pp. 792-798.

Matschinsky, F. M. (1996). Banting Lecture 1995. A lesson in metabolic regulation inspired by the glucokinase glucose sensor paradigm. *Diabetes,* Vol. 45,No. 2, pp. 223-241.

Matsumoto, K., Fukunaga, K., Miyazaki, J. et al. (1995). Ca2+/calmodulin-dependent protein kinase II and synapsin I-like protein in mouse insulinoma MIN6 cells. *Endocrinology,* Vol. 136,No. 9, pp. 3784-3793.

McClenaghan, N. H., Barnett, C. R.& Flatt, P. R. (1998). Na+ cotransport by metabolizable and nonmetabolizable amino acids stimulates a glucose-regulated insulin-secretory response. *Biochem Biophys Res Commun,* Vol. 249,No. 2, pp. 299-303.

Meier, J. J., Butler, A. E., Saisho, Y. et al. (2008). Beta-cell replication is the primary mechanism subserving the postnatal expansion of beta-cell mass in humans. *Diabetes,* Vol. 57,No. 6, pp. 1584-1594.

Melloul, D., Marshak, S.& Cerasi, E. (2002). Regulation of insulin gene transcription. *Diabetologia,* Vol. 45,No. 3, pp. 309-326.

Montanya, E., Nacher, V., Biarnes, M. et al. (2000). Linear correlation between beta-cell mass and body weight throughout the lifespan in Lewis rats: role of beta-cell hyperplasia and hypertrophy. *Diabetes,* Vol. 49,No. 8, pp. 1341-1346.

Navarro-Tableros, V., Sanchez-Soto, M. C., Garcia, S. et al. (2004). Autocrine regulation of single pancreatic beta-cell survival. *Diabetes,* Vol. 53,No. 8, pp. 2018-2023.

Newsholme, P., Gaudel, C.& McClenaghan, N. H. (2010). Nutrient regulation of insulin secretion and beta-cell functional integrity. *Adv Exp Med Biol,* Vol. 654,No. pp. 91-114.

Newsholme, P., Bender, K., Kiely, A. et al. (2007a). Amino acid metabolism, insulin secretion and diabetes. *Biochem Soc Trans,* Vol. 35,No. Pt 5, pp. 1180-1186.

Newsholme, P., Keane, D., Welters, H. J. et al. (2007b). Life and death decisions of the pancreatic beta-cell: the role of fatty acids. *Clin Sci (Lond),* Vol. 112,No. 1, pp. 27-42.

Nielander, H. B., Onofri, F., Valtorta, F. et al. (1995). Phosphorylation of VAMP/synaptobrevin in synaptic vesicles by endogenous protein kinases. *J Neurochem,* Vol. 65,No. 4, pp. 1712-1720.

Nolan, C. J., Madiraju, M. S., Delghingaro-Augusto, V. et al. (2006). Fatty acid signaling in the beta-cell and insulin secretion. *Diabetes,* Vol. 55 Suppl 2,No. pp. S16-23.

Norman, A. W. (2006). Minireview: vitamin D receptor: new assignments for an already busy receptor. *Endocrinology,* Vol. 147,No. 12, pp. 5542-5548.

Norman, A. W., Henry, H. L., Bishop, J. E. et al. (2001). Different shapes of the steroid hormone 1alpha,25(OH)(2)-vitamin D(3) act as agonists for two different receptors in the vitamin D endocrine system to mediate genomic and rapid responses. *Steroids,* Vol. 66,No. 3-5, pp. 147-158.

Odegaard, M. L., Joseph, J. W., Jensen, M. V. et al. (2010). The mitochondrial 2-oxoglutarate carrier is part of a metabolic pathway that mediates glucose- and glutamine-stimulated insulin secretion. *J Biol Chem,* Vol. 285,No. 22, pp. 16530-16537.

Olson, L. K., Redmon, J. B., Towle, H. C. et al. (1993). Chronic exposure of HIT cells to high glucose concentrations paradoxically decreases insulin gene transcription and alters binding of insulin gene regulatory protein. *J Clin Invest,* Vol. 92,No. 1, pp. 514-519.

Parnaud, G., Bosco, D., Berney, T. et al. (2008). Proliferation of sorted human and rat beta cells. *Diabetologia,* Vol. 51,No. 1, pp. 91-100.

Paul, P. K.& Duttagupta, P. N. (1976). The effect of an acute dose of biotin at a post-implantation stage and its relation with female sex steriods in the rat. *J Nutr Sci Vitaminol (Tokyo),* Vol. 22,No. 3, pp. 181-186.

Perl, S., Kushner, J. A., Buchholz, B. A. et al. (2010). Significant human beta-cell turnover is limited to the first three decades of life as determined by in vivo thymidine analog incorporation and radiocarbon dating. *J Clin Endocrinol Metab,* Vol. 95,No. 10, pp. E234-239.

Persaud, S. J., Muller, D.& Jones, P. M. (2008). Insulin signalling in islets. *Biochem Soc Trans,* Vol. 36,No. Pt 3, pp. 290-293.

Prentki, M., Vischer, S., Glennon, M. C. et al. (1992). Malonyl-CoA and long chain acyl-CoA esters as metabolic coupling factors in nutrient-induced insulin secretion. *J Biol Chem,* Vol. 267,No. 9, pp. 5802-5810.

Raum, J. C., Gerrish, K., Artner, I. et al. (2006). FoxA2, Nkx2.2, and PDX-1 regulate islet beta-cell-specific mafA expression through conserved sequences located between base pairs -8118 and -7750 upstream from the transcription start site. *Mol Cell Biol,* Vol. 26,No. 15, pp. 5735-5743.

Rhodes, C. J. (2005). Type 2 diabetes-a matter of beta-cell life and death? *Science,* Vol. 307,No. 5708, pp. 380-384.

Rodriguez-Melendez, R.& Zempleni, J. (2003). Regulation of gene expression by biotin (review). *J Nutr Biochem,* Vol. 14,No. 12, pp. 680-690.

Romero-Navarro, G., Cabrera-Valladares, G., German, M. S. et al. (1999). Biotin regulation of pancreatic glucokinase and insulin in primary cultured rat islets and in biotin-deficient rats. *Endocrinology,* Vol. 140,No. 10, pp. 4595-4600.

Rorsman, P.& Renstrom, E. (2003). Insulin granule dynamics in pancreatic beta cells. *Diabetologia,* Vol. 46,No. 8, pp. 1029-1045.

Russell, M. A.& Morgan, N. (2010). Expression and functional roles of guanylate cyclase isoforms in BRIN-BD11 beta-cells. *Islets,* Vol. 2,No. 6, pp. 23-31.

Salehi, A., Flodgren, E., Nilsson, N. E. et al. (2005). Free fatty acid receptor 1 (FFA(1)R/GPR40) and its involvement in fatty-acid-stimulated insulin secretion. *Cell Tissue Res,* Vol. 322,No. 2, pp. 207-215.

Schmidt, H. H., Warner, T. D., Ishii, K. et al. (1992). Insulin secretion from pancreatic B cells caused by L-arginine-derived nitrogen oxides. *Science,* Vol. 255,No. 5045, pp. 721-723.

Sharp, G. W. (1979). The adenylate cyclase-cyclic AMP system in islets of Langerhans and its role in the control of insulin release. *Diabetologia,* Vol. 16,No. 5, pp. 287-296.

Shibasaki, T., Takahashi, H., Miki, T. et al. (2007). Essential role of Epac2/Rap1 signaling in regulation of insulin granule dynamics by cAMP. *Proc Natl Acad Sci U S A,* Vol. 104,No. 49, pp. 19333-19338.

Simmins, P. H.& Brooks, P. H. (1983). Supplementary biotin for sows: effect on reproductive characteristics. *Vet Rec,* Vol. 112,No. 18, pp. 425-429.

Sone, H., Ito, M., Sugiyama, K. et al. (1999). Biotin enhances glucose-stimulated insulin secretion in the isolated perfused pancreas of the rat. *J Nutr Biochem,* Vol. 10,No. 4, pp. 237-243.

Sone, H., Ito, M., Shimizu, M. et al. (2000). Characteristics of the biotin enhancement of glucose-induced insulin release in pancreatic islets of the rat. *Biosci Biotechnol Biochem,* Vol. 64,No. 3, pp. 550-554.

Song, G., Ouyang, G.& Bao, S. (2005). The activation of Akt/PKB signaling pathway and cell survival. *J Cell Mol Med,* Vol. 9,No. 1, pp. 59-71.

Soria, B., Quesada, I., Ropero, A. B. et al. (2004). Novel players in pancreatic islet signaling: from membrane receptors to nuclear channels. *Diabetes,* Vol. 53 Suppl 1,No. pp. S86-91.

Srikanta, S., Ganda, O. P., Jackson, R. A. et al. (1983). Type I diabetes mellitus in monozygotic twins: chronic progressive beta cell dysfunction. *Ann Intern Med,* Vol. 99,No. 3, pp. 320-326.

Stagner, J. I., Samols, E.& Weir, G. C. (1980). Sustained oscillations of insulin, glucagon, and somatostatin from the isolated canine pancreas during exposure to a constant glucose concentration. *J Clin Invest,* Vol. 65,No. 4, pp. 939-942.

Strandell, E., Eizirik, D. L.& Sandler, S. (1990). Reversal of beta-cell suppression in vitro in pancreatic islets isolated from nonobese diabetic mice during the phase preceding insulin-dependent diabetes mellitus. *J Clin Invest,* Vol. 85,No. 6, pp. 1944-1950.

Straub, S. G.& Sharp, G. W. (2002). Glucose-stimulated signaling pathways in biphasic insulin secretion. *Diabetes Metab Res Rev,* Vol. 18,No. 6, pp. 451-463.

Straub, S. G.& Sharp, G. W. (2004). Hypothesis: one rate-limiting step controls the magnitude of both phases of glucose-stimulated insulin secretion. *Am J Physiol Cell Physiol,* Vol. 287,No. 3, pp. C565-571.

Thomas, H., Jaschkowitz, K., Bulman, M. et al. (2001). A distant upstream promoter of the HNF-4alpha gene connects the transcription factors involved in maturity-onset diabetes of the young. *Hum Mol Genet,* Vol. 10,No. 19, pp. 2089-2097.

Vilches-Flores, A., Tovar, A. R., Marin-Hernandez, A. et al. (2009). Biotin increases glucokinase expression via soluble guanylate cyclase/protein kinase G, adenosine triphosphate production and autocrine action of insulin in pancreatic rat islets. *J Nutr Biochem,* Vol. No. pp.

Wang, H., Iezzi, M., Theander, S. et al. (2005). Suppression of Pdx-1 perturbs proinsulin processing, insulin secretion and GLP-1 signalling in INS-1 cells. *Diabetologia,* Vol. 48,No. 4, pp. 720-731.

Watanabe, T. (1996). Morphological and biochemical effects of excessive amounts of biotin on embryonic development in mice. *Experientia,* Vol. 52,No. 2, pp. 149-154.

Weir, G. C.& Bonner-Weir, S. (2010). Dreams for type 1 diabetes: shutting off autoimmunity and stimulating beta-cell regeneration. *Endocrinology,* Vol. 151,No. 7, pp. 2971-2973.

Xu, G. G.& Rothenberg, P. L. (1998). Insulin receptor signaling in the beta-cell influences insulin gene expression and insulin content: evidence for autocrine beta-cell regulation. *Diabetes,* Vol. 47,No. 8, pp. 1243-1252.

Xu, J., Han, J., Long, Y. S. et al. (2008). The role of pyruvate carboxylase in insulin secretion and proliferation in rat pancreatic beta cells. *Diabetologia,* Vol. 51,No. 11, pp. 2022-2030.

Xu, X., D'Hoker, J., Stange, G. et al. (2008). Beta cells can be generated from endogenous progenitors in injured adult mouse pancreas. *Cell,* Vol. 132,No. 2, pp. 197-207.

Yaney, G. C.& Corkey, B. E. (2003). Fatty acid metabolism and insulin secretion in pancreatic beta cells. *Diabetologia,* Vol. 46,No. 10, pp. 1297-1312.

Zempleni, J. (2005). Uptake, localization, and noncarboxylase roles of biotin. *Annu Rev Nutr,* Vol. 25,No. pp. 175-196.

Zhang, C. L., Katoh, M., Shibasaki, T. et al. (2009). The cAMP sensor Epac2 is a direct target of antidiabetic sulfonylurea drugs. *Science,* Vol. 325,No. 5940, pp. 607-610.

6

Steady-State Cell Apoptosis and Immune Tolerance - Induction of Tolerance Using Apoptotic Cells in Type 1 Diabetes and Other Immune-Mediated Disorders

Chang-Qing Xia[1], Kim Campbell[2],
Benjamin Keselowsky[3] and Michael Clare-Salzler[1]
[1]*Department of Pathology, Immunology and Laboratory Medicine, University of Florida*
[2]*Therakos*
[3]*Department Bioengineering, University of Florida*
USA

1. Introduction

Type 1 diabetes (T1D) is also named insulin-dependent diabetes mellitus. Because T1D is more frequently seen in children, it is also called juvenile diabetes. Currently the standard treatment for T1D is the daily use of exogenous insulin. Because of the poor compliance with insulin use, T1D patients often suffer from hyperglycemia or hypoglycemia (1; 2). In addition, T1D patients are at high risk for experiencing ketoacidosis due to a variety of different reasons (3-5). Many T1D patients will inevitably develop serious, chronic complications in organs such as heart and kidney (6-9). Therefore, T1D is a devastating disease for young individuals. Thus far, there has been no cure for T1D, and the search for its cure is a long-term goal in T1D research.

Regarding the pathogenesis of T1D, it is clear that T1D is an autoimmune disease that is mediated by pathogenic T cell responses to pancreatic islet β cells (10-12). The fundamental problem in T1D is the breakdown of immune tolerance to self antigens. More specifically, β cell antigen-specific T cells, which are usually well controlled in healthy individuals through various self tolerance mechanisms, attack insulin-producing β cells. Thus, to cure T1D, restoration of immune tolerance against β cell antigens is necessary. Numerous investigators have expended tremendous energy and efforts in finding ways to prevent or cure T1D; however, much work still remains.

During fetal development, the majority of self-reactive T cell clones are deleted in the thymus. This process is referred to as central tolerance. Some self-reactive T cell clones do escape T cell deletion mechanisms and are exported to the periphery, leading to a potential risk for development of autoimmune diseases. In healthy individuals, self-reactive T cell clones are not pathogenic, because of well-functioning peripheral regulatory mechanisms (13; 14). One of the major mechanisms by which self tolerance is maintained is through the steady-state processing of apoptotic cells during normal tissue turnover (14). Evidence has shown that the impaired processing of apoptotic cells is associated with the pathogenesis of systemic lupus erythematosus (15; 16). In this chapter, we will focus on discussing the relationship between steady-state cell apoptosis and self-tolerance maintenance. In addition, we will discuss β cell apoptosis and T1D pathogenesis as well as the application of intravenous apoptotic cell delivery in restoring immune tolerance in T1D and other immune-mediated disorders.

2. Steady-state cell apoptosis and immune tolerance

2.1 Steady-state apoptosis

The effective clearance of apoptotic cells and subsequent regeneration of cells is crucial in organ development, tissue homeostasis, response to injury, and maintenance of the innate and adaptive immune system (17). In the spleen and liver, greater than 1 X 10^{11} circulating neutrophils are eliminated each day. The vast majority (95%) of thymocytes die by apoptosis due to negative selection. Another example exists in the retina where photoreceptor rods continuously renew their light-sensitive outer segments (17). The reality is that almost every cell in our bodies is replaced during a lifetime, and some types of cells turnover more than once. It was once thought that clearance of apoptotic cells was immunologically inert, but we now know that the uptake of apoptotic cells by phagocytes can induce immunosuppression or tolerance (discussed in greater detail below). Interestingly, some pathogens (*Plasmodium falciparum*) and tumors exploit the immune inhibitory pathways involved in apoptotic cell clearance to aid in their survival and perseverance in the body (17). Cell death and the ensuing removal of dying cells by phagocytes can have profound regulatory effects on the immune system.

2.2 Immature dendrite cells (DCs) and macrophages engulf apoptotic cells during tissue cell turnover

The fate of hundreds of millions of apoptotic tissue cells that die each day is to be engulfed as quickly as possible by antigen-presenting cells, especially immature dendritic cells and macrophages. DCs distributed in the peripheral tissues are able to sense "find-me" signals elicited by the apoptotic cells (18-23). DCs migrate toward the dying cells then bind the apoptotic cells through recognition of "eat-me" signals on their surface (20; 22; 24-26). After phagocytosing apoptotic cells, DCs home to the T cell zone of local draining lymph nodes where they present self tissue antigens in a tolerogenic fashion to self antigen-reactive T cells that have escaped from the thymus. The various mechanisms will be discussed in the following sections.

2.3 Dendritic cells acquire a tolerogenic phenotype following phagocytosis of apoptotic cells

DCs interact with apoptotic cells through specific receptors that can recognize molecules uniquely expressed on the apoptotic cell surface. Early studies demonstrated that DCs that had engulfed apoptotic cells were able to maintain an immature state as evidenced by low expression levels of major histocompatibility complex (MHC) molecules and co-stimulatory molecules such as CD80, CD86 (27; 28). More importantly, these DCs resisted maturation induction by lipopolysaccharide or CD40L. When these immature DCs presented antigens to the antigen-specific T cells, the latter became unresponsive to subsequent stimulation by the same antigens (29; 30). The mechanisms underlying this process were unclear, but the recent discovery of TAM (Tyro-3-Axl-Mer) receptors on DCs or macrophages that specifically recognize ligands on apoptotic cells may help unravel the mystery (31). TAM receptors directly or indirectly interact with apoptotic cell surface molecules and work together with cytokines to transduce suppressive signals in DCs or macrophages (31). TAM receptors play important roles in regulating innate immunity, helping to avoid unwanted autoimmunity. It is worth mentioning here that DCs interacting with apoptotic cells may become immunogenic under certain circumstances (32; 33). An elegant study demonstrated that DCs phagocytosing bacteria-infected apoptotic cells became fully mature, showing strong T cell stimulatory activity, and induced inflammatory Th17 cells; whereas, DCs that had engulfed non-infected apoptotic cells acquired tolerogenic properties, inducing Foxp3+ regulatory T cells (33). This study suggests that following phagocytosis of dead cells during infections or inflammatory conditions, DCs or other antigen-presenting cells may actually trigger activation of self-reactive T cells, which may lead to autoimmunity or autoimmune disorders. More details regarding immunogeneic and tolerogenic cell death were discussed recently (review by Green, et al) (32).

2.4 TGF-β is an important cytokine participating in immune tolerance induced by apoptotic cells

Several cytokines produced during the clearance of apoptotic cells are associated with the induction of tolerance. In particular, TGF-β is important in this process. TGF-β is an immunosuppressive cytokine that can be produced by apoptotic cells but more importantly, is secreted by DCs or macrophages that have phagocytosed apoptotic cells (34-37). Recently, TGF- β has been identified as an essential cytokine for the differentiation of adaptive Foxp3+ regulatory T cells (Tregs) (38; 39). Tregs play an important role in maintaining peripheral tolerance (40). Thus, increased levels of TGF-β produced during the processing of apoptotic cells likely contributes to apoptotic cell-induced tolerance through generation of Tregs. A recent report supplied evidence to support this idea by demonstrating that TGF-β is essential for anti-CD3 antibody treatment-induced autoantigen-specific tolerance in experimental autoimmune encephalomyelitis (EAE) (41). In this report, the authors clearly demonstrated that macrophages ingesting apoptotic T cells produced high levels of TGF-β, which subsequently induced Treg production, and consequently, EAE was prevented. However, under conditions where DCs and macrophages were depleted, the effect of anti-CD3 therapy was drastically compromised in preventing EAE because of the reduced levels of systemic TGF-β and Tregs (41). Hence, the local or systemic levels of TGF- β may be an important factor in determining the immunological outcomes associated with engulfment of apoptotic cells.

2.5 Phosphatidylserine on apoptotic cells mediates immunosuppression

The recognition of apoptotic cells by phagocytes involves highly specific receptor-ligand interactions. In the synapse between a phagocyte and an apoptotic cell, multiple Apoptotic Cell-Associated Molecular Patterns (ACMP) presented on the apoptotic cell surface interact with Pattern-Recognition Receptors (PRR) that are expressed by the phagocyte (42). One of the earliest events in apoptosis is the "flip-flop" and external exposure of the anionic phospholipid phosphatidylserine (PS), which is normally restricted to the inner leaflet of the plasma membrane. PS is an important "eat-me" signal that stimulates apoptotic cell phagocytosis by DCs or macrophages. PS recognition receptors can either bind PS directly or bind indirectly through soluble bridging molecules. Receptors that directly interact with PS include members of the TIM (T cell immunoglobulin domain and mucin domain) family (43-49), BAI1, the seven transmembrane brain angiogenesis inhibitor 1(50), and the atypical EGF-motif containing membrane protein Stabilin-2 (20). MFG-E8 has been identified as a bridging molecule that can simultaneously bind PS on apoptotic cells with high affinity (51-54) and engage integrin αvβ3 on phagocytes. Gas6 (growth arrest specific gene 6) and protein S bridge PS to TAM family of receptors on phagocytes (31). Additional membrane proteins important in binding apoptotic cells include CD36, CD14, CD68, and thrombospondins (55-58). It is believed that PS receptors not only help to physically tether the apoptotic cells to the phagocytes but also generate intracellular signals that stimulate endocytosis. Important for the induction of tolerance, binding of PS to its receptor MerTK on DCs or macrophages induces downstream signals which result in down-regulation of NF-kB and inhibition of pro-inflammatory cytokine production (59-61). It has also been reported that PS through the bridging molecule Gas6 protein binds to AXL/Mer family members to suppress NK-kB activation and inflammatory mediators such as IL-1 and iNOS (62). Recently, it was shown monocyte-derived DCs incubated with PS liposomes assumed immature DC characteristics and were unable to stimulate T cells (63; 64). Our data showed that water-soluble PS (C6) dramatically inhibited T cell proliferation in response to stimulatory anti-CD3 and anti-CD28 antibodies (Xia, unpublished data). We also discovered that PS could be released from apoptotic cells, as supernatants from apoptotic cells efficiently blocked anti-PS antibody binding to apoptotic cells (xia, unpublished data). Therefore, PS has proven to be an important factor in apoptotic cell-induced immunosuppression.

3. β cell apoptosis and type 1 diabetes pathogenesis

It has been widely accepted that diabetes, including T1D and T2D, is associated with excess death of pancreatic β cells. However, evidence that pancreatic β cells undergo a wave of cell death in the early age of normal individuals suggests that early β cell death may be beneficial for avoiding autoimmunity. In line with this, results from an animal study demonstrated that induction of β cell death at an early age in NOD mice protected the animals from developing T1D (65). Despite contradictions, β cell death may play distinct and different roles in autoimmune processes depending on the environment where β cell death occurs. The following will discuss β cell apoptosis and T1D pathogenesis in hopes of clarifying certain issues that are clouded in confusion.

3.1 Two waves of β cell death in T1D

Animal studies have shown that pancreatic β cells only undergo a single wave of β cell death at an early age in normal strains of animals, whereas, in T1D prone animals, there are two waves of β cell death. The first wave occurs at ages similar to normal strains, yet, the second wave of β cell death follows a few weeks later (66; 67). The second wave of β cell death is thought to be mediated by autoimmune attack (66; 68). However, it is still unclear whether the first wave of β cell death is associated with the second wave, and why the second wave of β cell death occurs only in T1D prone animals. A few lines of evidence show that inefficient processing of dead β cells at an early age might contribute to the development of autoimmune responses in the pancreatic islets (66; 67). Unfortunately, the role of early β cell death in T1D pathogenesis remains poorly understood.

3.2 β cell death in self tolerance or autoimmunity

While both environmental and genetic risk factors contribute to the susceptibility of an individual to T1D, the exact mechanisms that initiate T1D autoimmunity remain elusive (69). Accumulating evidence supports the idea that the exposure of β cell antigens resulting from early β cell death may be an initiating factor. If this is really the initiating factor, why does autoimmunity only occur in T1D prone animals but not in normal strains? As we discussed earlier, apoptotic cells are immediately processed by phagocytes in vivo in order to maintain self tolerance. A key in this process is the quick and efficient clearance of apoptotic cells after early stages of cell apoptosis, which prevents reactions to self-antigens. Otherwise, the apoptotic cells may advance to late stage apoptosis or to a necrotic stage at which point the dead cells may cause inflammatory responses and potentially lead to autoimmune disorders, such as SLE, as mentioned previously. It has been reported that in T1D animal models, phagocytes are defective in efficiently clearing apoptotic β cells during the first wave of islet β cell death (66). Failure to scavenge dead β cells could potentially initiate β cell antigen-specific autoimmunity, which subsequently leads to recruitment of additional inflammatory cells, including macrophages, DCs, and T cells to the islets to worsen autoimmune damage (68). This hypothesis, however, does not help explain the T1D protection mediated by streptozotocin-induced β cell death in NOD mice at young ages (65). In the study reported by Hugues et al, the authors demonstrated that NOD mice were protected from developing T1D when they were treated at 4 weeks of age with streptozotocin to induce cell death of a limited number of β cells (65). The data in the study also showed that there were more cells infiltrating the islets at an early time after streptozotocin administration, but the islet β cells were eventually protected. These findings suggest that β cell death induced by streptozotocin before autoimmunity begins may modulate autoimmune T cells to become tolerized, thereby protecting from T1D. The mechanisms underlying this protection were not well elucidated, but it is possible that early induction of β cell death creates a microenvironment that is more tolerogenic and characterized by increased TGF-β production by apoptotic β cells or the DCs and macrophages that phagocytose them. A recent report demonstrated that expression of TGF-β on islet β cells actually protected NOD mice from T1D (70), suggesting that local levels of TGF-β may play an essential role in the protection of β cells from autoimmune attack.

Regarding the relationship between β cell death and T1D pathogenesis, more attention has been focused on the investigation as to how innate and adaptive immunity induces β cell death leading to autoimmune diabetes. Based on histological analysis of the pancreas in T1D, DCs and macrophages appear first in the islets (66; 68). Thus, it is believed that DCs and macrophages are two important inflammatory cells in the initiation of autoimmunity. DCs and macrophages not only damage β cells directly through the secretion of pro-inflammatory cytokines such as TNF-α, IL-1, and IL-6, but more importantly, they present β cell antigens to antigen-specific CD4+ and CD8+ T cells, leading to adaptive autoimmune reactions against islet β cells. Preferentially induced Th1 cells in T1D can target β cells through direct killing or by secreting pro-inflammatory cytokines, such as IFN-γ (71). CD8+ cytotoxic T cells may kill β cells via the release of granzymes and perforin (72). Furthermore, soluble inflammatory mediators secreted by DCs, macrophages, or activated T cells, such as IL-1 and IFN-γ, can induce Fas expression on β cells (71; 73; 74). Pancreatic histology of new onset T1D patients has shown that Fas+ β cells are surrounded by FasL+ activated T cells, (75-77) indicating that activated T cells may induce β cell death through FasL-Fas ligation during T cell and β cell interaction. There is still some debate about whether the up-regulation of Fas on β cells is associated with β cell death. Specific deletion of Fas from β cells using Cre-Loxp genetic manipulation leads to normal or slightly reduced incidence of T1D (78). Similar results were obtained with β cells over-expressing a dominant negative form of Fas (79). Another important factor potentially involved in β cell death is oxidative stress occurring in β cells during active inflammation in the local islets. It has been documented that β cells are highly sensitive to oxidative stress because of their inefficiency in making antioxidants (80-82). Streptozotocin and alloxan drug-induced diabetes is thought to be due to overproduction of reactive oxygen species (ROS) induced by the drugs. Supporting the role of ROS in β cell death, a study showed that genetic overexpression of the antioxidant thioredoxin in β cells significantly prevented NOD mice from developing T1D (83). Overexpression of antioxidants such as catalase or metallothionein reduces the susceptibility of β cells to cytokine-induced death in vitro (84-86). Recently, it was demonstrated that ROS participated in inflammatory processes by activating inflammatory cytokines via inflammasome-dependent or inflammasome-independent pathways (87; 88). Inflammatory cytokines such as IL-1 are secondary to oxidative stress and exaggerate β cell damage. Based on what has been described above, it is likely that T1D is a disease caused by multiple factors working together. Once autoimmunity starts, a vicious cycle appears to be initiated until all β cells are destroyed, leading to diabetes.

In summary, β cell death can play completely opposing roles in T1D pathogenesis. Steady-state β cell death that occurs in normal individuals, normal strains of mice or young T1D-prone animals provides protection from T1D. On the other hand, β cell death that occurs under inflammatory conditions seems to accelerate disease progression through exaggerating inflammation. Therefore, any measures capable of breaking this vicious cycle will potentially offer opportunities to restore homeostasis, facilitate self tolerance, and hopefully attenuate or cure T1D.

4. Application of apoptotic cells in immune-mediated disorders

4.1 Extracorporeal photopheresis for the treatment of autoimmune disease

Intravenous delivery of apoptotic cells has been shown to have clinical efficacy in T-cell mediated autoimmune diseases. Extracorporeal photopheresis (ECP) is a novel immunotherapy that involves collecting peripheral blood mononuclear cells from patients and exposing them to a photoactivatable drug that induces programmed cell death or apoptosis. More specifically, the apheresis-based procedure involves connecting a patient through venous access to the THERAKOS™ UVAR™ XTS™ or CELLEX™ photopheresis medical device (shown below). Both photopheresis systems offer a point-of-care, patient connected, sterile, automated centrifugation platform that separates white blood cells from whole blood (89). Once white blood cells are concentrated into a collection bag, 8-methoxypsoralen (8-MOP), a naturally derived furocoumarin compound that readily intercalates into DNA (trade name=UVADEX®), is added and readily absorbs into the cells. 8-MOP-treated cells are then circulated across a photoactivation plate, which is exposed to 1.5-2 Joules/cm^2 of energy from an ultraviolet A (UVA) light source (90). Apoptotic processes are triggered in the treated cells, and they are returned to the patient. ECP is currently approved by the U.S. Food and Drug Administration for the palliative treatment of skin manifestations associated with Cutaneous T cell Lymphoma (CTCL) that is refractory to other forms of therapy. ECP is available worldwide (>150 medical centers) (91) and has been utilized for over 20 years for the treatment of both allo-immune (graft vs host disease, GVHD, and graft rejection) and autoimmune conditions (Crohn's disease, T1D). This therapy is associated with a very rare incidence of serious adverse events and is generally well-tolerated by patients with no significant side effects (90; 92). In a few European countries, an alternative method has been utilized for performing photopheresis. Mononuclear cells are collected with a standard cell separator and UVA irradiation is performed in a laboratory setting using a stand-alone irradiator; however, no commercially available UVA irradiator is compliant with European standards marking for the sale and use of medical devices for performing ECP. While there are chain-of-custody issues and potential risks of infection associated with these 'open' photopheresis systems, there are reports of similar clinical efficacy between both techniques; however, no head-to-head comparison studies have been reported to date (93).

ECP is most commonly used to treat CTCL and GVHD. CTCL is a rare lymphoproliferative disorder characterized by the accumulation of malignant T lymphocytes in the skin. While clinicians have been successfully treating some CTCL patients with ECP monotherapy (94), others use ECP in combination with other therapies to improve outcomes (92). On average, response rates in CTCL range from 33% to 88% with ECP monotherapy; whereas, multimodality ECP response rates are comparable (94). Collectively across 19 studies, a combined overall response rate of 55.7% was reported across all stages of CTCL with 17.6% achieving a complete response (95). ECP is also highly beneficial for the treatment of GVHD. In a prospective phase II study involving steroid-refractory acute GVHD patients, 82% of patients with cutaneous involvement, 61% with liver involvement, and 61% with gut involvement achieved responses after ECP treatments. Interestingly, ECP not only facilitated tapering and eventual discontinuation of corticosteroids in responders but ECP therapy also improved overall survival (96; 97). A retrospective analysis of 71 patients with severe chronic GVHD demonstrated that patients who had received ECP showed an overall response rate of 61%, and complete responses were observed in 20% of patients (98). ECP therapy has also been reported to provide positive clinical outcomes for the treatment of rejection episodes associated with cardiac and lung transplantation (99). In conclusion, published data demonstrate that patients with conditions characterized by overactive inflammation and dysregulation of T cells can realize significant clinical benefit from ECP treatments. ECP seems to restore immune homeostasis without causing general immunosuppression in patients with inflammatory diseases. In fact, ECP-treated patients can respond normally to novel and recall antigenic challenges (100).

4.2 Apoptotic cell infusion and the use of ECP in type 1 diabetes

Intravenous infusion of apoptotic cells can significantly prevent type 1 diabetes in non-obese diabetic mice (101-103). More specifically, weekly delivery of ECP-treated spleen cells significantly delayed the onset of diabetes. The disease protective effects were enhanced when apoptotic cells were injected in combination with β cell antigens as demonstrated by a reduction in insulitis and an increase in Foxp3+ Treg cells. Importantly, infusion of ECP-treated spleen cells did not induce global immunosuppression or exacerbate autoimmune responses in treated mice (101).

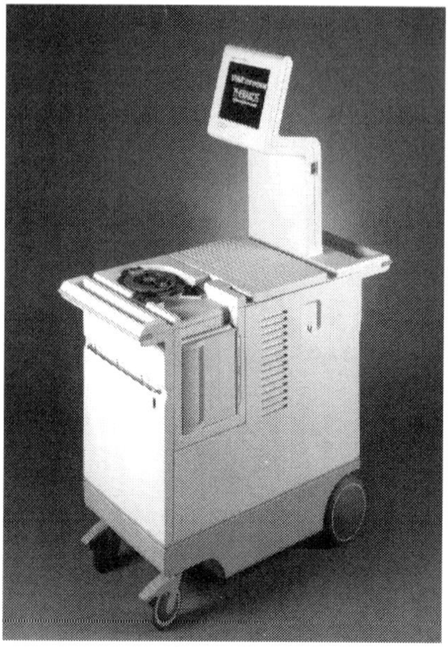

Fig. 1. THERAKOS™ XTS™ Photopheresis instrument

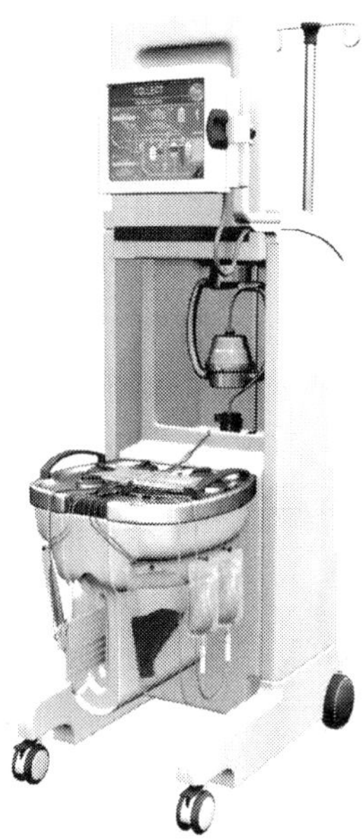

Fig. 2. THERAKOS™ CELLEX™ Photopheresis Instrument

In the clinical setting, positive outcomes have been reported when ECP was used to treat patients with various autoimmune diseases. For instance, ECP has positively modified the disease course in systemic sclerosis, rheumatoid arthritis, atopic dermatitis, and systemic lupus erythematosus due to its ability to modulate immune processes (104). Because T1D is an immune-mediated disease with a defined diagnosis that follows a relatively homogeneous course, Ludvigsson et al (105) conducted a double-blind, randomized, placebo-controlled, prospective study to assess the efficacy of ECP in children newly diagnosed with Type 1 diabetes. A total of 49 patients were enrolled in the study across 3 different pediatric sites in Sweden. A total of 19 kids completed treatment in the active ECP treatment group; whereas, 21 patients completed treatment in the control group. Photopheresis was delivered using the first-generation THERAKOS™ UVAR photopheresis system in combination with an oral formulation of 8-MOP. ECP or sham pheresis was delivered on 2 consecutive days with the first treatment given within 5-6 days after the initial clinical diagnosis, and treatments were repeated after 2, 4, 8 and 12 weeks so that a total of 10 treatments were delivered over a 3 month period. The patients were followed for at least 3 years. Blood glucose levels, C peptide, HbA1c values, and other blood measures were monitored throughout the treatment period as well as during follow-up. Results demonstrate that the group actively treated with ECP had higher C peptide concentrations in the urine during the follow up period compared to the control group. Regarding HbA1c values, the proportion of children with HbA1c <6% was similar in the two groups during the follow up period. Interestingly, insulin doses/kg body weight required for stable blood glucose levels were always lower in the ECP-treated group, except at month 1 when photopheresis treatments were just beginning. The control group was more seriously ill than the ECP group with more weight loss, more ketonuria, higher HbA1c values and lower pH, which provides additional support for the efficacy of ECP in Type 1 diabetes. Collectively, the results from this study show that ECP had a long-term effect on the disease processes associated with diabetes in children, and there was a low frequency of adverse events associated with ECP procedures in this study. While it cannot be argued that the effectiveness of ECP was lower compared to other immune response modifiers, the safety profile of this modality does make it an attractive candidate for treating children with T1D. Since the study was conducted, there have been advances in the formulation of 8-MOP, advances in photopheresis device technology, and advances in the understanding of treatment algorithms and of the mechanism of action of ECP. As a result, additional studies are warranted to determine the optimal utilization of this treatment modality in order to reach its full potential in the T1D clinical setting.

4.3 ECP therapy in rheumatoid arthritis

A pilot study was conducted at Yale University by Malawista et al to investigate the effect of ECP on rheumatoid arthritis (RA) (106). Seven RA patients were treated on 2 consecutive days with ECP at 4 week intervals for 6 months. Joint scores and counts improved in 4 patients after 3 to 4 months of therapy. Responses were maintained for 2 to 3 months after completion of the protocol and no serious or toxic adverse events were reported (106). In a single-blinded, controlled, parallel group multicenter phase III clinical trial, the effect of ECP on joint count, joint score, bilateral grip strength, and physician assessment were compared to treatment with gold. In all categories, the 17 patients treated with ECP showed improvement over the 11 patients treated with gold. Univariate analysis of the results suggests that ECP treated patients responded in a comparable fashion to patients treated with gold(107; 108).

4.4 ECP therapy in crohn's disease

Crohn's disease (CD) and ulcerative colitis (UC) are collectively known as inflammatory bowel disease (IBD) and are chronic inflammatory conditions affecting the gastrointestinal tract in which seemingly innocuous luminal antigens stimulate mucosal $CD4^+$ T cell mediated autoimmune responses in genetically susceptible individuals (109). A delicate balance of inflammation involving pro-inflammatory cytokines (TNF-α, IL-1, IL-6, IL-8, and IL-12) and anti-inflammatory cytokines (IL-4, IL-10, IL-11, and IL-13) occurs at the intestinal mucosa under normal conditions; however, once that balance is perturbed, chronic inflammation characterized by persistent T cell activation ensues. Current treatment guidelines recommend the use of aminosalicylates, glucocorticosteroids, and immunomodulators (azathioprine, 6-mercaptopurine, cyclosporine) to treat UC and CD; however, these medical approaches have limitations in efficacy and safety (110). Emerging therapeutic interventions targeting immunopathogenic mechanisms in CD include anti-TNF biologic therapies (eg. infliximab, etanercept, and adalimumab), inhibitors of proinflammatory cytokine receptors (anti-IL-6R), and anti-leukocyte adhesion therapies (natalizumab); however, long term safety still needs to be fully evaluated (110). Because of its safety and effectiveness in diseases mediated by pathogenic T cell populations, ECP has also been used to treat Crohn's disease.

Reinisch et al (111) reported results from a prospective, open label, single center pilot study conducted in 10 patients to assess the efficacy of ECP in the treatment of steroid-dependent Crohn's disease. Response was observed in 8 of 10 patients after a median time of 10 weeks (range 8-19 weeks), and remission was seen in 4 of these patients after a median time of 20 weeks (range 19-23 weeks). Steroid maintenance doses were significantly reduced from baseline, and improvements in clinical performance and quality of life were observed in responding patients. Mean C-reactive protein (CRP) declined and intestinal permeability in patients with ileal and ileocolonic Crohn's disease decreased after ECP.

Recently, a phase II study investigating ECP in 28 patients with moderately active CD who were refractory or intolerant to immunosuppressants and/or anti-TNF agents was completed (112). ECP was performed twice weekly for 4 weeks then twice weekly every other week until week 12. Primary efficacy assessment was a decrease in Crohn's Disease Activity Index (CDAI) of > 100 from baseline or CDAI <150 at week 12. A clinical response was obtained in 14 of 28 (50%) patients, 13 of whom responded by week 6. Remission was observed in 7 of 28 patients who also had a CDAI reduction of over 200 points. Seven of 14 patients who were intolerant or refractory to anti-TNF agents responded to ECP. ECP was well-tolerated with minor serious adverse events reported. The investigators concluded that ECP is safe and beneficial for patients with moderately active Crohn's Disease that is refractory to immunosuppression and/or anti-TNF therapies.

4.5 ECP therapy in other autoimmune conditions

In pilot studies, patients with atopic dermatitis, multiple sclerosis, pemphigus vulgaris, and systemic sclerosis have acheived promising results when treated with ECP (92); however, further investigation through large, prospective clinical studies is required in order to fully understand the utility of this complex therapeutic approach in treating autoimmune conditions.

5. Immunological consequences of apoptotic cell clearance

5.1 Apoptotic cells modulate dendritic cell function

To limit unnecessary collateral damage in healthy tissue, apoptotic cells are rapidly and efficiently removed or cleared by both professional (dendritic cells and macrophages) and non-professional (cells localized near the dying cell, eg., primary lens epithelial cells, astrocytes, microglia) phagocytes (113). As mentioned previously, apoptotic cells can potentially be immunogenic and prime immune responses. In this section, we will only focus on the role of apoptotic cells in the induction of tolerance.

Apoptotic cell clearance plays a critical role in the maintenance of central and peripheral self-tolerance because 1) removal of cell corpses prevents the release of potentially immunogenic intracellular materials from dying cells and 2) phagocytes present self-antigens derived from apoptotic cells to T cells in the draining lymph nodes, which leads to deletion or anergy of self-reactive T cells. Dendritic cells, in particular, play an important role in these ongoing self-tolerance mechanisms (114). While there are several factors involved in the induction of immunological tolerance, the generation of regulatory T cells by DCs that have ingested apoptotic cells is a critical aspect of peripheral self-tolerance (115-117).

Apoptotic cells exert immunosuppressive effects when they are engulfed by phagocytes by modulating cytokine secretion profiles, blocking maturation, and inducing Tregs (118). Voll et al (119) were the first to report that the presence of apoptotic cells during monocyte activation increases the ability of these cells to secrete anti-inflammatory cytokines (IL-10) and decreases their ability to release pro-inflammatory cytokines (TNF-α, IL-1, and IL-12). Our data demonstrate similar results can be obtained *in vitro* when human monocyte-derived dendritic cells are incubated with ECP-treated cells prior to or during activation (unpublished data). In a mouse model of allogeneic bone marrow engraftment, intravenous infusion of apoptotic cells exerted their immunoregulatory functions through TGF-β dependent Treg induction which required host macrophages (34; 41). In fact, TGF-β is mostly responsible for the immunomodulatory effects of apoptotic cells by creating a suppressive microenvironment (34; 120-122). Not only do apoptotic cells regulate TGF-β secretion but engulfment of apoptotic neutrophils has been shown to reduce the ability of DCs to secrete IL-23 (123), which is involved in the differentiation of Th17 lymphocytes and may reciprocally affect Treg cell expansion (124). In addition to modulating cytokine production, engulfment of apoptotic cells reduces the ability of DCs to stimulate effector immune responses by decreasing the levels of co-stimulatory surface molecule expression and by inhibiting maturation even after an inflammatory challenge. In humans, Lamioni et al showed that the apoptotic leukocytes are cleared by antigen-presenting cells *in vivo* leading to the differentiation of antigen-presenting cells towards a more tolerogenic phenotype (125). Collectively, evidence suggests that upon engagement and engulfment of apoptotic cells, there is an increase in anti-inflammatory cytokines, a reduction of pro-inflammatory cytokines, and a diminution in the stimulatory capacity by APCs, which results in suppression of inflammation and cell-mediated immunity, eliciting immune tolerance (89).

5.2 Apoptotic cell infusion leads to the generation of regulatory T cells

Regulatory T lymphocytes play a critical role in self-tolerance and homeostasis by actively suppressing immune responses (126-128). In the periphery, Tregs are present as either naturally occurring or induced, and the classic Treg phenotype is CD4+CD25+ cells expressing the molecular marker Foxp3, which is a member of the forkhead/winged-helix family of transcriptional regulators (129). There is evidence in both animal models and from clinical studies that apoptotic cell infusion induces Tregs. Wang et al showed that the survival of cardiac allografts was prolonged as a result of donor apoptotic cell infusion which induced Tregs (130). In another mouse model of cardiac allograft rejection, George et al showed that compared to untreated mice, the frequency of splenic CD4+CD25+Foxp3+ cells increased 2-fold in ECP-treated animals and graft survival was prolonged (131). In a murine model of contact hypersensitivity, Maeda *et al* demonstrated that intravenous infusion of ECP-treated leukocytes induced Tregs (132). These Tregs were shown to mediate suppression through IL-10 and were characterized as expressing glucocorticoid-induced TNF family-related receptor (GITR) and the surface molecule neuropilin-1 (133). In a murine model that closely reproduces the treatment of GVHD with ECP, the infusion of ECP-treated cells significantly reduced clinical GVHD scores and pathology, diminished mortality, and increased the number of Foxp3+ Tregs in the spleen and thymus (134) . Extending pre-clinical findings to humans, Lamioni *et al* observed that ECP treatments promote a significant increase in regulatory T cells in the blood of cardiac and lung transplant patients compared to untreated healthy individuals and patients who received traditional immunosuppressants (125). Treg function in both GVHD and CTCL patients was reported to be strengthened as a result of ECP treatments (135). The frequency of circulating CD4+CD25+GITR+CD62L+Foxp3+ Tregs with suppressive function increased in GVHD patients treated with ECP, suggesting an association between elevation in Tregs and response to ECP treatments (136). Lastly, a recent report from the pediatric ECP T1D trial suggested that ECP effectively inhibited autoimmune processes against islet cells by maintaining regulatory T cell activity (137). Collectively, these results suggest that infusion of apoptotic cells or ECP treatments can mediate an upregulation of Tregs via modulation of cytokines and dendritic cells, which may help explain why ECP has therapeutic effects in malignancy, alloimmune conditions, and autoimmunity; however, additional research and clinical studies are warranted in order to fully understand the full potential of apoptotic cells in the treatment of diseases.

6. References

[1] Borus JS, Laffel L: Adherence challenges in the management of type 1 diabetes in adolescents: prevention and intervention. *Curr Opin Pediatr* 22:405-411, 2010

[2] Hood KK, Rohan JM, Peterson CM, Drotar D: Interventions with adherence-promoting components in pediatric type 1 diabetes: meta-analysis of their impact on glycemic control. *Diabetes Care* 33:1658-1664, 2010

[3] Fasanmade OA, Odeniyi IA, Ogbera AO: Diabetic ketoacidosis: diagnosis and management. *Afr J Med Med Sci* 37:99-105, 2008

[4] Umpierrez GE, Kitabchi AE: Diabetic ketoacidosis: risk factors and management strategies. *Treat Endocrinol* 2:95-108, 2003

[5] Weber C, Kocher S, Neeser K, Joshi SR: Prevention of diabetic ketoacidosis and self-monitoring of ketone bodies: an overview. *Curr Med Res Opin* 25:1197-1207, 2009

[6] Ritz E, Haxsen V: Diabetic nephropathy and anaemia. *Eur J Clin Invest* 35 Suppl 3:66-74, 2005

[7] Toto RD: Heart disease in diabetic patients. *Semin Nephrol* 25:372-378, 2005

[8] Pop-Busui R, Roberts L, Pennathur S, Kretzler M, Brosius FC, Feldman EL: The management of diabetic neuropathy in CKD. *Am J Kidney Dis* 55:365-385, 2010

[9] Alicic RZ, Tuttle KR: Management of the diabetic patient with advanced chronic kidney disease. *Semin Dial* 23:140-147, 2010
[10] Wasserfall CH, Atkinson MA: Autoantibody markers for the diagnosis and prediction of type 1 diabetes. *Autoimmun Rev* 5:424-428, 2006
[11] Shoda LK, Young DL, Ramanujan S, Whiting CC, Atkinson MA, Bluestone JA, Eisenbarth GS, Mathis D, Rossini AA, Campbell SE, Kahn R, Kreuwel HT: A comprehensive review of interventions in the NOD mouse and implications for translation. *Immunity* 23:115-126, 2005
[12] Atkinson MA, Eisenbarth GS: Type 1 diabetes: new perspectives on disease pathogenesis and treatment. *Lancet* 358:221-229, 2001
[13] Sakaguchi S, Ono M, Setoguchi R, Yagi H, Hori S, Fehervari Z, Shimizu J, Takahashi T, Nomura T: Foxp3+ CD25+ CD4+ natural regulatory T cells in dominant self-tolerance and autoimmune disease. *Immunol Rev* 212:8-27, 2006
[14] Parish IA, Heath WR: Too dangerous to ignore: self-tolerance and the control of ignorant autoreactive T cells. *Immunol Cell Biol* 86:146-152, 2008
[15] Licht R, Dieker JW, Jacobs CW, Tax WJ, Berden JH: Decreased phagocytosis of apoptotic cells in diseased SLE mice. *J Autoimmun* 22:139-145, 2004
[16] Gaipl US, Voll RE, Sheriff A, Franz S, Kalden JR, Herrmann M: Impaired clearance of dying cells in systemic lupus erythematosus. *Autoimmun Rev* 4:189-194, 2005
[17] Erwig LP, Henson PM: Immunological consequences of apoptotic cell phagocytosis. *Am J Pathol* 171:2-8, 2007
[18] Mueller RB, Sheriff A, Gaipl US, Wesselborg S, Lauber K: Attraction of phagocytes by apoptotic cells is mediated by lysophosphatidylcholine. *Autoimmunity* 40:342-344, 2007
[19] Lauber K, Blumenthal SG, Waibel M, Wesselborg S: Clearance of apoptotic cells: getting rid of the corpses. *Mol Cell* 14:277-287, 2004
[20] Ravichandran KS: Find-me and eat-me signals in apoptotic cell clearance: progress and conundrums. *J Exp Med* 207:1807-1817, 2010
[21] Peter C, Waibel M, Radu CG, Yang LV, Witte ON, Schulze-Osthoff K, Wesselborg S, Lauber K: Migration to apoptotic "find-me" signals is mediated via the phagocyte receptor G2A. *J Biol Chem* 283:5296-5305, 2008
[22] Elliott MR, Chekeni FB, Trampont PC, Lazarowski ER, Kadl A, Walk SF, Park D, Woodson RI, Ostankovich M, Sharma P, Lysiak JJ, Harden TK, Leitinger N, Ravichandran KS: Nucleotides released by apoptotic cells act as a find-me signal to promote phagocytic clearance. *Nature* 461:282-286, 2009
[23] Chekeni FB, Elliott MR, Sandilos JK, Walk SF, Kinchen JM, Lazarowski ER, Armstrong AJ, Penuela S, Laird DW, Salvesen GS, Isakson BE, Bayliss DA, Ravichandran KS: Pannexin 1 channels mediate 'find-me' signal release and membrane permeability during apoptosis. *Nature* 467:863-867, 2010
[24] Gardai SJ, Bratton DL, Ogden CA, Henson PM: Recognition ligands on apoptotic cells: a perspective. *J Leukoc Biol* 79:896-903, 2006
[25] Grimsley C, Ravichandran KS: Cues for apoptotic cell engulfment: eat-me, don't eat-me and come-get-me signals. *Trends Cell Biol* 13:648-656, 2003
[26] Ravichandran KS: "Recruitment signals" from apoptotic cells: invitation to a quiet meal. *Cell* 113:817-820, 2003
[27] Inaba K, Turley S, Yamaide F, Iyoda T, Mahnke K, Inaba M, Pack M, Subklewe M, Sauter B, Sheff D, Albert M, Bhardwaj N, Mellman I, Steinman RM: Efficient

presentation of phagocytosed cellular fragments on the major histocompatibility complex class II products of dendritic cells. *J Exp Med* 188:2163-2173, 1998
[28] Steinman RM, Turley S, Mellman I, Inaba K: The induction of tolerance by dendritic cells that have captured apoptotic cells. *J Exp Med* 191:411-416, 2000
[29] Clayton AR, Prue RL, Harper L, Drayson MT, Savage CO: Dendritic cell uptake of human apoptotic and necrotic neutrophils inhibits CD40, CD80, and CD86 expression and reduces allogeneic T cell responses: relevance to systemic vasculitis. *Arthritis Rheum* 48:2362-2374, 2003
[30] Kushwah R, Wu J, Oliver JR, Jiang G, Zhang J, Siminovitch KA, Hu J: Uptake of apoptotic DC converts immature DC into tolerogenic DC that induce differentiation of Foxp3+ Treg. *Eur J Immunol* 40:1022-1035, 2010
[31] Lemke G, Rothlin CV: Immunobiology of the TAM receptors. *Nat Rev Immunol* 8:327-336, 2008
[32] Green DR, Ferguson T, Zitvogel L, Kroemer G: Immunogenic and tolerogenic cell death. *Nat Rev Immunol* 9:353-363, 2009
[33] Torchinsky MB, Garaude J, Martin AP, Blander JM: Innate immune recognition of infected apoptotic cells directs T(H)17 cell differentiation. *Nature* 458:78-82, 2009
[34] Kleinclauss F, Perruche S, Masson E, de Carvalho Bittencourt M, Biichle S, Remy-Martin JP, Ferrand C, Martin M, Bittard H, Chalopin JM, Seilles E, Tiberghien P, Saas P: Intravenous apoptotic spleen cell infusion induces a TGF-beta-dependent regulatory T-cell expansion. *Cell Death Differ* 13:41-52, 2006
[35] Zhang M, Xu S, Han Y, Cao X: Apoptotic cells attenuate fulminant hepatitis by priming Kupffer cells to produce interleukin-10 through membrane-bound TGF-beta. *Hepatology* 53:306-316, 2011
[36] Nacu N, Luzina IG, Highsmith K, Lockatell V, Pochetuhen K, Cooper ZA, Gillmeister MP, Todd NW, Atamas SP: Macrophages produce TGF-beta-induced (beta-ig-h3) following ingestion of apoptotic cells and regulate MMP14 levels and collagen turnover in fibroblasts. *J Immunol* 180:5036-5044, 2008
[37] Hodge S, Hodge G, Flower R, Reynolds PN, Scicchitano R, Holmes M: Up-regulation of production of TGF-beta and IL-4 and down-regulation of IL-6 by apoptotic human bronchial epithelial cells. *Immunol Cell Biol* 80:537-543, 2002
[38] Curotto de Lafaille MA, Lafaille JJ: Natural and adaptive foxp3+ regulatory T cells: more of the same or a division of labor? *Immunity* 30:626-635, 2009
[39] Horwitz DA, Zheng SG, Gray JD: Natural and TGF-beta-induced Foxp3(+)CD4(+) CD25(+) regulatory T cells are not mirror images of each other. *Trends Immunol* 29:429-435, 2008
[40] Sakaguchi S, Yamaguchi T, Nomura T, Ono M: Regulatory T cells and immune tolerance. *Cell* 133:775-787, 2008
[41] Perruche S, Zhang P, Liu Y, Saas P, Bluestone JA, Chen W: CD3-specific antibody-induced immune tolerance involves transforming growth factor-beta from phagocytes digesting apoptotic T cells. *Nat Med* 14:528-535, 2008
[42] Morelli AE, Larregina AT: Apoptotic cell-based therapies against transplant rejection: role of recipient's dendritic cells. *Apoptosis* 15:1083-1097, 2010
[43] Kobayashi N, Karisola P, Pena-Cruz V, Dorfman DM, Jinushi M, Umetsu SE, Butte MJ, Nagumo H, Chernova I, Zhu B, Sharpe AH, Ito S, Dranoff G, Kaplan GG, Casasnovas JM, Umetsu DT, Dekruyff RH, Freeman GJ: TIM-1 and TIM-4 glycoproteins bind phosphatidylserine and mediate uptake of apoptotic cells. *Immunity* 27:927-940, 2007

[44] Miyanishi M, Tada K, Koike M, Uchiyama Y, Kitamura T, Nagata S: Identification of Tim4 as a phosphatidylserine receptor. *Nature* 450:435-439, 2007
[45] Santiago C, Ballesteros A, Martinez-Munoz L, Mellado M, Kaplan GG, Freeman GJ, Casasnovas JM: Structures of T cell immunoglobulin mucin protein 4 show a metal-Ion-dependent ligand binding site where phosphatidylserine binds. *Immunity* 27:941-951, 2007
[46] Santiago C, Ballesteros A, Tami C, Martinez-Munoz L, Kaplan GG, Casasnovas JM: Structures of T Cell immunoglobulin mucin receptors 1 and 2 reveal mechanisms for regulation of immune responses by the TIM receptor family. *Immunity* 26:299-310, 2007
[47] Ichimura T, Asseldonk EJ, Humphreys BD, Gunaratnam L, Duffield JS, Bonventre JV: Kidney injury molecule-1 is a phosphatidylserine receptor that confers a phagocytic phenotype on epithelial cells. *J Clin Invest* 118:1657-1668, 2008
[48] DeKruyff RH, Bu X, Ballesteros A, Santiago C, Chim YL, Lee HH, Karisola P, Pichavant M, Kaplan GG, Umetsu DT, Freeman GJ, Casasnovas JM: T cell/transmembrane, Ig, and mucin-3 allelic variants differentially recognize phosphatidylserine and mediate phagocytosis of apoptotic cells. *J Immunol* 184:1918-1930, 2010
[49] Wong K, Valdez PA, Tan C, Yeh S, Hongo JA, Ouyang W: Phosphatidylserine receptor Tim-4 is essential for the maintenance of the homeostatic state of resident peritoneal macrophages. *Proc Natl Acad Sci U S A* 107:8712-8717, 2010
[50] Park D, Tosello-Trampont AC, Elliott MR, Lu M, Haney LB, Ma Z, Klibanov AL, Mandell JW, Ravichandran KS: BAI1 is an engulfment receptor for apoptotic cells upstream of the ELMO/Dock180/Rac module. *Nature* 450:430-434, 2007
[51] Hanayama R, Tanaka M, Miwa K, Shinohara A, Iwamatsu A, Nagata S: Identification of a factor that links apoptotic cells to phagocytes. *Nature* 417:182-187, 2002
[52] Hanayama R, Tanaka M, Miyasaka K, Aozasa K, Koike M, Uchiyama Y, Nagata S: Autoimmune disease and impaired uptake of apoptotic cells in MFG-E8-deficient mice. *Science* 304:1147-1150, 2004
[53] Hanayama R, Tanaka M, Miwa K, Nagata S: Expression of developmental endothelial locus-1 in a subset of macrophages for engulfment of apoptotic cells. *J Immunol* 172:3876-3882, 2004
[54] Miyasaka K, Hanayama R, Tanaka M, Nagata S: Expression of milk fat globule epidermal growth factor 8 in immature dendritic cells for engulfment of apoptotic cells. *Eur J Immunol* 34:1414-1422, 2004
[55] Savill J, Hogg N, Haslett C: Macrophage vitronectin receptor, CD36, and thrombospondin cooperate in recognition of neutrophils undergoing programmed cell death. *Chest* 99:6S-7S, 1991
[56] Balasubramanian K, Schroit AJ: Characterization of phosphatidylserine-dependent beta2-glycoprotein I macrophage interactions. Implications for apoptotic cell clearance by phagocytes. *J Biol Chem* 273:29272-29277, 1998
[57] Imachi H, Murao K, Hiramine C, Sayo Y, Sato M, Hosokawa H, Ishida T, Kodama T, Quehenberger O, Steinberg D, Takahara J: Human scavenger receptor B1 is involved in recognition of apoptotic thymocytes by thymic nurse cells. *Lab Invest* 80:263-270, 2000
[58] Mevorach D: Opsonization of apoptotic cells. Implications for uptake and autoimmunity. *Ann N Y Acad Sci* 926:226-235, 2000

[59] Eken C, Martin PJ, Sadallah S, Treves S, Schaller M, Schifferli JA: Ectosomes released by polymorphonuclear neutrophils induce a MerTK-dependent anti-inflammatory pathway in macrophages. *J Biol Chem* 285:39914-39921, 2010

[60] Wallet MA, Sen P, Flores RR, Wang Y, Yi Z, Huang Y, Mathews CE, Earp HS, Matsushima G, Wang B, Tisch R: MerTK is required for apoptotic cell-induced T cell tolerance. *J Exp Med* 205:219-232, 2008

[61] Yi Z, Li L, Matsushima GK, Earp HS, Wang B, Tisch R: A novel role for c-Src and STAT3 in apoptotic cell-mediated MerTK-dependent immunoregulation of dendritic cells. *Blood* 114:3191-3198, 2009

[62] Grommes C, Lee CY, Wilkinson BL, Jiang Q, Koenigsknecht-Talboo JL, Varnum B, Landreth GE: Regulation of microglial phagocytosis and inflammatory gene expression by Gas6 acting on the Axl/Mer family of tyrosine kinases. *J Neuroimmune Pharmacol* 3:130-140, 2008

[63] Shi D, Fu M, Fan P, Li W, Chen X, Li C, Qi X, Gao T, Liu Y: Artificial phosphatidylserine liposome mimics apoptotic cells in inhibiting maturation and immunostimulatory function of murine myeloid dendritic cells in response to 1-chloro-2,4-dinitrobenze in vitro. *Arch Dermatol Res* 299:327-336, 2007

[64] Chen X, Doffek K, Sugg SL, Shilyansky J: Phosphatidylserine regulates the maturation of human dendritic cells. *J Immunol* 173:2985-2994, 2004

[65] Hugues S, Mougneau E, Ferlin W, Jeske D, Hofman P, Homann D, Beaudoin L, Schrike C, Von Herrath M, Lehuen A, Glaichenhaus N: Tolerance to islet antigens and prevention from diabetes induced by limited apoptosis of pancreatic beta cells. *Immunity* 16:169-181, 2002

[66] O'Brien BA, Harmon BV, Cameron DP, Allan DJ: Apoptosis is the mode of beta-cell death responsible for the development of IDDM in the nonobese diabetic (NOD) mouse. *Diabetes* 46:750-757, 1997

[67] Maree AF, Kublik R, Finegood DT, Edelstein-Keshet L: Modelling the onset of Type 1 diabetes: can impaired macrophage phagocytosis make the difference between health and disease? *Philos Transact A Math Phys Eng Sci* 364:1267-1282, 2006

[68] Turley S, Poirot L, Hattori M, Benoist C, Mathis D: Physiological beta cell death triggers priming of self-reactive T cells by dendritic cells in a type-1 diabetes model. *J Exp Med* 198:1527-1537, 2003

[69] Todd JA: Genetic control of autoimmunity in type 1 diabetes. *Immunol Today* 11:122-129, 1990

[70] Wallberg M, Wong FS, Green EA: An islet-specific pulse of TGF-(beta) abrogates CTL function and promotes (beta) cell survival independent of Foxp3+ T cells. *J Immunol* 186:2543-2551, 2011

[71] Amrani A, Verdaguer J, Thiessen S, Bou S, Santamaria P: IL-1alpha, IL-1beta, and IFN-gamma mark beta cells for Fas-dependent destruction by diabetogenic CD4(+) T lymphocytes. *J Clin Invest* 105:459-468, 2000

[72] Mandrup-Poulsen T: Beta cell death and protection. *Ann N Y Acad Sci* 1005:32-42, 2003

[73] Suarez-Pinzon W, Sorensen O, Bleackley RC, Elliott JF, Rajotte RV, Rabinovitch A: Beta-cell destruction in NOD mice correlates with Fas (CD95) expression on beta-cells and proinflammatory cytokine expression in islets. *Diabetes* 48:21-28, 1999

[74] Yamada K, Takane-Gyotoku N, Yuan X, Ichikawa F, Inada C, Nonaka K: Mouse islet cell lysis mediated by interleukin-1-induced Fas. *Diabetologia* 39:1306-1312, 1996

[75] Moriwaki M, Itoh N, Miyagawa J, Yamamoto K, Imagawa A, Yamagata K, Iwahashi H, Nakajima H, Namba M, Nagata S, Hanafusa T, Matsuzawa Y: Fas and Fas ligand

expression in inflamed islets in pancreas sections of patients with recent-onset Type I diabetes mellitus. *Diabetologia* 42:1332-1340, 1999

[76] Imagawa A, Hanafusa T, Tamura S, Moriwaki M, Itoh N, Yamamoto K, Iwahashi H, Yamagata K, Waguri M, Nanmo T, Uno S, Nakajima H, Namba M, Kawata S, Miyagawa JI, Matsuzawa Y: Pancreatic biopsy as a procedure for detecting in situ autoimmune phenomena in type 1 diabetes: close correlation between serological markers and histological evidence of cellular autoimmunity. *Diabetes* 50:1269-1273, 2001

[77] Loweth AC, Williams GT, James RF, Scarpello JH, Morgan NG: Human islets of Langerhans express Fas ligand and undergo apoptosis in response to interleukin-1beta and Fas ligation. *Diabetes* 47:727-732, 1998

[78] Apostolou I, Hao Z, Rajewsky K, von Boehmer H: Effective destruction of Fas-deficient insulin-producing beta cells in type 1 diabetes. *J Exp Med* 198:1103-1106, 2003

[79] Allison J, Thomas HE, Catterall T, Kay TW, Strasser A: Transgenic expression of dominant-negative Fas-associated death domain protein in beta cells protects against Fas ligand-induced apoptosis and reduces spontaneous diabetes in nonobese diabetic mice. *J Immunol* 175:293-301, 2005

[80] Tiedge M, Lortz S, Drinkgern J, Lenzen S: Relation between antioxidant enzyme gene expression and antioxidative defense status of insulin-producing cells. *Diabetes* 46:1733-1742, 1997

[81] Thomas HE, McKenzie MD, Angstetra E, Campbell PD, Kay TW: Beta cell apoptosis in diabetes. *Apoptosis* 14:1389-1404, 2009

[82] Lenzen S, Drinkgern J, Tiedge M: Low antioxidant enzyme gene expression in pancreatic islets compared with various other mouse tissues. *Free Radic Biol Med* 20:463-466, 1996

[83] Hotta M, Tashiro F, Ikegami H, Niwa H, Ogihara T, Yodoi J, Miyazaki J: Pancreatic beta cell-specific expression of thioredoxin, an antioxidative and antiapoptotic protein, prevents autoimmune and streptozotocin-induced diabetes. *J Exp Med* 188:1445-1451, 1998

[84] Li X, Chen H, Epstein PN: Metallothionein protects islets from hypoxia and extends islet graft survival by scavenging most kinds of reactive oxygen species. *J Biol Chem* 279:765-771, 2004

[85] Chen H, Li X, Epstein PN: MnSOD and catalase transgenes demonstrate that protection of islets from oxidative stress does not alter cytokine toxicity. *Diabetes* 54:1437-1446, 2005

[86] Lortz S, Tiedge M, Nachtwey T, Karlsen AE, Nerup J, Lenzen S: Protection of insulin-producing RINm5F cells against cytokine-mediated toxicity through overexpression of antioxidant enzymes. *Diabetes* 49:1123-1130, 2000

[87] Naik E, Dixit VM: Mitochondrial reactive oxygen species drive proinflammatory cytokine production. *J Exp Med* 208:417-420, 2011

[88] Bulua AC, Simon A, Maddipati R, Pelletier M, Park H, Kim KY, Sack MN, Kastner DL, Siegel RM: Mitochondrial reactive oxygen species promote production of proinflammatory cytokines and are elevated in TNFR1-associated periodic syndrome (TRAPS). *J Exp Med* 208:519-533, 2011

[89] Peritt D: Potential mechanisms of photopheresis in hematopoietic stem cell transplantation. *Biol Blood Marrow Transplant* 12:7-12, 2006

[90] Hivelin M, Siemionow M, Grimbert P, Lantieri L: Extracorporeal photopheresis: from solid organs to face transplantation. *Transpl Immunol* 21:117-128, 2009

[91] Scarisbrick J: Extracorporeal photopheresis: what is it and when should it be used? *Clin Exp Dermatol* 34:757-760, 2009

[92] Knobler R, Barr ML, Couriel DR, Ferrara JL, French LE, Jaksch P, Reinisch W, Rook AH, Schwarz T, Greinix H: Extracorporeal photopheresis: past, present, and future. *J Am Acad Dermatol* 61:652-665, 2009

[93] Marshall SR: Technology insight: ECP for the treatment of GvHD--can we offer selective immune control without generalized immunosuppression? *Nat Clin Pract Oncol* 3:302-314, 2006

[94] Miller JD, Kirkland EB, Domingo DS, Scull H, Jekutis B, Dallas M, Cooper KD, Baron ED: Review of extracorporeal photopheresis in early-stage (IA, IB, and IIA) cutaneous T-cell lymphoma. *Photodermatol Photoimmunol Photomed* 23:163-171, 2007

[95] Zic JA: The treatment of cutaneous T-cell lymphoma with photopheresis. *Dermatol Ther* 16:337-346, 2003

[96] Greinix HT, Socie G, Bacigalupo A, Holler E, Edinger MG, Apperley JF, Schwarz T, Ullrich SE, Albert ML, Knobler RM, Peritt D, Ferrara JL: Assessing the potential role of photopheresis in hematopoietic stem cell transplant. *Bone Marrow Transplant* 38:265-273, 2006

[97] Greinix HT, Knobler RM, Worel N, Schneider B, Schneeberger A, Hoecker P, Mitterbauer M, Rabitsch W, Schulenburg A, Kalhs P: The effect of intensified extracorporeal photochemotherapy on long-term survival in patients with severe acute graft-versus-host disease. *Haematologica* 91:405-408, 2006

[98] Couriel DR, Hosing C, Saliba R, Shpall EJ, Anderlini P, Rhodes B, Smith V, Khouri I, Giralt S, de Lima M, Hsu Y, Ghosh S, Neumann J, Andersson B, Qazilbash M, Hymes S, Kim S, Champlin R, Donato M: Extracorporeal photochemotherapy for the treatment of steroid-resistant chronic GVHD. *Blood* 107:3074-3080, 2006

[99] Marques MB, Schwartz J: Update on extracorporeal photopheresis in heart and lung transplantation. *J Clin Apher* 2010 Dec 6 (Epub ahead of print)

[100] Suchin KR, Cassin M, Washko R, Nahass G, Berkson M, Stouch B, Vowels BR, Rook AH: Extracorporeal photochemotherapy does not suppress T- or B-cell responses to novel or recall antigens. *J Am Acad Dermatol* 41:980-986, 1999

[101] Xia CQ, Chernatynskaya A, Lai Y, Campbell KA, Clare-Salzler MJ: Experimental extracorporeal photopheresis therapy significantly delays the development of diabetes in non-obese diabetic mice. *Clin Immunol* 135:374-383, 2010

[102] Xia CQ, Qiu Y, Peng RH, Lo-Dauer J, Clare-Salzler MJ: Infusion of UVB-treated splenic stromal cells induces suppression of beta cell antigen-specific T cell responses in NOD mice. *J Autoimmun* 30:283-292, 2008

[103] Xia CQ, Peng R, Qiu Y, Annamalai M, Gordon D, Clare-Salzler MJ: Transfusion of apoptotic beta-cells induces immune tolerance to beta-cell antigens and prevents type 1 diabetes in NOD mice. *Diabetes* 56:2116-2123, 2007

[104] McKenna KE, Whittaker S, Rhodes LE, Taylor P, Lloyd J, Ibbotson S, Russell-Jones R: Evidence-based practice of photopheresis 1987-2001: a report of a workshop of the British Photodermatology Group and the U.K. Skin Lymphoma Group. *Br J Dermatol* 154:7-20, 2006

[105] Ludvigsson J, Samuelsson U, Ernerudh J, Johansson C, Stenhammar L, Berlin G: Photopheresis at onset of type 1 diabetes: a randomised, double blind, placebo controlled trial. *Arch Dis Child* 85:149-154, 2001

[106] Malawista SE, Trock D, Edelson RL: Photopheresis for rheumatoid arthritis. *Ann N Y Acad Sci* 636:217-226, 1991

[107] Zic JA, Miller JL, Stricklin GP, King LE, Jr.: The North American experience with photopheresis. *Ther Apher* 3:50-62, 1999

[108] Menkes CJ, Andreu G, Heshmati F, Hilliquin P: Extracorporeal photochemotherapy. *Br J Rheumatol* 31:789-790, 1992

[109] Laroux FS, Pavlick KP, Wolf RE, Grisham MB: Dysregulation of intestinal mucosal immunity: implications in inflammatory bowel disease. *News Physiol Sci* 16:272-277, 2001

[110] Lim WC, Hanauer SB: Controversies with aminosalicylates in inflammatory bowel disease. *Rev Gastroenterol Disord* 4:104-117, 2004

[111] Reinisch W, Nahavandi H, Santella R, Zhang Y, Gasche C, Moser G, Waldhor T, Gangl A, Vogelsang H, Knobler R: Extracorporeal photochemotherapy in patients with steroid-dependent Crohn's disease: a prospective pilot study. *Aliment Pharmacol Ther* 15:1313-1322, 2001

[112] Abreu MT, von Tirpitz C, Hardi R, Kaatz M, Van Assche G, Rutgeerts P, Bisaccia E, Goerdt S, Hanauer S, Knobler R, Mannon P, Mayer L, Ochsenkuhn T, Sandborn WJ, Parenti D, Lee K, Reinisch W: Extracorporeal photopheresis for the treatment of refractory Crohn's disease: results of an open-label pilot study. *Inflamm Bowel Dis* 15:829-836, 2009

[113] Parnaik R, Raff MC, Scholes J: Differences between the clearance of apoptotic cells by professional and non-professional phagocytes. *Curr Biol* 10:857-860, 2000

[114] Tanaka M, Asano K, Qiu CH: Immune regulation by apoptotic cell clearance. *Ann N Y Acad Sci* 1209:37-42, 2010

[115] Steinman RM, Hawiger D, Liu K, Bonifaz L, Bonnyay D, Mahnke K, Iyoda T, Ravetch J, Dhodapkar M, Inaba K, Nussenzweig M: Dendritic cell function in vivo during the steady state: a role in peripheral tolerance. *Ann N Y Acad Sci* 987:15-25, 2003

[116] Liu K, Iyoda T, Saternus M, Kimura Y, Inaba K, Steinman RM: Immune tolerance after delivery of dying cells to dendritic cells in situ. *J Exp Med* 196:1091-1097, 2002

[117] Mueller DL: Mechanisms maintaining peripheral tolerance. *Nat Immunol* 11:21-27, 2010

[118] Savill J, Dransfield I, Gregory C, Haslett C: A blast from the past: clearance of apoptotic cells regulates immune responses. *Nat Rev Immunol* 2:965-975, 2002

[119] Voll RE, Herrmann M, Roth EA, Stach C, Kalden JR, Girkontaite I: Immunosuppressive effects of apoptotic cells. *Nature* 390:350-351, 1997

[120] Fadok VA, Bratton DL, Konowal A, Freed PW, Westcott JY, Henson PM: Macrophages that have ingested apoptotic cells in vitro inhibit proinflammatory cytokine production through autocrine/paracrine mechanisms involving TGF-beta, PGE2, and PAF. *J Clin Invest* 101:890-898, 1998

[121] Fadok VA, McDonald PP, Bratton DL, Henson PM: Regulation of macrophage cytokine production by phagocytosis of apoptotic and post-apoptotic cells. *Biochem Soc Trans* 26:653-656, 1998

[122] Chen W, Frank ME, Jin W, Wahl SM: TGF-beta released by apoptotic T cells contributes to an immunosuppressive milieu. *Immunity* 14:715-725, 2001

[123] Stark MA, Huo Y, Burcin TL, Morris MA, Olson TS, Ley K: Phagocytosis of apoptotic neutrophils regulates granulopoiesis via IL-23 and IL-17. *Immunity* 22:285-294, 2005

[124] Bettelli E, Carrier Y, Gao W, Korn T, Strom TB, Oukka M, Weiner HL, Kuchroo VK: Reciprocal developmental pathways for the generation of pathogenic effector TH17 and regulatory T cells. *Nature* 441:235-238, 2006

[125] Lamioni A, Parisi F, Isacchi G, Giorda E, Di Cesare S, Landolfo A, Cenci F, Bottazzo GF, Carsetti R: The immunological effects of extracorporeal photopheresis unraveled: induction of tolerogenic dendritic cells in vitro and regulatory T cells in vivo. *Transplantation* 79:846-850, 2005

[126] Roncarolo MG, Bacchetta R, Bordignon C, Narula S, Levings MK: Type 1 T regulatory cells. *Immunol Rev* 182:68-79, 2001

[127] Groux H, O'Garra A, Bigler M, Rouleau M, Antonenko S, de Vries JE, Roncarolo MG: A CD4+ T-cell subset inhibits antigen-specific T-cell responses and prevents colitis. *Nature* 389:737-742, 1997

[128] Sakaguchi S, Sakaguchi N, Shimizu J, Yamazaki S, Sakihama T, Itoh M, Kuniyasu Y, Nomura T, Toda M, Takahashi T: Immunologic tolerance maintained by CD25+ CD4+ regulatory T cells: their common role in controlling autoimmunity, tumor immunity, and transplantation tolerance. *Immunol Rev* 182:18-32, 2001

[129] Hori S, Nomura T, Sakaguchi S: Control of regulatory T cell development by the transcription factor Foxp3. *Science* 299:1057-1061, 2003

[130] Wang Z, Larregina AT, Shufesky WJ, Perone MJ, Montecalvo A, Zahorchak AF, Thomson AW, Morelli AE: Use of the inhibitory effect of apoptotic cells on dendritic cells for graft survival via T-cell deletion and regulatory T cells. *Am J Transplant* 6:1297-1311, 2006

[131] George JF, Gooden CW, Guo L, Kirklin JK: Role for CD4(+)CD25(+) T cells in inhibition of graft rejection by extracorporeal photopheresis. *J Heart Lung Transplant* 27:616-622, 2008

[132] Maeda A, Schwarz A, Kernebeck K, Gross N, Aragane Y, Peritt D, Schwarz T: Intravenous infusion of syngeneic apoptotic cells by photopheresis induces antigen-specific regulatory T cells. *J Immunol* 174:5968-5976, 2005

[133] Maeda A, Schwarz A, Bullinger A, Morita A, Peritt D, Schwarz T: Experimental extracorporeal photopheresis inhibits the sensitization and effector phases of contact hypersensitivity via two mechanisms: generation of IL-10 and induction of regulatory T cells. *J Immunol* 181:5956-5962, 2008

[134] Gatza E, Rogers CE, Clouthier SG, Lowler KP, Tawara I, Liu C, Reddy P, Ferrara JL: Extracorporeal photopheresis reverses experimental graft-versus-host disease through regulatory T cells. *Blood* 112:1515-1521, 2008

[135] Rao V, Saunes M, Jorstad S, Moen T: Cutaneous T cell lymphoma and graft-versus-host disease: a comparison of in vivo effects of extracorporeal photochemotherapy on Foxp3+ regulatory T cells. *Clin Immunol* 133:303-313, 2009

[136] Biagi E, Di Biaso I, Leoni V, Gaipa G, Rossi V, Bugarin C, Renoldi G, Parma M, Balduzzi A, Perseghin P, Biondi A: Extracorporeal photochemotherapy is accompanied by increasing levels of circulating CD4+CD25+GITR+Foxp3+CD62L+ functional regulatory T-cells in patients with graft-versus-host disease. *Transplantation* 84:31-39, 2007

[137] Jonson CO, Pihl M, Nyholm C, Cilio CM, Ludvigsson J, Faresjo M: Regulatory T cell-associated activity in photopheresis-induced immune tolerance in recent onset type 1 diabetes children. *Clin Exp Immunol* 153:174-181, 2008

7

Innate Immunity in the Recognition of β-Cell Antigens in Type 1 Diabetes

Jixin Zhong[1,2], Jun-Fa Xu[3], Ping Yang[1], Yi Liang[3] and Cong-Yi Wang[1,2,3]

[1]*The Center for Biomedical Research, Tongji Hospital, Tongji Medical College, Huazhong University of Science and Technology, Wuhan,*
[2]*The Center for Biotechnology and Genomic Medicine, Medical College of Georgia, Augusta, GA,*
[3]*The Department of Clinical Immunology, Guangdong Medical College, Dongguan*
[1,3]*China*
[2]*USA*

1. Introduction

Diabetes is a chronic disease caused by the inability to produce enough insulin by the pancreatic β cells or inappropriately use insulin by the peripheral tissues, and therefore, patients with diabetes are unable to control blood glucose to a normal level. Along with the industrialization and economic development, diabetes has gradually become a global health challenge as manifested by that it affects 5-10% of the world population (Home, 2003). For example, in United States alone, approximately 21 million children and adults (around 7% of the total population) have diabetes. Despite the significant advances in the development of therapeutic approaches for this devastating disease, the long-term outcome of diabetes, however, remains unsatisfied, as many complications could occur during the process of diabetes. Transient improper control of blood glucose level will result in the dangerous short-term complications such as diabetic ketoacidosis, nonketotic hyperosmolar coma, and hypoglycemia., while the life threading condition is the development of various long-term complications such as cardiovascular disease, nerve damage, chronic renal failure, retinal damage, and poor wound healing (Zhong et al., 2011). Given the fact that the administrated exogenous insulin cannot regulate glucose levels as accurately as the endogenous insulin released by the functioning pancreatic islets, diabetic patients are highly prone to the development of those complications. For example, patients with diabetes are 17 times more prone to kidney diseases (World Health Organization (WHO), 1994; Home, 2003), and diabetes also has become the most common cause of blindness in developed countries as manifested by that nearly half of the diabetic patients developed retinopathy (Amos et al., 1997).

There are two types of diabetes, type1 and type 2. **Type 1 diabetes (T1D)**, also called Insulin Dependent Diabetes Mellitus (IDDM) or juvenile diabetes, which is characterized by the selective destruction of the insulin-secreting pancreatic β cells by the autoreactive immune cells. Therefore, T1D is characterized by the absolute deficiency of insulin, and patients require injection of exogenous insulin for survival, which renders the blood glucose unable to be regulated at a perfect level, leading to the persistent epigenetic changes which predispose to the change of gene expression and serve as risk factors for diabetic complications (El-Osta et al., 2008). Therefore, diverse complications are easily developed in patients with T1D. In contrast, **type 2 diabetes** is relevant to insulin resistance, usually caused by obesity. Insulin secretion in patients with type 2 diabetes could be normal, inadequate, or higher, but the peripheral tissues such as liver, muscle, and fat, have a low response to insulin.

It is believed that both genetic and environmental factors are implicated in the susceptibility of T1D. As one of the polygenic diseases, vulnerability to T1D involves more than 20 genetic intervals, among which loci within the HLA account for the most of genetic susceptibility (Bach et al., 2001; Onengut-Gumuscu & Concannon, 2002; Pociot & McDermott, 2002). In addition to genetic factors, a variety of environmental factors can affect T1D susceptibility. A majority of T1D are believed to be triggered by infections such as viral infection. Although less commonly, other environmental factors such as stress and certain chemical or drug exposure also appeared to be triggers for T1D.

Despite of extensive studies, the underlying mechanism of T1D is still not fully elucidated. Decades of clinical and experimental studies indicate that adaptive immune responses play a central role in the pathogenesis of T1D in both humans and NOD mice (Roep, 2003). As the major effector cells for β-cell destruction, T cells and T-cell-mediated adaptive immunity are considered to be the major factor for T1D. Autoreactive CD8+ T cells are confirmed to be critical for T1D pathogenesis in both patients and experimental animal models (Bottazzo et al., 1985; Conrad et al., 1994). Other than CD8+ T cells, self-antigen specific CD4+ T cells can also promote the production of autoantibodies against β cells by B lymphocytes. Therefore, most T1D related studies have been focused on adaptive immunity, while the role of innate immunity is overshadowed. Recently, accumulating evidence indicates that innate immunity also plays an essential role in the initiation and progression of T1D. For example, in addition to T cells, innate immune cells such as dendritic cells (DCs), macrophages, and natural killer (NK) cells are highly enriched in the insulitis lesion during diabetogenic process (Pietropaolo et al., 2007; Katz et al., 1995a; Rosmalen et al., 2000). Depletion of DCs and macrophages prevents the infiltration of lymphocytes into the pancreatic islets, and deletion of macrophages by silica almost completely prevents the development of diabetes and insulitis in diabetes-prone NOD mice and BB (BioBreeding) rats (Jun et al., 1999c; Lee et al., 1988d; Lee et al., 1988a; Oschilewski et al., 1985a). Furthermore, even temporary deletion of DCs and macrophages by clodronate-loaded liposomes for one week can tremendously postpone the onset of diabetes (Nikolic et al., 2005). Studies from our and other groups further provided strong evidence showing that diverse innate molecules such as high mobility group protein B1 (HMGB1) and heat shock proteins (HSPs) or innate receptors (e.g., Toll-like receptors and RAGE) are involved in T1D pathogenesis. Therefore, innate immunity has a key effect on the etiology of T1D.

2. Innate immunity and adaptive immunity

Given the fact that T1D is an autoimmune disorder, it would be logic to first introduce the immune system and its relevant defensive mechanisms, the innate and adaptive immune response. The **immune system** is defined as the collection of organs, tissues, cells, and molecules that protects host from various environmental threats such as tumor cells, pathogens, toxins, and other foreign molecules. It includes thymus, spleen, lymph nodes, bone marrow, tonsils, and various cells and molecules such as white blood cells, antibodies, and cytokines. The **immune response** is the defensive mechanism of immune system to protect body against those invasions, which is built on two separate foundation pillars: the innate and adaptive immune response. The **adaptive immune response** is an antigen-specific process by which the immune system discriminates non-self antigens. As suggested by its name, adaptive immune response is highly adaptable, antigen-specific, but its response is relatively slow. It recognizes an unlimited number of antigens by antigen receptors or immunoglobulins which went through somatic hypermutation to acquire their high diversity. In contrast, the **innate immune response** is the primary defensive mechanism against environmental threats in a non-specific manner, which is evolutionally older than its counterpart, the adaptive immune system. The innate immune system can be found in all classes of plants and animals and is the dominant immune system in insects, plants, fungi, and multicellular organisms. It distinguishes invading molecules from host component by recognizing conserved constituents of foreign molecules. The differences and similarities between innate and adaptive immune response are described in Table 1.

Properties	innate immunity	adaptive immunity
Specificity	non-specific	antigen specific
Action time	quick	slow,2-6 days later than innate immune response
Persistence	short	long
Memory	no	yes
Antigens	conserved microbe-specific molecules, such as LPS, glycans, microbial DNA	divers proteins, peptides, and carbohydrates
Receptors	germ-line encoded	encoded in gene segments, its diversity relies on rearrangement

Table 1. Comparison of innate and adaptive immunity

The major function for the immune system is to defend against environmental threats and protect the body against disease by distinguishing and eliminating foreign or dangerous substance including pathogens, tumor cells and even transplanted organs. When encountering antigens derived from the host, the immune system in a normal individual is able to recognize them as self and decide not to respond. Dysfunction of the immune system may cause various immune disorders such as immunodeficiency and autoimmune diseases. Immunodeficiency is manifested by unable to respond to foreign or harmful antigens which results in both opportunistic and normal infections. In contrast, an autoimmune disease is caused by interpreting self-antigens as foreign or harmful antigens. In this case, the immune system in the patients cannot tell the difference between body's own tissue and foreign antigens, resulting in an immune response that destroys their own tissues and cells. There are over 80 different types of autoimmune disorders including type 1 diabetes, systemic lupus erythematosus, multiple sclerosis, Grave's disease, rheumatoid arthritis and so on. Autoimmune responses can be initiated by the following conditions: (1) the release of an antigen that is usually expressed in a specific area and is not exposed to the immune system. For example, the fluid in the eyeball contains some antigens that are hidden from the immune system. Once the fluid is released into the bloodstream by injury, the immune system will recognized them as foreign antigens and react against them; (2) An antigen is altered. For example, antigens within the body can be altered by infections, drugs, and radiations. The altered antigens are then recognized by the immune system to initiate an autoimmune response; (3) Exposure of a foreign antigen with a similar conformation to the body's natural antigen may trigger an autoimmune response against the body's antigen as well as the foreign antigen; (4) Malfunction of the immune cells. For example, cancerous B lymphocytes may produce abnormal antibodies that attack body's own antigens (Breecher & Dworken, 1986).

Since T1D is caused by the autoimmune responses that progressively destroy the insulin producing β cells, the role of adaptive immune response has long been proposed in T1D pathogenesis. The idea that T1D is an autoimmune disease first came from the observation that it usually occurred in association with other classic autoimmune diseases such as Grave's disease, hypothyroidism, Addison's disease and pernicious anemia (Eisenbarth, 1984), and histological examination showed a large amount of T cells in the insulitis lesion (Gepts, 1965). Further studies confirmed that insulitis happens only in the islets containing β cells, indicating that the autoimmune reaction in T1D is driven by β-cell-derived antigens (Roep, 2003). Autoreactive T-cell is believed to be the major mediator of β-cell destruction in both primary T1D and recurrent β-cell loss after islet transplantation (Pinkse et al., 2005). Circulating autoreactive T cells against different β-cell-derived antigens were detected in newly-onset diabetic patients (Velthuis et al., 2010), suggesting its role in T1D development. Treatment of monoclonal CD3 antibody has been shown to be able to protect T1D patients from autoimmune mediated β-cell destruction and preserve insulin production (Herold et al., 2002; Herold et al., 2009; Killestein, 2002). In addition, circulating autoantibodies against β cells are produced by B lymphocytes, another important component of the adaptive immune system, have also been detected in T1D patient. Nevertheless, the production of autoantibodies seems to be a consequence of β-cell destruction (Baekkeskov et al., 1982; Rodacki et al., 2006). Due to the fact that T-cell is the major effector cell in mediating β-cell destruction, adaptive immune response in T1D has been extensively studied and its role in T1D pathogenesis has been well established. However, accumulating evidence suggests that innate immune response is also essential to the pathogenesis of T1D.

3. Immune recognition of antigens

Antigens can come from both environment and body's own tissues. However, the immune system reacts only to foreign or harmful substances under physiologic conditions. This is because each individual has its own identification molecules expressed on the surface of all cells, and the immune system is able to identify them during the recognition process. Major histocompatibility complex (MHC) is the most important identification molecule. MHC molecule in humans is also called human leukocyte antigens (HLA), while MHC in mice is termed histocompatibility-2 (H-2) (Kumanovics et al., 2003). In an effort to be identified in a large population, almost every individual has a unique set of MHC molecules different from others. Therefore, MHC molecules have an extremely large population diversity (Borghans et al., 2004). The diversity of MHC molecules comes from: (1) the polygenic of MHC locus; (2) the high polymorphic MHC locus, each MHC locus has many, even hundreds of different alleles; (3) the co-dominantly expression of MHC. Thus, the combination of MHC molecules in each individual is almost unique. After positive and negative selection, T cells are tolerant to cells with self MHC molecules and potent to attack cells possessing different MHC molecules (such as foreign cells and mutated cells).

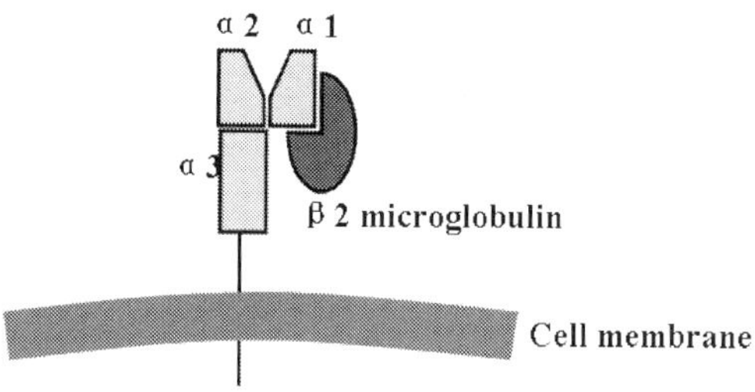

Fig. 1. **Molecular Structure of MHC Class I:** MHC class I protein is composed of two chains: α chain and β2 microglobulin. The α chain consists of a transmembrane region and three extracellular domains: α1, α2, and α3. MHC class I molecule is expressed on the membrane of all nucleated cells.

MHC regions are divided into three classes: class I, class II, and class III (Newton et al., 2004). MHC class I encodes heterodimeric peptide-binding proteins (the classical MHC class I molecules) and antigen-processing molecules (the non-classical MHC class I molecules). MHC class I protein has an immunoglobulin-like structure containing an α chain and a β2 microglobulin. The α chain consists of a transmembrane region and three extracellular domains (α1, α2, and α3) (Figure 1). MHC class I molecule is expressed in all nucleated cells. It presents cytosolic peptide (including self peptides and viral peptides synthesized by own cells) that is anchored to a cleft formed by α1 and α2 to TCR on CD8+ cytotoxic T cells. MHC class II is responsible for encoding peptide-binding proteins (the classical MHC class II molecules) as well as molecules modulating antigen loading (the non-classical MHC class II molecules). The MHC class II molecule also has an immunoglobulin-like structure and consists of two chains, one α chain and one β chain (Figure 2). Each chain contains a transmembrane region and two extracellular domains (α1 and α2 in α chain, β1 and β2 in β

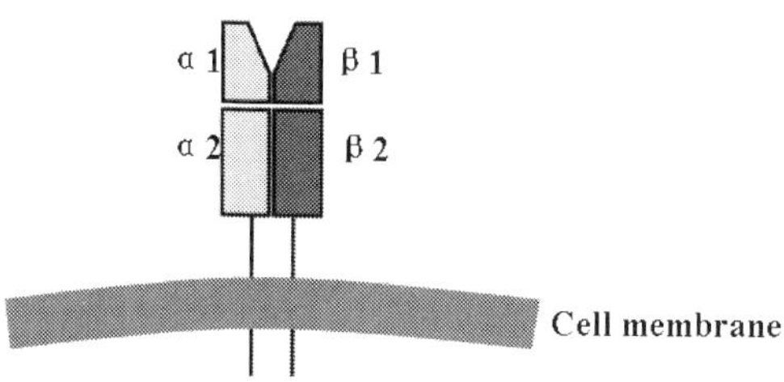

Fig. 2. **Molecular Structure of MHC Class II:** MHC class II molecule has an immunoglobulin-like structure. It consists of one α chain and one β chain. Each chain contains a transmembrane region and two extracellular domains (α1 and α2 in α chain, β1 and β2 in β chain). MHC class II protein is expressed on the membrane of APCs and is responsible for presenting extracellular antigens.

chain). The MHC class II protein is expressed on the membrane of antigen presenting cells (APCs). It loads processed extracellular peptide (e.g., peptides originating from microbes ingested in vesicles) on a cleft formed by α1 and β1 domain, and presents it to TCR on CD4+ helper T cells. MHC class III is responsible for encoding several secreted proteins such as complement components (C2, C4, and B factor), cytokines (TNFα, LTA, and LTB), and heat shock proteins. The function of MHC class III is different from class I and II, but MHC class III is located between them, so they are usually described together. In humans, the most intensely studied MHC class I genes are HLA-A, HLA-B, and HLA-C, while the most studied MHC class II genes are HLA-DP, HLA-DQ, and HLA-DR (Kindt et al., 2006).

The recognition of adaptive immune system is based on the interaction of T cell receptor (TCR) and peptide-MHC (p-MHC) complex (Figure 3). TCR on T-cell membrane can only detect antigens presented on the surface of MHC molecules. The property of this recognition is called MHC restriction. TCR recognizes the residues on the peptide and residues from

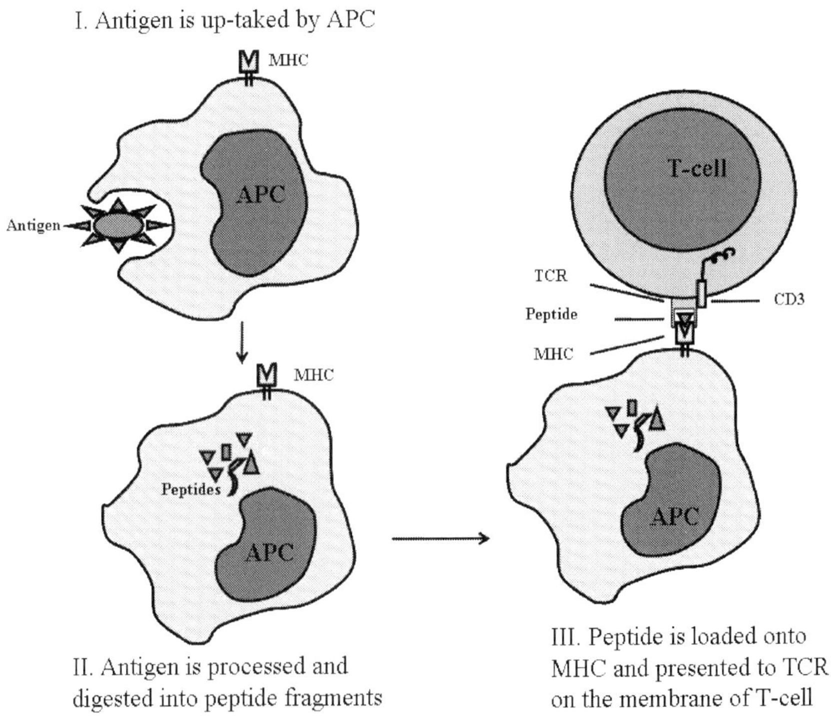

Fig. 3. **Recognition of p-MHC by TCR:** T cell cannot detect an antigen by itself. It can only recognize antigens presented by MHC on APC. APC uptakes foreign antigens and digests them into small peptides which are loaded onto the cleft of MHC molecules and then presented to TCR. Once they bind to p-MHC, TCR signal is transduced into T-cell via intracellular domain of associated CD3. T-cell is then activated and reacts to the invaders with corresponding antigen to clear them.

MHC molecules at the same time. TCR itself, however, lacks intracellular domain to transduce signal into T cells. On T-cell membrane, TCR forms a TCR/CD3 complex together with CD3. When binding to p-MHC, TCR signal is transduced into T cells via the intracellular domain of CD3 (Kuhns et al., 2006).

TCR consists of two chains, the α and β chain. Each chain is composed of two regions, the N-terminal variable (V) region and the C-terminal constant (C) region (Kuhns et al., 2006; Deng & Mariuzza, 2007). TCR is encoded by several segments, V, D, J, and C. The C region is encoded by C segment, while the V region is determined by V, D, and J segment. The V, D, and J segment have numerous copies. Despite of sharing the same genome, different T-cell clones have different TCR. The diversity of TCR originated from V region especially the complementary-determining regions (CDRs). Each TCR chain has three CDRs (CDR1, CDR2, and CDR3). CDR1 and CDR2 are encoded by V segment of the TCR gene, while CDR3 is generated from the V(D)J recombination (V_α and J_α segment recombination for α chain; and V_β, D, and J_β segment recombination for β chain) (Deng & Mariuzza, 2007; cha-Orbea et al., 1989). The diversity of TCR is believed to be generated by the following mechanisms: (1) the combination of α chain and β chain (each chain has two copies originated from father and mother, respectively); (2) V(D)J recombination (each TCR chain contains multiple gene segments, V, D, J segments, which need to be re-arranged by somatic gene re-arrangement during the development); (3) junctional diversity (additional bases will be inserted between segments during the V(D)J recombination, which results in the additional diversity of complementary-determining regions).

Normally, T cells do not provoke an immune response against self antigens, because autoreactive T cells are removed during the development of lymphocytes in the thymus (Deng & Mariuzza, 2007). Developing T cells are subjected to positive selection and negative selection in the thymus prior their presence in the periphery. Positive selection occurs in the cortex of thymus. The developing T cells that are unable to bind to MHC molecules on the thymic epithelial cells undergo programmed cell death (apoptosis), and as a result, only those cells with a high affinity to self MHC molecules on the thymic epithelial cells can survive. Those survived cells are next subjected to negative selection to get rid of autoreative T cells. The medulary thymic epithelial cells and dendritic cells in the thymus display self antigens on MHC molecules. T cells with a high affinity to self-peptide-MHC complex, which are also called autoreactive T cells, undergo apoptosis and thereby to be removed from the T cell repertoire. During this process, T cells develop tolerance to those antigens present on the thymic DCs and medulary thymic epithelial cells. The ectopic expression of organ-specific antigens such as insulin in those cells is regulated by a transcription factor called AIRE (the Autoimmune Regulator) (Kindt et al., 2006). Therefore, loss of AIRE function impairs ectopic expression of organ-specific autoantigens such as insulin and thereby interferes T-cell negative selection, predisposing to the development of type 1 diabetes (Anderson et al., 2002; Pugliese, 2005).

Other than the involvement in T-cell recognition and T-cell negative selection, components of the innate immune system are also directly implicated in the recognition of pathogenic antigens, which is called pattern recognition. As the first line of host defense, the innate immune system is the first component to take an action on invading microbes. Innate immune recognition occurs in advance to adaptive immune recognition and determines the responsive consequence to the antigens. Host immune system including innate and adaptive immune system relies on the innate recognition to make the decision to respond or not to respond to a particular antigen.

4. Pattern recognition

Innate immune recognition is also known as **pattern recognition**. It refers to the detection of common molecular structural motifs or pattern unique to microorganisms or other innate danger signals by the binding of pattern recognition receptors (PRRs) to their ligands (Zhong et al., 2011). Unlike the adaptive immune system which has diverse antigen receptors to identify a large number of foreign antigens, the innate immune system recognizes conserved microbe-derived molecules using a limited number of germline-encoded receptors - PRRs. Due to their limited number, every pattern recognition receptor can identify a large amount of pathogen specific molecules which share a certain structural motif. According to the originality, the ligands of PRR are divided into 2 classes: pathogen-associated molecular patterns (PAMPs) or damage-associated molecular patterns (DAMPs). PAMPs are conserved components among microorganisms that can be discriminated from host molecules such as flagellin, lipoteichoic acid from Gram positive bacteria, LPS from Gram negative bacterial, and peptidoglycan and dsRNA from virus. They are unique to microorganisms and important for the survival and/or expansion of microorganisms. Following the recognition, an immune reaction against the PAMPs is initiated to eliminate the invaded pathogens. **DAMPs** are small intracellular molecules released by cells during injury and served as a danger signal to initiate tissue repair. Using PRRs, the innate immune system can sense DAMPs and sequentially initiate noninfectious inflammatory responses. DAMPs are usually small molecules belonging to nuclear or cytosolic proteins. For example, HMGB1, ATP, HSP, and DNA are examples of DAMPs that can be released into the extracellular matrix in the damaged tissues. They are then recognized by PRRs to induce noninfectious inflammations to clear cellular debris, limit tissue injury, and promote tissue repair.

In contrast to adaptive immune recognition that is accomplished by the members of a single family - the Ig super-family, innate immune recognition is mediated by several protein families including C-type lectins, leucine-rich proteins, scavenger receptors, pentraxins, lipid transferases, and integrins (Medzhitov & Janeway, Jr., 1997). According to their function, localization, ligand specificity, and evolutionary relationships, PRRs can be classified into two groups: signaling PRRs and endocytic PRRs. Upon binding to the microbial molecules, signaling PRRs transmit a signal into the host innate immune cells and induce the synthesis of regulatory molecules that are crucial to initiate inflammatory and immune response, such as cytokines and costimulatory molecules. They include membrane-bound Toll-like receptors (TLRs) and cytoplasmic NOD-like receptors (NLRs). Endocytic PRRs are usually expressed on the cell surface of phagocytes and promote the attachment, engulfment and destruction of microbes by phagocytes, without inducing intracellular signals. They include mannose receptor (MMR), macrophage scavenger receptor (MSR), and opsonin receptors. Among those PRRs, TLRs are the best characterized PRRs. They play a major role in innate immune recognition and contribute to the initiation of inflammatory and immune responses.

TLRs belong to the evolutionarily conserved type I transmembrane proteins. There are a handful of members have been discovered so far, with 10 TLRs in humans (TLR1-10) and 12 TLRs in mice (TLR1-9, 11-13) (Beutler, 2004). The ligands for TLRs include various components of microbes that share the same motif. For example, TLR1/2/6, 4, 5, 9, and 11 can sense lipoprotein, LPS, flagellin, bacterial CpG DNA, and UPEC protein from bacteria; TLR3, 4, 7/8, 9 recognize dsDNA, RSV F protein, ssRNA, and viral CpG DNA from viruses;

whereas glycolipids, GIPLs, zymosan, and profilin-like protein derived from protozoa and fungi can be identified by TLR2/6 and TLR11 (West et al., 2006). Other than those PAMPs, certain DAMPs can also be recognized by TLRs (Johnson et al., 2003; Ohashi et al., 2000). For example, intracellular components as HMGB1 and HSP60 that are passively released from damaged cells can also bind to TLRs and induce TLR signaling (Ohashi et al., 2000; Erridge, 2010); oxidized beta2-GPI acts as another endogenous ligand of TLR to induce NF-κB activation and DC maturation (Buttari et al., 2005). TLRs consist of three domains: an N-terminal leucine-rich-repeat (LRR) domain, a single transmembrane domain, and a C-terminal intracellular TIR (Toll/IL-1 receptor) domain (Zhong et al., 2011; Takeda et al., 2003). The LRR domain is responsible for ligand binding, whereas the TIR domain is responsible for signaling. Upon the binding of PAMPs or DAMPs to LRR domain, TLRs initiate a cascade of signaling via TIR domain. By using a point mutation in TIR domain of TLR4 (P712H mutation), Poltorak and coworkers confirmed that TIR domain recruits downstream effectors and transduces intracellular signal for TLR (Poltorak et al., 1998). Binding of TLRs to their ligands induces diverse antimicrobial genes, proinflammatory cytokines, and chemokines. TLR signaling also can increase the expression of costimulatory molecules and promote antigen-presenting capability for APCs. Thus, innate recognition by TLR activates APCs to trigger inflammatory responses and initiates adaptive immune responses (Medzhitov & Janeway, Jr., 1997). TLR signaling is mediated via two types of pathways, the myeloid differentiation primary-response gene 88 (MyD88)-dependent and -independent pathway. Almost all TLRs except for TLR3 transmit intracellular signaling via MyD88-dependent pathway. Furthermore, MyD88-dependent pathway is the only pathway for TLR2, 5, 7/8, 9, and 11 (Zhong et al., 2011). Therefore, ligands for those TLRs such as peptidoglycans, flagellin, CpG DNA, ssRNA, and *toxoplasma* profilin-like protein cannot be sensed by MyD88 deficient cells (Takeda et al., 2003; Beutler et al., 2005; Adachi et al., 1998; Yarovinsky et al., 2005). Upon activation, MyD88 sequentially recruits IL-1 receptor-associated kinase-4 (IRAK-4) and IL-1 receptor-associated kinase-1 (IRAK-1) (Lin et al., 2010). Tumor necrosis factor receptor-associated factor-6 (TRAF-6) is subsequently recruited to MyD88/IRAK-4/IRAK-1 and then disassociate from the complex together with IRAK-1. TRAF-6 next sequentially activates c-Jun N-terminal kinase (JNK) and inhibitor of κB kinase (IKK), which in turn activates activator protein-1 (AP-1) and nuclear factor-kappa B (NF-κB) to initiate the transcription of diverse pro-inflammatory cytokine and chemokine genes (Beutler et al., 2006) (Figure 4). However, MyD88 cannot explain all downstream effect initiated by some TLRs as manifested by that TLR3 and TLR4 signaling are not completely blocked by the deficiency of MyD88, indicating that there must be MyD88-independent pathways for TLR signaling (Covert et al., 2005; Kawai et al., 1999). Studies have now indicated that TLR3 and TLR4 can signal through IRF3 and finally activate NF-κB in MyD88 deficient cells. In MyD88-independent pathway, TLR signal is mediated by TRIF (TIR domain-containing adaptor inducing IFN-β) and TRAM (TRIF-related adaptor molecule), and finally results in the activation of NF-κB, AP-1, or IRFs (Akira et al., 2001; Hoebe et al., 2003; Yamamoto et al., 2003a; Yamamoto et al., 2002; Yamamoto et al., 2003b; Fitzgerald et al., 2003). Upon activation, NF-κB, AP-1, or IRFs subsequently induces a series of events such as promoting proinflammatory cytokine and chemokine production, recruiting leucocytes, activating APCs, and initiating an adaptive immune response (Medzhitov, 2001; Takeda et al., 2003; Kawai & Akira, 2006; Akira, 2003).

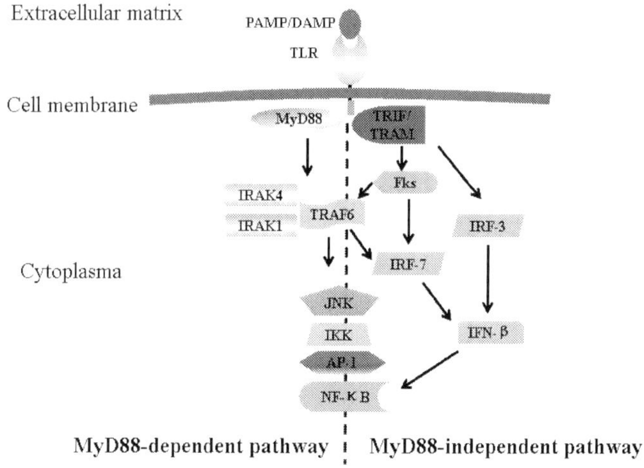

Fig. 4. **Signal Pathway of TLR:** TLRs transduce signal through MyD88-dependent and -independent pathway. Activation of MyD88 recruits IRAK-4, IRAK-1, and TRAF-6, and then sequentially activates JNK, IKK, AP-1, and NF-κB. MyD88-independent pathway is mediated by TRIF and TRAM, which finally leads to activation of NF-κB, AP-1, or IRFs.

NLR is another type of innate receptors. NLR proteins are a group of NOD domain containing intracellular receptors which detect the presence of PAMPs or DAMPs in the cytosol. NLRs are composed of an N-terminal protein interaction domain, a central nucleotide-binding oligomerization domain (NOD) and C-terminal leucine-rich repeat (LRR) domain(Chen et al., 2009). The N-terminal domain of the NLRs is critical for downstream signaling, and NOD domain mediates self-oligomerization that occurs during activation, whereas LRR domain is responsible for detecting PAMPs or DAMPs. Based on their N-terminal structure, NLRs are categorized into 5 subfamilies: NLRA which contains an acidic transactivation domain; NLRB which is characterized by the presence of a baculovirus inhibitor of apoptosis protein repeat (BIR); NLRC which possesses a caspase recruitment domain (CARD), NLRP which is manifested by a Pyrin domain; and NLRX whose N-terminal domain is unknown (Kawai & Akira, 2009). NLRs are expressed in epithelial, mesothelial, and immune cells including both APCs and lymphocytes. NOD1 and NOD2, members of NLRC, are the two well-characterized NLR proteins. They recognize peptidoglycan structure of pathogens. Recognition by NLRs induces self-oligomerization of NLRs and actiavates NF-κB and MAPK (Park et al., 2007; Hasegawa et al., 2008; Hitotsumatsu et al., 2008), which subsequently results in the release of IL-1 family of cytokines including IL-1β, IL-18, and IL-33 (Meylan et al., 2006; Fritz et al., 2006; Ting et al., 2006; Kanneganti et al., 2007; Yu & Finlay, 2008). There is feasible evidence supporting that NLRs play a role in the pathogenesis of autoimmune diseases. For example, NOD1 genetic variants modulate the host response to environmental bacteria and thus are associated with the development of allergic diseases such as asthma (Weidinger et al., 2005; Hysi et al., 2005; Eder et al., 2006). In addition, the polymorphisms of NLRs are also demonstrated to be associated with Crohn disease (Hugot et al., 2001). However, the role of NLRs in T1D pathogenesis is yet to be clarified (Eizirik et al., 2009).

In addition to TLRs and NLRs, other well-studied PRRs include Macrophage mannose receptor (MMR), macrophage scavenger receptor (MSR), and receptor for advanced glycation endproducts (RAGE) (Janeway, Jr. & Medzhitov, 2002; Kumagai et al., 2008; Li et al., 1996; Medzhitov & Janeway, Jr., 2000; Medzhitov, 2001; Medzhitov, 2007; Pearson, 1996). MMR is an important phagocytic receptor expressed on macrophages (Janeway, Jr. & Medzhitov, 2002). It is a member of the C-type lectin family and functions as a PPR to mediate phagocytosis of a variety of gram-positive, gram-negative bacteria, and fungal pathogens (Fraser et al., 1998). The microbial pathogens are then delivered into lysosomal compartment to be destroyed by lysosomal enzymes.

MSR is a member of scavenger receptor type A family. It also serves as a phagocytic pattern recognition receptor on macrophages. Blockade or genetic deletion of MSR on macrophages impairs the recognition of apoptotic cells by macrophages (Platt et al., 1996). The ligands for MSR include LPS, dsRNA, and liptocheic acid (LTA) (Pearson, 1996). Due to the defective LPS scavenging, loss of MSR increases the susceptibility to infection of various pathogens including Listeria monocytogenes, herpes simplex virus, and malaria (Thomas et al., 2000; Suzuki et al., 1997).

RAGE belongs to the immunoglobulin super-family. It is a 35kD multiligand transmembrane receptor (Neeper et al., 1992; Xie et al., 2008). Its major ligands are advanced glycation end products (AGE) and HMGB1. RAGE is composed of five domains: one cytosolic domain, one transmembrane domain, one variable domain, and two constant domains. The cytosolic domain is responsible for the signal transduction, and the variable domain is responsible for the binding of its ligand (Xie et al., 2008). RAGE signal activates NF-κB which sequentially induces the transcription of many pro-inflammatory genes. RAGE can also enhance the adhesion of leukocyte to endothelial cells and thus promote the recruitment of inflammatory cells (Chavakis et al., 2003).

5. Innate immune cells in the autoimmune response against β cells

Recent findings suggest that innate immune cells play an essential role in the initiation of β-cell-specific autoimmune response. Innate immune cells such as DCs, macrophages, and NK cells are found in a large number in the autoimmune diabetic pancreas in addition to lymphocytes. Furthermore, DCs and macrophages are the major population of infiltrating immune cells during the initial phase of autoimmune insulitis (Pietropaolo et al., 2007; Rosmalen et al., 2000; Charre et al., 2002; Delovitch & Singh, 1997; Jansen et al., 1994; Katz et al., 1995b; Lee et al., 1988c; Voorbij et al., 1989). Their presence at the pancreas precedes the infiltration of T and B lymphocytes. In addition to the early stage of autoimmunity, accumulation of innate immune cells is also observed during the later β-cell destructive insulitis process (Jansen et al., 1994). The density of DCs is much higher in diabetes-prone NOD mice immediately after birth than that of control non-diabetic strains. Therefore, the entry of macrophages and DCs is considered as the initial sign of autoimmunity in T1D pathogenesis (Medzhitov, 2001; Pearson, 1996; Takeda et al., 2003).

A wave of physiological β-cell death was found in newborns of both mice and humans, cumulating at early infancy (Finegood et al., 1995; Trudeau et al., 2000; Kassem et al., 2000). This physiological β-cell apoptosis, which is peaking at 14-17 days after birth in NOD mice, is proposed to be an initial stimulus for triggering islet-specific autoimmune response (Turley et al., 2003). Scavenger cells are believed to be responsible for the clearance of these apoptotic β cells. It was found that scavenger cells in the pancreas of NOD mice are abnormally higher than that of control strains and they persist in the NOD pancreas (Charre et al., 2002). This accumulation of scavenger cells is believed to be a result from the defective clearance of apoptotic β cells (Haskins et al., 2003; Mathis et al., 2001; Akirav et al., 2008).

It is proposed that the defective clearance of apoptotic β cells results in apoptotic β-cell accumulation which then leads to the secondary necrosis (Erridge, 2010). During the secondary necrosis process, β-cell-derived antigens could be released and then taken up and processed by APCs in the islets. After uptake of β-cell-derived antigens, APCs become matured and migrate into the immediate draining lymph nodes (pancreatic lymph nodes, PLNs). In the PLNs, naive β-cell-reactive T and B lymphocytes are primed and activated by APCs carrying the β-cell-derived antigens. Upon activation, T and B cells then migrate into the islets to attack the insulin producing β cells (Jansen et al., 1994). Depletion of macrophages by liposomal dichloromethylene diphosphonate, a substance known to be toxic to macrophages, in NOD mice results in the inability of T cells to differentiate into β-cell-cytotoxic T cells. During the initiation of β-cell-specific autoimmune response, APCs present β-cell-derived antigens to T cells and provide IL-12 to promote Th1 responses. T cells in a macrophages-depleted environment differentiate toward Th2 cells rather than Th1 cells. Of note, substantial administration of IL-12 restores the susceptibility to diabetes in macrophages-depleted NOD mice (Jun et al., 1999b). Consistently, many other groups also confirmed that depletion of macrophages dramatically prevents diabetes and insulitis in CY (cyclophosphamide)-treated NOD mice or BB rats (Lee et al., 1988e; Lee et al., 1988b; Oschilewski et al., 1985b).

In addition to activating lymphocytes, macrophages are also directly implicated in the final stage of autoimmune-mediated β-cell destruction. Adoptive transfer of monocyte-depleted diabetogenic T cells failed to induce diabetes. Moreover, activated macrophages can directly kill β cells in vitro (Calderon et al., 2006; Jun et al., 1999a). By using a transgenic model, Martin *et al.* provided direct evidence suggesting that macrophages are able to directly destroy β cells without T and B lymphocytes (Martin et al., 2008). Chemokines are a group of proteins produced in response to cell/tissue damage or inflammatory stimuli to attract immune cells. They are subdivided into 4 subgroups: C, CC, CXC, and CX3C family. Transgenic expression of CCL2 (also known as MCP-1), a chemokine belongs to the CC family, under the control of insulin promoter recruits circulating monocytes into the pancreas. When the RIP-CCL2 transgene was bred into the *Rag-1*$^{-/-}$ mice in which they are deficient for mature T and B lymphocytes, these mice developed insulitis and diabetes spontaneously, and showed a similar time course with immunocomponent RIP-CCL2 transgenic *Rag-1*$^{-/+}$ mice (Martin et al., 2008). This work demonstrates that macrophages are able to directly destroy β cells and play a more important role than what we thought. In addition, pro-inflammatory cytokines (e.g., IL-1β, TNFα, IL-6, and IL-12), as well as nitrogen and oxygen free radicals can be secreted into the pancreatic islets by activated APCs to directly destroy β cells (Beyan et al., 2003). Pro-inflammatory cytokines including TNFα and IL-1β produced by APCs and IFNγ produced by T cells can induce β cells to produce oxygen free radicals, nitric oxide, and peroxynitrite, which are highly cytotoxic to β cells themselves (Rabinovitch & Suarez-Pinzon, 1998). IL-12 secreted by macrophages in the pancreas is critical for T cells to differentiate into β-cell-cytotoxic T cells. Thus, macrophages can also promote T1D development by secreting IL-12 to enhance the differentiation of β-cell-targeting cytotoxic T cells. Deletion of macrophages decreases Th1 and Tc1 responses and thus prevents diabetes in NOD mice. In line with this observation, T cells can regain β-cell-cytotoxic potential with the return of macrophages or macrophage-derived IL-12 (Lee et al., 1988e; Jun et al., 1999b). Free radicals released by immune cells or β cells (induced by pro-inflammatory cytokines) can cause lipid peroxidation of membranes, DNA fragmentation, protein cross-linking, and thus, directly destroy β cells (Gewirtz, 1999; Dean et al., 1986).

NK cells are another type of innate immune cells presence in the lesion of insulitis. In a virus-induced diabetes model, Foldstrom and coworkers found that NK cells are critical for virus-induced autoimmune destruction of β cells (Flodstrom et al., 2002). Coxsackievirus B4 (CVB4) infection can induce autoimmune diabetes on SOSC-1-transgenic NOD mice. Depletion of NK cells can prevent β-cell loss on CVB4-infected SOSC-1-transgenic NOD mice and thereby blocks the development of diabetes (Flodstrom et al., 2002). Due to the ability to directly kill target cells and interact with APCs and T cells, the potential involvement of NK cells in T1D has been suggested in early 1980s. Splenic NK cells were shown to be able to destroy islet cells in both diabetes-prone BB rats and NOD mice (Flodstrom et al., 2002; MacKay et al., 1986; Koevary, 1988; Nakamura et al., 1990). Deletion of NK cells prevent T1D development in mice induced with virus, streptozotocin and cyclophosphamide (Flodstrom et al., 2002; Maruyama et al., 1991a; Maruyama et al., 1991b). Nevertheless, the role of NK cells in T1D seems only to modulate the intensity or aggressiveness of autoimmune destruction, as NK deletion failed to prevent spontaneous T1D in NOD mice or BB rats (Edouard et al., 1993; Ellerman et al., 1993; Sobel et al., 1995).

6. Innate molecules in the recognition of β-cell antigen

Given the involvement of innate immunity in T1D pathogenesis, innate recognition by PRRs, the first event of innate immune response, is suggested to be involved in triggering autoimmune reaction against β cells. In patients with T1D, TLR-2 and TLR-4 and their downstream molecules including MyD88, TRIF, and NFκB in monocytes are significantly upregulated, demonstrating that TLRs and their downstream signaling contribute to the development of T1D (Devaraj et al., 2008).

As mentioned earlier, there is a wave of physiological β-cell death after birth. Defective clearance of apoptotic β cells during β mass turnover has been suggested to be associated with the initiation of autoimmune response. The accumulated apoptotic β cells due to defective clearance undergo a secondary necrosis, which results in the passive release of innate inflammatory molecules to trigger an autoimmune response (Erridge, 2010). On the other hand, auto-antigens can be released from those necrotic β cells and then uptaken by APCs resided in the pancreas. It is believed that PRR signaling can promote uptake of auto-antigens by APCs (West et al., 2006; Doyle et al., 2004; Blander & Medzhitov, 2004). In support of this notion, stimulation of TLRs enhances antigen processing by up-regulating scavenger receptors via MyD88-dependent pathway. Doyle *et al.* found that TLR signaling can increase both the percentage of macrophage uptake of microbes and the number of microbes uptaken by each macrophage (Doyle et al., 2004). In addition, actin cytoskeleton mobilization, which can facilitate antigen processing and presentation by DCs, is also enhanced by TLR signaling (West et al., 2006).

Danger signals sensed by PRRs determine the consequence of antigens after its endocytosis (Matzinger, 2002; van & Geijtenbeek, 2006). Danger signals include exogenous signal (such as pathogens and toxins) and endogenous signal (such as mammalian DNA, RNA, HSPs, HMGB1, and interferons). A recent report demonstrated that APCs discriminate self and pathogenic antigens with the help of TLRs (Blander & Medzhitov, 2004). Blander and coworkers described that TLR signaling activated by bacteria regulates antigen internalization and phagosome maturation, and thus, promotes phagocytosis. Phagocytosis of bacteria but not apoptotic cells by macrophages was impaired in TLR2$^{-/-}$ and TLR4$^{-/-}$ or MyD88$^{-/-}$ mice (Blander & Medzhitov, 2004). Phagocytosis of bacterial induces DC maturation, whereas phagocytosis of apoptotic cells cannot. However, uptake of apoptotic cells along with LPS treatment can induce DC maturation, indicating that TLR signaling determines the fate of auto-antigen. Antigens derived from apoptotic cells cannot be efficiently presented by MHC class II. Nevertheless, co-administration with TLR ligand enhances antigen presentation and promotes antigen-specific CD4+ T cell response (West et al., 2006). Therefore, TLRs can sense danger signal and control the discrimination of self and non-self antigens. Normally, self antigens are excluded from antigen presentation due to the lack of TLR signaling. However, self antigens and TLR signals can co-exist under certain pathological circumstances. For example, defective clearance of apoptotic β cells, which is observed in diabetes-prone individuals, results in the release of both self antigen and endogenous danger signaling molecules (such as HMGB1, HSPs, and nucleic acids), while PRRs can bind to both exogenous and endogenous molecules (Matzinger, 2002). For example, TLR2 is the receptor for endogenous molecules HSP60 and HMGB1, as well as exogenous molecules of bacterial lipoproteins, Similarly, TLR4 is a receptor for HSP70, HMGB1, and LPS. Therefore, those endogenous danger signaling molecules (also called alarmins) released from necrotic β cells function as DAMPs to signal TLRs. With the presence of those TLR signals and auto-antigens, the tolerance to self antigens is broken down and an autoimmune response against β cells is then initiated. TLR2 has been suggested to be an important sensor for apoptotic or secondary necrotic β cells (Kim et al., 2007). Apoptotic β cells undergoing secondary necrosis can provoke a β-cell-specific autoimmune response in a TLR2-dependent manner. Therefore, autoimmune diabetes is significantly suppressed in TLR2$^{-/-}$ mice but not in TLR4$^{-/-}$ mice (Kim et al., 2007). Engagement of TLR3 by poly I:C is also reported to be able to accelerate diabetes in a dose-dependent manner (Sobel et al., 1992; Ewel et al., 1992).

As a multifactoral autoimmune disease, T1D is affected by both genetic and environmental factors. Viral infection, as an environmental perturbant, is believed to be the most common trigger for T1D development (Akerblom et al., 2002). TLRs have been shown to be implicated in the process of virus-induced diabetes. Kilham rat virus (KRV) can induce autoimmune diabetes on BioBreeding diabetes-resistant (BBDR) rats (Nair et al., 2008). KRV infection has been shown to be able to induce the production of pro-inflammatory cytokines such as IL-6 and IL-12 in BBDR rats, which can be abolished by TLR9 antagonists (Zipris et al., 2007). TLR9 blockade on KRV-infected BBDR rats decreased diabetes incidence (Zipris et al., 2007). Furthermore, engagement of TLR3, 4, 6, 7, and 8 was also found to significantly increase the incidence of KRV-induced diabetes on BBDR rats (Zipris et al., 2005). A lymphochoriomeningitis virus (LCMV)-induced diabetes model with RIP-GP transgenic mice was employed to dissect the role of virus infection in triggering diabetes (Ohashi et al., 1991). The islet cells of RIP-GP mice express LCMV-GP protein under the control of RIP promoter. Unlike LCMV, viral peptide failed to induce diabetes in RIP-GP mice (Lang et al., 2005; Ohashi et al., 1993). However, co-administration of TLR3 and 7 ligands with a viral peptide successfully induces diabetes in RIP-GP mice (Lang et al., 2005), indicating that TLR signals play a critical role in virus-induced autoimmune diabetes.

HMGB1, an evolutionarily conserved nuclear protein, has recently been found to be a "danger signal" to alert the immune system of tissue damage. It can be passively released from damaged cells during various pathogenic processes. For example, HMGB1 released from damaged cells during liver ischemia-reperfusion plays a critical role in mediating hepatic injury ((Tsung et al., 2005). In line with this result, we demonstrated that HMGB1 can be passively released during cardiac cold ischemic injury as well as in graft with acute rejection (Huang et al., 2007). In a model for syngenic heart transplantation, HMGB1 increased for a few days after surgery and dropped back to normal level thereafter, while HMGB1 steadily increased in allografts after transplantation along with acute allograft rejection, suggesting that HMGB1 is implicated in the pathogenesis of allograft rejection. In support of this notion, we characterized that allograft infiltrated immune cells actively secrete HMGB1. Therefore, administration of recombinant A box, a specific antagonist for the endogenous HMGB1, reduced pro-inflammatory cytokine production and Th1 response, and thus, prolonged cardiac allograft survival (Huang et al., 2007). Together, these data support a critical role for HMGB1 in mediating allo-immune response. Given the similarity between allograft rejection and autoimmune destruction of the pancreatic β cells in type 1 diabetes, we next proposed that HMGB1 might serve as an innate mediator implicated in β-cell specific autoimmune response during T1D development. By studies in NOD neonates, we demonstrated the accumulation of apoptotic β cells during neonate β mass turnover, which is associated with secondary β cell necrosis and passive release of HMGB1 into the extracellular milieu in the pancreatic islets (Zhang et al., 2009). The passively released HMGB1 could then serve as an innate alarmin for the initiation of autoimmune response in genetic predisposed subjects. To address the role of HMGB1 in T1D progression, we next confirmed that HMGB1 can be released from apoptotic β cells and thus served as a danger signal to enhance autoimmune response in T1D (Han et al., 2008). In addition to being passively released by the damaged β cells, HMGB1 can also be actively secreted by DCs and other islet-infiltrating immune cells. Upon LPS or TNFα/IFN-γ stimulation, HMGB1 translocated from the nucleus into the cytosol in DCs and then secreted into the extracellular matrix. In consistent with these results, *in situ* immunostaining confirmed the co-localization of HMGB1 and CD11c, a specific surface marker for DCs, in the pancreatic sections originated from diabetic NOD mice (Han et al., 2008). Therefore, with the presence of extracellular HMGB1, APCs efficiently uptake apoptotic β cells and become matured. Our subsequent studies further revealed that extracellular HMGB1 released by damaged cells or secreted by activated immune cells is potent in promoting inflammatory response. For example, treatment of DCs with HMGB1 significantly increased their pro-inflammatory cytokine production and allo-stimulatory capacity along with higher expression of MHC class II and costimulatory molecules. More important, this stimulatory effect can be abolished by the administration of HMGB1 blockades such as HMGB1 neutralizing antibodies. Therefore, treatment of NOD mice with a neutralizing HMGB1 Ab dramatically reduced insulitis progression and diabetes onset (Han et al., 2008). Consistent with our observations, Dumitriu *et al.* found that HMGB1 can be released from plasmacytoid DCs (pDCs) following TLR9 stimuli. Furthermore, pDCs express RAGE, a receptor for HMGB1. Disruption of HMGB1/RAGE signaling suppressed the maturation of pDCs (Dumitriu et al., 2005). In addition, HMGB1 was found to promote inflammatory response by enhancing DC migration, and as such, blockade of HMGB1 or RAGE, suppressed homing receptor expression on monocyte-derived DCs and inhibited their migration which is required for T-cell priming (Yang et al., 2007; Dumitriu et al., 2007).

7. Conclusion

Innate immune response, as one of the two pillars of the immune system and the mediator of adaptive immune response, plays an essential role in the pathogenesis of T1D. Pattern recognition receptors expressed on the innate immune cells sense the conserved pathogen specific molecules (PAMPs) or alarmins released by host cells (DAMPs) to initiate an immune response. In the normal condition, self antigens can be distinguished from foreign antigens and do not provoke an immune response. However, under certain circumstances, self antigens released from damaged host cells could be processed and presented to autoreactive T cells with the presence of PRR signaling. For the case of type 1 diabetes, defective clearance of apoptotic β cells during neonate β mass turnover by phagocytes results in the accumulation of apoptotic β cells in the pancreas, which then undergo a secondary necrosis along with the release of β-cell-derived autoantigens and danger signals (e.g., HMGB1, HSPs, and DNA). Danger signals subsequently activate PRRs and promote self antigen presentation by APCs. Furthermore, PRR signals also induce maturation and migration of APCs, which facilitate both innate and adaptive immune response to mediate the destruction of β cells. The effect of current therapeutic approaches for T1D is unsatisfied. A variety of severe complications developed in the relatively large proportion of T1D patients. Therefore, a clear understanding of the recognition of β-cell antigens and the initiation of autoreative immune response against β cells is essential to the development of better effective therapeutic approaches for this devastating disorder.

8. Acknowledgements

Jixin Zhong and Jun-Fa Xu contributed equally to this work. Correspondence should be addressed to Dr. Cong-Yi Wang (cwang@georgiahealth.edu). Our research is supported by grants from the Juvenile Diabetes Research Foundation International (JDRFI) and the EFSD/CDC/Lilly Program for Collaborative Diabetes Research between China and Europe, and by the Bridge Funding from Tongji Hospital of HUST to CYW. The authors declare that they have no competing financial interest.

9. References

Adachi, O., Kawai, T., Takeda, K., Matsumoto, M., Tsutsui, H., Sakagami, M., Nakanishi, K., & Akira, S. (1998). Targeted disruption of the MyD88 gene results in loss of IL-1- and IL-18-mediated function. *Immunity. 9*, 143-150.

Akerblom, H.K., Vaarala, O., Hyoty, H., Ilonen, J., & Knip, M. (2002). Environmental factors in the etiology of type 1 diabetes. *Am. J. Med. Genet. 115*, 18-29.

Akira, S. (2003). Toll-like receptor signaling. *J. Biol. Chem. 278*, 38105-38108.

Akira, S., Takeda, K., & Kaisho, T. (2001). Toll-like receptors: critical proteins linking innate and acquired immunity. *Nat. Immunol. 2*, 675-680.

Akirav, E., Kushner, J.A., & Herold, K.C. (2008). Beta-cell mass and type 1 diabetes: going, going, gone? *Diabetes 57*, 2883-2888.

Amos, A.F., McCarty, D.J., & Zimmet, P. (1997). The rising global burden of diabetes and its complications: estimates and projections to the year 2010. *Diabet. Med. 14 Suppl 5*, S1-85.

Anderson, M.S., Venanzi, E.S., Klein, L., Chen, Z., Berzins, S.P., Turley, S.J., von, B.H., Bronson, R., Dierich, A., Benoist, C., & Mathis, D. (2002). Projection of an immunological self shadow within the thymus by the aire protein. *Science 298*, 1395-1401.

Bach, J.F., Garchon, H.J., & van, E.P. (2001). Genetics of human type 1 diabetes mellitus. *Curr. Dir. Autoimmun. 4*, 1-30.

Baekkeskov, S., Nielsen, J.H., Marner, B., Bilde, T., Ludvigsson, J., & Lernmark, A. (1982). Autoantibodies in newly diagnosed diabetic children immunoprecipitate human pancreatic islet cell proteins. *Nature 298*, 167-169.

Beutler, B. (2004). Inferences, questions and possibilities in Toll-like receptor signalling. *Nature 430*, 257-263.

Beutler, B., Hoebe, K., Georgel, P., Tabeta, K., & Du, X. (2005). Genetic analysis of innate immunity: identification and function of the TIR adapter proteins. *Adv. Exp. Med. Biol. 560*, 29-39.

Beutler, B., Jiang, Z., Georgel, P., Crozat, K., Croker, B., Rutschmann, S., Du, X., & Hoebe, K. (2006). Genetic analysis of host resistance: Toll-like receptor signaling and immunity at large. *Annu. Rev. Immunol. 24*, 353-389.

Beyan, H., Buckley, L.R., Yousaf, N., Londei, M., & Leslie, R.D. (2003). A role for innate immunity in type 1 diabetes? *Diabetes Metab Res. Rev. 19*, 89-100.

Blander, J.M. & Medzhitov, R. (2004). Regulation of phagosome maturation by signals from toll-like receptors. *Science 304*, 1014-1018.

Borghans, J.A., Beltman, J.B., & De Boer, R.J. (2004). MHC polymorphism under host-pathogen coevolution. *Immunogenetics 55*, 732-739.

Bottazzo, G.F., Dean, B.M., McNally, J.M., MacKay, E.H., Swift, P.G., & Gamble, D.R. (1985). In situ characterization of autoimmune phenomena and expression of HLA molecules in the pancreas in diabetic insulitis. *N. Engl. J. Med. 313*, 353-360.

Breecher, M.M. & Dworken, A.M. (1986). The Merck Manual. *Med. Herit. 2*, 229-231.

Buttari, B., Profumo, E., Mattei, V., Siracusano, A., Ortona, E., Margutti, P., Salvati, B., Sorice, M., & Rigano, R. (2005). Oxidized beta2-glycoprotein I induces human dendritic cell maturation and promotes a T helper type 1 response. *Blood 106*, 3880-3887.

Calderon, B., Suri, A., & Unanue, E.R. (2006). In CD4+ T-cell-induced diabetes, macrophages are the final effector cells that mediate islet beta-cell killing: studies from an acute model. *Am. J. Pathol. 169*, 2137-2147.

cha-Orbea, H., Steinman, L., & McDevitt, H.O. (1989). T cell receptors in murine autoimmune diseases. *Annu. Rev. Immunol. 7*, 371-405.

Charre, S., Rosmalen, J.G., Pelegri, C., Alves, V., Leenen, P.J., Drexhage, H.A., & Homo-Delarche, F. (2002). Abnormalities in dendritic cell and macrophage accumulation in the pancreas of nonobese diabetic (NOD) mice during the early neonatal period. *Histol. Histopathol. 17*, 393-401.

Chavakis, T., Bierhaus, A., Al-Fakhri, N., Schneider, D., Witte, S., Linn, T., Nagashima, M., Morser, J., Arnold, B., Preissner, K.T., & Nawroth, P.P. (2003). The pattern recognition receptor (RAGE) is a counterreceptor for leukocyte integrins: a novel pathway for inflammatory cell recruitment. *J. Exp. Med. 198*, 1507-1515.

Chen, G., Shaw, M.H., Kim, Y.G., & Nunez, G. (2009). NOD-like receptors: role in innate immunity and inflammatory disease. *Annu. Rev. Pathol. 4*, 365-398.

Conrad, B., Weidmann, E., Trucco, G., Rudert, W.A., Behboo, R., Ricordi, C., Rodriquez-Rilo, H., Finegold, D., & Trucco, M. (1994). Evidence for superantigen involvement in insulin-dependent diabetes mellitus aetiology. *Nature 371*, 351-355.

Covert, M.W., Leung, T.H., Gaston, J.E., & Baltimore, D. (2005). Achieving stability of lipopolysaccharide-induced NF-kappaB activation. *Science 309*, 1854-1857.

Dean, R.T., Thomas, S.M., & Garner, A. (1986). Free-radical-mediated fragmentation of monoamine oxidase in the mitochondrial membrane. Roles for lipid radicals. *Biochem. J. 240*, 489-494.

Delovitch, T.L. & Singh, B. (1997). The nonobese diabetic mouse as a model of autoimmune diabetes: immune dysregulation gets the NOD. *Immunity. 7*, 727-738.

Deng, L. & Mariuzza, R.A. (2007). Recognition of self-peptide-MHC complexes by autoimmune T-cell receptors. *Trends Biochem. Sci. 32*, 500-508.

Devaraj, S., Dasu, M.R., Rockwood, J., Winter, W., Griffen, S.C., & Jialal, I. (2008). Increased toll-like receptor (TLR) 2 and TLR4 expression in monocytes from patients with type 1 diabetes: further evidence of a proinflammatory state. *J. Clin. Endocrinol. Metab 93*, 578-583.

Doyle, S.E., O'Connell, R.M., Miranda, G.A., Vaidya, S.A., Chow, E.K., Liu, P.T., Suzuki, S., Suzuki, N., Modlin, R.L., Yeh, W.C., Lane, T.F., & Cheng, G. (2004). Toll-like receptors induce a phagocytic gene program through p38. *J. Exp. Med. 199*, 81-90.

Dumitriu, I.E., Baruah, P., Bianchi, M.E., Manfredi, A.A., & Rovere-Querini, P. (2005). Requirement of HMGB1 and RAGE for the maturation of human plasmacytoid dendritic cells. *Eur. J. Immunol. 35*, 2184-2190.

Dumitriu, I.E., Bianchi, M.E., Bacci, M., Manfredi, A.A., & Rovere-Querini, P. (2007). The secretion of HMGB1 is required for the migration of maturing dendritic cells. *J. Leukoc. Biol. 81*, 84-91.

Eder, W., Klimecki, W., Yu, L., von, M.E., Riedler, J., Braun-Fahrlander, C., Nowak, D., Holst, O., & Martinez, F.D. (2006). Association between exposure to farming, allergies and genetic variation in CARD4/NOD1. *Allergy 61*, 1117-1124.

Edouard, P., Hiserodt, J.C., Plamondon, C., & Poussier, P. (1993). CD8+ T-cells are required for adoptive transfer of the BB rat diabetic syndrome. *Diabetes 42*, 390-397.

Eisenbarth, G.S. (1984). The immunoendocrinopathy syndromes. In Williams Texbook of Endocrinology.

Eizirik, D.L., Colli, M.L., & Ortis, F. (2009). The role of inflammation in insulitis and beta-cell loss in type 1 diabetes. *Nat. Rev. Endocrinol. 5*, 219-226.

El-Osta, A., Brasacchio, D., Yao, D., Pocai, A., Jones, P.L., Roeder, R.G., Cooper, M.E., & Brownlee, M. (2008). Transient high glucose causes persistent epigenetic changes and altered gene expression during subsequent normoglycemia. *J. Exp. Med. 205*, 2409-2417.

Ellerman, K., Wrobleski, M., Rabinovitch, A., & Like, A. (1993). Natural killer cell depletion and diabetes mellitus in the BB/Wor rat (revisited). *Diabetologia 36*, 596-601.

Erridge, C. (2010). Endogenous ligands of TLR2 and TLR4: agonists or assistants? *J. Leukoc. Biol. 87*, 989-999.

Ewel, C.H., Sobel, D.O., Zeligs, B.J., & Bellanti, J.A. (1992). Poly I:C accelerates development of diabetes mellitus in diabetes-prone BB rat. *Diabetes 41*, 1016-1021.

Finegood, D.T., Scaglia, L., & Bonner-Weir, S. (1995). Dynamics of beta-cell mass in the growing rat pancreas. Estimation with a simple mathematical model. *Diabetes 44*, 249-256.

Fitzgerald, K.A., Rowe, D.C., Barnes, B.J., Caffrey, D.R., Visintin, A., Latz, E., Monks, B., Pitha, P.M., & Golenbock, D.T. (2003). LPS-TLR4 signaling to IRF-3/7 and NF-kappaB involves the toll adapters TRAM and TRIF. *J. Exp. Med. 198*, 1043-1055.

Flodstrom, M., Maday, A., Balakrishna, D., Cleary, M.M., Yoshimura, A., & Sarvetnick, N. (2002). Target cell defense prevents the development of diabetes after viral infection. *Nat. Immunol. 3*, 373-382.

Fraser, I.P., Koziel, H., & Ezekowitz, R.A. (1998). The serum mannose-binding protein and the macrophage mannose receptor are pattern recognition molecules that link innate and adaptive immunity. *Semin. Immunol. 10,* 363-372.

Fritz, J.H., Ferrero, R.L., Philpott, D.J., & Girardin, S.E. (2006). Nod-like proteins in immunity, inflammation and disease. *Nat. Immunol. 7,* 1250-1257.

Gepts, W. (1965). Pathologic anatomy of the pancreas in juvenile diabetes mellitus. *Diabetes 14,* 619-633.

Gewirtz, D.A. (1999). A critical evaluation of the mechanisms of action proposed for the antitumor effects of the anthracycline antibiotics adriamycin and daunorubicin. *Biochem. Pharmacol. 57,* 727-741.

Han, J., Zhong, J., Wei, W., Wang, Y., Huang, Y., Yang, P., Purohit, S., Dong, Z., Wang, M.H., She, J.X., Gong, F., Stern, D.M., & Wang, C.Y. (2008). Extracellular high-mobility group box 1 acts as an innate immune mediator to enhance autoimmune progression and diabetes onset in NOD mice. *Diabetes 57,* 2118-2127.

Hasegawa, M., Fujimoto, Y., Lucas, P.C., Nakano, H., Fukase, K., Nunez, G., & Inohara, N. (2008). A critical role of RICK/RIP2 polyubiquitination in Nod-induced NF-kappaB activation. *EMBO J. 27,* 373-383.

Haskins, K., Bradley, B., Powers, K., Fadok, V., Flores, S., Ling, X., Pugazhenthi, S., Reusch, J., & Kench, J. (2003). Oxidative stress in type 1 diabetes. *Ann. N. Y. Acad. Sci. 1005,* 43-54.

Herold, K.C., Gitelman, S., Greenbaum, C., Puck, J., Hagopian, W., Gottlieb, P., Sayre, P., Bianchine, P., Wong, E., Seyfert-Margolis, V., Bourcier, K., & Bluestone, J.A. (2009). Treatment of patients with new onset Type 1 diabetes with a single course of anti-CD3 mAb Teplizumab preserves insulin production for up to 5 years. *Clin. Immunol. 132,* 166-173.

Herold, K.C., Hagopian, W., Auger, J.A., Poumian-Ruiz, E., Taylor, L., Donaldson, D., Gitelman, S.E., Harlan, D.M., Xu, D., Zivin, R.A., & Bluestone, J.A. (2002). Anti-CD3 monoclonal antibody in new-onset type 1 diabetes mellitus. *N. Engl. J. Med. 346,* 1692-1698.

Hitotsumatsu, O., Ahmad, R.C., Tavares, R., Wang, M., Philpott, D., Turer, E.E., Lee, B.L., Shiffin, N., Advincula, R., Malynn, B.A., Werts, C., & Ma, A. (2008). The ubiquitin-editing enzyme A20 restricts nucleotide-binding oligomerization domain containing 2-triggered signals. *Immunity. 28,* 381-390.

Hoebe, K., Du, X., Georgel, P., Janssen, E., Tabeta, K., Kim, S.O., Goode, J., Lin, P., Mann, N., Mudd, S., Crozat, K., Sovath, S., Han, J., & Beutler, B. (2003). Identification of Lps2 as a key transducer of MyD88-independent TIR signalling. *Nature 424,* 743-748.

Home, P. (2003). The challenge of poorly controlled diabetes mellitus. *Diabetes Metab 29,* 101-109.

Huang, Y., Yin, H., Han, J., Huang, B., Xu, J., Zheng, F., Tan, Z., Fang, M., Rui, L., Chen, D., Wang, S., Zheng, X., Wang, C.Y., & Gong, F. (2007). Extracellular hmgb1 functions as an innate immune-mediator implicated in murine cardiac allograft acute rejection. *Am. J. Transplant. 7,* 799-808.

Hugot, J.P., Chamaillard, M., Zouali, H., Lesage, S., Cezard, J.P., Belaiche, J., Almer, S., Tysk, C., O'Morain, C.A., Gassull, M., Binder, V., Finkel, Y., Cortot, A., Modigliani, R., Laurent-Puig, P., Gower-Rousseau, C., Macry, J., Colombel, J.F., Sahbatou, M., & Thomas, G. (2001). Association of NOD2 leucine-rich repeat variants with susceptibility to Crohn's disease. *Nature 411,* 599-603.

Hysi, P., Kabesch, M., Moffatt, M.F., Schedel, M., Carr, D., Zhang, Y., Boardman, B., von, M.E., Weiland, S.K., Leupold, W., Fritzsch, C., Klopp, N., Musk, A.W., James, A.,

Nunez, G., Inohara, N., & Cookson, W.O. (2005). NOD1 variation, immunoglobulin E and asthma. *Hum. Mol. Genet. 14,* 935-941.

Janeway, C.A., Jr. & Medzhitov, R. (2002). Innate immune recognition. *Annu. Rev. Immunol. 20,* 197-216.

Jansen, A., Homo-Delarche, F., Hooijkaas, H., Leenen, P.J., Dardenne, M., & Drexhage, H.A. (1994). Immunohistochemical characterization of monocytes-macrophages and dendritic cells involved in the initiation of the insulitis and beta-cell destruction in NOD mice. *Diabetes 43,* 667-675.

Johnson, G.B., Brunn, G.J., & Platt, J.L. (2003). Activation of mammalian Toll-like receptors by endogenous agonists. *Crit Rev. Immunol. 23,* 15-44.

Jun, H.S., Santamaria, P., Lim, H.W., Zhang, M.L., & Yoon, J.W. (1999a). Absolute requirement of macrophages for the development and activation of beta-cell cytotoxic CD8+ T-cells in T-cell receptor transgenic NOD mice. *Diabetes 48,* 34-42.

Jun, H.S., Yoon, C.S., Zbytnuik, L., van, R.N., & Yoon, J.W. (1999b). The role of macrophages in T cell-mediated autoimmune diabetes in nonobese diabetic mice. *J. Exp. Med. 189,* 347-358.

Jun, H.S., Yoon, C.S., Zbytnuik, L., van, R.N., & Yoon, J.W. (1999c). The role of macrophages in T cell-mediated autoimmune diabetes in nonobese diabetic mice. *J. Exp. Med. 189,* 347-358.

Kanneganti, T.D., Lamkanfi, M., & Nunez, G. (2007). Intracellular NOD-like receptors in host defense and disease. *Immunity. 27,* 549-559.

Kassem, S.A., Ariel, I., Thornton, P.S., Scheimberg, I., & Glaser, B. (2000). Beta-cell proliferation and apoptosis in the developing normal human pancreas and in hyperinsulinism of infancy. *Diabetes 49,* 1325-1333.

Katz, J.D., Benoist, C., & Mathis, D. (1995a). T helper cell subsets in insulin-dependent diabetes. *Science 268,* 1185-1188.

Katz, J.D., Benoist, C., & Mathis, D. (1995b). T helper cell subsets in insulin-dependent diabetes. *Science 268,* 1185-1188.

Kawai, T., Adachi, O., Ogawa, T., Takeda, K., & Akira, S. (1999). Unresponsiveness of MyD88-deficient mice to endotoxin. *Immunity. 11,* 115-122.

Kawai, T. & Akira, S. (2009). The roles of TLRs, RLRs and NLRs in pathogen recognition. *Int. Immunol. 21,* 317-337.

Kawai, T. & Akira, S. (2006). TLR signaling. *Cell Death. Differ. 13,* 816-825.

Killestein, J. (2002). Anti-CD3 monoclonal antibody in new-onset type 1 diabetes mellitus. *N. Engl. J. Med. 347,* 1116-1117.

Kim, H.S., Han, M.S., Chung, K.W., Kim, S., Kim, E., Kim, M.J., Jang, E., Lee, H.A., Youn, J., Akira, S., & Lee, M.S. (2007). Toll-like receptor 2 senses beta-cell death and contributes to the initiation of autoimmune diabetes. *Immunity. 27,* 321-333.

Kindt, T., Osborne, B., and Goldsby, R. (2006). *Kuby Immunology* (6th Ed.), W. H. Freeman, ISBN-13: 978-1429202114, New York.

Koevary, S.B. (1988). In vitro natural killer cell activity in the spontaneously diabetic BB/Wor rat: effects of serum on lysis of insulinoma cells. *Diabetes Res. 8,* 77-84.

Kuhns, M.S., Davis, M.M., & Garcia, K.C. (2006). Deconstructing the form and function of the TCR/CD3 complex. *Immunity. 24,* 133-139.

Kumagai, Y., Takeuchi, O., & Akira, S. (2008). Pathogen recognition by innate receptors. *J. Infect. Chemother. 14,* 86-92.

Kumanovics, A., Takada, T., & Lindahl, K.F. (2003). Genomic organization of the mammalian MHC. *Annu. Rev. Immunol. 21,* 629-657.

Lang, K.S., Recher, M., Junt, T., Navarini, A.A., Harris, N.L., Freigang, S., Odermatt, B., Conrad, C., Ittner, L.M., Bauer, S., Luther, S.A., Uematsu, S., Akira, S., Hengartner, H., & Zinkernagel, R.M. (2005). Toll-like receptor engagement converts T-cell autoreactivity into overt autoimmune disease. *Nat. Med. 11*, 138-145.

Lee, K.U., Amano, K., & Yoon, J.W. (1988b). Evidence for initial involvement of macrophage in development of insulitis in NOD mice. *Diabetes 37*, 989-991.

Lee, K.U., Amano, K., & Yoon, J.W. (1988a). Evidence for initial involvement of macrophage in development of insulitis in NOD mice. *Diabetes 37*, 989-991.

Lee, K.U., Kim, M.K., Amano, K., Pak, C.Y., Jaworski, M.A., Mehta, J.G., & Yoon, J.W. (1988c). Preferential infiltration of macrophages during early stages of insulitis in diabetes-prone BB rats. *Diabetes 37*, 1053-1058.

Lee, K.U., Pak, C.Y., Amano, K., & Yoon, J.W. (1988e). Prevention of lymphocytic thyroiditis and insulitis in diabetes-prone BB rats by the depletion of macrophages. *Diabetologia 31*, 400-402.

Lee, K.U., Pak, C.Y., Amano, K., & Yoon, J.W. (1988d). Prevention of lymphocytic thyroiditis and insulitis in diabetes-prone BB rats by the depletion of macrophages. *Diabetologia 31*, 400-402.

Li, Y.M., Mitsuhashi, T., Wojciechowicz, D., Shimizu, N., Li, J., Stitt, A., He, C., Banerjee, D., & Vlassara, H. (1996). Molecular identity and cellular distribution of advanced glycation endproduct receptors: relationship of p60 to OST-48 and p90 to 80K-H membrane proteins. *Proc. Natl. Acad. Sci. U. S. A 93*, 11047-11052.

Lin, S.C., Lo, Y.C., & Wu, H. (2010). Helical assembly in the MyD88-IRAK4-IRAK2 complex in TLR/IL-1R signalling. *Nature 465*, 885-890.

MacKay, P., Jacobson, J., & Rabinovitch, A. (1986). Spontaneous diabetes mellitus in the Bio-Breeding/Worcester rat. Evidence in vitro for natural killer cell lysis of islet cells. *J. Clin. Invest 77*, 916-924.

Martin, A.P., Rankin, S., Pitchford, S., Charo, I.F., Furtado, G.C., & Lira, S.A. (2008). Increased expression of CCL2 in insulin-producing cells of transgenic mice promotes mobilization of myeloid cells from the bone marrow, marked insulitis, and diabetes. *Diabetes 57*, 3025-3033.

Maruyama, T., Watanabe, K., Takei, I., Kasuga, A., Shimada, A., Yanagawa, T., Kasatani, T., Suzuki, Y., Kataoka, K., Saruta, & . (1991a). Anti-asialo GM1 antibody suppression of cyclophosphamide-induced diabetes in NOD mice. *Diabetes Res. 17*, 37-41.

Maruyama, T., Watanabe, K., Yanagawa, T., Kasatani, T., Kasuga, A., Shimada, A., Takei, I., Suzuki, Y., Kataoka, K., & Saruta, T. (1991b). The suppressive effect of anti-asialo GM1 antibody on low-dose streptozotocin-induced diabetes in CD-1 mice. *Diabetes Res. 16*, 171-175.

Mathis, D., Vence, L., & Benoist, C. (2001). beta-Cell death during progression to diabetes. *Nature 414*, 792-798.

Matzinger, P. (2002). The danger model: a renewed sense of self. *Science 296*, 301-305.

Medzhitov, R. (2001). Toll-like receptors and innate immunity. *Nat. Rev. Immunol. 1*, 135-145.

Medzhitov, R. (2007). Recognition of microorganisms and activation of the immune response. *Nature 449*, 819-826.

Medzhitov, R. & Janeway, C., Jr. (2000). Innate immune recognition: mechanisms and pathways. *Immunol. Rev. 173*, 89-97.

Medzhitov, R. & Janeway, C.A., Jr. (1997). Innate immunity: impact on the adaptive immune response. *Curr. Opin. Immunol. 9*, 4-9.

Meylan, E., Tschopp, J., & Karin, M. (2006). Intracellular pattern recognition receptors in the host response. *Nature 442*, 39-44.

Nair, A., Wolter, T.R., Meyers, A.J., & Zipris, D. (2008). Innate immune pathways in virus-induced autoimmune diabetes. *Ann. N. Y. Acad. Sci. 1150,* 139-142.

Nakamura, N., Woda, B.A., Tafuri, A., Greiner, D.L., Reynolds, C.W., Ortaldo, J., Chick, W., Handler, E.S., Mordes, J.P., & Rossini, A.A. (1990). Intrinsic cytotoxicity of natural killer cells to pancreatic islets in vitro. *Diabetes 39,* 836-843.

Neeper, M., Schmidt, A.M., Brett, J., Yan, S.D., Wang, F., Pan, Y.C., Elliston, K., Stern, D., & Shaw, A. (1992). Cloning and expression of a cell surface receptor for advanced glycosylation end products of proteins. *J. Biol. Chem. 267,* 14998-15004.

Newton, J.L., Harney, S.M., Wordsworth, B.P., & Brown, M.A. (2004). A review of the MHC genetics of rheumatoid arthritis. *Genes Immun. 5,* 151-157.

Nikolic, T., Geutskens, S.B., van, R.N., Drexhage, H.A., & Leenen, P.J. (2005). Dendritic cells and macrophages are essential for the retention of lymphocytes in (peri)-insulitis of the nonobese diabetic mouse: a phagocyte depletion study. *Lab Invest 85,* 487-501.

Ohashi, K., Burkart, V., Flohe, S., & Kolb, H. (2000). Cutting edge: heat shock protein 60 is a putative endogenous ligand of the toll-like receptor-4 complex. *J. Immunol. 164,* 558-561.

Ohashi, P.S., Oehen, S., Aichele, P., Pircher, H., Odermatt, B., Herrera, P., Higuchi, Y., Buerki, K., Hengartner, H., & Zinkernagel, R.M. (1993). Induction of diabetes is influenced by the infectious virus and local expression of MHC class I and tumor necrosis factor-alpha. *J. Immunol. 150,* 5185-5194.

Ohashi, P.S., Oehen, S., Buerki, K., Pircher, H., Ohashi, C.T., Odermatt, B., Malissen, B., Zinkernagel, R.M., & Hengartner, H. (1991). Ablation of "tolerance" and induction of diabetes by virus infection in viral antigen transgenic mice. *Cell 65,* 305-317.

Onengut-Gumuscu, S. & Concannon, P. (2002). Mapping genes for autoimmunity in humans: type 1 diabetes as a model. *Immunol. Rev. 190,* 182-194.

Oschilewski, U., Kiesel, U., & Kolb, H. (1985a). Administration of silica prevents diabetes in BB-rats. *Diabetes 34,* 197-199.

Oschilewski, U., Kiesel, U., & Kolb, H. (1985b). Administration of silica prevents diabetes in BB-rats. *Diabetes 34,* 197-199.

Park, J.H., Kim, Y.G., McDonald, C., Kanneganti, T.D., Hasegawa, M., Body-Malapel, M., Inohara, N., & Nunez, G. (2007). RICK/RIP2 mediates innate immune responses induced through Nod1 and Nod2 but not TLRs. *J. Immunol. 178,* 2380-2386.

Pearson, A.M. (1996). Scavenger receptors in innate immunity. *Curr. Opin. Immunol. 8,* 20-28.

Pietropaolo, M., Barinas-Mitchell, E., & Kuller, L.H. (2007). The heterogeneity of diabetes: unraveling a dispute: is systemic inflammation related to islet autoimmunity? *Diabetes 56,* 1189-1197.

Pinkse, G.G., Tysma, O.H., Bergen, C.A., Kester, M.G., Ossendorp, F., van Veelen, P.A., Keymeulen, B., Pipeleers, D., Drijfhout, J.W., & Roep, B.O. (2005). Autoreactive CD8 T cells associated with beta cell destruction in type 1 diabetes. *Proc. Natl. Acad. Sci. U. S. A 102,* 18425-18430.

Platt, N., Suzuki, H., Kurihara, Y., Kodama, T., & Gordon, S. (1996). Role for the class A macrophage scavenger receptor in the phagocytosis of apoptotic thymocytes in vitro. *Proc. Natl. Acad. Sci. U. S. A 93,* 12456-12460.

Pociot, F. & McDermott, M.F. (2002). Genetics of type 1 diabetes mellitus. *Genes Immun. 3,* 235-249.

Poltorak, A., He, X., Smirnova, I., Liu, M.Y., Van, H.C., Du, X., Birdwell, D., Alejos, E., Silva, M., Galanos, C., Freudenberg, M., Ricciardi-Castagnoli, P., Layton, B., & Beutler, B. (1998). Defective LPS signaling in C3H/HeJ and C57BL/10ScCr mice: mutations in Tlr4 gene. *Science 282,* 2085-2088.

Pugliese, A. (2005). The insulin gene in type 1 diabetes. *IUBMB. Life 57*, 463-468.

Rabinovitch, A. & Suarez-Pinzon, W.L. (1998). Cytokines and their roles in pancreatic islet beta-cell destruction and insulin-dependent diabetes mellitus. *Biochem. Pharmacol. 55*, 1139-1149.

Rodacki, M., Milech, A., & de Oliveira, J.E. (2006). NK cells and type 1 diabetes. *Clin. Dev. Immunol. 13*, 101-107.

Roep, B.O. (2003). The role of T-cells in the pathogenesis of Type 1 diabetes: from cause to cure. *Diabetologia 46*, 305-321.

Rosmalen, J.G., Martin, T., Dobbs, C., Voerman, J.S., Drexhage, H.A., Haskins, K., & Leenen, P.J. (2000). Subsets of macrophages and dendritic cells in nonobese diabetic mouse pancreatic inflammatory infiltrates: correlation with the development of diabetes. *Lab Invest 80*, 23-30.

Sobel, D.O., Azumi, N., Creswell, K., Holterman, D., Blair, O.C., Bellanti, J.A., Abbassi, V., & Hiserodt, J.C. (1995). The role of NK cell activity in the pathogenesis of poly I:C accelerated and spontaneous diabetes in the diabetes prone BB rat. *J. Autoimmun. 8*, 843-857.

Sobel, D.O., Newsome, J., Ewel, C.H., Bellanti, J.A., Abbassi, V., Creswell, K., & Blair, O. (1992). Poly I:C induces development of diabetes mellitus in BB rat. *Diabetes 41*, 515-520.

Suzuki, H., Kurihara, Y., Takeya, M., Kamada, N., Kataoka, M., Jishage, K., Ueda, O., Sakaguchi, H., Higashi, T., Suzuki, T., Takashima, Y., Kawabe, Y., Cynshi, O., Wada, Y., Honda, M., Kurihara, H., Aburatani, H., Doi, T., Matsumoto, A., Azuma, S., Noda, T., Toyoda, Y., Itakura, H., Yazaki, Y., Kodama, T., & . (1997). A role for macrophage scavenger receptors in atherosclerosis and susceptibility to infection. *Nature 386*, 292-296.

Takeda, K., Kaisho, T., & Akira, S. (2003). Toll-like receptors. *Annu. Rev. Immunol. 21*, 335-376.

Thomas, C.A., Li, Y., Kodama, T., Suzuki, H., Silverstein, S.C., & El, K.J. (2000). Protection from lethal gram-positive infection by macrophage scavenger receptor-dependent phagocytosis. *J. Exp. Med. 191*, 147-156.

Ting, J.P., Kastner, D.L., & Hoffman, H.M. (2006). CATERPILLERs, pyrin and hereditary immunological disorders. *Nat. Rev. Immunol. 6*, 183-195.

Trudeau, J.D., Dutz, J.P., Arany, E., Hill, D.J., Fieldus, W.E., & Finegood, D.T. (2000). Neonatal beta-cell apoptosis: a trigger for autoimmune diabetes? *Diabetes 49*, 1-7.

Tsung, A., Sahai, R., Tanaka, H., Nakao, A., Fink, M.P., Lotze, M.T., Yang, H., Li, J., Tracey, K.J., Geller, D.A., & Billiar, T.R. (2005). The nuclear factor HMGB1 mediates hepatic injury after murine liver ischemia-reperfusion. *J. Exp. Med. 201*, 1135-1143.

Turley, S., Poirot, L., Hattori, M., Benoist, C., & Mathis, D. (2003). Physiological beta cell death triggers priming of self-reactive T cells by dendritic cells in a type-1 diabetes model. *J. Exp. Med. 198*, 1527-1537.

van, K.Y. & Geijtenbeek, T.B. (2006). Toll-like receptors keep antigen sorting on the right track. *Immunity. 25*, 525-527.

Velthuis, J.H., Unger, W.W., Abreu, J.R., Duinkerken, G., Franken, K., Peakman, M., Bakker, A.H., Reker-Hadrup, S., Keymeulen, B., Drijfhout, J.W., Schumacher, T.N., & Roep, B.O. (2010). Simultaneous detection of circulating autoreactive CD8+ T-cells specific for different islet cell-associated epitopes using combinatorial MHC multimers. *Diabetes 59*, 1721-1730.

Voorbij, H.A., Jeucken, P.H., Kabel, P.J., De, H.M., & Drexhage, H.A. (1989). Dendritic cells and scavenger macrophages in pancreatic islets of prediabetic BB rats. *Diabetes 38,* 1623-1629.

Weidinger, S., Klopp, N., Rummler, L., Wagenpfeil, S., Novak, N., Baurecht, H.J., Groer, W., Darsow, U., Heinrich, J., Gauger, A., Schafer, T., Jakob, T., Behrendt, H., Wichmann, H.E., Ring, J., & Illig, T. (2005). Association of NOD1 polymorphisms with atopic eczema and related phenotypes. *J. Allergy Clin. Immunol. 116,* 177-184.

West, A.P., Koblansky, A.A., & Ghosh, S. (2006). Recognition and signaling by toll-like receptors. *Annu. Rev. Cell Dev. Biol. 22,* 409-437.

World Health Organization (WHO) (1994). Prevention of diabetes mellitus. Report of a WHO Study Group. *World Health Organ Tech. Rep. Ser. 844,* 1-100.

Xie, J., Reverdatto, S., Frolov, A., Hoffmann, R., Burz, D.S., & Shekhtman, A. (2008). Structural basis for pattern recognition by the receptor for advanced glycation end products (RAGE). *J. Biol. Chem. 283,* 27255-27269.

Yamamoto, M., Sato, S., Hemmi, H., Hoshino, K., Kaisho, T., Sanjo, H., Takeuchi, O., Sugiyama, M., Okabe, M., Takeda, K., & Akira, S. (2003a). Role of adaptor TRIF in the MyD88-independent toll-like receptor signaling pathway. *Science 301,* 640-643.

Yamamoto, M., Sato, S., Hemmi, H., Uematsu, S., Hoshino, K., Kaisho, T., Takeuchi, O., Takeda, K., & Akira, S. (2003b). TRAM is specifically involved in the Toll-like receptor 4-mediated MyD88-independent signaling pathway. *Nat. Immunol. 4,* 1144-1150.

Yamamoto, M., Sato, S., Mori, K., Hoshino, K., Takeuchi, O., Takeda, K., & Akira, S. (2002). Cutting edge: a novel Toll/IL-1 receptor domain-containing adapter that preferentially activates the IFN-beta promoter in the Toll-like receptor signaling. *J. Immunol. 169,* 6668-6672.

Yang, D., Chen, Q., Yang, H., Tracey, K.J., Bustin, M., & Oppenheim, J.J. (2007). High mobility group box-1 protein induces the migration and activation of human dendritic cells and acts as an alarmin. *J. Leukoc. Biol. 81,* 59-66.

Yarovinsky, F., Zhang, D., Andersen, J.F., Bannenberg, G.L., Serhan, C.N., Hayden, M.S., Hieny, S., Sutterwala, F.S., Flavell, R.A., Ghosh, S., & Sher, A. (2005). TLR11 activation of dendritic cells by a protozoan profilin-like protein. *Science 308,* 1626-1629.

Yu, H.B. & Finlay, B.B. (2008). The caspase-1 inflammasome: a pilot of innate immune responses. *Cell Host. Microbe 4,* 198-208.

Zhang, S., Zhong, J., Yang, P., Gong, F., & Wang, C.Y. (2009). HMGB1, an innate alarmin, in the pathogenesis of type 1 diabetes. *Int. J. Clin. Exp. Pathol. 3,* 24-38.

Zhong, J., Yang, P., & Wang, C. (2011). Environmental Triggers and Endogenous Alarmins Linking Innate Immunity to the Pathogenesis of Type 1 Diabetes. In: Aucoin L. & Prideux T., *Handbook of Type 1 Diabetes Mellitus: Etiology, Diagnosis and Treatment,* Nova Science Publishers, Inc., pp. 177-206.

Zipris, D., Lien, E., Nair, A., Xie, J.X., Greiner, D.L., Mordes, J.P., & Rossini, A.A. (2007). TLR9-signaling pathways are involved in Kilham rat virus-induced autoimmune diabetes in the biobreeding diabetes-resistant rat. *J. Immunol. 178,* 693-701.

Zipris, D., Lien, E., Xie, J.X., Greiner, D.L., Mordes, J.P., & Rossini, A.A. (2005). TLR activation synergizes with Kilham rat virus infection to induce diabetes in BBDR rats. *J. Immunol. 174,* 131-142.

8

The Role of Reg Proteins, a Family of Secreted C-Type Lectins, in Islet Regeneration and as Autoantigens in Type 1 Diabetes

Werner Gurr
Yale University, School of Medicine, New Haven, USA

1. Introduction

This chapter reviews literature regarding the role of Reg, a family of small C-type lectins, with a focus on the endocrine pancreas and introduces novel findings generated in our laboratory on the role of Reg as autoantigen in T1DM. It is not intended as a comprehensive literature review, but rather discusses a selection of articles in more detail in order to illustrate aspects that are important for the understanding of this protein family. In the author's view the scientific challenge consists in the development of a theory of Reg action that unifies seemingly disparate roles played by members of this family and provides the field of Reg research with a defined framework allowing unification of the many, to date, unconnected observations. Thus, although we focus on Reg and the endocrine pancreas, we also discuss findings obtained in other Reg research areas that appear to have little connection with the endocrine pancreas and T1DM. We choose this approach because we consider that the effects of Reg in the endocrine pancreas need to be understood in the context of a broader view of this protein family. The reader may easily find a large volume of additional literature on the effects of Reg referenced in the presented reports.

2. Nomenclature and classification of the Reg proteins and the origin of the family name

To act as a guide though the confusing nomenclature of this protein family we have prepared a phenogramm of the family incorporating Reg proteins from 5 different species (Fig. 1). In the text - as in the phenogramm- we use 'Reg', followed by a roman numeral designating the subfamily and a Greek letter that designates the member within the subfamily. Alternative names are used for those members where no Reg nomenclature exists and are otherwise indicated in brackets behind the standard name. 'Reg' is used without further classification when referring to the entire family. Reg stands for 'regenerating islet-derived', a name, which is not ideal since many Reg proteins are not or not solely associated with islet regeneration but function in different tissues and under quite diverse physiological conditions, as will be discussed in more detail later. In fact the first members of this family were described as a component of pancreatic stones in chronic pancreatitis or as constituent of normal pancreatic juice involved in the control of calcium carbonate crystal growth (Keim, Rohr et al. 1984; Multigner, De Caro et al. 1983; Sarles, Dagorn et al. 1990). Hence the names PAP or PSP (pancreatitis associated protein or pancreatic stone protein) or lithostathine remain in use for some of these proteins. Additional designations include 'pancreatic thread protein' (PTP), a name given to a bovine

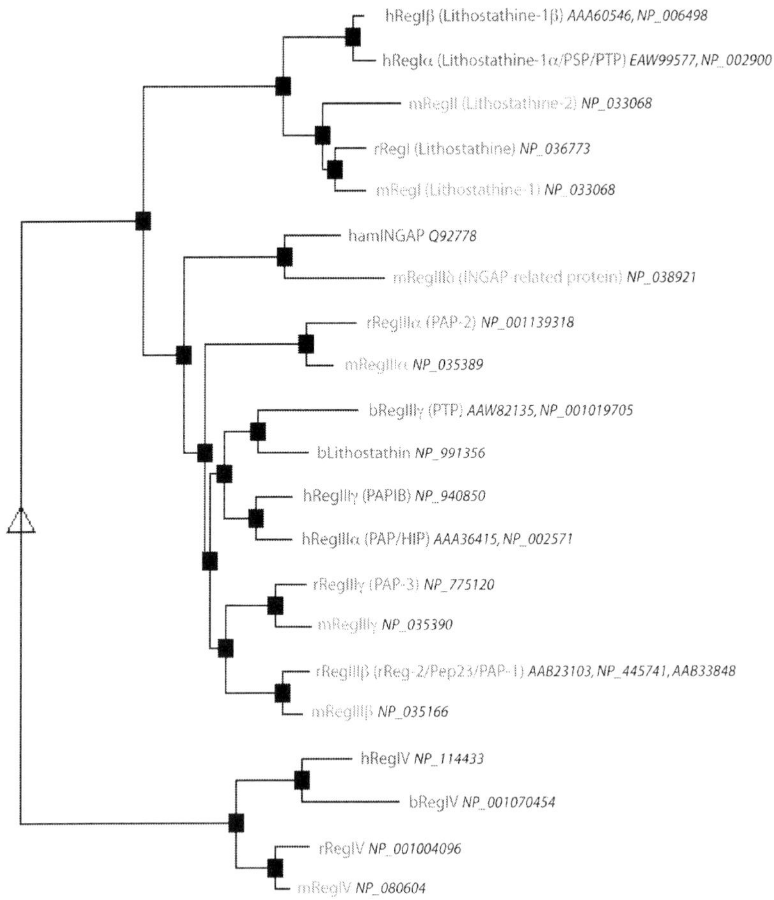

Fig. 1. Phenogramm of human (h), mouse (m), rat(r), hamster (ham), and bovine (b) Reg family members. 'Reg' followed by roman numerals and Greek letters was chosen as standard protein name whenever this nomenclature was found in the protein data bank. Otherwise the alternative names were used. These are indicated in brackets for members, which are found under both the standard and the alternative name in the data banks. Protein data bank accession numbers are given after each member. Abbreviations: Reg=regenerating islet-derived; INGAP=islet neogenesis associated protein; PTP=pancreatic thread protein; PAP=pancreatitis associated protein; HIP=hepatocellular carcinoma/intestine/pancreas; PSP=pancreatic stone protein

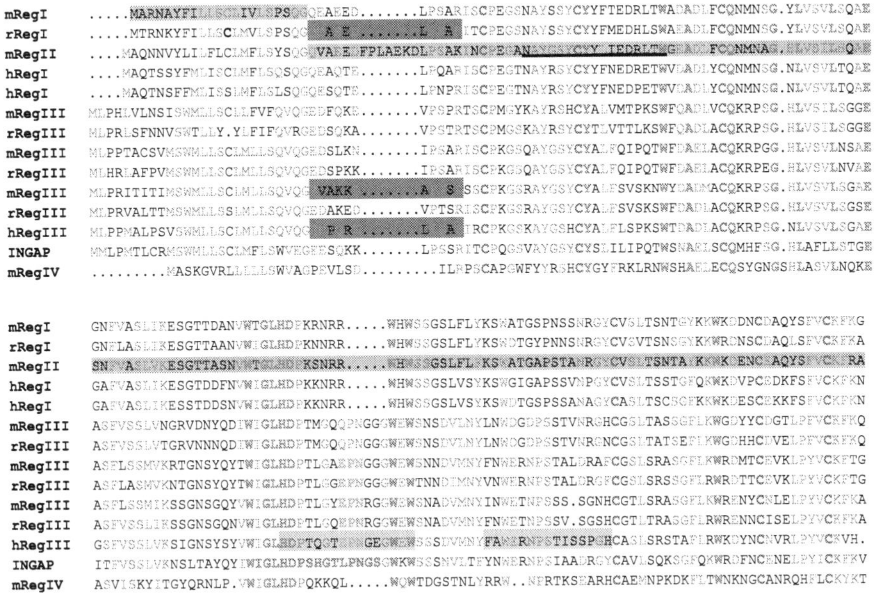

Fig. 2 Alignment of human, mouse, rat and hamster Reg family members. Features of Reg discussed in this review are highlighted. Blue background (mRegI): signal peptide; dark green background: prosegment (bactericidal effect/fibril formation. The arginine residue at the end of the prosegment is part of tryptic cleavage site); light blue background (mRegII): N-terminal fragment (acceleration of T1DM, activation of autoaggressive T-cells in NOD mice); lime green background: C-terminal fragment (delay of T1DM, T regulatory cells in NOD mice); light green letters: EPN motif (carbohydrate binding); gray background: loop 1 and loop 2 (carbohydrate binding); dark green letters: INGAP peptide (islet neogenesis/regeneration); blue letters denote the 6 cysteine residues that form the Reg C-type lectin domain.

pancreatic protein that precipitates at neutral pH in the form of double helical threads and was subsequently identified as a member of the Reg family (Gross, Brauer et al. 1985) and 'HIP' (for hepatocellular carcinoma, intestine, pancreas) – a name assigned to a human family member after Lasserre at al. found that it was overexpressed in a proportion of the hepatocellular carcinoma samples they had investigated (Lasserre, Christa et al. 1992). The designation 'Reg' was introduced because rat RegI (lithostathine) was rediscovered in a cDNA library constructed from *reg*enerating islets that had been isolated from the remaining pancreases of partially depancreatized, nicotinamide-treated rats (and was not expressed in normal islets) (Kobayashi, Akiyama et al. 2000). The investigators had previously shown that partial surgical removal of the pancreas followed by nicotinamide treatment induced a marked enlargement of the islets of Langerhans due to an increase in the number of β-cells. They write in their abstract: "The increase in expression of the gene was temporally correlated with the increase in size of regenerating islets…" and conclude "Thus the expression of the gene in regenerating and hyperplastic islets suggests a possible role for this gene in replication, growth and maturation of β-cells". Looking back on the years of Reg research, especially that performed with a focus on islet regeneration the authors of this manuscript might, in hindsight, have taken the trouble to remind their readers of an important scientific rule, namely, that correlation does not necessarily imply causation.

Although 'Reg' may not be an ideal designation the family is structurally well defined and a given protein sequence can unequivocally be assigned to it. To qualify as a member of the family a protein has to fulfill only one structural requirement; it must consist of a single C-type lectin domain of the type found in the first discovered Reg member, without additional attached domains. Any newly discovered protein was assigned to the family if it fulfilled this requirement and was assigned to a subfamily by primary sequence comparison with already existing Reg family members. This classification method resulted in the depicted phenogramm in which the three major subfamilies RegI and II, RegIII and RegIV each arise from a separate root. To illustrate the features of individual Reg members discussed in this review a primary sequence alignment is also shown (Fig. 2).

3. Studies investigating the role of reg in islet regeneration

Most studies that have investigated the role of Reg proteins have restricted themselves to one particular Reg member. Their basic approach *in vivo* and *in vitro* has been to either increase or decrease the concentration of the member under study or to add or eliminate it. Results of studies that increased Reg concentrations *in vivo* by administration of exogenous Reg protein include the finding that rRegI treatment can ameliorate surgically induced diabetes in rats (Watanabe, Yonemura et al. 1994). The same study also found that *in vitro* incubation with rRegI increased incorporation of radioactive thymidine into isolated rat islets. A corresponding approach was tested in NOD mice by i.p, administration of hRegIα with or without co-administration of linomide (Gross, Weiss et al. 1998). This study showed that Reg treatment of NOD mice that were still glucose tolerant could significantly reduce the incidence of diabetes and, when combined with linomide treatment, led to a reversal of glucosuria in glucose intolerant mice. In this study area the hamster INGAP protein deserves special mention. It was isolated from hamster pancreas using the cellophane wrapping procedure, which induces formation of new islets from pancreatic ducts (Rafaeloff, Pittenger et al. 1997). The results reported in this study draw attention to the actual definition of the process termed 'islet regeneration'. Should this term define β-cell proliferation taking place in pre-existing islets or should it rather describe a process that generates 'new' islets or β-cells from precursor cells? Although β-cell replication must presumably also take place at some stage in 'new' islets generated from precursor cells the investigators who discovered INGAP place their emphasis on neogenesis and argue that INGAP is associated with this process. Their designation for this Reg member, **i**slet **n**eo**g**enesis **a**ssociated **p**rotein, reflects this standpoint as does their demonstration that isolated primary duct cells thought to contain potential islet/β-cell progenitors respond with increased cell proliferation upon incubation with INGAP. The whole area of 'islet regeneration' is a subject of controversy. There are investigations that establish β-cell proliferation in preexisting islets as the predominant path to islet regeneration in rodents (Dor, Brown et al. 2004) whereas in other studies this process is attributed to the de novo formation of β-cells from endogenous progenitors (Xu, D'Hoker et al. 2008). 'Islet regeneration' should perhaps best be understood as the outcome of a combination of several processes including islet neogenesis, β-cell proliferation/size increase/maturation and islet destruction. As the cited studies show Reg seems to be at least involved in the first two processes and might also influence the third via its ability to protect from β-cell apoptosis (Bonner, Bacon et al. 2010; Simon, Pauloin et al. 2003).

INGAP is noteworthy from another aspect. The discoverers of this Reg member report in their initial publication that they were able to achieve duct cell proliferation not only by exposure to full length INGAP but also with a pentadecapeptide corresponding to amino acids 104–118 (Fig.2). The investigators seem to have derived this peptide without any hypothesis based on a possible effector mechanism of INGAP/Reg or any kind of peptide screening approach. We learn that "We included this region of the deduced protein because it differs from another related family of genes known to affect islet regeneration, Reg/PSP, in that it has a unique insertion of five amino acids and it precedes a potential N-glycosylation site situated at position 126, hence, a core of potential biological activity". Although the discovery of this peptide might have been taken as a peculiarity in the Reg field it has resulted in a string of subsequent investigations all showing some positive effect of a peptide with this sequence and corresponding peptides from other Reg members on diabetes and/or ductal cell proliferation. The findings finally led to a trial in humans, which again demonstrated positive effects in type 1 as well as in type 2 diabetic patients (Dungan, Buse et al. 2009; Levetan, Upham et al. 2008; Pittenger, Taylor-Fishwick et al. 2007; Rosenberg, Lipsett et al. 2004).

We have detailed the INGAP studies because they illustrate some important problems affecting the Reg field especially concerning diabetes/islet regeneration. No unequivocal effector mechanisms have been defined for this family and therefore it is not known if and how the differences between family members might manifest themselves clinically. It is not clear what process of 'islet regeneration' is preferentially impacted by Reg. Do all Reg members act as β-cell mitogens? Can all Reg members induce islet neogenesis and are all Reg members equally able to protect β-cells from apoptosis? Since these questions have not been answered we are left with a collection of observations lacking a basis (or a precise theory) from which they can be explained. As a consequence, it is difficult to generate testable hypotheses that would, for example, predict which cells should proliferate upon Reg stimulation and which should not, or that would allow improvement of the INGAP peptide sequence to produce a peptide with better mitogenic/anti inflammatory/anti-apoptotic/islet neogenesis-inducing properties.

Studies using overexpression or knockout mouse models to demonstrate Reg effects will be briefly considered here. As mentioned above there is no theory available that would predict which of the Reg members would be most promising for these studies and investigators have therefore tried different Reg candidates in these test systems. The first member to be tested in knockout experiments was RegI and this was also the first to be overexpressed in pancreatic islets under an insulin promoter (Unno, Nata et al. 2002). Overall, the results from these studies supported the observations obtained on exogenous administration of Reg. RegI ko mice had morphologically normal pancreatic islets and were euglycemic. However islets isolated from these mice incorporated less radioactive thymidine than islets from non-transgenic mice. Furthermore, stimulation with aurothioglucose, a method of inducing hyperplastic islets, failed to increase islet size in RegI ko mice to the same extent as it did in non transgenic mice, again supporting a mitogenic effect. A group that reported results on a knockout of RegIIIβ found that the mice were more sensitive to caeruleininduced pancreatitis but the report did not mention any deleterious effect of this genotype on islet size, insulin or glucose levels, suggesting that there may have been no difference between knockout mice and normal littermates (Gironella, Folch-Puy et al. 2007). Expression of transgenic mRegI under the insulin promoter in β-cells did not affect the size or morphology of islets compared to non-transgenic mice. However, when mRegI transgenic mice were crossed onto NOD mice the incidence of T1DM in the NOD RegI transgenic mice was significantly reduced compared to normal NOD mice (Unno, Nata et al. 2002). Subsequent mouse models tested the effects of transgenic expression of hamINGAP and mRegIIIβ targeted to islets via an insulin promoter (Chang, Weaver et al. 2010; Xiong, Wang et al. 2011). These studies found enhanced glucose tolerance, partial protection from streptozotocin (STZ)-induced diabetes and alterations in gene expression profiles when compared to non-transgenic mice. Overexpression of mRegII targeted to the exocrine pancreas with an elastase-1 promoter failed to provide protection from streptozotocin-induced diabetes (Li, Wang et al. 2010), whereas hamINGAP targeted to the exocrine pancreas with the same promoter did confer resistance to STZ-induced diabetes and increased the β-cell mass (expressed as insulin positive cells and the total pancreatic insulin/protein ratio) as well as the number of smaller islets compared to non transgenic littermates (Taylor-Fishwick, Bowman et al. 2006). The findings obtained from the two transgenic models with exocrine targeting of mRegII or hamINGAP were interpreted to indicate that different Reg members could have different effects. None of the more recent transgenic Reg models has so far been crossed onto the NOD background to study the impact of Reg overexpression in a T1DM model. The general conclusion from these studies is that Reg-induced effects appear to be pleiotropic probably impacting at least the three known processes mentioned above that contribute to 'islet regeneration'.

In our discussion of the effects induced by Reg, as derived from the presented findings, we place emphasis on a feature that was **not** observed in mice treated with exogenous Reg or in Reg transgenic mice. It is noteworthy that in the studies presented above euglycemia was maintained in the treated mice, hypoglycemia or excessive serum insulin levels were not observed and increases in islet mass were limited. This implies that the effects of exogenous (or transgenic) Reg as β-cell mitogen or stimulator of islet neogenesis did not lead to an expansion of the islet mass beyond what is physiologically normal. This feature is especially apparent in the transgenic models, where Reg is expressed from a constitutive promoter leading to sustained Reg overexpression from an early time-point. In this situation it is tempting to argue that the absence of documented effects in these studies suggests that the Reg proteins do not have any effects under normal physiological conditions. However, a different argument can be presented. The findings might indicate that the effects of Reg on 'islet regeneration' are tightly regulated and do not exceed the limits imposed by the target system, be it β-cells/islets or ductal precursor cells. In other words, when normal and transgenic mice are compared under normal, non-experimental conditions clinical differences are not found because the effect of the additional experimentally provided Reg input remains marginal. If this situation were expressed in the form of a hypothetical Reg effect curve where the X-axis represents the concentration and the Y-axis the effect, addition of exogenous or transgenic Reg would occur close to or at the point where the curve levels off i.e. adding more Reg at this stage would only have a marginal effect. In this model the system is kept close to the point of saturation due to the presence of endogenous Reg members and additionally due to the overlapping effect range of the various Reg members where one member can compensate at least to some extent for the loss of others. Thus knockout or overexpression of one Reg member shows little effect under normal conditions because the reduction/increase in the overall Reg concentration is small compared to the basal concentration that is provided by endogenous Reg members and keeps the system close to saturation. According to this interpretation it is possible that the effects of Reg are extremely important in the generation and maintenance of islet mass under normal conditions with an entire family of closely-related Reg members with overlapping functions rather than a single protein being necessary as a fail-safe mechanism to protect this function in a system that has to be kept at or close to saturation. Consequently this view would predict that, in order to better reveal the effects of Reg, a pronounced reduction in the Reg concentration by knocking out more than one and possibly all Reg members would be necessary.

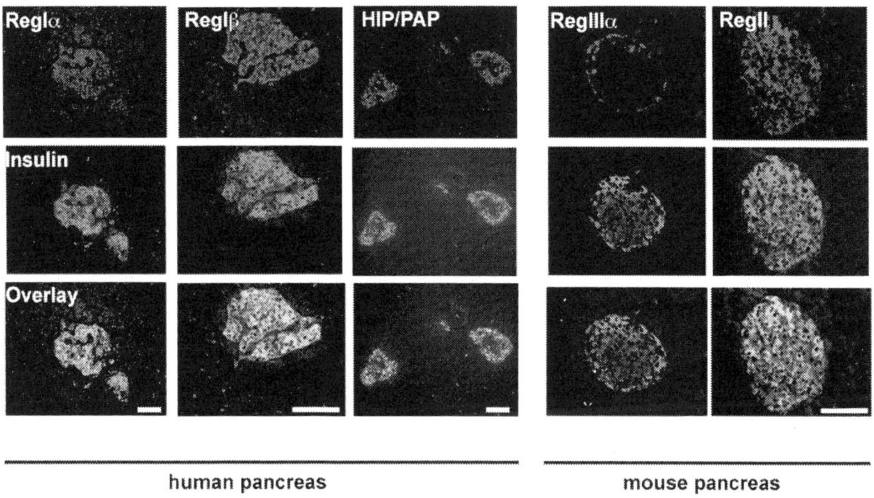

Fig. 3. Reg expression in human and murine islets. RegIα, RegIβ and RegIIIα (HIP/PAP) are expressed in human endocrine pancreas whereas RegII and RegIIIα are expressed in murine islets. (scale bar =50μm)

Such a multimember knockout model would be within the current technical capabilities because in the mouse all Reg family members except RegIV are located on one contiguous 75kb stretch of DNA (Kobayashi, Akiyama et al. 2000), and could therefore be knocked out as a whole. In such a model the effects of exogenous administration of Reg even under normal conditions might be quite spectacular or absolutely necessary for the survival of the animals with this genotype. Although this prediction might be considered a little extreme there are a few observations, which might support it. As we and others have shown, individual Reg family members seldom appear on their own. Wherever one family member is expressed others are likely to be found as well (see Fig. 3). Most importantly, the individual Reg members all contain the Reg C-type lectin domain, which is a strong indication that some of their functions may overlap and therefore generate redundancy. In terms of the hypothetical Reg effects graph mentioned above this means that the X-axis Reg concentration is unlikely to be derived from one single Reg member but is rather a result of the cumulative concentrations of all Reg members present at this site.

4. Studies in search of a reg receptor

The potentially pleiotropic effects of Reg emphasize the importance of defining if, where, when, and how the Reg members bind. A receptor for Reg, which are secreted proteins, might act as focal point for Reg action and might enable us to place the events taking place upon receptor binding and the subtype specific characteristics of the Reg family within a theoretical framework. There has only been one investigation that specifically set out to isolate an islet Reg receptor (Kobayashi, Akiyama et al. 2000). In this study an expression library of rat pancreatic islets was probed with rRegI. This led to the isolation of a cDNA that had significant sequence homology to those "of multiple exostoses (EXT) family genes especially to human EXT-like gene 3 (EXTL3)/ EXT-related gene 1 (EXTR1) (over 97% amino acid identity), indicating that the cDNA encodes a rat homolog to human EXTL3/EXTR1". EXTL genes are homologs of the EXT genes, which have been linked to hereditary multiple exostoses (HME), a rare medical condition in which multiple bony spurs or lumps (also know as exostoses or osteochondromas) develop on the bones of a child. However, EXTL genes are not linked to HME. EXT1 and 2 are thought to form Golgi-located hetero-oligomeric complexes and EXTL 1 and 3 contain a putative transmembrane domain with a short (31 amino acid for EXTL3 cytoplasmic domain) (Busse, Feta et al. 2007). All EXT family members are glycosyltransferases, which are involved in the biosynthesis of heparan sulfate and its analog heparin. EXT1 and 2 are essential for chain polymerization of heparan sulfate whereas EXTL3 most likely is involved in both chain initiation as well as elongation of heparan sulfate (Kim, Kitagawa et al. 2001). Heparan sulfate is a glycosaminoglycan found abundantly on the surface of most cells and in the extracellular space as proteoglycan. Heparan sulfate (HS) proteoglycans are involved in a wide range of biological processes such as cell adhesion, morphogenesis, cytokine effects and regulation of growth factors (Bernfield, Gotte et al. 1999). Regulation of HS proteoglycan biosynthesis would therefore be a good starting point to explain the pleiotropism of the Reg effects. However, the effects of Reg binding to EXTL3 are not known. Does this disrupt or enhance HS proteoglycan biosynthesis? How and where on the EXTL3 molecule does Reg bind and do different Reg members have different affinities? We do know that PANC-1 cells when incubated with a human version of the INGAP pentadecapeptide mentioned above respond with an accelerated translocation of the EXTL3 protein to the nuclear subcellular fraction (Levetan, Upham et al. 2008). Unfortunately, in this study, no alanine scans (mutated peptides each of which has an alanine replacing the naturally occurring residue at a different position in the sequence) or truncation or comparison studies with corresponding pentadecapeptides from other Reg members were performed. It is also known that islets contain HS (proteoglycans) and that heparinase treatment of isolated islets reduces their glucose responsiveness (glucose stimulated insulin secretion, GSIS). Furthermore islets of mice with a β-cell specific ablation of EXTL3 obtained with a rat insulin 2 promoter-Cre/loxP-system had reduced GSIS, a reduced number of insulin positive cells and, until the age of four weeks, fewer cells positive for the proliferating cell nuclear antigen. These mice also responded to glucose challenge with increased blood glucose levels and their plasma insulin levels were reduced. These findings demonstrate that β-cell specific EXTL3 knockout can affect the regulation of postnatal islet maturation via ablation or reduction or alteration of HS proteoglycan biosynthesis (Takahashi, Noguchi et al. 2009).

These encouraging data might lead to the formation of a basis from which the effects of Reg could be explained. However, large gaps in our knowledge remain. It is not clear if Reg binding to EXTL3 changes HS proteoglycan synthesis and if so how. Even if Reg binding to

EXTL3 were to cause an alteration in HS proteoglycan synthesis it is not clear if this would be sufficient to explain the effects seen in the models with transgenic expression or exogenous administration of Reg. There is therefore room for consideration of other potential Reg receptors. The methodology used in the experiments that discovered EXTL3 as Reg receptor involved screening of an islet cDNA library expressed in bacteria with rRegI. However proteins in a bacterial expression system are not subject to the same glycosylation that is introduced in a eukaryotic cell. Due to these limitations the screening assay could not detect Reg binding to carbohydrate structures found on glycoproteins or proteoglycans in eukaryotic cells. Reg-carbohydrate interaction however is an area that should definitely be covered by a search for potential Reg receptors because the family-defining structural feature of the Reg proteins is the C-type lectin domain. Lectins are proteins that bind to carbohydrate structures and C-type lectins do this better in the presence of calcium ions or their binding to carbohydrates is dependent on the presence of these cations. Surprisingly, despite the presence of a canonical C-type lectin fold, Reg-carbohydrate binding in the context of islet regeneration has so far not received any attention at all. A reason for this may possibly be that Reg proteins lack conserved amino acid residues that support Ca^{2+}-dependent carbohydrate binding in other C-type lectins (Drickamer 1999). However this in no way rules out the possibility that Reg proteins recognize carbohydrate epitopes. To uncover what is known about this property of Reg it is necessary to leave the area of islet regeneration and explore other fields of Reg research.

5. Reg effects in areas other than islet regeneration

5.1 Reg as a carbohydrate-binding bactericidal lectin and fibril-forming protein in degenerative processes afflicting the brain

Researchers studying the Reg family of proteins often work with a test system that involves the application of an artificial noxious stimulus thought to mimic a naturally occurring stress event. In a screen performed after application of the stimulus overexpression of one or more Reg members is observed. This was the case with the study that described the discovery of rRegI in regenerating pancreas and of INGAP. Recently a group of scientists investigating how gut microbial flora is maintained and controlled performed a study that compared gut epithelial cells from germ-free mice with those of mice that had been reconstituted with an intestinal microflora from conventional mice. They write "...To gain new insights into how intestinal surfaces cope with microbial challenges, we used DNA microarrays to identify Paneth cell antimicrobial factors whose expression is altered by bacteria. [....] The results of our screen revealed 149 transcripts whose expression was changed 2- to 45-fold by microbial colonization. One of the most prominent responses uncovered by our analysis was a 31-fold increase in the abundance of RegIIIγ transcripts in Paneth cells from conventionalized as compared with germ-free mice". Subsequently this group demonstrated that mRegIIIγ and hRegIIIα were bactericidal for Gram-positive bacteria. The bactericidal effect could be fully blocked by addition of chitotetraose ($GlcNAc_4$) and somewhat attenuated by the addition of soluble peptidoglycan fragments, chitobiose ($GlcNAc_2$), or N-acetylglucosamine. Interestingly, this assay revealed clear differences in susceptibility to glycan blocking between the mRegIIIγ and hRegIIIα. Precipitation experiments and binding studies revealed that both mRegIIIγ and hRegIIIα had affinity for peptidoglycans as well as mannan and chitin (Cash, Whitham et al. 2006). In a subsequent publication this group demonstrated that a short N-terminal peptide controlled the antibacterial activity of mRegIIIγ and hRegIIIα. This peptide spans the region between the end of the leader sequence and a canonical trypsin cleavage site that is conserved in all but the RegIV subfamily where the conserved arginine residue is followed by a proline thus blocking tryptic cleavage (see Fig. 2). The group found that removal of the prosegment by tryptic cleavage drastically increased the antibacterial properties of the two Reg members. They also showed that removal of the prosegment did not interfere with peptidoglycan binding, which is essential for the antibacterial effects and suggest that the prosegment exerts its blocking activity via a mechanism different from interference with Reg-peptidoglycan binding. The authors propose that this regulatory mechanism has evolved to give the host control over antibacterial activity and that the activation of Reg by cleavage of the small inhibitor peptide likely occurs in the lumen of the gut by two trypsin isozymes, which are expressed in gut epithelial cells (Mukherjee, Partch et al. 2009). It should be added that, as mentioned before, some Reg members are secreted by the exocrine pancreas under normal physiological conditions and this might therefore be another site of activation of Reg for release of antibacterial effects. A third publication of this group reports on the molecular basis for peptidoglycan recognition by mRegIIIγ and hRegIIIα. In this study the researchers used solution nuclear magnetic resonance to identify residues of hRegIIα involved in peptidoglycan binding. The three-dimensional structure of Reg is the C-type lectin fold containing a characteristic 'long loop' structure. In this long loop two subdomains can be distinguished which the scientists have designated loop 1 and loop 2. In other C-type lectins the loop 2 is involved in Ca^{2+}-dependent carbohydrate binding via specific amino acid residues (the EPN motif, Fig. 2). However the corresponding residues in hRegIIIα (HIP/PAP) are not found in loop 2 but in loop 1 and, as the authors of the study show, participate in carbohydrate binding. Also missing in hRegIIIα are two conserved residues in the β4 strand of the C-type lectin fold, which are necessary for carbohydrate binding in other C-type lectins. Thus although these Reg family members lack the canonical C-type lectin carbohydrate binding motifs they are nevertheless lectins. Interestingly, based on the presence of the EPN motif in loop 1 scientists were able to predict that mRegIIIβ should bind peptidoglycans whereas mRegIIIα, which lacks this motif should not. They were then able to confirm this prediction experimentally (Lehotzky, Partch et al. 2010). What conclusions can be derived from this? First, it should be appreciated that a C-type lectin domain can apparently bind carbohydrates via more than one mechanism. The domain functions as a three-dimensional scaffold within which changes affecting fine specificity are possible, allowing generation of diversity in carbohydrate binding. It is therefore quite conceivable that other Reg members also possess these properties despite lacking many or all of the residues that constitute the canonical C-type lectin carbohydrate binding motifs. These findings additionally give rise to new questions. All Reg members (except RegIV) contain the trypsin cleavage site, necessary for removal of the blocking peptide from hRegIIIα and mRegIIIγ. Would this mean that all Reg members are potentially bactericides or only those containing the EPN motif in loop 1? This would make RegIIIβ a bactericidal protein, while, as mentioned above, also protecting islets from STZ-induced diabetes when overexpressed (Xiong, Wang et al. 2011). What is the actual bactericidal mechanism of such Reg proteins? In studies on mRegIIIγ Mukherjee, et al. discovered that carbohydrate binding per se is insufficient to explain this effect. Removal by tryptic cleavage of the short N-terminal blocking peptide does not interfere with carbohydrate binding yet drastically increases the bactericidal effect of the two investigated RegIII members (hRegIIIα and mRegIIIγ). Is there a Reg effect that can manifest itself as bactericidal in the gut but as protective in pancreatic β-cells? Or can Reg proteins act in different ways depending on whether they are 'trypsin-activated' or not? It should also be noted that RegIV, which has a blocked tryptic cleavage site and can therefore not undergo the unblocking process leading to an active bactericidal Reg member and has a deleted EPN motif nevertheless does bind carbohydrates (Ho, Lou et al. 2010). Perhaps the carbohydrate-binding step is common to all Reg members, with effector mechanisms diverging downstream of this event.

In this context it is noteworthy that trypsin cleavage of Reg, which was discovered some years ago was reported to convert the previously soluble protein into a form that precipitates above pH6.5 and forms oligomeric fibrillar structures that combine into quadruple-helical filaments (QHF). It was also suggested that the small Reg prosegment inhibits formation of these fibrils. It was furthermore observed that rRegI is actually cleaved at the conserved trypsin site under conditions that rule out the presence of trypsin and other proteases thus suggesting that Reg may be subject to self-proteolysis at this site (Cerini, Peyrot et al. 1999) (Schiesser, Bimmler et al. 2001). Reg fibril formation may have profound consequences in degenerative processes in the central nervous system. These fibrils were found to be present in the pathological lesions of Alzheimer's disease and hRegIα was found to be overexpressed during very early stages of the disease before clinical signs appear (Duplan, Michel et al. 2001). Furthermore hRegIα (lithostathine-1) deposits were also observed in the blood vessels and in focal and multicentric plaques in the cerebellum of patients with Creutzfeldt-Jacob disease (Laurine, Gregoire et al. 2003). The authors of these studies suggest that Reg fibrils might represent a common component of amyloid deposits and may be a component of the material that coats amyloid fibrils observed clinically. This raises the question as to whether Reg could play a role as a link between brain injury and the later onset of neurodegenerative diseases. If indeed this protein possesses the ability to undergo a process of self-proteolysis promoting the tendency to fibril formation then overexpression of Reg members in response to traumatic brain injury, which is well-documented as discussed below, might under certain circumstances contribute or even act as trigger for subsequent degenerative processes.

To return to the bactericidal properties of Reg: fibril formation might actually be a process that contributes to its antibacterial effect. In such a scenario binding of Reg to bacterial carbohydrates would provide an anchorage and would be followed (or accompanied) by tryptic activation, which then leads to the formation of a Reg fibrillar coat on the surface of the bacteria. This coat could either inhibit bacterial movement or 'plug' channels in the bacterial cell wall or possibly cause perforation of the cell wall. A way to investigate this hypothesis would be to test if drugs that can dissociate Reg fibrils into individual protofilaments can actually reverse the bactericidal effect of Reg. Two remarks should end this section. The loop 1 of the C-type lectin domain that contains the EPN motif in mRegIIIγ and hRegIIIα, described above, overlaps to a large extent with the peptide of INGAP reported to stimulate islet neogenesis (although there is no EPN motif in INGAP, see Fig. 2). Thus the intuition of the discoverer of this peptide was correct in so far as the loop 1 indeed corresponds to "a core of potential biological activity". Although it should be added that a loop that has been cut at both ends no longer corresponds to a loop. These findings, together with the discovery by Christa et al. in 1994 that hRegIIIα (HIP/PAP) acted as a C-type lectin that bound to the disaccharide lactose (Christa, Felin et al. 1994) indicate that Reg proteins can bind carbohydrates despite the absence of the canonical binding motifs found to be essential for this task in other C-type lectins. This underlines the consideration that the rules governing carbohydrate binding in Reg C-type lectins are more complex than we currently understand.

5.2 Reg as regenerative factor in the nervous system and modulator of inflammatory responses

Involvement of the Reg family of proteins in nerve cell regeneration was observed while screening for genes overexpressed in an rat model that investigates motor neuron regeneration after crushing of the sciatic nerve. The authors write: "Within 24h of crushing the sciatic nerve, all motor neurons and a subpopulation of sensory neurons express high levels of rReg-2 (rRegIIIβ/PAP-1) mRNA and protein. This again exemplifies the standard process of discovery for this family. The authors observed that migration of rReg-2 along growing motor and sensory axons occurs via orthograde transport and that rReg-2 acts as mitogen to Schwann cells, the cells that create the support on which neuronal regrowth can take place. Intraneural injection of an antiserum, which blocks rReg-2 greatly reduced regeneration of neurons. Interestingly, the authors found that recombinant rReg-2 alone had only a weak mitogenic effect on Schwann cells. However this effect could be enhanced by addition of forskolin, an activator of adenylate cyclase. It should be noted that the discovery of rRegI in a model of islet regeneration mentioned before involved the treatment of rats with nicotinamide, an inhibitor of 3′-5′ cAMP phosphodiesterase. Thus forskolin and nicotinamide both increase the intracellular levels of cAMP leading to an amplification of Reg-induced mitogenic effects. The authors mention that enhancement of the mitogenic effect by forskolin is also seen with other Schwann cell mitogens such as glial growth factors and platelet derived growth factor. There it is attributed to cAMP-induced increase in receptor expression for those factors. In an attempt to trace the signal that induced overexpression of rReg-2 the authors investigated the effects of peripheral axotomy on Reg-2 expression in the neonatal period when motor neurons are particularly sensitive to this intervention. The sensitivity to axotomy is ascribed to the interruption of retrograde transport of peripherally-derived neurotrophic factors. Indeed they found that the intervention greatly reduced constitutive Reg-2 expression levels compared with uninjured motor neurons. This finding indicated that Reg-2 expression in developing motor neurons was dependent on contact with peripheral targets, which act as source of neurotrophic factors. The authors argued that these factors might be leukemia inhibitory factor or ciliary neurotrophic factor (LIF/CNTF) because these proteins are related to the IL-6 family of cytokines and rReg-2 and other Reg gene family members have IL-6 responsive elements in their promoter region. They could show that targeted disruption of gp130, which is a common component of the receptors for IL-6, LIF, CNTF and CT-1 indeed abolished Reg expression in developing motor and sensory neurons of the mutant mice thus demonstrating that the expression of the mouse Reg protein(s) at this site is dependent on the cytokines of the LIF family acting through the LIF receptor (Livesey, O'Brian et al. 1997).

This study was expanded subsequently by another group of scientists who showed that CNTF-related cytokines could induce rReg-2 expression in cultured motor neurons, which in turn acts as an autocrine/paracrine neurotrophic factor for a subpopulation of motor neurons by stimulating a survival pathway involving phophatidylinositol-3-kinase, Akt kinase and NF-κB. They also demonstrated that rReg-2 expression *in vivo* is controlled on a cell-by-cell basis and that not all neurons that have the LIF receptor express Reg-2. Since, by the time this report was prepared, the EXTL3 islet Reg receptor had already been identified the authors also performed rtPCR on motor neurons cultured with CNTF but failed to find mRNA for EXTL3. This resulted in the conclusion that "the Reg-2 receptor in motor neurons probably remains to be identified" (Nishimune, Vasseur et al. 2000). Over a decade later this receptor has still not been identified. In our opinion this is related to the little-appreciated fact that Reg proteins are lectins and therefore bind carbohydrates. Both studies presented again show pleiotropic effects of Reg impacting on the one hand Schwann cell mitogenesis and on the other hand motor neuron survival.

Before leaving this area two additional studies on the effects of Reg in the nervous system should be mentioned. The first provides an example of the observation that Reg family members are seldom found alone while the second introduces yet another role for mRegIIIβ, which has been identified as a potential bactericidal lectin, an islet regeneration factor and an inflammatory modulator in pancreatitis. The first study used a model that induces traumatic brain injury (TBI) by weight drop and then studied the expression of rat Reg members by quantitative real-time PCR and in situ hybridization in the cerebral cortex. This study reported a low level of rReg-2 (rRegIIIβ/PAP-1) and of rRegIIIγ (PAP-III) mRNA in normal animals. Upon surgery and TBI the mRNA levels of both rat Reg members increased dramatically. First rReg-2 mRNA increased 12hrs post TBI and remained elevated until day 5 post TBI. This was followed, at 24 hrs post TBI, by rRegIIIγ mRNA with a sharper temporal peak persisting until day 3 post TBI. The mRNA level of rReg-2 was also somewhat elevated in the cortex contralateral to TBI and the sham-operated ipsilateral side (Ampo, Suzuki et al. 2009). Two points here are relevant. First, low levels of Reg mRNA are detected in normal cortex, and as mentioned above, more than one Reg member is expressed. As shown in Fig. 3 this also correlates to the situation in pancreatic islets and would suggest redundancy due to overlap in the effector mechanisms mediated by different Reg members and a role for these proteins not only in response to stress but also under normal physiological conditions.

The second study described the generation of a mouse model in which the exons 2-5 of the gene encoding mRegIIIβ had been deleted and replaced with a lacZ reporter selection cassette. These mice were phenotypically indistinguishable from wild-type or heterozygous littermates. Interestingly, the knockout mice exhibited marked elevation of expression of mRegIIIα suggesting that the Reg system is designed to contain redundancies where one Reg member to some extent compensates for loss of another. The authors of this study provide evidence that, as in the case of rReg-2, expression of mRegIIIβ is restricted to certain neuronal populations and is also developmentally regulated. Peak RegIIIβ expression was observed on postnatal day 4 and had disappeared from all areas of the brain and spinal cord by postnatal day11. mRegIIIβ deletion did not affect the total number of motor neurons in the facial motor nucleus, suggesting that no neuronal cell death had resulted from the loss of mRegIIIβ. As in the aforementioned knockout studies, it was the application of a noxious stimulus that clearly revealed the effect of the knockout. When the scientists severed the facial motor nerve at postnatal day 3.5 and applied either saline or CNTF to the cut end of the nerve, more CNTF-treated motor neurons survived in the wild-type mice than in the knockout mice where CNTF treatment showed no improvement in survival over saline (Tebar, Geranton et al. 2008). In the latter case, as in pancreatic islets, knockout of a single Reg member causes no or only mild effects under normal physiological conditions. Only when a noxious stimulus is applied do the effects of the knockout become visible. As described above we attribute this to the presence of compensatory effects induced by other Reg members leading to saturation of the system under normal conditions, hence our advocacy of a multimember Reg knockout model and experiments designed to demonstrate the redundancies predicted to exist within the Reg family.

The neuronal role of Reg also extends to effects on macrophages. We previously mentioned publications that investigated the role of rReg-2 (rRegIIIβ/rPAP-1) and of mRegIIIβ in the neuronal context. As was to be expected more than one Reg member is involved in this process. rRegIIIγ is not only overexpressed in the cerebral cortex in response to traumatic brain injury as briefly mentioned above but also in the Schwann cells upon nerve injury (Namikawa, Fukushima et al. 2005). Injuries to axons in the peripheral nervous system induce the degeneration of distal axons, a process, which is accompanied by cellular responses. Among these responses the most striking is the invasion of the degenerating nerve by macrophages. They clear debris consisting of myelin components that inhibits axonal growth and secrete a number of soluble factors that can stimulate axonal growth. The influx of macrophages is ascribed to attractants that are released from the Schwann cells, which have undergone dedifferentiation as a consequence of loss of axon-Schwann cell contact. A number of such attractants have been described and include LIF and the monocyte chemoattractant protein-1 (MCP-1). Using a two-chamber cell migration assay Namikawa et al. could show that rRegIIIγ is equally effective as MCP-1 in promoting macrophage migration. The scientists produced a dose-response curve that showed an increase in the macrophage migration index at concentrations of rRegIIIγ between 0.1 and 10ng/ml. Doses above 10ng/ml did not further increase this index but rather led to a decrease with the effect completely disappearing at 500ng/ml, therefore revealing an effective concentration range typical for cytokines and chemokines. The authors also demonstrated that rRegIIIγ knock-down achieved with siRNA introduced into rat nerves by adenoviral gene transfer reduced the capacity of explanted nerve segments distal to the injury to attract macrophages (Namikawa, Okamoto et al. 2006). However, attraction is not the only effect on macrophages ascribed to Reg. rRegIIIα (PAP-2) is also able to modulate the inflammatory response in these cells. Viterbo et al. showed migration of macrophages to beads coated with rRegIIIα with subsequent agglutination. They also demonstrated that this Reg member binds to macrophages, but do not reveal whether this occurs via EXTL3 the islet Reg receptor, or via a different receptor. (We suggest that it occurs via carbohydrate binding). They then measured, by real-time PCR and ELISA, a range of cytokine responses in the macrophages during exposure to rRegIIIα. They reported upregulation of mRNAs for IL-1β, IL-6, TNFα and IL-1α most likely via the NF-κB pathway (Viterbo, Bluth et al. 2008).

Considering the roles of Reg introduced here the general conclusion may be drawn that Reg proteins are functionally placed well within the large family of endogenous lectins of which C-type lectins are a subgroup (Mascanfroni, Cerliani et al. 2011; Toscano, Ilarregui et al. 2007). These endogenous glycan-binding proteins have been implicated in a wide range of functions including first-line defense against pathogens (bactericidal effect of Reg) cell-trafficking (macrophage attraction of Reg), immune regulation (cytokine responses induced by Reg) neoplastic transformation (Reg expression in liver cancer). Reg is unique among the C-type lectin family in that it consists of a secreted lectin domain only. This feature makes its distribution wider than that of C-type lectins, which constitute part of receptors in the cell membrane. It is therefore possible that Reg can also act as a modulator of the interactions between lectins in receptors and their carbohydrate ligands (van Vliet, Garcia-Vallejo et al. 2008).

6. Reg as autoantigen in T1DM

Returning to the endocrine pancreas we now focus on studies performed in our laboratory that investigate the possibility that Reg might act as an autoantigen in T1DM. The insight that the pathogenesis of T1DM is driven by a disorder of the immune system has been well established by numerous animal experiments and clinical observations. That certain MHC alleles are associated with an increased risk of developing T1DM, that antibodies are present against β-cell self antigens and that lymphocyte infiltrates are observed in the endocrine pancreas all point to the adaptive immune system, i.e. B- and T-cells, as necessary elements in the process leading to islet damage/destruction and thus insulin dependency. Although insulin has received much attention in the search for potential cellular targets of the autoimmune process it has become evident that it is not the only β-cell component to which self-reactivity exists in T1DM. Our initial interest in the Reg proteins arose following our observation that one of its members, hRegIIIα, (HIP/PAP) was overexpressed in the remaining pancreatic islets of a patient who had died shortly after onset of the disease. This raised the question as to whether a vicious circle could become operational in a situation where a protein that becomes overexpressed as a result of the inflammatory process in the pancreatic islets, subsequently functions as an autoantigen (Gurr, Yavari et al. 2002). We therefore investigated if such a situation could occur during the pathogenesis of T1DM using the NOD mouse as model. We first defined Reg members present in mouse islets and found RegIIIα as well as RegII and, in more heavily infiltrated islets, also RegIIIδ. RegIIIα expression was restricted to non β-cells of the islets while RegII was found throughout the endocrine pancreas (Fig. 3). In the NOD model of T1DM autoantigens such as insulin and glutamic acid decarboxylase have been used as vaccine antigens to prevent or delay the onset of the disease. If a Reg member acted as autoantigen it might also have these properties and we therefore tested both RegII and RegIIIα as vaccines. While we could not prevent or even delay T1DM with RegIIIα we found a clear preventive effect with RegII vaccination. To ascertain that this effect was due to an immune-mediated process and not to the potential effects of Reg on islet regeneration we cleaved RegII into two fragments. The N-terminal fragment (NtfrII, residues 22-75) contained the first three cysteine residues of the Reg C-type lectin domain and the C-terminal fragment (CtfrII) contained the remainder of the protein (see Fig. 2). This, we argued, would inactivate possible direct effects of RegII on islet regeneration while retaining the function of Reg as autoantigen. On testing the two fragments we found that vaccination with the N-terminal fragment actually accelerated disease whereas vaccination with the C-terminal fragment delayed disease. This delay was more pronounced than that achieved with the full-length protein. In addition, it could be induced with late stage vaccinations, that is, delaying vaccination until shortly before onset of T1DM in NOD mice. We next demonstrated by adoptive transfer experiments that the clinical effects were mediated by T-cells. Both $CD4^+$ and $CD8^+$ T-cells from donors vaccinated with the N-terminal fragment could transfer disease to NOD-SCID mice - a strain that lacks B and T-cells and therefore does not develop T1DM. Similar experiments with T-cells obtained from donors vaccinated with CtfrII showed that $CD4^+$ T-cells from these mice could delay the onset of T1DM induced by diabetogenic T-cells. Taken together these experiments clearly demonstrated that the clinical effects seen after RegII vaccination were in fact immune-mediated and not a result of a direct effect of RegII on islet regeneration. They also identified the N-terminal fragment of RegII as the part of the protein that contained T-cell epitope(s) able to activate autoreactive T-cells, whereas it appeared that vaccination with the C-terminal fragment had activated T-regulatory cells. We had thus established that RegII could act as an autoantigen in T1DM of NOD mice (Gurr, Shaw et al. 2007). Another group had demonstrated in the meantime that 24.9% of patients with T1DM, 14.9% of patients with type 2 diabetes and 2.7 % of control subjects had autoantibodies against RegIα, thus confirming that Reg can also become a target of the autoimmune response in humans (Shervani, Takasawa et al. 2004). To add the second component of the vicious circle postulated above we had also shown that isolated human islets, when incubated with IL-6, secreted increased amounts of hRegIIIα (PAP/HIP). In a pancreatic islet under autoimmune attack this cytokine might be released by infiltrating macrophages leading to overexpression of Reg. Reg in turn then, since it acts as autoantigen, and as attractant for macrophages, as discussed above, enhances the inflammatory process thus leading to further overexpression and the operation of a vicious circle. However, we wanted to know if this process actually occurred *in vivo*. Autoantigens drain from the islets to the pancreatic lymph nodes where they are processed by antigen-presenting cells to generate peptides for display in the context of MHC molecules. Self-reactive T-cells are activated by these complexes, proliferate and migrate to the islets where they exert their deleterious effects. Since NtfrII activated self-reactive T-cells it had to contain one or more T-cell epitope(s). If at any time during the pathogenesis of T1DM a vicious circle operated then an increase in the NtfrII peptide MHC complexes should occur in the pancreatic lymph nodes. This should be followed by an increase in proliferation of T-cells specific for NtfrII. NOD mice only have one classII MHC molecule, namely I-A^{g7}. We therefore generated an antibody, termed D9 that was able to detect an NtfrII-derived peptide in context of I-A^{g7}. This antibody was phage-displayed, that is it was expressed, fused to a coat protein, on the surface of bacteriophages. The DNA strand carried by these phages encodes not only the antibody but also an antibiotic resistance gene. When bacteria are infected the phage DNA is transmitted and renders the bacteria resistant to the antibiotic. This allows estimation of the number of phages (colony forming units) in a given sample by infecting non-resistant bacteria with an aliquot of the phage-containing sample, spreading them out on an antibiotic containing agar plate and then counting the colonies that have grown after overnight incubation. This unique feature of phage-display allows the isolation of an antibody with a given specificity by selection of an antibody library constructed from appropriate source material on a given antigen. Non-binding phages are washed away while binding phages are retained and then eluted. Eluted phages serve to infect bacteria, producing a new batch of phages, which is then subjected to a new round of selection further amplifying specific binders. We used this technology to isolate antibody D9. In this case the antigen used for selection consisted of NOD antigen-presenting cells pulsed with NtfrII. The sequence of the NtfrII peptide recognized by D9 in context of I-A^{g7} was identified by pulsing antigen- presenting cells of NOD mice with short peptides covering NtfrII and analyzing if the pulsed cells could be stained with D9. We also determined that the complex formed by this peptide in context of I-A^{g7} NtfrII could activate autoreactive CD4^{+} T-cells. The complex therefore represented the link connecting Reg overexpression with the Reg specific immune attack on islets.

In order to establish a temporal profile of the I-A^{g7} NtfrII peptide complexes we collected pancreatic lymph nodes of NOD mice at different ages, prepared single cell suspensions and exposed them to the antibody. After washing, bound phages were detached, bacteria were infected and a colony count was obtained. As a control we used a mutated version of the antibody D9, which had a deletion in its heavy chain and only marginally bound to NOD antigen-presenting cells pulsed with NtfrII. The numbers of T-cells in the pancreatic lymph

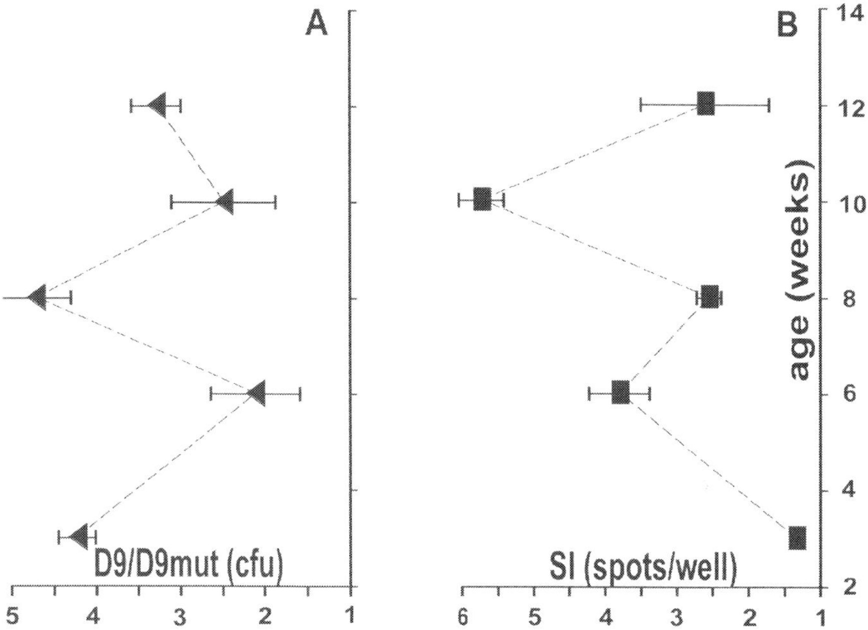

Fig. 4. Temporal profile of I-A^{g7} NtfrII peptide complexes (A) and spontaneous T-cell responses (B) in the pancreatic lymph nodes of NOD mice during the pathogenesis of T1DM. The y-axis in (A) displays the ratio of colony forming units (cfus) obtained with a binding antibody (D9) to colony forming units obtained with a mutated, non-binding antibody (D9mut); the y-axis in (B) displays the ratio (SI=stimulation index) of the number of spots obtained when cells of the pancreatic lymph nodes were incubated with NtfrII to the number of spots obtained when cells of the pancreatic lymph nodes were incubated without antigen (ELISPOT assay for IL-2). Both profiles show the same biphasic pattern but the T-cell pattern is shifted by two weeks i.e. the T-cell response in the pancreatic lymph nodes follows the temporal pattern of the I-A^{g7} NtfrII peptide complexes.

nodes that responded to stimulation with NtfrII were also counted. On plotting both curves (NtfrII peptide I-A^{g7} complexes and number of T-cells reactive for NtfrII) we observed that both curves had a biphasic profile and that the 'T-cell' curve followed the 'complex' curve with a delay of about two weeks (Fig. 4 A and B). This biphasic profile observed would clearly rule out the continuous operation of a vicious circle but suggests a temporary operation between 6 and 10 weeks of age. It also hints at the tight control of Reg expression. Reg does appear to become overexpressed in response to islet inflammation as manifested by the increase of I-A^{g7} NtfrII peptide complexes in the pancreatic lymph nodes. However, beyond a certain degree (or duration) of the inflammatory process (at ages >8 weeks Fig. 4A) this response ceases and the islets appear to actually reduce Reg expression. The existence of such control mechanisms can also be inferred from the observation that Reg acts as a macrophage chemoattractant. In this case an additional vicious circle may be constructed, involving IL-6 released from macrophages, which leads to up-regulation of Reg and more influx of macrophages. However, as demonstrated by the discoverers of the chemoattractant properties of Reg, the dose response curves do not level off but the attractant effect disappears above a certain Reg concentration. These observations exemplify two main levels of control that must be considered for the understanding of Reg action. One of the control levels is represented by the limits, which the target system imposes on Reg action - chemoattractant effect on macrophages - and the other by the limits, which the source system imposes on Reg production or release - I-A^{g7} NtfrII peptide complexes in pancreatic lymph nodes of NOD mice.

7. Concluding remarks and future research directions

The Reg family of proteins has been studied for over 25 years and today all mouse and human Reg members have been identified. However to date there is no unifying theory of Reg action and therefore the large body of work on the effects of Reg in different physiological systems remains a collection of unconnected observations. While it is important to accumulate more information on the role of individual Reg members, a framework needs to be developed within which this information can be placed and correlated. Such a unifying theory should be able to explain the seemingly very different effects induced by Reg such as, for example, Schwann or β-cell mitogenesis and bactericidal effects. Currently no such theory exists but its basic components should involve carbohydrate binding based on the fact that the unifying structure of the Reg family is a C-type lectin fold. It should additionally encompass fibril formation and possibly EXTL3 binding as well as up-regulation of Reg under a wide range of noxious stimuli (cytokine-mediated or other). Extracellular matrix remodeling might also play a role. These components then need to be placed and understood within the framework of regulatory constraints imposed by the systems impacted by Reg as well as by those that generate Reg. In this review we have drawn attention to areas of Reg research that introduce and exemplify some of these components. Development of a theory of Reg action would require a change in experimental approach away from 'what particular function is conveyed by a particular Reg member in a specific system?' to comparative studies concerned with 'what is common to all Reg members, how do they differ and what is the origin of these differences?' implemented with consideration of the basic components of the theory as outlined above. Consequently we argue that a model in which not one particular member but an entire subfamily or all Reg members have been knocked out would greatly further the development of this unifying theory. Such models might allow the characterization of the effects of Reg under normal conditions by eliminating the 'masking effects' of the likely redundancies that occur within the family. How the genomic organization of the Reg family would facilitate generation of these models is mentioned above. We are confident that they would also reveal that Reg proteins are necessary for islet (re)generation.

As far as the properties of Reg as autoantigen are concerned we are in the process of performing studies that evaluate if the antibodies specific for the Reg peptide MHC complexes generated in our laboratory may be useful as therapeutic agents for the treatment or prevention of T1DM. An important aim in the prevention and treatment of T1DM is the development of a specific immunotherapy, that is an intervention that targets and blocks/eliminates specifically self-reactive T-cells but does not affect T-cells, which are necessary for the normal functioning of the immune system. This aim can be achieved by intervening with the process that generates specificity in the immune system, namely the

binding of the T-cell receptor to its antigen, which is the complex formed by the T-cell epitope and the presenting MHC. An antibody that recognizes this complex, such as D9 introduced here, might interfere with the activation of the self-reactive T-cell recognizing the same complex and could represent a potential means to achieve specific immune suppression. A variant of this approach is the active vaccination with the receptor of a self-reactive T-cell in order to generate an immune response that targets only T-cells with this receptor but not others. This approach is known as anti-idiotypic vaccination and has been tested with some success in models of other autoimmune diseases. Which of these approaches might actually be practicable and effective in the treatment of T1DM will be the focus of future studies in our laboratory.
A successful therapy for T1DM will likely have two main components; one designed to support or enhance islet protection/regeneration and the other to control the aberrant immune response. Although more widely studied autoantigens like insulin or glutamic acid decarboxylase might be more suitable for addressing the control of the aberrant immune response, Reg is unique in that it represents an islet component that can play a role in relation to both therapeutic main approaches through its impact on islet regeneration on the one hand and its role as autoantigen on the other hand.

8. Acknowledgment

The work investigating the role of Reg as an autoantigen in T1DM was supported by funding from the Juvenile Diabetes Research Foundation (JDRF) and the American Diabetes Association (ADA). The author thanks Margaret Shaw and Yanxia Li for their efforts in carrying out the practical work. The author additionally thanks Professor Robert Sherwin for his overall support.

9. References

Ampo, K., A. Suzuki, et al. (2009). Induction of pancreatitis-associated protein (PAP) family members in neurons after traumatic brain injury. *J Neurotrauma* 26(10): pp. 1683-1693, ISSN 1557-9042

Bernfield, M., M. Gotte, et al. (1999). Functions of cell surface heparan sulfate proteoglycans. *Annu Rev Biochem* 68: pp. 729-777, ISSN 0066-4154

Bonner, C., S. Bacon, et al. (2010). INS-1 cells undergoing caspase-dependent apoptosis enhance the regenerative capacity of neighboring cells. *Diabetes* 59(11): pp. 2799-2808, ISSN 1939-327X

Busse, M., A. Feta, et al. (2007). Contribution of EXT1, EXT2, and EXTL3 to heparan sulfate chain elongation. *J Biol Chem* 282(45): pp. 32802-32810, ISSN 0021-9258

Cash, H. L., C. V. Whitham, et al. (2006). Symbiotic bacteria direct expression of an intestinal bactericidal lectin. *Science* 313(5790): pp. 1126-1130, ISSN 1095-9203

Cerini, C., V. Peyrot, et al. (1999). Biophysical characterization of lithostathine. Evidences for a polymeric structure at physiological pH and a proteolysis mechanism leading to the formation of fibrils. *J Biol Chem* 274(32): pp. 22266-22274, ISSN 0021-9258

Chang, T. J., J. R. Weaver, et al. (2010). Targeted expression of islet neogenesis associated protein to beta cells enhances glucose tolerance and confers resistance to streptozotocin-induced hyperglycemia. *Mol Cell Endocrinol*. ISSN 1872-8057

Christa, L., M. Felin, et al. (1994). The human HIP gene, overexpressed in primary liver cancer encodes for a C-type carbohydrate binding protein with lactose binding activity. *FEBS Lett* 337(1): pp. 114-118, ISSN 0014-5793

Dor, Y., J. Brown, et al. (2004). Adult pancreatic beta-cells are formed by self-duplication rather than stem-cell differentiation. *Nature* 429(6987): pp. 41-46, ISSN 1476-4687

Drickamer, K. (1999). C-type lectin-like domains. *Curr Opin Struct Biol* 9(5): pp. 585-590, ISSN 0959-440X

Dungan, K. M., J. B. Buse, et al. (2009). Effects of therapy in type 1 and type 2 diabetes mellitus with a peptide derived from islet neogenesis associated protein (INGAP). *Diabetes Metab Res Rev* 25(6): pp. 558-565, ISSN 1520-7560

Duplan, L., B. Michel, et al. (2001). Lithostathine and pancreatitis-associated protein are involved in the very early stages of Alzheimer's disease. *Neurobiol Aging* 22(1): pp. 79-88, ISSN 0197-4580

Gironella, M., E. Folch-Puy, et al. (2007). Experimental acute pancreatitis in PAP/HIP knock-out mice. *Gut* 56(8): pp. 1091-1097, ISSN 0017-5749

Gross, D. J., L. Weiss, et al. (1998). Amelioration of diabetes in nonobese diabetic mice with advanced disease by linomide-induced immunoregulation combined with Reg protein treatment. *Endocrinology* 139(5): pp. 2369-2374, ISSN 0013-7227

Gross, J., A. W. Brauer, et al. (1985). An unusual bovine pancreatic protein exhibiting pH-dependent globule-fibril transformation and unique amino acid sequence. *Proc Natl Acad Sci U S A* 82(17): pp. 5627-5631, ISSN 0027-8424

Gurr, W., M. Shaw, et al. (2007). RegII Is a {beta}-Cell Protein and Autoantigen in Diabetes of NOD Mice. *Diabetes* 56(1): pp. 34-40.

Gurr, W., R. Yavari, et al. (2002). A Reg family protein is overexpressed in islets from a patient with new-onset type 1 diabetes and acts as T-cell autoantigen in NOD mice. *Diabetes* 51(2): pp. 339-346.

Ho, M. R., Y. C. Lou, et al. (2010). Human RegIV protein adopts a typical C-type lectin fold but binds mannan with two calcium-independent sites. *J Mol Biol* 402(4): pp.682-695, ISSN 1089-8638

Keim, V., G. Rohr, et al. (1984). An additional secretory protein in the rat pancreas. *Digestion* 29(4): pp. 242-249, ISSN 0012-2823

Kim, B. T., H. Kitagawa, et al. (2001). Human tumor suppressor EXT gene family members EXTL1 and EXTL3 encode alpha 1,4- N-acetylglucosaminyltransferases that likely are involved in heparan sulfate/ heparin biosynthesis. *Proc Natl Acad Sci U S A* 98(13): pp. 7176-7181, ISSN 0027-8424

Kobayashi, S., T. Akiyama, et al. (2000). Identification of a receptor for reg (regenerating gene) protein, a pancreatic beta-cell regeneration factor. *J Biol Chem* 275(15): pp. 10723-10726.

Lasserre, C., L. Christa, et al. (1992). A novel gene (HIP) activated in human primary liver cancer. *Cancer Res* 52(18): pp. 5089-5095, ISSN 0008-5472

Laurine, E., C. Gregoire, et al. (2003). Lithostathine quadruple-helical filaments form proteinase K-resistant deposits in Creutzfeldt-Jakob disease. *J Biol Chem* 278(51): pp. 51770-51778, ISSN 0021-9258

Lehotzky, R. E., C. L. Partch, et al. (2010). Molecular basis for peptidoglycan recognition by a bactericidal lectin. *Proc Natl Acad Sci U S A* 107(17): pp. 7722-7727, ISSN 1091-6490

Levetan, C. S., L. V. Upham, et al. (2008). Discovery of a human peptide sequence signaling islet neogenesis. *Endocr Pract* 14(9): pp. 1075-1083, ISSN 1934-2403

Li, B., X. Wang, et al. (2010). Pancreatic acinar-specific overexpression of Reg2 gene offered no protection against either experimental diabetes or pancreatitis in mice. *Am J Physiol Gastrointest Liver Physiol* 299(2): pp. G413-421, ISSN 1522-1547

Lieu, H. T., M. T. Simon, et al. (2006). Reg2 inactivation increases sensitivity to Fas hepatotoxicity and delays liver regeneration post-hepatectomy in mice. *Hepatology* 44(6): pp. 1452-1464, ISSN 0270-9139

Livesey, F. J., J. A. O'Brien, et al. (1997). A Schwann cell mitogen accompanying regeneration of motor neurons. *Nature* 390(6660): pp. 614-618, ISSN 0028-0836

Mascanfroni, I. D., J. P. Cerliani, et al. (2011). Endogenous lectins shape the function of dendritic cells and tailor adaptive immunity: Mechanisms and biomedical applications. *Int Immunopharmacol.* ISSN 1878-1705

Mukherjee, S., C. L. Partch, et al. (2009). Regulation of C-type lectin antimicrobial activity by a flexible N-terminal prosegment. *J Biol Chem* 284(8): pp. 4881-4888, ISSN 0021-9258

Multigner, L., A. De Caro, et al. (1983). Pancreatic stone protein, a phosphoprotein which inhibits calcium carbonate precipitation from human pancreatic juice. *Biochem Biophys Res Commun* 110(1): pp. 69-74, ISSN 0006-291X

Namikawa, K., M. Fukushima, et al. (2005). Expression of Reg/PAP family members during motor nerve regeneration in rat. *Biochem Biophys Res Commun* 332(1): pp. 126-134, ISSN 0006-291X

Namikawa, K., T. Okamoto, et al. (2006). Pancreatitis-associated protein-III is a novel macrophage chemoattractant implicated in nerve regeneration. *J Neurosci* 26(28): pp. 7460-7467, ISSN 1529-2401

Nishimune, H., S. Vasseur, et al. (2000). Reg-2 is a motoneuron neurotrophic factor and a signalling intermediate in the CNTF survival pathway. *Nat Cell Biol* 2(12): pp. 906-914, ISSN 1465-7392

Pittenger, G. L., D. A. Taylor-Fishwick, et al. (2007). Intramuscular injection of islet neogenesis-associated protein peptide stimulates pancreatic islet neogenesis in healthy dogs. *Pancreas* 34(1): pp. 103-111, ISSN 1536-4828

Rafaeloff, R., G. L. Pittenger, et al. (1997). Cloning and sequencing of the pancreatic islet neogenesis associated protein (INGAP) gene and its expression in islet neogenesis in hamsters. *J Clin Invest* 99(9): pp. 2100-2109, ISSN 0021-9738

Rosenberg, L., M. Lipsett, et al. (2004). A pentadecapeptide fragment of islet neogenesis-associated protein increases beta-cell mass and reverses diabetes in C57BL/6J mice. *Ann Surg* 240(5): pp. 875-884, ISSN 0003-4932

Sarles, H., J. C. Dagorn, et al. (1990). Renaming pancreatic stone protein as 'lithostathine'. *Gastroenterology* 99(3): pp. 900-901, ISSN 0016-5085

Schiesser, M., D. Bimmler, et al. (2001). Conformational changes of pancreatitis-associated protein (PAP) activated by trypsin lead to insoluble protein aggregates. *Pancreas* 22(2): pp. 186-192, ISSN 0885-3177

Shervani, N. J., S. Takasawa, et al. (2004). Autoantibodies to REG, a beta-cell regeneration factor, in diabetic patients. *Eur J Clin Invest* 34(11): pp. 752-758.

Simon, M. T., A. Pauloin, et al. (2003). HIP/PAP stimulates liver regeneration after partial hepatectomy and combines mitogenic and anti-apoptotic functions through the PKA signaling pathway. *FASEB J* 17(11): pp. 1441-1450, ISSN 1530-6860

Takahashi, I., N. Noguchi, et al. (2009). Important role of heparan sulfate in postnatal islet growth and insulin secretion. *Biochem Biophys Res Commun* 383(1): pp. 113-118, ISSN 1090-2104

Taylor-Fishwick, D. A., A. Bowman, et al. (2006). Islet neogenesis associated protein transgenic mice are resistant to hyperglycemia induced by streptozotocin. *J Endocrinol* 190(3): pp. 729-737, ISSN 0022-0795

Tebar, L. A., S. M. Geranton, et al. (2008). Deletion of the mouse RegIIIbeta (Reg2) gene disrupts ciliary neurotrophic factor signaling and delays myelination of mouse cranial motor neurons. *Proc Natl Acad Sci U S A* 105(32): pp. 11400-11405, ISSN 1091-6490

Toscano, M. A., J. M. Ilarregui, et al. (2007). Dissecting the pathophysiologic role of endogenous lectins: glycan-binding proteins with cytokine-like activity? *Cytokine Growth Factor Rev* 18(1-2): pp. 57-71, ISSN 1359-6101

Unno, M., K. Nata, et al. (2002). Production and characterization of Reg knockout mice: reduced proliferation of pancreatic beta-cells in Reg knockout mice. *Diabetes* 51 Suppl 3: pp. S478-483, ISSN 0012-1797

van Vliet, S. J., J. J. Garcia-Vallejo, et al. (2008). Dendritic cells and C-type lectin receptors: coupling innate to adaptive immune responses. *Immunol Cell Biol* 86(7): pp. 580-587, ISSN 0818-9641

Viterbo, D., M. H. Bluth, et al. (2008). Pancreatitis-associated protein 2 modulates inflammatory responses in macrophages. *J Immunol* 181(3): pp. 1948-1958, ISSN 1550-6606

Watanabe, T., Y. Yonemura, et al. (1994). Pancreatic beta-cell replication and amelioration of surgical diabetes by Reg protein. *Proc Natl Acad Sci U S A* 91(9): pp. 3589-3592, ISSN 0027-8424

Xiong, X., X. Wang, et al. (2011). Pancreatic islet-specific overexpression of Reg3{beta} protein induced the expression of pro-islet genes and protected mice against streptozotocin-induced diabetes. *Am J Physiol Endocrinol Metab.* ISSN 1522-1555

Xu, X., J. D'Hoker, et al. (2008). Beta cells can be generated from endogenous progenitors in injured adult mouse pancreas. *Cell* 132(2): pp. 197-207, ISSN 1097-4172

9

Type I Diabetes and the Role of Inflammatory-Related Cellular Signaling

Lloyd Jesse[1], Kelleher Andrew[2], Choi Myung[1] and Keslacy Stefan[1]
[1]*Syracuse University, Department of Exercise Science, Syracuse NY*
[2]*Pennsylvania State College of Medicine Dept of Physiology H166, Hershey, PA*
United States of America

1. Introduction

Type 1 (T1DM) proceeds from a complete absence of insulin due to an autoimmune-associated degradation of the insulin-secreting pancreatic β-cell. An islet autoimmune response seems to be regulated by the T-helper lymphocyte and its cytokine products including IL-2, IFN-γ, and TNF-β, causing a cascade of inflammatory processes, known as insulitis and consequently gradual β-cell degradation (Rabinovitch and Suarez-Pinzon 2003). Therefore, T1DM etiology follows two stages. First, insulitis appears when various leukocytes attack the pancreas islets. Second, diabetes develops when most β-cells have been degraded, and there is no longer adequate insulin secretion to regulate blood glucose levels, leading to hyperglycemia (Mathis, Vence et al. 2001). Chronic hyperglycemia is believed to cause insulin resistance in T1DM (Patti, Maffettone et al. 1999). Thus, people can have concealed insulitis for years before it finally induces overt diabetes. Although most of diabetic patients suffer from T2DM, compelling evidence demonstrated that a proportion of people initially diagnosed with T2DM may in fact have a gradually progressing and less severe category of T1DM (Bell and Polonsky 2001). People affected by T1DM are constrained to insulin administration on a regular basis either through injections, pumps, or by inhalation. Outwardly, T1DM patients appear predominantly healthy; however failure to adhere to the appropriate treatment to effectively control blood glucose levels could lead to increased fatigue, neuropathies and long-term organ damages. The consequences of the autoimmunological destruction of pancreatic β-cells are clear, the causes are not, and the identification of the environmental factors that induce this destruction in genetically susceptible children, adolescents, and even adults still eludes us (Mathis, Vence et al. 2001).

2. Inflammation

In T1DM, it is suggested that inflammation contributes to the inhibition or stimulation of β-cell reformation and β-cell destruction, leading to peripheral insulin resistance (Eizirik, Colli et al. 2009). Inflammation is brought on by various cell mediators or cellular signals. Among them, cytokines, such as members of the interleukin family (IL-6, IL-1β), tumor necrosis super family (TNF-α), and the interferon family (INF-α, β, and γ), play an essential role in initiating and perpetuating the inflammatory process. Most of the T1DM-associated cytokines are involved in inflammation induced cellular apoptosis through the activation of a specific transcription factor: nuclear factor kappa-light-chain-enhancer of activated B cells (NF-κB).

2.1 Immunity and T1DM

In order to better understand the etiology of T1DM, plethora of research has been done to link the systematic destruction of β- cells and immunity. In all mammals there are two types of immune responses: adaptive and innate those mainly differ with regards to the types of receptors that recognize antigens. Innate responses are non-specific compare to adaptive which are fairly specialized based on the antigen. The key cellular players of innate immunity are dendritic cells, macrophages, mast cells and natural killer cells. They function through complex systems of T-cell surface receptors that recognize and destroy antigens produced from micro-organisms. Adaptive immunity is more specific, employing T and B cells that provide life-long immunity following the immunization process.

2.1.1 The role of innate immunity in T1DM

Activation of the receptors involved in innate immunity contributes to the development of autoimmune diseases including insulitis and T1DM. Pattern-recognition receptors (PRRs) are a class of receptors involved in the innate immune response and includes toll-like receptors (TLRs). It is possible that the binding of endogenous ligands to PRRs, specifically TLRs, may induce the inflammatory response that leads to β-cell destruction and T1DM. This theory is supported by animal models of autoimmune dysfunction; whereby TLRs contributed to an innate immune response to pancreatic β-cells and led to insulitis and T1DM (Zipris 2008). Specifically, TLR2 and TLR4 deficient mice were resistant to post-transplantation of islet cells induced T1DM and related inflammation (Goldberg, Parolini et al. 2007; Kim, Han et al. 2007). Although experiments such as these support a link between specific PRRs and T1DM development, other data suggest complex interactions between the immune system, genes, and other biochemical factors. For example, there was no difference in T1DM prevalence observed when TLR2 and TLR4 were genetically deleted from non-obese diabetic mice (NOD) (Wen, Ley et al. 2008). In that study, the nature of the animal's intestinal flora was thought to counter the effect of TLRs' absence. Other studies support that β-cell death can be caused by viral infections, most notably from enteroviruses, as viral antigens can elicit an acute inflammatory response. Enteroviruses infection occurred in half the subjects in a study assessing β-cells in patients with T1DM (Dotta, Censini et al. 2007). In addition, T1DM is characterized as an autoimmune disorder, as β-cells are also accessible to antigens-presenting cells: macrophages and dendritic cells. Therefore, macrophages are recruited to the pancreas of people suffering from T1DM and insulitis where they produce inflammatory cytokines such as IL-1β and TNF-α, involved in β-cell death (Uno, Imagawa et al. 2007). It has been also suggested that patients with T1DM have alterations in innate immunity in the peripheral blood, specifically in dendritic cells, mononuclear and plasmacytoid . These data support links between β-cell death, inflammation and innate immune responses and provide evidence that the innate immunity is a target of choice for T1DM treatments.

2.1.2 The role of adaptive immunity in T1DM

The nature of the biochemical reactions that occur during and following an acute inflammatory response may be key to determining whether autoimmunity develops with the potential to destroy β-cells and progress to T1DM. Altered expression of chemokines, signaling molecules that direct immune cells during inflammation, has been observed in several autoimmune disorders including T1DM. Certain chemokines such as CCL3, CCL4, CXCL10, have been shown to be elevated in T1DM patients (Shimada, Morimoto et al. 2001; Nicoletti, Conget et al. 2002; Hanifi-Moghaddam, Kappler et al. 2006). CCL3 has also been negatively correlated with C-peptide which is involved in insulin action (Pfleger, Kaas et al. 2008). Due to the difficulty accessing the pancreatic tissues to observe inflammatory markers, new methods have been developed to measure the response of immune cells from the systemic circulation in patients with T1DM. Using genetic microarray analysis, a T1DM "signature" pattern of chemokine and cytokine expression was revealed (Wang, Jia et al. 2008). Animal models of T1DM have displayed macrophages islet infiltration during the initial stages of the disease, responsible for chemokines production, namely CXCL10 and CCL2 (Martin, Rankin et al. 2008). Indeed, high levels of CCL2 in human islets have been associated with poor treatment prognosis after islet transplantation (Piemonti, Leone et al. 2002). Other chemokines have also been implicated in the development of autoimmune diabetes including CCL3 and CCL5 both of which have been positively correlated with insulitis and islet destruction in a murine model (Abdi, Smith et al. 2002). When exposed to inflammatory mediators during insulitis, it has been shown that the β-cells themselves can produce cytokines and chemokines (Eizirik, Moore et al. 2008). The expression of chemokines by β-cells is at mainly regulated by NF-κB, which also mediates β-cell death (Eldor, Yeffet et al. 2006). It is believed that dying β-cells may fuel the initial development of the autoimmune response which characterizes T1DM (Eizirik and Mandrup-Poulsen 2001; Cnop, Welsh et al. 2005). Proteins production resulting from an acute bout of islet inflammation, such as cytokines and chemokines, may facilitate the presentation of apoptosed β-cells to lymphocytes involved in the adaptive immune response (Filippi and von Herrath 2005). Another interesting mechanism by which β-cells fall victim to the adaptive immune system is through a stress response initiated by an accumulation of misfolded proteins in the β-cell endoplasmic reticulum (ER) (Cardozo, Ortis et al. 2005; Dogusan, Garcia et al. 2008). The presence of such proteins occurs as a result of inflammation in and around β-cells. Normally, the stress response to misfolded proteins restores balance to the ER by shuttling proteins out and preventing synthesis of new proteins into the ER. However, an error in this system can result in increased ER stress and β-cell apoptosis initiating the adaptive immune response (Cardozo, Ortis et al. 2005). Given the fact that insulin accounts for roughly half of the proteins produced by β-cells, therefore it is likely that the accumulation of misfolded insulin-related proteins could contribute to ER stress and the resulting response. As part of the dying β-cells, insulin could become a antigen recognized by effectors cells, thus explaining the autoimmune origin to β-cells apoptosis that occurs in T1DM. Ironically, the same inflammatory mediators involved in β-cell destruction may also contribute to β-cell proliferation and thus, the resolution of insulitis (Sarvetnick and Gu 1992; Sherry, Kushner et al. 2006). Although not yet observed in humans, β-cell proliferation has been seen in mice genetically modified to express high cytokine levels, and immunosuppression has also been shown to suppress β-cell generation (32).

2.1.3 At the frontier of inflammation and apoptosis: NF-κB signalling in T1DM

NF-κB, known as the "master regulator" of the inflammatory process, is a multi-protein complex transcription factor that mediates more than 200 genes. There are several internal and external factors associated with T1DM that affect the activation of NF-κB, most notably: reactive oxygen species (ROS), TNF-α, IL-1β, nitric oxide (NO) and inducible nitric oxide synthase (iNOS). Proper regulation of NF-κB is crucial for a healthy immune response. Conversely, a disruption in the NF-κB pathway often leads to the onset and/or progression of several types of cancers as well as viral infections, impaired immune function, and autoimmune disorders. It has been suggested that the ability to regulate specific cytokines, proteins or genes that activate the NF-κB cascade is crucial at slowing the progression of T1DM. For example, inflammation triggers NO production, an important transcription factor in iNOS gene expression, which then activates NF-κB in peripheral blood mononuclear cells (Igoillo-Esteve, Gurzov et al.). A recent study demonstrated an up-regulation of the expression of B-cell lymphoma-6 (Bcl-6), a sequence-specific repressor of transcription, in β-cells which decreased programmed cell death, iNOS expression, NO production, and NF-κB activation (Igoillo-Esteve, Gurzov et al.). This reveals the essential role that NF-κB signaling can play in β-cell damage and/or destruction. This notion has been demonstrated using transgenic mouse models where genes associated with NF-κB activation have been over expressed or knocked-down (Mathews, Suarez-Pinzon et al. 2005). ALR/Lt transgenic mice, which β-cells are engineered to resist apoptosis, showed resistance to stress induced by free radical damage. This resistance causes a failure in the production of pro-inflammatory cytokines (IL1-β, TNFα, and IFNγ) by inhibiting NF-κB activation. These outcomes coupled with decreased ROS accumulation leads to decreased β-cell death (Mathews, Suarez-Pinzon et al. 2005). More recently, the role of NF-κB has been associated with chromatin modifying enzymes, histone acetyltransferase, and histone deacetylase (HDAC). Positive effects associated with NF-κB expression on HDAC inhibition have been obtained for several inflammatory diseases (Keslacy, Tliba et al. 2007). HDAC inhibition lowered cytokine-mediated insulin resistance and increased iNOS levels, NO formation, and apoptosis. IL-1-β induced a biphasic phosphorylation of inhibitor protein IκBα with the second peak in the phase being sensitive to HDAC (Larsen, Tonnesen et al. 2007). These studies clearly demonstrate the contribution of NF-κB cascade activation to T1DM.

2.1.4 Transplantation of islet cells only promising because of inflammation?

Transplanting islet cells is a technique that has emerged in the past few years for treating individuals with T1DM. The current therapy is life-long exogenous insulin supplementation (Gillespie 2006). Although exogenous insulin administration is generally effective, it does not allow for physiological control over blood glucose levels resulting in micro and macrovascular consequences. Even when delivered in steady-controlled doses via insulin pumps, the results are not as effective as islet transplantation. Islet cells transplantation appears as a treatment of choice for T1DM, however, recent five-year follow-up studies showed that most of the islet cells that were transplanted were destroyed due to inflammation activation (Nanji and Shapiro 2004; Balamurugan, Bottino et al. 2006). Islet cells have a unique transplantation progression, as the rejection of the graft does not seem to follow the same rejection processes observed during other whole organ transplants. It has been shown that instead of the tissue itself, rejection was related to islet quality and vascularization, innate immunity, and coagulation (Swift, Clayton et al. 1998; Bach, Bendelac et al. 2004). Non-specific inflammation at the site of transplantation can occur in islet β-cells. In transplant models, stress as a result of the isolation procedure induced secretion of proinflammatory cytokines contributing to early islet graft loss after transplantation. This could represent one of the contributing factors for the destruction of the islet graft over time (Barbe-Tuana, Klein et al. 2006). A potential method of ensuring proper graft transplantation acceptance could result from CD40. It is a member of the TNF receptor family that binds to CD40L and is expressed in pancreatic β-cells. CD40 upregulates intracellular adhesion molecule-1 associated with inflammation at both transcriptional and translational levels. Inhibition of CD40 expression decreased in a dose dependent manner NF-κB-associated proinflammatory cytokines and protected human pancreatic duct cells (Vosters, Beuneu et al. 2008).

3. Insulin signaling: between treatment and etiology in T1DM

Inflammatory mediators from adaptive immune response are likely involved in the resolution or maintenance of insulitis that ultimately leading to T1DM. However, despite exhibiting the level of hyperglycemia recognized in T1DM diagnosis, some patients demonstrate higher insulin levels than would be expected with severe β-cell destruction. It has been hypothesized that the inflammatory mediators involved in β-cell dysfunction may also contribute to peripheral insulin resistance, thus resulting in the observed hyperglycemia (Strandell, Eizirik et al. 1990). Therefore, it is possible that the metabolic abnormalities of T1DM are the result of the associated development of progressive insulitis and insulin resistance. Though the consequences of progressive insulitis and T1DM can be dire, not all individuals who develop insulitis proceed to a full-fledged T1DM diagnosis (Eizirik, Sandler et al. 1993).

3.1 Underlying insulin signaling mechanisms on glucose transport

Insulin is the primary regulator of blood glucose level and a key signaling to better understand the pathology of T1DM. Biologically active human insulin consists of two polypeptide chains, the A chain (21 amino acids) and B chain (30 amino acids), joined by two interchain disulfide-linked bridges at A-Cys7/B-Cys7 and A-Cys20/B-Cys19 with an interconnnected disulfide bridge between A-Cys20/A-Cys11 (Steiner, 1985). Insulin triggers a wide variety of metabolic and mitogenic events by activating a series of intracellular signaling cascades (Zierath 2002; Wright, Ryals et al. 2004). The effect of insulin is mediated through binding to the heterotetrameric insulin receptor (IR) and activating intrinsic tyrosine kinase activity via autophosphorylation (Farese 2001). Phosphorylated tyrosine residues on the activated IR provide docking sites for insulin receptor substrates (IRSs) that contain SH2 (Src-homology 2) domains. IRS-1 and IRS-2 are widely expressed in tissues metabolically involved in glucose and lipid homeostasis (Sun, Rothenberg et al. 1991; Sun, Wang et al. 1995), and are therefore found in skeletal muscle, liver, fat, and pancreatic islets. While IRS-1 appears to play a more important role in skeletal muscle metabolism than IRS-2, it is thought that IRS-2 has a greater function in liver and islet β cells (Sun, Wang et al. 1995). Once phosphorylated by IR, IRS-1 activates a cellular cascade and binds to p85 regulatory subunit of phosphatidylinositol (PI) 3-kinase, which in turn activates the p110 catalytic subunit (Czech and Corvera 1999). To date, five isoforms of regulatory subunits of PI 3-kinase have been identified in skeletal muscle, including two classical isoforms (p85α and p85β) and three other isoforms (p55α, p55γ, and p50α) (Shepherd, Nave et al. 1997). Activated PI 3-kinase specifically phosphorylates the D3 position of the cellular phosphoinositides to produce phosphatidylinositol 3-monophosphate (PI-3-P), PI-3,4-bisphosphate (PIP2), and PI-3,4,5-triphosphate (PIP3) (Alessi, Deak et al. 1997; Alessi 2001).

These unique phospholipids serve as docking sites for cytoplasmic proteins with pleckstrin homology (PH) domains, including the serine/threonine kinases Akt/PKB and phosphoinositide-dependent kinase-1 (PDK1). The PH domain of Akt/PKB is displaced by 3-phosphoinositides and exposes regulatory phosphorylation sites in the catalytic/regulatory domain of the enzyme. Moreover, by recruiting both Akt and PDK1 to common membrane domains, the two enzymes come into closer proximity, promoting the phosphorylation of the Thr308 residue by PDK1. Ser473 phosphorylation is promoted by 3-phosphoinositides, through a second mechanism not involving the recruitment of Akt to the plasma membrane, which is required for Thr308 phosphorylation. The enzyme responsible for phosphorylating Ser473 site has not yet been cloned (Hresko, Murata et al. 2003; Murata, Hresko et al. 2003). To date, glucose transporter 4 (GLUT 4) translocation stimulated by Akt/PKB from intracellular compartments to the cell surface membrane in response to insulin in skeletal muscle and adipose tissue is not fully understood.

3.2 T1DM: to be or not to be insulin resistant, that is the question

As described previously, T1DM is characterized by hyperglycaemia, i.e., glucose toxicity, which leads to insulin resistance in T1DM patients (Patti, Maffettone et al. 1999). Since T1DM severity is correlated with the degradation of pancreatic β-cell, most T1DM patients are believed to have varying degree of insulin resistance. A series of studies have demonstrated 30-50% decreases in rates of insulin-stimulated glucose transport in T1DM patients (DeFronzo 1982; DeFronzo, Hendler et al. 1982; Yki-Jarvinen, Kiviluoto et al. 1986; Vuorinen-Markkola, Koivisto et al. 1992; Chillaron, Goday et al. 2009). One of potential trigger for disturbance of glucose uptake in T1DM results from elevated intramyocellular fat in human skeletal muscle (Krssak, Falk Petersen et al. 1999). In addition, it is well established that T1DM incidence may be related to overweight and obesity especially in children (Baum, Ounsted et al. 1975). More recently, several studies have demonstrated that obesity in childhood was highly related to the risk of subsequent T1DM (Kordonouri and Hartmann 2005; Ljungkrantz, Ludvigsson et al. 2008; Lammi, Moltchanova et al. 2009). Two factors are principally known to be the main components of the relationship between obesity and diabetes: insulin resistance and insulin deficiency (Felber and Golay 2002). These two factors are closely associated in a dual regulatory cycle in which high blood glucose levels promote insulin production which, in turn, reduces the increase in glycemia (Ferrannini and Camastra 1998). The effect of glucose is elicited by generating, stimulating, and amplifying signals in the β-cells (Henquin 2000). Chronic high levels of blood glucose create a glucotoxic milieu, impairing insulin sensitivity. Hence, genetic basis in the development of diabetes for people suffering from obesity could explain both insulin resistance and insulin deficiency (Gerich 1998). As peripheral insulin resistance increases, the adipose tissue produces more fatty acids, and in turn, impaired liver production of glucose. Thus, pancreatic β-cells may fail to maintain insulin homeostasis (Hegarty, Furler et al. 2003). Chronic hyperglycemia is an independent cause of insulin resistance with clinical importance in the treatment of T1DM (Vuorinen-Markkola, Koivisto et al. 1992). Obesity induces an elevation of delivery of fatty acids in the blood stream that can promote an accumulation of long chain fatty acyl-CoA (LCFACoA), diacylglycerol, and ceramides. These metabolically active molecules stimulate a serine/threonine kinase cascade leading to phosphorylation of serine/threonine sites on IRS-1 and IRS-2, which in turn decreases the capability of the IRSs to activate PI3 kinase (Dresner, Laurent et al. 1999; Itani, Ruderman et al. 2002). A more recent study indicated that intracellular LCFACoA is associated with an increased activation of PKCθ and a decrease in both IRS-1 tyrosine phosphorylation and IRS-1 associated PI3 kinase activity, which is involved in an increased IRS-1 Ser307 phosphorylation. Insulin signaling cascade is eventually altered, thereby impairing glucose uptake (Dresner, Laurent et al. 1999; Patti, Maffettone et al. 1999; Itani, Ruderman et al. 2002). In addition, a study from Thompson and Cooney (Thompson, Lim-Fraser et al. 2000) indicated that LCFACoAs decreased hexokinase activity in homogenates of human and rat soleus muscle in vitro. Hexokinase is the first enzyme of intracellular glucose metabolism and its suppression by LCFACoA might well account for a decrease in glucose influx into the muscle tissue. Furthermore, defects in Akt phosphorylation may also be associated with decreased glucose uptake in T1DM. A study demonstrated that Akt phosphoryation was significantly impaired in insulin-resistant hypoglycemic Goto-Kakizaki rats and this condition was normalized by a drug treatment, suggesting that Akt is a potential site of insulin resistance in T1DM patients (Krook, Kawano et al. 1997).

4. The consequences of T1DM on protein metabolism

T1DM patients exhibit overall changes in tissue protein metabolism. These changes are primarily the result of systemic hypoinsulinemia, changes in circulating hormones, intracellular signals, and catabolic factors also. T1DM-associated milieu disrupts tissue protein homeostasis and induces a net negative protein balance, particularly in skeletal muscle. Patients with T1DM often display profound skeletal muscle atrophy, which results in muscle weakness, fatigue, delayed recovery after illness, and has been linked with increased morbidity and mortality (Gordon, Serino et al.; Tisdale; Menconi, Fareed et al. 2007). Skeletal muscle atrophy associated with T1DM results from the upregulation of numerous catabolic factors, which increase protein degradation and decrease processes of protein synthesis. Therefore, understanding the mechanisms underlying T1DM-mediated skeletal muscle atrophy is important for developing potential strategies to preserve or reverse losses in protein, maintain skeletal muscle function and improve the quality of life of people suffering from T1DM. The protein content of a tissue is the result of protein synthesis and degradation (Nair 1995). Numerous pathological diseases disrupt the balance between protein synthesis and degradation resulting in tissue wasting conditions. Although the specific mechanisms underlying the cause of wasting are not completely understood, these conditions display decreased stimulation of protein synthesis and increased expression of catabolic factors that enhanced catabolic activity. T1DM milieu induces protein wasting where skeletal muscle tissue is rapidly degraded in order to provide amino acid substrates for gluconeogenesis in the liver.

4.1 Protein metabolism in the absence of insulin

Whole body protein metabolism is typically measured using an isotopically labeled amino acid tracer such as L-[1^{13}C] or [1^{14}C] leucine. Leucine is an essential amino acid whose appearance, disappearance, transamination to its ketoacid (α-ketoisocaproate or KIC), and oxidation can be measured to provide an indication of protein breakdown, synthesis, and metabolism (Charlton and Nair 1998). It has been demonstrated that whole-body leucine kinetics in T1DM patients indicated high levels of protein breakdown and metabolism with insulin deprivation relative to non-diabetic controls (Nair, Ford et al. 1995). These measures of protein breakdown, leucine transamination and oxidation are drastically decreased with insulin treatment indicating a decrease in catabolism and amino acid metabolism.

Interestingly, measures of whole body protein synthesis according to non-oxidative leucine flux were elevated in insulin-deprived T1DM patients above non-diabetic controls. When these patients were treated with insulin, a decrease in whole-body protein synthesis was observed (Nair, Ford et al. 1995; Charlton and Nair 1998). However, insulin treatment to fasted individuals without an increase in plasma amino acids caused a reduction in plasma amino acids (Charlton and Nair 1998). Several studies showed that when insulin treatment was administered to T1DM patients or healthy controls with an amino acid load increase in whole body protein synthesis occurred (Castellino, Luzi et al. 1987; Tessari, Inchiostro et al. 1987; Luzi, Castellino et al. 1990; Inchiostro, Biolo et al. 1992), although other studies were unable to measure an increase in protein synthesis (Flakoll, Kulaylat et al. 1989; Bennet, Connacher et al. 1991). In order to understand the underlying mechanisms of whole body protein metabolism with insulin treatment, it appears useful to evaluate the relative changes in individual tissues and cellular compartments. The primary responsive tissues to insulin-mediated changes in protein metabolism include hepatic, gastrointestinal, cardiac, and skeletal muscle. Numerous studies have measured the rates of protein synthesis and degradation using amino acid tracers (Charlton and Nair 1998). An increase in both protein degradation and protein synthesis has been observed in T1DM patients in the absence of insulin treatment (Charlton and Nair 1998; Herbert and Nair 2010). The rate of protein degradation in the absence of insulin treatment is higher than the rate of protein synthesis resulting in a net loss of whole body protein. T1DM patients in an insulin-deprived state display elevated skeletal muscle proteolysis and splanchnic bed protein synthesis. High rates of protein synthesis measured in the splanchnic bed may be related primarily to hepatic and/or gastrointestinal tissue activity. With insulin treatment, skeletal muscle proteolysis is inhibited while splanchnic bed protein synthesis is decreased. This decrease in splanchnic bed protein synthesis may be mediated by decreases in glucagon and gluconeogenic activity in hepatic tissue in response to insulin treatment (Herbert and Nair 2010). The splanchnic bed has a much higher rate of protein turnover than skeletal muscle which could account for the association between splanchnic bed and whole-body protein metabolism (Charlton and Nair 1998). Therefore, despite the larger total mass of skeletal muscle relative to total splanchnic mass, whole-body protein metabolism is likely to mimic that of the rapid protein turnover splanchnic bed in T1DM patients.

4.2 Lack of insulin in T1DM induces protein degradation

Insulin is considered a potent anabolic hormone. Insulin treatment promotes skeletal muscle protein accretion primarily through inhibition of mechanisms of protein degradation (Charlton, Balagopal et al. 1997; Fawcett, Permana et al. 2007). Although studies do not agree whether insulin alone stimulates protein synthesis in vivo, insulin treatment plays an important role in supporting mechanisms of protein synthesis. Evidence supports a necessity for the presence of insulin and amino acids, (leucine in particular) in order to maximally stimulate skeletal muscle protein synthesis with feeding (Anthony, Yoshizawa et al. 2000; Balage, Sinaud et al. 2001; Anthony, Lang et al. 2002; Anthony, Reiter et al. 2002). Insulin receptor binding signals through the PI3K/AKT/mTORC1 pathway and mediates control of the mRNA binding step of translation initiation (Kimball and Jefferson; Anthony, Lang et al. 2002). The mammalian target of rapamycin complex 1 (mTORC1) is a prominent signaling protein where multiple positive and negative signals converge to influence the phosphorylation of downstream regulators of translation initiation, p70 S6K1 and eIF4E-binding protein 4E-BP1 (Kimball and Jefferson). mTORC1 mediates phosphorylation and activation of protein kinase S6K1 which activates translation initiation and elongation factors leading to the activation of mRNA cap binding and mRNA joining to the 43 S preinitiation complex of the ribosome (Fenton and Gout; Kimball and Jefferson). In addition, mTORC1 mediated phosphorylation of 4E-BP1 decreases its affinity for binding translation initiation factor eIF4E, allowing it to interact with eIF4G in formation of the active mRNA cap-binding complex, eIF4F (Kimball and Jefferson; Anthony, Lang et al. 2002). Modulation of these two regulatory steps in translation initiation account for much of the increase in skeletal muscle protein synthesis with feeding in healthy non-diabetics (Kimball and Jefferson). Numerous animal studies have used chemical (streptozotocin, alloxan, diazoxide, and somatostatin) or procedures (pancreatecomy) to induce T1DM by abrogating the release of insulin from pancreatic β-cells. These agents allow for the study of insulin's influence on many physiological processes including protein metabolism. Using STZ-treated rats, we demonstrated a decrease in skeletal muscle mass (Kelleher). Skeletal muscle and liver protein synthesis are stimulated with increases in plasma amino acids and insulin (Yoshizawa, Kimball et al. 1998). The amino acid, leucine, is unique in its ability to stimulate skeletal muscle protein synthesis through the mTORC1 pathway (Anthony, Yoshizawa et al. 2000). Carbohydrate feeding without the supplementation of amino acids increases serum insulin, but does not increase skeletal muscle protein synthesis (Anthony, Anthony et al. 2000). Taken together, both amino acids (leucine) and insulin are required to stimulate muscle protein synthesis with feeding. In T1DM animal models, basal skeletal muscle protein synthesis is decreased relative to non-alloxan-treated controls, but increases proportionally with leucine gavage (Anthony, Reiter et al. 2002). Phosphorylation of 4E-BP1 and S6K1 were either attenuated or unresponsive to leucine or meal feeding in the absence of insulin, but responded to leucine gavage in a dose-dependent manner to insulin treatment (Gordon, Serino et al.; Balage, Sinaud et al. 2001; Anthony, Lang et al. 2002; Anthony, Reiter et al. 2002). When insulin-unresponsive neonatal pigs were treated with leucine, increases in skeletal muscle protein synthesis were associated with increased eIF4E availability for eIF4F formation (Escobar, Frank et al. 2005). Therefore, feeding-induced skeletal muscle protein synthesis appeared to be both insulin-dependent (phosphorylation of 4E-BP1 and S6K1) and insulin-independent (eIF4E availability) mechanisms (Anthony, Reiter et al. 2002). Thus, decreases in the rate of skeletal muscle protein synthesis in T1DM can be attributed to multiple factors. Hypoinsulinemia has been shown to decrease feeding-induced protein synthesis due to resistance to leucine stimulation of the translational regulators 4E-BP1 and S6K1 (Gordon, Serino et al.). Furthermore, the lack of circulating insulin reduces PI3K/AKT/mTORC1 pathway activation, a pathway which activates a multitude of anabolic signals and inhibits catabolic factors when stimulated (Price, Bailey et al. 1996). In T1DM the inflammatory and hormonal milieu increase protein degradation and decrease synthesis.

4.3 O-GlcNAcylation of proteins

Interestingly, hyperglycemia induced by the lack of insulin in T1DM is also capable of interfering with mechanisms of protein synthesis. Glucose can be converted to uridine diphosphate N-acetylglucosamine (UDP-GlcNAc) through the cellular energy sensor hexosamine biosynthetic pathway (Love and Hanover 2005). Hyperglycemia with less well-controlled diabetes can increase the amount of O-linked β--N-acetylglucosamine (O-

GlcNAc) (Park, Saudek et al.). Increased site-specific O-GlcNAcylation of proteins can be detrimental to protein function thus potentially contributing to the deleterious effects of hyperglycemia seen in T1DM on liver, β-cell, pancreatic, and red blood cell function (Issad, Masson et al.; Park, Saudek et al.). O-GlcNAcylation of proteins is involved with transcription, translation, ubiquitination, cell cycle, stress responses, and similar to phosphorylation can alter protein posttranslational function and cycle proteins on and off (Butkinaree, Park et al.; Love and Hanover 2005). In T1DM, there is a loss of regulation of O-GlcNAcylation and a crosstalk with protein phosphorylation can potentially underlying many of the abnormal protein functions and glucotoxicity exhibited by the disease. O-GlcNAcylation may compete with phosphorylation at key sites in the insulin signaling pathway (Love and Hanover 2005). High throughput studies have identified O-GlcNAcylation sites on translation factors and core ribosomal proteins that form active polysomes (Zeidan, Wang et al.). Thus modification of ribosomal proteins and signaling pathways by O-GlcNAcylation may play a role in T1DM-associated regulation of signal transduction and translation.

5. Hormonal influences on T1DM protein metabolism

The lack of circulating insulin resulting from β-cell destruction disrupts the production and release of other hormones. T1DM patients and animal models display increases in glucagon, glucocorticoids, catecholamines, and growth hormone which may influence changes in tissue specific protein metabolism independent of hypoinsulinemia. These hormones are the most prominent hormones affecting changes in protein metabolism when hypoinsulinemia results in their irregular production and release.

5.1 Glucagon

Basal energy expenditure was increased in T1DM following insulin withdrawal when compared to insulin treatment and non-diabetic control subjects (Nair, Halliday et al. 1984; Charlton and Nair 1998; Karakelides, Asmann et al. 2007). Insulin deprivation in T1DM patients displayed elevations in plasma glucagon which correlate with increased energy expenditure (Nair, Halliday et al. 1984). Evidence support that increased circulating glucagon the ability to increase leucine and phenylalanine oxidation, proteolysis, and whole-body oxygen consumption in T1DM (Nair 1987; Nair, Halliday et al. 1987; Charlton and Nair 1998). In addition to stimulating proteolysis, glucagon induced inhibition of muscle protein synthesis by reducing glucogenic plasma amino acids (Charlton, Adey et al. 1996). High circulating glucagon levels are likely to increase oxygen consumption by stimulating the energy-expensive process of gluconeogenesis, and macroautophagy in the liver of T1DM patients (Nair, Halliday et al. 1984; Mortimore, Poso et al. 1989; Chhibber, Soriano et al. 2000; Karakelides, Asmann et al. 2007). Enhanced hepatic glucose production along with increases in splanchnic region protein synthesis could be attributed to the increases in basal energy expenditure measured in insulin-deprived T1DM (Herbert and Nair 2010).

5.2 Catecholamines

Animal models of T1DM display increases in norepinephrine and IL-1-mediated epinephrine (Gwosdow, O'Connell et al. 1992; Baviera, Zanon et al. 2008). IL-1, a key mediator of inflammation, fever, and acute phase response plays an important role in the incidence of T1DM (Mandrup-Poulsen, Pickersgill et al.). IL-1 has been shown to stimulate catecholamine release and mediate a stimulatory effect on corticosterone release from the adrenal gland through an α-adrenergic receptor (Gwosdow, O'Connell et al. 1992). Catecholamines have been shown to inhibit muscle protein degradation via a cyclic adenosine monophosphate (cAMP) signaling cascade (Baviera, Zanon et al. 2007). Guanthidine-induced chemical sympathectomy of STZ-induced diabetes rats indicates that catecholamines inhibit protein degradation through both Ca2+-dependent and ATP-dependent pathways (Baviera, Zanon et al. 2008) that could provide prophylaxis in understanding the disruption of proteins homeostasis in T1DM.

5.3 Glucocorticoids

Catabolic doses of glucocorticoids have been implicated in a number of muscle wasting diseases including T1DM where increases in corticosterone production have been observed (Bailey, Wang et al. 1999; Menconi, Fareed et al. 2007). Circulating increases in TNF-α and IL-1 can stimulate the pituitary-adrenal axis to increase secretion of corticosterone (Gwosdow, Kumar et al. 1990; Hall-Angeras, Angeras et al. 1990). Insulinopenia, together with increased glucocorticoids have been shown to enhance muscle protein degradation through increased ubiquitin conjugation to proteins, proteolytic activity, and ubiquitin pathway component mRNA transcription (Price, Bailey et al. 1996; Bailey, Wang et al. 1999). Elevated levels of glucocorticoids have also been found to contribute to skeletal muscle atrophy through increased expression of ubiquitin pathway proteins, transcription factors CCAAT/enhancer-binding protein β and δ and Forkhead box O (Foxo), and nuclear cofactor p300/histone acetyl transferase (Menconi, Fareed et al. 2007). In addition to catabolic factors, glucocorticoids contribute to muscle atrophy through inhibition of anabolic factors, insulin signaling, and stimulation of protein synthesis (Shah, Kimball et al. 2000; Shah, Kimball et al. 2000; Hu, Wang et al. 2009). Glucocorticoids induce insulin and insulin-like growth factor (IGF-1) resistance through inhibition of the phosphoinositide-3-kinase(PI3K)/protein kinase B(AKT) pathway. This mechanism is believed to be caused by interference with PI3K-p85 subunit interaction, preventing activation of insulin receptor substrate-1 (IRS-1) and autoinhibition of the ribosomal protein S6 kinase (p70 S6K1) enzyme (Zheng, Ohkawa et al.; Shah, Iniguez-Lluhi et al. 2002; Hu, Wang et al. 2009). Increases in circulating glucocorticoids also contribute to the observed decreases in the rate of protein synthesis. In addition to their effects on protein degradation, glucocorticoids inhibit muscle protein synthesis through insulin, IGF-1, and leucine resistance. Despite no changes in heart, type I fiber, or liver protein synthesis with glucocorticoid administration for days, rates of skeletal type II muscle fiber protein synthesis were inhibited and maintained at a lower rate (Rannels and Jefferson 1980; Odedra, Bates et al. 1983). Inhibition of skeletal muscle protein synthesis is partially protected by increases in insulin administration in STZ-induced diabetic rats, but cannot produce positive accretion rates with increasing doses (Tomas, Murray et al. 1984) and even low doses of corticosterone induce muscle wasting with low doses of insulin administration in STZ-treated rats (Odedra and Millward 1982). Glucocorticoids appear to inhibit muscle protein synthesis through dephosphorylation and inhibition of 4E-BP1 and S6K and enhanced phosphorylation of eIF4E (Shah, Kimball et al. 2000; Shah, Kimball et al. 2000) along with mechanisms of anabolic factor resistance (Rieu, Sornet et al. 2004).

5.4 Growth hormone

Growth hormone inhibits leucine oxidation and stimulates skeletal muscle protein synthesis, but does not appear to affect mechanisms of protein degradation (Horber and Haymond 1990). Basal growth hormone levels in T1DM patients are normal or elevated when compared to non-diabetics controls depending on glycemic control. Interestingly, IGF-1 levels have been shown to be reduced in T1DM patients (de Sa, Nascif et al.). Alterations to the growth hormone-IGF-1 axis have been linked to hepatic resistance caused by reduced receptors expression and circulating growth hormone binding protein (Bereket, Lang et al. 1999). Poor metabolic control in T1DM alters the growth hormone/IGF-1 axis, but administration of insulin or insulin plus IGF-1 maintain the metabolism associated with this axis. T1DM-mediated hyperglycemia has not been shown to interfere with the rest of the hypothalamic-pituitary axis according to GH-, ACTH and cortisol-releasing mechanisms (de Sa, Nascif et al.; Moyer-Mileur, Slater et al. 2008).

6. Protein degradation, proteolysis, and pro-catabolic potential signals involved in T1DM

Tissue mass is the product of both anabolic and catabolic processes. In order to evaluate the fluctuation in tissue size, both rates of protein synthesis and protein degradation are important in order to understand the net protein flux. Protein degradation is important to control the rate-limiting and regulatory proteins in signaling pathways, remove mutated or damaged proteins, and to supply amino acids from muscle proteins for protein synthesis and gluconeogenesis (Price and Mitch 1998). There are four intracellular pathways utilized by eukaryotic cells to degrade proteins including the ATP-dependent ubiquitin-proteasome system, calcium-dependent protease, the lysosomal acid-activated protease, and the ATP-independent caspase pathways. T1DM is a pathological disease with considerable increases in protein degradation.

6.1 ATP and calcium-dependent proteolytic processes

Virtually all muscle wasting conditions such as T1DM exhibit increases in protein degradation through activation of the ubiquitin-proteasome system (Hu, Lee et al. 2007). Proteins are degraded in this ATP-dependent proteolytic process when conjugated by covalent attachment to an ubiquitin protein. With the aid of ATP hydrolysis, ubiquitin is transferred between several enzymes (E1, E2, and E3) prior to attachment at specific lysine residues on the target protein serving as a marker for proteolytic degradation. This process is repeated until several ubiquitin proteins are attached in a linear chain targeting the protein for degradation in the proteasome 26S. When targeted proteins meet the proteasome, they are unfolded and fed into the proteasome core where combinations of peptide sequence are recognized and hydrolyzed (Price and Mitch 1998). Calcium-dependent protein degradation has been shown to depend on the activity of a family of cysteine proteases called calpains (Costelli, Reffo et al. 2005). Calpains typically exist as inactive heterodimers in the cytoplasm. When the intracellular calcium concentration rises, calpains translocate to the plasma membrane where they are activated by phospholipids which induces a conformational change. This structural change removes regulatory constraints from the catalytic domain, and the catalytic subunit is released in an active state. Thus calpains might be involved in T1DM-related muscle wasting through their mechanism of myofibrillar degradation. Calpains attack the sarcomeric proteins of the Z-disk which leads to a disruption of the myofibrils and release of protein substrates for degradation by other proteolytic systems (Costelli, Reffo et al. 2005).

6.2 Ubiquitin-proteasome involvement in T1DM-induced muscle wasting

Two muscle protein degradation systems that operate independent of both ATP and calcium include the recruitment of caspases and the endosome-lysosome system and may be upregulated in T1DM. ATP-independent processes of protein degradation involve caspases, cysteine proteases commonly activated with the apoptotic response. A reduction in myonuclei associated with increases in apoptosis indicate that apoptosis plays a role in some models of muscle wasting. However, caspase-3 activation also can mediate skeletal muscle atrophy through actomyosin complex cleavage. Evidence suggests that caspase-3 activation is an initial step in the process of muscle protein degradation which cleaves larger actomyosin complexes into smaller fragments for other systems (ubiquitin-proteasome) to degrade (Du, Wang et al. 2004). The lysosomal acid-activated protease or endosome-lysosome system primarily degrades long-lived proteins using activated acid proteases in non-selective manner (Costelli, Reffo et al. 2005). This system is commonly incorporated in the recycling of substrates with autophagy. Although some of these proteases are abundant, lysomal degradation is not often involved in skeletal muscle wasting. Protein degradation studies on STZ-induced diabetes indicated increases in the ubiquitin-proteasome and calpain pathways that could be responsible for the skeletal muscle wasting observed with uncontrolled T1DM (Kettelhut, Pepato et al. 1994; Pepato, Migliorini et al. 1996). These studies measured the activity of these pathways in addition to the endosome-lysosomal system for 10 days post-STZ injection and observed variable changes in the systems over time. Within the first 3 days, the increase in skeletal muscle proteolysis was associated with activation of the ubiquitin-proteasome and calpain pathways, and increases in ubiquitin and proteasome subunit mRNA. At 5-10 days post-injection, the activity of these pathways decreased below non-diabetic control measures. The endosome-lysosomal system did not appear to be activated throughout the 10 days of diabetes, and caspase activity could not be measured at this point. After 24 hours of diabetes, rates of protein synthesis were reduced and continued to decrease for the remaining 10 days. Therefore, the STZ-treated animal model appears to develop muscle atrophy as a result of increased ubiquitin-proteasome and calpain pathway activation in addition to decreases in the rate of protein synthesis. In agreement with these two STZ-treatment studies above, increases in skeletal muscle protein degradation in patients and other animal models of T1DM is primarily associated with activation of the ubiquitin-proteasome system (Flakoll, Kulaylat et al. 1989; Smith, Wong et al. 1989; Price, Bailey et al. 1996). Uncontrolled STZ-induced diabetes in rats exhibits increases in both proteolytic capacity and activity (Kettelhut, Pepato et al. 1994; Pepato, Migliorini et al. 1996; Price, Bailey et al. 1996; Hu, Lee et al. 2007; Hu, Klein et al. 2008). In STZ-treated rats, the use of lysosomal and calcium-dependent degradation pathways inhibitors was unable to prevent skeletal muscle proteolysis (Price, Bailey et al. 1996). However, inhibition of the proteasome (MG132) or ATP synthesis decreased muscle proteolysis to similar levels compared to vehicle-treated controls. Therefore the ATP-dependent ubiquitin-proteasome pathway seems to mediate protein degradation in T1DM (Price, Bailey et al. 1996; Bailey, Wang et al. 1999).

6.2.1 Atrophy in T1DM

Additional evidence of the role of the ubiquitin-proteasome pathway in T1DM is the increased transcription of muscle atrophy-related genes in insulinopenic STZ-treated rats

(Price, Bailey et al. 1996). Muscle specific ubiquitin E3 ligases atrogin-1/MAFbx, muscle RING finger protein 1 (MuRF1), ubiquitin-conjugating enzyme E2 (14 kDa), and the C3, C5, and C9 proteasome subunits are important 'atrogenes' in the regulation of muscle mass and typically measured as indicators of muscle proteolytic capacity (Zheng, Ohkawa et al.; Wing and Bedard 1996; Bailey, Wang et al. 1999; Menconi, Fareed et al. 2007). Atrogene mRNAs are typically increased with insulin deficiency or resistance in conditions of muscle wasting and decreased or degraded with insulin and IGF-1 signaling (Wing and Bedard 1996; Price and Mitch 1998). Atrogin-1 and MuRF1 mRNA levels are common indicators of myofibrillar degradation because atrogin-1 targets eukaryotic initiation factor 3 subunit 5 that induces expression of muscle specific proteins and hypertrophy, and MuRF1 targets myosin in muscle (Tisdale). These gene products are atrophy-specific ubiquitin ligases transcribed with FOXO3a activation and nuclear translocation. Increases in atrogin-1 and MuRF1 transcription could indicate that the cell in T1DM is preparing for increases in muscle protein-specific proteolysis. In addition, transcription of atrogenes, expression levels of 26S proteasome and ubiquitin are measured as indicators of proteolytic capacity. Ubiquitin conjugation to proteins provides a way of analyzing which proteins are marked for proteolytic degradation. Finally, the chymotrypsin-like peptidase activity of homogenized tissue in the presence and absence of epoxomicin, a proteasome-specific inhibitor, provides a measure of ubiquitin-proteasome activity (Hu, Klein et al. 2008). According to such measurements, skeletal muscle tissue taken from uncontrolled T1DM patients and animal models, strongly indicate activation of the ubiquitin-proteasome system as the primary mode of protein degradation in T1DM. Insulin regulates proteolysis through multiple signals, but direct regulates proteolytic activity through a zinc metalloproteinase, insulin-degrading enzyme (IDE) (Duckworth, Bennett et al. 1998; de Tullio, Morelli et al. 2008). IDE co-purifies with the proteasome as part of a cytosolic complex (Duckworth, Bennett et al. 1994). If IDE-proteasome interaction is prevented or IDE activity inhibited, insulin's inhibitory effect on proteolytic activity is not observed (Bennett, Hamel et al. 1997; Duckworth, Bennett et al. 1998; Hamel, Bennett et al. 1998). Although insulin is the primary substrate for IDE, atrial natriuretic peptide, glucagon, proinsulin, IGF-1 and IGF-2 can also bind, get degraded by IDE, and have inhibitory effects on the chymotrypsin-like and trypsin-like catalytic activities of the proteasome (Bennett, Hamel et al. 1997). However, not all substrates equally inhibited proteolytic activity. Insulin analogues with various susceptibility to degradation by IDE showed a positive correlation between substrate degradation, proteolytic activity, and IDE-proteasome dissociation (Bennett, Fawcett et al. 2003). The mechanism by which insulin causes intracellular inhibition of proteolytic activity may be through fragments of degraded insulin or conformational changes in the IDE-proteasome complex (Bennett, Hamel et al. 1997; Hamel, Bennett et al. 1998; Bennett, Fawcett et al. 2003). Thus, increases in skeletal muscle proteolytic activity in uncontrolled T1DM are likely associated with a lack of IDE-mediated proteasome inhibition.

6.2.2 Cross-talk between anabolic-catabolic signaling

Extensive crosstalk between cellular signaling pathways regulates the processes of protein synthesis and degradation. Insulin, IGF-1, and leucine are among anabolic factors which signal through the PI3K/AKT/mTORC1 pathway, activating regulatory proteins associated with translation initiation and inhibiting mechanisms of protein degradation. Glucocorticoids and circulating proinflammatory cytokines are among catabolic factors which signal in opposition to insulin by inhibiting mechanisms of protein synthesis and increasing ubiquitin-proteasome pathway activity and apoptosis (Tisdale; Menconi, Fareed et al. 2007). A benefit of crosstalk between the protein synthetic and degradation pathways is that it can prevent energy expensive futile cycles. However, crosstalk can also create resistance to anabolic signals in conditions of muscle wasting (Rieu, Sornet et al. 2004). A strong reciprocal relationship exists between PI3K/AKT pathway activation and protein degradation in T1DM. Decreases in PTEN, the phosphatase which turns off PI3K signaling by inactivating phosphatidylinositol 3,4,5-triphosphate (PIP3) to phosphatidylinositol 4,5-bisphosphate (PIP2), was shown to suppress STZ-induced increases in proteolysis by maintaining PI3K signaling (Hu, Lee et al. 2007). PI3K/AKT pathway activation can be decreased in T1DM due to hypoinsulinemia in addition to an increase in circulating glucocorticoids. Glucocorticoids have been found to decrease IRS-1-mediated PI3K signaling due to increases in PI3K-glucocortioid receptor interaction (Hu, Wang et al. 2009). Glucocorticoid receptor stimulation contributes to muscle protein degradation through inhibition of insulin signaling and can activate muscle proteolysis independently of insulin signaling pathways. The lack of PI3K/AKT activation observed in T1DM models is coupled with increases in both ubiquitin-proteasome activity, and ATP-independent proteolysis in the activation of caspase-3 in skeletal and cardiac muscle (Hu, Lee et al. 2007; Hu, Klein et al. 2008). When the PI3K/AKT pathway is not activated, protein degradation pathways are activated through the dephosphorylation and activation of Foxo's (Sandri, Sandri et al. 2004; Baviera, Zanon et al. 2008). FOXO3a, a critical mediator between growth factor IRS-1/PI3K/AKT and IRS2/MEK/ERK signaling, induces the expression of ubiquitin, atrogin-1, and MuRF1 (Tisdale; Zheng, Ohkawa et al.; Sandri, Sandri et al. 2004). In addition to atrogenes, FOXO3a is responsible for apoptotic signaling leading to the loss of mitochondrial membrane permeability, degradation of nuclear DNA, cytochrome c release, Bad phosphorylation, downregulation of FLICE-inhibitory protein, and cleaved (active) caspase 1, 3, and 8 (Hou, Chong et al.; Shang, Chong et al.; Skurk, Maatz et al. 2004). Therefore, FOXO3a may represent a promising target for the treatment of T1DM-mediated skeletal muscle atrophy.

6.3 Inflammation and increases in protein degradation in T1DM

As discussed previously in this chapter, pro-inflammatory cytokine play a key role in the pathogenesis of T1DM. Increases in plasma cytokines can have detrimental effects on multiple tissues and is associated with skeletal muscle wasting. For example, aged rats with low grade inflammation resulted in an insensitivity to feeding-induced skeletal muscle protein synthesis (Balage, Averous et al.). Furthermore, inflammation is implicated in the increases in muscle protein degradation, reductions in muscle protein synthesis, and reduced intake of amino acids in a number of pathological conditions (Durham, Dillon et al. 2009). Circulating inflammatory cytokines can alter the release of hormones from the pituitary gland including inflammatory-suppressive glucocorticoids, or can have direct signaling effects on target tissues. The changes in protein metabolism associated with T1DM point towards TNF-α, and IL-1 as pro-inflammatory cytokines which play a role in skeletal muscle atrophy. TNF-α and IL-1 are capable of inducing both direct and indirect effects on skeletal muscle metabolism. TNF-α can inhibit skeletal muscle protein synthesis by inhibiting phosphorylation of 4E-BP1 (Tisdale 2005). This cytokine is further implicated as a mediator of skeletal muscle atrophy through the activation of NF-κB. NF-κB activation can inhibit synthesis of the muscle-specific differentiation factor MyoD and is posited to be the stimulator of ubiquitin-proteasome activity induced by cytokines, proteolytic-inducing factor (PIF), and reactive oxygen species (Libera and Vescovo 2004; Tisdale 2005; Durham, Dillon et al. 2009). However, it should be noted that these conclusions come from the literature associated with cancer cachexia and not T1DM, and increases in TNF-α administration or expression do not always show direct catabolic signaling. In septic rats, TNF-α increased myofibrillar breakdown rates with no changes in the rate of muscle protein synthesis (Zamir, Hasselgren et al. 1992). In healthy rats, TNF-α and IL-1α administration display increases in skeletal muscle proteolysis by different mechanisms (Zamir, Hasselgren et al. 1992). In these studies, TNF-α administration only increased muscle proteolysis when the effects of glucocorticoids were not inhibited (Hall-Angeras, Angeras et al. 1990; Zamir, Hasselgren et al. 1992). With glucocorticoid inhibition (adrenalectomy or receptor antagonist), TNF-α did not have any effect on protein turnover. IL-1α, on the other hand increased muscle proteolysis independently of glucocorticoid inhibition (Zamir, Hasselgren et al. 1992; Zamir, Hasselgren et al. 1993). Therefore, it was determined from these studies that TNF-α increased muscle proteolysis by stimulating the adrenal axis to increase release of glucocorticoids, while IL-1α can stimulate glucocorticoid release and signal muscle proteolysis independently of the mechanism of glucocorticoids (Gwosdow, Kumar et al. 1990; Hall-Angeras, Angeras et al. 1990). TNF-α is an important pro-inflammatory cytokine for understanding T1DM-associated skeletal muscle wasting because it can activate also apoptotic signaling pathways. TNF-α is capable of inducing production of a second messenger, sphingosine, which signals skeletal muscle cell apoptosis (Dalla Libera, Sabbadini et al. 2001). The interaction between TNF-α and TNF receptor 1 has been shown to cause rapid degradation of sphingomyelin which generated sphingosine inside the cell (Wiegmann, Schutze et al. 1992). Although this observation is more common to models of heart failure than STZ-treatment, the number of apoptotic nuclei is positively correlated with circulating TNF-α in T1DM, and the ensuing reduction in number of myonuclei may be responsible for skeletal muscle atrophy (Vescovo, Ambrosio et al. 2001). Therefore, wasting of skeletal muscle in T1DM may be linked to increases in pro-inflammatory regulators such as TNF-α and IL-1 which can influence mechanisms of protein degradation and apoptosis.

7. Conclusion

The focus of this chapter was on the various cellular signaling-associated with inflammation that could explain either the etiology or pathogenesis of T1DM. Although the exact cause of T1DM is still unknown, we have gained insight into the cellular mechanisms that are involved. T1DM is defined as an autoimmune disease, therefore inflammatory-related signaling cascades are critical to understand to discover new therapeutic treatment. Among the several transcription factors, NF-κB is of particular interest as it is involved in both the inflammatory and apoptosis process that could explain the degradation of β-cells. T1DM milieu influences also mechanisms of protein synthesis and protein degradation. A focus was placed on changes in the skeletal muscle due to the important of muscle in glucose metabolism. As treatments improve, more research is needed to help combat the consequences of T1DM on the quality of life.

8. References

Abdi, R., R. N. Smith, et al. (2002). "The role of CC chemokine receptor 5 (CCR5) in islet allograft rejection." Diabetes 51(8): 2489-95.

Alessi, D. R. (2001). "Discovery of PDK1, one of the missing links in insulin signal transduction. Colworth Medal Lecture." Biochem Soc Trans 29(Pt 2): 1-14.

Alessi, D. R., M. Deak, et al. (1997). "3-Phosphoinositide-dependent protein kinase-1 (PDK1): structural and functional homology with the Drosophila DSTPK61 kinase." Curr Biol 7(10): 776-89.

Anthony, J. C., T. G. Anthony, et al. (2000). "Orally administered leucine stimulates protein synthesis in skeletal muscle of postabsorptive rats in association with increased eIF4F formation." J Nutr 130(2): 139-45.

Anthony, J. C., C. H. Lang, et al. (2002). "Contribution of insulin to the translational control of protein synthesis in skeletal muscle by leucine." Am J Physiol Endocrinol Metab 282(5): E1092-101.

Anthony, J. C., A. K. Reiter, et al. (2002). "Orally administered leucine enhances protein synthesis in skeletal muscle of diabetic rats in the absence of increases in 4E-BP1 or S6K1 phosphorylation." Diabetes 51(4): 928-36.

Anthony, J. C., F. Yoshizawa, et al. (2000). "Leucine stimulates translation initiation in skeletal muscle of postabsorptive rats via a rapamycin-sensitive pathway." J Nutr 130(10): 2413-9.

Bach, J. F., A. Bendelac, et al. (2004). "The role of innate immunity in autoimmunity." J Exp Med 200(12): 1527-31.

Bailey, J. L., X. Wang, et al. (1999). "The balance between glucocorticoids and insulin regulates muscle proteolysis via the ubiquitin-proteasome pathway." Miner Electrolyte Metab 25(4-6): 220-3.

Balage, M., J. Averous, et al. "Presence of low-grade inflammation impaired postprandial stimulation of muscle protein synthesis in old rats." J Nutr Biochem 21(4): 325-31.

Balage, M., S. Sinaud, et al. (2001). "Amino acids and insulin are both required to regulate assembly of the eIF4E. eIF4G complex in rat skeletal muscle." Am J Physiol Endocrinol Metab 281(3): E565-74.

Balamurugan, A. N., R. Bottino, et al. (2006). "Prospective and challenges of islet transplantation for the therapy of autoimmune diabetes." Pancreas 32(3): 231-43.

Barbe-Tuana, F. M., D. Klein, et al. (2006). "CD40-CD40 ligand interaction activates proinflammatory pathways in pancreatic islets." Diabetes 55(9): 2437-45.

Baum, J. D., M. Ounsted, et al. (1975). "Letter: Weight gain in infancy and subsequent development of diabetes mellitus in childhood." Lancet 2(7940): 866.

Baviera, A. M., N. M. Zanon, et al. (2007). "Pentoxifylline inhibits Ca2+-dependent and ATP proteasome-dependent proteolysis in skeletal muscle from acutely diabetic rats." Am J Physiol Endocrinol Metab 292(3): E702-8.

Baviera, A. M., N. M. Zanon, et al. (2008). "Chemical sympathectomy further increases muscle protein degradation of acutely diabetic rats." Muscle Nerve 38(2): 1027-35.

Bell, G. I. and K. S. Polonsky (2001). "Diabetes mellitus and genetically programmed defects in beta-cell function." Nature 414(6865): 788-91.

Bennet, W. M., A. A. Connacher, et al. (1991). "Effects of insulin and amino acids on leg protein turnover in IDDM patients." Diabetes 40(4): 499-508.

Bennett, R. G., J. Fawcett, et al. (2003). "Insulin inhibition of the proteasome is dependent on degradation of insulin by insulin-degrading enzyme." J Endocrinol 177(3): 399-405.

Bennett, R. G., F. G. Hamel, et al. (1997). "Characterization of the insulin inhibition of the peptidolytic activities of the insulin-degrading enzyme-proteasome complex." Diabetes 46(2): 197-203.

Bereket, A., C. H. Lang, et al. (1999). "Alterations in the growth hormone-insulin-like growth factor axis in insulin dependent diabetes mellitus." Horm Metab Res 31(2-3): 172-81.

Butkinaree, C., K. Park, et al. "O-linked beta-N-acetylglucosamine (O-GlcNAc): Extensive crosstalk with phosphorylation to regulate signaling and transcription in response to nutrients and stress." Biochim Biophys Acta 1800(2): 96-106.

Cardozo, A. K., F. Ortis, et al. (2005). "Cytokines downregulate the sarcoendoplasmic reticulum pump Ca2+ ATPase 2b and deplete endoplasmic reticulum Ca2+, leading to induction of endoplasmic reticulum stress in pancreatic beta-cells." Diabetes 54(2): 452-61.

Castellino, P., L. Luzi, et al. (1987). "Effect of insulin and plasma amino acid concentrations on leucine metabolism in man. Role of substrate availability on estimates of whole body protein synthesis." J Clin Invest 80(6): 1784-93.

Charlton, M. and K. S. Nair (1998). "Protein metabolism in insulin-dependent diabetes mellitus." J Nutr 128(2 Suppl): 323S-327S.

Charlton, M. R., D. B. Adey, et al. (1996). "Evidence for a catabolic role of glucagon during an amino acid load." J Clin Invest 98(1): 90-9.

Charlton, M. R., P. Balagopal, et al. (1997). "Skeletal muscle myosin heavy chain synthesis in type 1 diabetes." Diabetes 46(8): 1336-40.

Charlton, M. R. and K. S. Nair (1998). "Role of hyperglucagonemia in catabolism associated with type 1 diabetes: effects on leucine metabolism and the resting metabolic rate." Diabetes 47(11): 1748-56.

Chhibber, V. L., C. Soriano, et al. (2000). "Effects of low-dose and high-dose glucagon on glucose production and gluconeogenesis in humans." Metabolism 49(1): 39-46.

Chillaron, J. J., A. Goday, et al. (2009). "Estimated glucose disposal rate in assessment of the metabolic syndrome and microvascular complications in patients with type 1 diabetes." J Clin Endocrinol Metab 94(9): 3530-4.

Cnop, M., N. Welsh, et al. (2005). "Mechanisms of pancreatic beta-cell death in type 1 and type 2 diabetes: many differences, few similarities." Diabetes 54 Suppl 2: S97-107.

Costelli, P., P. Reffo, et al. (2005). "Ca(2+)-dependent proteolysis in muscle wasting." Int J Biochem Cell Biol 37(10): 2134-46.

Czech, M. P. and S. Corvera (1999). "Signaling mechanisms that regulate glucose transport." J Biol Chem 274(4): 1865-8.

Dalla Libera, L., R. Sabbadini, et al. (2001). "Apoptosis in the skeletal muscle of rats with heart failure is associated with increased serum levels of TNF-alpha and sphingosine." J Mol Cell Cardiol 33(10): 1871-8.

de Sa, L. B., S. O. Nascif, et al. "Effects of ghrelin, growth hormone-releasing peptide-6, and growth hormone-releasing hormone on growth hormone, adrenocorticotropic hormone, and cortisol release in type 1 diabetes mellitus." Metabolism 59(10): 1536-42.

de Tullio, M. B., L. Morelli, et al. (2008). "The irreversible binding of amyloid peptide substrates to insulin-degrading enzyme: a biological perspective." Prion 2(2): 51-6.

DeFronzo, R. A. (1982). "Insulin secretion, insulin resistance, and obesity." Int J Obes 6 Suppl 1: 73-82.

DeFronzo, R. A., R. Hendler, et al. (1982). "Insulin resistance is a prominent feature of insulin-dependent diabetes." Diabetes 31(9): 795-801.

Dogusan, Z., M. Garcia, et al. (2008). "Double-stranded RNA induces pancreatic beta-cell apoptosis by activation of the toll-like receptor 3 and interferon regulatory factor 3 pathways." Diabetes 57(5): 1236-45.

Dotta, F., S. Censini, et al. (2007). "Coxsackie B4 virus infection of beta cells and natural killer cell insulitis in recent-onset type 1 diabetic patients." Proc Natl Acad Sci U S A 104(12): 5115-20.

Dresner, A., D. Laurent, et al. (1999). "Effects of free fatty acids on glucose transport and IRS-1-associated phosphatidylinositol 3-kinase activity." J Clin Invest 103(2): 253-9.

Du, J., X. Wang, et al. (2004). "Activation of caspase-3 is an initial step triggering accelerated muscle proteolysis in catabolic conditions." J Clin Invest 113(1): 115-23.

Duckworth, W. C., R. G. Bennett, et al. (1994). "A direct inhibitory effect of insulin on a cytosolic proteolytic complex containing insulin-degrading enzyme and multicatalytic proteinase." J Biol Chem 269(40): 24575-80.

Duckworth, W. C., R. G. Bennett, et al. (1998). "Insulin acts intracellularly on proteasomes through insulin-degrading enzyme." Biochem Biophys Res Commun 244(2): 390-4.

Durham, W. J., E. L. Dillon, et al. (2009). "Inflammatory burden and amino acid metabolism in cancer cachexia." Curr Opin Clin Nutr Metab Care 12(1): 72-7.

Eizirik, D. L., M. L. Colli, et al. (2009). "The role of inflammation in insulitis and beta-cell loss in type 1 diabetes." Nat Rev Endocrinol 5(4): 219-26.

Eizirik, D. L. and T. Mandrup-Poulsen (2001). "A choice of death--the signal-transduction of immune-mediated beta-cell apoptosis." Diabetologia 44(12): 2115-33.

Eizirik, D. L., F. Moore, et al. (2008). "Use of a systems biology approach to understand pancreatic beta-cell death in Type 1 diabetes." Biochem Soc Trans 36(Pt 3): 321-7.

Eizirik, D. L., S. Sandler, et al. (1993). "Repair of pancreatic beta-cells. A relevant phenomenon in early IDDM?" Diabetes 42(10): 1383-91.

Eldor, R., A. Yeffet, et al. (2006). "Conditional and specific NF-kappaB blockade protects pancreatic beta cells from diabetogenic agents." Proc Natl Acad Sci U S A 103(13): 5072-7.

Escobar, J., J. W. Frank, et al. (2005). "Physiological rise in plasma leucine stimulates muscle protein synthesis in neonatal pigs by enhancing translation initiation factor activation." Am J Physiol Endocrinol Metab 288(5): E914-21.

Farese, R. V. (2001). "Insulin-sensitive phospholipid signaling systems and glucose transport. Update II." Exp Biol Med (Maywood) 226(4): 283-95.

Fawcett, J., P. A. Permana, et al. (2007). "Regulation of protein degradation by insulin-degrading enzyme: analysis by small interfering RNA-mediated gene silencing." Arch Biochem Biophys 468(1): 128-33.

Felber, J. P. and A. Golay (2002). "Pathways from obesity to diabetes." Int J Obes Relat Metab Disord 26 Suppl 2: S39-45.

Fenton, T. R. and I. T. Gout "Functions and regulation of the 70kDa ribosomal S6 kinases." Int J Biochem Cell Biol 43(1): 47-59.

Ferrannini, E. and S. Camastra (1998). "Relationship between impaired glucose tolerance, non-insulin-dependent diabetes mellitus and obesity." Eur J Clin Invest 28 Suppl 2: 3-6; discussion 6-7.

Filippi, C. and M. von Herrath (2005). "How viral infections affect the autoimmune process leading to type 1 diabetes." Cell Immunol 233(2): 125-32.

Flakoll, P. J., M. Kulaylat, et al. (1989). "Amino acids augment insulin's suppression of whole body proteolysis." Am J Physiol 257(6 Pt 1): E839-47.

Gerich, J. E. (1998). "The genetic basis of type 2 diabetes mellitus: impaired insulin secretion versus impaired insulin sensitivity." Endocr Rev 19(4): 491-503.

Gillespie, K. M. (2006). "Type 1 diabetes: pathogenesis and prevention." CMAJ 175(2): 165-70.

Goldberg, A., M. Parolini, et al. (2007). "Toll-like receptor 4 suppression leads to islet allograft survival." FASEB J 21(11): 2840-8.

Gordon, C. S., A. S. Serino, et al. "Impaired growth and force production in skeletal muscles of young partially pancreatectomized rats: a model of adolescent type 1 diabetic myopathy?" PLoS One 5(11): e14032.

Gwosdow, A. R., M. S. Kumar, et al. (1990). "Interleukin 1 stimulation of the hypothalamic-pituitary-adrenal axis." Am J Physiol 258(1 Pt 1): E65-70.

Gwosdow, A. R., N. A. O'Connell, et al. (1992). "Interleukin-1-induced corticosterone release occurs by an adrenergic mechanism from rat adrenal gland." Am J Physiol 263(3 Pt 1): E461-6.

Hall-Angeras, M., U. Angeras, et al. (1990). "Interaction between corticosterone and tumor necrosis factor stimulated protein breakdown in rat skeletal muscle, similar to sepsis." Surgery 108(2): 460-6.

Hamel, F. G., R. G. Bennett, et al. (1998). "Regulation of multicatalytic enzyme activity by insulin and the insulin-degrading enzyme." Endocrinology 139(10): 4061-6.

Hanifi-Moghaddam, P., S. Kappler, et al. (2006). "Altered chemokine levels in individuals at risk of Type 1 diabetes mellitus." Diabet Med 23(2): 156-63.

Hegarty, B. D., S. M. Furler, et al. (2003). "The role of intramuscular lipid in insulin resistance." Acta Physiol Scand 178(4): 373-83.

Henquin, J. C. (2000). "Triggering and amplifying pathways of regulation of insulin secretion by glucose." Diabetes 49(11): 1751-60.

Herbert, S. L. and K. S. Nair (2010). "Protein and energy metabolism in type 1 diabetes." Clin Nutr 29(1): 13-17.

Horber, F. F. and M. W. Haymond (1990). "Human growth hormone prevents the protein catabolic side effects of prednisone in humans." J Clin Invest 86(1): 265-72.

Hou, J., Z. Z. Chong, et al. "FOXO3a governs early and late apoptotic endothelial programs during elevated glucose through mitochondrial and caspase signaling." Mol Cell Endocrinol 321(2): 194-206.

Hresko, R. C., H. Murata, et al. (2003). "Phosphoinositide-dependent kinase-2 is a distinct protein kinase enriched in a novel cytoskeletal fraction associated with adipocyte plasma membranes." J Biol Chem 278(24): 21615-22.

Hu, J., J. D. Klein, et al. (2008). "Cardiac muscle protein catabolism in diabetes mellitus: activation of the ubiquitin-proteasome system by insulin deficiency." Endocrinology 149(11): 5384-90.

Hu, Z., I. H. Lee, et al. (2007). "PTEN expression contributes to the regulation of muscle protein degradation in diabetes." Diabetes 56(10): 2449-56.

Hu, Z., H. Wang, et al. (2009). "Endogenous glucocorticoids and impaired insulin signaling are both required to stimulate muscle wasting under pathophysiological conditions in mice." J Clin Invest 119(10): 3059-69.

Igoillo-Esteve, M., E. N. Gurzov, et al. "The transcription factor B-cell lymphoma (BCL)-6 modulates pancreatic {beta}-cell inflammatory responses." Endocrinology 152(2): 447-56.

Inchiostro, S., G. Biolo, et al. (1992). "Effects of insulin and amino acid infusion on leucine and phenylalanine kinetics in type 1 diabetes." Am J Physiol 262(2 Pt 1): E203-10.

Issad, T., E. Masson, et al. "O-GlcNAc modification, insulin signaling and diabetic complications." Diabetes Metab 36(6 Pt 1): 423-35.

Itani, S. I., N. B. Ruderman, et al. (2002). "Lipid-induced insulin resistance in human muscle is associated with changes in diacylglycerol, protein kinase C, and IkappaB-alpha." Diabetes 51(7): 2005-11.

Karakelides, H., Y. W. Asmann, et al. (2007). "Effect of insulin deprivation on muscle mitochondrial ATP production and gene transcript levels in type 1 diabetic subjects." Diabetes 56(11): 2683-9.

Keslacy, S., O. Tliba, et al. (2007). "Inhibition of tumor necrosis factor-alpha-inducible inflammatory genes by interferon-gamma is associated with altered nuclear factor-kappaB transactivation and enhanced histone deacetylase activity." Mol Pharmacol 71(2): 609-18.

Kettelhut, I. C., M. T. Pepato, et al. (1994). "Regulation of different proteolytic pathways in skeletal muscle in fasting and diabetes mellitus." Braz J Med Biol Res 27(4): 981-93.

Kim, H. S., M. S. Han, et al. (2007). "Toll-like receptor 2 senses beta-cell death and contributes to the initiation of autoimmune diabetes." Immunity 27(2): 321-33.

Kimball, S. R. and L. S. Jefferson "Control of translation initiation through integration of signals generated by hormones, nutrients, and exercise." J Biol Chem 285(38): 29027-32.

Kordonouri, O. and R. Hartmann (2005). "Higher body weight is associated with earlier onset of Type 1 diabetes in children: confirming the 'Accelerator Hypothesis'." Diabet Med 22(12): 1783-4.

Krook, A., Y. Kawano, et al. (1997). "Improved glucose tolerance restores insulin-stimulated Akt kinase activity and glucose transport in skeletal muscle from diabetic Goto-Kakizaki rats." Diabetes 46(12): 2110-4.

Krssak, M., K. Falk Petersen, et al. (1999). "Intramyocellular lipid concentrations are correlated with insulin sensitivity in humans: a 1H NMR spectroscopy study." Diabetologia 42(1): 113-6.

Lammi, N., E. Moltchanova, et al. (2009). "Childhood BMI trajectories and the risk of developing young adult-onset diabetes." Diabetologia 52(3): 408-14.

Larsen, L., M. Tonnesen, et al. (2007). "Inhibition of histone deacetylases prevents cytokine-induced toxicity in beta cells." Diabetologia 50(4): 779-89.

Libera, L. D. and G. Vescovo (2004). "Muscle wastage in chronic heart failure, between apoptosis, catabolism and altered anabolism: a chimaeric view of inflammation?" Curr Opin Clin Nutr Metab Care 7(4): 435-41.

Ljungkrantz, M., J. Ludvigsson, et al. (2008). "Type 1 diabetes: increased height and weight gains in early childhood." Pediatr Diabetes 9(3 Pt 2): 50-6.

Love, D. C. and J. A. Hanover (2005). "The hexosamine signaling pathway: deciphering the "O-GlcNAc code"." Sci STKE 2005(312): re13.

Luzi, L., P. Castellino, et al. (1990). "Leucine metabolism in IDDM. Role of insulin and substrate availability." Diabetes 39(1): 38-48.

Mandrup-Poulsen, T., L. Pickersgill, et al. "Blockade of interleukin 1 in type 1 diabetes mellitus." Nat Rev Endocrinol 6(3): 158-66.

Martin, A. P., S. Rankin, et al. (2008). "Increased expression of CCL2 in insulin-producing cells of transgenic mice promotes mobilization of myeloid cells from the bone marrow, marked insulitis, and diabetes." Diabetes 57(11): 3025-33.

Mathews, C. E., W. L. Suarez-Pinzon, et al. (2005). "Mechanisms underlying resistance of pancreatic islets from ALR/Lt mice to cytokine-induced destruction." J Immunol 175(2): 1248-56.

Mathis, D., L. Vence, et al. (2001). "beta-Cell death during progression to diabetes." Nature 414(6865): 792-8.

Menconi, M., M. Fareed, et al. (2007). "Role of glucocorticoids in the molecular regulation of muscle wasting." Crit Care Med 35(9 Suppl): S602-8.

Mortimore, G. E., A. R. Poso, et al. (1989). "Mechanism and regulation of protein degradation in liver." Diabetes Metab Rev 5(1): 49-70.

Moyer-Mileur, L. J., H. Slater, et al. (2008). "IGF-1 and IGF-binding proteins and bone mass, geometry, and strength: relation to metabolic control in adolescent girls with type 1 diabetes." J Bone Miner Res 23(12): 1884-91.

Murata, H., R. C. Hresko, et al. (2003). "Reconstitution of phosphoinositide 3-kinase-dependent insulin signaling in a cell-free system." J Biol Chem 278(24): 21607-14.

Nair, K. S. (1987). "Hyperglucagonemia increases resting metabolic rate in man during insulin deficiency." J Clin Endocrinol Metab 64(5): 896-901.

Nair, K. S. (1995). "Muscle protein turnover: methodological issues and the effect of aging." J Gerontol A Biol Sci Med Sci 50 Spec No: 107-12.

Nair, K. S., G. C. Ford, et al. (1995). "Protein dynamics in whole body and in splanchnic and leg tissues in type I diabetic patients." J Clin Invest 95(6): 2926-37.

Nair, K. S., D. Halliday, et al. (1984). "Increased energy expenditure in poorly controlled Type 1 (insulin-dependent) diabetic patients." Diabetologia 27(1): 13-6.

Nair, K. S., D. Halliday, et al. (1987). "Hyperglucagonemia during insulin deficiency accelerates protein catabolism." Am J Physiol 253(2 Pt 1): E208-13.

Nanji, S. A. and A. M. Shapiro (2004). "Islet transplantation in patients with diabetes mellitus: choice of immunosuppression." BioDrugs 18(5): 315-28.

Nicoletti, F., I. Conget, et al. (2002). "Serum concentrations of the interferon-gamma-inducible chemokine IP-10/CXCL10 are augmented in both newly diagnosed Type I diabetes mellitus patients and subjects at risk of developing the disease." Diabetologia 45(8): 1107-10.

Odedra, B. R., P. C. Bates, et al. (1983). "Time course of the effect of catabolic doses of corticosterone on protein turnover in rat skeletal muscle and liver." Biochem J 214(2): 617-27.

Odedra, B. R. and D. J. Millward (1982). "Effect of corticosterone treatment on muscle protein turnover in adrenalectomized rats and diabetic rats maintained on insulin." Biochem J 204(3): 663-72.

Park, K., C. D. Saudek, et al. "Increased expression of beta-N-acetylglucosaminidase in erythrocytes from individuals with pre-diabetes and diabetes." Diabetes 59(7): 1845-50.

Patti, L., A. Maffettone, et al. (1999). "Long-term effects of fish oil on lipoprotein subfractions and low density lipoprotein size in non-insulin-dependent diabetic patients with hypertriglyceridemia." Atherosclerosis 146(2): 361-7.

Pepato, M. T., R. H. Migliorini, et al. (1996). "Role of different proteolytic pathways in degradation of muscle protein from streptozotocin-diabetic rats." Am J Physiol 271(2 Pt 1): E340-7.

Pfleger, C., A. Kaas, et al. (2008). "Relation of circulating concentrations of chemokine receptor CCR5 ligands to C-peptide, proinsulin and HbA1c and disease progression in type 1 diabetes." Clin Immunol 128(1): 57-65.

Piemonti, L., B. E. Leone, et al. (2002). "Human pancreatic islets produce and secrete MCP-1/CCL2: relevance in human islet transplantation." Diabetes 51(1): 55-65.

Price, S. R., J. L. Bailey, et al. (1996). "Muscle wasting in insulinopenic rats results from activation of the ATP-dependent, ubiquitin-proteasome proteolytic pathway by a mechanism including gene transcription." J Clin Invest 98(8): 1703-8.

Price, S. R. and W. E. Mitch (1998). "Mechanisms stimulating protein degradation to cause muscle atrophy." Curr Opin Clin Nutr Metab Care 1(1): 79-83.

Rabinovitch, A. and W. L. Suarez-Pinzon (2003). "Role of cytokines in the pathogenesis of autoimmune diabetes mellitus." Rev Endocr Metab Disord 4(3): 291-9.

Rannels, S. R. and L. S. Jefferson (1980). "Effects of glucocorticoids on muscle protein turnover in perfused rat hemicorpus." Am J Physiol 238(6): E564-72.

Rieu, I., C. Sornet, et al. (2004). "Glucocorticoid excess induces a prolonged leucine resistance on muscle protein synthesis in old rats." Exp Gerontol 39(9): 1315-21.

Sandri, M., C. Sandri, et al. (2004). "Foxo transcription factors induce the atrophy-related ubiquitin ligase atrogin-1 and cause skeletal muscle atrophy." Cell 117(3): 399-412.

Sarvetnick, N. E. and D. Gu (1992). "Regeneration of pancreatic endocrine cells in interferon-gamma transgenic mice." Adv Exp Med Biol 321: 85-9; discussion 91-3.

Shah, O. J., J. A. Iniguez-Lluhi, et al. (2002). "The activated glucocorticoid receptor modulates presumptive autoregulation of ribosomal protein S6 protein kinase, p70 S6K." J Biol Chem 277(4): 2525-33.

Shah, O. J., S. R. Kimball, et al. (2000). "Acute attenuation of translation initiation and protein synthesis by glucocorticoids in skeletal muscle." Am J Physiol Endocrinol Metab 278(1): E76-82.

Shah, O. J., S. R. Kimball, et al. (2000). "Glucocorticoids abate p70(S6k) and eIF4E function in L6 skeletal myoblasts." Am J Physiol Endocrinol Metab 279(1): E74-82.

Shang, Y. C., Z. Z. Chong, et al. "Wnt1, FoxO3a, and NF-kappaB oversee microglial integrity and activation during oxidant stress." Cell Signal 22(9): 1317-29.

Shepherd, P. R., B. T. Nave, et al. (1997). "Differential regulation of phosphoinositide 3-kinase adapter subunit variants by insulin in human skeletal muscle." J Biol Chem 272(30): 19000-7.

Sherry, N. A., J. A. Kushner, et al. (2006). "Effects of autoimmunity and immune therapy on beta-cell turnover in type 1 diabetes." Diabetes 55(12): 3238-45.

Shimada, A., J. Morimoto, et al. (2001). "Elevated serum IP-10 levels observed in type 1 diabetes." Diabetes Care 24(3): 510-5.

Skurk, C., H. Maatz, et al. (2004). "The Akt-regulated forkhead transcription factor FOXO3a controls endothelial cell viability through modulation of the caspase-8 inhibitor FLIP." J Biol Chem 279(2): 1513-25.

Smith, O. L., C. Y. Wong, et al. (1989). "Skeletal muscle proteolysis in rats with acute streptozocin-induced diabetes." Diabetes 38(9): 1117-22.

Strandell, E., D. L. Eizirik, et al. (1990). "Reversal of beta-cell suppression in vitro in pancreatic islets isolated from nonobese diabetic mice during the phase preceding insulin-dependent diabetes mellitus." J Clin Invest 85(6): 1944-50.

Sun, X. J., P. Rothenberg, et al. (1991). "Structure of the insulin receptor substrate IRS-1 defines a unique signal transduction protein." Nature 352(6330): 73-7.

Sun, X. J., L. M. Wang, et al. (1995). "Role of IRS-2 in insulin and cytokine signalling." Nature 377(6545): 173-7.

Swift, S. M., H. A. Clayton, et al. (1998). "The potential contribution of rejection to survival of transplanted human islets." Cell Transplant 7(6): 599-606.

Tessari, P., S. Inchiostro, et al. (1987). "Differential effects of hyperinsulinemia and hyperaminoacidemia on leucine-carbon metabolism in vivo. Evidence for distinct mechanisms in regulation of net amino acid deposition." J Clin Invest 79(4): 1062-9.

Thompson, A. L., M. Y. Lim-Fraser, et al. (2000). "Effects of individual fatty acids on glucose uptake and glycogen synthesis in soleus muscle in vitro." Am J Physiol Endocrinol Metab 279(3): E577-84.

Tisdale, M. J. "Reversing cachexia." Cell 142(4): 511-2.

Tisdale, M. J. (2005). "The ubiquitin-proteasome pathway as a therapeutic target for muscle wasting." J Support Oncol 3(3): 209-17.

Tomas, F. M., A. J. Murray, et al. (1984). "Interactive effects of insulin and corticosterone on myofibrillar protein turnover in rats as determined by N tau-methylhistidine excretion." Biochem J 220(2): 469-79.

Uno, S., A. Imagawa, et al. (2007). "Macrophages and dendritic cells infiltrating islets with or without beta cells produce tumour necrosis factor-alpha in patients with recent-onset type 1 diabetes." Diabetologia 50(3): 596-601.

Vescovo, G., G. B. Ambrosio, et al. (2001). "Apoptosis and changes in contractile protein pattern in the skeletal muscle in heart failure." Acta Physiol Scand 171(3): 305-10.

Vosters, O., C. Beuneu, et al. (2008). "N-acetylcysteine derivative inhibits CD40-dependent proinflammatory properties of human pancreatic duct cells." Pancreas 36(4): 363-8.

Vuorinen-Markkola, H., V. A. Koivisto, et al. (1992). "Mechanisms of hyperglycemia-induced insulin resistance in whole body and skeletal muscle of type I diabetic patients." Diabetes 41(5): 571-80.

Wang, X., S. Jia, et al. (2008). "Identification of a molecular signature in human type 1 diabetes mellitus using serum and functional genomics." J Immunol 180(3): 1929-37.

Wen, L., R. E. Ley, et al. (2008). "Innate immunity and intestinal microbiota in the development of Type 1 diabetes." Nature 455(7216): 1109-13.

Wiegmann, K., S. Schutze, et al. (1992). "Human 55-kDa receptor for tumor necrosis factor coupled to signal transduction cascades." J Biol Chem 267(25): 17997-8001.

Wing, S. S. and N. Bedard (1996). "Insulin-like growth factor I stimulates degradation of an mRNA transcript encoding the 14 kDa ubiquitin-conjugating enzyme." Biochem J 319 (Pt 2): 455-61.

Wright, D. E., J. M. Ryals, et al. (2004). "Diabetes-induced expression of activating transcription factor 3 in mouse primary sensory neurons." J Peripher Nerv Syst 9(4): 242-54.

Yki-Jarvinen, H., T. Kiviluoto, et al. (1986). "Insulin resistance is a prominent feature of patients with pancreatogenic diabetes." Metabolism 35(8): 718-27.

Yoshizawa, F., S. R. Kimball, et al. (1998). "Effect of dietary protein on translation initiation in rat skeletal muscle and liver." Am J Physiol 275(5 Pt 1): E814-20.

Zamir, O., P. O. Hasselgren, et al. (1992). "Tumour necrosis factor (TNF) and interleukin-1 (IL-1) induce muscle proteolysis through different mechanisms." Mediators Inflamm 1(4): 247-50.

Zamir, O., P. O. Hasselgren, et al. (1992). "Evidence that tumor necrosis factor participates in the regulation of muscle proteolysis during sepsis." Arch Surg 127(2): 170-4.

Zamir, O., P. O. Hasselgren, et al. (1993). "In vivo administration of interleukin-1 alpha induces muscle proteolysis in normal and adrenalectomized rats." Metabolism 42(2): 204-8.

Zeidan, Q., Z. Wang, et al. "O-GlcNAc cycling enzymes associate with the translational machinery and modify core ribosomal proteins." Mol Biol Cell 21(12): 1922-36.

Zheng, B., S. Ohkawa, et al. "FOXO3a mediates signaling crosstalk that coordinates ubiquitin and atrogin-1/MAFbx expression during glucocorticoid-induced skeletal muscle atrophy." Faseb J 24(8): 2660-9.

Zierath, J. R. (2002). "Invited review: Exercise training-induced changes in insulin signaling in skeletal muscle." J Appl Physiol 93(2): 773-81.

Zipris, D. (2008). "Innate immunity and its role in type 1 diabetes." Curr Opin Endocrinol Diabetes Obes 15(4): 326-31.

Part 2

Pathogenesis – Virus

10

Echovirus Epidemics, Autoimmunity, and Type 1 Diabetes

Oscar Diaz-Horta[1,3], Luis Sarmiento[2], Andreina Baj[3], Eduardo Cabrera-Rode[1] and Antonio Toniolo[3]
[1]*National Institute of Endocrinology, Havana*
[2]*"Pedro Kouri" Tropical Medicine Institute, Havana*
[3]*University of Insubria, Varese*
[1,2]*Cuba*
[3]*Italy*

1. Introduction

Type 1 diabetes mellitus [T1D] results from the autoimmune destruction of insulin-producing beta cells triggered by environmental factors (Hyoty & Taylor, 2002; Jun & Yoon, 2003). Genetic predisposition accounts for 36-50% of disease susceptibility as demonstrated in monozygotic twin studies (Barnett et al., 1981; Hemminki et al., 2010; Redondo et al., 2001). Differences in the incidence of T1D among countries are thought to be due to the proportions of HLA susceptibility haplotypes; however, other genes seem to be involved in conferring risk. On the other hand, the bulk of new T1D cases lack family history of the disease, altogether indicating that the contribution of exogenous factors to disease pathogenesis is important. Among examined environmental agents, human enteroviruses (HEVs) seem to play a prominent role (Hyoty & Taylor, 2002).

HEVs are common RNA viruses spreading through the fecal-oral route. The genus comprises over 100 different virus types (Simmonds, 2006). The positive sense single-stranded 7.5 kb RNA genome contains a single open reading frame flanked by two untranslated regions (termed 5` and 3` UTRs). A translated single poly-protein is cleaved generating four structural proteins (VP1, VP2, VP3 to VP4) and seven nonstructural proteins (2A, 2B, 2C and 3A, 3B, 3C, 3D). VP1 to VP4 proteins form the viral capsid comprising epitopes involved in virus neutralization; they are responsible for the type-specific protective immunity. Nonstructural proteins determine virus replication and cellular pathology (Agol, 2006).

Although prediction of T1D using genetic, immunologic, and biochemical markers is rather accurate (Hirai et al., 2008; Notkins, 2007), the cost-benefit ratio of periodical determinations appears not to justify large scale screening programs. Unfortunately, primary, secondary and tertiary prevention strategies evaluated so far have failed to prevent or halt the initiation or progression of the disease. For instance, attempts to induce disease regression by utilizing either immunosuppressive and/or cell replacement therapies have been successful only temporarily (Shapiro et al., 2006; Voltarelli et al., 2007).

A vaccine inducing neutralization of putative pathogenic HEVs may represent an ideal primary prevention means for T1D. Unfortunately, available data on sequence of HEV isolated from pancreases of patients who died at T1D onset are not sufficient to define the characteristics of diabetogenic viruses. Nucleic acid technology has shown HEV genomes in sera, plasma or peripheral blood mononuclear cells of patients with T1D at clinical onset (Yeung et al., 2011). However, complete or partial virus genotyping has not been possible so far. Over the years, indirect evidence indicated that HEVs infections are associated with islet autoimmunity and the development of T1D.

Since 1986, public health surveillance strategies have identified 3 meningitis epidemics in Cuba that were caused by echovirus type -4, -16, and -30. Cases of HEV infections were related to the appearance of autoantibodies towards pancreatic islet cells, the immunological hallmark of T1D. Infection-associated autoantibodies showed subtle differences among these epidemics in terms of titer and antigen specificity. In the epidemic of 1998, higher frequencies of neutralizing antibodies against echovirus 4 were found in T1D patients at onset as compared to controls. In the epidemic of 2006, molecular methods allowed detecting HEV RNA more frequently in T1D patients at onset than in non-diabetic controls. Finally, a case of T1D onset in strict association with a HEV infection was also reported.

Molecular homology between beta cell antigens and HEV proteins has been suggested to explain the participation of HEV in T1D pathogenesis. Indeed, we have shown that inoculation of rabbits with selected HEV types caused the appearance of GAD65 antibodies, an early marker of disease progression.

In this chapter, we provide epidemiological and experimental data indicating HEV as possible agents involved in islet cell associated autoimmunity and T1D. The genetic characteristics of the Cuban admixed population influencing T1D genetic susceptibility, the high HEV circulation and low T1D incidence paradox, and how the HEV-disease associations in the Cuban population is inserted into the worldwide landscape will be discussed.

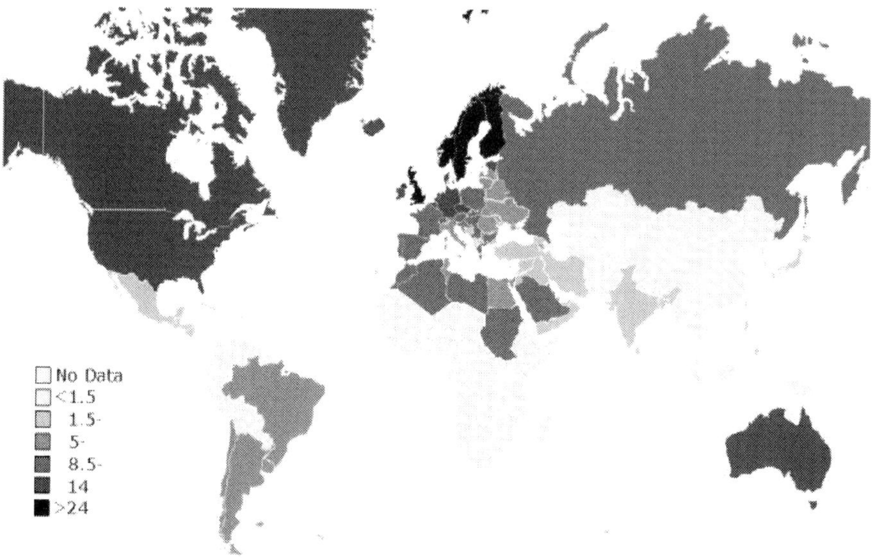

Fig. 1. Worldwide incidence of type 1 diabetes in children under 14 years of age. Incidence is given per 100,000 inhabitants per year (http://www.diabetesatlas.org/map).

2. Population genetic background influences T1D incidence

The incidence of T1D varies widely across nations [Figure 1]. In the year 2009, Nordic countries and UK appeared to show the highest rates [>24/100,000 per year], whereas other European and North-American countries show high to moderate rates [8.5-24/100,000 per year]. Latin-America and Asia exhibit the lowest incidence [usually <8.5/100,000 per year]. Worldwide variations of T1D incidence appear to derive from differences in genetic and/or environmental factors. Within the genetic component, the proportion of susceptibility/protection HLA haplotypes appears to have the highest influence (Concannon et al., 2009). In the late '80s, the presence of a non-aspartic aminoacid in the position 57 of the DQ beta chain (Morel et al., 1988) was proposed to be the most sensitive marker to assess T1D risk. Then, the frequency of this marker appeared to be strongly related with the incidence of T1D across studied populations (Dorman et al., 1990). However, subsequent studies including more populations showed that the accuracy of the marker was not as good as expected (Dorman & Bunker, 2000).

The peak of association between T1D and a gene has been shown to be 85 kb centromeric of HLA-DQB1 (Herr et al., 2000). However, the DR locus seems to confer risk to T1D *per se* (Fernando et al., 2008), not just as a result of linkage disequilibrium with DQ. In fact, effects of individual DR and DQ alleles on disease risk are modified by the haplotypes on which they are carried (She, 1996). Interestingly, a very accurate predictor of T1D susceptibility consists of the present of polar residues at beta 7 and beta 37 in both DR/DQ chains, representing an additional factor for disease progression the absence of aspartic acid at DQ beta 57 (Parry & Brooks, 2008).

Not all populations display the same HLA DR/DQ as T1D susceptibility haplotypes. For instance, considering two-locus haplotypes, DRB1*0301-DQB1*0201 and DRB1*0401-DQB1*0302 are positively associated with T1D in European populations, whereas DRB1*0405-DQB1*0401 and DRB1*0901-DQB1*0303 haplotypes are associated with the disease in most East Asian populations (Ikegami et al., 2008). In populations of European origin, the three-locus haplotypes DRB1*04-DQA1*0301-DQB1*0302 and DRB1*03-DQA1*0501-DQB1*0201 have been shown to play a predominant role in conferring disease susceptibility (Fernando et al., 2008) being heterozygosity for both haplotypes the greatest known genetic risk for T1D. For the Cuban population, these haplotypes are also represented in subjects with T1D and they display odds ratios of 26 and 7.6, respectively (Diaz-Horta et al., 2010). On the other hand, DRB1*1501-DQA1*0102-DQB1*0602 is the haplotype conferring the highest protection for T1D in both European and Cuban populations. This is in agreement with the genetic structure of the Cuban population (Cintado et al., 2009) which is composed mainly by individuals with Spanish descent (65.05%) followed by individuals with a variable degree of Spanish and West African admixed ancestry (23.84%) (http://en.wikipedia.org/wiki/Cubans). In a collaborative study, the frequency of HLA alleles in a sample of the healthy Cuban population was analyzed (Alegre et al., 2007). A neighbor-joining tree using HLA-DRB1 alleles showed that the Cuban population is grouped together with Mediterranean populations and well separated from Amerindian and Oriental populations. Similarly, genetic distances (based on HLA-DRB1-DQB1 allelic frequencies) between Cubans and other populations show that Cubans are close to Mediterranean and European populations. French, Berbers and Spaniards show the closest genetic distances to Cubans, followed by Russians, Algerians and Spanish Basques (Alegre et al., 2007).

It is important to notice that associations between genotype and outcome (e.g. T1D in the present analysis) may be confounded by unrecognized population stratification. In Cuba, population stratification exists because the population has been formed by admixture between subpopulations (mainly Spanish and West Africans) and admixture proportions (defined as the proportions of the genome that have ancestry from each subpopulation) vary between individuals (Hoggart et al., 2003). By utilizing ancestry informative markers, T1D-HLA associations were controlled for factors attributable to admixture or stratification of the population (Diaz-Horta et al., 2010). After controlling for individual admixture, HLA allele- and haplotype-T1D associations mentioned above remained significant indicating their consistence.

Altogether, these studies indicate that the large differences in incidence of T1D between the Cuban and the European population is difficult to explain on the basis of HLA alleles or haplotypes alone.

The HLA region is not the sole genetic factor associated with T1D. Other genes, many of them involved in the regulation of the immune response (e.g., expansion of self-reactive cells, regulation of immune functions, interference with immune regulation) and the beta-cell survival, contribute to disease risk (Liston, 2010). For instance, insulin has been suggested to be the first autoantigen to which the immune tolerance is lost (Nakayama et al., 2005). Coincidentally, the second highest odds ratio for a genetic marker after the HLA region is a variable nucleotide tandem repeat (VNTR) minisatellite located at the 50 end of the insulin gene. More recently, a polymorphism [IFIH1] of a gene encoding for a cytoplasmic helicase that mediates the induction of the interferon response to viral RNA (Nejentsev et al., 2009) has been linked to T1D. This particular association represents genetic evidence suggesting the participation of RNA viruses in the etiology of T1D.

Ethnicity has also been proposed to influence T1D incidence (Karvonen et al., 2000). Perhaps, one of the most illustrative examples of this phenomenon is the large difference of T1D incidence among the 3 principal ethnic groups living in the USA: European descendants, African Americans and American natives (Borchers et al., 2010). Other epidemiological study suggested that differences in T1D incidence among countries of Latin America could be explained by the proportion of the Amerindian population in those countries (Collado-Mesa et al., 2004). Using ancestry informative markers, we have recently shown that ancestral proportions do influence T1D development (Diaz-Horta et al., 2010). Studies of this type allow evaluating the influence of genetic background in disease incidence considering a homogeneous distribution of environmental factors across a given admixed population. In Cuba, individuals carrying high European ancestry proportions in their genome seem to be more prone to develop the disease than those with high African ancestry (figure 2). The size of this effect was estimated as 5.7 odds ratio (95% CI 1.2–36). This value embodies the odds ratio for T1D associated with a unit change in European admixture proportion (from 0 to 1).

Overall, these data indicate that genetic background does influence T1D risk/protection. However, the involved genetic determinants are not restricted to HLA alleles or haplotypes alone.

More recently, using a novel genomic analysis, it has been discovered that the genetic evidence linking virus infections and T1D is not limited to the IFIH1 polymorphism (Heinig et al., 2010). Indeed, it seems that an entire network of interferon response genes driven by the transcription factor IRF7 is associated with T1D. Taking in consideration that HEV infections are relatively frequent and that the latter genetic finding associates a robust antiviral response with T1D susceptibility, it is likely that the host response to certain virus infections is more pathogenic than the virus itself (Foxman & Iwasaki, 2011).

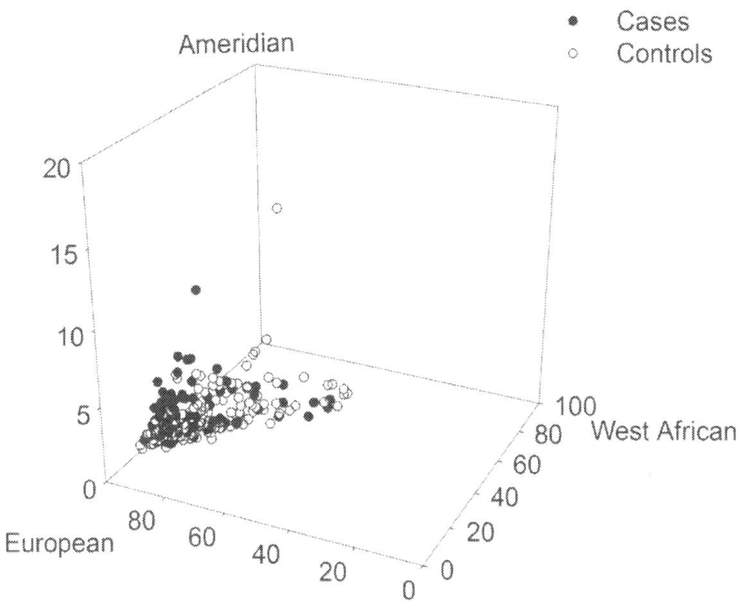

Fig. 2. Distribution of individual admixture estimates in 100 T1D cases and 129 matched non-diabetic subjects in a sample of the Cuban population (Diaz-Horta et al., 2010). Each of the three founder populations constitutes the axes of the graph. Each symbol represents a single subject and its position is determined by the ancestry proportions.

3. Environmental factors and T1D incidence

The finest epidemiological evidence indicating the large contribution of environmental factors in the pathogenesis of T1D is the pairwise T1D discordance of >60% among monozygotic twins (Knip et al., 2005; Redondo et al., 1999). Other studies of populations migrating to nations with dissimilar T1D incidences than that of their origins (Akerblom & Knip, 1998) are adequate examples, since they minimize the variability of genetic background. In addition, the constant and rapid increase of T1D incidence rates worldwide cannot be explained by changes in the genetic background of any particular populations.

A host of variants have been associated with T1D incidence and termed "environmental factors". Among them: geographic latitude, sun exposure, mean temperature, breast feeding rates, cow's milk consumption, national prosperity (infant mortality rate, life expectancy at birth, and national human development index), urban-rural status (Borchers et al., 2010). These and other associations, sometimes discrepant (Borchers et al., 2010), are obviously the reflection of underlying molecular events. Most of these events are unknown but some has been extensively discussed in previous reviews (Cooke, 2009; Feillet & Bach, 2004; von Herrath, 2009). A variety of associations with viruses have been reported for human T1D, including rubella, mumps, and cytomegalovirus infections. However, among investigated agents, HEVs appear to play a prominent role (Hyoty & Taylor, 2002).

The role of the adaptive immune system in triggering or protecting against virus-induced autoimmunity was addressed in a pioneer study of Notkins and Yoon (Notkins & Yoon, 1982). Two strains of encephalomyocarditis (EMC) virus were used to inoculate genetically susceptible mice: a diabetogenic (D) variant of the EMC virus and a non-diabetogenic (B) variant. Both derived from plaque purification of an M variant of the virus capable to induce a diabetes-like syndrome in susceptible mice. Note that EMC virus belongs to the picornavirus family and is classified as an animal cardiovirus. Interestingly, the two variants were antigenically indistinguishable but genome sequence analysis revealed 14 nucleotide differences between them (Bae et al., 1989). In a subsequent study, the analysis of several mutant viruses generated from the EMC-B and EMC-D variants, revealed that just one amino acid at position 776 (alanine) was responsible of the diabetogenic effects (Bae & Yoon, 1993). Finally, it was shown that protection for T1D was achieved in an antigen-dependent fashion by injection of the non-diabetogenic EMC-B variant prior to the inoculation of EMC-D diabetogenic variant.

Although certain pathogens (e.g. putative diabetogenic HEVs) may initiate or accelerate autoimmunity and T1D, it is also likely that exposure to common or non diabetogenic pathogens may protect against this process. For example, over the last fifty years (1950 to 2000), the decreasing incidence of prototypical infectious diseases such as hepatitis A, measles, mumps, rheumatic fever, tuberculosis has been linked to the increasing incidence of immune-mediated disorders (e.g., asthma, multiple sclerosis, Crohn's disease) (Bach, 2002). In addition, recognized HEV infections appear to be an infrequent event in countries exhibiting an elevated incidence of T1D (Viskari et al., 2005). In a study, authors measured the frequency of neutralizing antibodies (NtAb) against selected HEV types in pregnant women (mean age 25-30 years) from populations of high and low-intermediate incidence of T1D. The frequency of NtAb (titer ≥ 4) in the high T1D incidence country (Finland) was 40.5 - 65.0 % (minimum - maximun) for single NtAbs against different HEVs and 38.5 % for multiple NtAbs. In contrast, in the adjacent regions Estonia and Karelia which are characterized by low T1D incidence, the values were 71.9 – 90.6 % and 84.2 %, respectively. Interestingly, the frequencies of NtAbs (especially those against CA9, CB4 and CB5) in pregnant women from Estonia and Karelia (85.7, 71.9 and 90.6 %, respectively) are similar to

Groups	N	Age	Sex	Coxsackievirus (%)							Echovirus (%)			
		Mean	%(M)	CA9	CB1	CB2	CB3	CB4	CB5	CB6	**E4**	E6	E9	E11
Matched Controls	57	8.3	56.1	78.9	57.9	64.9	77.2	82.5	21.1	1.8	**1.8**	57.9	54.4	54.4
T1D onset	33	10.7	45.5	93.9	57.6	72.2	60.6	93.9	33.3	6.1	**21.2** *	66.7	72.7	57.6

Table 1. Frequency of HEV neutralizing antibodies in Cuban subjects at the clinical onset of T1D and nondiabetic subjects matched for age, sex, date of collection and location (Diaz-Horta et al., 2001). * $p<0.05$, Fisher's exact test.

those found in 7-11 year-old nondiabetic children from Cuba (78.9, 82.5 and 21.1 %, respectively) (Diaz-Horta et al., 2001). These data indicate that the circulation of enteroviruses is very high in both regions. It is also well known that the frequency of NtAbs against HEVs largely depends on the age of subjects, being much higher at older ages. This supports the hypothesis that the more a population is exposed to common HEV types the higher is its protection against subsequent exposure to diabetogenic HEVs.

In animal models of spontaneous T1D (i.e., the NOD mouse and the BB rat) it has been demonstrated that the incidence of the disease is much higher in those animals bred in specific pathogen-free environments than in conventional conditions (Bach, 2002). By just decontaminating the food in the latter conditions an increase in incidence was observed. More interesting, prevention of T1D in NOD mice has been achieved by treatment with a variety of immune enhancers, including complete Freund's adjuvant (McInerney et al., 1991), immunogenic but not tolerated peptides (Vaysburd et al., 1995), Mycobacterium avium (Martins & Aguas, 1996), Lactobacillus casei (Matsuzaki et al., 1997), Mycobacterium leprae (Nomaguchi et al., 2002), lymphocytic choriomeningitis virus (LCMV) (Christen et al., 2004). T1D prevention has also been achieved by exposure to helminthes or products from these organisms, however, it is important to recognize that not all infecting agents, parasites or their products are able to induce this effect (Cooke, 2009). Another important observation is the fact that the timing of exposure to these "protective" agents largely influences the outcome (Cooke, 2009). For example, if the exposure is performed before the appearance of the mononuclear infiltrate in the pancreas of NOD mice (generally around week 5) then protection is generally achieved. After that time, exposure to the protective agent is useless and fails to prevent T1D.

Thus, protection through infection or by stimulation of the immune system has allowed applying the term "hygiene hypothesis" to experiments in animals. The term was originally coined on the basis of epidemiologic studies of poliomyelitis. Several mechanisms have been proposed to explain this phenomenon. For example, a study conducted by von Herrath (von Herrath, 2009) clearly demonstrated that regulatory T-cells (CD4+ CD25+ Tregs) can invigorate by infection in a toll like receptor (TLR)-2 dependent fashion. These cells, instead of exerting effector functions such as killing infected cells or inducing interferon production, can turn off immune responses. The increment in TGF-β concentrations induced by the viral infection is associated with Treg invigoration (Aumeunier et al., 2010; von Herrath, 2009). Other cytokines induced simultaneously are the programmed cell death ligand 1 (PD-1L) and the tumor necrosis factor (TNF)-α which in turn may mediate the bystander death of auto-aggressive T-cells. The protective effect of viral infections and other immune modulators has also been associated with the induction of interferon gamma-induced protein 10 kDa (IP-10) and other pro-inflammatory cytokines (Christen et al., 2004).

Taken together, these data suggest that not only the adaptive immune response provides protection against exposure to diabetogenic viruses, but also the innate immune system. Multiple non-specific stimuli acting on the immune system during early childhood and before puberty are hoped to provide an effective strategy to reduce the increasing incidence of T1D (Petrovsky, 2010).

4. Classification of enteroviruses and properties of the echovirus group

HEVs are extremely common RNA viruses that spread mainly through the fecal-oral route. They are etiological agents of different clinical entities varying from asymptomatic to mild, severe, or fatal diseases. Overall, these agents cause millions new infections per year in the US (Khetsuriani et al., 2006). The enterovirus genus comprises over 100 antigenically different virus types (Simmonds, 2006). The single-stranded 7.5 kb RNA genome (figure 3) is positive sense and contains a single open reading frame flanked by two untranslated regions (5` and 3` UTRs). The coding region is translated into a single polyprotein (of approximately 2,200 amino acids) which is cleaved to generate four structural proteins (VP1 to VP4) and seven nonstructural proteins (2A to 2C and 3A to 3D). VP1-VP4 proteins are assembled to form the viral capsid whose external surface comprises the epitopes involved in virus neutralization that are responsible for the type-specific protective immunity. Nonstructural proteins have enzymatic functions and play essential roles in virus replication and cellular pathology. An important property of HEVs (common to all RNA viruses) is their high mutation and recombination rates. RNA replication is extremely error-prone, due to the lack of proofreading activity of the viral RNA-dependent RNA polymerase, taking the error rate to approximately one per genome replication (Savolainen-Kopra & Blomqvist, 2010).

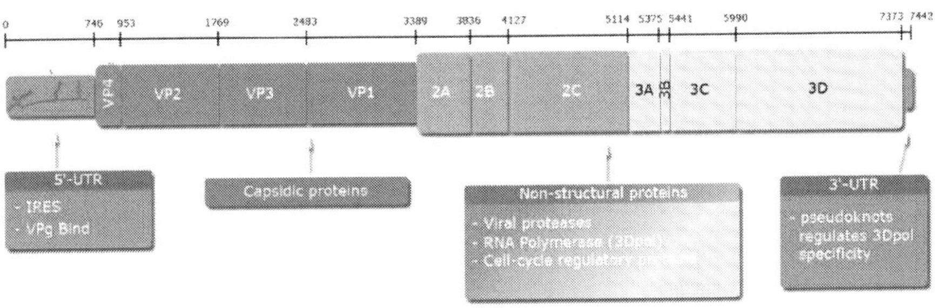

Fig. 3. HEV genome organization.

HEVs were originally classified on the basis of shared pathogenic properties in experimental animals. For example, polioviruses were described to cause a poliomyelitis resembling disease in primates; coxsackieviruses A and B, produced flaccid and spastic paralysis in newborn mice, respectively; echoviruses were not associated to any known clinical symptom or disease. Echoviruses received their name from the initials of "Enteric isolates", "Cytopathogenic in tissue culture", isolated from "Humans" and, "Orphans" because they were not apparently associated to any disease (Fields et al., 2007). Currently, many HEV types have been fully sequenced allowing their genetic classification. For example, considering the amino acid similarity of the capsid protein region P1 (comprising VP4, VP2, VP3 and VP1 proteins) HEVs are now grouped into species A, B, C and D (table 2).

As observed in table 2, there is some conflict between the classical subgroup division and the genetic classification of HEVs. For instance, although coxsakieviruses B, echoviruses (now within the species B) and polioviruses (species C) are rather genetically homogeneous, coxsackieviruses A distribute in species A, B and C. On the other hand, echoviruses took their name because they were not originally associated to any disease. Now, however, it is known that they are one of the main causes of aseptic meningitis as well as other diseases, and that these agents are widespread in the environment (Djikeng et al., 2009). Interestingly, the genetic subgrouping of enteroviruses is quite consistent regardless the zone of the genome being used for the analysis (Hyypia et al., 1997).

Species	Number of known serotypes	Serotypes
A	17	coxsackievirus A2 (CV-A2), CV-A3, CV-A4, CV-A5, CV-A6, CV-A7, CV-A8, CV-A10, CV-A12, CV-A14, CV-A16, enterovirus A71 (EV-A71), EV-A76, EV-A89, EV-A90, EV-A91, EV-114
B	58	coxsackievirus B1 (CV-B1), CV-B2, CV-B3, CV-B4, CV-B5, CV-B6, CV-A9, echovirus 1 (E-1), E-2, E-3, E-4, E-5, E-6, E-7, E-9, E-11, E-12, E-13, E-14, E-15, E-16, E-17, E-18, E-19, E-20, E-21, E-24, E-25, E-26, E-27, E-29, E-30, E-31, E-32, E-33, enterovirus B69 (EV-B69), EV-B73, EV-B74, EV-B75, EV-B77, EV-B78, EV-B79, EV-B80, EV-B81, EV-B82, EV-B83, EV-B84, EV-B85, EV-B86, EV-B87, EV-B88, EV-B93, EV-B97, EV-B98, EV-B100, EV-B101, EV-B106, EV-B107
C	20	poliovirus (PV) 1, PV-2, PV-3, coxsackievirus A1 (CV-A1), CV-A11, CV-A13, CV-A17, CV-A19, CV-A20, CV-A21, CV-A22, CV-A24, enterovirus C95 (EV-C95), EV-C96, EV-C99, EV-C102, EV-C104, EV-C105, EV-C109 and EV-C113.
D	4	EV-D68, EV-D70, EV-D94 and EV-D111

Table 2. Classification of human enteroviruses (Adapted from the Picornaviridae database http://www.picornaviridae.com/; Mars 2011).

	YEAR OF THE EPIDEMIC		
	1986	2000	2001
	(Uriarte et al., 1987)	(Cabrera-Rode et al., 2003; Sarmiento et al., 2001)	(Cabrera-Rode et al., 2005)
Echovirus serotype	4	16	30
Number of separate isolates obtained	14	47	43
Number of reported aseptic meningitis cases	~300,000	16,943	14,477
No. ICA-positive/No. echovirus-infected children	17/48	35/38	7/8
No. GADA-positive/No. echovirus-infected children	ND	11/38	0/8
No. IA2A-positive/No. echovirus-infected children	ND	0/38	0/8
No. IA-positive/No. echovirus-infected children	ND	17/38	0/8

Table 3. Summary of epidemiology and islet associated autoantibodies in echovirus epidemics in Cuba. ND= not done

5. Cuban epidemics of aseptic meningitis due to echoviruses

Since 1986, virus surveillance in Cuba has identified 3 different echoviruses (HEVs B) as the causing agents of 3 epidemics of aseptic meningitis (table 3). The predominant clinical manifestations in all three epidemics were vomiting, headache, and fever. No deaths related to aseptic meningitis were reported and all patients recovered completely. Cerebrospinal fluid (CSF), sera (during acute and convalescent stages of the disease) and feces were utilized for enterovirus detection using a specific RT-PCR technique. For enterovirus identification a neutralization test using the Lim–Benyesh–Melnick (LBM) antisera pools was used. Viral isolation was achieved by inoculating specimens on monolayers of human embryo fibroblasts (PhuE-1) and monkey kidney cells (Vero). Sera from infected children were matched with at least two control sera from healthy children for age, sex, date of collection, and location. All control subjects had no family history of diabetes, were screened for diabetes-associated antibodies (ICA, GADA, IAA, IA2A) and for neutralizing antibodies against different enterovirus serotypes.

The presence of islet cell antibodies (ICA) is considered the immunological hallmark of T1D. One of the most notable observations from these HEV epidemics is that in the convalescent but not in the acute stage of the infection, ICA seroconversion was demonstrated. On the other hand, in the epidemic caused by echovirus 16 we also detected the emergence of IAA, GADA and IA2A (Cabrera-Rode et al., 2003). The islet cell autoimmunity was clearly infection-associated, since no serum samples from uninfected subjects serologically negative for neutralizing antibodies to E16 and E30 had ICA. The seroconversion of T1D islet associated antibodies in subjects does not seem to be a general unspecific antibody response, since all infected subjects were negative for thyroid microsomal or parietal gastric cell autoantibodies. As for the echovirus 30 meningitis, we detected ICA seroconversion in a high percentage of patients but not GADA, IAA or IA2A seroconversion. From this and other studies (table 4), it can be observed that different echovirus types are associated with a variety pancreatic autoantibodies.

ICA	GADA	IA2A	IAA	Serotype	Reference
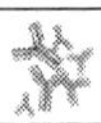	-	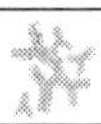	-	Echovirus 3	(Williams et al., 2006)
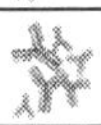	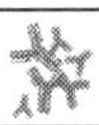	-	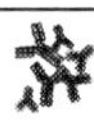	Echovirus 6	(Otonkoski et al., 2000)
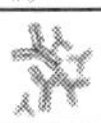	-	-	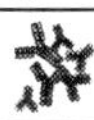	Echovirus 9	(Vreugdenhil et al., 2000)
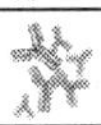	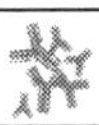	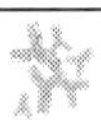	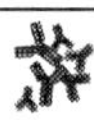	Echovirus 16	(Cabrera-Rode et al., 2003)
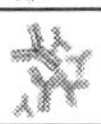	-	-	-	Echovirus 30	(Cabrera-Rode et al., 2005)
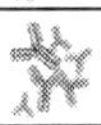	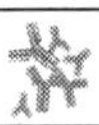	-	-	Non polio HEV	(Lonnrot et al., 2000b)
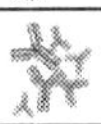	-	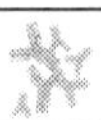	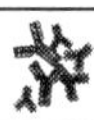	Non polio HEV	(Hyoty & Taylor, 2002)

Table 4. Patterns of T1D-associated autoantibodies in the course of echovirus infections.

During the echovirus 30 epidemic we reported an adolescent who developed pancreatic autoantibodies and T1D after infection (Cabrera-Rode et al., 2005). ICA and IA2A were detected post-infection and; the analysis of neutralizing antibodies to enterovirus serotypes most frequently isolated during the last 30 years in Cuba showed high titers of neutralizing antibodies only for E30 (titer 1:80) suggesting that this virus was the agent causing the aseptic meningitis. Interestingly, the patient carried the HLA DR15/DR7 and DQ2/DQ6 determinants that confer T1D protection.

It is important to notice that in mice inoculated with the echovirus 4 strain circulating during the late '80s in Cuba there was a reduction of the insulin concentration and overall protein synthesis in pancreatic islets (Szopa et al., 1992). Remarkably, Roivainen et al (Roivainen et al., 2002) showed that the capacity of an enterovirus to kill human beta cells or impair their function is not entirely defined by the serotype. For example, the prototype echovirus 30 strain (Bastianni) appear not to produce damage to beta cells while other isolates of echovirus 30 do. Similar results were obtained with echovirus 9 (Roivainen et al., 2002). Another interesting observation from echovirus epidemics in Cuba is that the titer of islet-associated autoantibodies correlates with the titer of neutralizing antibodies against echoviruses. This suggests that the extent of infection and the antiviral immune response could influence the intensity of the humoral response against host antigens (Figure 4).

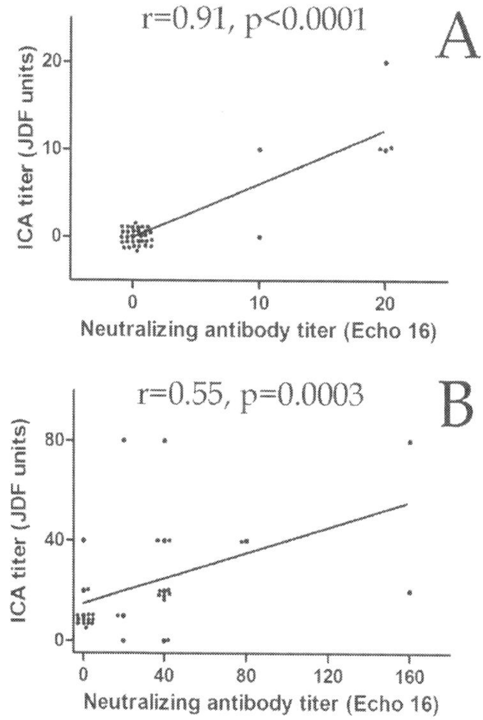

Fig. 4. Correlation between echovirus 16 neutralizing antibodies and ICA titers in sera of patients with aseptic meningitis in the acute (A) and convalescent (B) phase.

We also evaluated the induction of T1D associated antibodies by HEVs in experimental animals. In particular, rabbits were used since HEVs do not replicate in their cells (Fields et al., 2007). This minimizes the possibility of generating of humoral responses as consequence of beta-cell damage and subsequent autoantigen release. Strikingly, seroconversion to GAD65 antibodies was restricted to HEVs of the B species. Antibodies recognizing GAD65 were absent after inoculation with HEVs of the A and the C species (Sarmiento et al., 2007b). Antibodies against IA2 or insulin were undetected. Although indirect, this evidence suggests that different HEVs of the species B could share epitopes with GAD65. Thus, molecular mimicry might explain the induction of T1D/associated autoantibodies during HEV epidemics.
Taken together, these results show the association between echovirus epidemics and the induction of T1D associated autoantibodies. Other studies have shown similar results (Frisk & Tuvemo, 2004; Hiltunen et al., 1997; Lonnrot et al., 2000a; Moya-Suri et al., 2005; Oikarinen et al., 2011; Sadeharju et al., 2001; Salminen et al., 2003; Williams et al., 2006). Diabetogeneicity seems to be associated to HEVs of the B species although it is not restricted to one particular serotype or strain.

6. Detection of HEVs at T1D onset and in prediabetic stages

In 1999, neutralizing antibodies (NtAb) against different HEV types were measured in subjects with T1D at diagnosis and in controls matched for location, time of sampling, and age (Diaz-Horta et al., 2001). Both, patients and control subjects showed a high frequency of antibodies against a variety of HEV types (Table 1). Strikingly, the sole HEV serotype with NtAbs at higher frequency in cases vs. controls was echovirus 4, i.e., the same serotype that caused the huge epidemic of aseptic meningitis during the year 1987. More recently, HEV RNA was searched for in blood of T1D children at the time of diagnosis, in their first degree relatives with or without ICA and in matched non diabetic controls (Sarmiento et al., 2007a). As shown in table 5, subjects at diagnosis and subjects with ICA showed higher frequencies of HEV RNA than their matched controls. These and other results (Andreoletti et al., 1997; Clements et al., 1995; Craig et al., 2003; Moya-Suri et al., 2005; Nairn et al., 1999; Yin et al., 2002) strongly suggest the link between HEV detection and the early stages of T1D.

GROUP	N	HEV RNA+ (%)	P VALUE
T1D at clinical onset Matched controls	34 68	**9 (26,5)** 2 (2,9)	**0,0007**
First degree relatives of T1D patients (ICA+) Matched controls	32 64	**5 (15,6)** 0 (0,0)	**0,0033**
First degree relatives of T1D patients (ICA-) Matched controls	62 62	1 (1,6) 1 (1,6)	**NS**
First degree relatives of T1D patients (ICA+) First degree relatives of T1D patients (ICA-)	32 62	**5 (15,6)** 1 (1,6)	**0,0164**

Table 5. Frequency of enterovirus RNA in blood of subjects with T1D at clinical onset, their first degree relatives and controls matched for age, sex, date of collection and location (Sarmiento et al., 2007a). 1. p values were generated by the Fisher's exact test. NS = not significant.

The frequency of HEV genome positivity appeared to vary according to the specimen (Schulte et al., 2010a). In newly diagnosed T1D patients, the highest frequency of HEV RNA is detected in peripheral blood mononuclear cells (PBMC) followed by plasma or serum. Cerebrospinal fluid (CSF) and stool samples are the specimens with the lowest percent of HEV genome detection. Since HEVs primarily replicated in the gut, a recent study addressed the question of whether these agents could be detected in the small intestine of patients at clinical onset of T1D (Oikarinen et al., 2008). By *in situ* hybridization or immunohistochemistry, up to 50% of T1D patients were positive for HEVs. This finding is apparently in contrast with studies on feces (Schulte et al., 2010a)(and unpublished results). It is however known that enterovirus isolation from feces is difficult when virus titer is low. This finding suggests that an asymptomatic/low level infection takes place in children during the initial stages of the disease. In this regard, it should be pointed out that the amount of HEV genomes in serum/plasma and blood cells is extremely low and can only be evidence with highly sensitive methods (Sarmiento et al., 2007a; Schulte et al., 2010a). These findings indicate that small amounts of HEVs may derive from infected cells, e.g., cells of the islets of Langerhans islets or cell-debris (Schulte et al., 2010a; Schulte et al., 2010b). Though not yet demonstrated, virus low level persistence and/or low virus clearance are involved in T1D pathogenesis. In a recent study (Feuer et al., 2009), intracranial inoculation of BALB/c pups with Coxsackie B3 resulted in detection of the infecting virus at least for 10 days. At day 30, infectious virus was no longer present though viral RNA could be demonstrated by sensitive RT-PCR methods. Similar results have been reported for other target tissues, such as the myocardium (Kim et al., 2001; Klingel et al., 1992; Reetoo et al., 2000).

A recent meta-analysis by Craig and colleagues (Yeung et al., 2011) strongly indicates that HEVs (in terms of RNA detection) are unequivocally associated with T1D at the time of clinical presentation or at preclinical stages. Other data corroborate this association. Among them, the high frequency of IgM/IgG antibodies against HEVs (Banatvala et al., 1985; Elfaitouri et al., 2007; Helfand et al., 1995; King et al., 1983), the presence of interferon-α or dsRNA-dependent protein kinase R (indirect markers of virus infection) in serum and pancreas (Chehadeh et al., 2000; Foulis et al., 1987; Huang et al., 1995; Richardson et al., 2009), the demonstration of HEV capsid proteins in pancreatic islets (Dotta et al., 2007; Richardson et al., 2009; Tanaka et al., 2009).

7. Conclusion

The genetic background of a population influences the incidence of T1D. Although the HLA region confers the highest odds ratio, several other genes contribute to T1D susceptibility as suggested in our admixture study. The link between the IFIH1 polymorphism, and more recently the discovery of an entire network of interferon response genes driven by IRF7, corroborate the hypothesis that viruses have a role in T1D pathogenesis. These studies also evidence that HEV circulation is inversely proportional to T1D incidence. Upon exposure to a diabetogenic HEV, both the innate and adaptive immune response seem to have an influence on whether or not an individual will progress towards organ-specific autoimmunity and destruction of beta cells.

As indicated by studies of meningitis epidemics in Cuba, echoviruses - once thought to be harmless - appear to comprise a variety of pathogens causing slow and progressive disease. Current data indicate that different HEV types may be associated with the initial stages of

T1D. Technical improvements are however needed to unequivocally prove this hypothesis and to pave the way to viral vaccines as a preventing measure against T1D.

8. Acknowledgment

ODH has been supported by a research fellowship of the University of Insubria, Varese (Italy). The support of CARIPLO Foundation (Milan, IT) and Gianni Valcavi, Attorney at law (Varese, IT) is gratefully acknowledged. We also thank the VIDIS Group (London, UK) and the Enterovirus Foundation (San Francisco, CA) for inspiration and assistance.

9. References

Agol, V. I. (2006). Molecular mechanisms of poliovirus variation and evolution. *Curr Top Microbiol Immunol* 299, 211-59

Akerblom, H. K., and Knip, M. (1998). Putative environmental factors in Type 1 diabetes. *Diabetes Metab Rev* 14(1), 31-67

Alegre, R., Moscoso, J., Martinez-Laso, J., Martin-Villa, M., Suarez, J., Moreno, A., Serrano-Vela, J. I., Vargas-Alarcon, G., Pacheco, R., and Arnaiz-Villena, A. (2007). HLA genes in Cubans and the detection of Amerindian alleles. *Mol Immunol* 44(9), 2426-35

Andreoletti, L., Hober, D., Hober-Vandenberghe, C., Belaich, S., Vantyghem, M. C., Lefebvre, J., and Wattre, P. (1997). Detection of coxsackie B virus RNA sequences in whole blood samples from adult patients at the onset of type I diabetes mellitus. *J Med Virol* 52(2), 121-7

Aumeunier, A., Grela, F., Ramadan, A., Pham Van, L., Bardel, E., Gomez Alcala, A., Jeannin, P., Akira, S., Bach, J. F., and Thieblemont, N. (2010). Systemic Toll-like receptor stimulation suppresses experimental allergic asthma and autoimmune diabetes in NOD mice. *PLoS One* 5(7), e11484

Bach, J. F. (2002). The effect of infections on susceptibility to autoimmune and allergic diseases. *N Engl J Med* 347(12), 911-920

Bae, Y. S., Eun, H. M., and Yoon, J. W. (1989). Genomic differences between the diabetogenic and nondiabetogenic variants of encephalomyocarditis virus. *Virology* 170(1), 282-7

Bae, Y. S., and Yoon, J. W. (1993). Determination of diabetogenicity attributable to a single amino acid, Ala776, on the polyprotein of encephalomyocarditis virus. *Diabetes* 42(3), 435-43

Banatvala, J. E., Bryant, J., Schernthaner, G., Borkenstein, M., Schober, E., Brown, D., De Silva, L. M., Menser, M. A., and Silink, M. (1985). Coxsackie B, mumps, rubella, and cytomegalovirus specific IgM responses in patients with juvenile-onset insulin-dependent diabetes mellitus in Britain, Austria, and Australia. *Lancet* 1(8443), 1409-12

Barnett, A. H., Eff, C., Leslie, R. D., and Pyke, D. A. (1981). Diabetes in identical twins. A study of 200 pairs. *Diabetologia* 20(2), 87-93

Borchers, A. T., Uibo, R., and Gershwin, M. E. (2010). The geoepidemiology of type 1 diabetes. *Autoimmun Rev* 9(5), A355-65

Cabrera-Rode, E., Sarmiento, L., Molina, G., Perez, C., Arranz, C., Galvan, J. A., Prieto, M., Barrios, J., Palomera, R., Fonseca, M., Mas, P., Diaz-Diaz, O., and Diaz-Horta, O. (2005). Islet cell related antibodies and type 1 diabetes associated with echovirus 30 epidemic: a case report. *J Med Virol* 76(3), 373-7

Cabrera-Rode, E., Sarmiento, L., Tiberti, C., Molina, G., Barrios, J., Hernandez, D., Diaz-Horta, O., and Di Mario, U. (2003). Type 1 diabetes islet associated antibodies in subjects infected by echovirus 16. *Diabetologia* 46(10), 1348-53

Chehadeh, W., Weill, J., Vantyghem, M. C., Alm, G., Lefebvre, J., Wattre, P., and Hober, D. (2000). Increased level of interferon-alpha in blood of patients with insulin-dependent diabetes mellitus: relationship with coxsackievirus B infection. *J Infect Dis* 181(6), 1929-39

Christen, U., Benke, D., Wolfe, T., Rodrigo, E., Rhode, A., Hughes, A. C., Oldstone, M. B., and von Herrath, M. G. (2004). Cure of prediabetic mice by viral infections involves lymphocyte recruitment along an IP-10 gradient. *J Clin Invest* 113(1), 74-84

Cintado, A., Companioni, O., Nazabal, M., Camacho, H., Ferrer, A., De Cossio, M. E., Marrero, A., Ale, M., Villarreal, A., Leal, L., Casalvilla, R., Benitez, J., Novoa, L., Diaz-Horta, O., and Duenas, M. (2009). Admixture estimates for the population of Havana City. *Ann Hum Biol* 36(3), 350-60

Clements, G. B., Galbraith, D. N., and Taylor, K. W. (1995). Coxsackie B virus infection and onset of childhood diabetes. *Lancet* 346(8969), 221-3

Collado-Mesa, F., Barcelo, A., Arheart, K. L., and Messiah, S. E. (2004). An ecological analysis of childhood-onset type 1 diabetes incidence and prevalence in Latin America. *Rev Panam Salud Publica* 15(6), 388-94

Concannon, P., Rich, S. S., and Nepom, G. T. (2009). Genetics of type 1A diabetes. *N Engl J Med* 360(16), 1646-54

Cooke, A. (2009). Review series on helminths, immune modulation and the hygiene hypothesis: how might infection modulate the onset of type 1 diabetes? *Immunology* 126(1), 12-7

Craig, M. E., Howard, N. J., Silink, M., and Rawlinson, W. D. (2003). Reduced frequency of HLA DRB1*03-DQB1*02 in children with type 1 diabetes associated with enterovirus RNA. *J Infect Dis* 187(10), 1562-70

Diaz-Horta, O., Bello, M., Cabrera-Rode, E., Suarez, J., Mas, P., Garcia, I., Abalos, I., Jofra, R., Molina, G., Diaz-Diaz, O., and Dimario, U. (2001). Echovirus 4 and type 1 diabetes mellitus. *Autoimmunity* 34(4), 275-81

Diaz-Horta, O., Cintado, A., Fernandez-De-Cossio, M. E., Nazabal, M., Ferrer, A., Roca, J., Camacho, H., Benitez, J., Ale, M., Villarreal, A., Molina, G., Vera, M., Cabrera-Rode, E., and Novoa, L. (2010). Relationship of type 1 diabetes to ancestral proportions and HLA DR/DQ alleles in a sample of the admixed Cuban population. *Ann Hum Biol*

Djikeng, A., Kuzmickas, R., Anderson, N. G., and Spiro, D. J. (2009). Metagenomic analysis of RNA viruses in a fresh water lake. *PLoS One* 4(9), e7264

Dorman, J. S., and Bunker, C. H. (2000). HLA-DQ locus of the human leukocyte antigen complex and type 1 diabetes mellitus: a HuGE review. *Epidemiol Rev* 22(2), 218-27

Dorman, J. S., LaPorte, R. E., Stone, R. A., and Trucco, M. (1990). Worldwide differences in the incidence of type I diabetes are associated with amino acid variation at position 57 of the HLA-DQ beta chain. *Proc Natl Acad Sci U S A* 87(19), 7370-4

Dotta, F., Censini, S., van Halteren, A. G., Marselli, L., Masini, M., Dionisi, S., Mosca, F., Boggi, U., Muda, A. O., Prato, S. D., Elliott, J. F., Covacci, A., Rappuoli, R., Roep, B. O., and Marchetti, P. (2007). Coxsackie B4 virus infection of beta cells and natural killer cell insulitis in recent-onset type 1 diabetic patients. *Proc Natl Acad Sci U S A* 104(12), 5115-20

Elfaitouri, A., Berg, A. K., Frisk, G., Yin, H., Tuvemo, T., and Blomberg, J. (2007). Recent enterovirus infection in type 1 diabetes: evidence with a novel IgM method. *J Med Virol* 79(12), 1861-7

Feillet, H., and Bach, J. F. (2004). On the mechanisms of the protective effect of infections on type 1 diabetes. *Clin Dev Immunol* 11(3-4), 191-4

Fernando, M. M., Stevens, C. R., Walsh, E. C., De Jager, P. L., Goyette, P., Plenge, R. M., Vyse, T. J., and Rioux, J. D. (2008). Defining the role of the MHC in autoimmunity: a review and pooled analysis. *PLoS Genet* 4(4), e1000024

Feuer, R., Ruller, C. M., An, N., Tabor-Godwin, J. M., Rhoades, R. E., Maciejewski, S., Pagarigan, R. R., Cornell, C. T., Crocker, S. J., Kiosses, W. B., Pham-Mitchell, N., Campbell, I. L., and Whitton, J. L. (2009). Viral persistence and chronic immunopathology in the adult central nervous system following Coxsackievirus infection during the neonatal period. *J Virol* 83(18), 9356-69

Fields, B. N., Knipe, D. M., and Howley, P. M. (2007). "Fields' virology." 5th ed. / editors-in-chief, David M. Knipe, Peter M. Howley ; associate editors, Diane E. Griffin ... [et al.]. ed. Wolters Kluwer/Lippincott Williams & Wilkins, Philadelphia, Pa. ; London.

Foulis, A. K., Farquharson, M. A., and Meager, A. (1987). Immunoreactive alpha-interferon in insulin-secreting beta cells in type 1 diabetes mellitus. *Lancet* 2(8573), 1423-7

Foxman, E. F., and Iwasaki, A. (2011). Genome-virome interactions: examining the role of common viral infections in complex disease. *Nat Rev Microbiol* 9(4), 254-64

Frisk, G., and Tuvemo, T. (2004). Enterovirus infections with beta-cell tropic strains are frequent in siblings of children diagnosed with type 1 diabetes children and in association with elevated levels of GAD65 antibodies. *J Med Virol* 73(3), 450-9

Heinig, M., Petretto, E., Wallace, C., Bottolo, L., Rotival, M., Lu, H., Li, Y., Sarwar, R., Langley, S. R., Bauerfeind, A., Hummel, O., Lee, Y. A., Paskas, S., Rintisch, C., Saar, K., Cooper, J., Buchan, R., Gray, E. E., Cyster, J. G., Erdmann, J., Hengstenberg, C., Maouche, S., Ouwehand, W. H., Rice, C. M., Samani, N. J., Schunkert, H., Goodall, A. H., Schulz, H., Roider, H. G., Vingron, M., Blankenberg, S., Munzel, T., Zeller, T., Szymczak, S., Ziegler, A., Tiret, L., Smyth, D. J., Pravenec, M., Aitman, T. J., Cambien, F., Clayton, D., Todd, J. A., Hubner, N., and Cook, S. A. (2010). A trans-acting locus regulates an anti-viral expression network and type 1 diabetes risk. *Nature* 467(7314), 460-4

Helfand, R. F., Gary, H. E., Jr., Freeman, C. Y., Anderson, L. J., and Pallansch, M. A. (1995). Serologic evidence of an association between enteroviruses and the onset of type 1 diabetes mellitus. Pittsburgh Diabetes Research Group. *J Infect Dis* 172(5), 1206-11

Hemminki, K., Li, X., Sundquist, K., and Sundquist, J. (2010). Familial risks for type 2 diabetes in Sweden. *Diabetes Care* 33(2), 293-7

Herr, M., Dudbridge, F., Zavattari, P., Cucca, F., Guja, C., March, R., Campbell, R. D., Barnett, A. H., Bain, S. C., Todd, J. A., and Koeleman, B. P. (2000). Evaluation of fine mapping strategies for a multifactorial disease locus: systematic linkage and association analysis of IDDM1 in the HLA region on chromosome 6p21. *Hum Mol Genet* 9(9), 1291-301

Hiltunen, M., Hyoty, H., Knip, M., Ilonen, J., Reijonen, H., Vahasalo, P., Roivainen, M., Lonnrot, M., Leinikki, P., Hovi, T., and Akerblom, H. K. (1997). Islet cell antibody seroconversion in children is temporally associated with enterovirus infections. Childhood Diabetes in Finland (DiMe) Study Group. *J Infect Dis* 175(3), 554-60

Hirai, H., Miura, J., Hu, Y., Larsson, H., Larsson, K., Lernmark, A., Ivarsson, S. A., Wu, T., Kingman, A., Tzioufas, A. G., and Notkins, A. L. (2008). Selective screening of secretory vesicle-associated proteins for autoantigens in type 1 diabetes: VAMP2 and NPY are new minor autoantigens. *Clin Immunol* 127(3), 366-74

Hoggart, C. J., Parra, E. J., Shriver, M. D., Bonilla, C., Kittles, R. A., Clayton, D. G., and McKeigue, P. M. (2003). Control of confounding of genetic associations in stratified populations. *Am J Hum Genet* 72(6), 1492-1504

Huang, X., Yuang, J., Goddard, A., Foulis, A., James, R. F., Lernmark, A., Pujol-Borrell, R., Rabinovitch, A., Somoza, N., and Stewart, T. A. (1995). Interferon expression in the pancreases of patients with type I diabetes. *Diabetes* 44(6), 658-64

Hyoty, H., and Taylor, K. W. (2002). The role of viruses in human diabetes. *Diabetologia* 45(10), 1353-61

Hyypia, T., Hovi, T., Knowles, N. J., and Stanway, G. (1997). Classification of enteroviruses based on molecular and biological properties. *J Gen Virol* 78 (Pt 1), 1-11

Ikegami, H., Noso, S., Babaya, N., Hiromine, Y., and Kawabata, Y. (2008). Genetic Basis of Type 1 Diabetes: Similarities and Differences between East and West. *Rev Diabet Stud* 5(2), 64-72

Jun, H. S., and Yoon, J. W. (2003). A new look at viruses in type 1 diabetes. *Diabetes Metab Res Rev* 19(1), 8-31

Karvonen, M., Viik-Kajander, M., Moltchanova, E., Libman, I., LaPorte, R., and Tuomilehto, J. (2000). Incidence of childhood type 1 diabetes worldwide. Diabetes Mondiale (DiaMond) Project Group. *Diabetes Care* 23(10), 1516-26

Khetsuriani, N., Lamonte-Fowlkes, A., Oberst, S., and Pallansch, M. A. (2006). Enterovirus surveillance--United States, 1970-2005. *MMWR Surveill Summ* 55(8), 1-20

Kim, K. S., Hufnagel, G., Chapman, N. M., and Tracy, S. (2001). The group B coxsackieviruses and myocarditis. *Rev Med Virol* 11(6), 355-68

King, M. L., Shaikh, A., Bidwell, D., Voller, A., and Banatvala, J. E. (1983). Coxsackie-B-virus-specific IgM responses in children with insulin-dependent (juvenile-onset; type I) diabetes mellitus. *Lancet* 1(8339), 1397-9

Klingel, K., Hohenadl, C., Canu, A., Albrecht, M., Seemann, M., Mall, G., and Kandolf, R. (1992). Ongoing enterovirus-induced myocarditis is associated with persistent heart muscle infection: quantitative analysis of virus replication, tissue damage, and inflammation. *Proc Natl Acad Sci U S A* 89(1), 314-8

Knip, M., Veijola, R., Virtanen, S. M., Hyoty, H., Vaarala, O., and Akerblom, H. K. (2005). Environmental triggers and determinants of type 1 diabetes. *Diabetes* 54 Suppl 2, S125-36

Liston, A. (2010). How many genes in type 1 diabetes? *International Diabetes Monitor* 22(2), 90-93

Lonnrot, M., Korpela, K., Knip, M., Ilonen, J., Simell, O., Korhonen, S., Savola, K., Muona, P., Simell, T., Koskela, P., and Hyoty, H. (2000a). Enterovirus infection as a risk factor for beta-cell autoimmunity in a prospectively observed birth cohort: the Finnish Diabetes Prediction and Prevention Study. *Diabetes* 49(8), 1314-8

Lonnrot, M., Salminen, K., Knip, M., Savola, K., Kulmala, P., Leinikki, P., Hyypia, T., Akerblom, H. K., and Hyoty, H. (2000b). Enterovirus RNA in serum is a risk factor for beta-cell autoimmunity and clinical type 1 diabetes: a prospective study. Childhood Diabetes in Finland (DiMe) Study Group. *J Med Virol* 61(2), 214-20

Martins, T. C., and Aguas, A. P. (1996). Changes in B and T lymphocytes associated with mycobacteria-induced protection of NOD mice from diabetes. *J Autoimmun* 9(4), 501-7

Matsuzaki, T., Nagata, Y., Kado, S., Uchida, K., Kato, I., Hashimoto, S., and Yokokura, T. (1997). Prevention of onset in an insulin-dependent diabetes mellitus model, NOD mice, by oral feeding of Lactobacillus casei. *APMIS* 105(8), 643-9

McInerney, M. F., Pek, S. B., and Thomas, D. W. (1991). Prevention of insulitis and diabetes onset by treatment with complete Freund's adjuvant in NOD mice. *Diabetes* 40(6), 715-25

Morel, P. A., Dorman, J. S., Todd, J. A., McDevitt, H. O., and Trucco, M. (1988). Aspartic acid at position 57 of the HLA-DQ beta chain protects against type I diabetes: a family study. *Proc Natl Acad Sci U S A* 85(21), 8111-5

Moya-Suri, V., Schlosser, M., Zimmermann, K., Rjasanowski, I., Gurtler, L., and Mentel, R. (2005). Enterovirus RNA sequences in sera of schoolchildren in the general population and their association with type 1-diabetes-associated autoantibodies. *J Med Microbiol* 54(Pt 9), 879-83

Nairn, C., Galbraith, D. N., Taylor, K. W., and Clements, G. B. (1999). Enterovirus variants in the serum of children at the onset of Type 1 diabetes mellitus. *Diabet Med* 16(6), 509-13

Nakayama, M., Abiru, N., Moriyama, H., Babaya, N., Liu, E., Miao, D., Yu, L., Wegmann, D. R., Hutton, J. C., Elliott, J. F., and Eisenbarth, G. S. (2005). Prime role for an insulin epitope in the development of type 1 diabetes in NOD mice. *Nature* 435(7039), 220-3

Nejentsev, S., Walker, N., Riches, D., Egholm, M., and Todd, J. A. (2009). Rare variants of IFIH1, a gene implicated in antiviral responses, protect against type 1 diabetes. *Science* 324(5925), 387-9

Nomaguchi, H., Yogi, Y., Kawatsu, K., Okamura, H., Ozawa, Y., and Kasatani, T. (2002). Prevention of diabetes in non-obese diabetic mice by a single immunization with Mycobacterium leprae. *Nihon Hansenbyo Gakkai Zasshi* 71(1), 31-8

Notkins, A. L. (2007). New predictors of disease. Molecules called predictive autoantibodies appear in the blood years before people show symptoms of various disorders. Tests that detected these molecules could warn of the need to take preventive action. *Sci Am* 296(3), 72-9

Notkins, A. L., and Yoon, J. W. (1982). Virus-induced diabetes in mice prevented by a live attenuated vaccine. *N Engl J Med* 306(8), 486

Oikarinen, M., Tauriainen, S., Honkanen, T., Oikarinen, S., Vuori, K., Kaukinen, K., Rantala, I., Maki, M., and Hyoty, H. (2008). Detection of enteroviruses in the intestine of type 1 diabetic patients. *Clin Exp Immunol* 151(1), 71-5

Oikarinen, S., Martiskainen, M., Tauriainen, S., Huhtala, H., Ilonen, J., Veijola, R., Simell, O., Knip, M., and Hyoty, H. (2011). Enterovirus RNA in blood is linked to the development of type 1 diabetes. *Diabetes* 60(1), 276-9

Otonkoski, T., Roivainen, M., Vaarala, O., Dinesen, B., Leipala, J. A., Hovi, T., and Knip, M. (2000). Neonatal Type I diabetes associated with maternal echovirus 6 infection: a case report. *Diabetologia* 43(10), 1235-8

Parry, C. S., and Brooks, B. R. (2008). A new model defines the minimal set of polymorphism in HLA-DQ and -DR that determines susceptibility and resistance to autoimmune diabetes. *Biol Direct* 3, 42

Petrovsky, N. (2010). Immunomodulation with microbial vaccines to prevent type 1 diabetes mellitus. *Nat Rev Endocrinol* 6(3), 131-8

Redondo, M. J., Rewers, M., Yu, L., Garg, S., Pilcher, C. C., Elliott, R. B., and Eisenbarth, G. S. (1999). Genetic determination of islet cell autoimmunity in monozygotic twin, dizygotic twin, and non-twin siblings of patients with type 1 diabetes: prospective twin study. *BMJ* 318(7185), 698-702

Redondo, M. J., Yu, L., Hawa, M., Mackenzie, T., Pyke, D. A., Eisenbarth, G. S., and Leslie, R. D. (2001). Heterogeneity of type I diabetes: analysis of monozygotic twins in Great Britain and the United States. *Diabetologia* 44(3), 354-62

Reetoo, K. N., Osman, S. A., Illavia, S. J., Cameron-Wilson, C. L., Banatvala, J. E., and Muir, P. (2000). Quantitative analysis of viral RNA kinetics in coxsackievirus B3-induced murine myocarditis: biphasic pattern of clearance following acute infection, with persistence of residual viral RNA throughout and beyond the inflammatory phase of disease. *J Gen Virol* 81(Pt 11), 2755-62

Richardson, S. J., Willcox, A., Bone, A. J., Foulis, A. K., and Morgan, N. G. (2009). The prevalence of enteroviral capsid protein vp1 immunostaining in pancreatic islets in human type 1 diabetes. *Diabetologia* 52(6), 1143-51

Roivainen, M., Ylipaasto, P., Savolainen, C., Galama, J., Hovi, T., and Otonkoski, T. (2002). Functional impairment and killing of human beta cells by enteroviruses: the capacity is shared by a wide range of serotypes, but the extent is a characteristic of individual virus strains. *Diabetologia* 45(5), 693-702

Sadeharju, K., Lonnrot, M., Kimpimaki, T., Savola, K., Erkkila, S., Kalliokoski, T., Savolainen, P., Koskela, P., Ilonen, J., Simell, O., Knip, M., and Hyoty, H. (2001). Enterovirus antibody levels during the first two years of life in prediabetic autoantibody-positive children. *Diabetologia* 44(7), 818-23

Salminen, K., Sadeharju, K., Lonnrot, M., Vahasalo, P., Kupila, A., Korhonen, S., Ilonen, J., Simell, O., Knip, M., and Hyoty, H. (2003). Enterovirus infections are associated with the induction of beta-cell autoimmunity in a prospective birth cohort study. *J Med Virol* 69(1), 91-8

Sarmiento, L., Cabrera-Rode, E., Lekuleni, L., Cuba, I., Molina, G., Fonseca, M., Heng-Hung, L., Borroto, A. D., Gonzalez, P., Mas-Lago, P., and Diaz-Horta, O. (2007a). Occurrence of enterovirus RNA in serum of children with newly diagnosed type 1 diabetes and islet cell autoantibody-positive subjects in a population with a low incidence of type 1 diabetes. *Autoimmunity* 40(7), 540-5

Sarmiento, L., Cabrera-Rode, E., Mas-Lago, P., and Diaz-Horta, O. (2007b). Antibodies to human glutamic acid decarboxylase in sera from enterovirus-immunized rabbit. *Autoimmunity* 40(7), 546-7

Sarmiento, L., Mas, P., Goyenechea, A., Palomera, R., Morier, L., Capo, V., Quintana, I., and Santin, M. (2001). First epidemic of echovirus 16 meningitis in Cuba. *Emerg Infect Dis* 7(5), 887-9

Savolainen-Kopra, C., and Blomqvist, S. (2010). Mechanisms of genetic variation in polioviruses. *Rev Med Virol* 20(6), 358-71

Schulte, B. M., Bakkers, J., Lanke, K. H., Melchers, W. J., Westerlaken, C., Allebes, W., Aanstoot, H. J., Bruining, G. J., Adema, G. J., Van Kuppeveld, F. J., and Galama, J. M. (2010a). Detection of enterovirus RNA in peripheral blood mononuclear cells of type 1 diabetic patients beyond the stage of acute infection. *Viral Immunol* 23(1), 99-104

Schulte, B. M., Kramer, M., Ansems, M., Lanke, K. H., van Doremalen, N., Piganelli, J. D., Bottino, R., Trucco, M., Galama, J. M., Adema, G. J., and van Kuppeveld, F. J. (2010b). Phagocytosis of enterovirus-infected pancreatic beta-cells triggers innate immune responses in human dendritic cells. *Diabetes* 59(5), 1182-91

Shapiro, A. M., Ricordi, C., Hering, B. J., Auchincloss, H., Lindblad, R., Robertson, R. P., Secchi, A., Brendel, M. D., Berney, T., Brennan, D. C., Cagliero, E., Alejandro, R., Ryan, E. A., DiMercurio, B., Morel, P., Polonsky, K. S., Reems, J. A., Bretzel, R. G., Bertuzzi, F., Froud, T., Kandaswamy, R., Sutherland, D. E., Eisenbarth, G., Segal,

M., Preiksaitis, J., Korbutt, G. S., Barton, F. B., Viviano, L., Seyfert-Margolis, V., Bluestone, J., and Lakey, J. R. (2006). International trial of the Edmonton protocol for islet transplantation. *N Engl J Med* 355(13), 1318-30

She, J. X. (1996). Susceptibility to type I diabetes: HLA-DQ and DR revisited. *Immunol Today* 17(7), 323-9

Simmonds, P. (2006). Recombination and selection in the evolution of picornaviruses and other Mammalian positive-stranded RNA viruses. *J Virol* 80(22), 11124-40

Szopa, T. M., Ward, T., and Taylor, K. W. (1992). Disturbance of mouse pancreatic beta-cell function following echo 4 virus infection. *Biochem Soc Trans* 20(4), 315S

Tanaka, S., Nishida, Y., Aida, K., Maruyama, T., Shimada, A., Suzuki, M., Shimura, H., Takizawa, S., Takahashi, M., Akiyama, D., Arai-Yamashita, S., Furuya, F., Kawaguchi, A., Kaneshige, M., Katoh, R., Endo, T., and Kobayashi, T. (2009). Enterovirus infection, CXC chemokine ligand 10 (CXCL10), and CXCR3 circuit: a mechanism of accelerated beta-cell failure in fulminant type 1 diabetes. *Diabetes* 58(10), 2285-91

Uriarte, A., Cabrera-Rode, E., Ventura, R., and Vargas, J. (1987). Islet cell antibodies and Echo 4 virus infection. *Diabetologia* 30(A), 590

Vaysburd, M., Lock, C., and McDevitt, H. (1995). Prevention of insulin-dependent diabetes mellitus in nonobese diabetic mice by immunogenic but not by tolerated peptides. *J Exp Med* 182(3), 897-902

Viskari, H., Ludvigsson, J., Uibo, R., Salur, L., Marciulionyte, D., Hermann, R., Soltesz, G., Fuchtenbusch, M., Ziegler, A. G., Kondrashova, A., Romanov, A., Kaplan, B., Laron, Z., Koskela, P., Vesikari, T., Huhtala, H., Knip, M., and Hyoty, H. (2005). Relationship between the incidence of type 1 diabetes and maternal enterovirus antibodies: time trends and geographical variation. *Diabetologia* 48(7), 1280-7

Voltarelli, J. C., Couri, C. E., Stracieri, A. B., Oliveira, M. C., Moraes, D. A., Pieroni, F., Coutinho, M., Malmegrim, K. C., Foss-Freitas, M. C., Simoes, B. P., Foss, M. C., Squiers, E., and Burt, R. K. (2007). Autologous nonmyeloablative hematopoietic stem cell transplantation in newly diagnosed type 1 diabetes mellitus. *JAMA* 297(14), 1568-76

von Herrath, M. (2009). Can we learn from viruses how to prevent type 1 diabetes?: the role of viral infections in the pathogenesis of type 1 diabetes and the development of novel combination therapies. *Diabetes* 58(1), 2-11

Vreugdenhil, G. R., Schloot, N. C., Hoorens, A., Rongen, C., Pipeleers, D. G., Melchers, W. J., Roep, B. O., and Galama, J. M. (2000). Acute onset of type I diabetes mellitus after severe echovirus 9 infection: putative pathogenic pathways. *Clin Infect Dis* 31(4), 1025-31

Williams, C. H., Oikarinen, S., Tauriainen, S., Salminen, K., Hyoty, H., and Stanway, G. (2006). Molecular analysis of an echovirus 3 strain isolated from an individual concurrently with appearance of islet cell and IA-2 autoantibodies. *J Clin Microbiol* 44(2), 441-8

Yeung, W. C., Rawlinson, W. D., and Craig, M. E. (2011). Enterovirus infection and type 1 diabetes mellitus: systematic review and meta-analysis of observational molecular studies. *BMJ* 342, d35

Yin, H., Berg, A. K., Tuvemo, T., and Frisk, G. (2002). Enterovirus RNA is found in peripheral blood mononuclear cells in a majority of type 1 diabetic children at onset. *Diabetes* 51(6), 1964-71

Part 3

Pathogenesis – Environment

11

Environmental Triggers of Type 1 Diabetes Mellitus – Mycobacterium Avium Subspecies Paratuberculosis

Coad Thomas Dow[1] and Leonardo A. Sechi[2]
[1]*University of Wisconsin, Eye Research Institute*
[2]*University of Sassari*
[1]*USA*
[2]*Italy*

1. Introduction

Type 1 diabetes mellitus (T1DM) is an autoimmune disease. The etiology of T1DM is incompletely understood but environmental agent(s) are thought to trigger T1DM in the genetically at-risk. In the United States the prevalence of T1DM is increasing and is approximately 1 in 300 by 18 years of age. Research into risk factors for T1DM is an active area with attempts to identify genetic and environmental triggers that could potentially be targeted for intervention (Maahs et al., 2010).

The most important autoimmune diabetes triggering factors are thought to be infectious, dietary, perinatal, and/or psychosocial. Historically, enteroviruses (especially Coxsackie B virus) have been the most commonly regarded infectious triggering agents (Peng & Hagopian, 2006).

Evidence supports the critical role of exogenous factors in the development of T1DM: 1. less than 10% of individuals with HLA-conferred diabetes susceptibility progress to clinical disease, 2. pair-wise concordance of T1DM of less than 40% among monozygotic twins, 3. more than 10-fold difference in the disease incidence among Caucasians living in Europe, (annual rate Macedonia 3.2/100,000 vs. Finland 54/100,000) 4. several-fold increase in the incidence over the last 50 years, and 5. migration studies that indicate disease incidence increases in population groups who have moved from a low-incidence to a high-incidence region. (Knip et al., 2005).

The postulate that MAP plays a causal role in T1DM was presented at the 2005 Colloquium on Paratuberculosis (Dow, 2005) and published in 2006 (Dow, 2006). To understand the rationale of the hypothesis it is necessary to review MAP, the role MAP plays in animal disease and the proposed role MAP has in human disease.

2. Mycobacterium avium ss. paratuberculosis (MAP)

MAP is a gram-positive, acid-fast staining small rod-shaped bacterium. As with members of the Mycobacteriaceae genus, it has a unique cell wall structure rich in complex lipids (fig. 1). The thick and chemically distinctive cell wall of mycobacteria is responsible in large measure for the robust nature of these bacteria, both within the host cell and in the environment. The pathogenic potential of mycobacteria is correlated with their growth rate. Paradoxically, slow-growing mycobacteria are more virulent than fast-growing mycobacteria. With the exception of *Mycobacterium leprae* (the cause of leprosy in humans), which cannot be cultured in vitro, MAP has the slowest growth rate of pathogenic mycobacteria. After isolation from infected animals and grown under optimal conditions colonies of MAP are typically not visible for 3 months or more (Collins, 2003).

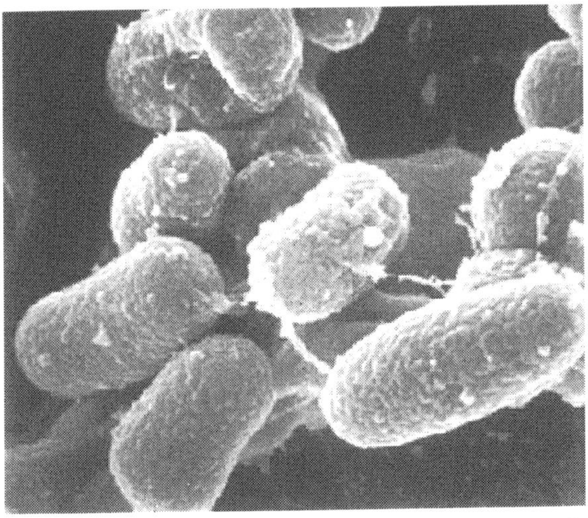

Fig. 1. Electron Microscopy of Mycobacterium avium ss. paratuberculosis (MAP).
Image courtesy of Dr. Mike Collins, University of Wisconsin - Madison.

Mycobacterium avium subspecies *paratuberculosis* (MAP) causes a chronic granulomatous inflammation of the intestines in ruminant animals called Johne's disease. Mostly studied in dairy cattle, goats and sheep, MAP also causes a chronic inflammation of the intestines in beef cattle and in a wide variety of other domestic and wild ruminants. MAP-induced enteric inflammation has been found in monogastric animals including dogs and pigs as well as four different types of subhuman primates - macaques, baboons, gibbons and cotton-top tamarins" (Hermon-Taylor et al., 2000). A majority of the dairy herds in the United States and Europe have infected animals within the herd (Stabel, 1998).

2.1 MAP and human exposure

The article, *Evolutionary bottlenecks in the agents for tuberculosis, leprosy and paratuberculosis* (Frothingham, 1999), indicates that these parasitic mycobacteria are different from the "environmental" mycobacteria and may reflect opportunities afforded the parasitic mycobacteria by human cohabitation with domesticated animals combined with consolidation of populations. More crowded conditions may have changed tuberculosis, leprosy, and paratuberculosis from sporadic to epidemic diseases.

Mycobacterium avium ss. *paratuberculosis* (MAP)is present in pasteurized milk (Millar et al., 1996; Ellingson et al., 2005), infant formula made from pasteurized milk (Hruska et al, 2005), surface water (Pickup et al., 2005; Whan et al., 2005; Pickup et al, 2006), soil (Pickup et al.,

2005), cow manure "lagoons" that can leach into surface water, cow manure in both solid and liquid forms that is applied as fertilizer to agricultural land (Grewal et al., 2006), and municipal tap water (Collins, 2003), providing multiple routes of transmission to humans. In a recent study in Ohio the DNA of MAP was detected in over 80% of domestic water samples (Beumer et al., 2010).

Normal water treatment processes such as filtration and chlorination amplify rather than eliminate mycobacteria organisms by killing off their competitors (Falkinham, 2003). In addition, mycobacteria organisms grow on tap water pipes (Falkinham & Norton, 2001), in biofilms (Vaerewijck et al., 2005) and on plastic water bottles (Tatchou-Nyamsi-Konig et al., 2009). It is estimated that mycobacteria may be present in drinking water in "massive numbers," on the level of up to 700,000 or 7 x 105 organisms per liter of water (Falkinham et al., 2001).

3. MAP and human disease – inflammatory bowel disease and sarcoidosis

Beyond Johne's disease of animals, MAP is the putative cause of the striking similar Crohn's disease of humans. Although there has been a century-long debate, the role of MAP in Crohn's has evolved from controversial to compelling (Chamberlin et al., 2007; Feller et al., 2007; Mendoza et al., 2010). The major source of the debate is that conventional methods of detecting bacteria - namely, culture and stain - are largely ineffective in detecting MAP. However, with newer laboratory techniques, primarily PCR, evidence of MAP is readily found in Crohn's tissues (Chiodini, 1989; McFadden et al, 1987); it can be visualized within the granulomas by in situ hybridization (Sechi, 2001): and, with extreme care and patience, MAP can be grown from the gut and blood of Crohn's patients (Naser et al., 2004, 2009; Sechi et al., 2005).

MAP has also been reported as a candidate pathogen in the causation irritable bowel syndrome (Scanu et al., 2007) and some suspect that MAP causes the spectrum of inflammatory bowel disease including Crohn's, ulcerative colitis and irritable bowel syndrome (Pierce, 2010). Irritable bowel syndrome is a widespread abdominal condition that affects about 10 to 15% of people in the industrialized economies of Europe, North America, Australasia, and Japan, with a rising prevalence among the populations in the developing economies of Asia. Some consider irritable bowel syndrome a *form fruste* of Crohn's disease (Olbe, 2008).

In addition to inflammatory bowel disease MAP has been historically linked is sarcoidosis; a multi-system inflammatory disease in which DNA evidence of MAP has been found (sporadically) in sarcoid granulomas (el-Zaatari, 1996).

4. Genetics and T1DM

Early studies indicated that the HLA region on chromosome 6p21 (commonly termed IDDM1, for insulin-dependent diabetes mellitus locus) is a critical susceptibility locus for T1DM (Nerup et al., 1974; Singal & Blajchman, 1973). A comprehensive review of the genetics of T1DM is beyond the scope of this chapter; instead, we will focus on genes that appear to be permissive to MAP (CARD15 and SLC11A1) and then to MAP and T1DM specifically (SLC11A1). Though we will focus on these genes, it is short sighted to expect that only one or two genes affect the susceptibility of humans to mycobacterial infections and autoimmune disease. Gene-gene interaction (epistasis) is known with regard to tuberculosis susceptibility (de Wit et al., 2010). For instance, there seems to be a role for vitamin D as well as the VDR gene (vitamin D receptor) (Hayes et al., 2003; Motohashi et al., 2003). In addition to regulation of bone and mineral metabolism, Vitamin D is a potent modulator of the immune system (Zella & DeLuca, 2003). Vitamin D activity occurs via the VDR. VDR is part of the steroid receptor super-family and is widely expressed in many cell types including lymphocytes, macrophages and the insulin producing pancreatic beta-cells (Hayes et al, 2003). Vitamin D and VDR, have been implicated in the susceptibility of TIDM: VDR gene polymorphisms have been described in TIDM in Taiwanese (Chang et al., 2000), Indian Asians (McDermot et al., 1997), Germans (Pani et al., 2000), Spaniards (Marti et al., 2004), Japanese (Ban et al., 2001) and Croatians (Skrabic et al., 2003). Additionally, calcitriol - the hormonal form of vitamin D - prevents or markedly suppress experimental TIDM (Deluca & Cantorna, 2001) and is active against tuberculosis (Jo, 2010).

4.1 Genetics – CARD15

The CARD15 gene is part of the ancestral innate immune system that senses and eliminates bacteria (Girardin et al., 2003; Hugot et al., 2002; Inohara et al., 2003); it is part of the newly recognized, larger CATERPILLER gene family that acts as sensors to detect pathogens and regulates inflammatory and apoptotic responses (Ting & Davis, 1985). Defects in the CARD15 gene are associated with Crohn's disease susceptibility (Hampe et al., 2002). In 2005, Sechi reported that more than 70 percent of people in Sardinia with Crohn's disease carry at least one of the susceptibility-associated NOD 2/CARD 15 alleles and were infected with MAP.

Insights into genetic susceptibility and MAP infection can be found in a rare inflammatory disease, Blau syndrome. Blau syndrome is an inherited granulomatous inflammatory disorder with clinical findings of uveitis, arthritis, and dermatitis (Blau, 1985). Although rare, Blau syndrome has been of interest in current medical literature because of the discovery that places its genetic defect on the same Crohn's susceptibility CARD15 gene (Hampe et al., 2002; Miceli-Richard et al., 2001). Linkage studies have placed the gene on chromosome 16; originally referred to as the NOD2 gene, it is now known as the CARD15 gene (Hugot et al., 2002). The Blau syndrome susceptibility component of the CARD15 gene is at the nucleotide binding site domain (Hampe et al., 2002; Wang et al., 2002) while the Crohn's susceptibility is at the N-terminal leucine-rich repeat domain (Hugot et al., 2002; Lesage et al., 2002). The CARD15 gene is part of the ancestral innate immune system that senses and eliminates bacteria (Girardin et al., 2003; Inohara et al., 2003).

The clinical findings of Blau syndrome are one and the same as juvenile sarcoidosis; and, indeed, de novo CARD15 defects are consistently found in cases of sporadic juvenile sarcoidosis - Blau syndrome (Kanazawa et al., 2005; Rose et al., 2005). For these reasons - the clinical appearance of sarcoidosis and a shared genetic susceptibility with Crohn's - it was proposed that MAP could have a role in Blau syndrome. The following results were presented at the 2005 Colloquium on Paratuberculosis (Dow) and published in 2010 (Dow & Ellingson, 2010):

> *Methods. Archival tissues of individuals with Blau syndrome were tested for the presence of MAP. Results. DNA evidence of MAP was detected in all of the tissues. Conclusions. This article finds that MAP is present in Blau syndrome tissue and postulates that it has a causal role. The presence of MAP in Blau syndrome – an autosomal dominant, systemic inflammatory disease – connects genetic and environmental aspects of "autoimmune" disease.*

The complexity of genetic susceptibility and microbial infection can be reflected in these two diseases (Crohn's and Blau), both having polymorphisms of the CARD15 gene. The proposed etiopathology is that with adequate MAP exposure, an individual with SNPs within one CARD15 location (nucleotide binding domain) will exhibit Blau syndrome and if the SNPs are within another location of the same gene (leucine-rich-repeat domain) they exhibit Crohn's disease. CARD15 defects of the leucine--rich-repeat domain, result in an aggressive phenotype of Crohn's disease (Lacher et al., 2010). Adding to the complexity is that there are several susceptibility genes associated with Crohn's (Franke et al., 2010).

4.2 Genetics - SLC11A1

One additional gene associated with Crohn's susceptibility is the SLC11A1 gene (Sechi et al., 2006). Natural resistance-associated macrophage protein 1 (NRAMP1) is now strictly referred to as SLC11A1 (solute carrier 11a1). The gene that encodes for this protein is recognized as having a role in the susceptibility of humans and animals to a number of infections, including mycobacterial infections, and is associated with a number of autoimmune diseases as well. In human beings, the SLC11A1 gene is located on chromosome 2q35. It encodes an integral membrane protein of 550 amino acids that is expressed exclusively in the lysosomal compartment of monocytes and macrophages (Canonne-Hergaux et al., 1999).

The product of the SLC11A1 gene modulates the cellular environment in response to activation by intracellular pathogens by acidifying the phagosome thus killing the pathogen (Lapham et al., 2004). As such, it plays a role in host innate immunity (Wyllie et al., 2002). Mutation of SLC11A1 impairs phagosome acidification yielding a permissive environment for the persistence of intracellular bacteria (Hackam et al., 1998).

5. SLC11A1 in infectious and autoimmune disease

Sarcoidosis, the previously mentioned systemic disease associated with MAP, is also associated with polymorphisms of the SLC11A1 gene (Dubaniewicz et al., 2005). Susceptibility to mycobacterial diseases tuberculosis, leprosy and Buruli's ulcer are associated with polymorphism of the SLC11A1 gene (Stienstra et al., 2006). Similar polymorphisms are associated with Johne's disease (paratuberculosis) in cattle (Ruiz-Larrañaga et al., 2010), goats (Korou et al., 2010), and sheep (Purdie et al., 2011). When researchers at the Belgium Pasteur Institute developed a murine model for MAP infection, they created an SLC11A1 defect mouse (Roupie et al., 2008).

Given the pivotal roles that SLC11A1 plays in innate immunity, it is not surprising that the relationship between polymorphisms in SLC11A1 and a number of mycobacterial as well as autoimmune diseases has been explored (Blackwell et al, 2003). Associations have been found with leprosy (Hatta et al., 2010), tuberculosis (Bellamy et al., 1998), rheumatoid arthritis (Ates et al., 2009), visceral leishmaniasis (Mohamed et al., 2004), multiple sclerosis (Kotze et al., 2001; Gazouli et al., 2008b), inflammatory bowel disease (Gazouli et al., 2008a; Kotlowski et al., 2008; Sechi et al., 2006) and type 1 diabetes mellitus (Paccagnini et al., 2009; Takahashi et al., 2004).

6. MAP and Type 1 diabetes

Type 1 diabetes mellitus (T1DM) is an autoimmune disease manifest by progressive T cell-mediated autoimmune destruction of insulin-producing beta cells in the pancreatic islets of Langherans (Eisenbarth, 1986). Dow in 2005 postulated a causative role for MAP in the T1DM, Sechi in 2007 found the DNA of MAP in the blood of autoimmune (type 1) patients but not non-autoimmune (type 2) diabetics (Rosu et al., 2009; Sechi, et al., 2007, 2008). Sechi also found an association of polymorphisms of the SLC11a1 gene and MAP in T1DM patients (Paccagnini et al., 2009).

While it may be intuitive to envision an occult presence of MAP as an infective agent producing a granulomatous lesion of Crohn's or sarcoidosis; it is broader divide to assign a role for MAP in T1DM. The link connecting MAP and T1DM comes from the concept of molecular mimicry: protein elements of the pathogen "look like" elements of the host to a degree that immune responses directed at the pathogen also attack the host.

One of the proposed links is the mimicry of mycobacterial heat shock protein of MAP (HSP65) and pancreatic glutamic acid decarboxylase(GAD) (Dow, 2006).

7. Molecular mimicry/ heat shock proteins - HSP65

Molecular mimicry has long been implicated as a mechanism by which microbes can induce autoimmunity (Oldstone, 1987; Raska & Weigl, 2005). Rheumatic fever is the classic example for molecular mimicry between an infecting agent—*Streptococcus pyogenes* (group A streptococcus) and a related autoimmune disease in humans (Guilherme et al., 2005; Kaplan & Svec, 1964; Kirvan et al., 2003). The disease is characterized by damage to the heart, joints, and the central nervous system (Sydenham's chorea). The activity of the host's immune system against the streptococcus generates a cross-recognition to human tissue causing an autoimmune reaction. Heart damage is the most serious consequence and is present in 30 to 45% of the cases - mostly causing damage to the heart valves.

Heat shock proteins (HSPs) are produced in response to environmental stress. They act in a protective capacity helping cells survive stressful conditions and promoting recovery (Parsell & Lindquist, 1993). During an active immune response to infection, both the host and the microorganisms synthesize HSPs. The increased expression of both self and infective stress proteins and the extensive sequence homology between microbial and human HSP (50–80% amino acid homology of mycobacterial HSP65 versus human HSP60) have led to the concept that HSPs are involved in the etiology and pathogenesis of many immune mediated disorders (Lamb & Young, 1990). Mycobacterial HSPs have been found in a myriad of autoimmune diseases (Jarjour et al., 1991). For example, the mycobacterial 65 kDa HSP has been implicated in the pathogenesis of rheumatoid arthritis (Moudgil et al.,1997; Quayle et al., 1992), autoimmune hepatitis (Miyata et al.,1995), primary biliary cirrhosis (Vilagut et al.,1997) and scleroderma (Danieli et al., 1992). HSP65 is implicated in multiple vasculitis-associated systemic autoimmune diseases such as Kawasaki disease (Yokota et al., 1993), Behcet's disease (Direskeneli & Saruhan-Direskeneli, 2003) and Takayasu's arteritis (Aggarwal et al., 1996).

8. Molecular mimicry and Type 1 diabetes mellitus

Individuals at-risk for T1DM produce anti-GAD antibodies. HSP65 was first associated with T1DM via GAD in 1990 (Jones et al., 1990). Mycobacteria produce HSP65 in response to stress. There is marked homology between mycobacterial HSP65 and human HSP60 (Jindal et al., 1989). Epitope homology between MAP/human HSP60/65 and pancreatic glutamic acid decarboxylase (GAD) likely triggers the anti-GAD antibodies that secondarily destroy the pancreas (Jones et al., 1993).

Mycobacterial HSP65 provides a well-described diabetogenic peptide, p277 (Liang et al., 2010). The critical role of immunity against hsp65 and its T-cell epitope, p277 was proven in two different experimental animal model systems: the spontaneous diabetes that develops in the diabetes model NOD (non-obese diabetic) mice, and the autoimmune diabetes induced by a very low dose of the toxin streptozotocin (STZ). Pre-diabetic NOD mice manifest spontaneous antibody formation and T cell responses to hsp60 and to peptide p277 prior to the onset of diabetes (Birk et al., 1996; Elias et al., 1990; Elias et al., 1991). A single administration of the peptide p277 conjugated to carrier molecules can induce diabetes in C57BL/6 mice and in other strains not genetically prone to develop diabetes (Elias et al., 1995). Conversely, a single injection of unconjugated peptide p277 in NOD mice could arrest the diabetogenic autoimmune process, even when it was advanced (Elias et al., 1991; Elias & Cohen, 1994; Elias & Cohen, 1995). Additionally, administration of peptide p277 could prevent the development of autoimmune diabetes induced by very low dose of STZ in 57BL/KsJ mice strain (Elias & Cohen, 1996).

9. T1DM and milk

We now have come full circle regarding MAP, exposure to MAP, MAP in animal and human disease, epitope homology between mycobacterial HSP65 (particularly p277) and pancreatic GAD. The observation regarding risk of T1DM and early life exposure to milk warrants discussion.

Several studies indicate an association between early exposure to dietary cow's milk and an increased risk of TIDM. (Akerblom & Knip, 1998; Gerstein, 1994; Gimeno & deSouza, 1997). These studies were prompted by the observation that children at risk for TIDM who were breast fed exclusively for more than six months were less likely to have TIDM later in life than similar risk children who were weaned onto cow's milk-based formula at an earlier age. This observation spawned a large study, the TRIGR study: Trial to Reduce IDDM in the Genetically at Risk (Akerblom et al., 2010). The postulate is that there is something about cow's milk protein that is an immunologic trigger for TIDM and that breaking the protein with hydrolysis may eliminate the trigger. The TRIGR study is an ongoing, 17-country study enlisting 6200 infants who are genetically at risk to develop TIDM. Children weaned early from breastfeeding are randomized into two groups; one receiving traditional cow's milk-based formula and the other receiving formula in which the protein has been hydrolyzed. A recent, smaller but somewhat parallel study shows that exposure to the hydrolyzed infant formula resulted in lessened incidence of T1DM (Knip et al., 2010). Antibodies against specie specific MAP proteins were found in Sardinian children involved in the TRIGR study (Sechi, personal communication) As previously mentioned, viable MAP has been found in infant formula powder (Hruska et al., 2005).

10. MAP and other autoimmune disease – thyroiditis and multiple sclerosis

Two recent articles link MAP to autoimmune (Hashimoto's) thyroiditis. The same molecular mimicry principle is suggested as the link between MAP (HSP65) and the organ-specific autoantigens of thyroiditis (D'Amore et al., 2010; Sisto et al., 2010). Another recent article implicates MAP in multiple sclerosis. Molecular mimicry and SLC11A1 associations are germane here as well (Cossu et al., 2011, Gazouli et al., 2008b).

11. MAP – the future

While evidence mounts that MAP is, indeed, a zoonotic agent, what policies and interventions might be employed to address curtailing MAP and the effects of its persistence in individuals? Presently, sound farm management practices and stringent culling are considered the best means to reduce the spread of MAP from animal to animal, as well as from farm to farm (Tavornpanich et al., 2008). However, because such practices have yet to eliminate MAP from food animals, other preventive or curative measures are needed. Industry has made an attempt to assess the risk of a positive MAP/Crohn's association (Groenendaal & Zagmutt, 2008).

TASF is a Swiss-based international forum for Transmissible Animal Diseases and Food Safety. TASF acknowledges the uncertainties of the zoonotic potential of MAP for Crohn's disease. TASF suggests that *"... a decision by food safety regulators to exercise the "precautionary principle", label MAP as a potential zoonotic agent, and adopt measures to limit as much as possible the levels of MAP contamination of raw milk and meat would go far to protect the coming generations of children from MAP exposure, possible infection, and potentially Crohn's disease."* (TAFS, white paper, 2009).

Preliminary studies with a probiotic of the Dietzia species have been shown effective in treating clinically ill adult cows with Johne's disease and in preventing Johne's in calves (Click & VanKampen, 2009; 2010). The use of Dietzia has also been suggested for individuals with inflammatory bowel disease (Click, 2011). Vaccines are effective in reducing the incidence of clinical Johne's disease (Kormendy, 1994; van Schaik et al., 1996) and attenuate pre-existing infection (Gwozdz et al., 2000). However, such whole killed vaccines do not eliminate subclinical MAP infection or its persistence in the gut. Additionally, about half of the animals receiving whole killed MAP vaccines become false positive using the conventional tuberculin skin test diagnostic for bovine tuberculosis (Mackintosh et al., 2005; Muskens et al., 2002). DNA vaccination may have an interesting application: Sechi et al., (2006) showed that lambs vaccinated with plasmids encoding mycobacterial antigens produced a Th1 immune response similar to that generated by natural infection by MAP. Moreover, lambs vaccinated with DNA mycobacterial antigens (expecially HSP65) were protected against MAP infection. Additionally, the unfolding knowledge regarding susceptibility polymorphism of genes such as the SLC11a1 gene described in this chapter may lead to breeding practices that would limit MAP infection in breeding lines thus keeping it from the human food chain.

In humans with MAP-associated disease recognition of both the need to treat as an infectious disease as well as the need to avoid further exposure is paramount. Aggressive anti-mycobacterial treatment has had beneficial effect in those who can tolerate the treatment (Borody et al., 2007; Hermon-Taylor, 2002). Vaccines against MAP for use in humans are being advocated and prototypes are being developed (Bull et al., 2007).

12. Conclusion

The controversy regarding MAP and human disease has been going for a century and will likely continue for a long time. T1DM has only recently been added to the discussion - and controversy. In addition to the human toll to individuals with T1DM, the dollar cost is extreme; the burden is passed along to all of society in the form of higher insurance premiums and taxes, reduced earnings, and reduced standard of living. Each year T1DM costs this country $14.4 billion (11.5–17.3) in medical costs and lost income. Were the disease eliminated by therapeutic intervention, an estimated $10.6 billion (7.2–14.0) incurred by a new cohort and $422.9 billion (327.2–519.4) incurred by the existing number of T1DM patients over their lifetime would be avoided (Tao et al., 2010). This alone should elevate the discussion, draw resources and bring a sense of urgency to the MAP/T1DM connection.

13. References

Aggarwal A, Chag M, Sinha N, Naik S. (1996) Takayasu's arteritis: Role of Mycobacterium tuberculosis and its 65 kDa heat shock protein. *Int J Cardiol* 1996 55(1):49–55.

Akerblom HK (2010) The TRIGR Study Group. The Trial to Reduce IDDM in the Genetically at Risk (TRIGR) study: recruitment, intervention and follow-up. *Diabetologia*. 2010 Dec 12.

Akerblom HK, Knip M. (1998) Putative environmental factors in Type 1 diabetes. *Diabetes Metab Rev* 1998 14(1):31–67.

Ates O, Dalyan L, Musellim B, Hatemi G, Turker H, Ongen G, Hamuryudan V, Topal-Sarikaya A. (2009)

NRAMP1 (SLC11A1) gene polymorphisms that correlate with autoimmune versus infectious disease susceptibility in tuberculosis and rheumatoid arthritis. *Int J Immunogenet* 2009; 36: 15-19

Ban Y, Taniyama M, Yanagawa T, Yamada S, Maruyama T, Kasuga A, et al. (2001) Vitamin D receptor initiation codon polymorphism influences genetic susceptibility to type 1 diabetes mellitus in the Japanese population. *BMC Med Genet* 2001 2:7 [Epub 2001 June 25].

Bellamy R, Ruwende C, Corrah T, McAdam KP, Whittle HC, Hill AV. (1998) Variations in the NRAMP1 gene and susceptibility to tuberculosis in West Africans. *N Engl J Med* 1998; 338: 640-644

Beumer A, King D, Donohue M, Mistry J, Covert T, Pfaller S. (2010) Detection of Mycobacterium avium subsp. paratuberculosis in drinking water and biofilms by quantitative PCR. *Appl Environ Microbio* 2010 Nov 76(21):7367-70. Epub 2010 Sep 3.

Birk OS, Elias D, Weiss AS, Rosen A, van-der Zee R, Walker MD, Cohen IR. (1996) NOD mouse diabetes: the ubiquitous mouse hsp60 is a beta-cell target antigen of autoimmune T cells. *J Autoimmun*. 1996 Apr;9(2):159-66.

Blackwell JM, Searle S, Mohamed H, White JK. (2003) Divalentcation transport and susceptibility to infectious and autoimmune disease: Continuation of the Ity/Lsh/Bcg/Nramp1/ Slc11a1 gene story. *Immunol Lett* 2003 85(2):197–203.

Blau B. (1985) Familial granulomatous arthritis, iritis, and rash, *Journal of Pediatrics*, vol. 107, no. 5, pp. 689–693, 1985.

Borody TJ, Bilkey S, Wettstein AR, Leis S, Pang G, Tye S. (2007) Anti-mycobacterial therapy in Crohn's disease heals mucosa with longitudinal scars. *Dig Liver Dis*. 2007 May 39(5):438-44. Epub 2007 Mar 21.

Bull TJ, Gilbert SC, Sridhar S, Linedale R, Dierkes N, Sidi-Boumedine K, Hermon-Taylor J. (2007) A novel multi-antigen virally vectored vaccine against Mycobacterium avium subspecies paratuberculosis. *PLoS One*. 2007 Nov 28 2(11):e1229.

Canonne-Hergaux F, Gruenheid S, Govoni G, Gros P. (1999) The Nramp1 protein and its role in resistance to infection and macrophage function. *Proc Assoc Am Physicians* 1999; 111: 283-289

Chamberlin W, Borody T, Naser S (2007) MAP-associated Crohn's disease MAP, Koch's postulates, causality and Crohn's disease. *Dig Liver Dis* 39:792–794.

Chang TJ, Lei HH, Yeh JI, et al. (2000) Vitamin D receptor gene polymorphisms influence susceptibility to type 1 diabetes mellitus in the Taiwanese population. *Clin Endocrinol (Oxf)* 2000 52(5):575–80.

Chiodini RJ. (1989) Crohn's disease and the mycobacterioses: a review and comparison of two disease entities. *Clin Microbiol Rev* 1989; 2: 90–117

Click RE, Van Kampen CL. (2010) Assessment of Dietzia subsp. C79793-74 for treatment of cattle with evidence of paratuberculosis. *Virulence.* 2010 May-Jun 1(3):145-55.

Click RE, Van Kampen CL.(2009) Short communication: progression of Johne's disease curtailed by a probiotic. *J Dairy Sci.* 2009 Oct 92(10):4846-51.

Click RE. (2011). Successful treatment of asymptomatic or clinically terminal bovine Mycobacterium avium subspecies paratuberculosis infection (Johne's disease) with the bacterium Dietzia used as a probiotic alone or in combination with dexamethasone: Adaption to chronic human diarrheal diseases. Virulence. 2011 Mar 1;2(2).

Cossu D, Cocco E, Paccagnini D, Masala S, Ahmed N, et al. (2011) Association of Mycobacterium avium subsp. paratuberculosis with Multiple Sclerosis in Sardinian Patients. PLoS ONE 6(4): e18482. doi:10.1371/journal.pone.0018482

Collins, MT. (2003) *International Handbook of Foodborne Pathogens* Edited by Marianne D. Miliotis and Jeffrey W. Bier CRC Press 2003

Collins MT. (2003) Paratuberculosis: review of present knowledge. *Acta Vet Scand* 44: 217–221.

D'Amore M, Lisi S, Sisto M, Cucci L, Dow CT.(2010) Molecular identification of Mycobacterium avium subspecies paratuberculosis in an Italian patient with Hashimoto's thyroiditis and Melkersson-Rosenthal syndrome. *J Med Microbiol.* 2010 Jan 59(Pt 1):137-9

Danieli MG, Candela M, Ricciatti AM, et al. Antibodies to mycobacterial 65 kDa heat shock protein in systemic sclerosis (scleroderma). *J Autoimmun* 1992 5(4):443–5.

Deluca HF, Cantorna MT. (2001) Vitamin D: its role and uses in immunology. *FASEB J* 2001 15(14): 2579–85

de Wit E, van der Merwe L, van Helden PD, Hoal EG. (2010) Gene-gene interaction between tuberculosis candidate genes in a South African population. Mamm Genome. 2010 Aug 27.

Direskeneli H, Saruhan-Direskeneli G. (2003) The role of heat shock proteins in Behcet's disease. *Clin Exp Rheumatol* 2003 21(Suppl. 30):S44–8.

Dow, CT. (2005) Paratuberculosis and Type I Diabetes -Mapping the TRIGR- In: *Proceedings of the 8th International Colloquium on Paratuberculosis.* August 2005, Denmark: Copenhagen; Available from: http://www.paratuberculosis.org/pubs/proc8/abst3b_o20.htm

Dow CT. (2006) Paratuberculosis and Type I diabetes: is this the trigger? *Med Hypotheses.* 2006 67(4):782-5. Epub 2006 Jul 7

Dow CT, Ellingson JL. (2010) Detection of Mycobacterium avium ss. Paratuberculosis in Blau Syndrome Tissues. *Autoimmune Dis.* 2010 Jun 20 2010:127692.

Dubaniewicz A, Jamieson SE, Dubaniewicz-Wybieralska M, Fakiola M, Nancy Miller E, Blackwell JM. (2005)Association between SLC11A1 (formerly NRAMP1) and the risk of sarcoidosis in Poland. *Eur J Hum Genet.* 2005 Jul 13(7):829-34.

Eisenbarth GS. (1986) Type I diabetes mellitus. A chronic autoimmune disease. N Engl J Med 1986 314(21):1360–8.

Elias D, Markovits D, Reshef T, van der Zee R, Cohen IR. (1990) Induction and therapy of autoimmune diabetes in the non-obese diabetic (NOD/Lt) mouse by a 65-kDa heat shock protein. *Proc Natl Acad Sci U S A.* 1990 Feb 87(4):1576-80.

Elias D, Reshef T, Birk OS, van der Zee R, Walker MD, Cohen IR. (1991) Vaccination against autoimmune mouse diabetes with a T-cell epitope of the human 65-kDa heat shock protein. *Proc Natl Acad Sci U S A.* 1991 Apr 15 88(8):3088-91

Elias D, Marcus H, Reshef T, Ablamunits V, Cohen IR. (1995) Induction of diabetes in standard mice by immunization with the p277 peptide of a 60-kDa heat shock protein. *Eur J Immunol.* 1995 Oct 25(10):2851-7.

Elias D, Cohen IR. (1994) Peptide therapy for diabetes in NOD mice. *Lancet.* 1994 Mar 19 343(8899):704-6.

Elias D, Cohen IR. (1995) Treatment of autoimmune diabetes and insulitis in NOD mice with heat shock protein 60 peptide p 277 *Diabetes.* 1995 Sep 44(9):1132-8.

Elias D, Cohen IR.(1996)The hsp60 peptide p277 arrests the autoimmune diabetes induced by the toxin streptozotocin. *Diabetes.* 1996 Sep 45(9):1168-72.

Ellingson JL, Anderson JL, Koziczkowski JJ, Radcliff RP, Sloan SJ, Allen SE, Sullivan NM. (2005) Detection of viable Mycobacterium avium subsp. paratuberculosis in retail pasteurized whole milk by two culture methods and PCR. *J Food Prot.* 2005 May 68(5):966-72.

el-Zaatari FAk, Naser SA, Markesich D C, Kalter DC, Engstand L, and Graham DY (1996) Identification of
Mycobacterium avium complex in sarcoidosis. *Journal of Clinical Microbiology,* vol. 34, no. 9, pp. 2240–2245, 1996.

Falkinham JO III. (2003) Factors influencing the chlorine susceptibility of Mycobacterium avium, Mycobacterium intracellulare, and Mycobacterium scrofulaceum. *Applied and environmental microbiology* 2003, 69:5685-5689.

Falkinham JO, III, Norton CD, LeChevallier MW (2001) Factors influencing numbers of Mycobacterium avium, Mycobacterium intracellulare, and other Mycobacteria in drinking water distribution systems. *Applied and environmental microbiology* 2001, 67:1225-1231.

Feller, M., K. Huwiler, R. Stephan, E. Altpeter, A. Shang, H. Furrer, G. E. Pfyffer, T. Jemmi, A. Baumgartner, and M. Egger. (2007) Mycobacterium avium subspecies paratuberculosis and Crohn's disease: a systematic review and meta-analysis. *Lancet Infect Dis* 7:607-613.

Franke A, et al. (2010) Genome-wide meta-analysis increases to 71 the number of confirmed Crohn's disease susceptibility loci. Nat Genet. 2010 Dec 42(12):1118-25.

Frothingham R. (1999) Evolutionary bottlenecks in the agents of tuberculosis, leprosy, and paratuberculosis. Med Hypotheses 1999 52(2):95–9

Gazouli M, Atsaves V, Mantzaris G, Economou M, Nasioulas G, Evangelou K, Archimandritis AJ, Anagnou NP. (2008a) Role of functional polymorphisms of NRAMP1 gene for the development of Crohn's disease. *Inflamm Bowel Dis* 2008; 14: 1323-1330

Gazouli M, Sechi L, Paccagnini D, Sotgiu S, Arru G, et al. (2008b) NRAMP1 polymorphism and viral factors in Sardinian multiple sclerosis patients. Can J Neurol Sciences 35: 491–494.

Gerstein HC. (1994) Cow's milk exposure and Type I diabetes mellitus. A critical overview of the clinical literature. *Diabetes Care* 1994; 17(1):13–9.

Gimeno SG, de Souza JM. (1997) DM and milk consumption. A case-control study in Sao Paulo, Brazil. Diabetes Care 1997 20(8): 1256–60.

Girardin S. E., Hugot J.-P., and Sansonetti P. J. (2003) Lessons from Nod2 studies: towards a link between Crohn's disease and bacterial sensing, *Trends in Immunology*, vol. 24, no. 12, pp. 652–658, 2003.

Grewal SK, Rajeev S, Sreevatsan S, Michel FC Jr. (2006) Persistence of Mycobacterium avium subsp. paratuberculosis and other zoonotic pathogens during simulated composting, manure packing, and liquid storage of dairy manure. *Appl Environ Microbiol* 72: 565–574.

Groenendaal H, Zagmutt FJ. (2008) Scenario analysis of changes in consumption of dairy products caused by a hypothetical causal link between Mycobacterium avium subspecies paratuberculosis and Crohn's disease.*J Dairy Sci.* 2008 Aug 91(8):3245-58.

Guilherme L, Faé K, Oshiro SE, Kalil J. (2005) Molecular pathogenesis of rheumatic fever and rheumatic heart disease. *Expert Rev Mol Med.* 2005 Dec 8;7(28):1-15.

Gwozdz JM, Thompson KG, Manktelow BW, Murray A, West DM. (2000) Vaccination against paratuberculosis of lambs already infected experimentally with Mycobacterium avium subspecies paratuberculosis. *Aust Vet J.* 2000 78:560–566.

Hackam DJ, Rotstein OD, Zhang W, Gruenheid S, Gros P, Grinstein S. (1998) Host resistance to intracellular infection: mutation of natural resistance-associated macrophage protein 1 (Nramp1) impairs phagosomal acidification. *J Exp Med* 1998 188(2):351–64.

Hampe J., Grebe J., Nikolaus S. et al., (2002) Association of NOD2 (CARD 15) genotype with clinical course of Crohn's disease: a cohort study, *Lancet*, vol. 359, no. 9318, pp. 1661–1665, 2002.

Hatta M, Ratnawati, Tanaka M, Ito J, Shirakawa T, Kawabata M. (2010) NRAMP1/SLC11A1 gene polymorphisms and host susceptibility to Mycobacterium tuberculosis and M. leprae in South Sulawesi, Indonesia. *Southeast Asian J Trop Med Public Health.* 2010 Mar 41(2):386-94.

Hayes CE, Nashold FE, Spach KM, Pedersen LB. (2003) The immunological functions of the vitamin D endocrine system. *Cell Mol Biol* (Noisy-le-grand) 2003. 49(2):277–300 [Review].

Hermon-Taylor J, Bull TJ, Sheridan JM, Cheng J, Stellakis ML, et al. (2000) Causation of Crohn's disease by Mycobacterium avium subspecies paratuberculosis. *Can J Gastroenterol* 14: 521–539.

Hermon-Taylor J. (2002) Treatment with drugs active against Mycobacterium avium subspecies paratuberculosis can heal Crohn's disease: more evidence for a neglected public health tragedy. *Dig Liver Dis.* 2002 Jan 34(1):9-12.

Hilborn ED, Covert TC, Yakrus MA, Harris SI, Donnelly SF, Rice EW, Toney S, Bailey SA, Stelma GN, Jr. (2006) Persistence of nontuberculous mycobacteria in a drinking water system after addition of filtration treatment. *Applied and environmental microbiology* 2006, 72:5864-5869.

Hruska K, Bartos M, Kralik P, Pavlik I. (2005) Mycobacterium avium subsp. paratuberculosis in powdered infant milk: paratuberculosis in cattle - the public health problem to be solved. *Vet. Med. 0 Czech*, 2005 50, (8); 327-335

Hugot J.-P., Chamaillard M., Zouali H., et al. (2001) Association of NOD2 leucine-rich repeat variants with susceptibility to Crohn's disease, *Nature*, vol. 411, no. 6837, pp. 599–603, 2001.

Inohara N., Ogura Y., Fontalba A., et al. (2003) Host recognition of bacterial muramyl dipeptide mediated through NOD2: implications for Crohn's disease, *Journal of Biological Chemistry*, vol. 278, no. 8, pp. 5509–5512, 2003.

Jarjour WN, Jeffries BD, Davis 4th JS, et al. (1991) Autoantibodies to human stress proteins. A survey of various rheumatic and other inflammatory diseases. *Arthritis Rheum* 1991 34(9):1133–8.

Jindal S, Dudani AK, Singh B, Harley CB, Gupta RS. (1989) Primary structure of a human mitochondrial protein homologous to the bacterial and plant chaperonins and to the 65-kilodalton mycobacterial antigen. *Mol Cell Biol* 1989 9(5):2279–83.

Jo EK. (2010) Innate immunity to mycobacteria: vitamin D and autophagy. *Cell Microbiol.* 2010 Aug 12(8):026-35. Epub 2010 Jun 14.

Jones DB, Hunter NR, Duff GW. (1990) Heat-shock protein 65 as a beta cell antigen of insulin-dependent diabetes. *Lancet.* 1990 Sep 8 336(8715):583-5.

Kanazawa N., Okafuji I., Kambe N. et al., (2005) Early-onset sarcoidosis and CARD15 mutations with constitutive nuclear factor-κB activation: common genetic etiology with Blau syndrome, *Blood*, vol. 105, no. 3, pp. 1195–1197, 2005.

Kaplan MH, SVEC KH. (1964) Immunologic relation of streptococcal and tissue antigens. III. Presence in human sera of streptococcal antibody cross-reactive with heart tissue. Association with streptococcal infection, rheumatic fever, and glomerulonephritis. *J Exp Med.* 1964 Apr 1;119:65166.

Kirvan CA, Swedo SE, Heuser JS, Cunningham MW. (2003) Mimicry and autoantibody-mediated neuronal cell signaling in Sydenham chorea. *Nat Med.* 2003 Jul 9(7):914-20.

Knip M, Virtanen SM, Seppä K, Ilonen J, Savilahti E, Vaarala O, Reunanen A, Teramo K, Hämäläinen AM, Paronen J, Dosch HM, Hakulinen T, Akerblom HK (2010) Dietary intervention in infancy and later signs of beta-cell autoimmunity. Finnish TRIGR Study Group. *N Engl J Med.* 2010 Nov 11;363(20):1900-8

Kormendy B. (1994) The effect of vaccination on the prevalence of paratuberculosis in large dairy herds. *Vet Microbiol.* 1994 41:117–125.

Korou LM, Liandris E, Gazouli M, Ikonomopoulos J. (2010) Investigation of the association of the SLC11A1 gene with resistance/sensitivity of goats (Capra hircus) to paratuberculosis. *Vet Microbiol.* 2010 Aug 26;144(3-4):353-8. Epub 2010 Jan 28.

Kotlowski R, Bernstein CN, Silverberg MS, Krause DO. (2008) Population-based case-control study of alpha 1-antitrypsin and SLC11A1 in Crohn's disease and ulcerative colitis. *Inflamm Bowel Dis* 2008; 14: 1112-1117

Kotze MJ, de Villiers JN, Rooney RN, Grobbelaar JJ, Mansvelt EP, Bouwens CS, Carr J, Stander I, du Plessis L. (2001) Analysis of the NRAMP1 gene implicated in iron transport: association with multiple sclerosis and age effects. *Blood Cells Mol Dis* 2001; 27: 44-53

Knip M, Veijola R, Virtanen SM, Hyöty H, Vaarala O, Akerblom HK. (2005) Environmental triggers and determinants of type 1 diabetes. *Diabetes*. 2005 Dec 54 Suppl 2:S125-36.

Lacher M, Helmbrecht J, Schroepf S, Koletzko S, Ballauff A, Classen M, Uhlig H, Hubertus J, Hartl D, Lohse P, von Schweinitz D, Kappler R. (2010) NOD2 mutations predict the risk for surgery in pediatric-onset Crohn's disease. J Pediatr Surg. 2010 Aug 45(8):1591-7.

Lamb JR, Young DB. T (1990) cell recognition of stress proteins. A link between infectious and autoimmune disease. *Mol Biol Med* 1990 7(4):311–21

Lapham AS, Phillips ES, Barton CH. (2004) Transcriptional control of Nramp1: a paradigm for the repressive action of c-Myc. *Biochem Soc Trans* 2004 32(Pt 6):1084–6.

Lesage S., Zouali H., C´ezard J.P., et al. (2002) CARD15/NOD2 mutational analysis and genotype-phenotype correlation in 612 patients with inflammatory bowel disease, *American Journal of Human Genetics*, vol. 70, no. 4, pp. 845–857, 2002.

Liang J, Aihua Z, Yu W, Yong L, Jingjing L. (2010) HSP65 serves as an immunogenic carrier for a diabetogenic peptide P277 inducing anti-inflammatory immune response in NOD mice by nasal administration. *Vaccine*. 2010 Apr 26;28(19):3312-7. Epub 2010 Mar 10.

Maahs DM, West NA, Lawrence JM, Mayer-Davis EJ. (2010) Epidemiology of type 1 diabetes. *Endocr Metab Clin North Am*, 2010 Sep 39(3):481-97.

Mackintosh CG, Labes RE, Griffin JF. (2005) The effect of Johne's vaccination on tuberculin testing in farmed red deer (Cervus elaphus). *N Z Vet J*. 2005 53:216

Marti G, Audi L, Esteban C, et al. (2004) Association of vitamin D receptor gene polymorphism with type 1 diabetes mellitusin two Spanish populations. *Med Clin (Barc)* 2004 123(8):286–90 [in Spanish].

McDermott MF, Ramachandran A, Ogunkolade BW, Aganna E, Curtis D, Boucher BJ, et al. (1997) Allelic variation in the vitamin D receptor influences susceptibility to IDDM in Indian Asians. *Diabetologia* 1997 40(8):971–5.

McFadden JJ, Butcher PD, Chiodini R, Hermon-Taylor J. (1987) Crohn's disease-isolated mycobacteria are identical to *M. para*, as determined by DNA probes that distinguish between mycobacterial species. *J Clin Microbiol* 1987; 25: 796–801.

Mendoza JL, San-Pedro A, Culebras E, Cíes R, Taxonera C, Lana R, Urcelay E, de la Torre F, Picazo JJ, Díaz-Rubio M. (2010) High prevalence of viable Mycobacterium avium subspecies paratuberculosis in Crohn's disease. *World J Gastroenterol*. 2010 Sep 28 16(36):4558-63

Miceli-Richard C., Lesage S., Rybojad M. et al. (2001) CARD15 mutations in Blau syndrome, *Nature Genetics*, vol. 29, no. 1, pp. 19–20, 2001.

Millar D, Ford J, Sanderson J, Withey S, Tizard M, et al. (1996) IS900 PCR to detect Mycobacterium paratuberculosis in retail supplies of whole pasteurized cows' milk in England and Wales. *Appl Environ Microbiol* 1996 62: 3446–3452.

Miyata M, Kogure A, Sato H, et al. (1995) Detection of antibodies to 65 KD heat shock protein and to human superoxide dismutase in autoimmune hepatitis-molecular mimicry between 65 KD heat shock protein and superoxide dismutase. *Clin Rheumatol* 1995 14(6):673–7.

Motohashi Y, Yamada S, Yanagawa T, et al. (2003) Vitamin D receptor gene polymorphism affects onset pattern of type 1 diabetes. J *Clin Endocrinol Metab*. 2003 88(7): 3137–40.

Moudgil KD, Chang TT, Eradat H, et al. (1997) Diversification of T cell responses to carboxy-terminal determinants within the 65 kD heat-shock protein is involved in regulation of autoimmune arthritis. *J Exp Med* 1997 185(7):1307–16.

Muskens J, van Zijderveld F, Eger A, Bakker D. (2002) Evaluation of the long-term immune response in cattle after vaccination against paratuberculosis in two Dutch dairy herds. *Vet Microbiol.* 2002 86:269–278.

Naser SA, Ghobrial G, Romero C, Valentine JF. (2004) Culture of Mycobacterium avium subspeciesparatuberculosis from the blood of patients with Crohn's disease. *Lancet.* 2004 Sep 18-24 364(9439):1039-44.

Naser SA, Collins MT, Crawford JT , Valentine JF. Culture of *Mycobacterium avium* subspecies *paratuberculosis* (MAP) from the Blood of Patients with Crohn's disease: A Follow-Up Blind Multi Center Investigation. The Open Inflammation Journal, 2009, *2*, 22-23

Nerup J, Platz P, Andersen OO, Christy M, Lyngsoe J. (1974) HL-A antigens and diabetes mellitus. *Lancet.* 2: 864–866, 1974.

Olbe L: Concept of Crohn's disease being conditioned by four main components, and irritable bowel syndrome being an incomplete Crohn's disease. *Scand J Gastroenterol* 2008, 43:234-241.

Oldstone MB. (1987) Molecular mimicry and autoimmune disease. *Cell* 1987 50(6):819–20.

Paccagnini D, Sieswerda L, Rosu V, Masala S, Pacifico A, Gazouli M, Ikonomopoulos J, Ahmed N, Zanetti S, Sechi LA. (2009) Linking chronic infection and autoimmune diseases: Mycobacterium avium subspecies paratuberculosis, SLC11A1 polymorphisms and type-1 diabetes mellitus. *PLoS One.* 2009 Sep 214(9):e7109.

Pani MA, Knapp M, Donner H, Braun J, Baur MP, Usadel KH, et al. (2000) Vitamin D receptor allele combinations influencegenetic susceptibility to type 1 diabetes in Germans. Diabetes 2000;49(3):504–7.

Parsell DA, Lindquist S. (1993) The function of heat shock proteins in stress tolerance: Degradation and reactivation of damaged proteins. *Annu Rev Genet* 1993 27:437–96.

Peng H, Hagopian W. (2006) Environmental factors in the development of Type 1 diabetes. *Rev Endocr Metab Disord.* 2006 Sep 7(3):149-62. Review.

Pickup RW, Rhodes G, Arnott S, Sidi-Boumedine K, Bull TJ, et al. (2005) Mycobacterium avium subsp. paratuberculosis in the catchment area and water of the River Taff in South Wales, United Kingdom, and its potential relationship to clustering of Crohn's disease cases in the city of Cardiff. *Appl Environ Microbiol* 71: 2130–2139.

Pickup RW, Rhodes G, Bull TJ, Arnott S, Sidi-Boumedine K, et al. (2006) Mycobacterium avium subsp. paratuberculosis in lake catchments, in river water abstracted for domestic use, and in effluent from domestic sewage treatment works: diverse opportunities for environmental cycling and human exposure. *Appl Environ Microbiol* 2006 72: 4067–4077.

Purdie AC, Plain KM, Begg DJ, de Silva K, Whittington RJ. (2011) Candidate gene and genome-wide association studies of Mycobacterium avium subsp. paratuberculosis infection in cattle and sheep: A review. *Comp Immunol Microbiol Infect Dis.* 2011 Jan 7.

Quayle AJ, Wilson KB, Li SG, et al. (1992) Peptide recognition, T cell receptor usage and HLA restriction elements of human heat-shock protein (hsp) 60 and mycobacterial

65 kDa hspreactive T cell clones from rheumatoid synovial fluid. *Eur J Immunol* 1992;22(5):1315–22.

Raska M, Weigl E. (2005) Heat shock proteins in autoimmune diseases. *Biomed Pap Med Fac Univ Palacky Olomouc Czech Repub* 2005 149(2):243–9.

Rose C. D., Doyle T. M., McIlvain-Simpson G. et al. (2005) Blau syndrome mutation of CARD15/NOD2 in sporadic early onset granulomatous arthritis, *Journal of Rheumatology*,vol. 32, no. 2, pp. 373–375, 2005.

Rosu V, Ahmed N, Paccagnini D, Gerlach G, Fadda G, Hasnain SE, Zanetti S, Sechi LA. (2009) Specific immunoassays confirm association of Mycobacterium avium Subsp. paratuberculosis with type-1 but not type-2 diabetes mellitus. *PLoS One.* 2009;4(2):e4386. Epub 2009 Feb 10.

Roupie V, Rosseels V, Piersoel V, Zinniel DK, Barletta RG, Huygen K. (2008) Genetic resistance of mice to Mycobacterium paratuberculosis is influenced by Slc11a1 at the early but not at the late stage of infection. *Infect Immun.* 2008 May 76(5):2099-105. Epub 2008 Feb 19.

Ruiz-Larrañaga O, Garrido JM, Manzano C, Iriondo M, Molina E, Gil A, Koets AP, Rutten VP, Juste RA, Estonba A. (2010) Identification of single nucleotide polymorphisms in the bovine solute carrier family 11 member 1 (SLC11A1) gene and their association with infection by Mycobacterium avium subspecies paratuberculosis. *J Dairy Sci.* 2010 Apr 93(4):1713-21

Scanu AM, Bull TJ, Cannas S, Sanderson JD, Sechi LA, Dettori G, Zanetti S, Hermon-Taylor J. (2007) Mycobacterium avium subspecies paratuberculosis infection in cases of irritable bowel syndrome and comparison with Crohn's disease and Johne's disease: common neural and immune pathogenicities. *J Clin Microbiol.* 2007 Dec 45(12):3883-90

Sechi LA, Mura M, Tanda F, Lissia A, Solinas A, Fadda G, Zanetti S. (2001) Identification of Mycobacterium avium subsp. paratuberculosis in biopsy specimens from patients with Crohn's disease identified by in situ hybridization. *J Clin Microbiol.* 2001 Dec 39(12):4514-7.

Sechi LA, Scanu AM, Molicotti P, Cannas S, Mura M, Dettori G, Fadda G, Zanetti S. (2005) Detection and Isolation of Mycobacterium avium subspecies paratuberculosis from intestinal mucosal biopsies of patients with and without Crohn's disease in Sardinia. *Am J Gastroenterol.* 2005 Jul 100(7):1529-36.

Sechi LA, Ruehl A, Ahmed N, Usai D, Paccagnini D, Felis GE, Zanetti S. (2007) Mycobacterium avium subspecies paratuberculosis infects and multiplies in enteric glial cells. *World J Gastroenterol.* 2007 Nov 21;13(43):5731-5.

Sechi LA, Gazouli M, Sieswerda LE, Molicotti P, Ahmed N, Ikonomopoulos J, Scanu AM, Paccagnini D, Zanetti S. (2006) Relationship between Crohn's disease, infection with Mycobacterium avium subspecies paratuberculosis and SLC11A1 gene polymorphisms in Sardinian patients. *World J Gastroenterol.* 2006 Nov 28;12(44):7161-4.

Sechi LA, Paccagnini D, Salza S, Pacifico A, Ahmed N, Zanetti S. (2008) Mycobacterium avium subspecies paratuberculosis bacteremia in type 1 diabetes mellitus: an infectious trigger? *Clin Infect Dis.* 2008 Jan 1;46(1):148-9. No abstract available.

Sechi LA, Rosu V, Pacifico A, Fadda G, Ahmed N, Zanetti S. (2008) Humoral immune responses of type 1 diabetes patients to Mycobacterium avium subsp.

paratuberculosis lend support to the infectious trigger hypothesis. (2008) *Clin Vaccine Immunol.* 2008 Feb 15(2):320-6. Epub 2007 Dec 12.

Sechi LA, Mara L, Cappai P, Frothingam R, Ortu S, Leoni A, Ahmed N, Zanetti S. (2006) Immunization with DNA vaccines encoding different mycobacterial antigens elicits a Th1 type immune response in lambs and protects against Mycobacterium avium subspecies paratuberculosis infection. *Vaccine.* 2006 Jan 16 24(3):229-35

Singal DP, Blajchman MA. Histocompatibility (1973) (HL-A) antigens, lymphocytotoxic antibodies and tissue antibodies in patients with diabetes mellitus. *Diabetes.* 22: 429–432, 1973.

Sisto M, Cucci L, D'Amore M, Dow TC, Mitolo V, Lisi S. (2010) Proposing a relationship between Mycobacterium avium subspecies paratuberculosis infection and Hashimoto's thyroiditis. *Scand J Infect Dis.* 2010 Oct 42(10):787-90.

Skrabic V, Zemunik T, Situm M, Terzic J.(2003) Vitamin D receptor polymorphism and susceptibility to type 1 diabetes in the Dalmatian population. *Diabetes Res Clin Pract* 2003 59(1):31–5.

Stabel JR. (1998) Johne's disease: a hidden threat. *J Dairy Sci.* 1998 Jan 81(1):283-8. Review.

Stienstra Y, van der Werf TS, Oosterom E, Nolte IM, van der Graaf WT, Etuaful S, Raghunathan PL, Whitney EA, Ampadu EO, Asamoa K, Klutse EY, te Meerman GJ, Tappero JW, Ashford DA, van der Steege G. (2006)Susceptibility to Buruli ulcer is associated with the SLC11A1 (NRAMP1) D543N polymorphism. *Genes Immun.* 2006 Apr 7(3):185-9.

Takahashi K, Satoh J, Kojima Y, Negoro K, Hirai M, Hinokio Y, Kinouchi Y, Suzuki S, Matsuura N,

Shimosegawa T, Oka Y. (2004) Promoter polymorphism of SLC11A1 (formerly NRAMP1) confers susceptibility to autoimmune type 1 diabetes mellitus in Japanese. *Tissue Antigens.* 2004 Mar 63(3):231-6.

Tao B, Pietropaolo M, Atkinson M, Schatz D, Taylor D. (2010) Estimating the cost of type 1 diabetes in the U.S.: a propensity score matching method. PLoS One. 2010 Jul 9;5(7):e11501.

Tatchou-Nyamsi-Konig JA, Dailloux M, Block JC (2009) Survival of Mycobacterium avium attached to polyethylene terephtalate (PET) water bottles. *J Appl Microbiol* 2009, 106:825-832.

Ting J. P.-Y., and Davis B. K. (2005) CATERPILLER: a novel gene family important in immunity, cell death, and diseases, *Annual Review of Immunology*, vol. 23, pp. 387–414, 2005. E

Tavornpanich, S., W. O. Johnson, R. J. Anderson, and I. A. Gardner. (2008) Herd characteristics and management practices associated with seroprevalence of *Mycobacterium avium* subspecies *paratuberculosis* infection in dairy herds. Am. J. Vet. Res. 69:904–911.

Vaerewijck MJ, Huys G, Palomino JC, Swings J, Portaels F (2005) Mycobacteria in drinking water distribution systems: ecology and significance for human health. *FEMS Microbiol Rev* 2005, 29:911-934.

van Schaik G, Kalis CH, Benedictus G, Dijkhuizen AA, Huirne RB. (1996) Cost-benefit analysis of vaccination against paratuberculosis in dairy cattle. *Vet Rec.* 1996 139:624–627.

Vilagut L, Pares A, Vinas O, et al. (1992) Antibodies to mycobacterial 65 kD heat shock protein cross-react with the main mitochondrial antigens in patients with primary biliary cirrhosis. Eur J Clin Invest 1997 27(8):667–72.

Wang X., Kuivaniemi H., Bonavita G., et al. (2002) CARD15 mutations in familial granulomatosis syndromes: a study of the original Blau syndrome kindred and other families with large-vessel arteritis and cranial neuropathy, *Arthritis and Rheumatism*, vol. 46, no. 11, pp. 3041–3045, 2002

Whan L, Ball HJ, Grant IR, Rowe MT. (2005) Occurrence of Mycobacterium avium subsp. paratuberculosis in untreated water in Northern Ireland. *Appl Environ Microbiol* 2006 71: 7107–7112.

Wyllie S, Seu P, Goss JA. (2002) The natural resistance-associatedmacrophage protein 1 Slc11a1 (formerly Nramp1) and iron metabolism in macrophages. *Microbes Infect* 2002 4 (3):351–9

Yokota S, Tsubaki S, Kuriyama T, et al. (1993) Presence in Kawasaki disease of antibodies to mycobacterial heatshock protein HSP65 and autoantibodies to epitopes of human HSP65 cognate antigen. *Clin Immunol Immunopathol* 1993 67:163–70.

Zella JB, DeLuca HF. (2003) Vitamin D and autoimmune diabetes. J *Cell Biochem* 2003 88(2):216–22

Part 4

Imaging

12

In Vivo Monitoring of Inflammation and Regulation in Type 1 Diabetes

Mi-Heon Lee[1,3], Sonya Liu[2], Wen-Hui Lee[1] and Chih-Pin Liu[1]
[1]*Department of Immunology, Department of Diabetes and Metabolic Diseases Research, Beckman Research Institute, City of Hope, Duarte, CA,*
[2]*Department of Biochemistry, University of California, Los Angeles, Los Angeles, CA,*
[3]*Department of Surgery, David Geffen School of Medicine at UCLA, Los Angeles, CA, USA*

1. Introduction

T1D is a tissue specific and T cell–mediated autoimmune disease characterized by the inflammation of pancreatic islets, namely insulitis, resulting in selective destruction of insulin-producing beta islet cells and development of overt diabetes (Atkinson & Leiter, 1999, Bach, 1994, Mathis et al., 2001, McDevitt, 2001, Nepom & Kwok, 1998, Quinn et al., 2001). The onset of T1D is preceded by at least two main inflammatory stages during insulitis development (Bach, 1994, Robles et al., 2003). In the first stage, termed peri-insulitis, a mixed population of leukocytes, including macrophages, dendritic cells, and T cells, migrate from draining lymph nodes to the peripheral space to the islets. In the second stage, the leukocytes further migrate and infiltrate into the islets, resulting in invasive insulitis. Overt T1D will develop when the majority of insulin-producing β cells in the islets are destroyed by the invading leukocytes and insufficient insulin is produced to control blood glucose levels in the body. Among leukocytes that infiltrate the islets, the autoantigen-specific diabetogenic T cells play a critical role in development of T1D. Recruitment or homing of these diabetogenic T cells into the islets is a critical component of insulitis leading to T1D. Thus inhibition of their homing to the islets would prevent the development of insulitis and T1D. Consequently, it is necessary to understand the homing or trafficking behavior of diabetogenic T cells during the formation of peri-insulitis and invasive insulitis. The knowledge gained from studies addressing those questions is imperative to the development of early diagnosis methods and immune modulatory approaches to treat T1D.

Due to the low number and frequency of T cells specific for an autoantigenic peptide, it has been difficult to identify and trace autoantigen-specific T cells in animals. We have previously addressed this problem by generating novel MHC class II tetramers that can stain T cells specific for a self peptide recognized presented by the MHC class II molecules such as the I-Ag7 in NOD mice (Liu et al., 2000, Chen et al., 2003, You et al., 2003). Using this approach, we have been able to successfully identify and trace autoantigen-specific T cells, such as the $CD4^+$ BDC2.5 (BDC) T cells. The tissue localization of various T cell populations at any given time point can be identified using techniques such as flow cytometry and immunofluorescence. However, these methods involve an invasive approach requiring tissue removal from animals, and therefore only provide terminal data. As such, these methods cannot help us assess real-time dynamic cell migration patterns *in vivo* as a longitudinal study. Therefore, it is desirable to address the above-mentioned questions using non-invasive *in vivo* imaging approaches.

Previous studies have shown that it is possible to monitor T cells and other immune cells in deep organs in small animals (Weissleder, 1999). In particular, positron-emission tomography imaging (PET) of radio-labeled cells (Oku et al., 1994, Koike et al., 1997, Kikkawa et al., 2000, Melder et al., 2002, Adonai et al., 2002) and magnetic resonance imaging (MRI) of probe-labeled cells (Lewin et al., 2000, Dodd et al., 2001, Moore et al., 2002) have been used to image cell trafficking in small animals. In addition, *in vivo* imaging of pancreatic infiltration of $CD8^+$ T cells labeled with nanoparticles using MRI (Moore et al., 2004) has been demonstrated. These techniques offer high resolution images. However, the intensity of the probes or radio-isotopes used for labeling cells is rapidly decreased over time. This is inappropriate for *in vivo* imaging that requires long-term monitoring and evaluation of T cell trafficking in various animal tissues. Therefore, the need for a non-invasive longitudinal imaging method for use in living animals is especially relevant to studies on a chronic autoimmune disease like T1D. Such methods may be used to reveal the T cell *in vivo* behavior, the kinetics of their appearance, and their persistence in various tissues over the course of the disease and in response to therapy. Using whole body *in vivo* imaging, one can develop imaging-guided assays that help investigators to determine the timing for tissue sampling, and ex vivo assays for functional and pathological assays. Whole body *in vivo* imaging assays help investigators assess whether novel T1D treatments may be effective in preventing or intervening T1D by modulating T cell trafficking in living animals. Therefore, other than PET and MRI, alternative imaging approaches need to be developed to better understand the trafficking behavior of diabetogenic T cells in pre-clinical animal studies and to evaluate the effects of various diabetes treatment regimens on the trafficking of these T cells.

Over the past decade, new imaging technologies for monitoring molecular and cellular changes in living animals have been developed. These methods were developed to help reveal the *in vivo* migratory behavior and/or paths of vitally important lymphocytes in response to altered immune conditions. In particular, bioluminescence imaging (BLI) technology has been a promising noninvasive imaging method that can be employed not only to image lymphocyte migration *in vivo* but also longitudinally monitor their behavior under various disease conditions (Hardy et al., 2001, Costa et al., 2001, Bhaumik and Gambhir, 2002, Scheffold et al., 2002, Edinger et al., 2003). These unique features are important for studies that need to investigate the *in vivo* roles of lymphocytes in chronic autoimmune diseases such as T1D. In our studies, we have used BLI to longitudinally monitor T cell trafficking in real time in living animals. To understand the *in vivo* behavior and tissue localization of T cells involved in T1D, we have established the experimental condition in which the trafficking of autoantigen-specific diabetogenic T cells in living animals can be successfully visualized using BLI. More importantly, aided by using the BLI approach, we have been able to examine the *in vivo* roles of nTreg cells on autoantigen-specific diabetogenic T cells during the pathogenesis of T1D. These studies also have helped us to uncover the tissue localization and potential site of action of nTreg cells during the induction of immune tolerance that prevents T1D development.

In the following sections, we will review some of the results obtained from *in vivo* BLI analyses of dynamic trafficking patterns of luciferase-expressing diabetogenic T cells under various disease conditions. We will focus our discussion on the findings from studies that have examined the *in vivo* behavior of autoantigen-specific diabetogenic T cells in pre-diabetic and newly diabetic animals, under conditions that either have or have no nTreg cells present in animals. We will also review the effect of nTreg cells on trafficking of pathogenic T cells *in vivo*, and the potential role and site of action of nTreg cells during the development of T cell-mediated insulitis leading to T1D.

2. *In vivo* imaging of pathogenic T cell-mediated insulitis during development of overt type 1 diabetes

In vivo tracking of autoreactive lymphocytes in intact micro-environment and macro-environment *in vivo* in real time has been a long sought-after goal of investigators who are developing imaging techniques in the context of autoimmunity. T1D is an organ-specific autoimmune disease in which both autoreactive CD4+ and CD8+ T cells participate in the destruction of pancreatic insulin-producing islet β cells. Development of clinical symptoms of overt diabetes is preceded by a prolonged period of chronic inflammation in the islets. This is characterized by mononuclear cell infiltration of the islets that involves the recruitment and differentiation of autoreactive T cells (Liblau et al., 2002). A study aiming at understanding the role of CD8+ T cells in T1D has demonstrated pancreatic infiltration of CD8+ T cells using MRI by labeling the T cells with nanoparticles (Moore et al., 2004). In addition, the small animal imaging systems using PET or MRI have made it possible to monitor not only T cells but also other immune cells in deep organs in rodents (Weissleder, 1999, Oku et al., 1994, Koike et al., 1997, Kikkawa et al., 2000, Melder et al., 2002, Adonai et al., 2002). Although considered as sensitive techniques, these approaches are not appropriate for a longitudinal study of chronic diseases such as T1D. In addition, although intravital microscopy provides greater spatial resolution than the other imaging approaches (Jain et al., 2002), this method involves invasive procedures. In order to better image ongoing immune response and T cell trafficking in living animals, several noninvasive imaging techniques have been employed to monitor leukocytes in various disease conditions using animal models (Moore et al., 2004, Denis et al., 2004, Hardy et al., 2001, Contag et al., 1998).

Despite extensive studies on the role of T cells in T1D, their *in vivo* behavior, trafficking pattern and tissue localization over the course of chronic insulitis development leading to T1D remain unclear. In order to address these important questions, we have performed longitudinal studies using *in vivo* BLI analyses in real time to noninvasively visualize autoantigen-specific diabetogenic T cell trafficking in mice under normal and diseased conditions. These studies were performed prior to and after the development of insulitis and overt diabetes in animal models. This approach of using BLI to image T cell trafficking offers the advantages of excellent temporal analyses, cell-labeling versatility, easily accessible instrumentation, and high sensitivity of signal detection (Cao et al., 2005, Cao et al., 2004, Wetterwald et al., 2002, Hardy et al., 2001, Contag et al., 1998). It is well known that the trafficking of diabetogenic CD4+ T cells such as BDC cells to the pancreas is necessary in order to induce insulitis and cause diabetes. Diabetogenic CD4+ T cells can also facilitate the homing of CD8+ T effector cells to the islets during insulitis and diabetes development (Thivolet et al., 1991). Therefore, these T cells play an important role during T1D development. However, the longitudinal trafficking behavior of diabetogenic CD4+ T cells to the pancreas during islet inflammation and diabetes development still remains largely unclear. Although we have been able to trace T cells such as BDC cells using antigen-specific tetramers (Liu et al., 2000, You et al., 2003), these methods are invasive, requiring tissue removal from animals; hence, only terminal data can be obtained. The data obtained from non-invasive imaging analyses can help guide investigators in making decisions on tissue sampling for the invasive assays. Whole-body *in vivo* imaging such as BLI will help the investigators perform longitudinal studies that examine the *in vivo* behavior of diabetogenic T cells. Additionally, they will be able to assess whether treatments to prevent diabetes or islet graft rejection can be mediated through modulating the systemic trafficking T cells in living animals, in addition to other cellular functions.

2.1 Real time bioluminescent imaging analyses

Previous studies have shown that BLI analyses can be used to view cell trafficking in small animals, using luciferase (Luc) as an *in vivo* reporter (Hardy et al., 2001, Costa et al., 2001, Bhaumik and Gambhir, 2002, Scheffold et al., 2002, Edinger et al., 2003). Luciferase provides excellent signal to noise ratios owing to the fact that there is almost no background luminescence from mammalian tissues. The photons emitted from Luc-expressing cells that are transmitted through tissues can be detected using charge-coupled device (CCD) cameras designed for lowlight imaging. BLI allows for long-term longitudinal studies of cell-trafficking patterns because the reporter is encoded in the genome of the cells and the signal is therefore replicated during cell division, and is not diluted (Nakajima et al., 2001, Costa et al., 2001). BLI modalities that use light-generating enzymes (e.g. luciferase) and low-light imaging devices based on exquisitely sensitive CCD cameras have been developed and refined during the past decade. This system is capable of noninvasively revealing the cellular and molecular features of normal and diseased conditions *in vivo*. This approach offers the advantages of excellent temporal analyses, cell-labeling versatility, easily accessible instrumentation, and high sensitivity of signal detection (Contag et al., 1998, Hardy et al., 2001, Cao et al., 2005, Cao et al., 2004, Wetterwald et al., 2002). This approach has also been proven to be very useful for longitudinally monitoring the *in vivo* behavior of the lymphocytes that cause chronic inflammation prior to development of autoimmune or inflammatory diseases.

2.2 Noninvasive real-time *in vivo* bioluminescence imaging of diabetogenic T cell trafficking patterns

The $CD4^+$ BDC2.5 (BDC) cells are islet antigen–specific and highly diabetogenic T cells (Haskins and McDuffie, 1990, Haskins et al., 1989). Activated BDC cells from BDC TCR transgenic NOD mice (BDC mice) induce an aggressive form of diabetes (Chen et al., 2006, Katz et al., 1995). To label T cells from these animals for trafficking studies, we crossed a transgenic reporter mouse line that expresses luciferase by a strong, ubiquitous, constitutive promoter with BDC mice for more than 8 generations (luc-BDC/NOD mice) (Cao et al., 2004). This synthetic hybrid promoter is composed of the chicken β-actin promoter and the immediate early enhancer from cytomegalovirus, and thus drives expression of Luc into virtually all cells in the mice (Cao et al., 2004). Therefore, transgenic expression of the Luc transgene in BDC mice results in stable expression of Luc in all BDC cells. Using these Luc-expressing BDC/NOD mice allows for long-term longitudinal *in vivo* imaging studies of Luc^+ BDC cell trafficking to the pancreas and the islets, as well as other lymphoid and nonlymphoid tissues relative to varied degrees of disease states in animals.

It is known that transferring CD4+ BDC cells alone into NOD/scid mice failed to induce diabetes. However, cotransfer of CD4+ cell-depleted splenocytes isolated from diabetic NOD mice with CD4+ BDC cells induced accelerated diabetes in recipient mice. It has also been observed that there can be a respectful degree of peri-insulitis or invasive insulitis (Katz et al., 1995, Katz et al., 1993, Peterson & Haskins, 1996). However, the mechanisms responsible for these novel observations were not clear. At least two non-mutually exclusive possibilities exist that may explain the effect of the non-CD4 splenocytes on CD4+ BDC cells during induction of expedited diabetes: (1) The non-CD4 splenocytes may cause an altered systemic trafficking pattern of BDC cells that prevents their homing to the islets, or (2) they may exert their effect on BDC cells locally at tissue levels. We have addressed these questions in our studies which will be discussed in more detail below.

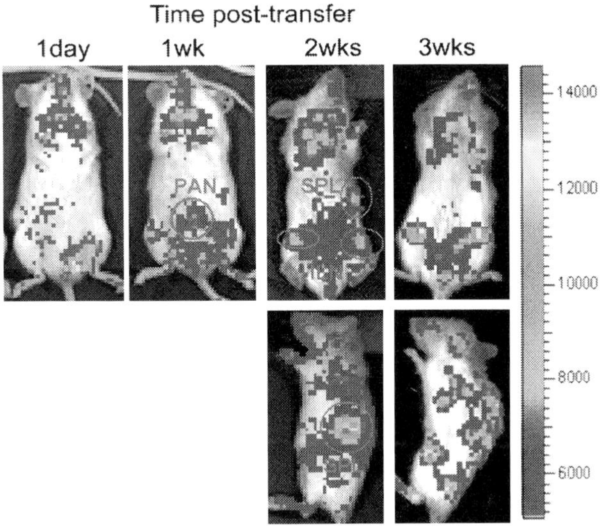

Fig. 1. Real-time *in vivo* bioluminescence imaging of luciferase-expressing primary CD4+ BDC cells. The CD4+ T cells were isolated from luc-BDC/NOD mice and i.v. injected into 9-wk old female NOD/scid mice (10x10^6 cells / mouse). The images were taken at different time points after cell transfer by a CCD camera. SPL: spleen, ILN: inguinal lymph nodes, PAN; pancreas.

We imaged BDC cells *in vivo* using BLI and compared their trafficking patterns in nondiabetic mice that received BDC cells alone with the trafficking patterns in prediabetic and newly diabetic recipients that were cotransferred with BDC cells plus CD4- splenocytes isolated from diabetic NOD mice. We also used these data to determine the best timing and the target tissues for further analyses using methods that would enable us to assess the effects of CD4+ cell-depleted splenocytes on the local patterns of BDC cells.

Using an adoptive transfer model, we have imaged Luc+ CD4+ BDC cells and examined their trafficking patterns in real time in NOD/scid mice recipients (Fig. 1). In order to monitor diabetogenic T cell trafficking patterns in real-time *in vivo* using noninvasive BLI, we first isolated CD4+ Luc+ BDC cells from Luc-BDC/NOD mice and adoptively transferred them into NOD/scid recipient mice for BLI analyses. Using this approach, we were able to visualize just the BDC cells that expressed luciferase. To perform longitudinal studies on the trafficking behavior of the $CD4^+$ BDC cells in recipient mice, the same living recipient mice were imaged at selected times over a period of 16 weeks following cell transfer. Initial signals from the transferred Luc^+ BDC cells in recipient mice were detected in their lungs on the first day after transfer. The BLI signals were then detected in other organs including the pancreas and the liver by day 3 (data not shown). We have also detected the BLI signals from Luc^+ BDC cells in lymphoid organs such as the spleen and lymph nodes within 1 week after the cell transfer (Fig. 1).

To quantify the bioluminescent signals detected from various tissues in the recipient mice, the total flux (photons/sec) was determined by drawing regions of interest (ROI) over the body corresponding to the designated organs. Based on these results, we have determined the total photon output per ROI to calculate the bioluminescence signal intensity. Each ROI was visually defined to be specific areas that correspond to selected organs from both recipient animals and control mice. The rates of increase in the *in vivo* bioluminescence signals detected in the ROI corresponding to the pancreas, spleen, and inguinal lymph nodes closely correlated with each other. These results indicate that the transferred BDC cells eventually accumulated and may also have proliferated in these tissues at the later time points, perhaps due to homeostatic expansion (Lee et al., 2007). Owing to the relatively low level of photon flux (photon/sec), especially in the pancreas at early time points, different colored bar scales were used for day 1 through day 15 (2,000–50,000) and for day 20 through day 113 (5,000–50,000). The data shown are from a representative mouse from at least 20 mice of four different experiments. The total photon flux was greatest in the spleen and lungs; the pancreas and mesenteric lymph nodes also showed significantly higher photon flux than the other tissues analyzed. The BLI signals from control mice were negligible. Quantification of luciferase activity in the dissected tissues is subject to oxygen availability in addition to levels of substrate and adenosine triphosphate. As such, it may not constitute a highly quantitative measurement. Additionally, although we cannot directly compare these *in vivo* BLI signals among different tissues without normalizing the tissue volume, we have also performed ex vivo BLI analyses by excising the tissues from the mice for BLI. The results from ex vivo BLI analyses on each tissue were confirmed by using the more quantitative FACS analyses by staining the BDC cells with BDC cell-specific I-Ag7-tetramers.

In summary, these noninvasive *in vivo* imaging studies revealed that, although BDC cells migrated to the pancreas rapidly after cell transfer, and the BLI signals of BDC cells detected in the pancreas ROI increased significantly with time, the recipient mice did not develop diabetes. Other than revealing in real time the rapid appearance of a large number of BDC cells in the pancreas without causing diabetes, these imaging results are also consistent with the idea that islet-antigen-specific diabetogenic T cells are able to traffic to the pancreas regardless of whether they induce diabetes. Therefore, these results support the notion that the recruitment and accumulation alone of a large number of diabetogenic T cells, like the BDC cells, are insufficient to induce overt diabetes.

2.3 Real time bioluminescent imaging of diabetogenic T cells during the development of insulitis leading to diabetes

The fact that a large number of Luc^+ $CD4^+$ BDC cells present in the islets did not induce diabetes in the recipient mice was not due to the introduction of luciferase transgene into

BDC mice. This is because purified Luc⁻ CD4⁺ BDC cells obtained from BDC mice of the same age in our mouse colony also did not induce diabetes in recipient mice (unpublished data). One possible explanation of these results is that the BLI analyses study was terminated before overt diabetes developed; however, the control mice receiving whole BDC mouse splenocytes develop diabetes within 6 weeks after cell transfer (Chen et al., 2006). This explanation seems unlikely because our additional studies have shown that recipient mice did not develop diabetes even at 23 weeks following the transfer of BDC cells alone (unpublished data). Alternatively, it is possible that BDC cells require the presence of other types of cells in the spleen in order to destroy the islets and induce diabetes.

It has been shown that transfer of T cells alone did not induce diabetes, and the presence of non-$CD4^+$ cells such as $CD8^+$ T cells are necessary (Bendelac et al., 1987, Christianson et al., 1993, Miller et al., 1988). Previous studies have also shown that cotransfer of the $CD4^+$ BDC cells with $CD4^+$ cell–depleted splenocytes from newly diabetic NOD mice induced accelerated diabetes in the recipient animals (Peterson and Haskins, 1996). In order to understand the trafficking behavior of BDC cells during islet inflammation that leads to diabetes, we co-transferred purified $CD4^+$ Luc^+ BDC cells and $CD4^+$ cell–depleted Luc^- splenocytes from newly diabetic NOD mice into NOD/scid recipient mice. Our results showed that the recipient mice receiving non-$CD4^+$ splenocytes alone did not develop diabetes. However, the mice that received both populations of cells developed diabetes as early as 9 days following cell transfer, and all recipient mice developed accelerated diabetes within 3 weeks.

In order to understand the behavior of BDC cells in these mice, BLI studies showed that the kinetics of Luc^+ BDC cells' trafficking in mice that were cotransferred with both $CD4^+$ Luc^+ BDC cells and $CD4^+$ cell–depleted Luc^- splenocytes from newly diabetic NOD mice were similar, at the level of the whole body and organs, to the kinetics in recipient mice that have BDC cells alone. In both types of recipients, the BDC cells migrated first to the lung in one day and then to the pancreas, inguinal lymph nodes, and spleen within one week. To further quantify and compare the changes in BLI signal intensity (total flux) in various tissues of the two different groups of recipient mice at the same time points, we imaged BDC cells and analyzed the ROI drawn on various tissues including the pancreas. The ROI analyses showed that the total BLI signal intensity gradually increased over time. A similar trend of signal intensity increase was also detected in the pancreas ROI in both cohorts, although the transferred Luc^+ BDC cells continued proliferating in the lymph organs in mice that received both cell types. Comparable levels of BLI intensity over time were detected in the lymphoid organs in both groups of mice before all the mice that received both types of cells became diabetic following a cotransfer of the cells. However, the BLI intensity in lymphoid organs increased at a faster rate in co-transferred mice during the post-diabetic period than that detected in nondiabetic mice that received BDC cells alone. Therefore, cotransfer of $CD4^-$ splenocytes led to diabetes but did not otherwise change the overall trafficking patterns of BDC cells to these tissues during the pre-diabetic stage. These results suggest that the co-transferred splenocytes may not help BDC cells to induce accelerated diabetes by modulating the trafficking and the total number of BDC cells in the pancreas. Instead, they may cause an increased proliferation of BDC cells in tissues other than the pancreas. BDC cells were able to induce insulitis in both groups of recipients, but only the co-transferred recipients developed diabetes. Therefore, it is likely that the total number of BDC cells present in the pancreas is not responsible for the development of diabetes. It may be that the cellular function of immune cells present within the islets and the microscopic localization of the cells within the tissue were the contributors to diabetes development in our studies.

Different degrees and types of insulitis may occur in the recipient animals after transfer of varied cell populations. Peri-insulitis does not lead to islet destruction, whereas invasive insulitis destroys islets and leads to diabetes. To further evaluate why the cotransferred $CD4^-$ splenocytes may help BDC cells induce accelerated diabetes, we examined whether these splenocytes promote infiltration of BDC cells into the islets and induce invasive insulitis. To make these distinctions, we performed microscopic imaging of the islets (since there is no macroscopic imaging method able to distinguish cell distribution differences at this resolution). Initial ex vivo BLI analyses of excised pancreases showed that comparable bioluminescent signals were detected in the pancreas of both groups of recipients (Lee et al., 2007). These results demonstrated that BDC cells can traffic to the pancreas independent on the presence of other splenocytes. Additonal histological analyses showed that mice co-transferred with both cell types developed more severe invasive insulitis than mice that received BDC cells alone. The islets in the pancreatic sections obtained from co-transferred mice on day 20 following cell transfer showed invasive insulitis and were severely damaged. Only peri-insulitis were detected in the islets from mice transferred with BDC cells alone and their islets remained intact. Therefore, the co-transferred splenocytes may help induce diabetes by enhancing the local infiltration of BDC cells into the islets.

We also performed FACS analyses to better understand the cellular component of the invasive insulitis found in the co-transferred mice. We found that the percentage of both $CD11b^+$ cells and $CD11c^+$ cells showed increase only in the islets of co-transferred mice (Lee et al., 2007). These results suggest that these innate immune cells are involved in promoting invasiveness of BDC cells into the islets. One possibility is that these cells help activation of BDC cells, leading to more activated BDC cells in the islets of co-transferred mice and resulting in accelerated diabetes. Investigation on the activation status of BDC cell present in the islets show that there was no difference in expression of activation markers, CD69 and CD62L, on BDC cells isolated from the islets of both cohorts. Overall, our results suggest that efficient trafficking of BDC cells alone to the pancreas is unable to induce T1D alone. The presence of $CD4^-$ splenocytes is necessary to help these pathogenic T cells locally infiltrate the islets without altering their activation status and systemic trafficking patterns.

In summary, these findings are possible because investigators have the ability to image T cell trafficking and tissue localization over a range of varied scales of techniques, from macroscopic imaging and whole-body BLI, to microscopic imaging via light microscopy of tissue sections and single cell analyses using FACS.

2.4 Application of BLI to understand the role of nTreg cells in regulating the *in vivo* behavior of diabetogenic T cells during T1D

The naturally-arised $Foxp3^+$ $CD4^+$ $CD25^+$ nTreg cells play a critical role in immune tolerance induction and autoimmune disease prevention (Sakaguchi and Powrie, 2007). It is well known that a deficiency in nTreg cells may contribute to development of insulitis and T1D in both humans and mice. Rebuilding a sufficient number of nTreg cells can re-induce immune tolerance, leading to inhibition of T1D (Herman et al., 2004, Tang et al., 2004, Tarbell et al., 2004, Brusko et al., 2005, Lindley et al., 2005, Tritt et al., 2008). Extensive studies have been performed to understand the role of nTreg cells during T1D. However, it is still largely unclear as to how these potent nTreg cells prevent destruction of the insulin-producing beta islet cells by pathogenic T cell-mediated immune responses.

As discussed in previous sections, the development of insulitis precedes development of overt T1D, and immune tolerance induced by nTreg cells often leads to prevention of insulitis in diabetes-free mice. It is conceivable that the development of insulitis involves at least four stages as outlined and depicted in Figure. 2. These include: (1) migration of antigen-presenting cells (APCs), such as macrophages and dendritic cells, to islet draining lymph nodes where the APCs can pick up islet antigens and present them to T cells; this leads to activation of autoreactive pathogenic T cells such as BDC cells in the lymph nodes, (2) expansion of activated pathogenic T cells, (3) migration of activated pathogenic T cells to the islets, and (4) infiltration of the pathogenic T cells into the islets, causing invasive insulitis and destruction of the islets. It is possible that in order to inhibit insulitis and T1D, nTreg cells may function by blocking pathogenic T cells at one of these four stages. For example, nTreg cells may modulate systemic trafficking behavior of pathogenic T effector cells such as BDC cells as well as APCs during the pre-diabetic stage. In addition to suppressing pathogenic T effector cell proliferation and expansion, nTreg cells may block

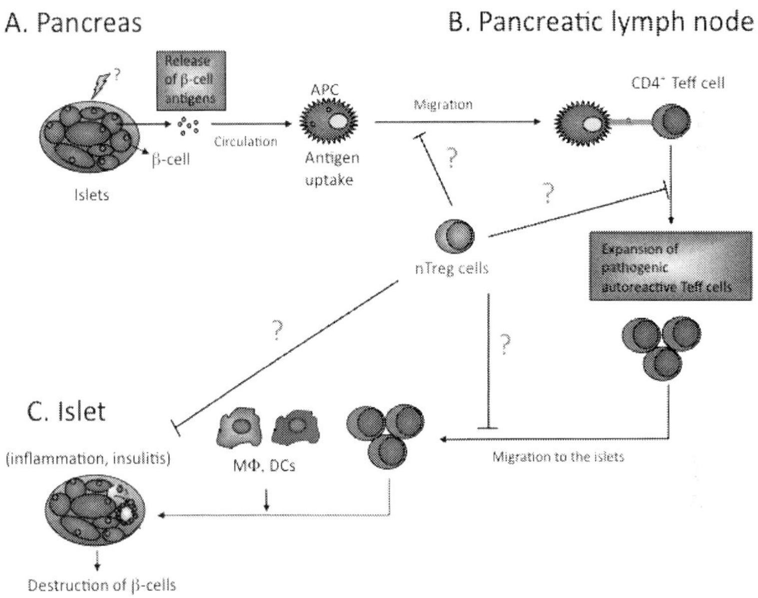

Fig. 2. Potential roles of nTreg cells in controlling T1D pathogenesis. Beta cell antigens are released from the islets into the circulation system. The islet antigens are taken up by the antigen presenting cells (APCs) that have migrated from the circulation to pancreatic draining lymph nodes. In the draining lymph nodes, islet antigen-specific pathogenic T effector cells are activated by islet antigen-loaded APCs, leading to expansion of pathogenic T cells. The expanded pathogenic T cells then traffic to the islets and induce insulitis. Another causative factor in insulitis development is the recruitment of innate immune cells such as macrophages and dendritic cells. This process eventually leads to destruction of islet beta cells and onset of overt diabetes. It is hypothesized that nTreg cells may prevent insulitis and T1D development at one of the four indicated stages.

the trafficking and homing of such T cells to the islets, resulting in inhibition of invasive insulitis that causes overt T1D. It is also possible that, in the absence of nTreg cells, the pathogenic T cells such as BDC cells may traffic more rapidly to and accumulate faster in the islets during pre-diabetic stage. This eventually leads to destruction of the insulin-producing islet beta cells and onset of diabetes.

In our studies to test these different hypotheses, we have performed several experiments, including real time imaging studies, to investigate whether BDC cells showed an altered trafficking pattern in nTreg cell-deficient mice compared to that in nTreg cell-sufficient mice. In order to examine the role of nTreg cells *in vivo* in T1D and distinguish their effects on T1D onset during the four stages of insulitis development, we have used the novel animal models described in the previous sections for imaging analyses. In these studies, as part of our approaches, we have performed noninvasive BLI-guided *in vivo* analyses of BDC cell trafficking in real-time under varied conditions in the presence or absence of nTreg cells (Lee et al., 2010). In particular, in these studies we performed experiments to address the following questions: (1) Compared to nTreg cell-deficient mice, can the trafficking and systemic tissue localization of BDC cells be modulated by nTreg cells during development of T1D? (2) Does the presence of nTreg cells affect the *in vivo* priming, activation, and expansion of BDC cells during the development of T1D? and (3) How does nTreg cells modulate BDC cell-mediated invasive insulitis during T1D?

As part of our studies to address these questions, we used a cell adoptive transfer model by transferring $CD4^+$ BDC cells into NOD/scid recipient mice. It is known that the transfer of $CD4^+$ $CD25^-$ (nTreg-deficient) BDC cells into NOD/scid mice induces aggressive T1D, whereas the transfer of $CD4^+$ (nTreg cell-sufficient) BDC cells does not cause onset of T1D in recipient mice. Therefore, to longitudinally monitor trafficking of the adoptively transferred BDC cells in mice with or without nTreg cells, we have isolated Luc^+ $CD4^+$ $CD25^-$ (nTreg-deficient) or Luc^+ $CD4^+$ (nTreg cell-sufficient) BDC cells from Luc-BDC/NOD mice. We then adoptively transferred these cells separately into NOD/scid recipient mice. Trafficking and tissue localization of the transferred Luc^+ BDC cells in the two cohorts were monitored until after the recipient mice that received Luc^+ $CD4^+$ $CD25^-$ (nTreg-deficient) BDC cells developed T1D (Lee et al., 2010).

We have performed initial macro imaging analyses using BLI on recipient mice during the pre-diabetic stages. Our *in vivo* BLI analyses results showed that, during the pre-diabetic stage on and before the fifth day after cell transfer, there was no significant difference in bioluminescence signal noted in any of the tissues examined between the two cohorts. These results suggest that the presence or absence of nTreg cells may not significantly affect the trafficking of BDC cells prior to development of T1D. On the other hand, an increased BLI signal was detected in several tissues in nTreg cell-deficient, but not control nTreg cell-sufficient mice, only at the postdiabetic stage after development of T1D on or after day 7. The reasons for this difference were unclear, but it could have been a result of a more rapid local expansion of BDC cells that migrated to and resided in these tissues in the absence of nTreg cells. These results demonstrated comparable trafficking and tissue localization of BDC cells during the prediabetic stage in both cohorts of mice. The imaging study results also suggest that nTreg cells may not prevent T1D by modulating the systemic trafficking behavior of pathogenic T cells or the expansion of such cells during the pre-diabetic stages.

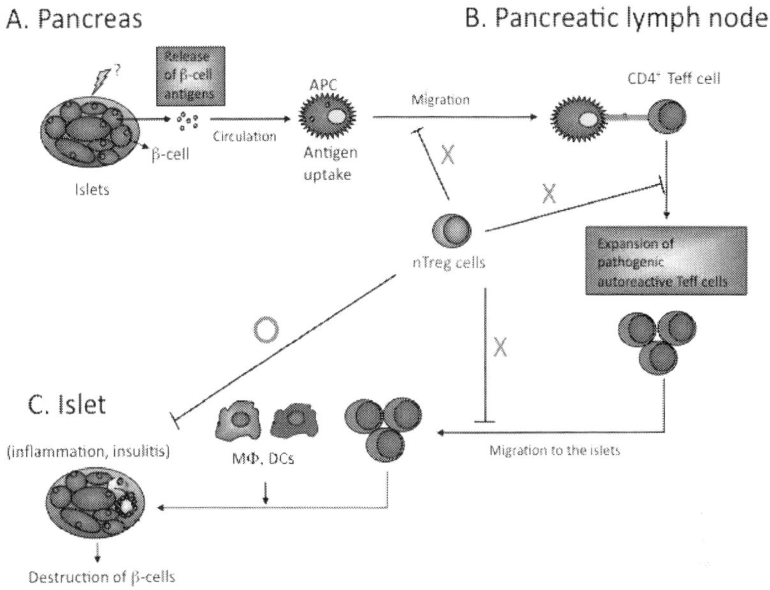

Fig. 3. The nTreg cells may prevent inulitis and T1D by functioning locally in the islets. They may negatively affect not only pathogenic T cells but also innate immune cells recruited to the islets.

In addition to macro imaging studies on systemic *in vivo* trafficking of T cells, we also determined whether nTreg cells may prevent T1D by modulating inflammatory processes locally in the islets. In particular, we performed micro imaging analyses and histological analyses of the islets. These studies showed that depletion of nTreg cells promoted progression and increased severity of insulitis in nTreg cell-deficient mice. Therefore, nTreg cell-deficient mice developed more severe invasive insulitis, compared to mostly peri-insulitis found in control nTreg cell-sufficient mice (Lee et al., 2010). However, despite these differences, the nTreg cell-deficiency did not affect the number and activation status of BDC cells during the pre-diabetic stage. These results suggested that cellular components other than or in addition to BDC T cells may be involved in the development from peri-insulitis to invasive insulitis leading to T1D. It is possible that nTreg cells helped maintain the steady-state of peri-insulitis in nTreg-sufficient mice. However, the steady-state of peri-insulitis in nTreg cell deficient mice may have been broken in the absence of nTreg cells. This in turn led to aggressive infiltration of immune cells from periphery space into the islets, resulting in invasive insulitis. Altogether, these results provide strong evidence supporting the notion that nTreg cells function locally in the islets.

Based on the results discussed above, one can hypothesize that nTreg cells can exert their function by preventing the infiltration of immune cells from the periphery space into the islets. In the absence of nTreg cells, one would expect that the cellular components of invasive insulitis would be altered in comparison to those found in peri-insulitis that are maintained by the presence of nTreg cells. In addition, the change in cellular components in the islets may be due to the nTreg cells' ability to regulate the local migration of immune cells. In studies to address these questions, we found that, compared to that in control nTreg cell-sufficient mice, the accelerated invasive insulitis in nTreg cell-deficient recipient NOD/scid mice was predominated by a population of $CD11c^+$ dendritic cells, instead of by the adoptively transferred $CD4^+$ BDC T cells (Lee et al., 2010). These results suggest that the presence of nTreg cells may inhibit islet-infiltration of $CD11c^+$ dendritic cells. Indeed, using an *in vitro* chemotaxis assay, we have found that the presence of nTreg cells were able to negatively regulate the chemotaxis of $CD11c^+$ dendritic cells isolated from the islets in NOD mice. Therefore, these novel results suggest that nTreg cells may function locally in the islets by preventing invasive islet-infiltration of innate immune cells such as $CD11c^+$ dendritic cells during development of overt T1D. In animals lacking nTreg cells, the deficiency may lead to enhanced islet infiltration of disease-promoting cells such as $CD11c^+$ dendritic cells, perhaps due to an altered response to chemokines.

In summary, using *in vivo* BLI-guided analyses, we have found that nTreg cells do not affect systemic localization of pathogenic T cells. Our results support the conclusion that nTreg cells can function locally in the islets to prevent inflammatory responses that cause invasive infiltration of innate immune cells, such as $CD11c^+$ dendritic cells, into the islets. The nTreg cells may exert such function, at least in part, by regulating their chemotaxis in the islets. Altogether, our study demonstrated that dendritic cell-dominated invasive insulitis may precede T1D onset, and nTreg cells can prevent T1D by inhibiting local invasiveness of DCs, not $CD4^+$ T cells, into the islets.

3. Conclusions and therapeutic implications

We have developed novel animal models that help investigators to perform *in vivo* BLI to visualize, in real time, the trafficking behavior of diabetogenic T cells in living animals under conditions that may or may not lead to diabetes. Based on the results obtained from these studies, we now have a better understanding of the kinetics, tissue localization, and relative cell numbers in various tissues in living animals during the development of islet inflammation and T1D. This approach is also used as an excellent initial assessment to understand the potential *in vivo* roles and site of action of nTreg cells during the development of T1D. By combining the sensitive imaging studies through performance of BLI analyses with other approaches, our studies obtained from experiments on *in vivo* nTreg cell function in adoptive transfer animal models have helped us to uncover the structural and kinetic features associated with islet destruction and T1D pathogenesis in mice. These results have demonstrated that non-invasive whole-body *in vivo* imaging-guided analyses, such as the use of BLI, is a useful and reliable tool for examining cell-trafficking patterns in animals during the onset of islet inflammation and diabetes. These methods are also useful for monitoring the potential outcomes or effects of various disease treatment regimens. For example, following treatment of chronic diseases like T1D, these approaches can help investigators to monitor the effects of the treatment on *in vivo* behavior of T cells in long-term longitudinal studies.

More importantly, these novel results demonstrate that, by combining micro and macro imaging analyses methods, the non-invasive *in vivo* imaging analyses can help guide the investigators to the times and tissues where the unique biology is taking place prior to and after development of inflammatory responses. These techniques will be a useful approach for monitoring the effects of various treatments that may regulate immune cell trafficking and inhibit diabetes. In summary, *in vivo* imaging approaches can help elucidate the temporal patterns, spatial distribution, and site of action of various immune cells in the body during the development of T1D. In addition, based on the results obtained from these *in vitro* and longitudinal *in vivo* assays, it is possible to better understand the important roles of nTreg cells during the regulation of autoimmunity and restoring of self-tolerance in the treatment for autoimmune diseases like T1D. Cell-based immunotherapy, such as the ones involving nTreg cells, has provided promising hope for treating diseases such as T1D and graft-vs-host-diseases (Roncarolo and Battaglia, 2007). The information gained from the combination of various imaging approaches, including the ones described in this chapter, should aid in the design of Treg-based novel immune therapies to treat these life-threatening diseases.

4. References

ADONAI, N., NGUYEN, K. N., WALSH, J., IYER, M., TOYOKUNI, T., PHELPS, M. E., MCCARTHY, T., MCCARTHY, D. W. & GAMBHIR, S. S. (2002). Ex vivo cell labeling with 64Cu-pyruvaldehyde-bis(N4-methylthiosemicarbazone) for imaging cell trafficking in mice with positron-emission tomography. *Proc Natl Acad Sci U S A*, 99, 3030-3035.

ATKINSON, M. A. & LEITER, E. H. (1999). The NOD mouse model of type 1 diabetes: as good as it gets? *Nat Med*, 5, 601-604.

BACH, J. F. (1994). Insulin-dependent diabetes mellitus as an autoimmune disease. *Endocr Rev*, 15, 516-542.

BENDELAC, A., CARNAUD, C., BOITARD, C. & BACH, J. F. (1987). Syngeneic transfer of autoimmune diabetes from diabetic NOD mice to healthy neonates. Requirement for both L3T4+ and Lyt-2+ T cells. *J Exp Med*, 166, 823-832.

BHAUMIK, S. & GAMBHIR, S. S. (2002). Optical imaging of Renilla luciferase reporter gene expression in living mice. *Proc Natl Acad Sci U S A*, 99, 377-382.

BRUSKO, T. M., WASSERFALL, C. H., CLARE-SALZLER, M. J., SCHATZ, D. A. & ATKINSON, M. A. (2005). Functional defects and the influence of age on the frequency of CD4+ CD25+ T-cells in type 1 diabetes. *Diabetes*, 54, 1407-1414.

CAO, Y. A., BACHMANN, M. H., BEILHACK, A., YANG, Y., TANAKA, M., SWIJNENBURG, R. J., REEVES, R., TAYLOR-EDWARDS, C., SCHULZ, S., DOYLE, T. C., FATHMAN, C. G., ROBBINS, R. C., HERZENBERG, L. A., NEGRIN, R. S. & CONTAG, C. H. (2005). Molecular imaging using labeled donor tissues reveals patterns of engraftment, rejection, and survival in transplantation. *Transplantation*, 80, 134-139.

CAO, Y. A., WAGERS, A. J., BEILHACK, A., DUSICH, J., BACHMANN, M. H., NEGRIN, R. S., WEISSMAN, I. L. & CONTAG, C. H. (2004). Shifting foci of hematopoiesis during reconstitution from single stem cells. *Proc Natl Acad Sci U S A*, 101, 221-226.

CHEN, C., LEE, W. H., YUN, P., SNOW, P. & LIU, C. P. (2003). Induction of autoantigen-specific Th2 and Tr1 regulatory T cells and modulation of autoimmune diabetes. *J Immunol*, 171, 733-744.

CHEN, C., LEE, W. H., ZHONG, L. & LIU, C. P. (2006). Regulatory T cells can mediate their function through the stimulation of APCs to produce immunosuppressive nitric oxide. *J Immunol*, 176, 3449-3460.

CHRISTIANSON, S. W., SHULTZ, L. D. & LEITER, E. H. (1993). Adoptive transfer of diabetes into immunodeficient NOD-scid/scid mice. Relative contributions of CD4+ and CD8+ T-cells from diabetic versus prediabetic NOD.NON-Thy-1a donors. *Diabetes,* 42, 44-55.

CONTAG, C. H. & ROSS, B. D. (2002). It's not just about anatomy: *in vivo* bioluminescence imaging as an eyepiece into biology. *J Magn Reson Imaging,* 16, 378-387.

CONTAG, P. R., OLOMU, I. N., STEVENSON, D. K. & CONTAG, C. H. (1998). Bioluminescent indicators in living mammals. *Nat Med,* 4, 245-247.

COSTA, G. L., SANDORA, M. R., NAKAJIMA, A., NGUYEN, E. V., TAYLOR-EDWARDS, C., SLAVIN, A. J., CONTAG, C. H., FATHMAN, C. G. & BENSON, J. M. (2001). Adoptive immunotherapy of experimental autoimmune encephalomyelitis via T cell delivery of the IL-12 p40 subunit. *J Immunol,* 167, 2379-2387.

DENIS, M. C., MAHMOOD, U., BENOIST, C., MATHIS, D. & WEISSLEDER, R. (2004). Imaging inflammation of the pancreatic islets in type 1 diabetes. *Proc Natl Acad Sci U S A,* 101, 12634-12639.

DODD, C. H., HSU, H. C., CHU, W. J., YANG, P., ZHANG, H. G., MOUNTZ, J. D., JR., ZINN, K., FORDER, J., JOSEPHSON, L., WEISSLEDER, R., MOUNTZ, J. M. & MOUNTZ, J. D. (2001). Normal T-cell response and *in vivo* magnetic resonance imaging of T cells loaded with HIV transactivator-peptide-derived superparamagnetic nanoparticles. *J Immunol Methods,* 256, 89-105.

EDINGER, M., CAO, Y. A., VERNERIS, M. R., BACHMANN, M. H., CONTAG, C. H. & NEGRIN, R. S. (2003). Revealing lymphoma growth and the efficacy of immune cell therapies using *in vivo* bioluminescence imaging. *Blood,* 101, 640-648.

HARDY, J., EDINGER, M., BACHMANN, M. H., NEGRIN, R. S., FATHMAN, C. G. & CONTAG, C. H. (2001). Bioluminescence imaging of lymphocyte trafficking *in vivo*. *Exp Hematol,* 29, 1353-1360.

HASKINS, K. & MCDUFFIE, M. (1990). Acceleration of diabetes in young NOD mice with a CD4+ islet-specific T cell clone. *Science,* 249, 1433-1436.

HASKINS, K., PORTAS, M., BERGMAN, B., LAFFERTY, K. & BRADLEY, B. (1989). Pancreatic islet-specific T-cell clones from nonobese diabetic mice. *Proc Natl Acad Sci U S A,* 86, 8000-8004.

HERMAN, A. E., FREEMAN, G. J., MATHIS, D. & BENOIST, C. (2004). CD4+CD25+ T regulatory cells dependent on ICOS promote regulation of effector cells in the prediabetic lesion. *J Exp Med,* 199, 1479-1489.

JAIN, R. K., MUNN, L. L. & FUKUMURA, D. (2002). Dissecting tumour pathophysiology using intravital microscopy. *Nat Rev Cancer,* 2, 266-276.

KATZ, J. D., BENOIST, C. & MATHIS, D. (1995). T helper cell subsets in insulin-dependent diabetes. *Science,* 268, 1185-1188.

KATZ, J. D., WANG, B., HASKINS, K., BENOIST, C. & MATHIS, D. (1993). Following a diabetogenic T cell from genesis through pathogenesis. *Cell,* 74, 1089-1100.

KIKKAWA, H., TSUKADA, H. & OKU, N. (2000). Usefulness of positron emission tomographic visualization for examination of *in vivo* susceptibility to metastasis. *Cancer,* 89, 1626-1633.

KOIKE, C., WATANABE, M., OKU, N., TSUKADA, H., IRIMURA, T. & OKADA, S. (1997). Tumor cells with organ-specific metastatic ability show distinctive trafficking *in vivo*: analyses by positron emission tomography and bioimaging. *Cancer Res,* 57, 3612-3619.

LEE, M. H., LEE, W. H., TODOROV, I. & LIU, C. P. (2010). CD4+ CD25+ regulatory T cells prevent type 1 diabetes preceded by dendritic cell-dominant invasive insulitis by affecting chemotaxis and local invasiveness of dendritic cells. *J Immunol,* 185, 2493-2501.

LEE, M. H., LEE, W. H., VAN, Y., CONTAG, C. H. & LIU, C. P. (2007). Image-guided analyses reveal that non-CD4 splenocytes contribute to CD4+ T cell-mediated inflammation leading to islet destruction by altering their local function and not systemic trafficking patterns. *Mol Imaging,* 6, 369-383.

LEWIN, M., CARLESSO, N., TUNG, C. H., TANG, X. W., CORY, D., SCADDEN, D. T. & WEISSLEDER, R. (2000). Tat peptide-derivatized magnetic nanoparticles allow *in vivo* tracking and recovery of progenitor cells. *Nat Biotechnol,* 18, 410-414.

LIBLAU, R. S., WONG, F. S., MARS, L. T. & SANTAMARIA, P. (2002). Autoreactive CD8 T cells in organ-specific autoimmunity: emerging targets for therapeutic intervention. *Immunity,* 17, 1-6.

LINDLEY, S., DAYAN, C. M., BISHOP, A., ROEP, B. O., PEAKMAN, M. & TREE, T. I. (2005). Defective suppressor function in CD4(+)CD25(+) T-cells from patients with type 1 diabetes. *Diabetes,* 54, 92-99.

LIU, C. P., JIANG, K., WU, C.-H., LEE, W.-H., LIN, W.-J. (2000). Detection of glutamic acid decarboxylase -activated T cells with I-Ag7 tetramers. *Proc. Natl. Acad. Sci. USA,* 97, 14596-14601.

MATHIS, D., VENCE, L. & BENOIST, C. (2001). beta-Cell death during progression to diabetes. *Nature,* 414, 792-798.

MCDEVITT, H. (2001). The role of MHC class II molecules in the pathogenesis and prevention of Type I diabetes. *Adv Exp Med Biol,* 490, 59-66.

MELDER, R. J., MUNN, L. L., STOLL, B. R., MARECOS, E. M., BAXTER, L. T., WEISSLEDER, R. & JAIN, R. K. (2002). Systemic distribution and tumor localization of adoptively transferred lymphocytes in mice: comparison with physiologically based pharmacokinetic model. *Neoplasia,* 4, 3-8.

MILLER, B. J., APPEL, M. C., O'NEIL, J. J. & WICKER, L. S. (1988). Both the Lyt-2+ and L3T4+ T cell subsets are required for the transfer of diabetes in nonobese diabetic mice. *J Immunol,* 140, 52-58.

MOORE, A., GRIMM, J., HAN, B. & SANTAMARIA, P. (2004). Tracking the recruitment of diabetogenic CD8+ T-cells to the pancreas in real time. *Diabetes,* 53, 1459-1466.

MOORE, A., SUN, P. Z., CORY, D., HOGEMANN, D., WEISSLEDER, R. & LIPES, M. A. (2002). MRI of insulitis in autoimmune diabetes. *Magn Reson Med,* 47, 751-758.

NAKAJIMA, A., SEROOGY, C. M., SANDORA, M. R., TARNER, I. H., COSTA, G. L., TAYLOR-EDWARDS, C., BACHMANN, M. H., CONTAG, C. H. & FATHMAN, C. G. (2001). Antigen-specific T cell-mediated gene therapy in collagen-induced arthritis. *J Clin Invest,* 107, 1293-1301.

NEPOM, G. T. & KWOK, W. W. (1998). Molecular basis for HLA-DQ associations with IDDM. *Diabetes,* 47, 1177-1184.

OKU, N., KOIKE, C., SUGAWARA, M., TSUKADA, H., IRIMURA, T. & OKADA, S. (1994). Positron emission tomography analysis of metastatic tumor cell trafficking. *Cancer Res,* 54, 2573-2576.

PETERSON, J. D. & HASKINS, K. (1996). Transfer of diabetes in the NOD-scid mouse by CD4 T-cell clones. Differential requirement for CD8 T-cells. *Diabetes,* 45, 328-336.

QUINN, A., KUMAR, V., JENSEN, K. P. & SERCARZ, E. E. (2001). Interactions of effectors and regulators are decisive in the manifestations of type 1 diabetes in nonobese diabetic mice. *Curr Dir Autoimmun,* 4, 171-192.

ROBLES, D. T., EISENBARTH, G. S., DAILEY, N. J., PETERSON, L. B. & WICKER, L. S. (2003). Insulin autoantibodies are associated with islet inflammation but not always related to diabetes progression in NOD congenic mice. *Diabetes,* 52, 882-886.

RONCAROLO, M. G. & BATTAGLIA, M. (2007). Regulatory T-cell immunotherapy for tolerance to self antigens and alloantigens in humans. *Nat Rev Immunol,* 7, 585-598.

SAKAGUCHI, S. & POWRIE, F. (2007). Emerging challenges in regulatory T cell function and biology. *Science,* 317, 627-629.

SCHEFFOLD, C., KORNACKER, M., SCHEFFOLD, Y. C., CONTAG, C. H. & NEGRIN, R. S. (2002). Visualization of effective tumor targeting by CD8+ natural killer T cells redirected with bispecific antibody F(ab')(2)HER2xCD3. *Cancer Res,* 62, 5785-5791.

TANG, Q., HENRIKSEN, K. J., BI, M., FINGER, E. B., SZOT, G., YE, J., MASTELLER, E. L., MCDEVITT, H., BONYHADI, M. & BLUESTONE, J. A. (2004). *In vitro*-expanded antigen-specific regulatory T cells suppress autoimmune diabetes. *J Exp Med,* 199, 1455-1465.

TARBELL, K. V., YAMAZAKI, S., OLSON, K., TOY, P. & STEINMAN, R. M. (2004). CD25+ CD4+ T cells, expanded with dendritic cells presenting a single autoantigenic peptide, suppress autoimmune diabetes. *J Exp Med,* 199, 1467-1477.

THIVOLET, C., BENDELAC, A., BEDOSSA, P., BACH, J. F. & CARNAUD, C. (1991). CD8+ T cell homing to the pancreas in the nonobese diabetic mouse is CD4+ T cell-dependent. *J Immunol,* 146, 85-88.

TRITT, M., SGOUROUDIS, E., D'HENNEZEL, E., ALBANESE, A. & PICCIRILLO, C. A. (2008). Functional waning of naturally occurring CD4+ regulatory T-cells contributes to the onset of autoimmune diabetes. *Diabetes,* 57, 113-123.

WEISSLEDER, R. (1999). Molecular imaging: exploring the next frontier. *Radiology,* 212, 609-614.

WETTERWALD, A., VAN DER PLUIJM, G., QUE, I., SIJMONS, B., BUIJS, J., KARPERIEN, M., LOWIK, C. W., GAUTSCHI, E., THALMANN, G. N. & CECCHINI, M. G. (2002). Optical imaging of cancer metastasis to bone marrow: a mouse model of minimal residual disease. *Am J Pathol,* 160, 1143-1153.

YOU, S., CHEN, C., LEE, W. H., WU, C. H., JUDKOWSKI, V., PINILLA, C., WILSON, D. B. & LIU, C. P. (2003). Detection and characterization of T cells specific for BDC2.5 T cell-stimulating peptides. *J Immunol,* 170, 4011-4020.

13

Imaging the Pancreatic Beta Cell

Ulf Ahlgren and Elena Kostromina
*Umeå Centre for Molecular Medicine, Umeå University, Umeå
Sweden*

1. Introduction

The development of advanced technologies for pancreatic beta-cell imaging intended for medical practice, preclinical testing and experimental diabetes research has become a field of intense study over the last decade. Insulin deficiency and hyperglycemia in type 1 diabetes (T1D) occurs as a result of selective T-cell-mediated autoimmune destruction of pancreatic beta-cells. During the first stage of T1D, known as insulitis, the islets of Langerhans are subjected to a massive invasion of a mixed population of leukocytes, followed by a selective destruction of pancreatic beta-cells. During the second stage of T1D, hyperglycemia develops as a result of impaired insulin production by damaged or disabled beta-cells (Mathis & Gaglia, 2010). In patients with T1D immune infiltration, the destruction of beta-cells and reduction in beta-cell mass (BCM) precede clinical manifestation of the disease. Furthermore, dynamic changes in BCM correlate with the time course of diabetes progression and the efficiency of anti-diabetic treatment. In clinical practice, the evaluation of islet inflammation is currently based on monitoring serum titers of antibodies directed against certain beta-cell antigens (Eisenbarth et al., 2002). The assessment of BCM is limited primarily to functional tests of insulin secretion in response to secretagogues (Robertson, 2007), the results of which reflect the specific mechanisms of beta-cell function. These diagnoses may however be affected by anti-diabetic treatments as well as other factors. Histological analyses provide the most accurate BCM determination in humans and are achieved by an examination of pancreas specimens obtained from patients undergoing pancreatic surgery. Due to the heterogeneous distribution of pancreatic islets within the pancreas, this procedure can provide BCM estimations within a specific pancreatic area rather than the whole organ (Meier et al., 2009). The analysis of BCM in whole pancreas samples, obtained during autopsy, is impractical. Hence, the development of non-invasive diagnostic techniques that enable detection of pancreatic islet inflammation in humans at risk for T1D and to estimate BCM would become powerful tools for both the early diagnosis and effective treatment of T1D.

Existing imaging technologies differ in terms of the type of energy that is used to generate visual information (e.g. positrons, photons, X-rays, sound and radiofrequency waves), the depth of penetration, spatial and temporal resolution, sensitivity, as well as the category of information that can be obtained using the technique (e.g., anatomical, physiological, cellular, or molecular). Extensive efforts are ongoing to create a non-invasive clinical imaging modality for beta-cell imaging based on the magnetic resonance imaging (MRI), positron emission tomography (PET) and single photon emission computed tomography (SPECT) platforms. Limited employment of beta-cell imaging in clinical practice has fostered great interest in using animal models of T1D at all stages of diabetes research. Adaptation of the modalities that are extensively used in clinical practice, such as MRI, PET and SPECT/CT for imaging animal models, allows the creation of experimental systems with high spacial resolution. Methods of optical imaging for the visualization of the pancreas from the molecular to the cellular level can be employed to test new therapeutic strategies as well as to develop new contrast agents for non-invasive T1D monitoring. These methodological approaches may eventually be applied to human T1D care in the early diagnosis of diabetes and the monitoring of disease progression and effectiveness of drug treatment. Since several recent reviews and book chapters focusing on nuclear imaging techniques using tracers for the visualization of specific tissue binding sites, such as PET and SPECT, and multimodality platforms PET/CT and SPECT/CT, as well as the application of these techniques for beta-cell imaging, have been recently published (Ahlgren & Gotthardt, 2010; Gotthardt, 2010; Hutton & Beekman, 2010; Ichise & Harris, 2010; Townsend, 2010), we will in this review focus on optical imaging techniques and MRI. In this chapter we will overview recent advances in beta-cell imaging using these imaging technologies with an emphasis on optical projection tomography (OPT), an advanced 3D imaging technology, developed to bridge the gap between MRI and microscopy techniques, employing optical sectioning approaches.

2. Magnetic resonance imaging

MRI has become one of the most practical, non-invasive imaging technologies over the last decades. MRI utilizes the principle of nuclear magnetic resonance and detects molecules containing nuclei with magnetic dipole properties or unpaired nuclear spins, such as hydrogen nuclei in water and other organic compounds (like lipids). In a strong static magnetic field produced within the MR scanner, hydrogen nuclei become aligned (either parallel or anti-parallel) to the magnetic field (these orientations correspond to the low- and high-energy states of the nuclei, accordingly). A temporary radiofrequency (RF) pulse, generated by a transmitter RF coil, changes the orientation of nuclear spins in the magnetic field, and is accompanied by absorbing energy. Following this pulse, nuclei return to their equilibrium (relaxation) state, emitting energy at resonance, or Larmor frequency, which can be detected by the receiver RF coil as an MRI signal (Rinck, 2001). The decaying signal is characterized by two relaxation time constants: T1 (the longitudinal relaxation time) and T2 (the transverse relaxation time), which depend on the physical and chemical properties of the tissue, the molecular environment of the nuclei and the strength of the static magnetic field. In different micro-environments, nuclear spins show different relaxation parameters that are detectable as different MRI signals at each point in the image. Differences in the relaxation behavior of tissues exposed to a magnetic field of a certain strength and RF pulses of a specific sequence determine image contrast and can be used for the monitoring of pathological processes in both organs and tissues (Budinger & Lauterbur, 1984). Detailed descriptions of MRI physics, engineering principles, instrumentation and contrast agent mechanisms have been presented in a number of publications (Gadian, 1995; Rinck, 2001; Artemov, 2003; Cassidy & Radda, 2005; Medarova & Moore, 2009).

In clinical practice, MRI has become a safe procedure because neither ionizing radiation nor a radiopharmaceutical agent is used for the scanning procedure. In comparison with other non-invasive imaging technologies, MRI possesses such advantages as high spatial resolution, unlimited penetration depth and high contrast for soft tissues which allows the collection of both anatomical and functional data. By applying contrast agents that can specifically label various cells types based on antigen expression levels, MRI can be used as a molecular imaging technique. Its key disadvantage is low sensitivity to molecular probes as compared with nuclear imaging methods such as PET and SPECT. This aspect has become a key challenge for the use of MRI in beta-cell imaging of both endogenous and transplanted islets. The introduction of a modified protocol for islet transplantation and immunosuppression, widely known as the Edmonton protocol, was followed by the successful replication of this procedure in many clinical centers around the world. Hereby islet transplantation from deceased donors has become a therapeutical option for patients with T1D, whose condition cannot be adequately managed (Shapiro et al., 2000). By utilizing this protocol, excellent metabolic control and independence from insulin injections could be achieved by 80% of the patients 1 year and ~20% 5 years after islet transplantation illustrating its promise for T1D treatment (Ryan et al., 2005). However, the long-term outcome of transplantation in many cases is influenced by substantial graft loss and damage of transplanted islets resulting from numerous adverse factors such as immune attack, glucose-induced deterioration, immunosuppression therapy etc., making the timely, non-invasive monitoring of islet grafts extremely important. To non-invasively resolve either native pancreatic islets of 100 to 400 micrometers in size and scattered throughout the pancreas, constituting approximately 1–2% of the total pancreatic volume under normal physiological conditions and considerably less in T1D, or islets transplanted into the liver, contrast agents with high beta-cell specificity are required.

2.1 MRI contrast agents for imaging pancreatic islets

Contrast agents used for MRI can be classified as positive, which primarily cause a reduction in T1 relaxation time and bright contrast, or negative, which cause a shortening in transverse T2 relaxation time and dark contrast. T1 contrast agents are usually compounds of small molecular weight, containing a paramagnetic metal, such as gadolinium or manganese, reduce T1 time, increasing the intensity of the signal in T1-weighted images. T2 contrast agents, e.g. superparamagnetic iron oxide (SPIO) nanoparticles, are usually iron-oxide nanocrystals covered by a polymer shell which cause a shortening of the T2 relaxation time, decreasing the signal intensity in MR images. T2 contrast agents are considered more sensitive than T1 contrast agents. (Rinck, 2001).

Imaging of beta-cells in native or transplanted islets is challenging because the magnetic properties of islets do not sufficiently differ from those of the surrounding tissues to be resolved non-invasively using existing contrast agents. However, *ex vivo* labeling of islets destined for transplantation with SPIO nanoparticles allows the MRI tracking of islet grafts within recipient organs. The potential for MRI to allow the direct visualization of the location and distribution of islet grafts labeled with the SPIO contrast agent ferucarbotran (approved for clinical application) and transplanted into the livers of streptozotocin (STZ)-treated and control recipient rats was first demonstrated by Jirak and co-authors (2004). The efficiency of islet transplantation was also evaluated by the restoration of normoglycemia in STZ-treated rats within 1 week of the procedure. *Ex vivo* co-labeling of human pancreatic islets with modified magnetic nanoparticles carrying the near-infrared fluorescent dye Cy 5.5 allowed both the MRI monitoring of prelabeled islets, transplanted either under the kidney capsules or into the livers of healthy and STZ-treated nonobese diabetic-severe combined immunodeficient (NOD-SCID) mice and the cross-evaluation of the islet grafts using optical imaging (Evgenov et al., 2006). Additionally, accumulation of nanoparticles in the endosomal structures of labeled islets did not affect glucose-induced insulin secretion *in vitro*.

By employing a transfection technique combining the electroporation and *ex vivo* labeling of rat and porcine islets with the SPIO contrast agent Feridex, complexed with poly-L-lysine, Tai and associates (2006) showed a good correlation between signal loss and increasing numbers of islets transplanted under the rat kidney capsule, imaged using a standard clinical 1.5 T scanner. Labeling of mouse and xenotransplanted human islets with T1 contrast agent-GdHPDO3A (Gd-gadolinium, HPDO3A-10-(2-hydroxypropyl)-1,4,7,10 tetraazacyclododecane-1,4,7-triacetic acid) was sufficient for direct MRI imaging with high spatial resolution and contrast of subrenal mouse islet grafts and intrahepatic human islet xenografts, respectively (Biancone et al., 2007).

To prevent the rejection of transplanted pancreatic islets by the immune system of a recipient, various immunoisolation techniques have been tested. One of the most widely used immunoisolation approaches employs the encapsulation of pancreatic islets within an immunoprotective alginate coating, which creates a semipermeable membrane around the transplanted islets and prevents antibody penetration into the capsule, while still allowing passage of glucose, insulin, and other metabolites (Lim & Sun, 1980, Sun et al., 1996). Chemically modified microcapsules can serve as multimodal contrast agents for the non-invasive monitoring of transplanted islets. Barnett et al. (2007) used MRI-detectable magnetocapsules, prepared with alginate containing Feridex, for the encapsulation of cadaveric human islets prior to transplantation into the livers of swine. Engrafted magnetocapsules were visualized by MRI as hypointense signal voids both immediately and 3 weeks after injection into the portal vein. There were functional *in vivo* and induced sustained human C-peptide levels. Incorporation of perfluorocarbons, hydrocarbons with most hydrogen atoms replaced by fluorine-19 (^{19}F), including perfluoropolyether (PEPE), in alginate capsules not only increases islet cell oxygenation and glucose-stimulated insulin secretion but also enables ^{19}F-MR imaging. Due to the absence of MRI detectable fluorine in the body, ^{19}F-labeling ensures high specificity of the signal and a lack of background signal (Barnett et al., 2011). Employment of a modified capsule coating could provide immunoprotection for xenografted islet cells, increasing the effectiveness of transplantation. It could also be used as a multimodal contrast agent for the monitoring of all steps of islet transplantation. To obtain better discrimination of labeled cells from the image background, Srinivas and co-authors (2007) applied *ex vivo* labeling of T cells using a PEPE agent and performed *in vivo* monitoring of T-cell migration to the pancreas after cells were transferred into non-obese diabetic (NOD) mice using spin density-weighted ^{19}F-MRI. Because of the negligible background, ^{19}F-MRI insures selective visualization only of labeled cells. Simultaneous acquisition of conventional ^{1}H images in the same session allows for a combination of images of labeled cells and images of anatomical structures.

In a pilot study, Toso et al. (2008) showed the feasibility and safety of MRI for the non-invasive monitoring of islet grafts prelabeled with SPIOs and transplanted into the livers of patients with T1D. Saudek and colleagues (2010) further developed this approach by implementing and optimizing new MR sequences using a scanner with a higher magnetic field strength (3T). Pancreatic islets labeled with ferucarbotran and transplanted into the livers of T1D patients with pre-transplant negative C-peptide levels were detected as hypointense areas on T2-, T2*-, and T2/T1-weighted images. These patients were followed for 24 weeks (Fig.1 (I)). Hence, MR imaging could play an important role not only in the monitoring and quantifying of transplanted islet engraftment and survival, but at all stages of islet transplantation, including screening of potential transplant recipients, for guiding the transplantation procedure and for monitoring post-transplantation complications in combination with other techniques for clinical imaging. (Low et al., 2010).

2.2 MRI based functional BCM monitoring

Imaging of endogenous pancreatic beta-cells in a living organism is more challenging, than the detection of *ex-vivo* labeled islet grafts, and requires highly specific beta-cell contrast agents to be applied. Prospective contrast agents for *in vivo* beta-cell imaging should meet the following requirements: 1) the agent should be sufficiently selective to beta-cells and not be taken up by adjacent cells and tissues, 2) it should provide a stable signal of high intensity, reflecting functional state and viability of beta-cells, 3) the agent should not have side toxic effects and should be retained by beta-cells during the entire period of time, required for scanning (Ahlgren & Gotthardt, 2010). It would obviously be of great practical value if a contrast agent for MRI could enable imaging of a parameter directly related to beta-cell function. A promising approach in this direction is based on the specific glucose-stimulated uptake of manganese ions by beta-cells. The paramagnetic manganese (Mn^{2+}) ion, a T1 relaxation-promoting contrast agent, has been tested by Antkowiak and co-authors (2009) for the non-invasive assessment of beta-cell function using MRI in control and STZ-treated C57BL/6J mice. Manganese mimics calcium by entering pancreatic beta-cells through voltage-gated Ca^{2+} channels after glucose challenge. Accumulated manganese in beta-cells represents integrated calcium signaling over time and can be detected as a brightening on T1-weighted images. Quantification of the normalized signal intensity showed a 51% increase in control mice after glucose infusion compared to the 9–20% increase in STZ-treated animals. These findings exhibit the potential of Mn^{2+}-enhanced MRI as a technique for the non-invasive monitoring of native beta-cell function, with sufficient sensitivity for the detection of functional BCM under normal physiological conditions and during progressively developing diabetes.

2.3 MR Imaging of microvascular changes and auto-immune inflammation in T1D

Endocrine cells in the pancreas are surrounded by a dense, glomerular-like capillary network and receive about 10% of total blood flow to the pancreas (Bonner-Weir & Orci, 1982, Svensson et al., 2003). The islet vasculature plays an important role in the regulation of endocrine cell function and glucose homeostasis is determined by both beta-cell secretory function and the microcirculation in the endocrine pancreas (Ballian & Brunicardi 2007, Kostromina et al., 2010). The development of T1D is commonly associated with progressive changes in the pancreatic islet microcirculatory system, including early augmented microvascular permeability, which allows transendothelial migration and the homing of T-cells, followed by a destruction of pancreatic beta-cells (Savinov et al., 2003, Savinov & Strongin, 2009). Microvascular alterations precede other symptoms of diabetes, including insulitis and hyperglycemia, as observed in various T1D animal models (Colantuoni et al., 1988, Enghofer et al., 1997) and patients with diabetes (Haller, 1997). Non-invasive detection of islet microvascular abnormalities as an early biomarker of pancreatic islet damage is considered a promising approach for the early diagnosis and monitoring of T1D.

Microvascular alterations associated with the onset and progression of insulitis were detected using MRI in a murine model of induced T1D (i.e., BDC2.5 T-cell receptor transgenic mice) after intravenous injection of long-circulating magnetofluorescent nanoparticles. It was demonstrated that accumulation of extravasated nanoparticles resulted from increased microvascular permeability and invading phagocytic macrophages, allowing probe uptake correlating with the aggressiveness of insulitis in these transgenic animals (Denis et al., 2004). Using the same, high-resolution, MRI approach, non-invasive real-time

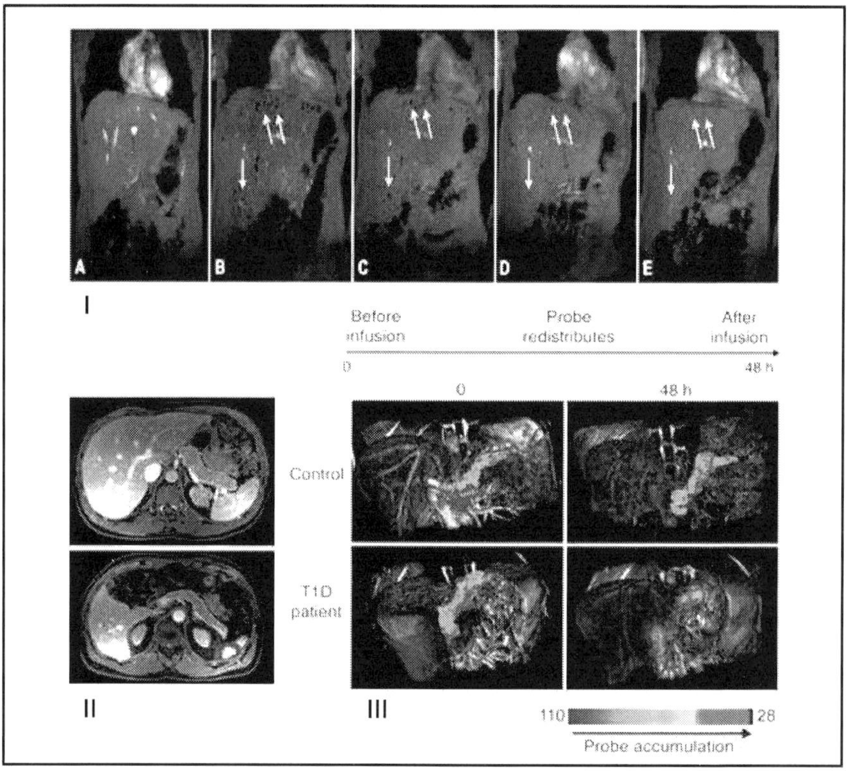

Fig. 1. I. Magnetic resonance imaging in a T1D patient on the day before transplantation (A), 1 day (B), 1 week (C), 4 weeks (D), and 24 weeks after transplantation (E). Typical areas of signal loss attributed to the detected islets are indicated by arrows (Saudek et al., 2010). Copyright © Lippincott Williams & Wilkins. Reproduced with permission of Wolters Kluwer Health/Lippincott Williams & Wilkins via Copyright Clearance Center.
II. Pancreas volume index (PVI) of recently diagnosed diabetes patients is less than that of controls. Representative single MR-VIBE (volumetric interpolated breath-hold examination) slices at the level of the body/tail of the pancreas are shown with the pancreas outlined in green. The control subject (upper panel) and the individual with recent onset T1D (lower panel) have total estimated pancreas volumes of 119 ml and 50 ml respectively.
III. Insulitis may be visualized by MRI. Shown are T2-pseudocolor reconstructions of the pancreas overlaid on 3D-VIBE images, measured before and 48 hours after MNP infusion. T2 values in the pancreas are similar between the patient and control subjects before infusion but different after infusion. (II & III adapted from Gaglia et al., 2011). © Copyright 2011 by American Society for Clinical Investigation. Reproduced with permission of American Society for Clinical Investigation.

quantification of microcirculatory changes, resulting from pancreatic inflammation during the progression of diabetes and after its reversal using anti-CD3 monoclonal antibody therapy in NOD mice, was performed (Turvey et al., 2005). Semi-quantitative assessment and direct visualization of microvascular changes in the pancreata of STZ-treated mice were performed using MRI after injection of a long-circulating contrast agent PGC-Gd-DTPA-F (a protected graft copolymer linked to gadolinium diethylenetriaminepentaacetic acid residues labeled with fluorescein isothiocyanate) (Medarova et al., 2007). A significantly greater accumulation of PGC-Gd-DTPA-F in the pancreata of diabetic animals was revealed compared with control mice. *Ex vivo* histological analysis confirmed not only extensive distribution of PGC-Gd-DTPA-F within pancreatic vasculature, but also a substantial leakage of the probe into the islet interstitium in diabetic animals whereas the fluorescent signal in control mice was determined predominantly in the vascular compartment.

Based on the results of experimental findings in animal models, MR imaging of magnetic nanoparticles has recently been successfully applied in a pilot clinical study to non-invasively visualize islet inflammation in recent-onset diabetic patients (Gaglia et al., 2011, Fig.1 (II&III)). It was presumed that magnetic nanoparticle retention in the pancreas emerged as a result of vascular leakage and uptake by macrophages, which were evaluated using local T2 changes, and was dependant on the aggressiveness of insulitis. This approach permitted the non-invasive detection of inflammatory events in the pancreas of patients at an early stage of diabetes and could be useful for monitoring the efficience of drug therapy.

3. Optical imaging

Optical imaging is based on the detection of photon transmission through biological tissues. The propagation of light through tissue is affected by two simultaneous processes: absorption and scattering. Both effects depend on the wavelength and depth of penetration (Ntziachristos, 2010). A significant part of our current knowledge about the pathogenesis of diabetes is based on analyses performed with conventional bright-field or epifluorescence microscopy, including the microscopic assessment of multiple histological sections, which has been widely used for analysis of experimental animal models of T1D for decades. Traditional microscopic examination of fixed tissue sections (normally 10-20 μm) ensures high quality of images because only a small part of photons are scattered.

3.1 Microscopy and morphometric analyses

Histological microscopic analysis is commonly used for the evaluation of progression and severity of insulitis in the pancreases of diabetic animals. The insulitis score is usually expressed in conventional units and reflects the degree of islet infiltration by mononuclear cells. In many experimental studies, this technique has been employed for the evaluation of the dynamics of islet infiltration as well as for the assessment of progressive BCM loss in relation to insulitis in animal models for T1D (Wicker et al., 1987; Signore et al., 1994). The ratio of islet area to the entire pancreatic area is considered a very informative indicator of pancreatic islet development and reflects the dynamics of BCM reduction with T1D progression (Li et al., 2000). For the quantification of this parameter, multiple sections or series of overlapping histological images can be acquired using a microscope equipped with a motorized stage (Zito et al., 2004). After the computerized "stitching" of multiple single planes, every composite image represents a histological section through the whole pancreas, containing a large number of islets. A similar quantitative approach is used for whole slide scanning, a recent technology that combines ultra-resolution digital scanning of glass slides with archiving, viewing, and image analysis of whole slide scans. After scanning the whole slide, all islets in the pancreatic section can be identified using either semi-automated or automated computer-assisted image analysis. This technology is widely used for the monitoring of pancreatic morphology in T1D animal models (Soltani et al., 2007).

Epifluorescence microscopy of the entire pancreas was performed by Kilimnik et al. (2009) for the assessment of pancreatic islet distribution *in situ* using transgenic mice that express green fluorescent protein (GFP) specifically in beta-cells under the control of the mouse insulin I promoter (MIP, Hara et al., 2003). After dissection, fixation and treatment with sucrose and glycerol, the pancreas was placed on a glass slide and examined at different depths. Integrated two-dimensional images obtained by forming a montage of single planes acquired along the Z-axis were processed and used for morphometric analyses. However, conventional epifluorescence microscopy has a limited ability to resolve the three-dimensional (3D) tissue architecture that provides both stereological data and 3D visualization.

3.2 Confocal laser scanning microscopy

In contrast to epifluorescence microscopy, confocal laser-scanning microscopy (CLSM), collects fluorescent photons from a single, illuminated, focused spot, excluding fluorescent signals from objects that are outside the focal plane. Single optical sections through fluorescent objects are generated after point-by-point scanning across the specimen. Parallel optical sections obtained by moving the focal plane along the Z-axis can be combined, assembling a 3D stack. The application of confocal microscopy for 3D analysis has become an important advance because it does not require sectioning and avoids the spatial distortion of biological structures, which is an inevitable result of tissue embedding, processing, and sectioning. A detailed comparative analysis of human pancreatic islets and islets isolated from non-human primates and mice of different strains, including their architectures and compositions using CLSM, have been performed by Brissova et al. (2005). Entire isolated islets were subjected to optical sectioning along the Z-axis at 1-μm intervals, after which optical sections were reconstructed into a 3D stack and analyzed using image analysis software. It was found that human islets were not only heterogeneous in terms of cell composition but also had a pattern of alpha, beta, and gamma cell distribution within the islets that differed from that of murine islets. Experimental studies performed by Cabrera et al. (2006) with the assistance of CLSM showed that human islets contained fewer beta-cells and more alpha cells than mouse islets, amounting to 60% and 30% of the total number of endocrine cells, respectively. Furthermore, all types of endocrine cells were found in close proximity to islet microvessels, but without any particular alignment along the microvasculature. A unique architecture and cellular composition of human islets is associated with a distinct physiology, as evaluated by oscillations in membrane potentials and intracellular Ca^{2+} responses to high glucose concentrations. A recent review on islet architecture and comparative anatomy of islets in different species of animals from an evolutionary point of view has been presented by Heller (2010).

3.3 Intravital microscopy

Intravital microscopy has become a powerful technique for studying the dynamics of biological processes and visualizing the cellular and sub-cellular events in the native environments of living animals. Due to a limited depth of penetration, application of the methods of *in vivo* microscopy to the imaging of most internal tissues, including the pancreas, requires special surgical tissue preparation methods. There are three main categories of tissue preparation which are based on the type of surgical method used: chronic-transparent windows (abdominal window, body window, dorsal skinfold chamber, etc.), exteriorized tissue preparation, and *in situ* preparations (Jain et al., 2005). Chronic abdominal window preparation, developed for direct intravital microscopy of the pancreas, is used mainly for studies of the growth of pancreatic tumors and the effects of anti-cancer therapies (Tsuzuki et al., 2001). A body window was designed for longitudinal *in vivo* imaging of islets, isolated from transgenic mice expressing proinsulin II tagged with a fluorescent reporter protein Timer, which changes colour from green to red in the first 24 h after synthesis, and transplanted under the kidney capsule (Bertera et al., 2003). By using this technique fluorescently labeled beta-cells and T cells can be simultaneously investigated through the window device placed and sutured over the site of islet transplantation after underlying skin and body wall are removed.

The dorsal skinfold chamber is a valid model for the intavital microscopic study of pancreatic islet grafts, in which the striated skin muscle serves as a bed for the transplants (Menger et al., 1992). After contrast enhancement is achieved by intravenous injection of fluorescently labeled dextran (FITC-dextran, TRITC-dextran), the microcirculatory bed of transplanted islets can be identified as a distinctive, glomerular-like vascular plexus and used for the quantitative analysis of all microvascular segments in individual islet grafts using traditional techniques (Menger et al., 1994). Intravital microscopy of the exteriorized pancreas, which is located deep in the area between the spleen, stomach and duodenum, is tightly connected with the surrounding tissues and possesses essential opacity, is extremely challenging and is not widely practiced compared with transparent and easily accessible organs, like the mesentery and a few skeletal muscles (Intaglietta & Messmer, 1983; Ley et al., 1986; Hudlicka, 1998; Segal, 2005). Exposure of the pancreas requires extreme care because this tissue is quite fragile and easily develops hemorrhages. Furthermore, to identify and locate islets that could be used for imaging, an additional contrast enhancement of the islets should be used. Pancreatic islets can be revealed after intravenous injection of dithizone (diphenylthiocarbazone, DTZ), a chelating agent that combines with zinc in islets to form a visible complex (Bunnag et al., 1963) that possesses fluorescent properties in the red spectrum (Denis et al., 2004, Martinic & Herrath, 2008). However, the fluorescence of DTZ complexes in the living pancreas fades rather quickly, so this type of staining cannot be used for long-lasting *in vivo* experiments. Generation of transgenic mice with pancreatic beta-cells genetically tagged with GFP, or with its yellow or cyan derivates that can be detected *in vivo*, has become a valuable tool for the real-time identification of pancreatic islets containing fluorescently labeled beta-cells (Hara et al., 2003). To visualize fluorescent protein-labeled beta-cells in the intact pancreas, Hara et al. (2006) developed an imaging technique that combines reflection and confocal microscopy. Visualization of the intact pancreas from MIP-GFP and red fluorescent protein (RFP) transgenic mice showed that the distribution of fluorescently labeled beta-cells within the pancreas was not even, as the majority of islets were located around large blood vessels, and some clusters of beta-cells were found around the pancreatic and common bile ducts. By crossing neurogenin-3-GFP mice with MIP-RFP mice the authors generated rainbow mice in which beta-cells and beta-cell progenitors were labeled with different fluorescent proteins and used for the study of pancreatic development at the molecular level.

Intravital microscopy of the pancreatic microcirculation has benefited greatly from genetically tagged fluorescence labeling of pancreatic beta-cells. The relationship between the pattern of blood flow through the pancreatic islets and islet cell composition and its influence on islet cell secretion has been a topic of many scientific discussions. Different orders of endocrine cell perfusion within an islet can have significant physiological consequences, because hormones secreted by one cell type can affect the secretory function of another cell type. Different hypotheses about the organization of blood flow in islets have been attributed to three models that describe the pattern of pancreatic islet blood flow: mantle-to-core, core-to-mantle and polar flow (Menger et al., 1994, Brunicardi et al., 1996, 1997). Most experimental data have been obtained using scanning electron microscopy-corrosion cast studies or intravital microscopy using fluorescent markers such as FITC-labeled red blood cells, FITC-dextran or fluorescent microspheres. To further investigate the relationship between pancreatic islet microcirculation and islet cell organization, dynamic optical imaging employing high-speed CLSM of the pancreases of IP-GFP mice has been used (Nyman et al., 2008, Fig.2). To assess 3D flow patterns in the islets, a time series of z stacks with an imaging rate of 70–72 frames per second after bolus injection of rhodamine dextran was acquired. Average fluorescence intensities were evaluated over time for selected regions of interest at different locations within the islet microvasculature using the 3D data. The analysis revealed two major directional blood flow patterns in the mouse islets: 1) the inner-to-outer type of perfusion, where the core of beta-cells is upstream of the non-beta-cell mantle, which was found in the majority of islets and 2) the top-to-bottom blood flow pattern, where the direction of blood flow is not dependant on cell type, which was found in 35% of islets. Due to the limited depth of penetration inherent in confocal microscopy, these results represent flow patterns obtained for islets located near the surface of the dorsal pancreas, revealing the predominance of the inner-to-outer type of islet perfusion, in which the products of beta-cell secretion likely have a regulatory effect on the secretory activity of non-beta-cells and ensuring the interaction of different types of endocrine cells in the regulation of blood glucose levels.

An intravital setup for islet monitoring, similar to those described above, relies on a different technology. Optical coherence tomography (OCT) is an interferometric technique that amplifies photons backscattered by the tissue. As such, it could be described as the optical equivalent of ultrasound imaging. Villiger et al., (2009) showed, by implementing an extended focus scheme (extended focus optical coherence microscopy, xfOCM, Leitgeb et al., 2006), that islets backscatter light stronger than the surrounding pancreatic tissue, allowing for the visualization of islets in the exteriorized pancreas of mice. Hence, although to some extent limited by its penetration depth (~300μm), this technique enables imaging of endogenous islets without the use of contrast agents.

3.4 TPLSM and MPLSM imaging

More recent advances in optical imaging platforms may further facilitate diabetes research and the development of new therapies for T1D, imaging of intracellular beta-cell metabolism and molecular probe generation. Examples of such approaches include the application of two- and multi-photon laser confocal scanning that enables 3D and longitudinal assessments of fluorescently labeled molecular structures in living pancreatic islets in both *in vitro* and intravital systems. Imaging of living cells and tissues with multi-photon microscopy provides important advantages over visualization performed using conventional confocal microscopy, including substantially increased depth of penetration and reduced phototoxicity in 3D imaging (Dunn & Young, 2006; Benninger et al., 2008).

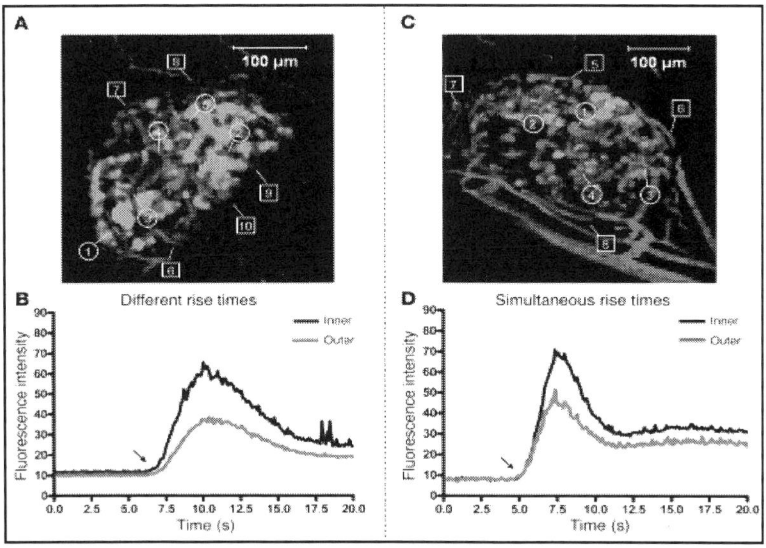

Fig. 2. Intravital laser-scanning confocal microscopic imaging of MIP-GFP mouse pancreases after injection of rhodamine dextran tracer into the vasculature. Temporal resolution analysis demonstrates different islet blood flow patterns. (**A** and **C**) Two different islets (single-plane images), shown with inner (circles) and outer (squares) vessel regions selected and marked for fluorescence intensity measurement after a bolus of rhodamine dextran. Scale bars: 100 µm. (**B** and **D**) Average inner vessel fluorescent intensity time courses (throughout the *z* plane) compared with average outer vessel fluorescence intensity time course for the islets in **A** and **C**, respectively. Arrows denote rise times. Average rise time for the inner vessels was either (**B**) before that of outer vessels, as demonstrated by increased fluorescence intensity shown first by inner vessels, or (**D**) no different from outer vessels, which demonstrates that different islets had different perfusion patterns (Nyman et al., 2008). © Copyright 2008 by American Society for Clinical Investigation. Reproduced with permission of American Society for Clinical Investigation.

Conventional fluorescence microscopy is based on the absorption of a single photon by a fluorescent molecule (fluorophore), which results in a transition of the molecule into an excited state with a higher energy level. Relaxation to the initial state leads to emission of a single photon of a wavelength longer than the excitation wavelength. High excitation intensity, which can be provided by ultra-short infrared pulsed lasers with twice the wavelength (or half the frequency) of the standard excitation beam within a shorter period of time than the time of fluorescence decay of the fluorescent molecule, can lead to the simultaneous absorption of two photons each with half the energy required for single-photon excitation. Focusing the excitation beam into a small volume is achieved using lenses with high numerical aperture. Due to this very precise focusing, the only location where the absorption takes place is in this focal volume, but not at other depths either below or above the focal plane through which the excitation light passes. However, fluorophores do not experience a two-photon effect, ensuring one of the most important two-photon LSM

(TPLSM) advantages - reduced photobleaching-which occurs only in the focal area but not within the surrounding tissue. The high excitation wavelength allows for deep tissue penetration. While in conventional confocal microscopy the scattering of excitation light induces fluorescence outside the focal plane, in TPLSM the scattered photons do not contribute to the fluorescence signal. Since fluorescence is derived only from the focal plane, the fluorescence signal can be achieved without a pinhole but with an external detector placed immediately after the objective, thus increasing the efficiency of signal collection. TPLSM therefore displays several important advantages over conventional confocal microscopy by allowing confocal images to be obtained with increased imaging depth and high light-gathering efficiency but with less photobleaching and specimen damage outside the focal volume. Hence, TPLSM makes it possible to undertake a number of studies related to beta-cell imaging at the cellular and sub-cellular level.

Coppieters and co-workers (2010) developed an approach based on intravital two-photon microscopy of the pancreas to study the dynamic interactions between individual T cells and pancreatic beta-cells in real time. An acute transfer model for autoimmune diabetes was employed by injection of fluorescently labeled splenocytes harboring diabetogenic T-cell receptor-transgenic CD8 T cells into reporter mice with beta-cells expressing both GFP and antigen. The authors were able to detect the transferred T cells around the islets, which were accessible for intravital examination by two-photon microscopy, and to track both T-cell motility and interactions with beta-cells.

Based on TPLSM, a platform for the non-invasive and longitudinal *in vivo* imaging of functional pancreatic islets transplanted into the anterior chamber of the eye at a single-cell resolution, has been developed. Non-invasive TPLSM monitoring of the islets isolated from mice expressing GFP under control of the rat insulin-1 promoter (RIP-GFP) and transplanted into the iris through the cornea was performed together with the visualization of the islet vascular network after injection of Texas Red-conjugated dextran (Speier et al., 2008a). Originally, the anterior chamber of the eye was chosen as a transplantation site because of its immune-privileged properties (Niederkorn, 2002). Being a natural body window, the anterior chamber of the eye can be easily accessed with LSM and TPLSM through the cornea, providing sub-cellular resolution in real time and the possibility for longitudinal monitoring of islet cytoarchitecture, vascularization and innervations as well as beta-cell metabolism, after islet engraftment on the iris (Speier et al., 2008b). Hence, this approach enables studies of beta-cell signal transduction, gene expression and mechanisms involved in exocytosis, to be conducted with fluorescent probes in a natural physiological environment with vascular and nervous supply re-established after transplantation (Leibiger et al., 2010).

3.5 Optical projection tomography

Optical projection tomography (OPT) Sharpe et al., (2002), is a relatively recent technique that was developed as a tool for 3D visualization of gene and protein expression patterns in biomedical specimen at the mm-cm scale. The technology in many ways bridges the gap between microscopy techniques utilizing optical sectioning such as CLSM (with a penetration depth limited to a few hundred micrometers) and non-optical techniques like MRI (commonly used for imaging at the level of the entire organism). The 3D images generated by OPT are volumetric data sets similar to those generated by other tomographic techniques and therefore the same visualization techniques may be used. Hence, OPT could be described essentially as computed tomography (CT), which instead of using x-rays employs light in the visible part of the spectrum (Sharpe, 2003). The basic OPT scanner setup includes a rotary stage driven by a stepper motor for positioning and holding the specimen, imaging lenses for focusing and magnifying the image, two types of illumination: a white light diffuser for the transmission imaging and an arrangement for imaging in the fluorescence mode and a charged coupled device (CCD) camera to capture the raw projection images. For OPT imaging, the specimen is embedded in an agarose gel and subjected to optical clearing. It is then attached onto a rotary stage of the scanner and immersed in an imaging chamber, filled with an organic solvent, most frequently, Murray's Clear (also referred to as BABB), prepared as a mixture of benzyl alcohol and benzyl benzoate. Placement of the sample in an index-matching medium reduces scattering of light and heterogeneity of refractive index within different parts of the specimen during scanning. While the specimen is rotated through 360°, light transmitted through the specimen is focused on the CCD chip by lenses and images are captured at each step-rotated position. For the reconstruction of raw projection data into a 3D voxel stack, a filtered back-projection algorithm is used (Sharpe, 2004). The technique has already contributed to addressing a broad range of biological questions in diverse systems such as human, mice, chicken, fly, zebrafish and plants (see e.g. Sarma et al., 2005; Kulandavelu et al., 2006; Fisher et al., 2008; McGurk et al., 2007; Bryson-Richardson & Currie 2004; and Lee et al 2006). However, due to inherent properties of pancreatic (and other) tissue (including strong endogenous autofluorescence and light scattering effects) in combination with difficulties in obtaining sufficient reagent penetration (primarily for antibodies), the technique was initially limited to studies of the embryonic pancreas. In this respect OPT has been a powerful resource for spatial and quantitative phenotypical analyses of pancreas development and in assessments of tissue interactions during pancreas organogenesis (Hecksher-Sørensen et al., 2004; Asayesh et al, 2006; Sand et al., 2011). By combined improvements in protocols for sample preparation, tomographic imaging and computational processing we could adapt the technique to also allow for imaging of the intact adult mouse pancreas (Alanentalo et al., 2007). By nature of the tomographic process, this enabled a practical approach to generate quantitative data (number and volume), spatial coordinates (x, y, z) and 3D reconstructions of individual molecularly labelled objects (e.g. insulin labelled islets of Langerhans) throughout the volume of the pancreas with close to cell level (~15μm) resolution. We further described how such global assessments of the pancreatic constitution (or disease state) could be used to guide confocal resolution regional assessments based on the expression of molecular markers, interacting cell types, spatial coordinates, morphology and volume of individual objects (e.g. an islet) throughout the volume of the gland Alanentalo et al., (2008). Hence, OPT imaging allows for detailed, spatial, quantitative and statistical analyses of the pancreatic BCM distribution down to the level of the individual islets with high molecular specificity and without the need for extrapolation of 2D data. Studies of dynamic events, such as the autoimmune induced destruction of beta-cells during T1D progression, highlights the added value of the OPT technique in such assessments. By allowing for the generation of full islet size distribution profiles, as opposed to average values such as mean islet volume, volume weighted mean, total islet volume and total islet count, important information regarding these processes may be revealed. As an example we recently addressed, by OPT, quantitative and spatial aspects of the autoimmune induced β-cell destruction during T1D progression in the NOD mouse. Although limited to "frozen moments in time" (OPT is due to the requirement for chemical processing of the tissue limited to ex-vivo assessments), we could hereby provide evidence for a preferential depletion of "smaller" islets during the initial phase of the autoimmune attack, a compensatory growth potential of the larger insulin positive islets during the later stages of the disease as well as new information on the insulitis process itself including its apparently random distribution at onset, local variations during its further development, and the formation of structures resembling tertiary lymphoid organs at later phases of insulitis progression (Alanentalo et al., 2010) (see Fig. 3). The possibility to extract this type of cross-relatable spatial and quantitative data suggests that OPT imaging may facilitate numerous diabetes related research areas encompassing those involving evaluations of strategies for therapy and restoration of BCM, interpretations of how metabolically induced phenotypes manifest as diabetic disorders, the screening for rare events or cell niches in genetically engineered mice, the effect of targeted gene ablation on BCM etc.

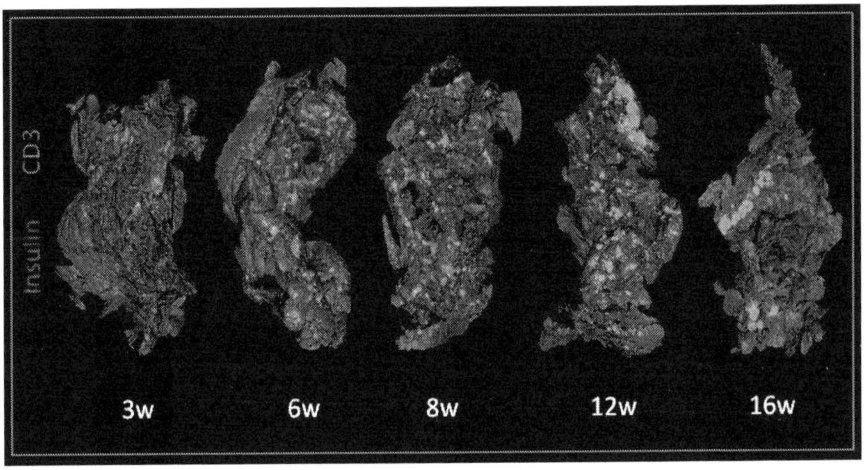

Fig. 3. Spatial assessment of the progression of autoimmune insulitis in the NOD mouse. Isosurface rendered OPT images of representative pancreata (duodenal) from NOD mice at 3, 6, 8, 12, and 16 weeks. Ins+ islets (red) are reconstructed based on the signal from insulin-specific antibodies and infiltrating T-cells (green) based on the signal from CD3-specific antibodies. A high-quality color representation of this figure with scale bars included is available in the online issue (Alanentalo et al., 2010) © Copyright 2010 by American Diabetes Association. Reproduced with permission of American Diabetes Association in the format other book via Copyright Clearance Center.

As with any tomographic imaging technology, OPT is associated with a number of technological hurdles. These most commonly relate to artifacts introduced by the tomographic reconstruction process itself or such that are of optical nature. Several recent reports have described improved reconstruction algorithms and/or other computational tools to further enhance OPT imaging (Birk et al., 2011; Walls et al., 2005, 2007.). As OPT will find its way into more research laboratories, studying different aspects the pancreas and/or T1D disease aetiology, improvements of this kind that more specifically address challenges associated with OPT imaging of organs on the pancreatic scale could be expected. OPT has an important advantage in that it can produce 3D images of both non-fluorescent and fluorescent specimen, i.e. it can operate in both transmission and emission mode (Sharpe, 2010). This holds the benefit of permitting visualization of pancreatic structures or cell types labeled with standard laboratory markers. Hence, in contrast to other imaging modalities, allowing for *in vivo* or *in vitro* imaging of the intact pancreas, OPT imaging may be performed with a huge selection of available or custom designed antibody markers pertinent to diabetes research. By the possibility to operate in emission mode, and thereby the option for the detection of markers at different fluorescent wavelengths, OPT thus appears well suited for "whole pancreas" monitoring of cellular ratios or cellular interactions under various genetic or pathologic conditions. Preliminary studies performed in our laboratory suggests that this potential may be further expanded by taking advantage of the increased channel separation and signal to noise ratio obtained by using wavelengths in the near infrared spectrum (U. Ahlgren, unpublished observation). An obvious drawback for OPT imaging, at least for studies of the adult rodent pancreas, is the non-existent capacity to perform longitudinal analyses. This is to some extent compensated for by the relative ease by which large number of specimen, e.g. at different stages of disease progression, may be investigated. Although current protocols for tissue processing and antibody labelling are relatively lengthy (~ 10-12 days), they require limited "hands on" and large series of pancreata may be run in parallel (Alanentalo et al., 2010). Further developments in automation of tomographic reconstruction and image processing may further increase the speed and accuracy by which post-scan processing of OPT data may be performed. It should be noted however that the large amount of digital data produced by OPT imaging impose specific challenges for storage capacity and for various aspects of image processing and analyses. A typical pancreas scan (projected and reconstructed images) on a commercial instrument produces in the range of 7-8 GB of data. Although the OPT technique does not allow for the visualization of diabetogenic processes in live mice, there is a potential application for the technique in attempts to develop new strategies for non-invasive beta-cell scoring by other imaging modalities. Preliminary data obtained in our laboratory suggests that by the possibility to detected multiple fluorescent markers, as is further facilitated by the adaptation of OPT to near infrared imaging, OPT could play an important role in the development of new contrast agents for non-invasive assessments of pancreatic cell types by nuclear imaging techniques such as MRI. In this respect, the uptake specificity and readout of essentially any contrast agent being developed for non-invasive imaging (of e.g. beta-cells), that may be also fluorescently labelled, should be possible to cross evaluate, *ex vivo*, by antibody staining (e.g. for insulin) imaged in another fluorescent channel. Finally, it should be emphasized that the potential use for OPT imaging in T1D research is not limited to assessments of the pancreas. By the adaptation of OPT to imaging of intact mouse organs (and larger tissue specimen) of adult mice (Alanentalo et al., 2007), it may well find important applications in experimental research on islet engraftment and in studies of vascular complications of diabetes.

4. Concluding remarks

A correlation between changes in BCM and the development of T1D is generally accepted. The development and refinement of imaging technologies that enables assessments of BCM dynamics and its distribution is therefore highly needed in both pre-clinical and clinical settings. To this end, a range of imaging platforms have been developed, with each one associated with strengths and weaknesses for parameters such as tissue penetration depth, spatial resolution, contrast agent specificity/availability etc. Together, these imaging modalities represent technologies for assessments of diabetogenic processes from the cellular and sub-cellular level, to the level of the whole organ or entire organism. Given the title of this chapter, it should be emphasized that the potential of these techniques for experimental diabetes research or in clinical applications goes far beyond the study of the beta-cells. Obviously, they have important applications for the study of other cells and tissues affected by- or mediating the disease, for example in the diagnostics of leukocyte infiltration. In this chapter, we have attempted an overview of the current status and future potential of MRI and a number of optical imaging modalities, including CLSM, M/TPLSM and OPT. Of these, the optical techniques have restricted possibilities for imaging of larger specimen due to their limited tissue penetration depth. However, by their generally speaking high spatial resolution, the abundant selection of available biomarkers and the possibility for simultaneous detection of different targets in the investigated tissue they are well suited for studying mechanistic aspects of T1D in experimental animal research. In contrast, MRI, PET and SPECT at present represent the technologies of choice for assessments of human subjects due to their "unlimited" penetration depth, non-invasive characteristics and the possibility to perform longitudinal studies. Although SPECT and PET are not covered by this chapter, it should again be emphasized that these techniques similarly to MRI hold great potential for the monitoring of BCM in clinical settings. Hereby, it should be noted that whereas MRI has the highest spatial resolution, with the potential of monitoring individual islets, it has the lowest sensitivity while the opposite is true for PET. Still, a number of technological hurdles, some of which are shared for all three modalities, for their routine use in clinical practice needs to be resolved. The perhaps major issue in this respect is the identification of suitable beta-cell ligands/ contrast agents. As discussed in section 3.5 of this chapter the development and/or identification of such agents may be facilitated by the use of *ex-vivo* optical techniques for whole organ imaging such as OPT. Given the dramatic technological and methodological advances that been presented during the past decade, it seems likely that many of the problems that currently impede beta cell and pancreas imaging, of spatial and quantitative nature, are to be resolved in an over-viewable future. Although, no technique can be expected to cover all the needs for imaging in diabetes research a palette of complementary techniques exist today that provides solutions for a vast variety of imaging tasks. Another important challenge for the future is the development of imaging strategies that also enables extraction of specific functional aspects of the native beta-cells. As development tends to progress in the direction of combinatorial/multimodal approaches, it seems likely that techniques for imaging-based multivariate analyses will be an important part of tomorrows toolbox for diabetes research and diabetes care.

5. Acknowledgements

We are grateful to Drs. U. Himmelreich and I. Jones for helpful comments on the manuscript.

6. Abbreviations

3D - three-dimensional

BCM - beta-cell mass

CLSM - Confocal laser scanning microscopy

DTZ - Dithizone

LSM - Laser scanning microscopy

MPLSM - Multi photon laser scanning microscopy

MNP - Magnetic nanoparticles

MRI - Magnetic resonance imaging

MR - Magnetic resonance

OCT - Optical coherence tomography

OPT - Optical projection tomography

PET - Positron emission tomography

SPECT - Single photon emission computed tomography

SPIO - Superparamagnetic iron oxide

STZ - Streptozotocin

T1D - Type 1 diabetes

TPLSM - Two photon laser scanning microscopy

xfOCM - extended focus optical coherence microscopy

7. References

Ahlgren, U., Gotthardt, M. (2010). Approaches for imaging islets: recent advances and future prospects. Adv Exp Med Biol. 2010; Vol. 654, pp. 39-57, ISSN - 0065-2598

Alanentalo, T., Asayesh, A., Morrison, H., Lorén, C.E, Holmberg, D., Sharpe, J & Ahlgren, U. (2007). Tomographic molecular imaging and 3D quantification within adult mouse organs. *Nature Methods*, Vol. 4, No. 1, (Jan 2007), pp. 31-33, ISSN 1548-7091

Alanentalo, T., Lorén, C.E., Larefalk, A., Sharpe, J., Holmberg, D. & Ahlgren, U. (2008). High-resolution three-dimensional imaging of islet-infiltrate interactions based on optical projection tomography assessments of the intact adult mouse pancreas. *J Biomed Opt.*, Vol. 13, No. 5, (Sep-Oct 2008), pp.054070, ISSN 1083-3668

Alanentalo, T., Hörnblad, A., Mayans, S., Nilsson, AK., Sharpe, J., Larefalk, A., Ahlgren, U.& Holmberg, D. (2010). Quantification and three-dimensional imaging of the insulitis-induced destruction of beta-cells in murine type 1 diabetes. *Diabetes*, Vol. 59, No. 7, (Jul 2010), pp. 1756-64, ISSN - 1939-327X

Antkowiak, P.F., Tersey, S.A., Carter, J.D., Vandsburger, M.H., Nadler, J.L., Epstein, F.H. & Mirmira, R.G. (2009). Noninvasive assessment of pancreatic beta-cell function in vivo with manganese-enhanced magnetic resonance imaging. *Am J Physiol Endocrinol Metab.*, Vol. 296, No.3, (Mar 2009), E573-578, ISSN 0193-1849

Artemov, D. (2003). Molecular magnetic resonance imaging with targeted contrast agents. *J Cell Biochem.*, Vol. 90, No.3, (Oct 2003), pp.518-524, ISSN 0730-2312

Asayesh, A., Sharpe, J., Watson, R.P., Hecksher-Sørensen, J., Hastie, N.D., Hill, R.E. & Ahlgren, U. (2006). Spleen versus pancreas: strict control of organ interrelationship revealed by analyses of Bapx1-/- mice. *Genes Dev.*, Vol. 20, No.16, (Aug 2006), pp. 2208-2213, ISSN 0890-9369

Ballian, N. & Brunicardi, F.C. (2007). Islet vasculature as a regulator of endocrine pancreas function. *World J Surg.*, Vol. 31, No. 4, (Apr 2007), pp. 705-714, ISSN 0364-2313

Barnett, B.P., Arepally, A., Karmarkar, P.V., Qian D., Gilson W.D., Walczak, P., Howland, V., Lawler, L., Lauzon, C., Stuber, M., Kraitchman, D.L. & Bulte J.W. (2007). Magnetic resonance-guided, real-time targeted delivery and imaging of magnetocapsules immunoprotecting pancreatic islet cells. *Nat Med.*, Vol. 13, No. 8, (August 2007), pp.986-991, ISSN - 1078-8956

Barnett, B.P, Ruiz-Cabello, J., Hota, P., Liddell, R., Walczak, P., Howland, V., Chacko, V.P., Kraitchman, D.L., Arepally, A. & Bulte, J.W. (2011). Fluorocapsules for improved function, immunoprotection, and visualization of cellular therapeutics with MR, US, and CT imaging. *Radiology*, Vol. 258, No. 1, (Jan 2011), pp. 182-191, ISSN 1527-1315

Benninger, R.K., Hao, M. & Piston, D.W. (2008). Multi-photon excitation imaging of dynamic processes in living cells and tissues. *Rev Physiol Biochem Pharmacol.*, Vol. 160, pp. 71-92, ISSN 0303-4240

Bertera, S., Geng, X., Tawadrous, Z., Bottino, R., Balamurugan, A.N., Rudert, W.A., Drain, P., Watkins, S.C. & Trucco, M. (2003). Body window-enabled in vivo multicolor imaging of transplanted mouse islets expressing an insulin-Timer fusion protein. *Biotechniques*, Vol. 35, No. 4, (Oct 2003), pp. 718-22, ISSN 0736-6205

Biancone, L., Crich, S.G., Cantaluppi, V., Romanazzi, G.M., Russo, S., Scalabrino, E., Esposito, G., Figliolini, F., Beltramo, S., Perin, P.C., Segoloni, G.P., Aime, S. & Camussi G. (2007). Magnetic resonance imaging of gadolinium-labeled pancreatic islets for experimental transplantation. *NMR Biomed.*, Vol. 20, No. 1, (Feb 2007), pp. 40-48, ISSN 0952-3480

Birk, U.J., Darrell, A., Konstantinides, N., Sarasa-Renedo, A. & Ripoll J. (2011). Improved reconstructions and generalized filtered back projection for optical projection tomography. *Appl Opt.*, Vol. 50, No. 4, (Feb 2011), pp. 392-398, ISSN 1539-4522

Bonner-Weir S. & Orci L. (1982). New perspectives on the microvasculature of the islets of Langerhans in the rat. *Diabetes*, Vol. 31, No. 10, (Oct 1982), pp. 883-889, ISSN 0012-1797

Brissova, M., Fowler, M.J., Nicholson, W.E., Chu, A., Hirshberg, B., Harlan, D.M. & Powers, A.C. (2005). Assessment of human pancreatic islet architecture and composition by laser scanning confocal microscopy. *J Histochem Cytochem.*, Vol. 53, No. 9, (Sep 2005), pp. 1087-1097, ISSN 0022-1554

Brunicardi, F.C., Stagner, J., Bonner-Weir, S., Wayland, H., Kleinman, R., Livingston, E., Guth, P., Menger, M., McCuskey, R., Intaglietta, M., Charles, A., Ashley, S., Cheung, A., Ipp, E., Gilman, S., Howard, T. & Passaro, E.Jr. (1996). Microcirculation of the islets of Langerhans. Long Beach Veterans Administration Regional Medical Education Center Symposium. *Diabetes*, Vol. 45, No. 4, (Apr 1996) pp. 385-92, ISSN 0012-1797

Brunicardi, F. C., Moldovan, S., Gilman, S., Livingston E. & Passaro,E. Jr (1997) An internet multicast symposium concerning the microcirculation of the islets of langerhans, *Transplantation Proceedings*, Vol. 29, Issue 4,(June 1997), pp. 2252-2254, ISSN 0041-1345

Bryson-Richardson, R.J. & Currie, P.D. (2004). Optical projection tomography for spatio-temporal analysis in the zebrafish. *Methods Cell Biol.*, Vol. 76, pp. 37-50, ISSN 0091-679X

Budinger, T.F. & Lauterbur, P.C. (1984). Nuclear magnetic resonance technology for medical studies. *Science,* Vol. 226, No.4672, (Oct 1984), pp.288-98, ISSN 0036-8075

Bunnag, S.C., Bunnag, S., Warner, N.E. (1963). Microcirculation in the islets of Langerhans of the mouse. *The Anatomical Record*, Vol. 146, No.6 (June 1963), pp. 117-23, ISSN 0003-276X

Cabrera, O., Berman, D.M., Kenyon, N.S., Ricordi, C., Berggren, P.O. & Caicedo A. (2006). The unique cytoarchitecture of human pancreatic islets has implications for islet cell function. *Proc Natl Acad Sci USA*, Vol. 103, No. 7, (February 2006), pp. 2334-2339, ISSN 0027-8424

Cassidy, P.J. & Radda G.K. (2005). Molecular Imaging Perspectives. *Journal of the Royal Society Interface*, Vol. 2, No. 3, (June 2005), pp. 133-144, ISSN 1742-5689

Colantuoni, A., Cimini, V., Coppini, G. & Bertuglia, S. (1988). Functional microangiopathy in alloxan-treated Syrian hamsters. *Int J Microcirc Clin Exp.*, Vol. 7, No. 2, (Mar 1988), pp.105-122, ISSN 0167-6865

Coppieters, K., Martinic, M.M., Kiosses, W.B., Amirian, N. & von Herrath M. (2010). A novel technique for the in vivo imaging of autoimmune diabetes development in the pancreas by two-photon microscopy. *PLoS One*, Vol. 5, No.12, (Dec 2010), ISSN 1932-6203

Denis, M.C., Mahmood, U., Benoist C., Mathis, D. & Weissleder, R. (2004). Imaging inflammation of the pancreatic islets in type 1 diabetes. *Proc Natl Acad Sci USA*, Vol. 101, No.34, (August 2004), pp. 12634-12639, ISSN - 0027-8424

Dunn, K.W., Young, P.A. (2006). Principles of multiphoton microscopy. *Nephron Exp Nephrol.*,Vol. 103, No. 2, (Mar 2006), pp.e33-40., ISSN 1660-2129

Eisenbarth, G.S, Moriyama, H., Robles, D.T., Liu, E., Yu, L., Babu, S., Redondo, M.J., Gottlieb, P., Wegmann, D., & Rewers, M. (2002). Insulin autoimmunity: prediction/precipitation/prevention type 1A diabetes, *Autoimmunity Reviews*, Vol. 1, Issue 3, (May 2002), pp. 139-145, ISSN 1568-9972

Enghofer, M., Usadel, K.H., Beck, O. & Kusterer, K. (1997). Superoxide dismutase reduces islet microvascular injury induced by streptozotocin in the rat. *Am J Physiol.*, Vol. 273, No. 2 (Pt 1), (Aug 1997), E376-382, ISSN 0002-9513

Evgenov, N.V., Medarova,Z., Dai, G., Bonner-Weir, S. & Moore, A. (2006). In vivo imaging of islet transplantation. *Nature Medicine*, Vol.12, No. 1, (January 2006), pp. 144-148, ISSN - 1078-8956

Fisher, M.E., Clelland, A.K., Bain, A., Baldock, R.A., Murphy, P., Downie, H., Tickle, C., Davidson, D.R. & Buckland, R.A. (2008). Integrating technologies for comparing 3D gene expression domains in the developing chick limb. *Dev Biol.*, Vol. 317, No. 1, (May 2008), pp.13-23, ISSN 1095-564X

Gadian, D.G. (1995). *NMR and its Applications to Living Systems* (2nd edition), Oxford University Press, ISBN 0-19-855803-1, Oxford

Gaglia, J.L., Guimaraes, A.R., Harisinghani, M., Turvey, S.E., Jackson, R., Benoist, C., Mathis, D. & Weissleder, R. (2011). Noninvasive imaging of pancreatic islet inflammation in type 1A diabetes patients. *J Clin Invest.*,Vol. 121, No1, (Jan 2011), pp.442-5, ISSN 1558-8238

Gotthardt, M. (2010). Beta cell imaging--why we need it and what has been achieved. *Curr Pharm Des.*, Vol. 16, No. 14, (May 2010), pp.1545-1546, ISSN 1873-4286

Haller, H. (1997). Postprandial glucose and vascular disease. *Diabet Med.*, Vol. 14, Suppl. 3, S50-56, (Aug 1997), ISSN 0742-3071.

Hara, M., Wang, X., Kawamura, T., Bindokas, V.P., Dizon, R.F., Alcoser, S.Y., Magnuson, M.A., Bell, G.I. (2003). Transgenic mice with green fluorescent protein-labeled pancreatic beta –cells. *Am J Physiol Endocrinol Metab.*, Vol.284, No.1, (January 2003), E177-E183, ISSN 0193-1849.

Hara, M., Dizon, R.F., Glick, B.S., Lee, C.S., Kaestner, K.H., Piston, D.W. & Bindokas VP (2006), Imaging pancreatic beta-cells in the intact pancreas, *Am J Physiol Endocrinol Metab.* Vol. 290, No 5, (May 2006), pp.E1041-1047, ISSN 0193-1849

Hutton, B.F. & Beekman, F.J. (2010). SPECT and SPECT/CT, In: *Molecular Imaging: Principles and Practice*, Ralph Weissleder, Brian D. Ross, Alnawaz Rehemtulla, Sanjiv Sam Gambhir, pp 40-53, People's Medical Publishing House–USA, ISBN 978-1-60795-005-9, Shelton, CT, USA

Hecksher-Sørensen, J., Watson, R.P., Lettice, L.A., Serup, P., Eley, L., De Angelis, C., Ahlgren, U. & Hill, R.E. (2004). The splanchnic mesodermal plate directs spleen and pancreatic laterality, and is regulated by Bapx1/Nkx3.2. *Development*, Vol.131, No.19, (Oct.2004), pp.4665-4675, ISSN 0950-1991

Heller, R.S.(2010). The comparative anatomy of islets. Adv Exp Med Biol. 2010; Vol.654, pp. 21-37, ISSN - 0065-2598.

Hudlicka, O. (1998). Is physiological angiogenesis in skeletal muscle regulated by changes in microcirculation? *Microcirculation,* Vol. 5, No.1, pp.7-23, ISSN 1073-9688

Ichise, M. & Harris, P.E. (2010). Imaging of B-cell mass and function. *J Nucl Med,* Vol.51, No.7, (Jul 2010), pp.1001-1004, ISSN 1535-5667

Intaglietta, M. & Messmer, K. (1983). Microangiodynamics, peripheral vascular resistance and the normal microcirculation. *Int J Microcirc Clin Exp.*, Vol. 2, No.1, (1983), pp.3-10, ISSN 0167-6865

Jain, R.K., Brown, E. B., Munn, L. L. & Fukumura, D. (2005). Intravital Microscopy of Normal and Diseased Tissues in the Mouse. In Live cell imaging: a laboratory manual/ edited Robert D Goldman, David Spector Cold Spring Harborr Laboratory Press, Cold Spring Harbor New York. , pp. 435-465, ISBN 0-87969-683-4

Jirák, D., Kríz, J., Herynek, V., Andersson, B., Girman, P., Burian, M., Saudek, F. and Hájek, M. (2004), MRI of transplanted pancreatic islets. *Magnetic Resonance in Medicine,* Vol.52, Issue 6, (December 2004), pp.1228–1233, ISSN 0740-3194

Kilimnik, G., Kim, A., Jo, J., Miller, K. & Hara M. (2009). Quantification of pancreatic islet distribution in situ in mice, *Am J Physiol Endocrinol Metab.* Vol.297, No.6, (Dec 2009), pp. E1331-8, ISSN 0193-1849

Kostromina, E., Gustavsson, N., Wang, X., Lim, C.Y., Radda, GK, Li, C. & Han W. (2010). Glucose intolerance and impaired insulin secretion in pancreas-specific STAT-3 knockout mice are associated with microvascular alterations in the pancreas. *Endocrinology,* Vol. 151, No.5, (May 2010), pp.2050-2059, ISSN 1945-7170

Kulandavelu, S., Qu, D., Sunn, N., Mu, J., Rennie, M.Y., Whiteley, K.J., Walls, J.R., Bock, N.A., Sun, J.C., Covelli A, Sled J.G. & Adamson S.L. (2006). Embryonic and neonatal phenotyping of genetically engineered mice. *ILAR J.*, Vol. 47, No. 2, pp.103-117, ISSN - 1084-2020

Lee, K., Avondo, J., Morrison, H., Blot ,L., Stark, M., Sharpe, J., Bangham, A. & Coen, E. (2006). Visualizing plant development and gene expression in three dimensions using optical projection tomography. *Plant Cell*, Vol. 18, No.9, (Sep 2006), pp.2145-56, ISSN 1040-4651

Leibiger, I.B., Brismar, K. & Berggren, P.O. (2010). Novel aspects on pancreatic beta-cellsignal-transduction. *Biochem Biophys Res Commun.*, Vol. 396, No.1, (May 2010), pp.111-5, ISSN 1090-2104

Leitgeb, R.A., Villiger, M., Bachmann, A.H., Steinmann, L.& Lasser, T. (2006). Extended focus depth for Fourier domain optical coherence microscopy. *Opt Lett.* Vol. 31, No. 16, (Aug 2006), pp.2450-2452, ISSN 0146-9592

Ley, K, Pries, A.R. & Gaehtgens, P. (1986). Topological structure of rat mesenteric microvessel networks. *Microvasc Res.*, Vol.32, No.3, (Nov 1986), pp.315-32, ISSN 0026-2862

Li, Z, Karlsson, F.A. & Sandler S. (2000) Islet loss and alpha cell expansion in type 1 diabetes induced by multiple low-dose streptozotocin administration in mice. *J Endocrinol.*, Vol. 165, No.1, (Apr.2000), pp.93-9, ISSN 0022-0795

Lim, F. & Sun A.M. (1980). Microencapsulated islets as bioartificial endocrine pancreas. *Science*, Vol. 210, No. 4472, (Nov 1980), pp.908-10, ISSN 0036-8075

Low, G., Hussein, N., Owen, R.J., Toso, C., Patel, V.H., Bhargava, R. & Shapiro A.M. (2010). Role of imaging in clinical islet transplantation. *Radiographics*, Vol. 30, No.2, (Mar 2010), pp.353-66, ISSN 1527-1323

Martinic, M.M. & von Herrath M.G. (2008). Real-time imaging of the pancreas during development of diabetes. *Immunol Rev.*, Vol. 221, (Feb 2008), pp.200-13, ISSN 1600-065X

Mathis, D. & Gaglia, J. (2010). Autoimmune Diabetes, In: *Molecular Imaging: Principles and Practice*, Ralph Weissleder, Brian D. Ross, Alnawaz Rehemtulla, Sanjiv Sam Gambhir, PP 1130-1146 , People's Medical Publishing House–USA, ISBN 978-1-60795-005-9, Shelton, CT, USA

McGurk, L., Morrison,H., Keegan, L.P., Sharpe, J. & O'Connell, M.A. (2007). Three-dimensional imaging of Drosophila melanogaster. *PLoS One*, Vol. 2, Issue 9, (Sep 2007), e834, ISSN 1932-6203

Medarova, Z., Castillo, G., Dai, G., Bolotin, E., Bogdanov, A. & Moore A. (2007). Noninvasive magnetic resonance imaging of microvascular changes in type 1 diabetes. *Diabetes*, Vol. 56, No. 11, (Nov 2007), pp.2677-82, ISSN 1939-327X

Medarova, Z. & Moore A. (2009). MRI as a tool to monitor islet transplantation. *Nat Rev Endocrinol.*, Vol. 5, No. 8, (Aug 2009), pp. 444-52, ISSN 1759-5037

Meier, J.J., Menge BA, Breuer TG, Müller CA, Tannapfel A, Uhl W, Schmidt WE,Schrader H. (2009). Functional assessment of pancreatic beta-cell area in humans. *Diabetes*, Vol. 58, No.7, (Jul 2009), pp.1595-603, ISSN 1939-327X

Menger, M.D., Vajkoczy, P., Leiderer, R., Jäger, S. & Messmer K. (1992) Influence of experimental hyperglycemia on microvascular blood perfusion of pancreatic islet isografts. *J Clin Invest.*, Vol.90, No. 4, (Oct 1992), pp.1361-9, ISSN 0021-9738

Menger, M.D., Vajkoczy, P., Beger, C. & Messmer.K. (1994). Orientation of microvascular blood flow in pancreatic islet isografts. *J Clin Invest.*, Vol.93, Issue 5 (May 1994), pp. 2280–2285, ISSN 0021-9738

Niederkorn, J.Y. (2002). Immunology and immunomodulation of corneal transplantation. *Int Rev Immunol.*, Vol.21, No.2-3, (Mar-Jun 2002), pp.173-96, ISSN 0883-0185

Ntziachristos V. (2010). Going deeper than microscopy: the optical imaging frontier in biology. *Nat Methods*, Vol. 7, No.8, (Aug 2010), pp.603-14, ISSN 1548-7105

Nyman, L.R., Wells, K.S., Head W.S., McCaughey, M., Ford, E., Brissova, M., Piston, D.W. & Powers, A.C. (2008). Real-time, multidimensional in vivo imaging used to investigate blood flow in mouse pancreatic islets. *J Clin Invest.*, Vol.118, No.11, (Nov. 2008), pp.3790-7, ISSN 0021-9738

Rinck, P.A. (2001). *Magnetic resonance in medicine.* The basic textbook of the European Magnetic Resonance Forum, 4th completely revised edition, Blackwell, ISBN 0-632-05986-9, Berlin Vienna.

Robertson, R.P. (2007) Estimation of beta-cell mass by metabolic tests: necessary, but how sufficient? Vol. 56, No. 10 (October 2007), pp.2420-4, ISSN 1939-327X

Ryan, E.A., Paty, B.W., Senior, P.A., Bigam, D., Alfadhli, E., Kneteman, N.M., Lakey, J.R., Shapiro, A.M. (2005). Five-year follow-up after clinical islet transplantation. *Diabetes*, Vol. 54, No.7, (Jul 2005), pp.2060-9, ISSN 0012-1797

Sand, F.W., Hörnblad, A., Johansson, J.K., Lorén, C., Edsbagge, J., Ståhlberg, A., Magenheim, J., Ilovich, O., Mishani, E., Dor, Y., Ahlgren, U. & Semb, H. (2011). Growth-limiting role of endothelial cells in endoderm development. *Dev Biol.*, Vol. 352, No.2, (Apr 2011), pp.267-77, ISSN 1095-564X

Sarma, S., Kerwin, J., Puelles, L., Scott, M., Strachan, T., Feng, G., Sharpe, J., Davidson, D., Baldock, R. & Lindsay, S. (2005). 3D modelling, gene expression mapping and post-mapping image analysis in the developing human brain. *Brain Res Bull.*, Vol. 66, No. 4-6, (Sep 2005) pp.449-53, ISSN 0361-9230

Saudek, F., Jirák, D., Girman, P., Herynek, V., Dezortová, M., Kríz, J., Peregrin, J., Berková, Z., Zacharovová, K. & Hájek M. (2010). Magnetic resonance imaging of pancreatic islets transplanted into the liver in humans. *Transplantation*, Vol.90, No.12, (Dec 2010), pp. 1602-6, ISSN 1534-6080

Savinov, A.Y., Wong, F.S., Stonebraker, A.C. & Chervonsky, A.V. (2003). Presentation of antigen by endothelial cells and chemoattraction are required for homing of insulin-specific CD8+ T cells. *J Exp Med.*, Vol. 197, No.5, (Mar 2003), pp.643-56, ISSN 0022-1007

Savinov, A.Y. & Strongin, A.Y. (2009). Matrix metalloproteinases, T cell homing and beta-cell mass in type 1 diabetes. *Vitam Horm.*, Vol. 80,(2009), pp.541-62, ISSN 0083-6729

Segal, S.S. (2005). Regulation of blood flow in the microcirculation. *Microcirculation*, Vol.12, No.1, (Jan-Feb 2005), pp.33-45, ISSN 1073-9688

Shapiro, A.M., Lakey, J.R., Ryan, E.A., Korbutt, G.S., Toth, E., Warnock, G.L., Kneteman, N.M. & Rajotte, R.V. (2000). Islet transplantation in seven patients with type 1 diabetes mellitus using a glucocorticoid-free immunosuppressive regimen. *N Engl J Med.*, Vol. 343, No.4, (Jul 2000), pp. 230-238, ISSN 0028-4793

Sharpe, J., Ahlgren, U., Perry, P., Hill, B., Ross, A., Hecksher-Sørensen, J., Baldock, R. & Davidson, D. (2002). Optical projection tomography as a tool for 3D microscopy and gene expression studies. *Science*, Vol. 296, No.5567, (Apr 2002), pp.541-5, ISSN 1095-9203

Sharpe, J. (2003). Optical projection tomography as a new tool for studying embryo anatomy. *J Anat*, Vol. 202, No. 2, (Feb 2003), pp.175-81, ISSN 0021-8782

Sharpe, J. (2004). Optical projection tomography. *Annu Rev Biomed Eng.*, Vol. 6, (2004), pp.209-28, ISSN 1523-9829

Sharpe, J. (2010). Optical Projection Tomography, In: *Molecular Imaging: Principles and Practice,* Ralph Weissleder, Brian D. Ross, Alnawaz Rehemtulla, Sanjiv Sam Gambhir, pp.244-261, People's Medical Publishing House–USA, ISBN 978-1-60795-005-9, Shelton, CT, USA

Signore, A., Procaccini, E., Toscano, A.M., Ferretti, E., Williams, A.J., Beales, P.E., Cugini, P. & Pozzilli, P. (1994). Histological study of pancreatic beta-cell loss in relation to the insulitis process in the non-obese diabetic mouse. *Histochemistry,* Vol. 101, No.4, (Apr 1994), pp.263-9, ISSN 0301-5564

Soltani, N., Kumar, M., Glinka, Y., Prud'homme, G.J. & Wang, Q. (2007). In vivo expression of GLP-1/IgG-Fc fusion protein enhances beta-cell mass and protects against streptozotocin-induced diabetes. *Gene Ther.*, Vol. 14, No. 12, (Jun 2007), pp.981-8, ISSN 0969-7128

Speier, S., Nyqvist, D., Cabrera, O., Yu, J., Molano, R.D., Pileggi, A., Moede, T., Köhler, M., Wilbertz, J., Leibiger, B., Ricordi, C., Leibiger, I.B., Caicedo, A. & Berggren, P.O. (2008a). Noninvasive In Vivo Imaging of Pancreatic Islet Cell Biology. Nature Medicine, Vol.14, No.5, (May 2008), pp.574-578, ISSN 1546-170X

Speier, S., Nyqvist, D., Köhler, M., Caicedo, A., Leibiger, I.B. & Berggren, P.O. (2008b). Noninvasive High-Resolution In Vivo Imaging of Cell Biology in the Anterior Chamber of the Mouse Eye. *Nature Protocols,* Vol.3, No.8, (August 2008), pp. 59-64, ISSN 1750-2799

Srinivas, M., Morel, P.A., Ernst, L.A., Laidlaw, D.H. & Ahrens, E.T.(2007). Fluorine-19 MRI for visualization and quantification of cell migration in a diabetes model. *Magn Reson Med.*Vol. 58, No.4, (Oct 2007), pp. 725-34, ISSN 0740-3194

Sun, Y., Ma, X., Zhou, D., Vacek, I., Sun, A.M. (1996). Normalization of diabetes in spontaneously diabetic cynomologus monkeys by xenografts of microencapsulated porcine islets without immunosuppression. *J Clin Invest.* Sep 15; Vol. 98, No. 6 (Sep 1996), pp.1417-22, ISSN - 0021-9738

Svensson, A.M., Sandler, S. & Jansson, L. (2003). Role of superoxide anion in pancreatic islet blood flow regulation in anesthetized rats. *Eur J Pharmacol.* Vol. 459, No. 1, (Jan 2003), pp. 59-64. ISSN 0014-2999

Tai, J.H., Foster, P., Rosales, A., Feng, B., Hasilo, C., Martinez, V., Ramadan, S., Snir, J., Melling, C.W., Dhanvantari, S., Rutt, B. & White, D.J. (2006). Imaging islets labeled with magnetic nanoparticles at 1.5 Tesla. *Diabetes,* Vol. 55, No. 11, (Nov 2006), pp.2931-2938, ISSN 0012-1797

Toso, C., Vallee, J.P., Morel, P., Ris, F., Demuylder-Mischler, S., Lepetit-Coiffe, M., Marangon, N., Saudek, F., Shapiro, J.A.M, Bosco, D., Berney, T. (2008). Clinical magnetic resonance imaging of pancreatic islet grafts after iron nanoparticle labeling. *Am J Transplant.*, Vol. 8, No. 3, (Mar 2008), pp.701-706, ISSN 1600-6143

Townsend, D. (2010). Imaging of structure and function with PET/CT, In: Molecular Imaging: Principles and Practice, Ralph Weissleder, Brian D. Ross, Alnawaz

Rehemtulla, Sanjiv Sam Gambhir, People's Medical Publishing House - USA, Shelton, CT, pp. 10-28, ISBN 978-1-60795-005-9.

Tsuzuki, Y, Mouta Carreira C, Bockhorn, M, Xu L, Jain, R.K, Fukumura, D. (2001). Pancreas microenvironment promotes VEGF expression and tumor growth: novel window models for pancreatic tumor angiogenesis and microcirculation. *Lab Invest.*, Vol. 81, No. 10, (Oct 2001), pp.1439-1451, ISSN 0023-6837

Turvey, S.E., Swart, E., Denis, M.C., Mahmood, U., Benoist, C., Weissleder, R. & Mathis, D. (2005). Noninvasive imaging of pancreatic inflammation and its reversal in type 1 diabetes, *J Clin Invest.*, Vol. 115, No.9, (September 2005), pp.2454–2461, ISSN 0021-9738

Villiger, M, Goulley, J, Friedrich, M, Grapin-Botton, A, Meda, P, Lasser, T, Leitgeb, R.A. (2009). In vivo imaging of murine endocrine islets of Langerhans with extended-focus optical coherence microscopy. *Diabetologia,* Vol. 52, No.8, (Aug 2009), 1599-1607, ISSN 1432-0428

Walls, J.R., Sled, J.G., Sharpe, J., Henkelman, R.M. (2005). Correction of artefacts in optical projection tomography. *Phys Med Biol.*, Vol. 50, No. 19, (Oct 2005), pp. 4645-65, ISSN 0031-9155

Walls, J.R., Sled, J.G., Sharpe, J, Henkelman, R.M. (2007). Resolution improvement in emission optical projection tomography. *Phys Med Biol.*, Vol. 52, No. 10, (May 2007), pp.2775-90, ISSN 0031-9155

Wicker, L.S., Miller, B.J., Coker, L.Z., McNally, S.E., Scott, S., Mullen, Y. & Appel, M.C. (1987). Genetic control of diabetes and insulitis in the nonobese diabetic (NOD) mouse. *J Exp Med.*, Vol.165, No.6, (June 1987), pp.1639-54, ISSN 0022-1007

Zito, F.A., Marzullo, F., D'Errico, D., Salvatore, C., Digirolamo, R., Labriola, A. & Pellecchia A. (2004). Quicktime virtual reality technology in light microscopy to support medical education in pathology. *Mod Pathol.*, Vol. 17, No. 6, (Jun 2004), pp.728-31, ISSN 0893-3952

Part 5

Therapy

14

Present Accomplishments and Future Prospects of Cell-Based Therapies for Type 1 Diabetes Mellitus

Preeti Chhabra[1], Clark D. Kensinger[1,2], Daniel J. Moore[3] and Kenneth L. Brayman[1,2]
[1]Department of Surgery, University of Virginia,
[2]Division of Transplantation, Department of Surgery, University of Virginia,
[3]Department of Pediatrics, Division of Endocrinology and Diabetes, Vanderbilt Children's Hospital,
[1,2]Charlottesville,
[3]Nashville,
USA

1. Introduction

Type 1 diabetes mellitus is a classical autoimmune disease that results from immune-mediated destruction of pancreatic β-cells, primarily by T cells specific for β-cell antigens, leading to an absolute loss of insulin production (Gillard and Mathieu et al., 2011; van Belle et al. 2011). While the disease can become clinically apparent at any age, it commonly starts during childhood, and may appear later in adulthood in approximately 30-40% of affected individuals (Fändrich and Ungefroren, 2010; Knip, 1997). A combination of a genetic predisposition and autoimmune processes contribute to its development resulting in the gradual destruction of the insulin-producing β-cells. Daily insulin delivery by injection or pump to manage hyperglycemia by no means represents a cure, often resulting in hypoglycemic episodes (Leitão et al.,2008; Noguchi, 2009). Current strategies to prevent or reverse diabetes are broadly based on the concepts of β-cell regeneration, replacement or protection from T-cell-mediated autoimmune destruction. While transplantation of both, whole pancreas as well as islets of Langerhans, is able to restore endocrine function and glucose homeostasis, islet transplantation offers added advantage in terms of being minimally invasive, preventing the incidence of severe hypoglycemic episodes and significantly lowering hypoglycemic unawareness, thereby improving the quality of life of the transplant recipients (Bretzel et al, 2007; Langer, 2010; Noguchi et al, 2009). Furthermore, manipulation of islets *in vitro*, prior to transplantation, provides an opportunity for the development of various therapeutic manipulations aimed at achieving better transplant outcomes. However, despite islet transplantation being an excellent "proof of principle" for β-cell replacement therapy, its wide-spread applicability is limited by the scarcity of donor organs resulting in inadequate number of islets available for transplant as well as the harmful side-effects of immunosuppressive therapy (Huang et al., 2008). To overcome these limitations, generating a large quantity of β-cells that would allow transplantation of sufficient β-cell mass to achieve normoglycemia, along with restoration of immunologic tolerance, represents a highly attractive alternative. To this end, proposed mechanisms for islet regeneration consist of replication of pre-existing β-cells, neogenesis from ductal and non β-cell progenitors, transdifferentiation of fully differentiated acinar cells and directed-differentiation of stem cells (putative β-cell progenitors/pancreatic stem cells; embryonic, mesenchymal, hematopoietic and umbilical cord blood-derived stem cells etc). While several studies demonstrate these mechanisms in mice, proving the occurrence of these phenomena in humans is hard to achieve. In this review, we will focus on various approaches to obtain an expandable mass of functional, insulin-secreting β-cells, emphasizing the major cell candidates for β-cell regeneration, the specific factors and stimuli involved in β-cell differentiation and expansion and alternate strategies that may enhance the effective β-cell mass and function. The basic science driving these discoveries and the obstacles that hinder clinical translation of these avenues will be highlighted from the perspective of islet transplantation.

2. Endocrine pancreas plasticity in physiological conditions

Although the formation of new islets in adults has primarily been demonstrated in response to pancreatic injury (eg. pancreatic duct ligation (PDL), β-cell ablation, partial pancreactomy etc.) and metabolic stress, there is ample evidence that β-cell replication from existing cells occurs throughout adulthood (Brennand et al, 2007; Dor et al., 2004; Levetan, 2010; Nir et al., 2007; Teta et al., 2007). This has been observed in several physiologic situations including amongst others, late pregnancy and obesity (Bernard-Kargar and Ktorza, 2001). In both these cases, increases in β-cell mass have been observed in response to insulin resistance and contribute to insulin oversecretion. Several studies have demonstrated a doubling of β-cell mass by the end of pregnancy that decreased progressively after parturition, a good illustration of the plasticity of the endocrine pancreas (Karnik et al., 2007; Rieck & Kaestner, 2010; Scaglia et al., 1995). As in pregnancy, euglycemia is maintained in obesity by increased insulin secretion, due not only to enhanced individual β-cell activity but also to β-cell growth. This increase in β-cell mass approximates 50% in obese, non-diabetic humans and seems consigned to β-cells, with α, δ and PP cell mass remaining unchanged (Bernard-Kargar & Ktorza, 2001). In addition to β-cell expansion based on self-duplication, there is evidence indicating the contribution of stem cell differentiation towards pancreatic β-cell maintenance (Bonner-Weir et al.,2004, 2006,2010). The mechanism of islet regeneration remains controversial, making identification of β-cell progenitors and the in-depth understanding of the underlying mechanisms that trigger β-cell regeneration and expansion absolutely critical in order to apply this strategy in a clinical scenario.

2.1 β-cell progenitors within the pancreas

The exocrine tissue of the pancreas consists of acinar cells that secrete digestive enzymes into a branched ductal network that drains into the gastrointestinal tract. The endocrine cells consist of α, β, δ, ε, and PP cells that are grouped into islets of Langerhans and secrete insulin and other polypeptide hormones into the bloodstream. Numerous studies propose that in addition to replication of pre-existing β-cells, new β-cells can be produced from differentiated adult cells by interconversions amongst different pancreatic cell compartments as well as neogenesis from ductal and circulating progenitors and putative pancreatic stem cells (Bonner-Weir et al., 2004,2006; Gao et al., 2003, 2005; Granger and

Kushner, 2009; Juhl et al., 2010; Kikugawa et al.,2009; Pittenger et al., 2009). However, while these strategies demonstrate the generation of insulin-producing cells, the major challenge encountered is the inability to generate sufficient amounts of 'glucose-responsive' β-cells to normalize hyperglycemia. True mature β-cells are defined by the ability to store large amounts of insulin and secrete it in a regulated manner in response to glucose challenge. This inability to mature into 'glucose responsive' β-cells may indicate an underlying inability to dedifferentiate completely to a progenitor state or to efficiently redifferentiate/transdifferentiate into β-cells. Therefore, while these studies outline the therapeutic potential of various regenerative strategies for β-cell expansion, they also highlight the importance of elucidating the underlying mechanisms required to form islets that perform similar to primary islets used in clinical applications.

2.1.1 Can β-cells be derived from the exocrine pancreas - the plasticity of the pancreatic acinar cell.

The exocrine tissue consisting of acinar and ductal cells, comprises approximately 95% of the adult pancreas and shares a common progenitor with endocrine cells, namely, pancreatic and duodenal homeobox 1(Pdx1)-expressing cells (Gu et al, 2002). Several studies indicate the capability of acinar cells to transdifferentiate into insulin positive cells (IPCs) either directly (Minami et al., 2005; Minami and Seino S, 2008) or via a ductal intermediate (Means et al., 2005), usually accompanied by a corresponding increase in functional β-cell mass. However, other studies using cultured, genetically marked, murine acinar cells indicate that these cells are only able to rapidly transdifferentiate into a amylase-negative, keratin 19- and mucin-antigens positive ductal phenotype and not into functional β-cells (Blaine et al., 2010). Using a mouse model that develops hyperplastic ducts containing IPCs in response to the transforming growth factor (TGF-α), Blaine et al. performed genetic lineage tracing experiments and demonstrated that hyperplastic ductal cells arose largely from acinar cells that transdifferentiated into ductal cells, while IPCs adjacent to acinar-derived ductal cells arose from pre-existing IPCs, suggesting that islet endocrine cells can intercalate into hyperplastic ducts as they develop. Thus, the apparent pancreatic plasticity resulted from both, the ability of acinar cells to transdifferentiate and of endocrine cells to reorganize in association with duct structures. Enthusiasm was further curbed by a Cre/loxP-based lineage tracing study suggesting that transdifferentiation of acinar to β-cells was unlikely a part of the normal β-cell turnover, even after injury such as pancreatectomy, ductal ligation, or pancreatitis (Desai et al., 2007). A recent time-specific lineage tracing study indicated that in mice containing genetically marked ductal and acinar cells carrying the mucin gene Muc1, the Muc1 positive cells only gave rise to β-cells and other islet cells *in utero* (Kopinke & Murtaugh, 2010). From birth onwards, Muc1 lineage-labeled cells were confined to the exocrine compartment with no detectable contribution to islet cells. In contrast, other studies showed that differentiated exocrine cells were capable of reverting to a partially dedifferentiated state with the capacity to transdifferentiate into different phenotypes, including ductal cells (Rooman et al., 2000), hepatocyte-like cells (Lardon et al., 2004) and IPCs (Baeyens et al., 2005, 2008). Treatment of rat exocrine pancreatic cells *in vitro* with epidermal growth factor (EGF) and leukaemia inhibitory factor (LIF) resulted in an 11-fold increase of the β-cell mass in a 3 day culture period with the newly-formed cells secreting insulin in response to glucose, containing insulin immunoreactive secretory granules, immunoreactive for C-peptide-I, Pdx-1 and Glucose transporter-2 (Glut-2) and able to restore normoglycemia upon transplantation into alloxan-diabetic mice. Interestingly, the cells were immunoreactive for amylase and cytokeratin-20, characteristics of exocrine cells. Similar results were obtained using adult mouse pancreatic acinar cells cultured in suspension in the presence of EGF and nicotinamide. Analysis using a Cre/loxP-based direct cell lineage tracing system indicated that newly made cells originated from amylase/elastase-expressing pancreatic acinar cells and had insulin-containing secretory granules (Minami et al., 2005). Insulin secretion was stimulated by glucose, sulfonylurea, and carbachol; potentiation by glucagon-like peptide-1 (GLP-1) was also observed. In addition, enzymatic dissociation of pancreatic acini itself lead to activation of EGF signaling and inhibition of EGF receptor kinase blocked transdifferentiation, suggesting that activation of EGF signaling was required for transdifferentiation of pancreatic acinar cells into insulin-secreting cells with secretory properties similar to native pancreatic β-cells (Minami & Seino, 2008). Using a different approach, Melton and coworkers demonstrated that a specific combination of transcription factors Neurogenin3 (Ngn3), Pdx1 and MafA could reprogram differentiated, pancreatic exocrine cells in adult mice into cells that were indistinguishable from endogenous islet β-cells in size, shape and ultrastructure and expressed genes essential for β-cell function (Zhou et al., 2008). These cells increased by 20% after the triple adenoviral transduction and were capable of ameliorating hyperglycemia by remodeling local vasculature and secreting insulin, providing proof that 1) exocrine cells can assume an insulin-secreting phenotype and 2) that cellular reprogramming of exocrine pancreatic tissue using defined factors in an adult organ was possible without reverting to a pluripotent stem cell state or involving activation of the cell cycle. The drawback of this study however, was that these cells did not form islets nor became incorporated into them. Also, the use of viruses raises concerns about insertional mutagenesis and tumor initiation. A more clinically suitable study through induction of acinar-to-islet transdifferentiation was the expansion of adult, human islet tissue via a duct epithelial-like intermediate using a combination of gastrin, hepatocyte growth factor (HGF), and the Reg family member INGAP, islet neogenesis gene associated protein (Lipsett et al., 2007). A 6-fold increase in total dithizone (DTZ) positivity and approximately 15-fold increase in neoislets compared with untreated control tissue cultures was observed. However, these cells were not as efficient as native islets in the production of insulin and the success of this process depended heavily on the reorganization of the extracellular matrix begging definition of the role of extracellular scaffolding in increasing the output of islet-like cells or their insulin-secreting function(Okuno et al., 2007). Thus, transdifferentiation into insulin-secreting cells with low insulin expression levels and secretory response, absence of transcription factors essential for β-cell development and the inability to fully mature remain serious concerns.

2.1.2 The feasibility of β-cell regeneration through neogenesis from pancreatic ductal cells

Morphological observations of islet-ductal complexes comprising IPCs within or near adult pancreatic ducts in instances such as pregnancy or obesity, damage or disease, supported by various lineage-tracing studies in both human and rodent pancreata, suggest that differentiated pancreatic ductal cells act as *in vivo* progenitors for pancreatic β-cells (Bonner-Weir et al., 2008; Inada et al., 2008; Suarez-Pinzon et al.,2005; Xu et al., 2008, Xia et al. 2009). This is particularly impressive in the pancreata of individuals with a clinical diagnosis of chronic pancreatitis or with asymptomatic pancreatic fibrosis wherein immunophenotypical characterization of duct-associated islet-like cells revealed positivity for both ductal and endocrine markers (Gianani et al., 2006, 2011). The presence of insulin- and cytokeratin-positive cells has also been reported in transplanted pancreata of individuals with recurrence of β-cell autoimmunity (Martin-Pagola et al., 2008). Transient expression of the Ngn3 marks progenitor cells in the pancreas as they differentiate into islet cells. Using lineage-tracing and pancreatic ductal ligation in adult mice, Xu et al. revealed the appearance of facultative Ngn3+ Cytokeratin19+ progenitors in the ductal lining of the regenerating portion but not in the non-injured pancreas during the robust β-cell expansion that followed pancreatic duct ligation (PDL), suggesting that endogeneous duct cells represented an obvious target for therapeutic regeneration of β-cells in diabetes (Xu et al., 2008). Concerns raised about using Ngn3 expression as a marker of endocrine progenitors and neogenesis were allayed in a very recent study that developed a transgenic mouse line that could monitor Ngn-3 expression, and thus islet cell genesis, by surrogate markers that secreted alkaline phosphatase (SeAP) and enhanced green florescent protein (EGFP) (Shimajiri et al., 2011). They demonstrated that in transgenic embryos, cells expressing EGFP lined the pancreatic ducts while SeAP was readily detectable in embryos, in the media of cultured embryonic pancreases and in the serum of adult animals. Duct ligation in adult mice caused an increase in circulating SeAP levels. A genetic lineage tracing study using a human carbonic anhydrase II (CA2) promoter fragment to express Cre and CreER in differentiated duct cells showed that a significant proportion of adult pancreatic ductal cells retain the potential to differentiate into other pancreatic cell types including β-cells. Impressively, two weeks after duct ligation, 42% of islets and 24% of β-cells expressed the lineage marker (Inada et al., 2008). In fact, dedifferentiation of ductal epithelial cells is often associated with the epithelial-mesenchymal transition (EMT)(Fanjul et al., 2010). An interesting study by Seaberg et al reported the identification of multipotent precursor cells from the adult mouse pancreatic islet and ductal populations (Seaberg et al., 2004) that proliferated *in vitro* to form clonal colonies coexpressing neural and pancreatic precursor markers. Upon differentiation, individual clonal colonies produced distinct populations of neurons and glial cells, pancreatic endocrine β-, α-and δ-cells and pancreatic exocrine and stellate cells. The newly generated β-like cells demonstrated glucose-dependent Ca(2+) responsiveness and insulin release, representing a previously unidentified, intrinsic, pancreatic precursor population that is a promising candidate for cell-based therapeutic strategies. Taken together, these data show that the ductal epithelium in human as well as rodent pancreata is capable of producing IPCs, however whether these cells are mature β-cells with the full complement of molecules necessary for maintaining optimal glucose homeostasis remains to be seen. Despite these advances, the ductal origin hypothesis of pancreatic regeneration is under attack (Kushner et al., 2010). While some reports suggest that β-cell replication rather than neogenesis is the main source of regenerating islets in the murine pancreas (Dor et al., 2004), others using genetic labeling to fate map embryonic and adult pancreatic duct cells have demonstrated that pancreatic ductal epithelial cells do not contribute to endocrine or acinar cells postnatally (Solar et al., 2009). The latter study demonstrated that as the embryonic Hnf1β+ epithelium gradually acquires the anatomical configuration of the pancreatic ductal network, it sequentially sets aside cells for the acinar and endocrine lineages and finally takes on a differentiated pancreatic duct phenotype. The embryonic ducts give rise to both differentiated endocrine and ductal cells but once the pancreatic duct epithelium acquires a differentiated phenotype, it does not contribute significantly to new β-cells that are formed in diverse physiological or regenerative settings. However, certain caveats have not been addressed in this study; amongst them being low labeling efficiency during embryonic development and variable expression of Hnf1β in ductal progenitors with the cells that do become marked, representing a population of duct cells with a higher activity of Hnf1 β transcription or greater accessibility to Cre recombinase. Thus, taking into account possible low levels of leakiness of the Cre-lox system over time with the strong insulin promoter, the small proportion of the islets counted, limited (only 30%) labeling of the β-cells and the lack of examination of the new lobes after pancreatectomy, neogenesis in the adult cannot be ruled out by negative data of a lack of dilution of labeled β-cells (Kushner et al., 2010). The observed discrepancies warrant rigorous investigation with definitive experiments, using lineage tracing studies with additional markers that label either ducts or other candidate precursor cells to tease out the underlying mechanisms. Until then, however, the identification of differentiated pancreatic duct epithelium represents an expandable source of facultative progenitor cells for generating β-cells with major implications for replenishment therapy for diabetes.

2.1.3 Replication of pre-existing β-cells: contribution to β-cell growth and regeneration

Following stimuli such as pregnancy, obesity, glucose infusion, manipulating growth-hormone expression, toxigene-mediated β-cell ablation and partial pancreatectomy, self-renewal by β-cell replication has emerged as a dominant mechanism for homeostatic maintenance of β-cell mass postnatally. This was elegantly demonstrated in a study by Melton and coworkers wherein, using lineage-tracing highly specific for β-cells (double transgenic mice bearing a tamoxifen-dependent Cre-recombinase construct under the control of a rat insulin promoter together with a reporter Z/AP gene) they showed that pre-existing terminally differentiated β-cells, rather than pluripotent stem cells, were the major source of new β-cells retaining significant proliferative capacity *in vivo* during adult life, even after pancreatectomy (Dor et al., 2004). This conclusion was supported by the observation that forced cell-cycle arrest of β-cells by transgenic expression of the cyclin-dependent kinase inhibitor p27 blocked β-cell proliferation, severely restricting postnatal but not embryonic β-cell mass, indicating that non β-cells were unable to compensate (Nir & Dor, 2005). Deletion of cyclin-dependent kinase 4 (Cdk4) showed similar results that could be rescued by β-cell-specific expression of *Cdk4*, suggesting that the underlying proliferative defect in *Cdk4*-null mice lay in β-cells (Martin et al., 2003; Rane et al., 1999, Uchida et al., 2005). A recent *in vivo* pulse-chase labeling assay investigating the replication dynamics of adult mouse β-cells indicated that replicated β-cells were able to re-enter the cell division cycle shortly after mitosis and regained their normal proliferative potential after a short quiescence period of several days (Salpeter et al., 2010). Metabolic demand was a key determinant of cell cycle re-entry as quiescence period was lengthened with advanced age, but shortened during injury-driven β-cell regeneration and following treatment with a pharmacological activator of glucokinase. Their results implicated glucose control of cyclin D2 expression in regulating the capacity of β-cells to re-enter the cell cycle post-mitosis. A novel DNA analog-based lineage-tracing technique to detect multiple rounds of cell division *in vivo* indicated that β-cells rather than specialized progenitors contributed to adult β-cells, slowed by a replication refractory period that prevented β-cells from immediately redividing (Teta et al., 2007). Also, label-retaining experiments, clonal analysis and sequential thymidine analogue labeling indicated that all β-cells replicated homogeneously, contributing equally to islet growth and maintenance in healthy adult mice as well as during periods of increased replication such as pregnancy, neonatal growth and following pancreatectomy (Brennand et al., 2007, Teta et al., 2007). By counting accumulated mitotic figures following colchicine treatment (Bonner-weir et al., 1989), 5-bromo-2'-deoxyuridine (BrdU) incorporation (Montana et al., 1994), tritiated thymidine incorporation (Kaung, 1994) or expression of the cell cycle marker Ki67 (Meier et al., 2008), it has been shown that β-cell replication rates in rodents and human beings *in vivo* are a function of age, highest during late embryonic development and the neonatal period and declining significantly throughout adulthood (Brennand & Melton, 2009). However, hyperglycemia and hyperinsulinemia can induce a robust increase in β-cell replication even in older mice. Unfortunately human β-cell replication is difficult to demonstrate compared to murine pancreas (Butler et al., 2003, 2010; Menge et al., 2008). Although there have been reports of human β-cell proliferation in the presence of HGF (Kayali et al., 2007) or by overexpression of Cdk6 (Fiaschi-Taesch et al., 2010), the results were questionable, since insulin expression was lost after 5 doublings in the former study and the investigators in the latter study did not measure β-cell mass or number thereby raising doubts whether their approach did induce proliferation of β-cells. While β-cell replication offers an attractive mechanism for postnatal homeostatic maintenance of β-cells, the complete absence of β-cells in patients with type 1 diabetes and a declining ability to replicate with age are questions that need to be addressed.

2.1.4 Intra-Islet cells: role of α and δ cells in β-cell regeneration

Several studies using the streptozotocin (STZ)-induced diabetic model have indicated the presence of intra-islet precursor cells with the potential to differentiate into neo islets/pancreatic β-cells upon appropriate stimulation (Banerjee & Bhonde, 2003; Guz et al., 2001; Kodama et al., 2005). While some studies indicate that administration of betacellulin improved STZ-induced hyperglycemia by promoting neoformation of β-cells mainly from somatostatin-positive islet cells (Li et al., 2003), others suggested that differentiation of multipotent nestin-positive stem cells isolated from adult pancreatic islets resulted in pancreatic endocrine, exocrine, and hepatic phenotypes *ex vivo* (Zulewski et al., 2001). By conditional and ectopic expression of Pax4 using different cell-specific promoters, Collombat et al have demonstrated that Pax4 forces endocrine precursor cells as well as mature α-cells to adopt a β-cell destiny (Collombat et al., 2009). Upon Pax4 ectopic expression, the resulting glucagon deficiency provoked a compensatory and continuous glucagon-positive cell neogenesis requiring the re-expression of the proendocrine gene Ngn3, with the newly-formed α-cells acquiring a β-cell phenotype. Thus, ectopic expression of Pax4 in α-cells caused a cycle of neogenesis and redifferentiation capable of restoring a functional β-mass and restoring normoglycemia in animals that had been chemically depleted of β-cells. In an elegant experiment using alloxan damage to eliminate all pre-existing β-cells followed by PDL to stimulate β-cell neogenesis, Fred Levine and coworkers demonstrated β-cell neogenesis from α-cells (Chung et al., 2010a,2010b). They showed that virtually all β-cells that appeared after treatment were neogenic, mostly arising from adult α-cells within 14 days. At one week, 58% of IPCs coexpressed glucagon and β-cell-specific transcription factors such as Pdx1 and Nkx6.1. By two weeks, these MafB-expressing immature IPCs demonstrated a predominant mature phenotype defined by MafA expression and lack of glucagon. Furthermore, in this PDL plus alloxan model, in response to environmental cues, α-cells could a) replicate first, forming a potential reservoir of β-cell progenitors; b) could directly differentiate into β-cells without intervening replication; or c) replicate first and then convert to β-cells. β-cell regeneration from α-cells was also demonstrated using a transgenic model of diphtheria-toxin-induced, acute, selective, near-total β-cell ablation (Thorel et al., 2010). Administration of insulin resulted in β-cell mass augmentation with time and lineage-tracing to label the glucagon-producing α-cells before β-cell ablation tracked large fractions of regenerated β-cells as derived from α-cells. Transdifferentiation of glucagon-expressing cells into insulin-expressing cells on menin inactivation, without the necessity of Pdx1, MafA, Pax4, and Ngn3 expression, has also been demonstrated albeit in a scenario relating to islet tumorigenesis (Lu et al., 2010). The lack of Ngn3, Pdx1, and MafA expression in these cells makes them more similar to the immature MafB+Ins+ cells that have been documented during development, however, further investigation will be required to clarify the similarities and the differences. Taken together, these results demonstrate that adult α-cells can serve as *in vivo* source for generating β-cells. There are only a few published records of this phenomenon in human pancreata. Gianani et al. reported the presence of insulin–glucagon double-positive cells in fibrotic pancreata and speculated that in conditions like chronic pancreatitis and pancreatic fibrosis, α-cells increased through neogenesis from ductal cells followed by transdifferentiation into insulin-producing cells (Gianani et al., 2006, 2011). This theory is supported by experiments demonstrating insulin–glucagon double-positive cells intermixed with a severe insulitic islet infiltrate in the pancreata of a subset of NOD mice that remain non-diabetic despite the total loss of insulin-producing cells. Since α-cells appear to be capable of resisting immune-mediated destruction in autoimmune diabetes, with residual α-cells persisting long after the onset of disease, this scenario is particularly attractive in terms of potential therapy. Other studies indicating the presence of intra-islet β-cell precursors include the development of a tissue culture platform wherein isolated adult human pancreatic islets formed proliferative duct-like structures expressing ductal and progenitor markers. Short-term treatment with INGAP induced these structures to reform islet-like structures that resembled freshly isolated islets with respect to the frequency and distribution of the four endocrine cell types, islet gene expression and hormone production, insulin content, and glucose-responsive insulin secretion (Hanley & Rosenberg, 2009). Similar results were obtained by dedifferentiation of fresh human islets into a duct cell phenotype with further redifferentiation into β-cells in appropriate conditions *in vivo* (Gao et al., 2005). While the plasticity of adult human islets has significant implications for islet regeneration, until the maximum extent of neogenesis achieved using intra-islet cells can be determined, significant investment in developing regenerative strategies based on these cells should be reconsidered.

3. Stem cells strategies for β-cell regeneration

Obtaining a large source of β-cells for cellular therapy is a major challenge in the treatment of diabetes. While efforts thus far are based on deriving maximal utilization of all the unwanted tissue from the donor organ, the insignificant yield of differentiated β-cells, diminished function and insignificant amounts of insulin secreted both *in vitro* and *in vivo*, make it necessary to seek alternative approaches. Regeneration of β-cells from a self renewing, expandable stock of stem/progenitor cells via processes that include dedifferentiation, proliferation, tissue-specific directed differentiation and genetic reprogramming offer an attractive alternate source towards achieving insulin independency in diabetic patients. Based on their origins, stems cells from blastocyst-stage embryos can be classified as pluripotent embryonic stem cells (ESCs), whilst those obtained from niches of mature adult tissues and bone marrow as adult multipotent stem cells. The tissue-specific differentiation of ESCs, pancreas-derived multipotent progenitor/stem cells, extra-pancreatic adult stem cells (bone-marrow (BM) derived stem cells, neural progenitor cells, umbilical cord blood (UCB)-derived stem cells, etc.) or induced pluripotent stem cells (iPSCs) established from adult differentiated cells, into unprecedented quantities of cells with an insulin expressing phenotype *in vitro* has tremendous potential in β-cells replacement therapy(Aguayo-Mazzucato & Bonner-Weir, 2010; Furth etal., 2009; Guo et al., 2009; Santana et al., 2006; Sordi et al., 2008; Stanley et al., 2008; Tang 2004). Additionally, the immunosuppressive, anti-inflammatory properties of stem cells shared among ESCs and several types of non-haematopoietic stem cells (HSCs) such as BM-derived mesenchymal stem cells (BM-MSCs) and UCB-derived stem cells are an added advantage. Better yet is the ability of iPSCs to generate an unlimited supply of clinically compliant, functional β-cells derived from a patient's own somatic cells, and therefore not subject to allograft rejection, providing a framework for a solution to the cited limits of islet transplantation, tissue supply and chronic immunosuppression.

3.1 Potential stem/progenitor cell sources for regeneration of insulin-producing β-cells

3.1.1 Regeneration of β-cells from embryonic stem cells

ESCs are pluripotent with high self-renewal potential and a limitless capacity of proliferation. There are several elegant strategies to induce β-cell generation from ESCs, based on sequential exposure of human ESCs to epigenetic signals that mimic *in-vivo* pancreatic development, beginning with the formation of definite endoderm, followed by pancreatic endoderm, endocrine tissue and finally β-cell maturation (Aguayo-Mazzucato & Bonner-Weir, 2010). These differentiated β-cells display architecture consistent with mature islets, contain islet hormones, respond successfully to glucose challenge in glucose-tolerance tests (GTT) and reverse hyperglycemia in diabetic mice. While several growth factors, such as activin A, fibroblast growth factor 10 (FGF10) and retinoic acid (RA) drive differentiation of hESCs into cells expressing Pdx1, recent efforts have focused on the identification of efficient, less expensive, small molecule inducers capable of controlling differentiation by modulating signal transduction pathways, gene expression or metabolism (Borowiak et al., 2009). For eg. induce definitive endoderm (IDE) 1 and 2 have been shown to induce the formation of large amounts of definitive endoderm expressing multiple endodermal markers from mouse and human ESCs with a 70–80% efficiency, higher than Activin A or Nodal. Further development of these endodermal cells into pancreatic progenitors *in vitro* has been shown to occur in response to FGF10, RA, inhibitors of hedgehog signaling and more recently small molecule indolactam V (Aguayo-Mazzucato & Bonner-Weir, 2010; Chen et al., 2009). While these hESC-derived β-cells resemble human islets, in that they are capable of synthesizing insulin, glucagon, somatostatin, pancreatic polypeptide and ghrelin (D'Amour et al., 2006; Kroon et al., 2008) and prolong graft survival, the lack of glucose-stimulated insulin secretion (GSIS) is one of the main drawbacks. In an elegant study utilizing a five-stage hESC differentiation protocol, Kroon et al assessed the competence of hESC–derived pancreatic endoderm to produce functional endocrine cells *in vivo*. Direct engraftment of hESC derived pancreatic endoderm from the penultimate fourth stage of the five-step differentiation protocol into immunodeficient mice generated 'glucose-responsive' endocrine cells with maximal insulin secretion which developed during a 3 month period post implant. These glucose-responsive cells had insulin secretory properties similar in kinetics and magnitude to ~ 3000 adult human islets similarly engrafted, expressed critical β-cell transcription factors, demonstrated appropriate processing of proinsulin and the presence of mature endocrine secretory granules. 92% of the mice receiving hESC–derived pancreatic endoderm implants achieved insulin levels sufficient to fully protect against STZ-induced hyperglycemia, providing definitive and compelling evidence that hESCs are competent to generate glucose-responsive, insulin-secreting cells and serve as a renewable source of mature functional islets for diabetes cell-replacement therapies. This study also demonstrates the contribution of *in vivo* factors for the final stages of maturation and the need to identify these factors for efficient *in vitro* differentiation in order to produce sufficient amounts of functional β-cells.

3.1.2 Islet-derived stem/precursor cells as a source for insulin-producing β-cell regeneration

While ESCs have tremendous potential in tissue engineering, their use is hampered by ethical, legal and scientific considerations. On the contrary, non-embryonic adult stem cells are multipotent and can be derived from several sources including bone marrow, umbilical cord tissue, amniotic fluid, fat tissue, skin, retina and central nervous system (Chhabra et al., 2009). The existence of putative pancreatic stem cells that express low amounts of insulin mRNA *in vitro* with clonogenic potential and multipotency has been described previously(Bonner-Weir & Weir, 2005; Seaberg et al., 2004). Suzuki et al also demonstrated the existence of a possible pancreatic stem/progenitor cell candidate that expressed HGF c-Met receptor, did not express hematopoietic and vascular endothelial antigens such as CD45, TER119, c-Kit, and Flk-1, formed clonal colonies *in vitro*, differentiated into multiple pancreatic lineage cells and expanded with self-renewing cell divisions in culture (Suzuki et al., 2004). Following transplantation, these cells differentiated into pancreatic endocrine and acinar cells *in vivo*. A recent study reported the isolation, culture and functional characterization of islet-derived stem/precursor cells from purified human islet preparations (Carlotti et al.,2011). The cultured stem/precursor cells did not express the genes for endocrine hormones and when transferred to serum-free medium, aggregated to form clusters expressing insulin, glucagon, and somatostatin genes. They were not of hematopoietic, endothelial, or of ductal origin, expressed MSC markers CD105, CD90, CD73, CD44, CD29, and CD13 as well as nestin and vimentin and pericyte markers CD146, NG2, αSMA and PDGF-Rβ. Immuno-flowcytometry and confocal microscopic analyses revealed 2.0±0.8% of CD105/CD90 double-positive cells resided within the human islets, supporting the presence of a distinct MSC-like stem cell population in isolated human islets.

3.1.3 Mesenchymal stem cells: stopping immune destruction and promoting β-cell regeneration

Whole bone marrow contains a mixture of multiple types of stem cells, including BM-HSCs, BM-MSCs, endothelial progenitor cells (EPCs), multipotent adult progenitor cells and side population (SP) cells. BM-MSCs are plastic-adherent cells, typically expressing surface markers such as CD90, CD73, CD105, CD44 and CD29. They lack hematopoietic lineage markers such as CD34, CD45, CD14 and HLA-DR and can differentiate into cells of connective tissue lineages, including bone, fat, cartilage and muscle (Volarevik et al., 2011). These multipotent cells can be isolated and expanded with high efficiency in culture, are non-immunogenic and display immunosuppressive properties, for eg. inhibiting the proliferation and function of major immune cell populations, including T cells, B cells and natural killer (NK) cells as well as modulating the activities of dendritic cells (DCs) and inducing regulatory T cells (Tregs) both *in vivo* and *in vitro* (Shi et al.,2011). They also express a number of growth factors (GF) such as vascular endothelial growth factor (VEGF), HGF and insulin-like growth factor-1 (IGF-1), secrete tolerogenic cytokines as well as display significant anti-inflammatory and anti-apoptotic features (Uccelli et al., 2011). Thus, non-immunogenic BM-MSCs can enhance repair and regeneration, not only by repopulating damaged tissue, but also by reducing inflammation. These cells also do not possess cell surface human leukocyte antigen (HLA) or major histocompatibility complex (MHC) class II molecules, thereby allowing transplantation across MHC barriers. The possible therapeutic effect of BM-MSCs in type 1 diabetes was suggested by their capacity to generate insulin-producing cells and to abrogate immune injury (Chen et al., 2004; Sun et al., 2007; Tang et al., 2004; Volarevic et al., 2011; Xie et al., 2009). These insulin producing cells expressed multiple genes related to the development or function of pancreatic β-cells including high expression of pdx1, insulin, and glucagon and were able to release insulin in a glucose-dependent manner that led to amelioration of diabetic conditions in STZ-treated nude mice. Bouzama et al. also showed that administration of *in vitro*-expanded syngeneic BM-MSCs in STZ-induced diabetic rats promoted Pdx1 and insulin expression in the islets, altered T cell cytokine pattern toward IL-10/IL-13 production, preserved CD4(+)/CD8(+) Foxp3(+) Tregs in the periphery and induced sustained normoglycemia, thereby establishing a tissue microenvironment that supported β-cell activation/survival in the pancreas (Boumaza et al., 2009). While an increase in pancreatic islets and β-cells producing mouse insulin was observed with intracardiac infusion of human MSCs into STZ-induced diabetic NOD/scid mice, nearly 3% of the infused human MSCs engrafted into the pancreas and 11% in the kidney, the two organs sustaining most damage, effectively demonstrating the homing and tissue repair potential of MSCs (Lee et al., 2006). A recent study (Y. Zhang et al., 2010) demonstrated the effective differentiation of human first-trimester fetal BM-MSCs under a novel four-step induction procedure into functional pancreatic islet-like cell clusters (ILCs) that contained 62±14% IPCs, expressed a broad gene profile related to pancreatic islet β-cell development, and released high levels of insulin (2.245±0.222 pmol/100 clusters per 30 min) and C-peptide (2.200 ± 0.468 pmol/100 clusters per 30 min) in response to glucose challenge *in vitro*. The pancreatic ILCs normalized the blood glucose level of diabetic model mice for at least 9 weeks when xenografted and examination of the grafts indicated that the transplanted cells survived in recipients and produced human insulin and C-peptide *in situ*. Most studies suggest the requirement of *in vivo* hyperglycemia or transplantation into a diabetic model for BM-MSCs to differentiate into IPCs able to produce and release insulin in a glucose-dependent manner and normalize hyperglycemia (Chen et al., 2004; Karnieli et al., 2007; Tang et al., 2004). An added benefit is that MSC and islet co-transplantation has been shown to improve islet graft function and survival in diabetic rats by promoting graft revascularization, suppressing inflammation and maintaining islet organization and morphology (Figliuzzi et al., 2009; Ito et al., 2010; Rackham et al., 2011). In fact, engraftment might not be a necessary prerequisite for human MSCs to enhance tissue repair as MSCs embolized in the lung were shown to improve myocardial infarction by secreting anti-inflammatory factors (Lee et al., 2009). Due to these findings, MSCs offer an attractive avenue of research in diabetic stem cell therapy and may have the potential to enhance β-cell repair mechanisms even if the infused cells do not contribute significantly to the β-cell pool. However, in order to efficiently use MSCs therapeutically, problems of poor engraftment, limited differentiation under *in vivo* conditions and possible malignant transformation needs to be overcome.

3.1.4 Umbilical cord blood (UCB)-derived stem cells: Potential therapeutic tool in β-cell regeneration

Human UCB-derived stem cells represent a readily available source of MSCs and blood stem cells, both of which are potential sources of IPCs. hUCB-derived mononuclear cells (MNCs) possess MSC-like characteristics (expression of CD44, CD90 and CD105) (McGuckin et al., 2005) and have the ability to differentiate into mature adipocytes, osteoblasts, chondrocytes, skeletal myocytes, cardiomyocytes, neurons, and endothelial cells (Fan et al., 2011; Kogler et al., 2004; Parekh et al., 2009; Yoshida et al., 2005). *In vitro* differentiation of UCB-derived stem cells into insulin- and C-peptide-producing cells has been demonstrated using different approaches (Koblas et al., 2009; Gao et al., 2008). While some differentiated Oct-4 and SSEA-4 expressing hUCB cells by a protocol consisting of nicotinamide and extracellular matrix proteins (ECMs) laminin and fibronectin (Szymczak et al., 2010), others used RA, nicotinamide, exendin-4 and extracellular matrix proteins to differentiate hUCB-MSCs (Gao et al, 2008). In fact recently, 'cryopreserved' human UCB-derived MSCs were induced to differentiate into ILCs expressing nestin, Pdx-1, Ngn3, Ils-1, Pax6, Pax4, Nkx2.2, Nkx6.1, Glut-2 and insulin genes (Phuc et al., 2011). Unfortunately, despite differentiation into insulin producing cells, these cells seemed immature in terms of glucose sensing and/or secretory machinery required for glucose stimulated insulin secretion (GSIS) (D'Amour et al., 2006). *In vivo* differentiation of hUCB cells into β-cells has also been demonstrated following transplantation into STZ-induced diabetic immunocompromised (Kogler et al., 2004; Parekh et al., 2009; Zhao et al., 2006) or NOD mice (Koblas et al.,2009; Yoshida et al.,2005), though at a low rate. Detailed characterization of freshly isolated hUCB-MNCs indicate the ability to maintain as islet-progenitor cells expressing pdx1 and GLP1R for at least 5 passages of *in vitro* expansion. Transplantation of these cells into immune-incompetent mice resulted in their differentiation into insulin producing cells, more frequently during partial pancreatectomy, that were immature in terms of GSIS response (Parekh et al., 2009). Thus, it appears that the diabetic status, wherein a demand for neogenesis of insulin producing cells is induced in response to the decreased β-cells mass, results in a higher rate of compensatory hUCB cell differentiation (Yoshida et al., 2005). Kadam et al reported islet neogenesis from constitutively nestin-expressing human umbilical cord matrix stem cells (hUC-MSCs) (Kadam & Bhonde, 2010). These hUC-MSCs expressed CD29, CD44, CD73, CD90, CD105, smooth muscle actin, nestin, vimentin, proliferation marker Ki67 and embryonic markers Oct4, SSEA4, exhibited high proliferating capacity for an extended period and when subjected to a cocktail of specific differentiating factors, differentiated into fat, cartilage, bone, neurons and ILCs. These ILCs stained positive for DTZ, expressed human C-peptide, insulin and glucagon and demonstrated abundance of Pdx-1, Ngn3, insulin, glucagon and somatostatin transcripts. Transplantation into diabetic mice restored normoglycemia and exhibited normal glucose tolerance test, demonstrating the potential of constitutively-expressing nestin-positive progenitors from hUC as a novel source for islet neogenesis and their usage in cell replacement therapy for diabetes. Interestingly, treatment with CD4(+)CD62L(+) Tregs that were modulated by hUCB derived stem cells was able to simultaneously overcome autoimmunity via systemic and local immunomodulations as well as the shortage of insulin producing cells via stimulation of β-cell regeneration (Zhao et al., 2010). A number of studies indicate the use of these cells for autologous transplantantion in type 1 diabetes subjects. An initial trial with promising results of autologous cord blood has been attempted for diabetes reversal in patients with new onset diabetes who had banked cord blood (Haller et al., 2008). However, although the potential of UCB derived stem cells in the future of T1D interventional therapies is immense, the reality remains that multiple therapeutic avenues need to be combined in order to achieve the dream of permanently reversing/preventing T1D.

3.1.5 Generation of insulin producing β-cells from induced pluripotent stem cells

Efforts to create pluripotent stem cells (iPSCs) that are molecularly and functionally similar to ES cells by reprogramming somatic cells have tremendous therapeutic potential. Fibroblasts, B lymphocytes, liver, stomach epithelial cells, UCBs, human fetal and newborn epithelia etc. have all been dedifferentiated by the stable genomic integration and overexpression of various combinations of defined transcription factors that participate in determining pluripotency in cells, for instance, oct3/4, sox2, klf4, c-myc or oct3/4, sox2, nanog, lin28 (Hochedlinger & Plath, 2009). However, the use of oncogenes (c-myc, klf4) and retroviral and lentiviral vectors have raised concerns about the risk of potential tumorigenicity. Various novel alternatives directed towards making reprogrammed cells safer and more practical for therapeutic use have been explored. For e.g. iPSCs generated by viral integration of only three transcription factors, Oct4/Sox2/Klf4 have exhibited reduced tumorigenicity in chimeras and progeny mice (Nakagawa et al., 2008), albeit with substantially lower reprogramming efficiency. Interestingly, the addition of two factors p53 siRNA and UTF1 enhanced the efficiency of iPSC generation upto 100-fold (Zhao et al., 2008). Furthermore, a combination of two small molecules, BIX-01294 (a G9a histone methyltransferase inhibitor) and BayK8644 (a L-channel calcium agonist) was able to compensate for viral transduction of Sox2, enabling reprogramming of Oct4/Klf4-transduced mouse embryonic fibroblasts, which do not endogenously express the factors essential for reprogramming (Shi et al., 2008). Similarly, valproic acid (VPA), a histone deacetylase inhibitor has been shown to enable reprogramming of primary human fibroblasts with only two factors, Oct4 and Sox2, without the need for the oncogenes c-Myc or Klf4 (Huangfu et al., 2008). In fact, the generation of iPSCs from hUCBs with only Oct4 and Sox2 has also been demonstrated recently (Giorgetti et al.,2010). These two factor-induced human iPSCs resemble human ES cells in pluripotency, global gene expression profiles and epigenetic states, highlighting an important new trend in this field, the replacement of viral-mediated gene transfer with drug therapies such as small molecule gene inducers. However, finding small molecules that induce specified gene targets is not always possible. Alternatively, it is possible to engineer cell-penetrating protein therapies wherein a protein of interest can directly be transferred into the target cell. This approach has been applied in a study that reported the generation of protein-induced pluripotent stem cells (piPSCs) from murine embryonic fibroblasts using recombinant cell-penetrating reprogramming proteins (Zhou et al.,2009). These piPSCs were capable of long-term self-renewal and were pluripotent *in vitro* and *in vivo*. Addition of a transportation tag consisting of 11 linked copies of arginine to four proteins c-Myc, Klf4, Oct4 and Sox2 has also been shown to facilitate translocation across cell and nuclear membranes (Baker, 2009) with addition of valproic acid further boosting reprogramming rates. In fact, when proteins were administered four times over six days at 36-hour intervals, cells over 30 passages were morphologically indistinguishable from ES cells and expressed similar markers. Mixing in these cells with normal mouse embryos and allowing development in a surrogate mother resulted in the reprogrammed cells contributing to the germlayers in 13.5-day-old embryos. Interestingly, UCB-derived iPSCs have also been generated by lentiviral overexpression of oct4, sox2, nanog and lin28 with reprogramming efficiency similar to that of keratinocytes and fibroblasts. Towards development of a reliable protocol for induction of mature insulin-producing cells from iPSCs, a highly efficient strategy involving a) the use of activin A and wortmannin to induce definitive endoderm formation followed by b) priming with FGF10, KAAD-cyclopamine and c) addition of RA, NOGGIN and FGF7 to induce pancreatic specialization and d) EGF to regulate progenitor expansion has been demonstrated (Zhang et al., 2009). Using this stepwise induction strategy, most human iPSC lines could be induced into Pdx1-positive progenitor cells and further differentiated into cells expressing islet cell specific marker genes including Pdx1, MafA, Glut2 and insulin. Various marker genes were expressed at different induction stages: Sox17 on day 4, Pdx1 on day 8, Sox9 on day 13, amylase, Pdx1 and insulin on day 20. Additionally, co-expression of Pdx1 and C-peptide further confirmed insulin-producing cells suggesting that human iPSCs could be efficiently differentiated into pancreatic lineage cells. In a very recent study, a similar stepwise induction protocol was utilized with the exception that the pancreatogenic cocktail was enriched with Indolactam V/GLP-1 (Thatava et al., 2011). Under feeder-free conditions, fate specification of human iPSCs was initiated with activin A and Wnt3a that triggered engagement into definitive endoderm, followed by priming with FGF10 and KAAD-cyclopamine. Addition of RA, boosted by the pancreatic endoderm inducer indolactam V (ILV), yielded pancreatic progenitors expressing Pdx1, Ngn3 and NeuroD1 markers. Further differentiation under IGF-1, HGF and N-[N-(3,5-Difluorophenacetyl)-L-alanyl]-S-phenylglycine t-butyl ester (DAPT) was enhanced by GLP-1 to generate islet-like cells that expressed pancreas-specific markers including insulin and glucagon. Sustained expression of Pdx and functional responsiveness to glucose challenge, secreting up to 230pM of C-peptide, was observed in progeny. Thus, a proficient means for lineage spefication of human iPSCs into functional glucose-responsive hormone-producing progeny has further refined the development of a personalized platform for islet-like cell generation. Whilst these studies generate proof of concept that iPSCs may be an appropriate source for the generation of clinically compliant, immunologically quiescent, therapeutic β-cells from an autologous, non-embryonic origin, progress towards clinical application is hampered by a number of factors. Determining the somatic cell candidate for dedifferentiation depends on factors such as relative availability and ease of isolation, definitive identification and characterization markers, *ex vivo* expansion potential as well as safety upon transplantation. For future consideration, extensive characterization of *in vitro* differentiated iPSC will be critical and must be investigated. While the use of small molecule gene inducers and cell-penetrating protein therapies address the issues of poor efficiency and slow kinetics of the reprogramming process by viral transfection of the nuclear factors, these methodologies require substantial improvement before they could be used in clinical applications.

Similarly, the use of non-viral gene delivery vectors that can obviate safety concerns regarding the risk of mutagenesis, terratoma and tumor formation that prevail in the use of oncogenes and viral transduction need to be stringently addressed. Last but not least, studies thus far have demonstrated that the induction of the insulin-secreting phenotype is still incomplete with differentiated cells making multiple hormones or inadequate amounts of insulin or lacking response to glucose challenge to be clinically useful. Extensive, in-depth investigation into the underlying mechanisms involved is therefore of critical importance. Thus, while iPSCs derived from autologous somatic cells represent an exciting and important avenue to replenish islet supply while simultaneously obviating immune concerns such as rejection and chronic immunosuppression, until the accompanying risks are completely obviated, other avenues of β-cell replacement need to be judiciously explored.

3.2 Identifying stem cells with insulin-generating capability and tracking differentiated β-cells - the necessity for cellular markers.

Nestin, which is detected at low levels in human pancreatic tissue *in vitro,* has long since been debated as a cellular marker for ESC differentiation into IPCs (Baharvand et al., 2006). The existence of multipotential nestin-positive cells with unusually extended proliferative capacity that might participate in neogenesis of islet endocrine cells has been demonstrated in rat and human pancreatic islets and ducts (Zulewski et al., 2001). Upon confluence, these cells differentiated into cells that expressed liver and exocrine pancreas markers such as α-fetoprotein and pancreatic amylase, and displayed a ductal/endocrine phenotype with expression of CK19, neural-specific cell adhesion molecule, insulin, glucagon, and the pancreas/duodenum specific homeodomain transcription factor, IDX-1. While others dispute that nestin-positive cells residing in the pancreas are a potential source for regenerating or expanding islets (Gao et al., 2003), multipotential stem cells with β-cell generative capacity may be identified by this marker. Very recently, Kadam et al. isolated and characterized hUC-MSCs that constitutively expressed nestin and differentiated into functional ILCs capable of restoring normoglycemia in experimental diabetic mice (Kadam & Bhonde 2010). An effective multistep protocol to efficiently induce pancreatic ductal and β-cell differentiation *in vitro* from multipotent, nestin-positive rat bone-marrow stem cells in a serum-free system has recently been described (Milanesi et al., 2011). In this procedure, trichostatin A, a regulator of chromatin remodeling and 5-aza 2' deoxycytidine, an inhibitor of DNA methylase were used to enhance the induction and differentiation toward pancreatic lineage, followed by all-trans RA to promote pancreatic differentiation. Important transcription factor genes, such as Pdx1, Ngn3, and Pax6 were sequentially induced following the *in vivo* development timeline. Lastly, nicotinamide, was used to induce expression of islet and ductal-specific markers. The differentiated cells displayed glucose-responsive insulin secretion and expressed Glut2, indicating the clinical relevance of 'nestin-positive' bone-marrow stem cells. In further characterization of candidate nestin-positive islet progenitors (NIPs), Lechner *et al.* proposed that some islet cell progenitors possess characteristics of both neural origin, exemplified by nestin, as well as of bone-marrow progenitors, exemplified by the so-called side-positive (SP) cell phenotype (Lechner et al., 2002). This phenotype is characterized by the ability to exclude the vital dye Hoechst through the action of the ATP-binding cassette transporter ABCG2 (BCRP1). The presence of this molecular marker potentially allows for purification of these cells thereby providing an efficient progenitor cell for islet differentiation. These studies prompted investigation into the possibility that pancreatic SP cells possessed β-cell regenerative potential (Zhang et al., 2005). SP cells were shown to be capable of insulin, glucagon, Glut2 and Pdx1 expression induced by a variety of growth factors, concomitant with a decreased expression of progenitor cell markers such as nestin and Ngn3. These differentiated cells also released insulin in response to high glucose concentrations, though in notably lesser amounts when compared to primary β-cells, calling for continued investigation into standardizing the the conditions required for inducing complete differentiation of SP cells into fully functional β-cells.

As necessary as it is to have markers that identify progenitor cells amenable to the islet pathway, it is of equal importance to have makers that can rapidly identify the small number of successfully differentiated cells. With an aim to improve the efficiency of analyzing and sorting β-like insulin-producing cells from undifferentiated cells, Fukazawa *et al.* designed a novel β-cell specific and glucose-responsive artificial promoter system designated pGL3.hINS-363 3x (Fukazawa et al., 2006). This system exhibited significant luciferase activity not only in insulin-producing MIN6 m9 cells but also in isolated human islets. The pGL3.hINS-363 3x construct showed no activity in non-insulin producing cells in low glucose conditions (2mM glucose) but demonstrated significant activity with β-cell specificity in high glucose conditions (16mM glucose). Furthermore, pGL3.hINS-363 3x showed significant promoter activity in differentiated AR42J cells that could produce insulin after activin A and betacellulin treatment. Detection of small numbers of newly formed β-cells by this approach could significantly enhance the production of differentiated, insulin-positive, β-cells for transplantation. Growing evidence suggests that microRNAs (miRNA) play an important role in insulin production, secretion and action and that diabetes changes miRNA expression profiles in many tissues (Baroukh et al., 2007; Correa-Medina et al.,2009; Joglekar et al.,2007,2009; Li et al., 2009; Poy et al., 2004,2009; Tang et al., 2009). miRNAs are a novel group of highly conserved, endogenous, 22–23 nucleotide non-coding RNAs that regulate biological functions very precisely by negatively modulating the gene expression either by promoting mRNA degradation or through translational repression of proteins. Very recently, Chen et al. have described an approach wherein they isolated miRNAs from human embryonic stem cell (hES-T3 cells) -derived pancreatic ILCs (T3Pi) that expressed insulin, glucagon and somatostatin and showed that these miRNAs negatively regulated the expression of protein-coding mRNAs (Chen et al., 2011; Sebastiani et al., 2011). T3pi clusters showed very high expression of miRNAs, miR-186, miR-199a and miR-339, that down-regulated the expression of LIN28, PRDM1, CALB1, GCNT2, RBM47, PLEKHH1, RBPMS2 and PAK6 indicating that these miRNAs and their target genes very likely played important regulatory roles in the development of pancreas and/or differentiation of islet cells. Using this approach, differentiated T3Pi cells with high miRNA expression can be identified and miRNAs may possibly even be manipulated to increase the proportion of β-cells and insulin synthesis for cellular therapy in type I diabetics. Another recent study indicates that miR-24, miR-26,miR-182 or miR-148 act as positive regulators of insulin transcription in cultured β-cells or in isolated primary islets by reducing the expression of insulin transcriptional repressors (Melkman-Zehavi et al.,2011). MiRNAs may also provide a new class of biomarkers for diabetes and progress in the development and use of synthetic miRNAs such as antagomirs (Krutzfeldt et al., 2005) to silence miRNAs such as miR-375 in case of diabetes may provide a novel therapeutic tool for the treatment of diabetes and other diseases in the future. Furthermore, mechanistic studies on the role of miRNAs in the modulation of the immune system may help identify potential therapeutic targets to ameliorate responses to islet transplantation.

4. Role of transcription factors, growth factors and other cellular targets in enhancing β-cell differentiation and proliferation

Pancreatic development includes the generation of endoderm/gut endothelium, pancreatic differentiation, endocrine specification, and ultimately β-cell differentiation. Therefore, in order to efficiently promote β-cell differentiation and expansion, it is of vital importance to understand the factors that contribute to islet development. A number of signaling molecules and transcriptional regulators including Wnt, TGF-β, FGF, Notch and Hedgehog control various aspects of pancreas and endocrine cell development, proliferation and differentiation (Evans-Molina et al., 2009; Jun et al.,2010; Mishra et al., 2010). During development, it is the definitive endoderm that gives rise to the pancreas and genes such as Wnt/β -catenin, Nodal, GATA4/6, FoxA, Sox17 and Mix amongst others participate in its formation. Pdx1 represents a marker of all pancreatic lineages (endocrine, exocrine and ductal), mediating β-cell function, growth, and proliferation and its inactivation prevents both islet and acinar cell differentiation. Pdx1 regulation is mediated by the IRS2/Akt/FoxO1 pathway, maintaining the ability of β-cells to proliferate and function properly. The notch signaling pathway in turn regulates the expansion and differentiation of the pancreatic progenitor cells by the expression of the 'pro-endocrine' gene, Ngn3. Transcription factors such as Pdx-1, Isl1, Ngn-3, Nkx2.2, Nkx6.1, NeuroD, Hlxβ9, Pax-4, MafA and Pax-6 all participate in islet differentiation with Ngn-3 acting as a key transcription factor required for islet cell development. Amongst these transcription factors, Pdx-1 is the most extensively utilized factor, driving both β-cell neogenesis as well as transdifferentation of pancreatic and extra-pancreatic cells into insulin-producing β-cells.

Various factors such as pregnancy, diabetogenic stimuli, growth factors such as HGF, a combination of epidermal growth factor (EGF) and gastrin, clonophylline, betacellulin, GLP-1 or its long-lasting homolog exendin-4, members of the regenerating protein family such as Reg protein and INGAP can stimulate replication and proliferation of β-cells (Jun et al., 2010; Mishra et al., 2010). Herein, we describe a few of the candidates that are used to attain maximal β-cell expansion by targeting pathways that augment mature β-cell proliferation, inhibit apoptosis, or simultaneously target both. Betacellulin is a member of the EGF family, and is known to increase the rate of native β-cell self-duplication and enhance Pdx1-positive progenitor differentiation. It also induces proliferation and differentiation of insulinoma cells as well as converts an exocrine pancreatic cell line (AR42J) into an insulin-expressing phenotype when combined with activin A. This combined treatment potentiates β-cell self-duplication, ductal cell proliferation and δ-cell transdifferentation into new β-cells (Li et al., 2004). Similarly, activin promotes regeneration and differentiation of newly formed β-cells and together with growth differentiation factors participates in endocrine and exocrine lineage specification (Mishra et al., 2010). The incretin GLP-1 is produced from gut endocrine cells and has been shown to stimulate β-cell proliferation and neogenesis, inhibit β-cell apoptosis and have a profound effect on stimulating the release of insulin and suppression of glucagon from the pancreas. Rapid degradation by dipeptidyl peptidase IV (DPPIV) is responsible for its short biological half life. To overcome this, exenatide/Exendin-4 (AC2993), a long acting GLP-1 receptor (GLP-1R) agonist and other such stable GLP-1 analogs that are resistant to degradation (liraglutide) and inhibitors of DPPIV(sitagliptin, vidaglitpin) are being investigated for treatment of diabetes (Geelhoed-Duijvestijn, 2007). Injections of GLP-1 or exendin-4, have been shown to increase the β-cell mass and improve hyperglycemia. Combination of GLP-1 and gastrin or EGF with gastrin restores β-cell mass and inhibits autoimmune destruction of islet cells (Suarez-Pinzon et al., 2005, 2008). Administration of GLP-1 and gastrin restores normoglycemia by expanding β-cell mass and by downregulating immune response in autoimmune diabetic NOD mice. Diabetic immunodeficient NOD*scid* mice recipients treated with this combination therapy together with transplantation of human islets demonstrated expanded β-cell mass largely derived from cytokeratin 19-positive pancreatic duct cells. Several growth factors play important roles in β-cell differentiation, proliferation and islet survival. For instance, HGF acts by targeting the protein kinase B/Akt involved in an intracellular signaling cascade linked to improving islet cell survival and function. It also upregulates Glut-2, glucokinase, and insulin gene expression in β-cells and has been shown to increase longitudinal and functional graft survival. Keratinocyte growth factor promotes differentiation of IPCs and VEGF regulates insulin gene expression and β-cell proliferation through laminin and maintains adult islet function. IGF1 expression in β-cells of transgenic mice regenerates the endocrine pancreas during type 1 diabetes. Though the IGF-I-mediated mechanism(s) of restoring β-cell mass is not fully understood, early studies indicate that IGF-I modulates cell cycle proteins and increases replication of pre-existing β-cells after damage (Agudo et al., 2008). The Reg gene family belongs to the calcium-dependent lectin (C-type lectin) gene superfamily and is divided into subclasses based on the primary structures of the encoded proteins. Several Reg family genes, such as Reg2, -3α, and -3β, are upregulated to induce β-cell regeneration, growth and protection and also during the progression of autoimmune diabetes. INGAP, one of the Reg family gene products has been used in numerous studies to facilitate β-cell differentiation and expansion. In addition, heparan sulfate, by regulating ligand-receptor interactions, plays an important role in embryonic development and regulation of postnatal islet maturation. Dicer1 (a ribonuclease required by the RNA interference and miRNA pathways to produce the active small RNA component that represses gene expression) maintains the adult pancreas and regulates the differentiation of endocrine precursor cells. Interestingly, Dicer1-deficient β-cells mostly retain their identity including the expression of typical β-cell markers involved in glucose sensing and insulin transcription but show an increase in repressors of insulin transcription (Melkman-Zehavi et al., 2011). Similarly miRNAs reinforce insulin expression by reducing the expression of insulin transcriptional repressors. Before utilizing these factors as treatment options, safety concerns regarding the risk of cancerous transformation and participation in other cellular processes should be investigated in depth.

β-cell proliferation is not only affected by factors that that induce expansion and differentiation, but is also tightly regulated by factors that impede/inhibit proliferation. Modulation of these factors therefore represents another alternative to enhance β-cell proliferation. For instance deletion of p27Kip1, a key cell cycle inhibitor, increased the frequency of cellular replication and proliferation during β-cell development and in the early neonatal period (Rachdi et al., 2006). Improved glucose tolerance and hyperinsulinemia associated with increased islet mass and proliferation was observed in p27-deficient mice, while induction of p27 expression resulted in severe glucose intolerance and reduced β-cell mass. Additionally, p27(-/-) mice showed decreased susceptibility to develop STZ-induced diabetes compared to controls that displayed elevated blood glucose levels (Georgia & Bhushan, 2006). In mice that developed STZ-induced diabetes, β-cells retained the ability to reenter the cell cycle at a far greater frequency in the p27(-/-) mice than in wild-type littermates. These studies establish the role of p27 in maintaining the quiescent state of newly differentiated β-cells generated during embryogenesis and indicate p27 as a key regulator in the establishment of β-cell mass and thus as an important target in regenerative therapies for diabetes. The success of this therapy however would depend on the ability of the cell to reactivate p27 to stop uncontrolled proliferation when metabolic demands for insulin are met. Apart from the risk of tumorigenesis, another drawback is the dedifferentiation and loss of insulin secretion commonly observed with repeated cell division of β-cells. Another key regulator of β-cell replication and expansion is glycogen synthase kinase-3 (GSK3), known to negatively regulate insulin-mediated glycogen synthesis and glucose homeostasis (Rayasam et al 2009). Islet β-cell growth is controlled by endogenous GSK-3β activity via feedback inhibition of the insulin receptor/PI3K/Akt signalling pathway (Liu et al., 2010). In fact, glucose regulates steady-state levels of Pdx1 via the reciprocal actions of GSK3 and AKT kinases. Glucose-stimulated activation of AKT and inhibition of GSK3 decreased Pdx1 phosphorylation and delayed Pdx1 degradation demonstrating the important role of AKT-GSK3 axis in glucose modulation of Pdx1 stability (Humphrey et al., 2010). Similarly, direct pharmacologic inhibition of AKT destabilized, while inhibition of GSK3 increased Pdx1 protein stability. Increased expression and activity of GSK3 has been reported in type II diabetics and obese animal models and consequently, inhibitors of GSK3 have been demonstrated to have anti-diabetic effects *in vitro* and in animal models. However, the use of GSK3 inhibitors poses a challenge as achieving selectivity of an over achieving kinase involved in various pathways with multiple substrates may lead to side effects and toxicity.

5. Prolonging long term survival, growth and function of β-cells *in vitro*

Despite the promising results of β-cell regenerative strategies, maintaining functional islet cells in long-term cultures with persistent insulin-secreting capabilities has proven challenging. The efficacy of various cell culture medium supplements in prolonging the survival and function of newly generated β-cells and enhancing their survival in long-term cultures for optimal expansion has been investigated. For e.g. human islets were cultured *in vitro* for more than a year during which time, using multilabeling immunohistochemical and immunoelectron microscopic analyses with islet cell markers (antibodies to hormones, neuron-specific enolase, chromogranin A) and ductal cell markers (cytokeratins 7 and 19, carbonic anhydrase II, DU-PAN2, CA19-9, and MUC1), islet cells gradually transdifferentiated into ductal, acinar, and undifferentiated cells, considered pancreatic precursor (stem) cells (Schmied et al., 2001). Although endocrine cells remained detectable at day 60, hormone secretion ceased after day 28. Eventually all endocrine and exocrine cells were replaced by undifferentiated cells that expressed neuron-specific enolase, chromogranin A, laminin, vimentin, cytokeratin 7 and 19, α-1-antitrypsin, TGF-α, and EGF-receptor. While this study successfully demonstrated the possibility of culturing human islets for long periods, it brings into focus the formidable challenge of overcoming the loss of insulin-secreting capabilities and transdifferentiation of β-cells. The efficacy of supplementing culture medium with growth hormone (GH) and prolactin (PRL) as well as co-culturing islets with fibroblasts on stimulating long term cell proliferation as well as maintenance of insulin-synthesizing and -secreting capacity has also been investigated (Gartner et al., 2006). The supportive role of FGF2 in maintaining functional β-cells in culture has been previously demonstrated (Hardikar et al, 2003). FGF2, acting as a paracrine chemoattractant, stimulates clustering of human islet-derived precursor cells, leading to islet-like cell aggregate formation necessary for the early stages of islet cell differentiation. An impressive protocol that combined bFGF, leukemia inhibitory factor (LIF), and bone morphogenetic protein-4 (BMP-4) proved that islet progenitor-like cells can be derived from islet-enriched fractions under serum-free defined culture conditions and induced to stably express high levels of Pdx1 and Notch pathway-associated genes, characteristic of embryonic pancreatic progenitor cells, for more than 6 months and maintain endodermal and pancreatic phenotypes. Unfortunately, insulin expression remained minimal. Based on the hypothesis that loss of the trophic support provided by surrounding non-endocrine pancreatic cell populations underlies the decline in β-cell mass and insulin secretory function observed in human islets following isolation and culture, the effect of co-culturing islets with ductal epithelial cells on islet structural integrity, β-cell mass and insulin secretory capacity was investigated (Murray et al., 2009). Ten days following isolation, the results showed that co-culturing islets with ductal epithelial cells led to preserved islet morphology and sustained β-cell function, with the presence of ductal epithelial cells beneficial for maintenance of β-cell mass. While reinforcing the possibility of maintaining islets in long-term cultures under appropriate cell culture conditions, the study highlights the necessity for further characterization of regulatory influences in order to realize the promise of its therapeutic potential. The importance of a three-dimensional (3D) environment incorporating extracellular matrix (ECM) components in providing favorable conditions to preserve human islets in long-term culture has also been demonstrated (Daoud et al., 2010). The loss of the ECM basement membrane during isolation contributes to eventual apoptosis *in vitro*. While collagen I/IV and fibronectin induce adhesion, fibronectin is the only ECM protein capable of maintaining islet structural integrity and insulin content distribution in cultures. Although in this study islet phenotype was eventually lost, insulin gene expression was highest in islets cultured on collagen I and IV. Insulin release peaked with fibronectin along with a decrease in SUR1 expression, while glucose metabolism along with Glut2 and GCK expression was highest on collagen I and IV surfaces. A very recent study consisting of long-term and highly uniform human islet culture within a micro-fabricated scaffold with collagen 1 gel supplemented with ECM components fibronectin and collagen IV with controlled pore structures, displayed an insulin release profile similar to freshly isolated islets, yielding a stimulation index of approximately 1.8 (Daoud et al., 2011). Gene expression was markedly increased for all pancreatic genes, giving approximately 50-fold elevation of insulin gene expression with respect to suspension culture. The level of pancreatic hormones was also highly elevated. These findings provide the groundwork for, 1) establishing a modified 3D construct to culture pancreatic islets, and 2) for understanding the underlying mechanisms of islet interactions with its surroundings, in order to provide a platform for long-term maintenance and preservation of human pancreatic islets *in vitro*.

6. Hepatocytes and Xenogeneic islets - prospects and barriers as alternative sources

Reprogramming adult mammalian cells is an attractive approach for generating β-cells for replacement therapy. The common embryonic origin of liver and pancreas, the similarity of glucose-sensing systems, the large group of mutually expressed, specific transcription factors and the high level of developmental plasticity exhibited by adult human liver cells suggest that liver stem cells/hepatocytes are a potential source of pancreatic progenitor tissue. For instance, persistent expression of the Pdx1 or its super-active form Pdx1-VP16 fusion protein in hepatic cells reprograms these cells into pancreatic β-cell precursors under condition of hyperglycemia or hepatic regeneration (Yang et al., 2006). Also, most hepatocytes of Ad-pdx-1-infected mice demonstrated positivity for Pdx-1 expression but expressed insulin and somatostatin only in STZ-treated or in STZ-treated plus partial hepatectomy mice vs. nontreated mice. A corresponding amelioration of hyperglycemia and along with expression of other β-cell markers like Glut2 glucokinase was also observed (Kim etal., 2007). Similarly *ex vivo* lentiviral-mediated Pdx1 expression in isolated adult liver cells resulted in expression of insulin in the transduced cells at both mRNA and protein levels, dependent on the presence of glucose and sulfonylurea (Fodor etal., 2007). Expression of β-cell genes, including those encoding solute carrier family 2 (facilitated glucose transporter), member 2 (Slc2a2), glucokinase (Gck), ATP-binding cassette, sub-family C (CFTR/MRP), member 8 (Abcc8), the potassium inwardly-rectifying channel, subfamily J, member 11 (Kcnj11) and proprotein convertase subtilisin/kexin type 1 (Pcsk1) were also observed. The PDX1-transduced hepatocytes expressed several pancreatic transcription factors related to early pancreatic endocrine development (endogenous Pdx1, NeuroD1, and Nkx6.1) as well as the late-stage pancreatic transcription factors (Pax4, Pax6, and MafA). Transplantation of these transdifferentiated liver cells in STZ-induced diabetic *scid* mice resulted in improvement in hyperglycemia. This capacity of Pdx-1 to activate the pancreatic lineage in mature liver has been independently confirmed in numerous studies (Imai et al., 2005, Horb et al., 2003, Li et al., 2005; Miyatsuka et al., 2003; Zalzman et al., 2005). Also the effects of additional pancreatic transcription factors alone or combined with Pdx-1 expression on this process have been analyzed (Sapir et al., 2005; Kaneto et al., 2005a, 2005b; Kojima et al., 2003; Meivar-Levy et al., 2006). For instance, a recent study indicates the dominant role of Nkx6.1, expressed in mature β-cells, in altering the hepatic developmental fate along the pancreatic lineage and function (Gefen-Halevi et al., 2010; Wang, 2007). Nkx6.1 activated immature pancreatic markers such as Ngn-3 and Isl-1 but not pancreatic hormones gene expression in human liver cells, suggesting a potential role for Nkx6.1 in promoting Pdx-1 reprogrammed cells maturation along the β-cell-like lineage. Complementation of Nkx6.1 by ectopic Pdx-1 expression substantially and specifically promoted insulin expression while addition of glucose augmented processed hormone secretion without increasing the number of reprogrammed cells. Other studies demonstrate that combinations of overexpressed MafA with NeuroD and Ngn3 or NeuroD and betacellulin in diabetic mice markedly induced insulin gene transcription and ameliorated glucose tolerance without producing hepatitis (Kaneto et al.., 2005a, 2005b; Kojima et al., 2003). Transient transfection of human hepatoma cells (Li et al., 2005) or hepatic WB cells (Tang et al., 2006) with super-active version Pdx1-VP16 resulted in transdifferentiation into pancreatic cells, characterized by induction of both pancreatic exocrine cells (by detection of amylase protein) and endocrine cells (by detecting insulin, glucagon and somatostatin proteins) and suppression of the hepatic phenotype.

Transdifferentiated β-cells were responsive to physiological stimuli, exhibiting 1) functional β-cell markers including prohormone convertase 1/3 (PC1/3), insulin C-peptide and GLP-1R, 2) increased insulin mRNA expression after treatment of cells with GLP-1 and betacellulin and c) elevated insulin secretion after glucose challenge. Thus, reprogramming with multiple pancreatic transcription factors using first generation, non-toxic, transiently-expressed adenoviral vectors along with appropriate conditions (hyperglycemia and/or partial hepatectomy) can reprogram liver stem/adult liver cells into functional insulin-producing cells. The use of adult human liver cells for generating functional insulin-producing tissue may pave the way to autologous transplantation, circumventing both the shortage in tissue availability, the need for immunosuppressive therapy and the ethical issues associated with ESC therapy. Additionally the ability of the liver to regenerate itself after surgical removal of a portion to use for transdifferentiation without significant harm to the patient is an added bonus.

Xenotransplantation using porcine cells, tissues, or organs may offer a potential solution for the shortage of allogeneic human organs (Denner et al., 2009). However, prior to their clinical use the hurdles of immunologic rejection and risk of transmission of porcine pathogens needs to be overcome. Immunologic rejection in pig to primate xenotransplants consists of hyperacute rejection, acute humoral xenograft rejection (AHXR), acute cellular rejection and chronic rejection (Elliott et al., 2011). Hyperacute rejection results from the activation of the complement cascade that converts graft endothelial cells from an anticoagulant to a procoagulant phenotype. Apart from old world primates and man, all animals possess a cell surface antigen containing the epitope - Galα1-3Galβ1-4GlcNAc-R ('α-gal') to which humans have complement fixing antibodies that cause immediate rejection of animal cells when transplanted into humans. This can be prevented by reducing or inhibiting functional 'α-gal' activity using knock-out or knock-in procedures involving human alpha-1, 2-Ft or GnT-111 gene expression as well as by depletion of anti-pig antibodies or complement from serum. Adult porcine islets do not express Gal, reducing the antibody-mediated response to them after transplantation. However, fetal and neonatal islets do, and therefore the use GT knockout (α1,3-galactosyltransferase gene-knockout [GTKO]) pigs as the as the sources of all islets (fetal, neonatal and adult) is likely to be advantageous. Similarly, genetically-engineered pigs expressing thrombomodulin, tissue factor (TF) pathway inhibitor, CD39 or other mechanisms that prevent the coagulation dysfunction; or expressing human complement-regulatory proteins, CD46 [membrane cofactor protein] or CD55 [human decayacceleratingfactor] or CD59 or all three in pig islets (Ekser & Cooper, 2010); or expressing anticoagulant and antiplatelet molecules within the graft, may afford some protection (Cowan & d'Apice, 2008). Recombinant antithrombin III may also ameliorate both early graft damage and the development of systemic coagulation disorders in pig-to-human xenotransplantation. This strategy, in parallel with physical methods such as encasing islets in a protective layer, holds promise for reducing the thrombogenicity of pig islet xenografts. Ideally, genetically engineered GTKO/CD46 pigs whose organs and cells are protected from the coagulation dysregulation that include modifications that prevent tissue factor activity on the graft and as well as activation of recipient platelets to express TF and initiate consumptive coagulopathy are required. AHXR or delayed xenograft rejection results from vascular endothelial cell activation and injury caused by the complement and cellular components of the innate immune system. There is increasing evidence that primate neutrophils, natural killer (NK) cells and macrophages play a role in AHXR, particularly seen following the development of a T-cell dependent elicited antibody response. Administration of CD39, heme oxygenase, thrombomodulin and TF pathway inhibitor have been used in its treatment (Cowan & d'Apice, 2008). Acute cellular rejection involving T- and B-cell infiltration of the graft, T-cell activation and a T-cell-dependent elicited antibody response is believed to be stronger following xenotransplantation than the alloresponse. However, potent pharmacologic agents can largely prevent acute cellular rejection, which is therefore typically not observed with intense immunosuppressive drug regimens. Ekser et al. have obtained promising results using an immunosuppressive regimen consisting of induction therapy with antithymocyte globulin (ATG), and maintenance with an anti-CD154 monoclonal antibody and Mycophenolate mofetil (MMF) (Ekser & Cooper, 2010). A clinically acceptable regimen of ATG, CTLA4-Ig and MMF has also been found to be particularly effective in preventing T-cell activation in the xenotransplantation setting. Chronic rejection symptoms in the form of chronic vasculopathy has been observed in pig to primate graft that survived for more than a few weeks, similar to the chronic rejection seen in long-surviving allografts. The risk of development of xenozoonosis in the recipient of a pig graft (particularly with regard to porcine endogenous retroviruses (PERV), is of concern. However, the stable long-term expression of anti-PERV siRNAs has been shown to be effective in knocking down PERV expression in cells. Breeding of designated pathogen-free pigs can prevent transmission of most porcine microbes (Dieckhoff et al., 2008; Ramsoondar et al., 2009). Another hurdle includes sensitization to pig antigens (e.g., swine leukocyte antigens), resulting in an increase in antibodies to HLA. Fortunately current evidence indicates that antibodies that develop after exposure to a pig xenograft are not crossreactive against HLA, and so would not be detrimental to a subsequent allograft (Cooper et al., 2004). However this does not preclude patients with a high level of HLA-reactive antibodies who may still be at greater risk of rejecting a pig xenograft. Clinical attempts to treat type 1 diabetes with implanted porcine islets are underway and showing promising early results. Immune-suppression, sertoli cell co-transplantation and intraperitoneal implantation of micro-encapsulated neonatal islets have been tried in type 1 diabetic humans with some clinical benefit reported from the latter two. In a very recent study by Elliot et al using the microencapsulation technique, transitory insulin independence of several months duration was observed (Elliott et al., 2011). Interestingly, the treatment appeared to significantly decrease severe hypoglycemic episodes and reduce/abolish hypoglycemic unawareness episodes, even in the absence of insulin independence. Evidence of xenosis in the xenotransplants recipients though diligently sought could not be found, given the credentials of the designated pathogen free source herd used. Virus safety in xenotransplantation is a fast-developing field, and new findings may contribute to improved outcomes.

7. The role of gene therapy in enhancing islet function

While not routinely achieving long-term normoglycemia, islet transplantation does afford substantial benefits in the form of reduced incidences of debilitating hypoglycemic episodes and hypoglycemic unawareness, lower daily insulin requirements, a detectable level of c-peptide, and improved A1c levels. The major limitation of this procedure is the inadequate numbers of donor islets available for transplantation. While we have discussed the various approaches to generate and expand islet β-cells, strategies aimed at increasing the efficiency of islet function in terms of insulin synthesis and secretion are of equal importance since it would reduce the number of islets required for restoring glucose homeostasis following transplantation. Towards this end, gene therapy has been proposed. A simple conceptual approach to create hyper-functional islets would consist of augmentation of the regulated insulin secretory capacity of an islet graft by insulin gene transfer to the graft before transplantation. Deng et al. demonstrated that Ad-Ins-transduced islets showed superior function in terms of insulin production and secretion as well as GSIS (Deng et al., 2003). The amount of basal insulin secretion and the overall pattern of insulin secretion from the Ad-Ins-transduced islet appeared completely normal and following transplantation, recipients remained normoglycemic for more than 100 days without evidence of deterioration in graft function. Histological examination of the grafts showed normal islet graft morphology and the presence of abundant insulin. Interestingly, although transfer of an exogenous insulin gene under control of a powerful viral promoter forced β-cells to produce more insulin, transplantation of a large number of these islets did not result in recipient hypoglycemia, confirming that Ad-Ins-transduced islets secreted insulin in an appropriately regulated manner. Furthermore, only 25% of the previously needed islet mass was required to reverse diabetes suggesting that four times as many transplants could be performed compared to the unmodified islets. The use of insulin promoter instead of the CMV promoter would have further increased insulin secretion from Ad-Ins-transduced islets in response to changes in blood glucose concentration in a highly regulated manner. Furthermore, the islet gene transfer was carried out using an islet-virus co-culture technique resulting in only partial islet transduction (37% expressing transgene). The authors speculate that Ad-Ins-vector delivery by vascular perfusion of the pancreas, would achieve maximal transgene expression in nearly all islet endocrine cells making it possible to reverse diabetes with islets isolated from only a portion of the perfused pancreas. The consideration of live donors as a source of islets is not unreasonable since laparoscopic-assisted distal pancreatectomy and nephrectomy has been performed successfully in three living donors since December 2007 with minimal peri-operative mortality and acceptable morbidity and the distal pancreas has been used successfully as a segmental vascularised graft (Gruessner et al., 2001; Maruyama et al., 2010; Tan et al., 2005). The uneventful postoperative course and normal functioning of the grafts indicate the technique to be minimally invasive and safe, making the consideration of live related donors for providing islet tissue supply a reasonable solution to the problem of organ shortage until other strategies such as stem-cell derivation of β-cells or xenogeneic sources of islet tissue can be refined. In order to avoid the potential side effects associated with the use of viral vectors, Chen et al. demonstrated targeting of plasmid DNA to the pancreas *in vivo* using ultrasound-targeted microbubble destruction (UTMD) (Chen et al., 2010). Intravenous microbubbles carrying plasmids were destroyed within the pancreatic microcirculation by ultrasound, achieving local gene expression that was further targeted to β-cells by a modified rat insulin promoter (RIP3.1). Delivery of RIP3.1-NeuroD1 two days after STZ-induced diabetes to rats pretreated with the JNK inhibitor SP600125 successfully blocked β-cell apoptosis and resulted in *in vivo* islet regeneration, restoration of β-cell mass and normalization of blood glucose level, insulin and C-peptide in rats. The key pancreatic transcription factor Pdx1, possesses a protein transduction domain (PTD) that facilitates its entry into cells (Koya et al., 2008). Reversal of STZ-induced diabetes in mice by cellular transduction with recombinant Pdx1 represents a novel protein transduction domain-based therapy. The potential use of a non-viral, systemic, carrier-based delivery of Fas siRNA gene therapy through intravenous administration using a polymeric carrier, polyethylenimine

(PEI) offers yet another novel approach (Jeong et al., 2010). Another alternative for obtaining hyper-functional islets lies in hyperinsulinemia. Genetic conditions that include mutations in the potassium channel, the sulfonylurea receptor and the energy-sensing mechanisms of β-cells result in hyperinsulinemia. In diffuse congenital hyperinsulinism of infancy, near-total pancreatectomy (98%) has to be performed as a life-saving procedure in order to achieve glycemic control, demonstrating the extreme potency of these cells when compared to a normal islet (Lovvorn et al., 1999; Pierro et al., 2011). Use of these hyperfunctional islets in islet transplantation, preferably along with normal islet tissue, is an interesting proposition, although the use of diseased tissue would raise several concerns and challenges.

8. Increasing post-transplant islet survival - an ummunological approach

From 1999 to 2007, clinical islet transplantation at established centers has resulted in a remarkable reduction in the occurrence of severe hypoglycemia and a success rate of 70% in achievement of insulin independence persisting for 2 years or more in 50% of those achieving insulin independence, or 35% of all islet alone graft recipients. These results are consistent throughout the 8 years of follow-up included in the Collaborative Islet Transplant Registry (Alejandro et al., 2008). Approximately 60% of transplanted islets are lost in the first 10–14 days post-transplantation (Evgenov et al., 2006) most likely due to local hypoxic injury caused by lack of islet vascularity and the deleterious effects of the innate immune response which induces apoptosis, necrosis, coagulation, and complement fixation (Huang et al., 2008). This non-specific inflammatory response results in the production and release of a number of proinflammatory cytokines (e.g. TNF-α, IL-1β, IFN-γ) that further enhance local inflammatory activity, stimulate adaptive immunity and exert deleterious effects on islet β-cell function by inducing apoptosis and cell death (Donath et al., 2008). Islet cells themselves, upon transplantation, possess the ability to receive signals that result in the activation of multiple signaling factors including STAT1, AP-1 and NFkB (Eizirik & Mandrup-Poulsen, 2001). Lisofylline has demonstrated significant ability in down-regulating the systemic inflammatory response by interference with STAT4 signaling resulting in improved islet transplant survival (Yang et al., 2005). Suppression of these pathways has also been attempted through gene therapy approaches (Moore et al., 2006). Currently, islet-directed anti-inflammatory therapy mostly focuses on Toll-like receptor (TLR) signaling pathways within the islets (Huang et al., 2008). Fortifying the β-cell with protection against islet-destructive cytokines represents another avenue to defend against the immune response. For instance, adenoviral transduction of islet cells with a construct expressing IRAP, the interleukin-1 receptor antagonist protein, resulted in improved islet survival and replication caused mainly due to interference in the activation of the IL-1 mediated apoptotic pathway (Tellez et al., 2005). Other strategies that overexpress anti-apoptotic proteins such as the TNF-α inducible transcription factor A20 or bcl-2 demonstrate beneficial effects on islet survival. While immunomodulatory therapies (e.g. monoclonal antibody therapies, CTLA4Ig, anti-thymocyte globulin (ATG), IL-1 receptor antagonist therapy, cellular therapies, etc.) act by either providing immunoregulatory cytokines such as IL-4, IL-10 or TGF-β or by altering the balance between TH1 and TH2 cells, immunosuppressive regimens act by either suppressing the immune response by binding to specific cytoplasmic proteins that inhibit IL-2 secretion and subsequent T cell expansion (Calcineurin inhibitors CNIs; cyclosporine and tacrolimus) or by suppressing IL-2R signaling thereby inactivating T cells (sirolimus) or by suppressing cell division of lymphocytes (Azathioprine) (Winter & Schatz, 2003). Therefore, combinations of CNIs and steroid-sparing or -free regimens with drugs that demonstrate powerful immunosuppressive/anitinflammatory potency in the absence of nephrotoxicity and diabetogenicity are being investigated. A triple therapy approach that combined rapamycin plus agonist IL-2-related and antagonist-type mutant IL-15-related Ig cytolytic fusion proteins(IL-2.Ig and mutIL-15.Ig) demonstrated a striking ability to reverse diabetes and ameliorate inflammation, mainly due to augmentation of the pro-regulatory effects of IL-2 and inhibition of the proinflammatory mediator IL-15, creating a favorable balance between regulation and inflammation (Koulmanda et al., 2007). Currently, targeted antigen specific/non-specific and antibody-specific immunotherapies that readjust the underlying immunologic imbalance in order to stop or reverse the β-cell-specific autoimmune and inflammatory process within islets and maintain immune tolerance are being combined with islet regeneration therapies in a variety of clinical studies and hold great therapeutic promise for islet transplantation outcomes. These include islet transplantation followed with ATG /alemtuzumab (Campath -1H, monoclonal anti CD52 Ab) / hOKT3 γ induction therapy / anti-CD25 (daclizumab) induction therapy along with a sirolimus-based, prednisone-free maintenance regimen in combination with MMF and low Tacrolimus (Bellin et al., 2008; Gillard et al., 2010; Herold et al. 2005; Magliocca & Knechtle, 2006). Short term ATG treatment in T1DM of recent onset has been shown to contribute to the preservation of residual C-peptide production and to lower insulin requirement following diagnosis. Because Tregs strongly suppress the immune response in syngeneic islet transplantation and improve graft survival and function, several approaches are now emerging to induce/increase host Tregs activity in the transplant setting, including amongst others, systemic TGF-β1 therapy (W. Zhang et al., 2010). Other β-cell therapies currently in Phase II or III stages of development include Otelixizumab (anti-CD3), Teplizumab (anti-CD3), rituximab(anti-CD20), abatacept (CTLA4Ig), DiapPep 277 (heat shock protein) and GAD, Oral Insulin amongst others. Parenteral administration of anti-CD3 mAb for transplantation in humans and for treatment of autoimmune diabetes has been approved. Various combination interventions such as costimulatory blockade with anti-CD4 monoclonal antibodies plus CTLA4Ig and ATG plus CTLA4Ig (Suzuki et al., 2010) as well as combinations of anti-lymphocyte serum (ALS) plus anti-CD3mAb are under investigation. As discussed earlier, GLP-1R agonists like exendin-4 stimulate β-cell proliferation and neogenesis and inhibit β-cell apoptosis while DPPIV inhibitors increase cell insulin content, and therefore are of immense benefit in the above mentioned combination therapies (GLP-1 agonists plus anti-CD3mAB, anti-CD3mAb plus exendin-4, ALS plus exendin-4 etc.) for preserving and expanding β-cell mass following transplantation. Other avenues include encapsulating islets with nanofibre scaffolds or biomatrices synthesized to contain immunosuppressive drugs or drugs that stimulate vasculogenesis/angiogenesis as well as 'bioartificial pancreas'. Stem cells of embryonic, mesenchymal (prochymal), cord blood and haematopoietic (and some neural stem cell) origin, besides their use for regenerative purposes, also possess potent immunomodulatory functions and have great therapeutic potential in increasing post-transplant survival either alone or in combination with the therapies discussed above. Thus, depending on the time of the therapeutic intervention, various immunological approaches may be employed as monotherapy or in combination with short-term tolerance promoting immunoregulatory drugs or drugs promoting preservation, differentiation, expansion or insulin secretion to increase the functional and longitudinal survival of islets post-transplantation. However, while assessing the efficacy of these therapies, it is important to keep in mind that both CNIs as well as corticosteroids contribute to an increased risk of developing post-transplant hyperglycemia and to the differential diagnosis of graft rejection (Cantarovich &Vistoli, 2011; Egidi et al., 2005). Conducting large randomized trials to establish guidelines that minimize the adverse effects of immunosuppressive regimens for pancreas transplantation will be useful in achieving long-term, functional graft survival.

9. Conclusion

The possibility of transplanting sufficient quantities of functional, viable islets to induce life-long euglycemia depends on the successful outcomes of the various strategies discussed herein, namely regeneration of β-cells utilizing every kind cell from the pancreas, stem cells as well as cells from alternate sources, preserving and expanding their number *ex vivo*, and ensuring their maximal survival after transplantation through protection from hypoxic and immune insults. The possibility of generating a β-cell with a hyperfunctional phenotype would also significantly expand the functional β-cell pool. The evidence presented here indicates that while the challenges are many and accomplishing this task seems formidable, considerable inroads have already been made in each step highlighted in this review, drawing us a step closer to the possibility of widespread applicability of islet transplantation for the reversal of diabetes. Islet transplantation represents a definitive intervention for patients with Type 1 diabetes and with the significant progress achieved in the fields of stem cell therapy, immunomodulation, and gene therapy, the prospect of translating this new found knowledge into clinical applications that promote successful long term outcomes of islet transplantation is looking very promising.

10. References

Aguayo-Mazzucato C, Bonner-Weir S.(2010). Stem cell therapy for type 1 diabetes mellitus. *Nat Rev Endocrinol*, Vol.6, No.3, pp.139-148, ISSN 1759-5037.

Agudo J, Ayuso E, Jimenez V, Salavert A, Casellas A, Tafuro S, Haurigot V, Ruberte J, Segovia JC, Bueren J, Bosch F. (2008). IGF-I mediates regeneration of endocrine pancreas by increasing beta cell replication through cell cycle protein modulation in mice. *Diabetologia,* Vol.51, No.10, pp.1862-1872, ISSN 0012-186X.

Alejandro R, Barton FB, Hering BJ, Wease S; Collaborative Islet Transplant Registry Investigators. (2008). 2008 Update from the Collaborative Islet Transplant Registry.*Transplantation*, Vol.86, No.12, pp.1783-1788, ISSN1534-6080.

Baeyens L, Bouwens L. (2008).Can beta-cells be derived from exocrine pancreas? *Diabetes Obes Metab,* Vol. 10, Suppl. 4, pp.170-178, ISSN 1463-1326.

Baeyens L, De Breuck S, Lardon J, Mfopou JK, Rooman I, Bouwens L. (2005). In vitro generation of insulin-producing beta cells from adult exocrine pancreatic cells. *Diabetologia*, Vol.48, No.1, pp. 49-57, ISSN 0012-186X.

Baharvand H, Jafary H, Massumi M, Ashtiani SK. (2006). Generation of insulin-secreting cells from human embryonic stem cells. *Dev Growth Differ*, Vol.48, No.5, No.323-332, ISSN 0012-1592

Baker M. (2009). Stem cells: Fast and furious. *Nature*,Vol.458, No.7241, pp.962-965, ISSN 1476-4687.

Bai MD, Rong LQ, Wang LC, Xu H, Fan RF, Wang P, Chen XP, Shi LB, Peng SY. (2008). Experimental study on operative methods of pancreaticojejunostomy with reference to anastomotic patency and postoperative pancreatic exocrine function. *World J Gastroenterol*, Vol.14, No.3, pp. 441-447, ISSN 1007-9327.

Banerjee M & Bhonde RR. (2003). Islet generation from intra islet precursor cells of diabetic pancreas: in vitro studies depicting in vivo differentiation. *JOP*, Vol.4, No.4, pp. 137-145, ISSN 1590-8577.

Baroukh N, Ravier MA, Loder MK, Hill EV, Bounacer A, Scharfmann R, Rutter GA, Van Obberghen E. (2007). MicroRNA-124a regulates Foxa2 expression and intracellular signaling in pancreatic beta-cell lines. *J Biol Chem*, Vol.282, No.27, pp. 19575-19588, ISSN 0021-9258.

Bellin MD, Kandaswamy R, Parkey J, Zhang HJ, Liu B, Ihm SH, Ansite JD, Witson J, Bansal-Pakala P, Balamurugan AN, Papas KK, Sutherland DE, Moran A, Hering BJ.(2008).Prolonged insulin independence after islet allotransplants in recipients with type 1 diabetes. *Am J Transplant*, Vol.8, No.11, pp.2463-2470, ISSN 1600-6143.

Bernard-Kargar C and Ktorza A. (2001). Endocrine pancreas plasticity under physiological and pathological conditions. *Diabetes* Vol.50, Suppl.1, pp.S30-35, ISSN 0012-1797.

Blaine SA, Ray KC, Anunobi R, Gannon MA, Washington MK, Means AL. (2010). Adult pancreatic acinar cells give rise to ducts but not endocrine cells in response to growth factor signaling. *Development*, Vol.137, No.14, pp. 2289-2296, ISSN 1477-9129.

Bonner-Weir S, Deery D, Leahy JL, Weir GC.(1989). Compensatory growth of pancreatic beta-cells in adult rats after short-term glucose infusion. Diabetes, Vol.38, No.1, pp.49-53, ISSN 0012-1797.

Bonner-Weir S, Inada A, Yatoh S, Li WC, Aye T, Toschi E, Sharma A. (2008). Transdifferentiation of pancreatic ductal cells to endocrine beta-cells. *Biochem Soc Trans*, Vol.36, Pt 3, pp. 353-356, ISSN 0300-5127.

Bonner-Weir S, Li WC, Ouziel-Yahalom L, Guo L, Weir GC, Sharma A. (2010). Beta-cell growth and regeneration: replication is only part of the story. *Diabetes*, Vol.59, No.10, pp. 2340-2348. ISSN 1939-327X.

Bonner-Weir S, Sharma A.(2006). Are there pancreatic progenitor cells from which new islets form after birth? *Nat Clin Pract Endocrinol Metab*, Vol.2, No.5, pp.240-241, ISSN 1745-8366.

Bonner-Weir S, Toschi E, Inada A, Reitz P, Fonseca SY, Aye T, Sharma A. (2004). The pancreatic ductal epithelium serves as a potential pool of progenitor cells. Pediatr Diabetes, Vol.5,Suppl. 2, pp.16-22, ISSN 1399-543X.

Bonner-Weir S, Weir GC. (2005). New sources of pancreatic beta-cells.*Nat Biotechnol*, Vol.23, No.7, pp.857-861, ISSN 1087-0156.

Borowiak M, Maehr R, Chen S, Chen AE, Tang W, Fox JL, Schreiber SL, Melton DA. (2009).Small molecules efficiently direct endodermal differentiation of mouse and human embryonic stem cells. *Cell Stem Cell*,Vol.4, No.4, pp.348-358, ISSN 1875-9777.

Boumaza I, Srinivasan S, Witt WT, Feghali-Bostwick C, Dai Y, Garcia-Ocana A, Feili-Hariri M. (2009). Autologous bone marrow-derived rat mesenchymal stem cells promote PDX-1 and insulin expression in the islets, alter T cell cytokine pattern and preserve regulatory T cells in the periphery and induce sustained normoglycemia. *J Autoimmun*, Vol.32, No.1, pp. 33-42, ISSN 0896-8411.

Brennand K, Huangfu D, Melton D. (2007). All beta cells contribute equally to islet growth and maintenance. *PLoS Biol,* Vol. 5, No.7, pp.e163, ISSN 1545-7885.

Brennand K, Melton D.(2009). Slow and steady is the key to beta-cell replication. *J Cell Mol Med,* Vol.13, No.3, pp.472-487, ISSN 1582-4934.

Bretzel RG, Jahr H, Eckhard M, Martin I, Winter D, Brendel MD. (2007). Islet cell transplantation today. *Langenbecks Arch Surg.* Vol. 392, No.3, pp. 239-253, ISSN 1435-2443.

Butler AE, Cao-Minh L, Galasso R, Rizza RA, Corradin A, Cobelli C, Butler PC. (2010).Adaptive changes in pancreatic beta cell fractional area and beta cell turnover in human pregnancy. *Diabetologia,* Vol.53, No.10, pp.2167-2176, ISSN 1432-0428.

Butler AE, Janson J, Bonner-Weir S, Ritzel R, Rizza RA, Butler PC. (2003). Beta-cell deficit and increased beta-cell apoptosis in humans with type 2 diabetes. *Diabetes,* Vol.52, No.1, pp.102-110, ISSN 0012-1797.

Cantarovich D, Vistoli F. (2009). Minimization protocols in pancreas transplantation. *Transpl Int,* Vol.22, No.1, pp.61-68, ISSN 0934-0874.

Carlotti F, Zaldumbide A, Loomans CJ, van Rossenberg E, Engelse M, de Koning EJ, Hoeben RC. (2010). Isolated human islets contain a distinct population of mesenchymal stem cells. Islets, Vol.2, No.3, pp.164-173, ISSN 1938-2022.

Chhabra P, Mirmira RG, Brayman KL.(2009). Regenerative medicine and tissue engineering: contribution of stem cells in organ transplantation. *Curr Opin Organ Transplant,* Vol.14, No.1, pp.46-50, ISSN 1531-7013.

Chen BZ, Yu SL, Singh S, Kao LP, Tsai ZY, Yang PC, Chen BH, Shoei-Lung Li S. (2011). Identification of microRNAs expressed highly in pancreatic islet-like cell clusters differentiated from human embryonic stem cells. *Cell Biol Int,* Vol.35, No.1, pp. 29-37, ISSN 1095-8355.

Chen LB, Jiang XB and Yang L (2004). Differentiation of rat marrow mesenchymal stem cells into pancreatic islet beta-cells. *World J Gastroenterol,* Vol.10, No.20, pp. 3016-3020, ISSN 1007-9327.

Chen S, Borowiak M, Fox JL, Maehr R, Osafune K, Davidow L, Lam K, Peng LF, Schreiber SL, Rubin LL, Melton D.(2009). A small molecule that directs differentiation of human ESCs into the pancreatic lineage. *Nat Chem Biol,*Vol.5, No.4, pp.258-265, ISSN 1552-4469.

Chen S, Shimoda M, Wang MY, Ding J, Noguchi H, Matsumoto S, Grayburn PA. (2010). Regeneration of pancreatic islets in vivo by ultrasound-targeted gene therapy. *Gene Ther,* Vol.17, No.11, pp.1411-1420, ISSN 1476-5462.

Chung CH, Hao E, Piran R, Keinan E, Levine F. (2010). Pancreatic beta-cell neogenesis by direct conversion from mature alpha-cells. *Stem Cells,* Vol.28, No.9, pp. 1630-1638, ISSN 1549-4918.

Chung CH & Levine F. (2010). Adult pancreatic alpha-cells: a new source of cells for beta-cell regeneration. *Rev Diabet Stud,* Vol.7, No.2, pp. 124-131, ISSN 1614-0575.

Collombat P, Xu X, Ravassard P, Sosa-Pineda B, Dussaud S, Billestrup N, Madsen OD, Serup P, Heimberg H, Mansouri A. (2009). The ectopic expression of Pax4 in the mouse pancreas converts progenitor cells into alpha and subsequently beta cells. *Cell,* Vol.138, No.3, pp. 449-462, ISSN 1097-4172.

Cooper DKC, Tseng Y-L, Saidman SL. (2004). Alloantibody and xenoantibody cross-reactivity in transplantation. *Transplantation,* pp. 77:1–5, ISSN 0041-1337.

Correa-Medina M, Bravo-Egana V, Rosero S, Ricordi C, Edlund H, Diez J, Pastori RL. (2009). MicroRNA miR-7 is preferentially expressed in endocrine cells of the developing and adult human pancreas. *Gene Expr Patterns,* Vol.9, No.4, pp. 193-199, ISSN 1567-133X.

Cowan PJ, d'Apice AJ. (2008)The coagulation barrier in xenotransplantation: incompatibilities and strategies to overcome them. *Curr Opin Organ Transplant,* Vol.13, No.2, pp.178-183, ISSN 1531-7013.

D'Amour KA, Bang AG, Eliazer S, Kelly OG, Agulnick AD, Smart NG, Moorman MA, Kroon E, Carpenter MK, Baetge EE, (2006) Production of pancreatic hormone-expressing endocrine cells from human embryonic stem cells. *Nat Biotechnol,* Vol.24, No.11, pp. 1392-1401, ISSN 1087-0156.

Daoud J, Petropavlovskaia M, Rosenberg L, Tabrizian M. (2010). The effect of extracellular matrix components on the preservation of human islet function in vitro. *Biomaterials,* Vol.31, No. 7, pp. 1676-1682, ISSN 1878-5905.

Daoud JT, Petropavlovskaia MS, Patapas JM, Degrandpré CE, Diraddo RW, Rosenberg L, Tabrizian M. (2011). Long-term in vitro human pancreatic islet culture using three-dimensional microfabricated scaffolds. *Biomaterials,* Vol.32, No.6,pp. 1536-1542, ISSN 1878-5905.

Deng S, Vatamaniuk M, Lian MM, Doliba N, Wang J, Bell E, Wolf B, Raper S,Matschinsky FM, Markmann JF. (2003). Insulin gene transfer enhances the function of human islet grafts. *Diabetologia,* Vol.46, No.3, pp.386-393, ISSN 0012-186X.

Denner J, Schuurman HJ, Patience C. (2009). The International Xenotransplantation Association consensus statement on conditions for undertaking clinical trials of porcine islet products in type 1 diabetes--chapter 5: Strategies to prevent transmission of porcine endogenous retroviruses. *Xenotransplantation,* Vol.16, No.4, pp.239-248, ISSN 1399-3089.

Desai BM, Oliver-Krasinski J, De Leon DD, Farzad C, Hong N, Leach SD, Stoffers DA. (2007). Preexisting pancreatic acinar cells contribute to acinar cell, but not islet beta cell, regeneration. *J Clin Invest,* Vol.117, No.4, pp.971-977, ISSN 0021-9738.

Dieckhoff B, Petersen B, Kues WA, Kurth R, Niemann H, Denner J. (2008). Knockdown of porcine endogenous retrovirus (PERV) expression by PERV-specific siRNA in transgenic pigs. *Xenotransplantation,* Vol.15, pp.36–45, ISSN 1399-3089.

Donath MY, Størling J, Berchtold LA, Billestrup N, Mandrup-Poulsen T.(2008). Cytokines and beta-cell biology: from concept to clinical translation. *Endocr Rev,* Vol.29,No.3, pp.334-350, ISSN 0163-769X.

Dor Y, Brown J, Martinez OI, Melton DA. (2004). Adult pancreatic beta-cells are formed by self-duplication rather than stem-cell differentiation. *Nature,* Vol.429, No.6987, pp. 41-46, ISSN 1476-4687.

Dor Y & Melton DA (2004). How important are adult stem cells for tissue maintenance? *Cell Cycle,* Vol. 3, No. 9, pp. 1104-1106, ISSN 1551-4005.

Egidi FM.(2005). Management of hyperglycaemia after pancreas transplantation: are new immunosuppressants the answer? *Drugs,* Vol.65, No.2,pp.153-166, ISSN 0012-6667.

Eizirik DL, Mandrup-Poulsen T.(2001).A choice of death--the signal-transduction of immune-mediated beta-cell apoptosis. *Diabetologia,* Vol.44, No.12, pp.2115-2133, ISSN 0012-186X

Ekser B, Cooper DK.(2010). Overcoming the barriers to xenotransplantation: prospects for the future. *Expert Rev Clin Immunol,* Vol.6, No.2, pp.219-230, ISSN 1744-666X.

Elliott RB. (2011). Towards Zenotransplantation of pig islets in the clinic. *Curr Opin Organ Transplant,* Vol.16, No.2, pp.195-200, ISSN 1531-7013.

Evans-Molina C, Vestermark GL, Mirmira RG.(2009). Development of insulin-producing cells from primitive biologic precursors. *Curr Opin Organ Transplant,* Vol.14, No.1, pp.56-63, ISSN1531-7013.

Evgenov NV, Medarova Z, Pratt J, Pantazopoulos P, Leyting S, Bonner-Weir S, Moore A.(2006). In vivo imaging of immune rejection in transplanted pancreatic islets. *Diabetes,* Vol.55, No.9,pp.2419-2428, ISSN 0012-1797.

Fan CG, Zhang QJ, Zhou JR. (2011). Therapeutic potentials of mesenchymal stem cells derived from human umbilical cord. *Stem Cell Rev,* Vol.7, No.1, pp. 195-207, ISSN 1558-6804.

Fändrich F, Ungefroren H. (2010). Customized cell-based treatment options to combat autoimmunity and restore beta-cell function in type 1 diabetes mellitus: current protocols and future perspectives. *Adv Exp Med Biol.* Vol.654, pp. 641-665, ISSN 0065-2598.

Fanjul M, Gmyr V, Sengenès C, Ratovo G, Dufresne M, Lefebvre B, Kerr-Conte J, Hollande E. (2010). Evidence for epithelial-mesenchymal transition in adult human pancreatic exocrine cells. *J Histochem Cytochem,* Vol.58, No.9, pp. 807-823, ISSN 1551-5044.

Fiaschi-Taesch NM, Salim F, Kleinberger J, Troxell R, Cozar-Castellano I, Selk K, Cherok E, Takane KK, Scott DK, Stewart AF.(2010). Induction of human beta-cell proliferation and engraftment using a single G1/S regulatory molecule, cdk6. *Diabetes,* Vol.59, No.8, pp.1926-1936, ISSN 1939-327X.

Figliuzzi M, Cornolti R, Perico N, Rota C, Morigi M, Remuzzi G, Remuzzi A, Benigni A. (2009). Bone marrow-derived mesenchymal stem cells improve islet graft function in diabetic rats. *Transplant Proc,* Vol.41, No.5, pp. 1797-1800, ISSN 1873-2623.

Fodor A, Harel C, Fodor L, Armoni M, Salmon P, Trono D, Karnieli E. (2007). Adult rat liver cells transdifferentiated with lentiviral IPF1 vectors reverse diabetes in mice: an ex vivo gene therapy approach. *Diabetologia,*Vol.50, No.1, pp.121-130, ISSN 0012-186X .

Fukazawa T, Matsuoka J, Naomoto Y, Nakai T, Durbin ML, Kojima I, Lakey JR, Tanaka N. (2006). Development of a novel beta-cell specific promoter system for the identification of insulin-producing cells in in vitro cell cultures. *Exp Cell Res,* Vol.312, No.17, pp. 3404-3412, ISSN 0014-4827.

Furth ME & Atala A (2009). Stem cell sources to treat diabetes. *J Cell Biochem,* Vol.106, No.4, pp. 507-511, ISSN 1097-4644.

Gao R, Ustinov J, Pulkkinen MA, Lundin K, Korsgren O, Otonkoski T. (2003). Characterization of endocrine progenitor cells and critical factors for their differentiation in human adult pancreatic cell culture. *Diabetes,* Vol.52, No.8, pp. 2007-2015, ISSN 0012-1797.

Gao R, Ustinov J, Korsgren O, Otonkoski T.(2005). In vitro neogenesis of human islets reflects the plasticity of differentiated human pancreatic cells. *Diabetologia,* Vol.48, No.11, pp.2296-2304, ISSN 0012-186X.

Gao F, Wu DQ, Hu YH, Jin GX, Li GD, Sun TW, Li FJ.(2008).In vitro cultivation of islet-like cell clusters from human umbilical cord blood-derived mesenchymal stem cells. *Transl Res,*Vol.151, No.6, pp.293-302, ISSN 1931-5244.

Gartner W, Koc F, Nabokikh A, Daneva T, Niederle B, Luger A, Wagner L. (2006). Long-term in vitro growth of human insulin-secreting insulinoma cells. *Neuroendocrinology,* Vol. 83,No.2, pp.123-130, ISSN 0028-3835.

Geelhoed-Duijvestijn PH.(2007). Incretins: a new treatment option for type 2 diabetes? *Neth J Med.* Vol.65, No.2, pp.60-64, ISSN0300-2977.

Gefen-Halevi S, Rachmut IH, Molakandov K, Berneman D, Mor E, Meivar-Levy I, Ferber S. (2010). NKX6.1 promotes PDX-1-induced liver to pancreatic β-cells reprogramming. *Cell Reprogram,* Vol.12, No.6,pp.655-664, ISSN 2152-4998.

Georgia S, Bhushan A. (2006). p27 Regulates the transition of beta-cells from quiescence to proliferation. *Diabetes,* Vol.55, No.11, pp.2950-2956, ISSN 0012-1797.

Gianani R. (2011). Beta cell regeneration in human pancreas. Semin Immunopathol, Vol.33, No.1, pp.23-27,ISSN1863-2300.

Gianani R, Putnam A, Still T, Yu L, Miao D, Gill RG, Beilke J, Supon P, Valentine A, Iveson A, Dunn S, Eisenbarth GS, Hutton J, Gottlieb P, Wiseman A. (2006). Initial results of screening of nondiabetic organ donors for expression of islet autoantibodies. *J Clin Endocrinol Metab,* Vol.91, No.5, pp.1855-1861, ISSN 0021-972X.

Gillard P, Keymeulen B, Mathieu C.(2010). Beta-cell transplantation in type 1 diabetic patients: a work in progress to cure.*Verh K Acad Geneeskd Belg,* Vol.72No.1-2, pp.71-98, ISSN 0302-6469.

Gillard P, Mathieu C. (2011) .[Epub ahead of print] Immune and cell therapy in type 1 diabetes: too little too late? *Expert Opin Biol Ther,* ISSN 1744-7682.

Giorgetti A, Montserrat N, Rodriguez-Piza I, Azqueta C, Veiga A, Izpisúa Belmonte JC. Generation of induced pluripotent stem cells from human cord blood cells with only two factors: Oct4 and Sox2. Nat Protoc, Vol.5, No.4, pp.811-820, ISSN 1750-2799.

Granger A, Kushner JA. (2009). Cellular origins of beta-cell regeneration: a legacy view of historical controversies. *J Intern Med.* Vol.266, No.4, pp.325-338, ISSN1365-2796.

Gruessner RW, Kandaswamy R, Denny R. (2001). Laparoscopic simultaneous nephrectomy and distal pancreatectomy from a live donor. *J Am Coll Surg,* Vol.193, No.3, pp.333-337, ISSN 1072-7515.

Gu G, Dubauskaite J, Melton DA. (2002). Direct evidence for the pancreatic lineage: NGN3+ cells are islet progenitors and are distinct from duct progenitors. *Development,* Vol.129, No.10, pp. 2447-2457, ISSN 0950-1991.

Guo T & Hebrok M (2009). Stem cells to pancreatic beta-cells: new sources for diabetes cell therapy. *Endocr Rev.* Vol.30, No.3, pp. 214-227. ISSN 1945-7189.

Guz Y, Nasir I, Teitelman G. (2001). Regeneration of pancreatic beta cells from intra-islet precursor cells in an experimental model of diabetes. *Endocrinology,*Vol.142, No.11, pp. 4956-4968, ISSN 0013-7227.

Haller MJ, Viener HL, Wasserfall C, Brusko T, Atkinson MA, Schatz DA.(2008) Autologous umbilical cord blood infusion for type 1 diabetes. *Exp. Hematol*, Vol.36, No.6, pp.710-715, ISSN 0301-472X.

Hanley S & Rosenberg L. (2009). Islet-derived progenitors as a source of in vitro islet regeneration. *Methods Mol Biol*, Vol.482:371-385, ISSN 1064-3745.

Hardikar AA, Marcus-Samuels B, Geras-Raaka E, Raaka BM, Gershengorn MC.(2003). Human pancreatic precursor cells secrete FGF2 to stimulate clustering into hormone-expressing islet-like cell aggregates. *Proc Natl Acad Sci U S A*, Vol.100, No.12, pp. 7117-7122, ISSN 0027-8424.

Herold KC, Gitelman SE, Masharani U, Hagopian W, Bisikirska B, Donaldson D, Rother K, Diamond B, Harlan DM, Bluestone JA.(2005).A single course of anti-CD3 monoclonal antibody hOKT3gamma1(Ala-Ala) results in improvement in C-peptide responses and clinical parameters for at least 2 years after onset of type 1 diabetes. *Diabetes*,Vol.54, No.6, pp.1763-1769, ISSN 0012-1797.

Hochedlinger K, Plath K.(2009). Epigenetic reprogramming and induced Pluripotency. *Development*,Vol.136, NO.4, pp.509-523, ISSN 0950-1991.

Horb ME, Shen CN, Tosh D, Slack JM. (2003). Experimental conversion of liver to pancreas. *Curr Biol*, Vol.13, No.2, pp.105–115, ISSN 0960-9822.

Huang X, Moore DJ, Ketchum RJ, Nunemaker CS, Kovatchev B, McCall AL, Brayman KL. (2008). Resolving the conundrum of islet transplantation by linking metabolic dysregulation, inflammation, and immune regulation. *Endocr Rev*, Vol.29, No.5, pp.603-630, ISSN 0163-769X.

Huangfu D, Osafune K, Maehr R, Guo W, Eijkelenboom A, Chen S, Muhlestein W, Melton DA. (2008). Induction of pluripotent stem cells from primary human fibroblasts with only Oct4 and Sox2. *Nat Biotechnol*, Vol.26, No.11, pp.1269-1275, ISSN 1546-1696.

Humphrey RK, Yu SM, Flores LE, Jhala US.(2010) Glucose regulates steady-state levels of PDX1 via the reciprocal actions of GSK3 and AKT kinases. *J Biol Chem*, Vol.285, No.5, pp.3406-3416, ISSN 1083-351X.

Imai J, Katagiri H, Yamada T, Ishigaki Y, Ogihara T,Uno K, Hasegawa Y, Gao J,Ishihara H, Sasano H, Mizuguchi H, Asano T, Oka Y. (2005). Constitutively active PDX1induced efficient insulin production in adult murine liver. *Biochem Biophys Res Commun*, Vol.326, No.2,pp. 402–409, ISSN 0006-291X.

Inada A, Nienaber C, Katsuta H, Fujitani Y, Levine J, Morita R, Sharma A, Bonner-Weir S. (2008). Carbonic anhydrase II-positive pancreatic cells are progenitors for both endocrine and exocrine pancreas after birth. *Proc Natl Acad Sci U S A*, Vol.105, No.50, pp. 19915-19919. ISSN 1091-6490.

Ito T, Itakura S, Todorov I, Rawson J, Asari S, Shintaku J, Nair I, Ferreri K, Kandeel F, Mullen Y. (2010). Mesenchymal stem cell and islet co-transplantation promotes graft revascularization and function. *Transplantation*, Vol.89, No.12, pp. 1438-1445, ISSN 1534-6080.

Jeong JH, Kim SH, Lee M, Kim WJ, Park TG, Ko KS, Kim SW. (2010). Non-viral systemic delivery of Fas siRNA suppresses cyclophosphamide-induced diabetes in NOD mice. *J Control Release*, Vol.143, No.1, pp.88-94, ISSN 1873-4995.

Joglekar MV, Joglekar VM, Hardikar AA. (2009). Expression of islet-specific microRNAs during human pancreatic development. *Gene Expr Patterns,* Vol.9, No.2, pp. 109-113, ISSN 1567-133X.

Joglekar MV, Parekh VS, Mehta S, Bhonde RR, & Hardikar AA. (2007). MicroRNA profiling of developing and regenerating pancreas reveal post-transcriptional regulation of neurogenin3. *Dev Biol,* Vol.311, No.2, pp. 603-612, ISSN 1095-564X.

Juhl K, Bonner-Weir S, Sharma A. (2010). Regenerating pancreatic beta-cells: plasticity of adult pancreatic cells and the feasibility of in-vivo neogenesis. *Curr Opin Organ Transplant,* Vol.15, No.1, pp. 79-85, ISSN1531-7013.

Jun HS. (2010). In vivo regeneration of insulin-producing beta-cells. *Adv Exp Med Biol,* Vol.654, pp.627-640, ISSN 0065-2598.

Kadam SS & Bhonde RR. (2010). Islet neogenesis from the constitutively nestin expressing human umbilical cord matrix derived mesenchymal stem cells. *Islets,* Vol.2, No.2, pp. 112-120. ISSN 1938-2022.

Kaneto H, Matsuoka TA, Nakatani Y, Miyatsuka T, Matsuhisa M,Hori M,Yamasaki Y. (2005a). A crucial role of MafA as a novel therapeutic target for diabetes. *J Biol Chem* , Vol.280, No.15, pp.15047–15052, ISSN 0021-9258.

Kaneto H, Nakatani Y, Miyatsuka T, Matsuoka TA, Matsuhisa M,Hori M,Yamasaki Y. (2005b). PDX-1/VP16 fusion protein, together with NeuroD or Ngn3, markedly induces insulin gene transcription and ameliorates glucose tolerance. *Diabetes,* Vol.54, No.4,pp.1009–1022, ISSN 0012-1797.

Karnieli O, Izhar-Prato Y, Bulvik S, Efrat S. (2007). Generation of insulin-producing cells from human bone marrow mesenchymal stem cells by genetic manipulation. *Stem Cells,* Vol.25, No.11, pp. 2837-2844, ISSN 1549-4918.

Karnik SK, Chen H, McLean GW, Heit JJ, Gu X, Zhang AY, Fontaine M, Yen MH,Kim SK. (2007). Menin controls growth of pancreatic beta-cells in pregnant mice andpromotes gestational diabetes mellitus. *Science,* Vol.318, No.5851, pp.806-809, ISSN 1095-9203.

Kaung HL.(1994). Growth dynamics of pancreatic islet cell populations during fetal and neonatal development of the rat. *Dev Dyn,* Vol.200, No.2,163-175, ISSN 1058-8388.

Kayali AG, Flores LE, Lopez AD, Kutlu B, Baetge E, Kitamura R, Hao E, Beattie GM, Hayek A.(2007). Limited capacity of human adult islets expanded in vitro to redifferentiate into insulin-producing beta-cells.*Diabetes,* Vol.56, No.3, pp703-708, ISSN 0012-1797.

Kikugawa R, Katsuta H, Akashi T, Yatoh S, Weir GC, Sharma A, Bonner-Weir S. (2009). Differentiation of COPAS-sorted non-endocrine pancreatic cells into insulin-positive cells in the mouse. *Diabetologia,* Vol.52, No.4, pp. 645-652, ISSN1432-0428.

Kim S, Shin JS, Kim HJ, Fisher RC, Lee MJ, Kim CW. (2007). Streptozotocin-induced diabetes can be reversed by hepatic oval cell activation through hepatic transdifferentiation and pancreatic islet regeneration. *Lab Invest,* Vol.87, No.7, pp.702-712, ISSN 0023-6837.

Knip M. (1997) Disease-associated autoimmunity and prevention of insulin-dependent diabetes mellitus. *Ann Med,* Vol. 29, No.5, pp. 447-451, ISSN 0785-3890.

Koblas T, Zacharovová K, Berková Z, Leontovic I, Dovolilová E, Zámecník L, Saudek F.(2009). In vivo differentiation of human umbilical cord blood-derived cells into insulin-producing beta cells. Folia Biol (Praha), Vol.55, No.6, pp.224-232, ISSN 0015-5500.

Kodama S, Toyonaga T, Kondo T, Matsumoto K, Tsuruzoe K, Kawashima J, Goto H, Kume K, Kume S, Sakakida M, Araki E. (2005). Enhanced expression of PDX-1 and Ngn3 by exendin-4 during beta cell regeneration in STZ-treated mice. *Biochem Biophys Res Commun,* Vol.327, No.4, pp. 1170-1178, ISSN 0006-291X.

Kogler G, Sensken S, Airey JA, Trapp T, Muschen M, Feldhahn N, Liedtke S, Sorg RV, Fischer J, Rosenbaum C, Greschat S, Knipper A, Bender J, Degistirici O, Gao J, Caplan AI, Colletti EJ, Almeida-Porada G, Müller HW, Zanjani E, Wernet P. (2004). A new human somatic stem cell from placental cord blood with intrinsic pluripotent differentiation potential. *J Exp Med,* Vol.200, No.2, pp. 123-135, ISSN 0022-1007

Kojima H, Fujimiya M, Matsumura K, Younan P,Imaeda H, Maeda M,Chan, L. (2003). NeuroD-betacellulin gene therapy induces islet neogenesis in the liver and reverses diabetes in mice. *Nat Med,* Vol.9, No.5, pp.596–603, ISSN 1078-8956.

Kopinke D & Murtaugh LC. (2010). Exocrine-to-endocrine differentiation is detectable only prior to birth in the uninjured mouse pancreas. *BMC Dev Biol,* Vol.10, pp. 38, ISSN 1471-213X.

Koulmanda M, Budo E, Bonner-Weir S, Qipo A, Putheti P, Degauque N, Shi H, Fan Z, Flier JS, Auchincloss H Jr, Zheng XX, Strom TB.(2007). Modification of adverse inflammation is required to cure new-onset type 1 diabetic hosts. *Proc Natl Acad Sci U S A,* Vol.104, No.32, pp.13074-13079, ISSN 0027-8424.

Koya V, Lu S, Sun YP, Purich DL, Atkinson MA, Li SW, Yang LJ. (2008). Reversal of streptozotocin-induced diabetes in mice by cellular transduction with recombinant pancreatic transcription factor pancreatic duodenal homeobox-1: a novel protein transduction domain-based therapy. *Diabetes,* Vol.57, No.3, pp.757-769, ISSN 1939-327X.

Kroon E, Martinson LA, Kadoya K, Bang AG, Kelly OG, Eliazer S, Young H, Richardson M, Smart NG, Cunningham J, Agulnick AD, D'Amour KA, Carpenter MK, Baetge EE. (2008). Pancreatic endoderm derived from human embryonic stem cells generates glucose-responsive insulin-secreting cells in vivo. *Nat Biotechnol,* Vol.26, No.4, pp. 443-452, ISSN 1546-1696.

Krutzfeldt J, Rajewsky N, Braich R, Rajeev KG, Tuschl T, Manoharan M, Stoffel M. (2005). Silencing of microRNAs in vivo with 'antagomirs'. *Nature,* Vol.438, No. 7068, pp. 685-689, ISSN 1476-4687.

Kushner JA, Weir GC, Bonner-Weir S. (2010). Ductal origin hypothesis of pancreatic regeneration under attack. Cell Metab. Vol.11, No.1, pp.:2-3, ISSN 932-7420.

Langer RM. (2010) Islet transplantation: lessons learned since the Edmonton breakthrough. *Transplant Proc,* Vol.42, No.5, pp. 1421-1424, ISSN 1873-2623.

Lardon J, De Breuck S, Rooman I, Van Lommel L, Kruhøffer M, Orntoft T, Schuit F, Bouwens L.(2004). Plasticity in the adult rat pancreas: transdifferentiation of exocrine to hepatocyte-like cells in primary culture. *Hepatology,*Vol.39, No.6, pp.1499-1507, ISSN 0270-9139.

Lechner A, Leech CA, Abraham EJ, Nolan AL, & Habener JF. (2002). Nestin-positive progenitor cells derived from adult human pancreatic islets of Langerhans contain side population (SP) cells defined by expression of the ABCG2 (BCRP1) ATP-binding cassette transporter. *Biochem Biophys Res Commun,* Vol.293, No.2, pp. 670-674, ISSN 0006-291X.

Lee RH, Pulin AA, Seo MJ, Kota DJ, Ylostalo J, Larson BL, Semprun-Prieto L, Delafontaine P, Prockop DJ. (2009). Intravenous hMSCs improve myocardial infarction in mice because cells embolized in lung are activated to secrete the anti-inflammatory protein TSG-6. *Cell Stem Cell,* Vol.5, No.1, pp. 54-63, ISSN 1875-9777.

Lee RH, Seo MJ, Reger RL, Spees JL, Pulin AA, Olson SD, Prockop DJ. (2006). Multipotent stromal cells from human marrow home to and promote repair of pancreatic islets and renal glomeruli in diabetic NOD/scid mice. *Proc Natl Acad Sci U S A,* Vol.103, No.46, pp. 17438-17443, ISSN 0027-8424.

Leitão CB, Tharavanij T, Cure P, Pileggi A, Baidal DA, Ricordi C, Alejandro R. (2008). Restoration of hypoglycemia awareness after islet transplantation. *Diabetes Care,* Vol.31, No.11, pp.2113-2115, ISSN 1935-5548.

Levetan C. (2010). Distinctions between islet neogenesis and β-cell replication: implications for reversal of Type 1 and 2 diabetes. *J Diabetes.* Vol.2, No.2, pp.76-84, ISSN 1753-0407.

Li L, Seno M, Yamada H, Kojima I. (2003). Betacellulin improves glucose metabolism by promoting conversion of intraislet precursor cells to beta-cells in streptozotocin-treated mice. *Am J Physiol Endocrinol Metab,* Vol.285, No.3, pp. E577-583, ISSN 0193-1849.

Li L, Yi Z, Seno M, Kojima I.(2004). Activin A and betacellulin: Effect on regeneration of pancreatic beta-cells in neonatal streptozotocin-treated rats. *Diabetes,* Vol.53,No.3,pp.608-615, ISSN 0012-1797.

Li WC, Horb ME, Tosh D, Slack JM. (2005). In vitro transdifferentiation of hepatoma cells into functional pancreatic cells. *Mech Dev,* Vol. 122, No.6, pp. 835–847, ISSN 0925-4773.

Li Y, Song YH, Li F, Yang T, Lu YW, Geng YJ. (2009). MicroRNA-221 regulates high glucose-induced endothelial dysfunction. *Biochem Biophys Res Commun,* Vol.381, No.1, pp. 81-83, ISSN 1090-2104.

Lipsett MA, Castellarin ML, Rosenberg L. (2007). Acinar plasticity: development of a novel in vitro model to study human acinar-to-duct-to-islet differentiation. *Pancreas,* Vol.34, No.4, pp.452-457, ISSN 1536-4828.

Liu Y, Tanabe K, Baronnier D, Patel S, Woodgett J, Cras-Méneur C, Permutt MA. (2010). Conditional ablation of Gsk-3β in islet beta cells results in expanded mass and resistance to fat feeding-induced diabetes in mice. *Diabetologia,* Vol.53, No.12, pp. 2600-2610, ISSN 1432-0428.

Lovvorn HN 3rd, Nance ML, Ferry RJ Jr, Stolte L, Baker L, O'Neill JA Jr, Schnaufer L, Stanley CA, Adzick NS. (1999). Congenital hyperinsulinism and the surgeon: lessons learned over 35 years. *J Pediatr Surg.* Vol.34, No.5, pp.786-792; discussion 792-793, ISSN 0022-3468.

Lu J, Herrera PL, Carreira C, Bonnavion R, Seigne C, Calender A, Bertolino P, Zhang CX. (2010). Alpha cell-specific Men1 ablation triggers the transdifferentiation of glucagon-expressing cells and insulinoma development. *Gastroenterology,* Vol.138, No.5, pp. 1954-1965, ISSN 1528-0012.

Magliocca JF, Knechtle SJ. (2006).The evolving role of alemtuzumab (Campath-1H) for immunosuppressive therapy in organ transplantation. *Transpl Int,* Vol.19, No.9,pp.705-714, ISSN 0934-0874.

Martín J, Hunt SL, Dubus P, Sotillo R, Néhmé-Pélluard F, Magnuson MA, Parlow AF, Malumbres M, Ortega S, Barbacid M. (2003). Genetic rescue of Cdk4 null mice restores pancreatic beta-cell proliferation but not homeostatic cell number. *Oncogene,* Vol.22, No.34, pp. 5261-5269, ISSN 0950-9232.

Martin-Pagola A, Sisino G, Allende G, Dominguez-Bendala J, Gianani R, Reijonen H, Nepom GT, Ricordi C, Ruiz P, Sageshima J, Ciancio G, Burke GW, Pugliese A.(2008). Insulin protein and proliferation in ductal cells in the transplanted pancreas of patients with type 1 diabetes and recurrence of autoimmunity. *Diabetologia,* Vol.51,No.10,pp.1803-1813, ISSN 0012-186X

Maruyama M, Kenmochi T, Akutsu N, Saigo K, Iwashita C, Otsuki K, Ito T, Asano T. (2010). Laparoscopic-assisted distal pancreatectomy and nephrectomy from a live donor. *J Hepatobiliary Pancreat Sci,*Vol.17, No.2, pp.193-196, ISSN 1868-6982. McGuckin CP, Forraz N, Baradez MO, Navran S, Zhao J, Urban R, Tilton R, Denner L.(2005). Production of stem cells with embryonic characteristics from human umbilical cord blood. *Cell Prolif.* Vol.38, No.4, pp.245-55, ISSN 0960-7722.

Means AL, Meszoely IM, Suzuki K, Miyamoto Y, Rustgi AK, Coffey RJ Jr, Wright CV, Stoffers DA, Leach SD. (2005). Pancreatic epithelial plasticity mediated by acinar cell transdifferentiation and generation of nestin-positive intermediates. *Development,* Vol.132, No.16, pp. 3767-377,. ISSN 0950-1991.

Meier JJ, Butler AE, Saisho Y, Monchamp T, Galasso R, Bhushan A, Rizza RA, Butler PC.(2008). Beta-cell replication is the primary mechanism subserving the postnatal expansion of beta-cell mass in humans. *Diabetes,* Vol.57, No.6, pp.1584-1594, ISSN1939-327X.

Meivar-Levy I, Ferber S. (2006). Regenerative medicine: using liver to generate pancreas for treating diabetes. *Isr Med Assoc J,* Vol.8, No.6, pp.430-434, ISSN 1565-1088.

Melkman-Zehavi T, Oren R, Kredo-Russo S, Shapira T, Mandelbaum AD, Rivkin N, Nir T, Lennox KA, Behlke MA, Dor Y, Hornstein E. (2011) miRNAs control insulin content in pancreatic β-cells via downregulation of transcriptional repressors. *EMBO J,* Vol.30,No. 5, pp.835-845, ISSN1460-2075.

Menge BA, Tannapfel A, Belyaev O, Drescher R, Müller C, Uhl W, Schmidt WE, Meier JJ.(2008). Partial pancreatectomy in adult humans does not provoke beta-cell regeneration. *Diabetes,* Vol.57, No.1,pp.142-149, ISSN 1939-327X.

Milanesi A, Lee JW, Xu Q, Perin L, Yu JS. (2011). Differentiation of Nestin-Positive Cells Derived from Bone Marrow into Pancreatic Endocrine and Ductal Cells in vitro. *J Endocrinol,* ISSN 1479-6805.

Minami K, Okuno M, Miyawaki K, Okumachi A, Ishizaki K, Oyama K, Kawaguchi M, Ishizuka N, Iwanaga T, Seino S. (2005). Lineage tracing and characterization of insulin-secreting cells generated from adult pancreatic acinar cells. *Proc Natl Acad Sci U S A,* Vol.102, No.42, pp. 15116-15121, ISSN 0027-8424.

Minami K & Seino S. (2008). Pancreatic acinar-to-beta cell transdifferentiation in vitro. *Front Biosci,* Vol.13, pp.5824-5837, ISSN 1093-4715.

Mishra PK, Singh SR, Joshua IG, Tyagi SC.(2010). *Front Biosci,* Vol.15, pp.461-477, ISSN 1093-4715.

Miyatsuka T, Kaneto H, Kajimoto Y, et al. (2003). Ectopically expressed PDX-1 in liver initiates endocrine and exocrine pancreas differentiation but causes dysmorphogenesis. *Biochem Biophys Res Commun,* Vol.310, No.3, pp.1017–1025, ISSN0006-291X.

Montaña E, Bonner-Weir S, Weir GC. (1994). Transplanted beta cell response to increased metabolic demand. Changes in beta cell replication and mass. *J Clin Invest,* Vol.93, No.4, pp.1577-1582, ISSN.0021-9738.

Moore DJ, Markmann JF, Deng S.(2006). Avenues for immunomodulation and graft protection by gene therapy in transplantation. *Transpl Int,*Vol.19,No.6, pp.435-445, ISSN 0934-0874.

Murray HE, Paget MB, Bailey CJ, Downing R. (2009). Sustained insulin secretory response in human islets co-cultured with pancreatic duct-derived epithelial cells within a rotational cell culture system. *Diabetologia,* Vol.52, No.3, pp.477-485, ISSN 1432-0428.

Nakagawa M, Koyanagi M, Tanabe K, Takahashi K, Ichisaka T, Aoi T, Okita K,Mochiduki Y, Takizawa N, Yamanaka S. (2008). Generation of induced pluripotent stem cells without myc from mouse and human fibroblasts. *Nat Biotechnol* ,Vol.26, No.1, pp.101-106, ISSN 1546-1696.

Nir T & Dor Y. (2005). How to make pancreatic beta cells--prospects for cell therapy in diabetes. *Curr Opin Biotechnol,* Vol.16, No.5, pp. 524-529, ISSN 0958-1669.

Nir T, Melton DA, Dor Y. (2007). Recovery from diabetes in mice by beta cell regeneration. *J Clin Invest* 117, No.9, pp. 2553-2561, ISSN 0021-9738.

Noguchi H. (2009). Pancreatic islet transplantation. *World J Gastrointest Surg.* Vol.1, No.1, pp.16-20, ISSN 1948-9366.

Okuno M, Minami K, Okumachi A, Miyawaki K, Yokoi N, Toyokuni S, Seino S. (2007). Generation of insulin-secreting cells from pancreatic acinar cells of animal models of type 1 diabetes. *Am J Physiol Endocrinol Metab,* Vol.292, No.1, pp.E158-65, ISSN 0193-1849.

Parekh VS, Joglekar MV, Hardikar AA. (2009). Differentiation of human umbilical cord blood-derived mononuclear cells to endocrine pancreatic lineage. *Differentiation,* Vol.78, No.4, pp. 232-240, ISSN 1432-0436.

Phuc PV, Nhung TH, Loan DT, Chung DC, Ngoc PK (2011). Differentiating of banked human umbilical cord blood-derived mesenchymal stem cells into insulin-secreting cells. *In Vitro Cell Dev Biol Anim,* Vol.47, No.1, pp. 54-63, ISSN 1543-706X.

Pierro A, Nah SA. (2011). Surgical management of congenital hyperinsulinism of infancy. *Semin Pediatr Surg,* Vol.20, No. 1, pp. 50-53, ISSN 1532-9453.

Pittenger GL, Taylor-Fishwick D, Vinik AI. (2009). A role for islet neogenesis in curing diabetes. *Diabetologia.* Vol.52, No.5, pp.735-738, ISSN 1432-0428.

Poy MN, Eliasson L, Krutzfeldt J, Kuwajima S, Ma X, Macdonald PE, Pfeffer S, Tuschl T, Rajewsky N, Rorsman P, Stoffel M. (2004). A pancreatic islet-specific microRNA regulates insulin secretion. *Nature,* Vol.432, No.7014, pp. 226-230, ISSN 1476-4687.

Poy MN, Hausser J, Trajkovski M, Braun M, Collins S, Rorsman P, Zavolan M, Stoffel M. (2009). miR-375 maintains normal pancreatic alpha- and beta-cell mass. *Proc Natl Acad Sci U S A,* Vol.106, No.14, pp. 5813-5818, ISSN 1091-6490.

Rachdi L, Balcazar N, Elghazi L, Barker DJ, Krits I, Kiyokawa H, Bernal-Mizrachi E. (2006). Differential effects of p27 in regulation of beta-cell mass during development, neonatal period, and adult life. *Diabetes*, Vol.55, No.12, pp.3520-3528, ISSN 0012-1797.

Rackham CL, Chagastelles PC, Nardi NB, Hauge-Evans AC, Jones PM, King AJ. (2011). Co-transplantation of mesenchymal stem cells maintains islet organisation and morphology in mice. *Diabetologia*, ISSN 1432-0428.

Ramsoondar J, Vaught T, Ball S, et al. (2009). Production of transgenic pigs that express porcine endogenous retrovirus small interfering RNAs. *Xenotransplantation*, Vol.16, pp.164–180, ISSN 1399-3089.

Rane SG, Dubus P, Mettus RV, Galbreath EJ, Boden G, Reddy EP, Barbacid M. (1999). Loss of Cdk4 expression causes insulin-deficient diabetes and Cdk4 activation results in beta-islet cell hyperplasia. *Nat Genet*, Vol.22, No.1, pp. 44-52, ISSN 1061-4036.

Rayasam GV, Tulasi VK, Sodhi R, Davis JA, Ray A. (2009). Glycogen synthase kinase 3: more than a namesake. *Br J Pharmacol*, Vol.156, No.6, pp.885-898, ISSN 1476-5381.

Rieck S, Kaestner KH. (2010). Expansion of beta-cell mass in response to pregnancy. *Trends Endocrinol Metab*, Vol.21, No.3, pp.151-158, ISSN 1879-3061.

Rooman I, Heremans Y, Heimberg H, Bouwens L. (2000). Modulation of rat pancreatic acinoductal transdifferentiation and expression of PDX-1 in vitro. *Diabetologia*, Vol. 43, No.7, pp.907-914, ISSN 0012-186X.

Salpeter SJ, Klein AM, Huangfu D, Grimsby J, Dor Y. (2010). Glucose and aging control the quiescence period that follows pancreatic beta cell replication. *Development*, Vol.137, No.19, pp. 3205-3213, ISSN 1477-9129.

Santana A, Ensenat-Waser R, Arribas MI, Reig JA, Roche E (2006). Insulin-producing cells derived from stem cells: recent progress and future directions. *J Cell Mol Med*, Vol.10, No.4, pp. 866-883, ISSN 1582-1838.

Sapir T, Shternhall K, Meivar-Levy I, et al. (2005). From the cover: cell replacement therapy for diabetes. Generating functional insulinproducing tissue from adult human liver cells. *Proc Natl Acad Sci USA*, Vol.102, No.22, pp.7964–7969, ISSN 0027-8424.

Scaglia L, Smith FE, Bonner-Weir S. (1995). Apoptosis contributes to the involution of beta cell mass in the post partum rat pancreas. *Endocrinology*, Vol.136, No.12, pp.5461-5468, ISSN 0013-7227.

Schmied BM, Ulrich A, Matsuzaki H, Ding X, Ricordi C, Weide L, Moyer MP, Batra SK, Adrian TE, Pour PM. (2001). Transdifferentiation of human islet cells in a long-term culture. *Pancreas*. Vol.23, No.2, pp.157-171, ISSN 0885-3177.

Seaberg RM, Smukler SR, Kieffer TJ, Enikolopov G, Asghar Z, Wheeler MB, Korbutt G, van der Kooy D. (2004). Clonal identification of multipotent precursors from adult mouse pancreas that generate neural and pancreatic lineages. *Nat Biotechnol*, Vol.22, No.9, pp. 1115-1124, ISSN 1087-0156.

Sebastiani G, Vendrame F, Dotta F. (2011). MicroRNAs as New Tools for Exploring Type 1 Diabetes: Relevance for Immunomodulation and Transplantation Therapy. *Transplant Proc*, Vol.43, No.1, pp.330-332, ISSN 1873-2623.

Shi M, Liu ZW, Wang FS.(2011). Immunomodulatory properties and therapeutic application of mesenchymal stem cells. *Clin Exp Immunol*, Vol.164, No.1,pp.1-8, ISSN 1365-2249.

Shi Y, Desponts C, Do JT, Hahm HS, Scholer HR, Ding S. (2008) Induction of pluripotent stem cells from mouse embryonic fibroblasts by Oct4 and Klf4 with small-molecule compounds. *Cell Stem Cell*, Vol.3, No.5, pp.568-574, ISSN 1875-9777.

Shimajiri Y, Kosaka Y, Scheel DW, Lynn FC, Kishimoto N, Wang J, Zhao S, German MS. (2011). A mouse model for monitoring islet cell genesis and developing therapies for diabetes. *Dis Model Mech,* Vol.4, No.2, pp. 268-276, ISSN 1754-8411.

Solar M, Cardalda C, Houbracken I, Martín M, Maestro MA, De Medts N, Xu X, Grau V, Heimberg H, Bouwens L, Ferrer J. (2009). Pancreatic exocrine duct cells give rise to insulin-producing beta cells during embryogenesis but not after birth. *Dev Cell,* Vol.17, No.6, pp. 849-860, ISSN 1878-1551.

Sordi V, Bertuzzi F, Piemonti L. (2008). Diabetes mellitus: an opportunity for therapy with stem cells? *Regen Med,* Vol.3, No.3, pp. 377-397, ISSN 1746-076X.

Stanley EG & Elefanty AG. (2008). Building better beta cells. *Cell Stem Cell,* Vol.2, No.4, pp. 300-301, ISSN 1875-9777.

Suarez-Pinzon WL, Lakey JR, Brand SJ, Rabinovitch A. (2005). Combination therapy with epidermal growth factor and gastrin induces neogenesis of huan islet {beta}-cells from pancreatic duct cells and an increase in functional {beta}-cell mass. *J Clin Endocrinol Metab,* Vol.90, No.6, pp. 3401-3409, ISSN 0021-972X.

Suarez-Pinzon WL, Power RF, Yan Y, Wasserfall C, Atkinson M, Rabinovitch A. (2008).Combination therapy with glucagon-like peptide-1 and gastrin restores normoglycemia in diabetic NOD mice. *Diabetes,*Vol.57,No.12, pp.3281-3288,ISSN1939-327X.

Sun Y, Chen L, Hou XG, Hou WK, Dong JJ, Sun L, Tang KX, Wang B, Song J, Li H, Wang KX. (2007). Differentiation of bone marrow-derived mesenchymal stem cells from diabetic patients into insulin-producing cells in vitro. *Chin Med J (Engl),* Vol.120, No.9, pp. 771-776, ISSN 0366-6999.

Suzuki A, Nakauchi H, Taniguchi H.(2004). Prospective isolation of multipotent pancreatic progenitors using flow-cytometric cell sorting. *Diabetes,*Vol.53, No.8, pp.2143-2152, ISSN 0012-1797.

Suzuki J, Ricordi C, Chen Z. (2010). Immune tolerance induction by integrating innate and adaptive immune regulators. *Cell Transplant,* Vol.19, No.3, pp.253-268, ISSN 1555-3892.

Szymczak P, Wojcik-Stanaszek L, Sypecka J, Sokolowska A, Zalewska T.(2010). Effect of matrix metalloproteinases inhibition on the proliferation and differentiation of HUCB-NSCs cultured in the presence of adhesive substrates. *Acta Neurobiol Exp (Wars),*Vol.70, No.4, pp.325-336, ISSN 1689-0035.

Tan M, Kandaswamy R, Sutherland DE, Gruessner RW. (2005). Laparoscopic donor distal pancreatectomy for living donor pancreas and pancreas-kidney transplantation. *Am J Transplant,*Vol.5, No.8, pp.1966-1970, ISSN 1600-6135.

Tang DQ, Cao LZ, Burkhardt BR, Xia CQ, Litherland SA, Atkinson MA, Yang LJ. (2004). In vivo and in vitro characterization of insulin-producing cells obtained from murine bone marrow. *Diabetes,* Vol.53, No.7, pp. 1721-1732, ISSN 0012-1797.

Tang DQ, Lu S, Sun YP, Rodrigues E, Chou W, Yang C, Cao LZ, Chang LJ, Yang LJ. (2006). Reprogramming liver-stem WB cells into functional insulin-producing cells by persistent expression of Pdx1- and Pdx1-VP16 mediated by lentiviral vectors. *Lab Invest,*Vol.86, No.1, pp.83-93, ISSN 0023-6837.

Tang X, Muniappan L, Tang G, Ozcan S (2009). Identification of glucose-regulated miRNAs from pancreatic {beta} cells reveals a role for miR-30d in insulin transcription. *RNA,* Vol.15, No.2, pp. 287-293. ISSN 1469-9001.

Tellez N, Montolio M, Biarnes M, Castano E, Soler J, Montanya E. (2005). Adenoviral overexpression of interleukin-1 receptor antagonist protein increases beta-cell replication in rat pancreatic islets. *Gene Ther*,Vol.12, No.2, pp.120-128, ISSN 0969-7128.

Teta M, Rankin MM, Long SY, Stein GM, & Kushner JA. (2007). Growth and regeneration of adult beta cells does not involve specialized progenitors. *Dev Cell*, Vol.12, No.5, pp. 817-826, ISSN 1534-5807.

Thatava T, Nelson TJ, Edukulla R, Sakuma T, Ohmine S, Tonne JM, Yamada S, Kudva Y, Terzic A, Ikeda Y. (2011). Indolactam V/GLP-1-mediated differentiation of human iPS cells into glucose-responsive insulin-secreting progeny. *Gene Ther*, Vol.18, No.3, pp.283-293, ISSN 476-5462.

Thorel F, Népote V, Avril I, Kohno K, Desgraz R, Chera S, Herrera PL. (2010). Conversion of adult pancreatic alpha-cells to beta-cells after extreme beta-cell loss. *Nature*, Vol.464, No.7292, pp. 1149-1154, ISSN 1476-4687.

Uchida T, Nakamura T, Hashimoto N, Matsuda T, Kotani K, Sakaue H, Kido Y, Hayashi Y, Nakayama KI, White MF, Kasuga M. (2005). Deletion of Cdkn1b ameliorates hyperglycemia by maintaining compensatory hyperinsulinemia in diabetic mice. *Nat Med*, Vol.11, No.2, pp. 175-182, ISSN 1078-8956.

Uccelli A, Benvenuto F, Laroni A, Giunti D.(2011). Neuroprotective features of mesenchymal stem cells. Best Pract Res Clin Haematol. Vol.24, No.1, pp.59-64, ISSN 1532-1924.

van Belle TL, Coppieters KT, von Herrath MG. (2011). Type 1 diabetes: etiology, immunology, and therapeutic strategies. *Physiol Rev*, Vol.91, No.1 pp.79-118, ISSN 1522-1210.

Volarevic V, Arsenijevic N, Lukic ML, Stojkovic M (2011). Concise review: Mesenchymal stem cell treatment of the complications of diabetes mellitus. *Stem Cells*, Vol.29, No.1, pp. 5-10, ISSN 1549-4918.

Wang AY, Ehrhardt A, Xu H, Kay MA. (2007).Adenovirus transduction is required for the correction of diabetes using pdx-1 or neurogenin-3 in the liver. *Mol Ther*,Vol.15, No.2. pp.255-263, ISSN 1525-0016.

Winter WE, Schatz D. (2003). Prevention strategies for type 1 diabetes mellitus: current status and future directions. *BioDrugs*, Vol.17, No.1, pp.39-64, ISSN 1173-8804.

Xia B, Zhan XR, Yi R, Yang B. (2009). Can pancreatic duct-derived progenitors be a source of islet regeneration? *Biochem Biophys Res Commun*, Vol.383, No.4, pp. 383-385, ISSN 1090-2104.

Xie QP, Huang H, Xu B, Dong X, Gao SL, Zhang B, Wu YL. (2009). Human bone marrow mesenchymal stem cells differentiate into insulin-producing cells upon microenvironmental manipulation in vitro. *Differentiation*, Vol.77, No.5, pp. 483-491, ISSN 1432-0436

Xu X, D'Hoker J, Stangé G, Bonné S, De Leu N, Xiao X, Van de Casteele M, Mellitzer G, Ling Z, Pipeleers D, Bouwens L, Scharfmann R, Gradwohl G, Heimberg H. (2008). Beta cells can be generated from endogenous progenitors in injured adult mouse pancreas. *Cell*, Vol.132, No.2, pp. 197-207, ISSN 1097-4172.

Yang LJ. (2006). Liver stem cell-derived beta-cell surrogates for treatment of type 1 diabetes. *Autoimmun Rev*, Vol.5, No.6, pp.409-413, ISSN 1568-9972.

Yang Z, Chen M, Ellett JD, Carter JD, Brayman KL, Nadler JL.(2005).Inflammatory blockade improves human pancreatic islet function and viability. *Am J Transplant,* Vol.5, No.3, pp.475-483, ISSN 1600-6135.

Yoshida S, Ishikawa F, Kawano N, Shimoda K, Nagafuchi S, Shimoda S, Yasukawa M, Kanemaru T, Ishibashi H, Shultz LD, Harada M. (2005). Human cord blood--derived cells generate insulin-producing cells in vivo. *Stem Cells,* Vol.23, No.9, pp. 1409-1416, ISSN 1066-5099.

Zalzman M, Anker-Kitai L, Efrat S. (2005). Differentiation of human liver derived, insulin-producing cells toward the (beta)-cell phenotype.*Diabetes,*Vol.54, No.9, pp.2568-2575, ISSN 0012-1797.

Zhang D, Jiang W, Liu M, Sui X, Yin X, Chen S, Shi Y, Deng H. (2009). Highly efficient differentiation of human ES cells and iPS cells into mature pancreatic insulin producing cells. *Cell Res,*Vol.19, No.4, pp.429-438, ISSN 1748-7838.

Zhang L, Hu J, Hong TP, Liu YN, Wu YH, Li LS. (2005). Monoclonal side population progenitors isolated from human fetal pancreas. *Biochem Biophys Res Commun,* Vol.333, No.2, pp. 603-608, ISSN 0006-291X.

Zhang W, Zhang D, Shen M, Liu Y, Tian Y, Thomson AW, Lee WP, Zheng XX.(2010).Combined administration of a mutant TGF-beta1/Fc and rapamycin promotes induction of regulatory T cells and islet allograft tolerance. *J Immunol,*Vol.185, No.8,4750-4759, ISSN 1550-6606.

Zhang Y, Shen W, Hua J, Lei A, Lv C, Wang H, Yang C, Gao Z, Dou Z. (2010). Pancreatic islet-like clusters from bone marrow mesenchymal stem cells of human first-trimester abortus can cure streptozocin-induced mouse diabetes. *Rejuvenation Res,* Vol.13, No.6, pp. 695-706, ISSN 1557-8577.

Zhao Y, Lin B, Dingeldein M, Guo C, Hwang D, Holterman MJ.(2010). New type of human blood stem cell: a double-edged sword for the treatment of type 1 diabetes. *Transl Res.* Vol.155, No.5, pp.211-216, ISSN1878-1810.

Zhao Y, Wang H, Mazzone T. (2006). Identification of stem cells from human umbilical cord blood with embryonic and hematopoietic characteristics. *Exp Cell Res,* Vol.312, No.13, pp.2454-2464, ISSN 0014-4827.

Zhao Y, Yin X, Qin H, Zhu F, Liu H, Yang W, Zhang Q, Xiang C, Hou P, Song Z, Liu Y, Yong J, Zhang P, Cai J, Liu M, Li H, Li Y, Qu X, Cui K, Zhang W, Xiang T, Wu Y, Zhao Y, Liu C, Yu C, Yuan K, Lou J, Ding M, Deng H. (2008). Two supporting factors greatly improve the efficiency of human iPSC generation. *Cell Stem Cell,* Vol.3, No.5, pp. 475-479, ISSN 1875-9777.

Zhou H, Wu S, Joo JY, Zhu S, Han DW, Lin T, Trauger S, Bien G, Yao S, Zhu Y,Siuzdak G, Scholer HR, Duan L, Ding S. (2009). Generation of induced pluripotent stem cells using recombinant proteins, *Cell Stem* Cell, Vol.4, No.5, ISSN 1875-9777.

Zhou Q, Brown J, Kanarek A, Rajagopal J, Melton DA.(2008). In vivo reprogramming of adult pancreatic exocrine cells to beta-cells. *Nature,* Vol.455, No.7213, pp.627-632, ISSN 1476-4687.

Zulewski H, Abraham EJ, Gerlach MJ, Daniel PB, Moritz W, Müller B, Vallejo M, Thomas MK, Habener JF. (2001). Multi-potential nestin-positive stem cells isolated from adult pancreatic islets differentiate ex vivo into pancreatic endocrine, exocrine, and hepatic phenotypes. Diabetes, Vol.50, No.3, pp. 521-533, ISSN 0012-1797.

Part 6

Immunotherapy

15

Peptides and Proteins for the Treatment and Suppression of Type-1 Diabetes

Ahmed H. Badawi, Barlas Büyüktimkin, Paul Kiptoo and Teruna J. Siahaan
Department of Pharmaceutical Chemistry, The University of Kansas, USA

1. Introduction

Type-1 diabetes (T1D) is an autoimmune disease in which self-reactive immune cells infiltrate the islets in the pancreas to destroy β-cells. One of many possible causes is that self-reactive T cells that are normally eliminated can escape from the thymus along with normal T cells. The escaped T cells can be activated in response to a low level of secondary self-antigens, which can lead to a major step for tissue self-recognition. For activation, T cells interact with antigen-presenting cells (APC) via formation of the immunological synapse, which has a "bull's eye" structure at the membrane interface between both cells (Grakoui et al., 1999). The immunological synapse is composed of two segregated clusters of Signal-1 and Signal-2 molecular complexes. Signal-1 is generated by interaction between T-cell receptors (TCR) and antigen/multi histocompatibility complex-II (Ag/MHC-II). Signal-2 (costimulatory signal) can be delivered by a positive signal via B7/CD28 interactions or a negative signal via B7/CTLA-4 interactions. In addition, the CD40/CD154 costimulatory interaction between APC and T cells was found to induce an inflammatory immune response (Baker et al., 2008; Munro et al., 2007). Cell adhesion molecule interactions such as ICAM-1/LFA-1 interactions have also been categorized as a positive signal (Bromley et al., 2001; Grakoui et al., 1999). The positive costimulatory signal assists the induction of T-cell activation while the negative costimulatory signal suppresses T-cell activation (Bour-Jordan et al., 2011; Manikwar et al., 2011). The formation of the immunological synapse involves translocation of Signal-1 and Signal-2. Prior to the translocation process, Signal-1 is clustered at the periphery and Signal-2 is clustered at the center. Then, Signal-1 and Signal-2 switch places to establish the immunological synapse where Signal-1 is at the center (called central zone supramolecular activation complex or cSMAC) and Signal-2 is at the periphery (peripheral zone supramolecular activation complex or pSMAC) (Bromley et al., 2001; Grakoui et al., 1999).

TCR on T cells recognize self-antigens presented on MHC-II molecules on the surface of APC for activation of self-reactive T cells to initiate autoimmune diseases. In T1D, glutamic acid decarboxylase-65 (GAD65), is one of the important self-antigens in humans, and is a reliable marker in overt diabetes (Tisch et al., 1998). Administration of GAD peptides in complete Freund's adjuvant (CFA) into non-obese diabetes (NOD) mice triggers insulitis and destruction of β-cells to cause diabetes (Liu et al., 1999; Tisch et al., 1999; Yoon et al., 1999). There is a correlation between islet expression of GAD enzymes and the development of T1D. Different types of MHC-II molecules such as I-A^{g7} and I-A$^{g7.PD}$ recognize different epitopes of GAD65 (Table 1) (Chao et al., 1999). Administration of GAD65/67 antisense gene suppresses GAD enzyme expression and eliminates T1D development in NOD mice (Yoon et al., 1999)

Aly *et al.* suggested that there are several stages in treating patients with T1D (Aly et al., 2005). First, T1D could be treated prior to detection of autoantibodies in patients in high-risk populations. Second, patients could be treated after autoantibody detection but prior to the onset of clinical diabetes. Third, patients could be treated to prevent further destruction of β-islet cells and ameliorate the disease. Finally, treatment could be developed for curing the disease by islet cell transplantation. Many new and novel treatments of T1D have been proposed with the hope of not just treating the symptoms but halting or reversing the disease. Proteins and peptides have been evaluated as therapeutic agents for T1D; they include antibodies to cell adhesion molecules (i.e., anti-ICAM-1, anti-LFA-1, anti-VCAM-1, and anti-VLA-4 monoclonal antibodies (mAbs))(Chowdhury et al., 2002; Moriyama et al., 1996; Tsukamoto et al., 1995), anti-CD3 mAb (Bresson et al., 2006; You et al., 2007), and anti-TNF-α mAb (Ryba et al., 2010). GAD peptides (Tisch et al., 1999) and bifunctional peptide inhibitor (BPI) molecules (Murray et al., 2007) have also been investigated to induce immunotolerance in T1D by altering the balance from effector to regulatory immune cells.

Early diagnosis of T1D is necessary for prevention of irreversible damage to the β-cells. The detection of islet cell antibody (ICA) as a common marker for disease progression is critical for individuals with a high risk of developing T1D (Honeyman et al., 1995). Unfortunately, not all patients with ICA progress to clinical diabetes; therefore, there is still an urgent need to find other markers or factors that can predict the rate of progression of T1D. The presence of certain HLA genes can influence the rate of destruction of β-cells by the immune system. For example, a high risk of acquiring T1D in caucasians has been associated with the expression of DR3-DQ2 and DR4-DQ8 HLA class II. Other identifiers for relatives who are most likely predisposed to T1D are class II antigens DR3, DR4, DQ2, and DQ8. An individual with DR4 within a family has a higher probability to become diabetic compare than an individual with DR3. An additional independent risk factor is class I antigens such as HLA-A24, which are found significantly more frequently in ICA-positive relatives who developed T1D than in those who did not (Honeyman et al., 1995). In Japanese subjects, however, T1D has been correlated with the haplotype of DR4-DQ9, and the presence of A24 has been correlated to T1D in young Japanese patients.

2. Animal models of T1D to evaluate potential peptide and protein therapeutics

The *in vivo* efficacies of potential therapeutic agents for T1D are usually evaluated in spontaneous diabetes or GAD peptide/CFA-induced diabetes in NOD mice as well as in the BioBreeding (BB) diabetic rat model (Aly et al., 2005; Calcinaro et al., 1997). T cells could respond to β-cell antigens such as GAD65, GAD67, peripherin, carboxypeptidase H, insulin, and HSP60; however, not all of these antigens become targets of the immune cells (Tisch et al., 1993). GAD is the initial and criticial antigen for the development of T1D; however, participation of other antigens during the development of diabetes cannot be ruled out. Histology analysis of the pancreas of NOD mice treated with GAD65 shows significant reduction in intra-insulitis. Mice treated with intrathymic injections of GAD65 did not develop diabetes and had significant reduction of IFN-γ production. It should also be noted that IFA or CFA could inhibit the development of diabetes in young NOD mice; this was due to the change in population of destructive autoimmune cells surrounding the islets. In this case, a higher proportion of IL-4-producing cells compared to IFN-γ-producing cells were around the islets (Calcinaro et al., 1997; Liddi et al., 2000). Environmental factors such as the presence of retrovirus influence the development of T1D in NOD mice. Young NOD mice (below 2 months of age) infected with retrovirus are protected from developing T1D, and female sex hormones increase the incidence of T1D in NOD mice.

Progression of the disease occurs by means of lymphocyte infiltration of the pancreatic islets followed by destruction of insulin-producing β-cells. In NOD mice, early infiltration of leukocytes occurs at 3 weeks of age with intial infiltration of APC followed by $CD4^+$ and $CD8^+$ T cells (Solomon et al., 2004). Then, the β-cell destruction by $CD8^+$ T cells begins to show after 14 weeks (Qin et al., 2004a). Th17 and Th1 cells have been shown to participate in T1D (Bradshaw et al., 2009), multiple sclerosis (MS) (Hedegaard et al., 2008), and rheumatoid arthritis (RA) (Ziolkowska et al., 2000). Naïve CD4 T cells can be converted to Th-17 cells by IL-21 and TGF-β. In T1D patients, IL-1β and IL-6 cytokines produced by $CD14^+CD16^-$ and $CD14^+CD16^+$ monocytes stimulate the production of Th17 cells (Bradshaw et al., 2009). However, the role of Th17 cells has not yet fully elucidated. It has been reported that Th17 cells reverted to a Th1-like profile when transferred into NOD.Scid receipients and treatment with IL-17 neutralizing antibody did not prevent onset of T1D (Bending et al., 2009). NOD mice with depleted macrophages cannot develop T1D because macrophages are necessary for differentiation of β-cell-specific cytotoxic T cells. B cell-deficient NOD mice do not develop T1D because B cells play a role as antigen-presenting cells. The balance between self-reactive and regulatory T cells (T-regs) influences the development and progress of T1D. T-regs that express FoxP3 have a major role in tolerance in T1D as well as other autoimmune diseases (Chen et al., 2005) with no statistical difference between the number of T-regs in NOD and other autoimmune diseased mice (Waid et al., 2008). Adoptive transfer experiments were also used to elucidate the involvement of both $CD4^+$ and $CD8^+$ T cells in the etiology of T1D (Hartemann et al., 1999). The development of T1D is initiated by prolonged insulitis followed by induction of cytotoxic T cells (CTL) for β-cell destruction, which eventually leads to overt diabetes. Knockout Fas or FasL NOD as well as perforin-deficient NOD mice have a lower incidence of T1D, sugesting that apotosis of β-cells is due to the interaction of Fas ligand (FasL) on CTL and Fas on the surface of target cells (Qin et al., 2004a). Using different animal models, there are many efforts to investigate peptide and protein drugs as potential therapeutics for autoimmune diseases by tipping the balance from inflammatory to regulatory immune cells.

3. The role of cytokines and cellular mechanisms

It is not simple to correlate the role of each cytokine in the development of T1D; this is due to the influence of other factors in T1D development (Solomon et al., 2004). Diabetic patients have higher levels of IL-6, TNF-α, TNF-β, IL-1α, IL-1β, IFN-γ, IL-2, and IL-12, and the presence of Th1 cells is evident in T1D patients. Diabetogenic Th1 cells secrete IFN-γ, and the treatment of NOD mice with anti-IFN-γ mAb halts T1D development (Bradley et al., 1999; Hartemann et al., 1999). However, the disease progression does not correlate with the number of IFN-γ-secreting cells, suggesting that β-cell destruction may be independent of the IFN-γ-triggering mechanism. Thus, it supports the idea that $CD8^+$ CTL has an important role in the destruction of β-cells (Hartemann et al., 1999). In the early events of T1D development, CD4$^+$ Th1 cells enter and accumulate in the pancreas quicker than Th2 cells. This is due to the presence of LFA-1 and $\alpha_V\beta_4$-integrin on Th1 cells and the upregulation of adhesion molecules such as ICAM-1, VCAM-1, PNAd, and MAdCAM-1 on pancreatic vessels (Bradley et al., 1999). There is a high presence of activated CD4$^+$ Th1 cells in islets and splenocytes of diabetic NOD mice; although Th2 cells are present in the islets, they are in a resting state (Hartemann et al., 1999). Adoptive transfer of Th1 T cells into neonatal NOD mice induced T1D, while transfer of Th2 cells did not, confirming the Th1 cells had a more important role than Th2 cells in the destruction of β-cells (Bradley, 1999; Pakala et al., 1997). The production of RNA for multiple chemokines such as lymphotactin suggests the recruitment of Th1 cells into the pancreas during the T1D progress. The increase in MCP-1 chemokine produced by Th1 cells infers the recruitment of macrophages and monocytes into the pancreas (Bradley et al., 1999).

It has been proposed that T-regs have a protective effect to maintain tolerance and that a deficiency in T-regs can lead to T1D in NOD mice (Chen et al., 2005; Lawson et al., 2008). Adoptive transfer of T-regs in NOD mice can suppress the development of T1D by controlling the aggressiveness of autoreactive effector T cells in the target organ (Buckner, 2010). However, T-regs have no influence in the initial priming and activation in the draining lymph nodes. It is interesting to find that there is no significant difference in the number of CD4$^+$CD25^{hi} cells and the level of FoxP3 in patients with long-standing diabetes compared to control subjects. It was proposed that individuals with newly diagnosed T1D had reduced T-reg function compared to control individuals (Lawson et al., 2008). However, this proposal is still controversial because some studies found that there was no significant difference in the level of CD4$^+$CD25$^+$FOXP3$^+$ T-regs between T1D and normal individuals. It is possible that the function and persistence of generating T-regs are lacking in T1D patients (Buckner, 2010).

Th2 cells that secrete IL-4 are also important in suppressing T1D and treatment with IL-4 prevents the development of diabetes in NOD mice (Hartemann et al., 1999; Tisch et al., 1999). On the other hand, Pakala *et al.* have shown that co-transfer of a tenfold excess of Th2 over Th1 cells could not prevent diabetes, indicating that Th2 might not be the only cellular regulator of T1D (Pakala et al., 1997). Therefore, Th2 and T-regs may control the development of diabetes; this is reflected by the involvement of IL-4 and IL-10 in NOD mice (Hartemann et al., 1999; Solomon et al., 2004). Treatment of NOD mice with anti-IL-4 and anti-IL-10 mAbs causes a loss of β-cells along with generation of glucose intolerance (Calcinaro et al., 1997). An increase in the number of IL-4 secreting cells does not always indicate the presence of Th2-suppressive cells in the islets. Besides Th1, Th2 cells could transfer T1D in NOD.Scid mice, and Th2-mediated diabetes had a lower disease incidence and a longer prediabetic phase of the disease (Pakala et al., 1997). It has also been reported that transfer of Th2 cells into young NOD mice induced T1D (Dobbs et al., 2001). The lesions induced by Th2 cells were predominantly due to eosinophilic infiltration, islet necrosis and abscesses, and severe destruction of exo- and endocrine tissue.

4. Potential new therapies for T1D

Many potential therapies derived from peptides and proteins have been developed to control self-reactive T cells and induce the production of regulatory cells for generating immunotolerance (Masteller et al., 2002). Because incomplete or partial signaling in Signal 1 and/or Signal-2 can lead to regulatory responses, many of these theraputic agents are being developed to modulate these signals separately or simultaneously.

4.1 Activity of GAD Peptides to Suppress T1D:

In NOD mice, subpopulations of T cells recognize primary and secondary antigens (Sercarz et al., 1993; Tisch et al., 1999). In early stages of T1D, T cells are associated with the primary antigen causing damage to self-tissue (Lehmann et al., 1993). After the disease is in an advanced stage, T cells recognize secondary antigens; this process is called antigen spreading. B cells are effective promoters of antigenic spreading, and this is a way of increasing the immune response because a minimal number of antigenic peptide epitopes is sufficient to generate a strong immune response. Unfortunately, antigenic spreading could involve cross-reactivity with other antigens such as carboxypeptidase H, insulin, and HSP65, which are normally observed at the late stage of T1D.

Antigen-specific therapy could selectively inactivate autoreactive T cells without altering the remaining immune cells. Administering the whole GAD65 protein prevented the progress of T1D in older NOD mice that already developed insulitis (Tisch et al., 1998; Tisch et al., 1999). GAD65-treated mice had high levels of IL-4 and reduced levels of IFN-γ compared to control animals. It was proposed that prevention of T1D was due to the suppression of Th1 cells and upregulation of Th2 and T-reg cells (Awasthi et al., 2008; Tisch et al., 1998). A shift into the Th2 phenotype could be maintained for a long time, and the capacity of different epitopes to induce Th2 cells depended on the frequency of the clonotype T cells (Tisch et al., 1999).

$P_{208-217}$ peptide from the GAD sequence (Table 1) suppressed the progress of T1D in NOD mice due to deviation of T-cell differentiation from inflammatory to regulatory cells (Kim et al., 2004; McDevitt, 2004; Tisch et al., 1998). Different GAD65 epitopes are recognized by I-A^{g7} and I-$A^{g7.PD}$, and the selectivity of recognition is due to the specificity of MHC-II for a certain epitope as well as the specificity of TCR recognition of the MHC-peptide complex by a subpopulation of T cells (Chao et al., 1999). It was found that $P_{201-220}$ and $P_{231-250}$ peptides have high affinity for DQ8 while $P_{121-140}$ and $P_{471-490}$ peptides have poor binding properties to DQ8. The poor binding of peptides $P_{121-140}$ and $P_{471-490}$ to class II DQ8 is compensated by high efficiency presentation on B cells (Liu et al., 1999). It was proposed that antigenic peptides with low affinity may elicit a Th2 response to produce IL-4 and IL-5 rather than a Th1 response (Honeyman et al., 1995).

Adoptive transfer of T cells isolated from mice treated with $P_{206-220}$ and $P_{221-235}$ peptides from GAD65 (Table 1) suppressed T1D in the recepient mice, and these cells were peptide-specific regulatory cells that coproduced IL-4 and IL-10 (Chen et al., 2003). T1D suppression is presumably due to the inhibition of diabetogenic T cell migration into the lymph nodes. Transgenic mice (G286) expressing a T-cell receptor (TCR) specific for GAD65 epitope 286-300 ($P_{286-300}$) were used to investigate the role of GAD65-specific T cells in pathogenesis diabetes (Tarbell et al., 2002). During 30 weeks observation, 80% of the non-transgenic developed diabetes with severe insulitis while none of the transgenic mice (G286) developed diabetes with only 10% insulitis. The observed protection in G286 mice may be due to suppression of islet-specific cellular response and not to the absence of a pathogenic repertoire (Tarbell et al., 2002). In addition, $GAD_{206-220}$ was incorporated in the sequence of an immunoglobulin and tested for the treatment of T1D (Jain et al., 2008). It was shown that treatment with Ig-$GAD_{206-220}$ molecules leads to proliferation of pancreatic β-islet cells and restored normoglycemia in hyperglycemic mice.

Adoptive transfer of splenocytes from G286 failed to induce diabetes to NOD.Scid mice. Transfer of G286 splenocytes with diabetogenic cells resulted in a significant delay in diabetes transfer (McDevitt, 2003; Tarbell et al., 2002). The development of diabetes could be

Name	Sequence
GAD Peptides and GAD-BPI	**Suppression of Type 1 Diabetes**
$P_{208-217}$	EIAPVFVLLE
$P_{201-220}$	NTNMFTYEIAPVFVLLEYVT
$P_{231-250}$	PGGSGDGIFSPGGAISNMYA
$P_{121-140}$	YVVKSFDRSTKVIDFHYPNE
$P_{471-490}$	VDKCLELAEYLYNIIKNREG
$P_{206-220\ (g7)}$	TYELAPVFVLLEYVT
$P_{221-235\ (g7)}$	LKKMRFIIGWPGGSG
$P_{286-300\ (g7)}$	KKGAAAIGIGTDSVI
$P_{401-415\ (g7)}$	PLOCSALLVREEGLM
$P_{561-575\ (g7)}$	ISNPAATHQDIDFLI
$P_{331-345\ (g7.PD)}$	LVSATAGTTVYGAFD
$P_{456-470\ (g7.PD)}$	WLMWRAKGTTGFEAH
$P_{551-565\ (g7.PD)}$	GDKVNFFRMVISNPA
GAD-BPI	EIAPVFVLLE-(AcpGAcpGAcp)-ITDGEATDSG
PLP Peptide and PLP-BPI	**Suppression of EAE**
$PLP_{139-151}$	HSLGKWLGHPDKF
PLP-BPI	HSLGKWLGHPDKF-AcpGAcpGAcp-ITDGEATDSG
Ac-PLP-BPI-NH_2-2	Ac-HSLGKWLGHPDKF-$(AcpGAcpGAcp)_2$-ITDGEATDSG-NH_2
Ac-PLP-BPI-PEG6	Ac-HSLGKWLGHPDKF-$(C_2H_5O)_3$-G-$(C_2H_5O)_3$-ITDGEATDSG-NH_2
CII Peptides and CII-BPI	**Suppression of Rheumatoid Arthritis**
CII-1	PPGANGNPGPAGPPG
CII-BPI-1	Ac-PPGANGNPGPAGPPG-$(AcpGAcpGAcp)_2$-ITDGEATDSG-NH_2
CII-2	Ac-GEPGIAGFKGEQGPK-NH_2
CII-BPI-2	Ac-GEPGIAGFKGEQGPK-$(AcpGAcpGAcp)_2$-ITDGEATDSG-NH_2
CII-3	Ac-QYMRADEADSTLR-NH_2
CII-BPI-3	Ac-QYMRADEADSTLR-$(AcpGAcpGAcp)_2$-ITDGEATDSG-NH_2

Table 1. The sequence of different types of BPI molecules and antigenic peptides, which suppress EAE, RA, and T1D.

due to faster division or a longer lifespan of pathogenic cells compared to those of protective cells from G286 mice. The pathogenic cells overpowered the G286 cells over time. The *in vitro* activation of $CD4^+$ T cells from G286 mice increases the level of CTLA-4 compared to those from non-transgenic mice. The increase in negative costimulatory signal or upregulation of CTLA-4 could be one possible mechanism for diabetes protection observed in G286 mice (Tarbell et al., 2002).

4.2 Design of novel GAD-BPI for suppressing T1D

In T1D, recruitment of leukocytes into the islet of pancreas involves a multistep process, which includes rolling, firm adhesion, and migration across the endothelium (Huang et al., 2005). β_2-integrins on leukocytes such as $\alpha_L\beta_2$ (LFA-1), $\alpha_M\beta_2$ (Mac-1), $\alpha_x\beta_2$ (p150/95), and $\alpha_D\beta_2$ have a major role in adhesion and transmigration of leukocytes (Yusuf-Makagiansar et al., 2000). As indicated previously, both Th1 and Th2 can increase the expression of adhesion molecules, including ligands for β_2-integrins (i.e., ICAM-1, -2, and -3), on the vascular endothelium in the pancreas to enhance islet infiltration (Bradley et al., 1999). Blocking of ICAM-1/LFA-1-mediated T-cell adhesion can suppress diabetes progression in NOD mice (Huang et al., 2005; Moriyama et al., 1996). Linear and cyclic LABL peptides derived from the I-domain of the α_L-subunit of LFA-1 bind to D1 of ICAM-1 and inhibit ICAM-1/LFA-1-mediated (a) homotypic T-cell adhesion, (b) heterotypic T-cell adhesion to epithelial and endothelial cell monolayers, and (c) mixed lymphocyte reaction (MLR) (Tibbetts et al., 1999; Tibbetts et al., 2000; Yusuf-Makagiansar et al., 2001a; Yusuf-Makagiansar et al., 2001b; Yusuf-Makagiansar et al., 2001c). cLABL peptide can block T-cell adhesion but not monocyte adhesion to islet microvascular endothelium (Huang et al., 2005). This is because T-cell adhesion is via $\alpha_L\beta_2$ while monocyte adhesion is via $\alpha_M\beta_2$ (Mac-1); thus, cLABL peptide can selectively differentiate between α_L and α_M binding to ICAM-1.

Siahaan *et al.* developed bifunctional peptide inhibitor (BPI) molecules, which were assembled by conjugating an antigenic peptide to a cell adhesion peptide (i.e., LABL) via a linker (Table 1). The estimated length of the linker was determined by measuring the distance between the N-terminal of LABL peptide and the C-terminal of the antigenic peptide when they were docked to domain-1 (D1) of ICAM-1 (Bella et al., 1998; Casasnovas et al., 1998; Xu et al., 2002) and MHC-II (Corper et al., 2000), respectively. In this case, both ICAM-1 and MHC-II receptors were modeled as if they were protruding from the cell membranes into the extracellular space. In the case of GAD-BPI, it is a conjugate between $P_{208-217}$ peptide and LABL peptide (Table 1) (Tibbetts et al., 1999; Tibbetts et al., 2000). Using the distance estimate, a combination of glycine (G) and amino caproic acid (Acp) was used to connect LABL to GAD peptides. In general, BPI molecules are effective in suppressing different autoimmune diseases; for example, GAD-BPI, PLP-BPI, and CII-BPI molecules (Table 1) have excellent efficacy to suppress T1D (Murray et al., 2007), EAE (Kobayashi et al., 2008; Kobayashi et al., 2007; Ridwan et al., 2010; Zhao et al., 2010), and RA, respectively.

The central hypothesis is that binding of BPI molecules simultaneously to MHC-II and ICAM-1 on the surface of APC blocks the immunological synapse formation at the interface of APC-T cells. In other words, BPI molecules inhibit the translocation of Signal-1 and Signal-2 to prevent the segregation of each signal. As a result, the naïve T cells differentiate to T-reg or Th2 cells, and this process suppresses the differentiation and proliferation of Th1 and Th17 cells. This process alters the immune cell balance from inflammatory to regulatory phenotypes in an antigenic-specific manner without affecting the general immune response.

This is in contrast to the mechanism of Signal-2 or cell adhesion inhibitors that normally suppress the general immune response.

GAD-BPI can effectively suppress T1D in NOD and NOD.Scid mice. Subcutaneous (s.c.) administrations of GAD-BPI (80 nmol/injection/day) to NOD mice on days 0 and 7 after T1D stimulation with GAD peptide in CFA on day 0 effectively suppressed insulitis in NOD mice compared to PBS-treated mice (Murray et al., 2007). The majority of the islets (about 83%) in GAD-BPI-treated mice were normal or without insulitis. In contrast, only a low population of islets (about 35%) in PBS-treated mice was normal and the remaining islets (65%) had moderate to severe insulitis. The splenocytes of GAD-BPI-treated NOD mice had high levels of IL-4 compared to those of PBS-treated animals, indicating that GAD-BPI treatment increased Th2 cell differentiation and proliferation (Murray et al., 2007).

T cells isolated from splenocytes of GAD-BPI- and PBS-treated NOD mice were adoptively transferred into NOD.Scid mice that had received diabetogenic cells from NOD mice (Gonzales et al., 2001). Only 28% of NOD.Scid mice treated with T cells from GAD-BPI-treated mice had hyperglycemia (*i.e.*, blood glucose ≥250 mg/dl) at weeks 7 or 12 while 83% of NOD.Scid mice treated with T cells from PBS-treated NOD mice had hyperglycemia (Murray et al., 2007). In parallel, lower insulitis was observed in NOD.Scid mice receiving T cells of GAD-BPI-treated NOD mice than in NOD.Scid mice receiving T cells from PBS-treated NOD mice (Murray et al., 2007). This result indicates that GAD-BPI alters the composition of CD4+ T cells from effector to regulatory or suppressor cells, which have protective effects in limiting the invasion and destruction of the islets.

To evaluate whether GAD-BPI could simultaneously bind to MHC-II and ICAM-1 on the surface of APC, a colocalization study was carried out using B cells isolated from the spleens of NOD female mice (6 weeks of age). GAD-BPI, unlinked GAD + LABL peptide, and PBS were added to the B cell suspension. After washing, the cells were incubated with antibodies to MHC-II (I-A^{g7}) and ICAM-1 with two different fluorescence labels. The decoration of B cell surface by each antibody that corresponds to the fluorescence label was observed with confocal microscopy. The effect of each molecule to colocalize MHC-II and ICAM-1 on the surface of B cells was determined by merging the two different fluorescence signals from anti-MHC-II and anti-ICAM-1 mAbs. The result showed that B cells treated with GAD-BPI had about 60% of colocalization signals from both antibodies compared to about 12% of colocalization signals from B cells treated with unlinked GAD and LABL peptides (Murray et al., 2007). To further evaluate the binding properties of GAD-BPI, antibody inhibition studies were carried out. GAD-BPI inhibited binding of anti-I-A^{g7} and anti-ICAM-1 mAbs to MHC-II and ICAM-1, respectively. In addition, GAD-BPI inhibited binding of both antibodies in a cooperative manner. Therefore, colocalization and antibody inhibition studies both suggest that GAD-BPI could bind simultaneously to MHC-II and ICAM-1 on the surface of B cells.

As mentioned above, the BPI type of molecule has been used to suppress RA and EAE in animal models. EAE is an animal model for multiple sclerosis (MS). PLP-BPI derivatives are able to suppress EAE better than the parent PLP peptide ($PLP_{139-151}$), indicating that the presence of LABL peptide alters the mechanisms of action of PLP-BPI compared to PLP peptide alone (Kobayashi et al., 2008; Kobayashi et al., 2007; Ridwan et al., 2010; Zhao et al., 2010). Cytokine studies indicated that PLP-BPI treatment induced the differentiation and proliferation of T-reg and Th2 cells and suppressed the proliferation of Th17 cells. Using the same concept, CII-BPI-1 and CII-BPI-2 molecules could effectively suppress rheumatoid arthritis better than the respective antigenic peptides (CII-1 and CII-2) in the collagen-induced arthritis (CIA) mouse. The CII-BPI molecules could also lower the production of inflammatory cells. The results indicate the BPI molecules with appropriate antigenic peptides can effectively suppress autoimmune diseases.

4.3 Blocking ICAM-1/LFA-1 interactions

Interactions between adhesion molecules such as LFA-1 (CD11a/CD18) and ICAM-1 have an important role in insulitis in NOD mice and humans (Mysliwiec et al., 1999). ICAM-1/LFA-1 interactions are involved in leukocyte adhesion to vascular endothelium prior to infiltration of the islet. Individuals with overt diabetes have high levels of CD11a on their monocytes and lymphocytes (Mysliwiec et al., 1999). Administration of anti-LFA-1 and anti-ICAM-1 mAbs to female NOD mice at 2 weeks of age completely prevented the development of spontaneous diabetes and formation of insulitis until 30 weeks of age (Moriyama et al., 1996). In contrast, T1D was observed in 60% of mice treated with control mAbs, indicating that LFA-1/ICAM-1 interactions are critical for T-cell-mediated cellular responses as well as T-cell differentiation and extravasation. However, administration of these mAbs to NOD mice at 5 weeks of age did not induce this long-lasting protection, suggesting that the mechanism of action of these mAbs is in the early onset of the disease (Moriyama et al., 1996). Anti-ICAM-1 alone could significantly inhibit T1D development; however, it could not prevent significant infiltration of mononuclear cells into the islets. The conclusion is that blocking the ICAM-1/LFA-1 pathway can induce tolerance against pancreatic β-cells.

Adoptive transfer of spelenocytes from acutely diabetic mice into NOD.Scid mice followed by treatment with anti-LFA-1/anti-ICAM-1 and anti-CD8 mAbs prevented the development of T1D. In this case, 40% of the mAb-treated recipients became diabetic and exhibited moderate-to-severe insulitis around 12 to 35 weeks after transfer (Chowdhury et al., 2002). It is suggested that the mechanism of action of anti-ICAM-1 and anti-LFA-1 mAbs to induce tolerance is due to suppression of T-cell activation and not to clonal deletion or anergy. However, other mechanisms are plausible, such as the mAbs inhibiting the infiltration of autoreactive T cells that destroy β-cells.

4.4 Modulation of B7 and CD28 functions

Modulating costimulatory signals can induce immunotolerance and influence T-cell immunodominance; B7/CD28 is one of the costimulatory signals involved in the development of T1D in NOD mice (Lenschow et al., 1996; Salomon et al., 2001; Salomon et al., 2000). CD28-deficient and B7-1/B7-2-deficient NOD mice develop a more severe diabetes than control NOD mice. In CD28-deficient mice, the diabetes is due to a decrease in or absence of T-regs; transfer of T-regs from the control NOD mice to the CD28-deficient mice prevents the development of T1D (Salomon et al., 2000). B7-1, working together with self-antigen presentation by MHC-II on B cells, can induce T-cell activation during T1D development (Bour-Jordan et al., 2007). B7-1-mediated costimulatory signal promotes epitope-spreading in T1D in NOD mice. In contrast to the blocking of ICAM-1/LFA-1 interactions, inhibition of CD28/B7 interaction suppresses the production of Th2 cytokines (IL-4 and IL-5) (Labuda et al., 1998; Salomon et al., 1998). The homeostasis of T-reg is influenced by B7/CD28 signal. Although administration of CTLA4-Ig or anti-B7-2 mAbs to NOD mice did not prevent insulitis, it prevented the onset of diabetes in animals 2-4 weeks of age (Lenschow et al., 1995). In contrast, after the animals were past 10 weeks of age,

CTLA-4Ig and anti-B7-1 mAbs could not prevent T1D development. The results suggest that these molecules block the disease between insulitis and full-blown diabetes. Administration of anti-B7-1 mAb at the onset of insulitis resulted in a more severe infiltration and rapid onset of disease in both male and female NOD mice (Lenschow et al., 1995). T cells from anti-B7-1-treated mice were highly activated as reflected in the high levels of CD69 expression. It has been suggested that B7-1 costimulatory signal regulates the development of insulitis while B7-2 costimulatory signal is necessary for full development of T1D.

4.5 Modulation of CD3 function

T1D patients treated with anti-CD3 mAb called Otelixixumab have shown improvement in clinical trials (Keymeulen et al., 2010). This monoclonal antibody suppress the function of effector T cells and upregulate the regulatory T cells. In NOD mice, administration of anti-CD3 mAb prevented the onset of T1D by downregulating Th1 response and increasing T-reg response (Masteller et al., 2002). However, treatment of T1D with the anti-CD3 mAb, Otelixixiumab, can affect other non-self-reactive T cells; therefore along with another mAb known as Teplizumab, both antibodies were pulled from clinical trials due to their severe side effects caused by their general immuno-suppression. Thus, using antigen-specific therapeutics becomes a more attractive option for treating T1D. Because T cells recognize antigens presented on MHC molecules, treating with soluble TCR ligands is also an attractive option (Masteller et al., 2002). Treatment with a soluble peptide-MHC complex is similar to anti-TCR-CD3 mAb treatment, except that it target only those T cells that are self-reactive.

4.6 Modulation of cytokines

TNF-α can negatively or positively regulate the peripheral tolerance of T cells to β-islet antigens, depending on the age of NOD mice (Lee et al., 2005). Administration of TNF-α at a non-toxic dose to female NOD mice for 21 days after birth produced an early onset T1D (Lee et al., 2005). In this case, TNF-α activates macrophages and increases the expression of maturation markers such as CD86, CD40, CD54, MHC class II, and CD119 on $CD11c^+CD11b^+$ subpopulations. In contrast, administration of anti-TNF-α mAb for 21 days after birth prevented the development of T1D for a 1-year period. However, administration of anti-TNF-α to CD28-deficient and B7-1/B7-2-deficient NOD mice lead to more severe disease than the control NOD mice (Salomon et al., 2000). B7-deficient mice lack both CD28 and CTLA-4; CTLA-4 plays a critical role in regulating autoimmune disease. TNF-α mAb could not prevent T1D development when delivered at 3-4 weeks of age (Lee et al., 2005). Anti-TNF-α increases in $CD8\alpha^+CD11c^+$ dendritic cells (DC) compared to TNF-α. Because hyperglycemia has a direct effect on the expression of TNF-α, it is thought that TNF-α induces the maturation of DC and accelerates the migration of $CD\alpha^+CD11c^+$ DCs into the lymph nodes from the pancreas.

In response to GAD recognition as antigen, NOD mice increase the production of IFN-γ specifying the involvement Th1 cells, which are predominantly found in the islets regardless of mouse age. IFN-γ-producing cells are present even after the transfer of suppressor T cells (Hartemann et al., 1999). The number of IFN-γ-secreting cells does not correlate with NOD disease progression, which suggests that there is no absolute shift in the immune response leading to β-cell destruction. Although IL-4 secreting T cells are not detected, Th2-type cells are still present in the islet, but they are in a resting state. Therefore, an increase in the number of IL-4 secreting cells does not indicate the presence of Th2 suppressive cells in the islets. It is suggested that the destruction of β-cells may depend on either an IFN-γ-independent triggering event or the number of IFN-γ-secreting cells that reach a certain threshold in islets (Hartemann et al., 1999).

4.7 Adjuvant treatment to suppress T1D

Several studies have shown that adjuvant-containing mycobacterial preparations such as CFA or BCG effectively prevent onset and recurrence of T1D in NOD mice (Qin et al., 2004b; Qin et al., 1997). Adoptive transfer studies showed that BCG immunization of diabetic NOD mice impaired the ability of splenocytes to transfer diabetes. Histological examination indicated that splenocytes from BCG-immunized diabetic mice induced less insulitis in recipient NOD.Scid mice than did splenocytes from the saline-treated group. BCG immunization significantly decreased the proportions of CD4, CD8, and CD45RB^{low} T cells by inducing apoptosis and increased CD11b positive macrophages in time-course studies (Qin et al., 2004b). In comparison to control, the total number of TNF-α- or IFN-γ-positive splenocytes and IL-4 expression were significantly increased in BCG-immunized mice. Mechanistically, *in vivo* administration of anti-IFN-γ mAb reversed the immune regulatory effect of BCG to down-regulate CD45RB^{low} CD4 T cells and increase apoptosis of CD4 T cells (Qin et al., 2004b). BCG immunization also significantly increased Fas^{high}, FasL, and TNFR expression on CD4 and CD8 T cells. Furthermore, administration of anti-FasL or anti-TNFR1 mAb resulted in a significant decreased in T-cell apoptosis and increased in T-cell proliferative response. This suggests that BCG immunization down-regulates destructive autoimmunity by TNF-α-/IFN-γ-induced apoptosis of diabetogenic T cells through both Fas-FasL- and TNFR-TNF-α-mediated signaling pathways (Qin et al., 2004b).

5. Conclusions

The use of peptides and proteins for treating autoimmune diseases, including T1D, has been increasing steadily. Other than insulin, many monoclonal antibodies are being investigated as disease-modifying agents to treat T1D by tipping the balance of immune cells from effector to suppressor or regulatory cells and preventing further damage to β-cells. Recently, antigenic peptides and bifunctional peptide inhibitors (BPI) have been explored for altering the differentiation and proliferation of T cells to regulatory cells to prevent the development of diabetes. These molecules are developed to affect immune cells in an antigenic-specific manner; thus, they do not suppress the general immune response for fighting infections. However, further studies on the mechanisms of action of antigenic peptides and BPI molecules are still needed for improving the therapeutic index.

6. References

Aly T. et al. (2005). Immunotherapeutic approaches to prevent, ameliorate, and cure type 1 diabetes. *American Journal of Therapeutcs*, Vol. 12, No. 6, pp. 481–490.

Awasthi A. et al. (2008). Interplay between effector Th17 and regulatory T cells. *Journal of Clinical Immunology*, Vol. 28, No. 6, pp. 660–670.

Baker R.L. et al. (2008). CD40 on NOD CD4 T cells contributes to their activation and pathogenicity. *Journal of Autoimmunity*, Vol. 31, No. 4, pp. 385-392.

Bella J. et al. (1998). The structure of the two amino-terminal domains of human ICAM-1 suggests how it functions as a rhinovirus receptor and as an LFA-1 integrin ligand. *Proceedings of the National Academy of Sciences of the United States of America,* Vol. 95, No. 8, pp. 4140–4145.

Bending D. et al. (2009). Highly purified Th17 cells from BDC2.5NOD mice convert into Th1-like cells in NOD/SCID recipient mice. *Journal of Clinical Investigation,* Vol. 119, No. 3, pp. 565-572.

Bour-Jordan H. et al. (2011). Intrinsic and extrinsic control of peripheral T-cell tolerance by costimulatory molecules of the CD28/B7 family. *Immunological Reviews,* Vol. 241, No. 1, pp. 180-205.

Bour-Jordan H. et al. (2007). Constitutive expression of B7-1 on B cells uncovers autoimmunity toward the B cell compartment in the nonobese diabetic mouse. *Journal of Immunology,* Vol. 179, No. 2, pp. 1004–1012.

Bradley L.M. et al. (1999). Islet-specific Th1, but not Th2 cells secrete multiple chemokines and promote rapid induction of autoimmune diabetes. *Journal of Immunology,* Vol. 162, No. 5, pp. 2511–2520.

Bradshaw E.M. et al. (2009). Monocytes from patients with type 1 diabetes spontaneously secrete proinflammatory cytokines inducing Th17 cells. *Journal of Immunology,* Vol. 183, No. 7, pp. 4432–4439.

Bresson D. et al. (2006). Anti-CD3 and nasal proinsulin combination therapy enhances remission from recent-onset autoimmune diabetes by inducing Tregs. *Journal of Clinical Investigation,* Vol. 116, No. 5, pp. 1371–1381.

Bromley S.K. et al. (2001). The immunological synapse and CD28-CD80 interactions. *Nature Immunology,* Vol. 2, No. 12, pp. 1159–1166.

Buckner J.H. (2010). Mechanisms of impaired regulation by CD4(+)CD25(+)FOXP3(+) regulatory T cells in human autoimmune diseases. *Nature Reviews: Immunology,* Vol. 10, No. 12, pp. 849–859.

Calcinaro F. et al. (1997). Protection from autoimmune diabetes by adjuvant therapy in the non-obese diabetic mouse: the role of interleukin-4 and interleukin-10. *Immunology and Cell Biology,* Vol. 75, No. 5, pp. 467–471.

Casasnovas J.M. et al. (1998). A dimeric crystal structure for the N-terminal two domains of intercellular adhesion molecule-1. *Proceedings of the National Academy of Sciences of the United States of America,* Vol. 95, No. 8, pp. 4134–4139.

Chao C.C. et al. (1999). The role of MHC class II molecules in susceptibility to type I diabetes: identification of peptide epitopes and characterization of the T cell repertoire. *Proceedings of the National Academy of Sciences of the United States of America,* Vol. 96, No. 16, pp. 9299-9304.

Chen C. et al. (2003). Induction of autoantigen-specific Th2 and Tr1 regulatory T cells and modulation of autoimmune diabetes. *Journal of Immunology,* Vol. 171, No. pp. 733–744.

Chen Z. et al. (2005). Where CD4+CD25+ T reg cells impinge on autoimmune diabetes. *The Journal of Experimental Medicine,* Vol. 202, No. 10, pp. 1387–1397.

Chowdhury S.A. et al. (2002). Tolerance mechanisms in murine autoimmune diabetes induced by anti-ICAM-1/LFA-1 mAb and anti-CD8 mAb. *Kobe Journal Medical Sciences,* Vol. 48, No. 5–6, pp. 167–175.

Corper A.L. et al. (2000). A structural framework for deciphering the link between I-Ag7 and autoimmune diabetes. *Science*, Vol. 288, No. 5465, pp. 505–511.

Dobbs C.M. et al. (2001). Comparison of a T cell clone and of T cells from a TCR transgenic mouse: TCR transgenic T cells specific for self-antigen are atypical. *Journal of Immunology*, Vol. 166, No. 4, pp. 2495-2504.

Gonzales A. et al. (2001). Damage control, rather than unresponsiveness, effected by protective DX5+ T cells in autoimmune diabetes. *Nature Immunology*, Vol. 2, No. pp. 1117–1125.

Grakoui A. et al. (1999). The immunological synapse: a molecular machine controlling T cell activation. *Science*, Vol. 285, No. 5425, pp. 221-227.

Hartemann A.H. et al. (1999). Absence of significant Th2 response in diabetes-prone non-obese diabetic (NOD) mice. *Clinical and Experimental Immunology*, Vol. 116, No. 2, pp. 225–230.

Hedegaard C.J. et al. (2008). T helper cell type 1 (Th1), Th2 and Th17 responses to myelin basic protein and disease activity in multiple sclerosis. *Immunology*, Vol. 125, No. 2, pp. 161–169.

Honeyman M.C. et al. (1995). Analysis of families at risk for insulin-dependent diabetes mellitus reveals that HLA antigens influence progression to clinical disease. *Molecular Medicine*, Vol. 1, No. 5, pp. 576–582.

Huang M. et al. (2005). Alpha L-integrin I domain cyclic peptide antagonist selectively inhibits T cell adhesion to pancreatic islet microvascular endothelium. *Americn Journal of Physiology Gastrointestinal Liver Physiology*, Vol. 288, No. 1, pp. G67–73.

Jain R. et al. (2008). Innocuous IFNγ induced by adjuvant-free antigen restores normoglycemia in NOD mice through inhibition of IL-17 production. *Journal of Experimental Medicine*, Vol. 205, No. 1, pp. 207-218.

Keymeulen B. et al. (2010). Four-year metabolic outcome of a randomised controlled CD3-antibody trial in recent-onset type 1 diabetic patients depends on their age and baseline residual beta cell mass. *Diabetologia*, Vol. 53, No. 4, pp. 614–623.

Kim S.K. et al. (2004). Prevention of type I diabetes transfer by glutamic acid decarboxylase 65 peptide 206-220-specific T cells. *Proceedings of the National Academy of Sciences of the United States of America*, Vol. 101, No. 39, pp. 14204–14209.

Kobayashi N. et al. (2008). Prophylactic and therapeutic suppression of experimental autoimmune encephalomyelitis by a novel bifunctional peptide inhibitor. *Clinical Immunology*, Vol. 129, No. 1, pp. 69–79.

Kobayashi N. et al. (2007). Antigen-specific suppression of experimental autoimmune encephalomyelitis by a novel bifunctional peptide inhibitor. *The Journal of Pharmacology and Experimental Therapeutics*, Vol. 322, No. 2, pp. 879–886.

Labuda T. et al. (1998). ICAM-1 costimulation induces IL-2 but inhibits IL-10 production in superantigen-activated human CD4+ T cells. *Immunology*, Vol. 94, No. 4, pp. 496–502.

Lawson J.M. et al. (2008). Increased resistance to CD4+CD25hi regulatory T cell-mediated suppression in patients with type 1 diabetes. *Clinical and Experimental Immunology*, Vol. 154, No. 3, pp. 353–359.

Lee L.F. et al. (2005). The role of TNF-alpha in the pathogenesis of type 1 diabetes in the nonobese diabetic mouse: analysis of dendritic cell maturation. *Proceedings of the*

National Academy of Sciences of the United States of America, Vol. 102, No. 44, pp. 15995–16000.

Lehmann P.V. et al. (1993). Determinant spreading and the dynamics of the autoimmune T-cell repertoire. *Immunology Today,* Vol. 14, No. 5, pp. 203–208.

Lenschow D.J. et al. (1996). CD28/B7 regulation of Th1 and Th2 subsets in the development of autoimmune diabetes. *Immunity,* Vol. 5, No. pp. 285.

Lenschow D.J. et al. (1995). Differential effects of anti-B7-1 and anti-B7-2 mAb treatment on the development of diabetes in the NOD mouse. *Journal of Experimental Medicine,* Vol. 181, No. 3, pp. 1145–1155.

Liddi R. et al. (2000). Incomplete Freund's adjuvant reduces diabetes in the non-obese diabetic mouse. *Hormone and Metabolic Research,* Vol. 32, No. 6, pp. 201–206.

Liu J. et al. (1999). Major DQ8-restricted T-cell epitopes for human GAD65 mapped using human CD4, DQA1*0301, DQB1*0302 transgenic IA(null) NOD mice. *Diabetes,* Vol. 48, No. 3, pp. 469–477.

Manikwar P. et al. (2011). Antigen-specific blocking of CD4-specific immunological synapse formation using BPI and current therapies for autoimmune diseases. *Medicinal Research Reviews,* Vol. E-pub., No. Mar. 23, pp. 00–00.

Masteller E.L. & Bluestone J.A. (2002). Immunotherapy of insulin-dependent diabetes mellitus. *Current Opinion in Immunology,* Vol. 14, No. 5, pp. 652-659.

McDevitt H. (2003). The T cell response to glutamic acid decarboxylase 65 in T cell receptor transgenic NOD mice. *Annals of the New York Academy of Sciences,* Vol. 1005, pp. 75–81.

McDevitt H. (2004). Specific antigen vaccination to treat autoimmune disease. *Proceedings of the National Academy of Sciences of the United States of America,* Vol. 101, pp. 14627–14630.

Moriyama H. et al. (1996). Induction of tolerance in murine autoimmune diabetes by transient blockade of leukocyte function-associated antigen-1/intercellular adhesion molecule-1 pathway. *Journal of Immunology,* Vol. 157, No. 8, pp. 3737–3743.

Murray J.S. et al. (2007). Suppression of type 1 diabetes in NOD mice by bifunctional peptide inhibitor: modulation of the immunological synapse formation. *Chemical Biology and Drug Design,* Vol. 70, No. 3, pp. 227–236.

Munroe M.E. et al. (2007). A costimulatory function for T cell CD40. *Journal of Immunology,* Vol. 178, No. 2, pp. 671-682.

Mysliwiec J. et al. (1999). CD11a expression and soluble ICAM-1 levels in peripheral blood in high-risk and overt type 1 diabetes subjects. *Immunology Letters,* Vol. 70, No. 1, pp. 69–72.

Pakala S.V. et al. (1997). T helper 2 (Th2) T cells induce acute pancreatitis and diabetes in immune-compromised nonobese diabetic (NOD) mice. *Journal of Experimental Medicine,* Vol. 186, No. 2, pp. 299–306.

Qin H. et al. (2004a). Progression of spontaneous autoimmune diabetes is associated with a switch in the killing mechanism used by autoreactive CTL. *International Immunology,* Vol. 16, No. 11, pp. 1657–1662.

Qin H.Y., Chaturvedi P. & Singh B. (2004b). In vivo apoptosis of diabetogenic T cells in NOD mice by IFN-gamma/TNF-alpha. *International Immunology,* Vol. 16, No. 12, pp. 1723–1732.

Qin H.Y. & Singh B. (1997). BCG vaccination prevents insulin-dependent diabetes mellitus (IDDM) in NOD mice after disease acceleration with cyclophosphamide. *Journal of Autoimmunity*, Vol. 10, No. 3, pp. 271–278.

Ridwan R. et al. (2010). Antigen-specific suppression of experimental autoimmune encephalomyelitis by a novel bifunctional peptide inhibitor: structure optimization and pharmacokinetics. *The Journal of Pharmacology and Experimental Therapeutics*, Vol. 332, No. 3, pp. 1136–1145.

Ryba M. et al. (2010). Regulatory T lymphocytes expressing L-selectin in children and adolescents with type 1 diabetes mellitus. *Pediatric Endocrinology, Diabetes, and Metabolism*, Vol. 16, No. 1, pp. 12–16.

Salomon B. & Bluestone J.A. (1998). LFA-1 interaction with ICAM-1 and ICAM-2 regulates Th2 cytokine production. *Journal of Immunology*, Vol. 161, No. 10, pp. 5138–5142.

Salomon B. & Bluestone J.A. (2001). Complexities of CD28/B7: CTLA-4 costimulatory pathways in autoimmunity and transplantation. *Annual Review of Immunology*, Vol. 19, pp. 225–252.

Salomon B. et al. (2000). B7/CD28 costimulation is essential for the homeostasis of the CD4+CD25+ immunoregulatory T cells that control autoimmune diabetes. *Immunity*, Vol. 12, No. 4, pp. 431–440.

Sercarz E.E. et al. (1993). Dominance and crypticity of T cell antigenic determinants. *Annual Review of Immunology*, Vol. 11, No. pp. 729–766.

Solomon M. & Sarvetnick N. (2004). The pathogenesis of diabetes in the NOD mouse. *Advances in Immunology*, Vol. 84, pp. 239–264.

Tarbell K.V. et al. (2002). CD4(+) T cells from glutamic acid decarboxylase (GAD)65-specific T cell receptor transgenic mice are not diabetogenic and can delay diabetes transfer. *Journal of Experimental Medicine*, Vol. 196, No. 4, pp. 481–492.

Tibbetts S.A. et al. (1999). Peptides derived from ICAM-1 and LFA-1 modulate T cell adhesion and immune function in a mixed lymphocyte culture. *Transplantation*, Vol. 68, No. 5, pp. 685–692.

Tibbetts S.A. et al. (2000). Linear and cyclic LFA-1 and ICAM-1 peptides inhibit T-cell adhesion and function. *Peptides*, Vol. 21, No. 8, pp. 1161–1167.

Tisch R. et al. (1998). Induction of GAD65-specific regulatory T-cells inhibits ongoing autoimmune diabetes in nonobese diabetic mice. *Diabetes*, Vol. 47, No. 6, pp. 894–899.

Tisch R. et al. (1999). Induction of glutamic acid decarboxylase 65-specific Th2 cells and suppression of autoimmune diabetes at late stages of disease is epitope dependent. *Journal of Immunology*, Vol. 163, No. 3, pp. 1178–1187.

Tisch R. et al. (1993). Immune response to glutamic acid decarboxylase correlates with insulitis in non-obese diabetic mice. *Nature*, Vol. 366, No. 6450, pp. 72–75.

Tsukamoto K. et al. (1995). Administration of monoclonal antibodies against vascular cell adhesion molecule-1/very late antigen-4 abrogates predisposing autoimmune diabetes in NOD mice. *Cellular Immunology*, Vol. 165, No. 2, pp. 193–201.

Waid D.M. et al. (2008). Disruption of the homeostatic balance between autoaggressive ($CD4^+CD40^+$) and regulatory ($CD4^+CD25^+FoxP3^+$) T cells promotes diabetes. *Journal of Leukocyte Biology*, Vol. 84, No. 2, pp. 431-439.

Xu C.R. et al. (2002). Structural and ICAM-1-docking properties of a cyclic peptide from the I-domain of LFA-1: An inhibitor of ICAM-1/LFA-1-mediated T-cell adhesion. *Journal of Biomolecular Structure Dynamics,* Vol. 19, No. 5, pp. 789–799.

Yoon J.W. et al. (1999). Control of autoimmune diabetes in NOD mice by GAD expression or suppression in beta cells. *Science,* Vol. 284, No. 5417, pp. 1183–1187.

You S. et al. (2007). Adaptive TGF-beta-dependent regulatory T cells control autoimmune diabetes and are a privileged target of anti-CD3 antibody treatment. *Proceedings of the National Academy of Sciences of the United States of America,* Vol. 104, No. 15, pp. 6335–6340.

Yusuf-Makagiansar H. et al. (2000). Modulation of adhesion molecules in lymphocyte activation and cell-cell interaction. *Current Topics in Biochemistry Research,* Vol. 2, No. pp. 33–49.

Yusuf-Makagiansar H. et al. (2001a). Synergistic inhibitory activity of alpha- and beta-LFA-1 peptides on LFA-1/ICAM-1 interaction. *Peptides,* Vol. 22, No. 12, pp. 1955–1962.

Yusuf-Makagiansar H. et al. (2001b). Inhibition of the adherence of T-lymphocyte to epithelial cells by a cyclic peptide derived from inserted domain of lymphocyte function-associated antigen-1. *Inflammation,* Vol. 25, No. 3, pp. 203–214.

Yusuf-Makagiansar H. & Siahaan T.J. (2001c). Binding and internalization of an LFA-1-derived cyclic peptide by ICAM receptors on activated lymphocyte: a potential ligand for drug targeting to ICAM-1-expressing cells. *Pharm. Res.,* Vol. 18, No. 3, pp. 329–335.

Zhao H. et al. (2010). Immune response to controlled release of immunomodulating peptides in a murine experimental autoimmune encephalomyelitis (EAE) model. *Journal of Controlled Release,* Vol. 141, No. 2, pp. 145–152.

Ziolkowska M. et al. (2000). High levels of IL-17 in rheumatoid arthritis patients: IL-15 triggers in vitro IL-17 production via cyclosporin A-sensitive mechanism. *Journal of Immunology,* Vol. 164, No. 5, pp. 2832–2838.

16

Immunotherapy for Type 1 Diabetes – Preclinical and Clinical Trials

Alice Li[1] and Alan Escher[2]
[1]*Center for Transplant Immunology Research, Loma Linda University, Loma Linda, CA,*
[2]*SEKRIS Corporation, Redlands, CA, USA*

1. Introduction

According to the American Diabetes Association (http://www.diabetes.org/diabetes-basics/diabetes-statistics), 2-3 million individuals in the United States have type 1 diabetes and about 1 in every 400 to 600 children and adolescents was affected by the disease in 2007. Similar to other autoimmune diseases, allergies, and asthma, the incidence of type 1 diabetes is on the increase at an alarming rate in industrialized countries for unknown reasons. The disease is immune-mediated and thought to be caused by a combination of genetic and environmental factors that ultimately leads to loss of insulin secreting beta cells in pancreatic islets and high levels of blood glucose. High sugar levels and autoimmunity cause acute complications, such as ketoacidosis, as well as a wide variety of late complications, for example, atherosclerosis, retinopathy, kidney failure, neuropathy, and infection. Injection of insulin is a life saving treatment rather than a cure, and individuals suffering from type 1 diabetes and receiving insulin still show an unacceptable 15 year reduction in life expectancy and complications of the disease according to the Juvenile Diabetes Research Foundation (JDRF) (http://www.jdrf.org.uk/page.asp?section=163&sectionTitle=FAQs+about+type+1+diabetes). The requirement for insulin injection can be alleviated by transplantation of pancreas or pancreatic islets, but the procedure is limited by the low number of donors, the out lived usefulness of immunosuppression, and the pre-existing autoimmunity which still cause ~85% of islet transplants to fail 10 years post-transplantation.

The mammalian immune system is the main line of defense to protect from attacks by infection, cancer, and pathological autoimmunity. Leukocytes normally do not destroy host tissues or cells because immune cells targeting self-antigens are either deleted in the thymus and bone marrow, i.e., central tolerance; or they are under the control of regulatory T cells in peripheral tissues, i.e., peripheral tolerance. However, defects in either of these immune control systems can result in pathological autoimmunity and large bodies of evidence indicate that defects in central as well as peripheral tolerance can contribute to type 1 diabetes (Geenen et al., 2010). Type 1 diabetes is an organ-specific autoimmune disease resulting from the selective destruction of pancreatic insulin secreting beta cells by autoreactive CD4 and CD8 effector T lymphocytes which normally play an important role in self-protection by killing infected and tumor cells. On the other hand, CD4 and CD8 T lymphocytes also include regulatory cells that control the activity of effector cells, and can be drawn upon to ameliorate type 1 diabetes. In the past decade, these regulatory cells, especially CD4 T regulatory cells, have become a major immunotherapeutic target for the treatment of type 1 diabetes and other autoimmune diseases. In addition, antigen-presenting cells like dendritic cells, which present protein-derived antigens to T lymphocytes on their major histocompatibility complex molecules, have also received much attention not only because they can contribute to disease onset, but also because they can be used to induce T regulatory cells (Paul, 1999, Nikolic et al., 2009).

In addition to direct cell-to-cell interaction, immune cells modulate immune responses by secreting small molecular proteins, called cytokines, into their environment. Cytokines promote the development and differentiation of immune cells with different functions and therefore play an important role in directing immune responses. Several cytokines have been used alone and together with other immunotherapeutics for treatment of type 1 diabetes in animal model systems. One of the largest groups of cytokine is the interleukin group, which consists of more than 30 different proteins with interleukin-1, interleukin-2, interleukin-4, interleukin-10, and interleukin-15, among others, being potential targets for treatment. Other cytokines like tumor necrosis factor-alpha can also be used for type 1 diabetes treatment.

Antibodies are another important group of therapeutic molecules that have been investigated for type 1 diabetes. Antibodies, or immunoglobulins (Ig), are large Y-shaped proteins produced by B lymphocytes found in blood and other bodily fluids of vertebrates where their function includes binding to protein antigens and neutralizing pathogens. In the case of type 1 diabetes, the therapeutic antibodies that have been developed target self-antigens synthesized by cells that participate in the inflammatory response and cause the disease.

Under the effect of both genetic and environmental factors, immune cells like CD4 T lymphocytes and CD8 cytotoxic T lymphocytes infiltrate pancreatic islets resulting in different levels of insulitis (**Figure 1**). Insulitis ultimately results in the selective destruction of pancreatic beta cells as the result of regulatory dysfunction of CD4 T lymphocytes, and/or of dendritic cells and other cell types.

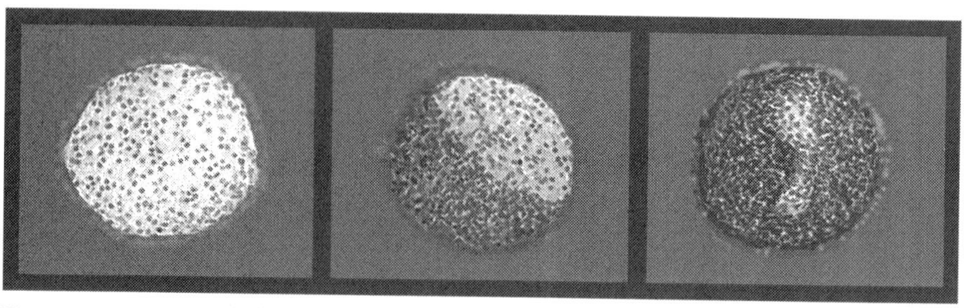

Fig. 1. **Graphic Representation of Mouse Islets with Lymphocyte Infiltration.** A. Normal islet; B. Islet partially infiltrated by lymphocytes; C. Islet fully infiltrated by lymphocytes.

Since there is no cure for clinical type 1 diabetes, novel immunotherapeutic approaches aimed at preserving and restoring functional endogenous beta cell mass as well as protecting transplanted islets are needed to rebuild immune tolerance to beta cells and improve the condition of type 1 diabetic patients. One of the animal models closest to human type 1 diabetes and most often used for studying the disease is the non-obese diabetic (NOD) female mouse, which is a spontaneous diabetes model that has helped to dissect the various stages of disease progression in human (Zhang et al., 2008, Ridgway, 2003). A variety of immunotherapies are being investigated in non-obese diabetic mice to treat type 1 diabetes. They can be divided into four main categories: first, non-antigen-specific therapies such as antibody therapies targeting effector cells; second, antigen-specific therapies such as protein and DNA vaccines targeting diabetic autoantigens; third, other immunotherapies such as bacille Calmette-Guérin (BCG), vitamin D3, and fourth, combinational therapies which combine antigen specific and non-specific therapies (**Figure 2**). Bench-to-bedside translation of these different approaches has already identified a number of promising therapies, which will be the main focus of this chapter. The strong impetus to develop prophylactic and therapeutic approaches for the disease is reflected by the activity of organizations like TrialNet (http://www.diabetestrialnet.org/) and the Immune Tolerance Network (http://www.immunetolerance.org/). TrialNet is an expansion of the Diabetes Prevention Trial (DPT-1) network, but with an emphasis not only on diabetes prevention but also on trials to prevent further destruction of islet beta cells in patients with type 1 diabetes.

2. Antibody therapies

Intervention studies using antibodies for type 1 diabetes in the 1980s demonstrated a potential for preserving insulin C-peptide level which serves as an indication of insulin secretion by beta cells. However, they were eventually abandoned due to the adverse side effect profiles of the agents being used (You et al., 2008). Pilot studies of new immunosuppressive and immunomodulatory agents with decreased side-effect profiles have recently shown promise in preserving C-peptide in new-onset type 1 diabetic patients. Some of these agents are specifically designed monoclonal antibodies targeting immune effector cells, e.g., anti-CD3, anti-CD20, anti-CD25 (daclizumab), and anti-thymocyte globulin are being tested in clinical trials for type 1 diabetes. Other antibodies, such as anti-CD154 (MR1) have been tested in the female non-obese diabetic mouse.

The first anti-CD3 antibody used clinically was a murine monoclonal IgG2 antibody, OKT3, which was identified while antibodies were investigated as lymphocytic mitogens (Kaufman & Herold, 2009). CD3 is a protein complex found on the cell surface of T cells and is involved in transduction of signals originating from the antigen receptor to start a cascade of events initiating activation of the T cell. The binding between anti-CD3 antibody and CD3 on T cells can inhibit lysis of targets by T cells. Along with potent mitogenic activity, OKT3 was found to be a potent inducer of cytokines, specifically, tumor necrosis factor-alpha, interleukin-2, and interferon-gamma. Among these induced cytokines, interleukin-2 is necessary for T regulatory cell proliferation and tumor necrosis factor-alpha and interferon-gamma are considered as regulatory cytokines. These characteristics made anti-CD3 a potential therapeutic agent for both transplantation medicine and anti-tumor activity in the clinic. Unfortunately, the toxic side effects of OKT3 became clear after patients receiving the drug immediately developed chills, fever, hypotension, and in some cases, dyspnea. The toxicity was thought to be associated with a cytokine, specifically tumor necrosis factor-alpha from T cells in response to the drug. This effect was attributed to the anti-CD3 mediated cross-linking of T cells, i.e., the anti-CD3 antibody causing linkage of T cells bearing CD3 molecules and cells bearing the Fc (fragmental crystallizable region of the antibody molecule) receptor. This cross-linking is thought to activate both the T cell and the Fc receptor-bearing cells, leading to the massive release of cytokines. These toxic side effects severely limited the clinical application of anti-CD3 to type 1 diabetes.

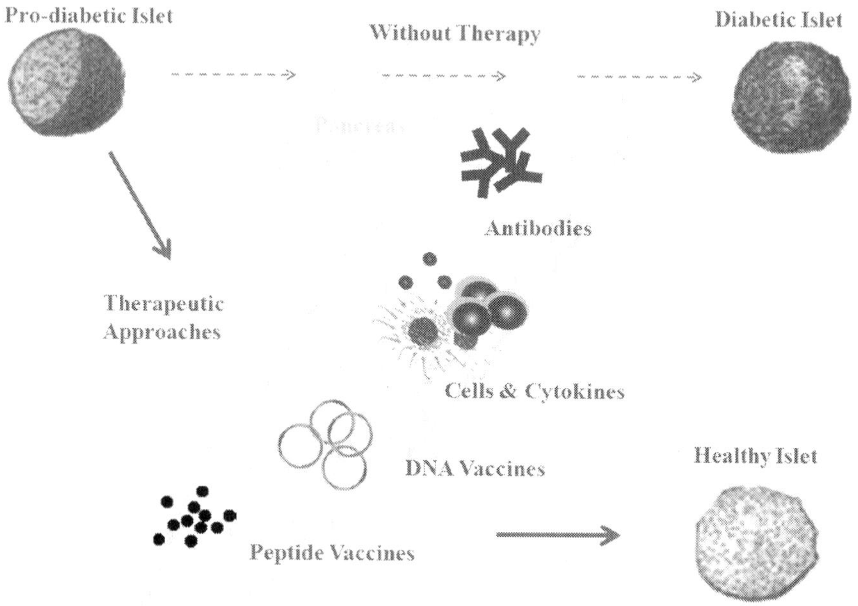

Fig. 2. **Immunotherapies for Type 1 Diabetes.** Without immunotherapy (top), pro-diabetic islets ultimately become diabetic islets after destruction of insulin-secreting beta-cells. Immunotherapies for type 1 diabetes can protect pro-diabetic islets from further destruction and permit them to regain function. A variety of immunotherapies, either alone or in combination, has been shown to stop pathological autoimmunity and protect islets to ameliorate type 1 diabetes.

To circumvent these problems, new antibodies were engineered to reduced Fc receptor binding after amino acid substitutions in the Fc portions of the antibody (Kaufman & Herold, 2009). Although reduced Fc receptor binding was predicted to eliminate T cell activation and cytokine release, the new anti-CD3 antibodies are still mildly mitogenic, i.e., T cell proliferation can be shown *in vitro* and even mild cytokine release has been observed. Nevertheless, it is important to note that the new anti-CD3 monoclonal antibodies differ greatly from OKT3 in their induction of T cell activation *in vivo*, and that the toxic side effects have been significantly reduced. In addition, the anti-CD3 antibodies derived from mouse generally are fully humanized to minimize the potential immunogenicity associated with heterogenic antibody isotype between mouse and human.

The modified anti-CD3 antibodies have been shown to be as effective as the full-length molecule but with reduced morbidity (Chatenoud et al., 1994). Using this treatment, 64–80% of treated diabetic non-obese diabetic mice returned to a euglycemic state without glycosuria while none of the non-obese diabetic mice treated with control immunoglobin recovered. In addition, the new antibodies could also protect transplanted allogeneic pancreatic islets in diabetic non-obese diabetic mice (Chatenoud et al., 1997). The mice could still reject allogeneic skingrafts and remain resistant to adoptive transfer of diabetogenic T cells, suggesting that their immune system was intact and that only beta cell specific immune responses were affected. However, results indicated that treatment of 4- and 8-week old mice did not prevent diabetes, but did protect 12-week-old mice, which indicated that the anti-CD3 was only effective when used after the onset of the disease.

Humanized non-Fc receptor binding anti-CD3 monoclonal antibodies include otelixizumab, teplizumab, and visilizumab. Teplizumab was shown to preserve C-peptide production up to five years after a single course of twelve days of treatment of new-onset type 1 diabetic patients in phase I/II clinical trials (Herold et al., 2009). Insulin is synthesized in the pancreas firstly as pro-insulin consisting of the A, C, and B peptide moieties. Mature active insulin is obtained after excision of the C peptide and folding/assembly of the A chain and B chain. Thus levels of C-peptide can be used as an indication of insulin secretion activity by β-cells. There may be several therapeutic mechanisms involved: induction of regulatory T cells, increased proportion of CD8+ T cells, increased expression of Foxp3 in CD8+ T cells, as well as induction of apoptotic cells. Similarly, otelixizumab could preserve residual beta-cell function for at least 18 months in patients with recent onset type 1 diabetes who were under treatment for six consecutive days (Keymeulen et al., 2005). However, anti-CD3 based approaches have suffered a setback because of the announced suspension of Phase III clinical trials for type 1 diabetes by MacroGenics and Eli Lilly as well as by Tolerx and GlaxoSmithKline due to lack of efficacy (GEN news, 2010; GSK Press Release, 2011). Previously, ulcerative colitis Phase II/III trials of visilizumab (trade name Nuvion) by PDL BioPharma Inc. had also been stopped due to inefficacy and poor safety profile (Lawler, 2009), which constitutes another setback.

Anti-CD25 IgG1 antibody (daclizumab) is another humanized recombinant monoclonal antibody which targets T cells. It is approximately 10% murine and 90% human, and activates T regulatory cells *in vivo* since the antibody inhibit initial T cell proliferation and differentiation but not initial activation (Egan et al., 2001). When used with the immunosuppressants rapamycin and tacrolimus, daclizumab maintains normal islet function in human recipients of transplanted allogeneic islet grafts. This glucocorticoid-free regimen appears to be highly beneficial for islet survival and function, as all patients were insulin independent (Shapiro et al., 2000). Daclizumab has also been used with success in human pancreas transplantation (Sutherland et al., 2001).

Monoclonal antibodies against CD154, also known as CD40 ligand, have also been used for treatment of type 1 diabetes. The CD154 protein is primarily synthesized by activated CD4 T cells, and binds to the CD40 receptor on antigen-presenting cells. CD40 receptor engagement induces activation through co-stimulation in antigen-presenting cells like dendritic cells, macrophages and B cells. Anti-CD154 monoclonal antibodies will bind to CD154 on the surface of CD4 T lymphocytes, and block stimulation of antigen-presenting cells (Howard & Miller, 2004). The application of anti-CD154 antibodies was shown to prevent expansion of CD40 expressing T cells, later called T helper 40 cells, which are highly pathogenic in the non-obese diabetic mouse model and human diabetes (Waid, et al., 2004). In addition, anti-CD154 monoclonal antibodies induced islet allograft tolerance involving a dominant mechanism associated with intragraft regulatory cells, and prevented autoimmune diabetes in non-obese diabetic mice, possibly because it inhibits effector T cells by expending regulatory T cell (Rigby et al., 2008).

Anti-thymocyte globulin (ATG) consists of antibodies from horse and rabbit against human T-lymphocytes. Its administration as intraperitoneal injections of 500 micrograms antibodies stops new-onset diabetes and induces long-term tolerance in non-obese diabetic mice (Simon et al., 2008). Treatment was associated with increased frequency and activity of $CD4^{+}CD25^{+}$ T regulatory cells, as well as altered alteration of dendritic cell profile and function (Bresson and von Herrath, 2011). However, the treatment was efficacious only when administered late in the prediabetic phase (12-week of age) or after recent-onset. Another report showed that the antibodies failed to protect diabetes in a more stringent virus (RIP-LCMV) induced diabetes model due at least partially to the inability to maintain or increase a sufficient $CD4^{+}CD25^{+}$ T regulatory cell frequency.

Human clinical trials of anti-thymocyte globulin suggest that short term therapy (9 mg/kg followed by 3 consecutive doses of 3 mg/kg/day intravenously) in eleven recent onset patients, i.e., within 4 weeks of diagnosis and with residual post-glucagon C-peptide levels still over 0.3 nmol/l, contributed to the preservation of residual C-peptide production and to lower insulin requirements in the first year following diagnosis (Saudek et al, 2004). Nevertheless, significant adverse effects consisting mainly of transient fever and moderate symptoms of serum sickness were observed during the first month of treatments. Two other clinical trials are ongoing, which include a phase II trial to determine whether thymoglobulin treatment can halt the progression of newly diagnosed type 1 diabetes when given within 12-weeks of disease diagnosis (Gitelman. 2007); and a phase I/II trial to determine if giving a combination therapy consisting of Thymoglobulin (anti-thymocyte globulin) and Neulasta (granulocyte colony-stimulating factor, GCSF) given to established type 1 diabetes patients is safe and preserves insulin production (Haller, 2010).

Although type 1 diabetes is considered a T cell-mediated disease, recent data have indicated a role for antigen presentation by B lymphocytes in disease pathogenesis. In fact, anti-CD20 monoclonal antibody treatment of 5-week-old non-obese diabetic female mice reduces B cell numbers by approximately 95%, decreases insulitis, and prevents diabetes in >60% of mice (Xiu et al., 2008). Furthermore, anti-CD20 monoclonal antibody treatment of 15-week old female non-obese diabetic mice significantly delays diabetes onset. A recent clinical trial delivering a four-dose course of anti-CD20 antibody (rituximab) 3 months after diagnosis of diabetes onset showed a significant improvement in beta cell function in 23% of patients at 1 year (Pescovitz et al., 2009). No beneficial effects were noted in placebo-treated subjects. These patients also showed significant improvements in clinical parameters like hemoglobin A1c level, which is a indicator of average blood glucose level, and decreased insulin use. After 3 months, however, there was a parallel decline in beta cell function in the drug and placebo treated subjects.

Clearly, antibody therapies can be effective in controlling diabetes. However, they cannot always be combined with other therapies in the clinic. For example, clinical trials of the combined application of daclizumab (anti-CD25) with either intensive insulin therapy or mycophenolate mofetil reported failure in preserving beta-cell function in clinic (Rother et al., 2009b; Gottlieb et al., 2010), and the anti-diabetic effects of anti-CD3 are negated by rapamycin in non-obese diabetic mice (Valle et al., 2009). In addition, antibodies act systemically in a non-specific manner and can interfere with normal immune function. For example, anti-CD20 and anti-CD3 monoclonal antibodies have caused treatment-related adverse events in some patients during clinical trials (Pescovitz et al., 2009; Keymeulen et al., 2005; Herold et al., 2005). The recent announcement by Biogen and Roche that clinical trials of an anti-CD20 monoclonal antibody for rheumatoid arthritis and systemic lupus had to be stopped due to death from opportunistic infection illustrates further the potential risks of certain monoclonal antibody treatments for autoimmune diseases.

3. Cellular and cytokine therapies

The main sign of pathosis in diabetic pancreatic islets is leukocyte infiltration or insulitis (**Figure 1**). Studies of islet-infiltrating cells have yielded clues to new therapeutic approaches by identifying immune cells and their associated molecules, such as cytokines, to suppress the disease. Preclinical and clinical trials of cellular therapies and cytokine therapies are currently ongoing, and will be discussed in this section.

3.1 Cellular therapies

Type 1 diabetes-associated deficiencies have been observed in several immune cell populations, such as CD4 T cells, CD8 T cells, B cells, dendritic cells, macrophages and NK cells in both non-obese diabetic mice and humans (Sgouroudis & Piccirillo, 2009; Luczyński et al., 2009). Regardless of whether diabetes is the result of increased effector cell activity or decreased regulatory cell function, the goal of cellular and many other therapies is to increase the regulatory function of cells like T regulatory lymphocytes and dendritic cells. Both cell types are important not only for therapeutic purposes, but are also suspected to play a determining role in the development of diabetes. T regulatory cellular therapies are currently at the preclinical stage and human T regulatory cell expansion strategies performed *in vitro* are under development.

T regulatory cells play a vital role as suppressive cells that regulate and control the effector arm of the immune system. In the past decade, an overwhelming body of literature has confirmed that $CD4^+CD25^+FoxP3^+$ and other T regulatory cells comprise a dominant mechanism regulating autoimmunity as well as responding to infection and cancer. These findings are further confirmation that T regulatory cell dysregulation is implicated in autoimmune disorders like type 1 diabetes. In the non-obese diabetic model system, the defects of T regulatory cells result in the loss of control of autoaggressive T cells and diabetes progression (Tang & Bluestone, 2006). In humans, defects in polyclonal regulatory T cell have also been proposed as a mechanism by which individuals develop type 1 diabetes (Kukreja et al., 2002). Here T regulatory cell numbers decrease in child (age 9.4 ± 2.16 years) and adult (age 45.2 ± 9.7 years) patients. Another report showed that while the T regulatory cell numbers remain normal, they are associated with functional deficiency in adult patients (age 32.3 ± 6.8 years) (Lindley et al., 2005). Therefore, control of pathological autoimmunity through the induction of functional T regulatory cells is a highly promising approach.

Surprisingly, central tolerance mechanisms associated with regulatory cells are generally intact in non-obese diabetic mice (Feuerer et al., 2007), and the frequency and function of single positive $CD4^+Foxp3^+$ T regulatory cells in the thymus of these animals is comparable to that of diabetes-resistant C57/BL6 mice (Tritt et al., 2008). The results suggest that a defect in the regulatory T cell population most likely happens in the peripheral immune system after a certain age. T regulatory cells are diverse in their phenotype and mechanisms of function, and as such investigators are developing various types of induced T cell precursors (e.g. antigen targeting specificities) with a variable degree of regulatory potential. It is possible to induce and expand islet antigen-specific T regulatory cells *in vitro* from both non-obese diabetic mice and humans. T regulatory cells from non-obese diabetic mice could be efficiently expanded *in vitro* using interleukin-2 and beads coated with a recombinant islet peptide mimic, a MHC class II molecule, and anti-CD28 monoclonal antibody. The expanded cells expressed normal surface markers like CD4, CD25, Foxp3, CD62L, GITR, and CTLA-4 in mice; and CD4, CD127^{lo}, CD25, and FOXP3 in humans. Once activated by the islet specific antigen, the T regulatory cells could suppress T effectors with other specificities both *in vitro* and *in vivo*. This feature is important for controlling type 1 diabetes in which numerous self-antigens are targeted by pathogenic effector cells. Importantly, the islet antigen specific T regulatory cells were more efficient than non-specific polyclonal T regulatory cells in suppressing autoimmune diabetes (Masteller et al., 2005; Putnam et al., 2009).

Results from T regulatory cell analysis of type 1 diabetic patients are varied, with either decreased cell frequency, unaltered T regulatory cell frequency with marked decrease in suppressive activity *in vitro*, or no difference compared to healthy controls (Kukreja et al., 2002; Lindley et al., 2005; Putnam et al., 2005). These variable results could be caused by different factors including different methods of T regulatory cell isolation and purification, the lack of functional tests for islet specific T regulatory cells in the blood, or simply different disease etiologies. Furthermore, studies in murine models indicate that T regulatory cells exert their function within the target organ undergoing autoimmune attack rather than solely in the lymph node draining sites. Thus, subtle functional differences in the T regulatory cell pool within sites of inflammation may not be adequately reflected in the peripheral blood and lymph node compartments, which are the main source of samples for human clinical data (Sgouroudis et al., 2009). A remaining question is whether changes in T regulatory cell function are the cause of diabetes onset or the uncontrolled activation and expansion of diabetogenic T effector cells are the cause of diabetes onset.

Similar to cells in mice, human T regulatory cells can be expanded *in vitro*. T regulatory cells from recent onset type 1 diabetic patients were expanded using anti-CD3 and anti-CD28 coated microbeads and interleukin-2 cytokine. Importantly, suppressive function, lineage markers such as FOXP3, and cytokine productions were similar to the T regulatory cells from healthy control subjects (Putnam et al., 2009). A phase I clinical trial of CD4^{+}CD127^{lo}/-CD25^{+} polyclonal T regulatory cells expanded using anti-CD3/anti-CD28 beads plus interleukin-2 started in 2010. The primary purpose of the trial is to assess the safety and feasibility of intravenous infusion of *ex vivo* selected and expanded autologous polyclonal regulatory cells in patients with type 1 diabetes to support dose selection for a future efficacy trial. The study also aims to assess the effect of T regulatory cells on beta cell function as well as on other measures of diabetes severity and the autoimmune response underlying type 1 diabetes (Gitelman & Bluestone, 2010).

In addition to T regulatory cells, dendritic cells can be cultured *in vitro* for *in vivo* applications. Dendritic cells are known as the most potent antigen-presenting cells and play a vital role in the control of immune homeostasis. Dendritic cells initiate T cell-mediated immunity and maintain immune tolerance in the periphery through activation of T regulatory cells and other mechanisms. Dendritic cells are the only professional antigen-presenting cells, as their main function is to prime naive T cells. They are the exclusive antigen-presenting cell subset capable of potentiating T regulatory cell proliferative and suppressive functions both *in vitro* and *in vivo*. As such, dendritic cells are at the crossroad of pathogenesis and therapy of autoimmune diseases like type 1 diabetes. Together with T regulatory cells, dendritic cells have been a main target for both *in vitro* and *in vivo* approaches to treat type 1 diabetes. The exact mechanism of tolerance induction by dendritic cells in diabetes remains to be established, but it likely includes inhibition and killing of effector T cells and induction of regulatory T cells (Feili-Hariri et al., 2006; Nikolic et al., 2009).

A dendritic cell clinical phase I safety trial is currently being conducted with type 1 diabetic patients (Phillips et al., 2009). The proposed studies describe a randomized trial to evaluate the safety of a new diabetes-suppressive cell vaccine, consisting of autologous monocyte-derived dendritic cells treated *ex vivo* with antisense phosphorothioate modified oligonucleotides targeting the primary transcripts of the dendritic cell co-stimulatory molecules CD40, CD80, and CD86 (immunoregulatory dendritic cells; iDC). Fifteen patients exhibiting fully-established, insulin-dependent type 1 diabetics, without any diabetes-related complications, infectious disease, or other medical anomaly, have been enrolled to establish safety of the approach. 7/15 patients have been administered autologous control dendritic cells and 8/15 patents have been administered immunoregulatory dendritic cells. The study is anticipated to be complete within a twelve month period.

Solely expanding cell population *in vitro* may not be sufficient as a therapy for an organ specific autoimmune disease, since it will be a systemic treatment and may be inducing significant off-target effects, such as general immuno-suppression that will compromise beneficial immune responses to infections and cancers. In addition, current methodologies are limited in terms of the capacity to isolate and expand a sufficient quantity of endogenous antigen specific human cells for therapeutic intervention at low cost. Even a T regulatory cell induced with antigen specificity possesses bystander suppressive function (Brusko et al., 2010; Masteller et al., 2005), and the induced antigen specific T regulatory cells could quickly revert to Foxp3 negative CD4 T cells in a Foxp3 transgenic mouse model (Koenecke et al., 2009). Therefore, significant improvements may have to be made before cellular therapies can be safely applied to humans.

3.2 Cytokine therapies

Several immunotherapies for type 1 diabetes have used cytokines and other molecules such as fusion proteins targeting the costimulatory pathway (http://en.wikipedia.org/wiki/Co-stimulation). For example, cytokines like interleukin-2 provides vital survival signals to regulatory cells and can trigger the death of effector T cells, and impede interleukin-15 driven expansion of memory cells. In addition, interleukin-4, tumor necrosis factor-alpha, interferon-alpha, and lymphotoxin cytokines can exert selective effects upon crucial lymphocyte subset populations *in vivo* that may also enable translation into potent therapies. Preclinical trials and a few clinical trials of cytokine therapies will be addressed in this section.

Pro-inflammatory cytokines may impair islet viability and function by activating inflammatory pathways. Interleukin-1 beta is a master inflammatory cytokine that is synthesized early during inflammation by a wide variety of cells. Interleukin-1 receptor-deficient non-obese diabetic mice have a reduced development incidence of diabetes (Thomas et al., 2004). Anakinra, which is a clinically approved recombinant human interleukin-1 receptor antagonist, can block the effects of interleukin-1 beta on rat islet cultured *in vitro*, and inhibits the activation of interleukin-1 beta dependent inflammatory pathways to protect islets from apoptotic impairment (Schwarznau et al., 2009). In addition, short term treatment with anakinra resulted in reduced ability of mononuclear cells to traffic to sites of inflammation in a small group of patients with type 1 diabetes. This suggests that mechanistic studies from large scale trials using interleukin-1 blockade in type 1 diabetes should focus on changes in monocyte trafficking and the interleukin-8 pathway (Sanda et al., 2010). Moreover, an adenoviral vector encoding interleukin-1 beta receptor antagonist together with another anti-inflammatory factor, i.e., hepatocyte growth factor, can reduce apoptosis of transplanted islets, and improve their survival in streptozotocin induced diabetes leading to lower blood glucose levels, as well as increased serum insulin and C-peptide levels (Panakanti & Mahato, 2009). Nevertheless, initial clinical data do not suggest that interleukin-1 blockade alone can prevent or reverse type 1 diabetes (Donath & Mandrup-Poulsen, 2008).

Interleukin-2 is another significant cytokine which has an important role in promoting T regulatory cell survival. Defective interleukin-2 or interleukin-2 receptor signaling in CD4 T-cells of type 1 diabetic subjects contributes to decreased persistence of FOXP3 expression that may impact establishment of tolerance (d'Hennezel et al., 2010). Therefore, interleukin-2 could be used as a therapeutic target for the restoration of Foxp3$^+$ regulatory T cell function in organ specific autoimmunity. Indeed, administration of a low dose of interleukin-2 in prediabetic non-obese diabetic mice results in restoration of CD25 expression, survival of intra islet T regulatory cells and prevention of type 1 diabetes, which are associated with enhanced synthesis of T regulatory cell associated proteins and suppression of interferon-gamma (Grinberg-Bleyer et al, 2010). Moreover, a cytolytic interleukin-2 and Fc fusion protein binding specifically to the interleukin-2 receptor is capable of suppressing induced diabetes in non-obese diabetic mice (Zheng et al., 1999). Co-administration of interleukin-2 and rapamycin to 10-week old non-obese diabetic mice synergistically prevents diabetes development for 13 weeks post therapy. Furthermore, the treatment could also synergistically protect transplanted syngeneic islet in diabetic non-obese diabetic mice most likely due to the decreasing numbers of leukocytes, which were associated with increasing apoptosis of these cells, and a shift from T helper-1 (pathogenic) to T helper-2 and T helper-3 (protective) lymphocytes (Rabinovitch et al., 2002).

It has been hypothesized that manipulating the levels of interleukin-2 or interleukin-15 available to activated effector and regulatory T cells may provide a means to govern the balance of cytopathic T cells and regulatory T cells *in vivo*. Interleukin-15 is a cytokine that can induce massive apoptosis of recently activated pathogenic cells but not regulatory T cells. The combined therapy of interleukin-2 and immunoglobin fusion protein, mutated interleukin-15 and immunoglobin fusion protein plus rapamycin restores euglycemic state in recent-onset diabetes, and prolongs transplanted syngeneic islet survival in diabetic non-obese diabetic mice. It also decreases inflammatory gene expression in pancreatic draining lymph nodes and other tissues (Koulmanda et al., 2007). Based on the results of these preclinical studies, the Immune Tolerance Network is conducting a trial of interleukin-2 and rapamycin in a Phase I clinical trial with new onset type 1 diabetic human patients starting 2007 (http://clinicaltrials.gov/ct2/show/NCT00525889).

In addition to interleukin-1, both tumor necrosis factor-alpha and interferon-gamma have a direct cytotoxic effect on beta cells, and are postulated to be a direct cause of pancreatic islet beta cell destruction. Nevertheless, tumor necrosis factor-alpha has a more complex role in diabetes progression, and sometime appears more like a regulating instead of a pathological molecule. Tumor necrosis factor-alpha may prevent development of insulitis and diabetes, and even the adoptive transfer of diabetes by lymphocytes into young non-obese diabetic mice (Jacob et al., 1990). Moreover, neutralization of tumor necrosis factor-alpha accelerated diabetes in older mice, but prevented disease at a younger age. Tumor necrosis factor-alpha or its agonists selectively kill autoreactive CD8, but not CD4 T cells derived from the blood of human type 1 diabetic patients (Ben et al, 2008). Most recently, a report from a small pilot trial (Phase I/II) of newly diagnosed pediatric patients found that administration of the soluble tumor necrotic factor receptor, etanercept, resulted in lower hemoglobin A1c level, and increased endogenous insulin production, suggesting preservation of beta-cell function in diabetic patients (Mastrandrea et al., 2009).

Interferon-alpha administered orally to non-obese diabetic mice caused decreased insulitis, increased mitogen-induced production of interleukin-4, interleukin-10 (T helper-2 like cytokines), and interferon-gamma secretion in splenocytes. The administered dose was 10 units daily from 9-week old, and suppressed diabetes from 100% diabetic mice in controls down to 10% in 24-week old mice. In addition, adoptive transfer of thirty million splenocytes intraperitoneally into 8-week old non-obese diabetic mice suppressed diabetes (Brod et al., 1998). In Phase I clinical trials of interferon-alpha, 10 newly diagnosed type 1 diabetic patients (ages 10-25, daily or every other day for 1 year) received an oral dose of 30,000 units of the cytokine within 1 month of diagnosis. The treatment induced at least a 30% increase in stimulated C-peptide levels at 0, 3, 6, 9, and 12 months compared to baseline (Brod et al., 2001). A phase I/II trial of safety and efficacy treated 31 new-onset patients (ages 3-25, daily for 1 year), and found that patients in the 5,000 units treatment group maintained increased beta-cell function 1 year after study enrollment compared with individuals in the placebo group (Rother et al., 2009a). In contrast, the effect was not observed in the 30,000 units treatment group.

Other cytokines, such as interleukin-4 and interleukin-10, have been reported to suppress type 1 diabetes at varying levels in animal models when delivered as part of a plasmid or virus vector (Wolfe et al., 2002; Goudy et al., 2001). Nonetheless, similar to antibodies, cytokine approaches are also systemic and associated with undesirable side-effects because of non-specificity *in vivo*.

4. Protein vaccine immunotherapies

It is now well established that loss of tolerance to beta-cell self-antigens, i.e., autoantigens, plays a determining role in the pathogenesis of type 1 diabetes. Autoantigens are self-molecules that become the target of the immune system under non-homeostatic conditions, which result from the combinations of genetic abnormalities with unknown environmental factors that ultimately lead to loss of immune tolerance for self-antigens. The autoantigens associated with type 1 diabetes covered in this chapter are heat shock protein 60, insulin, and glutamic acid decarboxylase 65, because they are therapeutic targets in ongoing clinical trials for type 1 diabetes. Nevertheless, there are others autoantigens like tyrosine phosphatase IA2, which is a target of humoral response in humans similar to insulin and glutamic acid decarboxylase 65, as well as the islet-specification efflux transporter znT8 and chromogranin A (Wenzlau et al., 2007; Stadinski et al., 2010), which will not be covered in this chapter.

The goal of autoantigen delivery as an immunotherapy is to re-establish at least some degree of immune tolerance activity for a target tissue to suppress pathological inflammation and ameliorate disease (Ludvigsson, 2009). This is not a new concept as it was used early in the 20th century to treat allergies to normally harmless foreign antigens (Krishna & Huissoon, 2011). In recent years, immunoregulatory vaccination, also sometimes referred to as "negative" or "inverse" vaccination, has become increasingly attractive as an immunotherapy principally because of the revival of the suppressor T cell concept, now named T regulatory cells. We know that T regulatory cells like $CD4^+CD25^+Foxp3^+$ cells that are natural, i.e., thymus derived, or adaptive, i.e., induced in the periphery, are fundamental for immune tolerance because deleterious mutations in the *Foxp3* gene causes systemic autoimmunity in both mice and humans (Mercer & Unutmaz, 2009). Accordingly, it is anticipated that approaches that modulate T regulatory cells activity will provide the means to mimic the immune system and finally control inflammation in a tissue specific manner. Two particularly apparent properties of T regulatory cells raise the hopes that development of T regulatory cells inducing immunoregulatory vaccines could lead to potent means of controlling inflammation (Tang & Bluestone, 2008). The first property is by-stander suppression, which is the capacity of T regulatory cells induced by a specific antigen to directly suppress effector cells induced by other antigens at the site of inflammation. The second property is infectious tolerance, which is the ability of a T regulatory cell clone to induce T regulatory cells of different antigen specificities. Therefore, T regulatory cells are naturally equipped to amplify in a targeted manner an immunoregulatory response induced by an immunoregulatory vaccine.

The first immunoregulatory vaccine to be successfully translated to the clinic was a peptide vaccine. Peptide vaccines are short polymers of amino acids derived from full-length proteins characterized as autoantigens. They are chosen based on their ability to bind as epitopes to major histocompatibility complex molecules on antigen-presenting cells. The bound peptide is then presented to the receptor of a restricted number of T lymphocytes, preferably T regulatory cells in the case of type 1 diabetes. The advantage of a peptide vaccine compared to the full-length parent protein is that it can focus the desired immune response by activating only a small number of T cell clones instead of multiple clones that may not be all relevant. The disadvantage of a peptide vaccine is that its activity will vary depending on the MHC molecules synthesized by a given individual. In this case, polypeptide vaccines are more advantageous because they ensure that all treated patients will present an epitope. Both peptide and polypeptide vaccines have been used with varying outcomes in type 1 diabetes.

4.1 Heat-shock protein 60 peptide vaccine (Diapep277)

Diapep277 was the first peptide vaccine successfully used in clinical trials for type 1 diabetes. Irun Cohen and colleagues identified peptide p277 derived from heat shock protein 60 and found that subcutaneous injection of 100 micrograms of the peptide in incomplete Freund's adjuvant inhibited the development of spontaneous diabetes in non-obese diabetic mice (Elias & Cohen, 1995). The main function of eukaryotic heat shock protein 60 is as a mitochondrial chaperone that assists in protein folding and translocation in the mitochondrial matrix (Fischer et al., 2010). From an immunological standpoint, mammalian heat shock proteins like HSP60 can also act as damage associated molecular patterns that are released or presented by dying cells and can activate antigen-presenting cells of the innate immune system (Chen et al., 1999). Heat shock proteins activate macrophages and dendritic cells through Toll-like receptor 4, which belongs to a class of membrane-bound proteins that act as sensors for immune cell activation, and promote proinflammatory effector immune responses. Paradoxically, heat shock proteins can also have T cell mediated anti-inflammatory effects through Toll-like receptor 2, and DiaPep277 peptide functions through a Toll-like receptor 2-mediated mechanism (Eldor et al., 2009).

Heat shock protein 60 has been found to be a possible autoantigen in type 1 diabetic children and murine models. It is found located on the membranes of the beta cell insulin secretary granules in pancreatic islets, and shares significant homology to bacterial heat shock protein 65. Epitope scanning of heat shock protein 60 with antibodies identified the peptide Diapep277 with the amino sequence VLGGGVALLRVIPALDSLTPANED as an immunodominant epitope in type 1 diabetic children (Brudzynski et al., 1992; Horváth et al., 2002).

As mentioned previously, in contrast with full-length heat shock protein 60, DiaPep277 has no effect on Toll-like receptor 4 and activates anti-inflammatory effectors through Toll-like receptor 2. Toll-like receptor 2 promotes cell adhesion, inhibits migration, and modulates cytokine secretion resulting in a deviation to a T helper-2 cytokine profile that is associated with a shift from an inflammatory to a regulatory response. Indeed, the peptide inhibits diabetes by shifting T cell responses from a T helper-1 to a T helper-2 like activity as indicated by the presence of pep277-specific antibodies of the IgG1, but not of the IgG2a isotype, and production of interleukin-4 and interleukin-10 in spleens of non-obese diabetic mice (Elias et al., 1997). The peptide also causes a decrease in the number of interferon-gamma producing islet T cells, which is concomitant with increased islet numbers and the arrest of type 1 diabetes when administered to 12-week old non-obese diabetic mice (Ablamunits et al., 1998). Moreover, the peptide induces islet protective T cells that can be adoptively transferred to protect non-obese diabetic-SCID mice from diabetes (Ablamunits et al., 1999).

Clinical trials of the peptide vaccine DiaPep277 have been ongoing and results have been reported since 2001. Patients were treated with 0.2, 1, and 2.5 mg doses of the peptide (Pfleger et al., 2010). The results showed that increased T helper-1 related cytokine responses (interferon-gamma) were associated with lower beta cell function whereas T helper-2 (interleukin-5, interleukin-13) and T regulatory activity (interleukin-10) related cytokine responses were positively associated with beta-cell function in adults and children. DiaPep277 also acts as an inhibitor of human T cells response. The signal transduction cascade induced by the p277 peptide involves suppression of both cytokine signaling 3 (SOCS3) expression and signal transducer and activator of transcription 3 (STAT3) (Zanin-Zhorov et al., 2005). This inhibition of T cell mediated inflammation by the peptide is due to down-regulation of T cell chemotaxis and reduced secretion of proinflammatory cytokines.

A randomized, double blind, phase Ib/II study of DiaPep277 tested its safety and efficacy, which was undertaken with recent onset type 1 diabetes patients with remaining insulin production (Huurman et al., 2007). Forty-eight adult patients were administered subcutaneous injections of 0.2, 1.0 or 2.5 mg DiaPep277 (12 patients per dosage) at entry, 1, 6, and 12 months, or they received four placebo injections (12 patients). C-peptide levels decreased in all groups with the exception of patients receiving the 2.5 mg dose, and decreased C-peptide production was attenuated in treated patients versus placebo. The main conclusion was that the treatment was safe, and may have a beneficial effect on C-peptide levels over time, although this was not supported by lower hemoglobin A1c levels as an indicator of diabetic control or daily insulin requirement.

Another phase II trial studies the effects of DiaPep277 in 2 stages (Lazar et al., 2007). In the first stage, 17 patients received four injections of 1 mg DiaPep277 at months 0, 1, 6, and 12, and 18-month, and preservation of endogenous insulin secretion was observed up to 18 months. In the second stage, which was only for those who completed stage 1 including placebo with C-peptide above 0.1 nmol/L, patients continued treatment with DiaPep277 (six patients, 1 mg DiaPep277 at months 0, 3, 6, and 9), and those switched from placebo to DiaPep277 (thirteen patients, 1 mg DiaPep277 at months 0, 3, 6, and 9) manifested a trend towards a greater preservation of beta-cell function compared to five patients maintained on and seven patients switched to placebo (Raz et al., 2007). Conversely, a trial with recent onset diabetic children (7-14 years old) showed no beneficial effect in preserving beta-cell function or improving metabolic control.

Phase III trials of DiaPep277 are currently ongoing. The first Phase III study has begun in 2005 in 40 centers worldwide (Fischer et al., 2010). The inclusion criteria include type 1 diabetes for less than 3 months, ages 16 - 45, and C-peptide > 0.22 nmol/L. The treatment regimen includes nine injections of 1 mg DiaPep277 or placebo over 21 months and 3 additional months of follow-up. At the end of recruitment in September 2009, 457 patients were randomly assigned to one of the groups and results are expected in September 2011. After an interim analysis, the Independent Data Monitoring Committee (IDMC) concluded that there were no safety concerns and that the study could be continued without modification. In addition, there is a clear treatment effect in different sub-group populations. Two additional phase III trials are ongoing and will end in August and December of 2013.

Immunological studies of the effects of DiaPep277 in human patients have revealed that the treatment is immunologically effective, specific and safe, when comparing T cell responses to specific antigen DiaPep277, related autoantigens heat shock protein 60, glutamic acid decarboxylase 65, and non-related third party antigen tetanus toxoid, between treatment and placebo (Huurman et al., 2008). Cytokine production in response to therapy was dominated by interleukin-10, and decreasing autoantigen specific T cell proliferation was associated with beta cell preservation. The investigators concluded that declining or temporary T cell proliferation in response to DiaPep277 may serve as an immunological biomarker for clinical efficacy.

4.2 Insulin peptide vaccines

Insulin is a hormone which is mainly responsible for regulating sugar and fat metabolism in the body. Insulin permits cells in the liver, muscle, and fat tissue to take up sugar from blood and store it as glycogen in the liver and muscle. Chronic high blood glucose, or hyperglycemia, can cause severe complications by damaging and impairing tissues via molecular mechanisms like protein glycosylation (Aronson, 2008). Since the onset of diabetes is the result of low levels of and ultimately no insulin secretion from pancreatic beta cells, injection of the insulin protein has been used as a replacement therapy to treat diabetes after its beneficial effects were discovered by Canadian scientists Frederick Grant Banting and Charles Best in 1921.

The current standard means of delivering insulin as replacement therapy is subcutaneous injection because of its lower cost and ease of self-delivery compared to other methods. Other routes such as oral administration and intramuscular injection are not chosen because of loss of insulin function in the digestive tract and rapid dispersion of the hormone, respectively. These limitations are not a concern when using insulin as a vaccine because only structural aspects of the molecule are needed, i.e., antigenicity instead of function.

Various clinical trials have been conducted to test whether delivering insulin protein as a vaccine via different delivery routes can prevent or ameliorate type 1 diabetes. The Diabetes Prevention Trial network (DPT-1) screened 103,391 healthy individuals who were under 45 years of age, islet antibody positive, and relatives of type 1 diabetic patients. Individuals at high risk of developing type 1 diabetes, i.e., at least 50% probability of developing type 1 diabetes within 5 years, received insulin both short-term intravenously and long-term subcutaneously (Schatz & Bingley 2001). In addition, individuals at moderate risk of developing type 1 diabetes, i.e., 25-50% probability of developing the disease within 5 years, received oral delivery of insulin. Results showed that subcutaneous injection of insulin did not slow type 1 diabetes onset, and that oral insulin did not delay or prevent the disease. Further studies of a subgroup with higher insulin autoantibody levels indicated that although oral insulin did not reduce insulin autoantibody levels, there was a possible delay in diabetic progression for approximately 4.5 years (Skyler et al., 2005, Barker et al., 2007). Accordingly, larger trials with more participants and similar standards of the oral insulin study are ongoing (Skyler 2008).

In addition to insulin polypeptide, the B:(9-23) B chain peptide or its altered form contains a major epitope recognized by the immune system and could delay or prevent diabetes when administered subcutaneously and intranasally in non-obese diabetic mice (Daniel & Wegmann, 1996; Kobayashi et al., 2007). A phase I/II clinical trial of insulin B-chain in incomplete Freund's adjuvant (IBC-VS01), i.e., non-inflammatory, was conducted using a single intramuscular injection in a small group (12 patients) with recently diagnosed type 1 diabetes (Orban et al., 2010). After two years, the patients developed robust insulin-specific humoral and T cell responses including insulin B-chain specific CD4 T regulatory cells, but did not show statistically different levels of C-peptide compared to the control group. Nevertheless, the results are meaningful because there is a growing body of evidence suggesting that autoimmunity observed in type 1 diabetes is the result of an imbalance between autoaggressive and regulatory cell subsets. Therefore, therapeutics that supplement or enhance the existing regulatory T cell subset could be beneficial.

Over the years, multiple studies have shown that mucosal administrations of insulin orally and intranasally retard development of autoimmune diabetes in the non-obese diabetic mice (Bergerot et al., 1994; Harrison et al., 1996). Accordingly, a trial using intranasal delivery of insulin (Humulin) to 38 children (median age 10.8 years) at risk for type 1 diabetes was undertaken as part of the Melbourne Pre-Diabetes Family Study in Australia (Harrison et al., 2004). The results suggested that intranasal insulin induced immune changes consistent with mucosal tolerance to insulin, and did not accelerate loss of β-cell function. Conversely, additional trials with 224 infant and 40 sibling relatives with HLA-DQB1 susceptibility allele genotypes and two or more autoantibodies at three university hospitals in Finland did not prevent or delay type 1 diabetes (Näntö-Salonen et al., 2008).

Altogether, results from these different clinical trials indicate that the pre-clinical success of insulin as an immunoregulatory vaccine in non-obese diabetic mice has not yet successfully translated in humans. Interestingly, evidence suggests that insulin may be the initiator autoantigen in type 1 diabetes, in other words, loss of tolerance to insulin could be the trigger of the disease (Harrison, 2008). Hypothetically, this loss of tolerance mechanisms for insulin could explain the difficulty in inducing tolerance in humans using therapeutic insulin vaccines. On the other hand, insulin may be a target of choice to prevent disease when mechanisms of tolerance to insulin are still in place in pre-diabetic individuals.

4.3 Glutamic acid decarboxylase 65 protein vaccine

In contrast with clinical trials using insulin polypeptide and peptide vaccines, the first human trials with glutamic acid decarboxylase 65 autoantigen as a therapeutic vaccine have shown beneficial therapeutic results (Ludvigsson & Linköping Diabetes Immune Intervention Study Group, 2009). Glutamic acid decarboxylase 65 is an enzyme that catalyzes the synthesis of gamma-aminobutyric acid (GABA), which acts as a neuroinhibitor as well as an immunoregulatory molecule. Several observations suggest that glutamic acid decarboxylase 65 may have a critical early role in mediating islet beta cell destruction. Detection of anti glutamic acid decarboxylase antibodies in the sera of prediabetic patients is a reliable predictive marker for the progression to overt diabetes, and anti glutamic acid decarboxylase reactivity can be detected in non-obese diabetic mice very early in the disease process (Ludvigsson & Linköping Diabetes Immune Intervention Study Group, 2009; Tisch et al., 1994).

Evidence for a role for the protein in disease etiology came from experiments reporting that delivery of glutamic acid decarboxylase 65 either intravenously or intrathymically into female non-obese prediabetic mice can prevent insulitis and diabetes (Kaufman et al., 1993; Tisch et al., 1993). Additional reports showed that intravenous delivery of glutamic acid decarboxylase 65 once every three days for a total of four injections of 200 micrograms from age 12-week can prevent diabetes from 70% in controls down to 20% in treated animals at week 35 through induction of glutamic acid decarboxylase 65 specific CD4 T regulatory cells (Tisch et al., 1998). Furthermore, injection of glutamic acid decarboxylase 65, but not heat shock protein pep277 or insulin B-chain, can increase survival of syngeneic islets transplanted into diabetic mice through modulation of T-helper 1/T-helper 2 balances (Tian et al, 1996).

The first results of phase I/II clinical trials using subcutaneous delivery of 4, 20, 100, and 500 micrograms of alum-formulated human recombinant glutamic acid decarboxylase 65 to eight patients with Latent Autoimmune Diabetes in Adults (LADA) were reported in 2005. Data showed that only the 20 microgram dose could increase both stimulated and fasting C-peptide levels and T regulatory cells from baseline over the 24-week period. A 5-year follow up study found that the 20 microgram dose, and to a lesser extent the 4 and 100 microgram doses, could maintain C-peptide levels compared to the placebo group (Agardh et al., 2005; Agardh et al., 2009).

In addition, seventy children and adolescents aged 10–18 years with recent onset type 1 diabetes participated in a phase II trial (Ludvigsson et al., 2011). Participants received either a subcutaneous injection of 20 microgram of the alum formulated glutamic acid decarboxylase 65, or placebo at baseline and 1 month later. Although there was no statistical significant differences in fasting C-peptide levels between the glutamic acid decarboxylase 65 and the placebo groups, those patients who were treated within 6 months of diabetes diagnosis had fasting C-peptide levels that decreased significantly less in the glutamic acid decarboxylase 65 group after 4 years compared with the placebo group. These results are significant because they indicate that, in contrast with Diapep277, glutamic acid decarboxylase vaccination is applicable to diabetic children who represent a large segment of the population with type 1 diabetes. However, in May 2011 it was reported that a European Phase III study with the antigen did not meet the primary efficacy endpoint of preserving beta cell function at 15 months, although a small positive effect was seen.

With regard to immune responses induced by alum-formulated glutamic acid decarboxylase 65 in human, a reduced percentage of IgG1 and increased IgG3/IgG4 antibodies were detected in treated children after 3 months, which suggested a T helper-2 deviation in the immune system. In addition, levels of IA-2A, IgE and tetanus toxoid antibodies as well as glutamic acid decarboxylase enzyme activity were unaffected, which suggested specificity of the treatment (Chéramy et al., 2010; Ortqvist et al., 2010). Importantly, injection of the glutamic acid decarboxylase 65 protein vaccine enhances the percentage of $CD4^{+}CD25^{high}FOXP3^{+}$ T regulatory cells, and induces secretion of interleukin-5, interleukin-

10, and interleukin-13 correlating with the expression of $CD4^{+}CD25^{high}FOXP3^{+}$ cells 21 to 30 months after treatment in 35 patients aged 10–18 years (Hjorth et al., 2011).
Vaccination with polypeptides/peptides to prevent and treat type 1 diabetes appears to be well-tolerated and safe in humans; however, the possibility of adverse events cannot be completely ignored. For example, insulin allergy occurs in less than 1% of diabetic patients treated with insulin peptide (Zhang et al., 2008). In these patients, different methods have been used for the treatment of insulin allergy including use of different insulin or insulin formulations. Allergic reactions range in severity from erythema and pruritus to life-threatening anaphylaxis. Indeed, vaccines inducing T helper-2 like responses can induce lethal anaphylaxis in non-obese mice (Overbergh et al., 2003, Pedotti et al., 2003), and may be less preferable compared to vaccines inducing regulatory cells like Foxp3 and T regulatory-1 T lymphocytes.

5. DNA vaccine based immunotherapies

DNA vaccines generally consist of bacterial plasmid DNA engineered to synthesize an antigen and other gene products after injection into a recipient. Compared to polypeptide/peptide vaccine immunotherapies, DNA vaccines bear several unique advantages, such as rapid development and standardized production, lower cost of storage, and synthesis over time of the chosen antigen in its native conformation.
The first DNA vaccines were designed to induce immunogenic responses to pathogens and cancer but have increasingly been applied to induce immune tolerance for autoimmune diseases like type 1 diabetes. DNA vaccines and other gene-based vaccines belong to a third generation of vaccines following live and attenuated whole organism vaccine and recombinant protein vaccines. Recent reports of beneficial results in different clinical trials indicate that DNA vaccination is reaching a stage where we are likely to see accelerated development of a therapeutic future of DNA vaccines for a variety of diseases. In the case of type 1 diabetes, early results using a DNA vaccine encoding insulin have shown promise in clinical trials, confirming the notion that DNA vaccines may be particularly well suited for promoting immune tolerance in humans compared to effects desired for infectious diseases and cancer. In addition, DNA vaccines encoding heat shock protein 60 or 65 and glutamic acid decarboxylase 65 have also shown efficacy in mice and are reviewed in this chapter.

5.1 Heat shock protein 60 or 65 DNA vaccines

As mentioned previously, Pep277 derived from mammalian heat shock protein 60 has shown protective effects in both pre-clinical and clinical trials. With regard to DNA vaccination, two 100 microgram intramuscular injections of plasmid DNA coding for mammalian heat shock protein 60 into 4-week old non-obese diabetic mice can prevent cyclophosphamide accelerated diabetes, i.e., 30% of treated mice develop diabetes compared with 60% diabetic in vector treated controls (Quintana et al., 2002). Disease prevention is associated with reduced T cell proliferation, an increase in interleukin-10 and interleukin-5 secretion, and a decrease in interferon-gamma secretion, which suggests a shift from a T helper-1 like toward a T helper-2 like immune response.
Furthermore, plasmid DNA encoding mycobacterial 65-kDalton heat shock protein caused decreased insulitis when injected intramuscularly in three doses (100 micrograms each) administered at 2-week intervals into 6- to 8-week-old, streptozotocin-induced diabetic C57BL/6 mice (Santos et al., 2009). The treatment was associated with the appearance of a

regulatory cell population in the spleen, with higher production of interleukin-10 in spleen and islets, and with a decreased infiltration of CD8 T lymphocytes in the islets. The same DNA vaccine with the same dose and delivery reduced the occurrence of diabetes from 100% to 33% in 28-week old non-obese diabetic mice when injected at 4-week of age, and was associated with a reduction in CD4 and CD8 T cells infiltration, appearance of CD25 cells, and increased levels of interleukin-10 in the islets (Santos et al., 2007).

5.2 Insulin DNA vaccines

Insulin-encoding plasmid DNA is the only type of DNA vaccine that has been tested in both preclinical and clinical trials for type 1 diabetes. The initial report demonstrating feasibility of this concept used a virus-induced diabetic mouse model system to show that intramuscular inoculation of plasmid DNA encoding the insulin B chain reduces the incidence of diabetes (blood glucose > 350 mg/dl) from 100 to 50% (Coon et al., 1999). DNA vaccination induced CD4 T regulatory cells that reacted with the insulin B chain, secreted interleukin-4, and locally reduced autoreactive activity of cytotoxic T lymphocytes in the pancreatic draining lymph nodes. The DNA vaccine also protected non-obese diabetic mice reducing diabetes onset from 80% down to 25% depending on the presence of interleukin-4 (Bot et al, 2001).

Rodent animals synthesize two isoforms of insulin, I in islets and II in both islets and thymus that are the products of non-allelic genes while humans have only one form of insulin. The pancreatic beta cells synthesize proinsulin before converting it to functional insulin (Sizonenko & Halban, 1991). Intranasal delivery of plasmid DNA encoding mouse proinsulin II (3 50 micrograms doses over a 2-week interval starting at 4 weeks of age) together with an anti-CD154 antibody (3 doses of 300 microgram over 2-week interval from 4 weeks of age) prevented type 1 diabetes by reducing the incidence in 40-week old mice from 100% diabetic animals down to 0%. On the other hand, intranasal delivery of the DNA vaccine alone did not prevent disease, but did induce regulatory T cells (Every et al., 2006). In contrast to prototypic $CD4^+$ $CD25^+$ T regulatory cells, the CD4 T regulatory cells induced by the proinsulin DNA vaccine alone were both $CD25^+$ and $CD25^-$, and were not defined by markers such as glucocorticoid-induced TNFR-related protein (GITR), CD103, or Foxp3.

Another report showed that co-delivery of a DNA vaccine encoding human proinsulin (50 microgram) and insulin peptide (100 microgram) intramuscularly twice over 2-week intervals starting when the mice were 6 weeks of age prevents diabetes in non-obese diabetic mice until 24 weeks of age, but not the DNA or peptide vaccine alone (Zhang et al., 2010). Results also indicated that the induction of transforming growth factor-beta producing $CD4^+CD25^-$ islet specific T regulatory cells was observed only in the co-immunization group, but not in the DNA or the protein vaccine alone group, which confirmed a synergistic effect.

Among the most promising reports of insulin DNA vaccination is a plasmid DNA vaccine encoding mouse proinsulin II, which reduces the incidence of diabetes in non-obese diabetic mice when administered intramuscularly to prediabetic 8-week old mice, and to diabetic mice older than 12-week old with blood glucose > 170 mg/dL (Solvason et al., 2008). The efficacy of the vaccine was improved by increasing the level of expression of insulin, frequency of dosing, dosage, and subcellular localization modification of the autoantigen to the intracellular compartment instead of secretion. In the prophylactic setting, the DNA vaccine decreased the incidence of diabetes from 80% in the control group down to 45% in 25-week old mice receiving weekly administration of 50

micrograms of the vaccine. The treatment caused increased numbers of interferon-gamma-secreting cells and a decrease in insulin autoantibodies. In the therapeutic setting, the DNA vaccine reduced progression to overt diabetes from 100% in the control groups down to 25% in treated mice (observation made at 25 weeks post treatment initiation). Treatment consisted of weekly delivery of 50 microgram of the vaccine for a total of 9 injections. The treatment induced increased numbers of insulin-specific interferon-gamma-producing T cells and levels of interleukin-10, which suggested induction of T regulatory-1 cells. Adoptive transfer experiments indicated that the protection was not mediated by induction of $CD4^{+}CD25^{+}$ T regulatory cells.
Importantly, a similar vaccine was used in the only human trial of a DNA vaccine for diabetes conducted to date (Gottlieb et al., 2008). The plasmid DNA vaccine (BHT-3021) has undergone a Phase I/II trial using four doses of plasmid DNA, i.e., 0.3, 1, 3 and 6 milligrams, administered intramuscularly once a week for 12 weeks. The interim results for the 1 mg dose showed pancreatic beta-cell preservation, demonstrated by a mean 17% increase in C-peptide levels with BHT-3021 by week 15 after enrollment, whereas placebo patients experienced a mean 42% decrease in C-peptide. Evidence for immune tolerance was suggested by a mean 17% reduction in anti-insulin antibodies, and 25% reduction in anti-glutamic acid decarboxylase 65 antibodies by week 15 after enrollment, whereas placebo patients experienced a mean 6% and 4% increase, respectively. The most recent report of the trial claimed that BHT-3021 preserves C-peptide levels for at least six months and one year in some of the patients from the point of initiation of the therapy (Garren, 2009). These results together with its favorable side-effects profile appear to be comparable to those reported with anti-CD3 monoclonal antibody and the glutamic acid decarboxylase 65 protein vaccines for type 1 diabetes.

5.3 Glutamic acid decarboxylase DNA vaccines

DNA vaccines encoding glutamic acid decarboxylase 65 are currently at the preclinical stage. The first report of a beneficial effect in non-obese diabetic mice showed that plasmid DNA encoding wild-type intracellular or engineered secreted glutamic acid decarboxylase, i.e., a fusion of the interleukin-2 signal peptide with a truncated form of human glutamic acid decarboxylase 65, causes decreased insulitis compared to plasmid vector alone when delivered intramuscularly, and is accompanied by higher secretion of interleukin-4 by splenocytes (Liu et al., 1999). A subsequent report indicated that only the DNA vaccine encoding secreted glutamic acid decarboxylase could suppress cyclophosphamide-accelerated diabetes in 4-week old female non-obese diabetic mice with a tendency to increase T helper-2 like activity when 2 x 400 micrograms were delivered intramuscularly over 2 days (Filippova et al., 2001).
Another report published the same year corroborated the notion that secretion of glutamic acid decarboxylase encoded by a DNA vaccine is important to ameliorate diabetes in mice (Weaver et al., 2001). In this report, plasmid DNA was engineered to encode a secreted fusion protein of a truncated form of glutamic acid decarboxylase 65 and an IgG Fc fragment as well as interleukin-4. Intramuscular injection of 50 micrograms of the vaccine effectively prevented diabetes in non-obese diabetic mice treated at early (4-week old, 3 times weekly) or late (12-week old, 4 times weekly) preclinical stages of diabetes. Diabetic onset reduction went from 75% in controls down to 25% at week 50+ and from 70% to 20% at week 55+. Protection was dependent on the vaccine-encoded interleukin-4 and endogenous interleukin-4, and was associated with induction of glutamic acid decarboxylase 65 specific

regulatory T helper-2 cells (Tisch et al., 2001). However, when the same vaccination strategy was applied using insulin, the vaccine encoding insulin B chain/IgG Fc fusion protein and interleukin-4 caused accelerated progression of insulitis and diabetes, which was correlated with an increased number of interferon-gamma secreting T cells in response to insulin B chain specific peptides (Weaver et al., 2001).

In addition, a study reported that a DNA vaccine encoding full-length intracellular human glutamic acid decarboxylase 65 could prevent spontaneous diabetes when delivered at week 4 or week 10 of age using intramuscular injection of 2 x 50 micrograms in non-obese diabetic mice (Balasa et al., 2001). Notably, disease prevention was associated with CD28/B7 costimulation because co-expression of B7-1 or B7-2 and glutamic acid decarboxylase 65 by the same DNA vaccine abrogated protection.

With regard to DNA vaccination and the effects of interleukin-4, a virus-induced murine diabetes model was used to study the relationship between different endogenous expression levels of islet autoantigen in beta-cells and the efficacy of DNA vaccination (Wolfe et al., 2002). Lower expression levels of a model autoantigen in beta-cells support immune regulation resulting in induction of autosuppressive regulatory cells characterized by increased interleukin-4 production (T helper-2 like). In contrast, higher levels of the autoantigen favor T helper-1 like autoaggressive responses characterized by increase interferon-gamma generation. Immunization with a DNA vaccine coding the autoantigen and interleukin-4 reduced the risk of augmenting autoaggression and thus increased the safety margin of this immune-based therapy.

DNA vaccines encoding secreted glutamic acid decarboxylase and anti-inflammatory interleukins have also been applied to transplantation for type 1 diabetes. Survival of syngeneic neonatal pancreata transplanted under the kidney capsule of non-obese diabetic mice is promoted by intramuscular injection of a DNA vaccine encoding the secreted glutamic acid decarboxylase 65/IgG Fc fusion and interleukin-4 plus interleukin-10 (Seifarth et al., 2003). The treatment consisted of 50 micrograms of the vaccine delivered weekly for four weeks from the age of 10 weeks with transplantation performed one week after the final DNA vaccination. The DNA vaccination protected the syngeneic islet transplanted mice from 100% diabetic mice in controls down to 20% diabetes incidence in treated animals at 30 weeks of age, 15 weeks post transplant, but required co-delivery of both interleukin-4 and interleukin-10. Increased islet survival correlated with a marked reduction in interferon-gamma reactivity that is glutamic acid decarboxylase 65 specific, and an increase in interleukin-10-secreting T cells. These results made apparent the increased difficulty in protecting exogenous syngeneic islet compared with endogenous islets, and the need for more stringent conditions of vaccination in the transplantation setting.

Intramuscular injection has traditionally been used for DNA vaccination because it permits delivery of larger amounts of DNA, and is commonly used in the clinic. Nonetheless, other routes of delivery may be more advantageous to induce tolerogenic responses. A report compared intramuscular, intradermal, and oral delivery of plasmid DNA coding for the intracellular or secreted form of glutamic acid decarboxylase for prevention of diabetes in a 4-week-old non-obese diabetic mouse model system (Li & Escher, 2003). Results showed that both intradermal and oral deliveries were more effective than intramuscular delivery for delaying the disease, and cytokine-specific ELISpot analysis indicated that immune responses induced by the DNA vaccines were more dependent on the cellular localization of glutamic acid decarboxylase antigen than on the delivery route. In contrast, ELISA indicated that intradermal delivery of DNA was most likely to induce a T helper-2 like response.

In addition to route of delivery, the method used to administer a DNA vaccine can be beneficial by directly improving immune responses and permitting lower vaccine dosage. For example, dermal delivery of plasmid DNA using gene gun technology, which consists in shooting microscopic metal particles covered with the vaccine, can improve protection from diabetes. In this regard, gene-gun delivery of 1 microgram of a DNA vaccine encoding the secreted glutamic acid decarboxylase 65/IgG Fc fusion polypeptide into 10-week old non-obese diabetic mice was compared with intramuscular injection of 50 micrograms of the same vaccine (Goudy et al., 2008). Results showed that in both cases gene expression peaked at week 8 post deliveries, and was maintained until at least week 35 with more than 40% higher expression from the gene-gun delivery. However, only gene-gun delivery could protect from diabetes with 90% diabetic in controls down to 50% diabetic at 35 weeks of age that was associated with induction of interleukin-4 secreting CD4 T cells. In contrast, intradermal gene-gun administration of plasmid-DNA encoding intracellular glutamic acid decarboxylase 65 to 3-week old non-obese diabetic mice does not suppress diabetes in non-obese diabetic mice (Joussemet et al., 2005). The different results might be attributed to the different subcellular localizations of the autoantigen.

So far in this section we have described how DNA vaccines can be engineered to enhance tolerogenic-like immune responses by co-delivering cytokine-encoding DNA, engineering subcellular localization of a target autoantigen, and choosing an effective route and method of delivery. The results obtained by different laboratories illustrate the promising potential of DNA vaccination as a safe, low-cost and patient-friendly means to treat autoimmune diabetes and other immune-mediated inflammatory disorders. Yet, as with all immunotherapies that seek safe means of improving the life of diabetic individuals, there is a pressing need to improve treatment efficacy. We strongly believe that one of the solutions to this problem is to mimic how the immune system maintains immune tolerance in peripheral tissues. DNA vaccination is particularly well-suited to achieve this goal because of the ability of plasmid DNA to deliver genetic instructions directly *in situ* for a limited time span and with low levels of danger signals known to activate proinflammatory immune responses. Here, we briefly discuss vaccine-induced apoptosis as a possible means to mimic physiological immune tolerance and to approach the "Holy Grail" of immunotherapy, namely, the ability to suppress inflammation in a homeostatic manner (**Figure 3**).

Apoptosis is a constantly on-going form of cell death that produces fifty to seventy billion dead cells on a daily basis in the average human adult (Reed, 1999). Upon a given intrinsic or extrinsic signal, cells initiate the process of apoptosis and become membrane-bound cellular fragments, or apoptotic bodies, which are rapidly engulfed and processed by surrounding living cells. For many years it was believed that these apoptotic bodies had little effect on the immune system. Today, it is becoming increasingly clear that apoptotic cells play a fundamental role in both establishing and maintaining peripheral immune tolerance as they not only serve as a source of self-antigens to maintain immune tolerance, but also recruit antigen-presenting cells, secrete anti-inflammatory cytokines, and display tolerogenic molecules (Birge and Ucker, 2008). The remarkable capacity of apoptotic cells to induce either tolerogenic immune responses or immunogenic responses depending on signals received makes them attractive candidates to intervene in many disorders like infectious diseases, cancer, and autoimmune diseases.

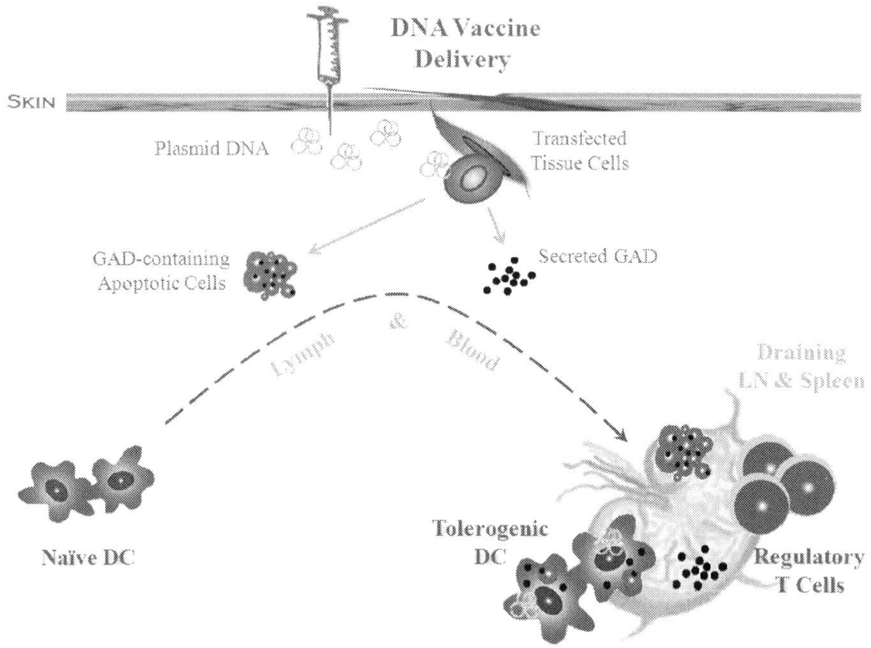

Fig. 3. **Possible events following intradermal injection of a pro-apoptotic DNA vaccine coding for secreted pancreatic autoantigen glutamic acid decarboxylase (GAD).** The plasmid DNA vaccine can transfect a variety of cell types at the chosen site of vaccine delivery, e.g., fibroblasts and keratinocytes in the case of intradermal injection. Dendritic cells (DC) recruited by vaccine-induced apoptotic cells can uptake and process GAD-containing apoptotic cells induced by the vaccine as well as vaccine-encoded secreted GAD, and present GAD on major histocompatibility complex class I and II molecules. The dendritic cells then migrate to lymph nodes and spleen where they can induce tolerogenic immune responses.

An important feature of pro-apoptotic DNA vaccination is that it permits the manipulation of physiological apoptosis both *de novo* and *in situ*. This is important because apoptotic cells synthesize a variety of immune molecules with levels that are most likely physiologically relevant in the context of a microenvironment. The concept of immunological microenvironment is also crucial to immune responses induced by dendritic cells, which are equipped to sense and act upon changes in their immediate vicinity. Therefore, induction of apoptosis by DNA vaccination could be a way to have access to homeostasis and maintain non-responsiveness to self.

The first report of DNA vaccines designed for pro-apoptotic immunoregulation, i.e., anti-inflammatory, used plasmid DNA coding for the pro-apoptotic BAX protein and intracellular or secreted glutamic acid decarboxylase, to prevent diabetes in the non-obese diabetic mouse (Li et al., 2004). Results indicated that intramuscular injection of the BAX cDNA recruited dendritic cells carrying vaccine-encoded protein in both spleen and lymph nodes. Furthermore, delivery of 2 x 150 micrograms plasmid DNA coding for secreted glutamic acid decarboxylase and BAX at a 3 days interval into 4-week old mice could prevent diabetes, i.e, reduce the incidence from 93% in controls down to 47% in treated animals. In contrast, the vaccines coding for BAX or secreted glutamic acid decarboxylase DNA alone or intracellular glutamic acid decarboxylase and BAX did not prevent diabetes. Notably, ELISA results indicated that co-delivery of BAX suppressed T helper-2 like activity which indicated that another cell type was responsible for disease suppression. Indeed, a subsequent report showed that delivery of both secreted glutamic acid decarboxylase and BAX were required to induce $CD4^+CD25^+FoxP3^+$ cells with contact dependent regulatory activity that was independent of transforming growth factor-beta and interleukin-10 (Li et al., 2006).

Importantly, additional studies revealed that increased CpG methylation of the DNA vaccine together with delivery of secreted glutamic acid decarboxylase and BAX DNA acted synergistically to ameliorate recent onset of diabetes in non-obese diabetic mice (Li et al., 2010). Mice receiving a weekly intradermal injection of 50 micrograms of the vaccine over eight weeks following early diabetes ameliorated diabetes from 90% diabetic in controls down to 20% in treated mice at 40 weeks of age. It is hypothesized that increased CpG methylation of plasmid DNA makes the DNA vaccine appear more mammalian-like to the immune system, as it is known that bacterial DNA has low levels of CpG methylation that can act as an inflammatory signal (Krieg, 2002). Taken together these results indicate that apoptosis-inducing DNA vaccination is a promising approach for treatment of type 1 diabetes.

5.4 Comparing DNA vaccines and polypeptide/peptide vaccines

Compared to polypeptide/peptide vaccine, the main advantages of DNA vaccines are: 1) known process of manufacturing, i.e., plasmid DNA can be isolated using a standard procedure while different polypeptides may require different protocols that have to be optimized for a specific antigen; 2) Cost-effective shipment and storage because plasmid DNA does not require refrigeration; 3) A more sustained expression of the antigen in its native conformation, or shape, instead of a purified antigen that can adopt different non-native conformations; and 4) Expression of the whole protein rather than specific epitopes in the case of peptides to ensure delivery of full antigenic signals that can be recognized by different major histocompatibility complex molecules in an outbred human population.

6. Other immunotherapies

There are currently other ongoing immunotherapies, such as the applications of Bacille Calmette-Guérin (BCG), Vitamin D3, nicotinamide, immunosuppressants, nanoparticles, and antisense oligonucleotides, etc., which have certain effects in suppressing type 1 diabetes in non-obese diabetic mice. Bacille Calmette-Guérin is a vaccine that is prepared from a strain of attenuated live bovine tuberculosis bacillus that has lost its virulence in human, which has been used as a vaccine to prevent tuberculosis. Although it has shown efficacy in animal models, clinical trials in recent onset diabetic children have been disappointing (Elliott et al., 1998; Allen et al., 1999).

Several clinical trials of vitamin D3 have been conducted since the 1990s, and results showed either temporary effects (Pitocco et al., 2006; Li et al., 2009), or no effects (Walter et al., 2010;

Bizzarri et al., 2010) on protecting pancreatic beta-cell function in child or adult type 1 diabetic patients.

Nicotinamide is a molecule belonging to the vitamin B group, i.e., vitamin B3, and has anti-inflammatory effects *in vivo*. The first report of clinical trials on type 1 diabetes was published in the mid 1980s (Vague et al., 1987), followed by multiple trials conducted worldwide with complex results. When using 25 mg/kg or 1.2 g/m^2 body surface/day of the vitamin B, most of the recent reports showed that nicotinamide has no protective effect on type 1 diabetes in new-onset patients or high-risk relatives (Pitocco et al., 2006; Skyler, 2008), even though it induces decreased spontaneous and *in vitro* autoantigen-induced interferon-gamma secretion in high-risk relatives who develop type 1 diabetes and may play a role in immune regulation (Hedman et al., 2006). Only one of the reports showed that nicotinamide treatment results in higher C-peptide values at 3 months and lower insulin requirement at 1 year in pancreatic interleukin-2 accumulated diabetic patients post 1 year treatment (Chianelli et al., 2008).

The immunosuppressant cyclosporin A was employed in the first trials showing effects of immune therapies on T1D. Continuous cyclosporin A treatment initiated soon after diagnosis eliminated the need for exogenous insulin (Bougneres et al., 1988; Stiller et al., 1984). Nevertheless, the lack of lasting effects and renal toxicity of the drug diminished enthusiasm for this approach and other broad-spectrum immune modulating agents such as azathioprine and prednisone (Bougneres et al., 1990; Silverstein et al., 1988).

The Major Histocompatibility Complex (MHC) genomic region is found in most vertebrates and encodes protein molecules playing an important role in immunity and recognition of antigens by T cells. It has been shown that nanoparticles loaded with diabetes relevant peptide-major histocompatibility complexes prevent and treat diabetes when administered intravenously in non-obese diabetic mice (Tsai et al., 2010). The treatment prevented diabetes from 75% in control down to 25% in 30-week-old non-obese diabetic mice (4-week old mice received 7.5 mg every 2 weeks until the 3rd injection and every 3 weeks thereafter), and restored normoglycemia in diabetic mice (blood glucose higher than 11 mM mice received 7.5 mg twice a week for 5 week). The treatment expanded CD8+ regulatory T cells which suppressed local presentation of autoantigens in an interferon-gamma, indoleamine 2,3-dioxygenase, and perforin dependent manner. Furthermore, adoptive transfer of CD8+ but not CD4+ splenocytes suppressed diabetes and restored normoglycemia in a humanized diabetic mouse model.

Antisense oligonucleotides are single strands of DNA or RNA that are complementary to chosen sequences of target messenger RNAs. Antisense DNA oligonucleotides for messenger RNAs coding for CD40, CD80, and CD86 were delivered subcutaneously into 5- to 8-week old non-obese diabetic mice using 50 micrograms of a 1:1:1 mixture of each antisense oligonucleotides administered weekly for eight consecutive weeks (Phillips et al., 2008). The treatment prevented disease in 25 % of mice compared to 100 % diabetes in control animals. A similar treatment was given to diabetic mice with blood glucose higher than 300 mg/dL three times a week maintained blood glucose lower than 200 mg/dl for 50+ days compared to higher than 200 mg/dL in control mice. The treatment decreased CD40, CD80, and CD86 cell surface expressions on dendritic cells in spleen, and augmented Foxp3$^+$ T regulatory cells numbers with hyporesponsiveness to self-antigen but not to alloantigen. In addition, spleen T-cells adoptive transfer from treated mice could suppress diabetes, confirming the induction of regulatory T cell activity.

7. Combinatorial approaches - the future of immunotherapy?

Combination immunotherapies are increasingly being considered, since none of the immunotherapies alone have reported thus far long term remission of type 1 diabetes (Li et al., 2008; Luo et al., 2010; Bluestone et al., 2010). This is especially true in view of the announcements in 2011 of failure of the anti-CD3 and glutamic acid decarboxylase protein vaccine therapeutic phase III trials for type 1 diabetic patients. Type 1 diabetes is an autoimmune disease correlated with multiple autoantigens and autoantibodies, and possible dysfunction in several cell types and associated cytokines. Therefore it is reasonable to anticipate a variety of synergistic effects that may be induced by combination therapies, as demonstrated in animal model systems. For example, a novel combination treatment with anti-CD3 epsilon specific antibody and intranasal delivery of proinsulin peptide can reverse recent onset diabetes in non-obese diabetic mice and a virus-induced diabetic mouse model with much higher efficacy than with monotherapy using anti-CD3 or the peptide alone (Bresson et al., 2006). Protection is associated with expansion of $CD25^+$ $Foxp3^+$ and insulin specific T regulatory cells producing cytokines, such as interleukin-10, transforming growth factor-beta, and interleukin-4. In addition, these cells can transfer dominant tolerance to immunocompetent recent onset diabetic recipients, and suppress heterologous autoaggressive CD8 T cell responses.

As mentioned previously, another synergistic effect was reported with prime boosting using DNA vaccine encoding proinsulin plus insulin protein vaccine to prevent new onset diabetes in non-obese diabetic mice. The induction of the transforming growth factor-beta producing $CD4^+CD25^-$ islet specific T regulatory cells against the onset of diabetes was observed only in the combination therapeutic group, but not in the monotherapy groups (Zhang et al., 2010).

Standard clinical complex therapeutic protocol for controlling allo organ transplant rejection may be used as an example of combinatorial therapy where various drugs can be used in combination or alone at different times to increase allograft survival. Single therapy alone has its limits, ranging from targeting a single arm of the immune process, lower efficacy, and higher possible adverse effect due to higher dose requirement. Combination therapies could be used to overcome these problems. The combinations could include antibody or cytokine therapy combined with polypeptide/peptide and DNA vaccine, DNA vaccination combined with polypeptide/peptide vaccine and cellular therapy, as well as other combinations (**Figure 4**).

Considering the number of approaches that have been developed for the treatment of type 1 diabetes over the years, there is a significant number of possible combinations of different therapies. Yet we cannot exclude the possibility that platform technologies that provide access to a wide array of possible gene-based therapeutic enhancements could still perform satisfactorily on their own at lower cost. Our work with pro-apoptotic DNA vaccination does indicate that combining different properties of DNA vaccines alone can result in potent synergistic effects (Li et al., 2010). In addition, different combinations of autoantigens and vaccine technologies could still yield significant therapeutic improvements in the clinic. For example, the fact that GAD65 polypeptide appears to be a better therapeutic vaccine than insulin polypeptide/peptide vaccines combined with the promising results of the DNA vaccine encoding pro-insulin suggests the possibility that GAD65 might be a better autoantigen than insulin for therapy of T1D, and that plasmid DNA could improve efficacy of vaccination compared to an equivalent protein vaccine. Therefore, a DNA vaccine coding for GAD65 could be particularly beneficial for treatment of T1D.

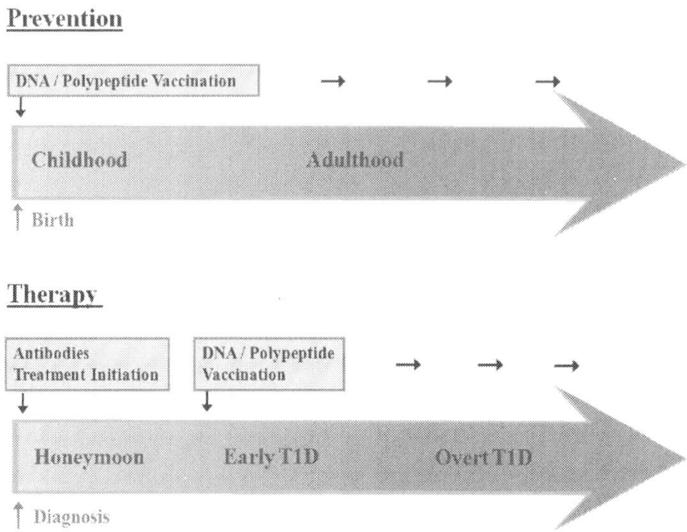

Fig. 4. **Hypothetic Models of Combinatorial Immunotherapies for Type 1 Diabetes**. Because of their increased safety compared to other approaches, antigen-based vaccines are the most likely to be applied to type 1 diabetes prevention. Combinatorial approaches for disease prevention could use prime-boosting with DNA and polypeptide vaccines. A body of evidence has shown the beneficial effects of this type of approach for infectious diseases and cancer, and initial results suggest that it is also applicable to type 1 diabetes. Antibodies like anti-CD3 may not be readily applicable to diabetes prevention for reasons of safety and efficacy, but could be used as induction therapy followed by prime-boost with DNA/polypeptide vaccines.

Clearly, the immunotherapeutic tools that have been generated over the past decade offer renewed hope for type 1 diabetic patients, as well as for the increasing number of individuals suffering from other chronic inflammatory disorders. We expect that in the near future, the development of novel therapeutic and preventive approaches, novel methods of delivery, and a better understanding of immunological mechanisms translated from animal models to human clinical studies and practices, will render the possibility of immunotherapy for type 1 diabetes a clinical reality.

8. References

Ablamunits V, Elias D, Cohen IR. (1999). The pathogenicity of islet-infiltrating lymphocytes in the non-obese diabetic (NOD) mouse. *Clinical and experimental immunology*. Vol.115(No.2): 260-7.

Ablamunits V, Elias D, Reshef T, Cohen IR. (1998). Islet T cells secreting IFN-gamma in NOD mouse diabetes: arrest by p277 peptide treatment. *Journal of Autoimmunity*. Vol.11(No.1): 73-81.

Agardh CD, Cilio CM, Lethagen A, Lynch K, Leslie RD, Palmér M, Harris RA, Robertson JA, Lernmark A. (2005). Clinical evidence for the safety of GAD65 immunomodulation in adult-onset autoimmune diabetes. *Journal of diabetes and its complications*. Vol.19(No.4): 238-46.

Agardh CD, Lynch KF, Palmér M, Link K, Lernmark A. (2009). GAD65 vaccination: 5 years of follow-up in a randomised dose-escalating study in adult-onset autoimmune diabetes. *Diabetologia*. Vol.52(No.7): 1363-8.

Allen HF, Klingensmith GJ, Jensen P, Simoes E, Hayward A, Chase HP. (1999). Effect of Bacillus Calmette-Guerin vaccination on new-onset type 1 diabetes. A randomized clinical study. *Diabetes Care*. Vol.22(No.10): 1703-7.

Aronson D. (2008). Hyperglycemia and the pathobiology of diabetic complications. *Advances in Cardiology*. Vol.45: 1-16.

Balasa B, Boehm BO, Fortnagel A, Karges W, Van Gunst K, Jung N, Camacho SA, Webb SR, Sarvetnick N. (2001). Vaccination with glutamic acid decarboxylase plasmid DNA protects mice from spontaneous autoimmune diabetes and B7/CD28 costimulation circumvents that protection. *Clinical Immunology*. Vol.99(No. 2): 241-52.

Ban L, Zhang J, Wang L, Kuhtreiber W, Burger D, Faustman DL. (2008). Selective death of autoreactive T cells in human diabetes by TNF or TNF receptor 2 agonism. *Proceedings of the National Academy of Sciences of the United States of America*. Vol.105(No.36): 13644-9.

Barker JM, McFann KK, Orban T. (2007). Effect of oral insulin on insulin autoantibody levels in the Diabetes Prevention Trial Type 1 oral insulin study. *Diabetologia*. Vol.50(No.8): 1603-6.

Bergerot I, Fabien N, Baguer V, Thivolet C. (1994) Oral administration of human insulin to NOD mice generates CD4 T cells that suppress adoptive transfer of diabetes. *Journal of Autoimmunity*. Vol.7(No.5): 655–663.

Bizzarri C, Pitocco D, Napoli N, Di Stasio E, Maggi D, Manfrini S, Suraci C, Cavallo MG, Cappa M, Ghirlanda G, Pozzilli P; IMDIAB Group. (2010). No protective effect of calcitriol on beta-cell function in recent-onset type 1 diabetes: the IMDIAB XIII trial. *Diabetes Care*. Vol.33(No.9): 1962-3.

Bluestone JA, Herold K, Eisenbarth G. (2010). Genetics, pathogenesis and clinical interventions in type 1 diabetes. *Nature*. Vol.464(No.7293): 1293-300.

Bot A, Smith D, Bot S, Hughes A, Wolfe T, Wang L, Woods C, von Herrath M. (2001). Plasmid vaccination with insulin B chain prevents autoimmune diabetes in nonobese diabetic mice. *Journal of immunology*. Vol.167(No.5): 2950-5.

Bougneres PF, Carel JC, Castano L, Boitard C, Gardin JP, Landais P, Hors J, Mihatsch MJ, Paillard M, Chaussain JL, et al. (1988). Factors associated with early remission of type I diabetes in children treated with cyclosporine. *New England Journal of Medicine*. Vol.318(No.11): 663-70.

Bougnères PF, Landais P, Boisson C, Carel JC, Frament N, Boitard C, Chaussain JL, Bach JF. (1990). Limited duration of remission of insulin dependency in children with recent overt type I diabetes treated with low-dose cyclosporin. *Diabetes*. Vol.39(No.10): 1264-72.

Bresson D, Togher L, Rodrigo E, Chen Y, Bluestone JA, Herold KC, and von Herrath M. (2006). Anti-CD3 and nasal proinsulin combination therapy enhances remission from recent-onset autoimmune diabetes by inducing Tregs. *Journal of Clinical Investigation*. Vol.116(No.5): 1371-81.

Bresson D, von Herrath MG. (2011). Anti-thymoglobulin (ATG) treatment does not reverse type 1 diabetes in the acute virally induced rat insulin promoter-lymphocytic choriomeningitis virus (RIP-LCMV) model. *Clinical and Experimental Immunology*. Vol.163(No.3): 375-80.

Birge RB, Ucker DS. (2008). Innate apoptotic immunity: the calming touch of death. *Cell Death and Differentiation*. Vol.15(No.7): 1096-102.

Brod SA, Atkinson M, Lavis VR, Brosnan PG, Hardin DS, Orlander PR, Nguyen M, Riley WJ. (2001). Ingested IFN-alpha preserves residual beta cell function in type 1 diabetes. *Journal of Interferon Cytokine Research*. Vol.21(No.12): 1021-30.

Brod SA, Malone M, Darcan S, Papolla M, Nelson L. (1998). Ingested interferon alpha suppresses type I diabetes in non-obese diabetic mice. *Diabetologia*. Vol.41(No.10): 1227-32.

Brudzynski K, Martinez V, Gupta RS. (1992). Secretory granule autoantigen in insulin-dependent diabetes mellitus is related to 62 kDa heat-shock protein (hsp60). *Journal of Autoimmunity*. Vol.5(No.4): 453-63.

Brusko TM, Koya RC, Zhu S, Lee MR, Putnam AL, McClymont SA, Nishimura MI, Han S, Chang LJ, Atkinson MA, Ribas A, Bluestone JA. (2010). Human antigen-specific regulatory T cells generated by T cell receptor gene transfer. *Public Library of Science one*. Vol.5(No.7): e11726.

Chatenoud L, Thervet E, Primo J, Bach JF. (1994). Anti-CD3 antibody induces long-term remission of overt autoimmunity in nonobese diabetic mice. *Proceedings of the National Academy of Sciences of the United States of America*. Vol.91(No.1): 123-7.

Chatenoud L, Primo J, Bach JF. (1997). CD3 antibody-induced dominant self tolerance in overtly diabetic NOD mice. *Journal of immunology*. Vol.158(No.6): 2947-54.

Chen W, Syldath U, Bellmann K, Burkart V, Kolb H. (1999). Human 60-kDa heat-shock protein: a danger signal to the innate immune system. *Journal of Immunology*. Vol.162(No.6): 3212-9.

Chéramy M, Skoglund C, Johansson I, Ludvigsson J, Hampe CS, Casas R. (2010). GAD-alum treatment in patients with type 1 diabetes and the subsequent effect on GADA IgG subclass distribution, GAD65 enzyme activity and humoral response. Clinical Immunology. Vol.137(No.1): 31-40.

Chianelli M, Parisella MG, Visalli N, Mather SJ, D'Alessandria C, Pozzilli P, Signore A; IMDIAB study group. (2008). Pancreatic scintigraphy with 99mTc-interleukin-2 at diagnosis of type 1 diabetes and after 1 year of nicotinamide therapy. *Diabetes/Metabolism Research and Reviews*. Vol.24(No.2): 115-22.

Coon B, An LL, Whitton JL, von Herrath MG. (1999). DNA immunization to prevent autoimmune diabetes. *Journal of Clinical Investigation*. Vol.104(No.2): 189-94.

d'Hennezel E, Kornete M, Piccirillo CA. (2010). IL-2 as a therapeutic target for the restoration of Foxp3+ regulatory T cell function in organ-specific autoimmunity: implications in pathophysiology and translation to human disease. *Journal of translational medicine*. Vol.8: 113.

Daniel D, Wegmann DR. (1996). Protection of nonobese diabetic mice from diabetes by intranasal or subcutaneous administration of insulin peptide B-(9–23). *Proceedings of the National Academy of Sciences of the United States of America*. Vol.93(No.2): 956–960.

Donath MY, Mandrup-Poulsen T. (2008). The use of interleukin-1-receptor antagonists in the treatment of diabetes mellitus. *Nature Clinical Practice. Endocrinology & Metabolism*. Vol.4(No.5): 240-1.

Egan CA, Brown M, White JD, Yancey KB. (2001). Treatment of epidermolysis bullosa acquisita with the humanized anti-Tac mAb daclizumab. *Clinical Immunology*. Vol.101(No.2): 146-51.

Eldor R, Kassem S, Raz I. (2009). Immune modulation in type 1 diabetes mellitus using DiaPep277: a short review and update of recent clinical trial results. *Diabetes/Metabolism Research and Reviews*. Vol.25(No.4): 316-20.

Elias D, Cohen IR. (1995). Treatment of autoimmune diabetes and insulitis in NOD mice with heat shock protein 60 peptide p277. *Diabetes*. Vol.44(No.9): 1132-8.

Elias D, Meilin A, Ablamunits V, Birk OS, Carmi P, Könen-Waisman S, Cohen IR. (1997). Hsp60 peptide therapy of NOD mouse diabetes induces a Th2 cytokine burst and downregulates autoimmunity to various beta-cell antigens. Diabetes. Vol.46(No.5): 758-64.

Elliott JF, Marlin KL, Couch RM. (1998). Effect of bacille Calmette-Guérin vaccination on C-peptide secretion in children newly diagnosed with IDDM. *Diabetes Care*. Vol.21(No.10): 1691-3.

Every AL, Kramer DR, Mannering SI, Lew AM, Harrison LC. (2006). Intranasal vaccination with proinsulin DNA induces regulatory CD4+ T cells that prevent experimental autoimmune diabetes. Journal of Immunology. Vol.176(No.8): 4608-15.

Feili-Hariri M, Flores RR, Vasquez AC, Morel PA. (2006). Dendritic cell immunotherapy for autoimmune diabetes. *Immunologic research*. Vol.36(No.1-3): 167-73.

Feuerer M, Jiang W, Holler PD, Satpathy A, Campbell C, Bogue M, Mathis D, Benoist C. (2007). Enhanced thymic selection of FoxP3+ regulatory T cells in the NOD mouse model of autoimmune diabetes. *Proceedings of the National Academy of Sciences of the USA*. Vol.104(No.46):18181-6.

Filippova M, Liu J, Escher A. (2001). Effects of plasmid DNA injection on cyclophosphamide-accelerated diabetes in NOD mice. *DNA and Cell Biology*. Vol.20(No.3): 175-81.

Fischer B, Elias D, Bretzel RG, Linn T. (2010). Immunomodulation with heat shock protein DiaPep277 to preserve beta cell function in type 1 diabetes - an update. *Expert Opinion on Biological Therapy*. Vol.10(No.2): 265-72.

Garren H. (2009). DNA vaccines for autoimmune diseases. *Expert Review of Vaccines*. Vol.8(No.9): 1195-203.

Geenen V, Mottet M, Dardenne O, Kermani H, Martens H, Francois JM, Galleni M, Hober D, Rahmouni S, Moutschen M. (2010). Thymic self-antigens for the design of a negative/tolerogenic self-vaccination against type 1 diabetes. *Current Opinion in Pharmacology*. Vol.10(No.4): 461-72.

GEN News Highlights. (2010). MacroGenics and Lilly ponder future of diabetes mAb after phase III flop. URL: http://www.genengnews.com/gen-news-highlights/macrogenics-and-lilly-ponder-future-of-diabetes-mab-after-phase-iii-flop/81244098/

Gitelman S. (2007). Study of Thymoglobulin to Arrest Newly Diagnosed Type 1 Diabetes (START). URL: http://www.clinicaltrials.gov/ct2/show/NCT00515099?term=ATG+type+1+diabetes&rank=2

Gitelman S, Bluestone J. (2010). T1DM Immunotherapy Using CD4+CD127lo/-CD25+ Polyclonal Tregs. URL: http://www.clinicaltrials.gov/ct2/show/NCT01210664?term=NCT01210664&rank=1

Gottlieb P, Eisenbarth G, Kipnes M, Ratner R, Rockell J, Wagner R, Solvason N, Tersini K, Valone F, Woody K, Steinman L, Garren H. (2008). Interim Results of a Phase I/II Clinical Trial of a DNA Plasmid Vaccine (BHT-3021) for Type 1 Diabetes. URL: http://www.bayhilltx.com/abstracts.html

Gottlieb PA, Quinlan S, Krause-Steinrauf H, Greenbaum CJ, Wilson DM, Rodriguez H, Schatz DA, Moran AM, Lachin JM, Skyler JS; Type 1 Diabetes TrialNet MMF/DZB Study Group. (2010). Failure to preserve beta-cell function with mycophenolate mofetil and daclizumab combined therapy in patients with new- onset type 1 diabetes. *Diabetes Care*. Vol.33(No.4): 826-32.

Goudy K, Song S, Wasserfall C, Zhang YC, Kapturczak M, Muir A, Powers M, Scott-Jorgensen M, Campbell-Thompson M, Crawford JM, Ellis TM, Flotte TR, Atkinson MA. (2001). Adeno-associated virus vector-mediated IL-10 gene delivery prevents type 1 diabetes in NOD mice. *Proceedings of the National Academy of Sciences of the United States of America*. Vol.98(No.24): 13913-8.

Goudy KS, Wang B, Tisch R. (2008). Gene gun-mediated DNA vaccination enhances antigen-specific immunotherapy at a late preclinical stage of type 1 diabetes in nonobese diabetic mice. Clinincal Immunology. Vol.129(No.1):49-57.

Grinberg-Bleyer Y, Baeyens A, You S, Elhage R, Fourcade G, Gregoire S, Cagn ard N, Carpentier W, Tang Q, Bluestone J, Chatenoud L, Klatzmann D, Salomon BL, Piaggio E. (2010). IL-2 reverses established type 1 diabetes in NOD mice by a local effect on pancreatic regulatory T cells. *Journal of Experimental Medicine*. Vol.207(No.9): 1871-8.

GSK Press Release. (2011). GlaxoSmithKline and Tolerx announce phase III DEFEND-1 study of otelixizumab in type 1 diabetes did not meet its primary endpoint. URL: http://www.gsk.com/media/pressreleases/2011/2011_pressrelease_10039.htm

Haller MJ. (2010). Reversing Type 1 Diabetes After it is Established. URL: http://www.clinicaltrials.gov/ct2/show/NCT01106157?term=ATG+type+1+diabetes&rank=1

Harrison LC, Dempsey-Collier M, Kramer DR, Takahashi K. (1996). Aerosol insulin induces regulatory CD8 gamma delta T cells that prevent murine insulin-dependent diabetes. *Journal of Experimental Medicine*. Vol.184(No.6): 2167–2174.

Harrison LC, Honeyman MC, Steele CE, Stone NL, Sarugeri E, Bonifacio E, Couper JJ, Colman PG. (2004). Pancreatic beta-cell function and immune responses to insulin after administration of intranasal insulin to humans at risk for type 1 diabetes. *Diabetes Care*. Vol.27(No.10): 2348-55.

Harrison LC. (2008). Vaccination against self to prevent autoimmune disease: the type 1 diabetes model. Immunology and cell biology. Vol.86(No.2): 139-45.

Hedman M, Ludvigsson J, Faresjö MK. (2006). Nicotinamide reduces high secretion of IFN-gamma in high-risk relatives even though it does not prevent type 1 diabetes. *Journal of Interferon & Cytokine Research*. Vol.26(No.4): 207-13.

Herold KC, Gitelman S, Greenbaum C, Puck J, Hagopian W, Gottlieb P, Sayre P, Bianchine P, Wong E, Seyfert-Margolis V, Bourcier K, Bluestone JA; Immune Tolerance Network ITN007AI Study Group. (2009). Treatment of patients with new onset Type 1 diabetes with a single course of anti-CD3 mAb Teplizumab preserves insulin production for up to 5 years. *Clinical Immunology*. Vol.132(No.2): 166-73.

Herold KC, Gitelman SE, Masharani U, Hagopian W, Bisikirska B, Donaldson D, Rother K, Diamond B, Harlan DM, Bluestone JA. (2005). A single course of anti-CD3 monoclonal antibody hOKT3 gamma1(Ala-Ala) results in improvement in C-peptide responses and clinical parameters for at least 2 years after onset of type 1 diabetes. *Diabetes*. Vol.54(No.6): 1763-9.

Hjorth M, Axelsson S, Rydén A, Faresjö M, Ludvigsson J, Casas R. (2011). GAD-alum treatment induces GAD65-specific CD4+CD25highFOXP3+ cells in type 1 diabetic patients. *Clinical Immunology*. Vol.138(No.1): 117-26.

Horváth L, Cervenak L, Oroszlán M, Prohászka Z, Uray K, Hudecz F, Baranyi E, Madácsy L, Singh M, Romics L, Füst G, Pánczél P. (2002). Antibodies against different epitopes of heat-shock protein 60 in children with type 1 diabetes mellitus. *Immunology Letters*. Vol.80(No.3): 155-62.

Howard LM, Miller SD. (2004). Immunotherapy targeting the CD40/CD154 costimulatory pathway for treatment of autoimmune disease. *Autoimmunity*. Vol.37(No.5): 411-8.

Huurman VA, Decochez K, Mathieu C, Cohen IR, Roep BO. (2007). Therapy with the hsp60 peptide DiaPep277 in C-peptide positive type 1 diabetes patients. *Diabetes/Metabolism Research and Reviews*. Vol.23(No.4): 269-75.

Huurman VA, van der Meide PE, Duinkerken G, Willemen S, Cohen IR, Elias D, Roep BO. (2008). Immunological efficacy of heat shock protein 60 peptide DiaPep277 therapy in clinical type I diabetes. *Clinical and Experimental Immunology*. Vol.152(No.3): 488-97.

Jacob CO, Aiso S, Michie SA, McDevitt HO, Acha-Orbea H. (1990). Prevention of diabetes in nonobese diabetic mice by tumor necrosis factor (TNF): similarities between TNF-alpha and interleukin 1. *Proceedings of the National Academy of Sciences of the United States of America. Proceedings of the National Academy of Sciences of the United States of America*. Vol.87(No.3): 968-72.

Joussemet B, Vu AT, Sai P, Bach JM. (2005). Gene-gun biolistic immunization encoding glutamic acid decarboxylase: a model for studying Langerhans cell abnormalities and mimicry in the nonobese diabetic mouse. *Annals of the New York Academy of Sciences*. Vol.1051: 613-25.

Kaufman DL, Clare-Salzler M, Tian J, Forsthuber T, Ting GS, Robinson P, Atkinson MA, Sercarz EE, Tobin AJ, Lehmann PV. (1993). Spontaneous loss of T-cell tolerance to glutamic acid decarboxylase in murine insulin-dependent diabetes. *Nature*. Vol.366(No.6450): 69-72.

Kaufman A, Herold KC. (2009). Anti-CD3 mAbs for treatment of type 1 diabetes. *Diabetes/Metabolism Research and Reviews*. Vol.25(No.4): 302-6.

Keymeulen B, Vandemeulebroucke E, Ziegler AG, Mathieu C, Kaufman L, Hale G, Gorus F, Goldman M, Walter M, Candon S, Schandene L, Crenier L, De Block C, Seigneurin

JM, De Pauw P, Pierard D, Weets I, Rebello P, Bird P, Berrie E, Frewin M, Waldmann H, Bach JF, Pipeleers D, Chatenoud L. (2005). Insulin needs after CD3-antibody therapy in new-onset type 1 diabetes. *New England journal of medicine*. Vol.352(No.25): 2598-608.

Kobayashi M, Abiru N, Arakawa T, Fukushima K, Zhou H, Kawasaki E, Yamasaki H, Liu E, Miao D, Wong FS, Eisenbarth GS, Eguchi K. (2007). Altered B:9 23 insulin, when administered intranasally with cholera toxin adjuvant, suppresses the expression of insulin autoantibodies and prevents diabetes. *Journal of Immunology*. Vol.179(No.4): 2082–2088.

Koenecke C, Czeloth N, Bubke A, Schmitz S, Kissenpfennig A, Malissen B, Huehn J, Ganser A, Förster R, Prinz I. (2009) Alloantigen-specific de novo-induced Foxp3+ Treg revert in vivo and do not protect from experimental GVHD. *European Journal of Immunology*. Vol.39(No.11): 3091-6.

Koulmanda M, Budo E, Bonner-Weir S, Qipo A, Putheti P, Degauque N, Shi H, Fan Z, Flier JS, Auchincloss H Jr, Zheng XX, Strom TB. (2007). Modification of adverse inflammation is required to cure new-onset type 1 diabetic hosts. *Proceedings of the National Academy of Sciences of the USA*. Vol.104(No.32): 13074-9.

Krieg AM. (2002). CpG motifs in bacterial DNA and their immune effects. *Annual Review of Immunology*. Vol.20: 709-60.

Krishna MT, Huissoon AP. (2011). Clinical immunology review series: an approach to desensitization. *Clinical and Experimental Immunology*. Vol.163(No.2): 131-46.

Kukreja A, Cost G, Marker J, Zhang C, Sun Z, Lin-Su K, Ten S, Sanz M, Exley M, Wilson B, Porcelli S, Maclaren N. (2002). Multiple immuno-regulatory defects in type-1 diabetes. *Journal of Clinical Investigation*. Vol.109(No.1): 131-40.

Lawler B. (2009). PDL Lands in a Hazard. URL: http://www.fool.com/investing/high-growth/2007/08/29/pdl-lands-in-the-hazard.aspx

Lazar L, Ofan R, Weintrob N, Avron A, Tamir M, Elias D, Phillip M, Josefsberg Z. (2007). Heat-shock protein peptide DiaPep277 treatment in children with newly diagnosed type 1 diabetes: a randomized, double-blind phase II study. *Diabetes/Metabolism Research And Reviews*. Vol.23(No.4): 286-91.

Li AF, Escher A. (2003). Intradermal or oral delivery of GAD-encoding genetic vaccines suppresses type 1 diabetes. *DNA and Cell Biology*. Vol.22(No.4): 227-32.

Li AF, Hough J, Henderson D, Escher A. (2004). Co-delivery of pro-apoptotic BAX with a DNA vaccine recruits dendritic cells and promotes efficacy of autoimmune diabetes prevention in mice. *Vaccine*. Vol.22(No.13-14): 1751-63.

Li A, Ojogho O, Franco E, Baron P, Iwaki Y, Escher A. (2006). Pro-apoptotic DNA vaccination ameliorates new onset of autoimmune diabetes in NOD mice and induces foxp3+ regulatory T cells in vitro. *Vaccine*. Vol.24(No.23): 5036.

Li A, Chen J, Hattori M, Franco E, Zuppan C, Ojogho O, Iwaki Y, Escher A. (2010). A therapeutic DNA vaccination strategy for autoimmunity and transplantation. *Vaccine*. Vol.28(No.8): 1897-904.

Li L, Yi Z, Tisch R, Wang B. (2008). Immunotherapy of type 1 diabetes. *Archivum Immunologiae et Therapiae Experimentalis*. Vol.56(No.4): 227-36.

Li X, Liao L, Yan X, Huang G, Lin J, Lei M, Wang X, Zhou Z. (2009). Protective effects of 1-alpha-hydroxyvitamin D3 on residual beta-cell function in patients with adult-onset latent autoimmune diabetes (LADA). *Diabetes/Metabolism Research and Reviews*. Vol.25(No.5): 411-6.

Lindley S, Dayan CM, Bishop A, Roep BO, Peakman M, Tree TI. (2005). Defective suppressor function in CD4(+)CD25(+) T-cells from patients with type 1 diabetes. *Diabetes*. Vol.54(No.1): 92-9.

Liu J, Filippova M, Fagoaga O, Nehlsen-Cannarella S, Escher A. (1999). Intramuscular injection of plasmid DNA encoding intracellular or secreted glutamic acid decarboxylase causes decreased insulitis in the nonobese diabetic mouse. *Gene Therapy and Molecular Biology*. Vol 3: 197-206. (This article is not available online, updated 2011)

Luczyński W, Stasiak-Barmuta A, Urban R, Urban M, Florys B, Hryszko M. (2009). Lower percentages of T regulatory cells in children with type 1 diabetes - preliminary report. *Pediatric endocrinology, diabetes, and metabolism*. Vol.15(No.1): 34-8.

Ludvigsson J. (2009). Adequate doses of autoantigen administered using the appropriate route may create tolerance and stop autoimmunity. *Diabetologia*. Vol.52(No.1): 175-6.

Ludvigsson J, Hjorth M, Chéramy M, Axelsson S, Pihl M, Forsander G, Nilsson NÖ, Samuelsson BO, Wood T, Aman J, Ortqvist E, Casas R. (2011). Extended evaluation of the safety and efficacy of GAD treatment of children and adolescents with recent-onset type 1 diabetes: a randomised controlled trial. *Diabetologia*. Vol.54(No.3): 634-40.

Ludvigsson J; Linköping Diabetes Immune Intervention Study Group. (2009). The role of immunomodulation therapy in autoimmune diabetes. *Journal of Diabetes Science and Technology*. Vol.3(No.2): 320-30.

Luo X, Herold KC, Miller SD. (2010). Immunotherapy of type 1 diabetes: where are we and where should we be going? *Immunity*. Vol.32(No.4): 488-99.

Masteller EL, Warner MR, Tang Q, Tarbell KV, McDevitt H, Bluestone JA. (2005). Expansion of functional endogenous antigen-specific CD4+CD25+ regulatory T cells from nonobese diabetic mice. *Journal of Immunology* Vol.175(No.5):3053-9.

Mastrandrea L, Yu J, Behrens T, Buchlis J, Albini C, Fourtner S, Quattrin T. (2009). Etanercept treatment in children with new-onset type 1 diabetes: pilot randomized, placebo-controlled, double-blind study. Diabetes Care. Vol.32(No.7): 1244-9.

Mercer F, Unutmaz D. (2009). The biology of FoxP3: a key player in immune suppression during infections, autoimmune diseases and cancer. *Advances in Experimental Medicine and Biology*. Vol.665: 47-59.

Näntö-Salonen K, Kupila A, Simell S, Siljander H, Salonsaari T, Hekkala A, Korhonen S, Erkkola R, Sipilä JI, Haavisto L, Siltala M, Tuominen J, Hakalax J, Hyöty H, Ilonen J, Veijola R, Simell T, Knip M, Simell O. (2008). Nasal insulin to prevent type 1 diabetes in children with HLA genotypes and autoantibodies conferring increased risk of disease: a double-blind, randomised controlled trial. *Lancet*. Vol.372(No.9651): 1746-55.

Nikolic T, Welzen-Coppens JM, Leenen PJ, Drexhage HA, Versnel MA. (2009). Plasmacytoid dendritic cells in autoimmune diabetes - potential tools for immunotherapy. Immunobiology. Vol.214(No.9-10): 791-9.

O'Brien BA, Huang Y, Geng X, Dutz JP, Finegood DT. (2002). Phagocytosis of apoptotic cells by macrophages from NOD mice is reduced. *Diabetes*. Vol.51(No.8): 2481-8.

Orban T, Farkas K, Jalahej H, Kis J, Treszl A, Falk B, Reijonen H, Wolfsdorf J, Ricker A, Matthews JB, Tchao N, Sayre P, Bianchine P. (2010). Autoantigen-specific regulatory T cells induced in patients with type 1 diabetes mellitus by insulin B-chain immunotherapy. *Journal of Autoimmunity*. Vol.34(No.4): 408-15.

Ortqvist E, Brooks-Worrell B, Lynch K, Radtke J, Bekris LM, Kockum I, Agardh CD, Cilio CM, Lethagen AL, Persson B, Lernmark A, Reichow J, Oak S, Palmer JP, Hampe CS. (2010). Changes in GAD65Ab-specific antiidiotypic antibody levels correlate with changes in C-peptide levels and progression to islet cell autoimmunity. *Journal of Clinical Endocrinology and Metabolism*. Vol.95(No.11): E310-8.

Overbergh L, Decallonne B, Branisteanu DD, Valckx D, Kasran A, Bouillon R, Mathieu C. (2003). Acute shock induced by antigen vaccination in NOD mice. *Diabetes*. Vol.52(No.2): 335-41.

Panakanti R, Mahato RI. (2009). Bipartite adenoviral vector encoding hHGF and hIL-1Ra for improved human islet transplantation. *Pharmaceutical research*. Vol.26(No.3): 587-96.

Paul WE. (1999). *Fundamental Immunology*. Lippincott – Raven Publishers, Philadelphia, PA.

Pedotti R, Sanna M, Tsai M, DeVoss J, Steinman L, McDevitt H, Galli SJ. (2003). Severe anaphylactic reactions to glutamic acid decarboxylase (GAD) self peptides in NOD mice that spontaneously develop autoimmune type 1 diabetes mellitus. *BioMed Central Immunology*. Vol.4: 2.

Pescovitz MD, Greenbaum CJ, Krause-Steinrauf H, Becker DJ, Gitelman SE, Goland R, Gottlieb PA, Marks JB, McGee PF, Moran AM, Raskin P, Rodriguez H, Schatz DA, Wherrett D, Wilson DM, Lachin JM, Skyler JS; Type 1 Diabetes TrialNet Anti-CD20 Study Group. (2009). Rituximab, B-lymphocyte depletion, and preservation of beta-cell function. *New England journal of medicine*. Vol.361(No.22): 2143-52.

Pfleger C, Meierhoff G, Kolb H, Schloot NC; p520/521 Study Group. (2010). Association of T-cell reactivity with beta-cell function in recent onset type 1 diabetes patients. *Journal of Autoimmunity*. Vol.34(No.2): 127-35.

Phillips B, Giannoukakis N, Trucco M. (2009). Dendritic cell-based therapy in Type 1 diabetes mellitus. *Expert review of clinical immunology*. Vol.5(No.3):325-39. URL: http://clinicaltrials.gov/ct2/results?term=NCT00445913

Phillips B, Nylander K, Harnaha J, Machen J, Lakomy R, Styche A, Gillis K, Brown L, Lafreniere D, Gallo M, Knox J, Hogeland K, Trucco M, Giannoukakis N. (2008). A microsphere-based vaccine prevents and reverses new-onset autoimmune diabetes. *Diabetes*. Vol.57(No.6): 1544-55.

Pitocco D, Crinò A, Di Stasio E, Manfrini S, Guglielmi C, Spera S, Anguissola GB, Visalli N, Suraci C, Matteoli MC, Patera IP, Cavallo MG, Bizzarri C, Pozzilli P; IMDIAB Group. (2006). The effects of calcitriol and nicotinamide on residual pancreatic beta-cell function in patients with recent-onset Type 1 diabetes (IMDIAB XI). *Diabetic medicine : a journal of the British Diabetic Association*. Vol.23(No.8): 920-3.

Putnam AL, Brusko TM, Lee MR, Liu W, Szot GL, Ghosh T, Atkinson MA, Bluestone JA. (2009). Expansion of human regulatory T-cells from patients with type 1 diabetes. *Diabetes*. Vol.58(No.3): 652-62.

Putnam AL, Vendrame F, Dotta F, Gottlieb PA. (2005). CD4+CD25high regulatory T cells in human autoimmune diabetes. *Journal of Autoimmunity*. Vol.24(No.1): 55-62.

Quintana FJ, Carmi P, Cohen IR. (2002). DNA vaccination with heat shock protein 60 inhibits cyclophosphamide-accelerated diabetes. *Journal of Immunology*. Vol.169(No.10): 6030-5.

Rabinovitch A, Suarez-Pinzon WL, Shapiro AM, Rajotte RV, Power R. (2002). Combination therapy with sirolimus and interleukin-2 prevents spontaneous and recurrent autoimmune diabetes in NOD mice. *Diabetes*. Vol.51(No.3): 638-45.

Raz I, Avron A, Tamir M, Metzger M, Symer L, Eldor R, Cohen IR, Elias D. (2007). Treatment of new-onset type 1 diabetes with peptide DiaPep277 is safe and associated with preserved beta-cell function: extension of a randomized, double-blind, phase II trial. *Diabetes/Metabolism Research and Reviews*. Vol.23(No.4): 292-8.

Reed JC. (1999). Dysregulation of apoptosis in cancer. *Journal of Clinical Oncology*. Vol.17(No.9): 2941-53.

Ridgway WM. (2003). The non obese diabetic (NOD) mouse: a unique model for understanding the interaction between genetics and T cell responses. *Reviews In Endocrine & Metabolic Disorders*. Vol.4(No.3): 263-9.

Rigby MR, Trexler AM, Pearson TC, Larsen CP. (2008). CD28/CD154 blockade prevents autoimmune diabetes by inducing nondeletional tolerance after effector t-cell inhibition and regulatory T-cell expansion. *Diabetes*. Vol.57(No.10): 2672-83.

Rother KI, Brown RJ, Morales MM, Wright E, Duan Z, Campbell C, Hardin DS, Popovic J, McEvoy RC, Harlan DM, Orlander PR, Brod SA. (2009a). Effect of ingested interferon-alpha on beta-cell function in children with new-onset type 1 diabetes. *Diabetes Care*. Vol.32(No.7): 1250-5.

Rother KI, Spain LM, Wesley RA, Digon BJ 3rd, Baron A, Chen K, Nelson P, Dosch HM, Palmer JP, Brooks-Worrell B, Ring M, Harlan DM. (2009b). Effects of exenatide alone and in combination with daclizumab on beta-cell function in long-standing type 1 diabetes. *Diabetes Care*. Vol.32(No.12): 2251-7.

Sanda S, Bollyky J, Standifer N, Nepom G, Hamerman JA, Greenbaum C. (2010). Short-term IL-1beta blockade reduces monocyte CD11b integrin expression in an IL-8 dependent fashion in patients with type 1 diabetes. *Clinical immunology*. Vol.136(No.2): 170-3.

Santos Júnior RR, Sartori A, Bonato VL, Coelho Castelo AA, Vilella CA, Zollner RL, Silva CL. (2007). Immune modulation induced by tuberculosis DNA vaccine protects non-obese diabetic mice from diabetes progression. *Clinical and Experimental Immunology*. Vol.149(No.3): 570-8.

Santos RR Junior, Sartori A, Lima DS, Souza PR, Coelho-Castelo AA, Bonato VL, Silva CL. (2009). DNA vaccine containing the mycobacterial hsp65 gene prevented insulitis in MLD-STZ diabetes. *Journal of Immune Based Therapies and Vaccines*. Vol.7(No.1): 4.

Saudek F, Havrdova T, Boucek P, Karasova L, Novota P, Skibova J. (2004). Polyclonal anti-T-cell therapy for type 1 diabetes mellitus of recent onset. *Review of Diabetic Studies*. Vol.1(No.2): 80-8.

Schatz DA, Bingley PJ. (2001). Update on major trials for the prevention of type 1 diabetes mellitus: the American Diabetes Prevention Trial (DPT-1) and the European Nicotinamide Diabetes Intervention Trial (ENDIT). *Journal of Pediatric Endocrinology & Metabolism*. Vol.14 Suppl 1: 619-22.

Schwarznau A, Hanson MS, Sperger JM, Schram BR, Danobeitia JS, Greenwood KK, Vijayan A, Fernandez LA. (2009). IL-1beta receptor blockade protects islets against pro-inflammatory cytokine induced necrosis and apoptosis. *Journal of cellular physiology.* Vol.220(No.2): 341-7.

Seifarth C, Pop S, Liu B, Wong CP, Tisch R. (2003). More stringent conditions of plasmid DNA vaccination are required to protect grafted versus endogenous islets in nonobese diabetic mice. *Journal of Immunology.* Vol.171(No.1): 469.

Sgouroudis E, Piccirillo CA. (2009). Control of type 1 diabetes by CD4+Foxp3+ regulatory T cells: lessons from mouse models and implications for human disease. *Diabetes/metabolism research and reviews.* Vol.25(No.3): 208-18.

Shapiro AM, Lakey JR, Ryan EA, Korbutt GS, Toth E, Warnock GL, Kneteman NM, Rajotte RV. (2000). Islet transplantation in seven patients with type 1 diabetes mellitus using a glucocorticoid-free immunosuppressive regimen. *New England Journal of Medicine.* Vol.343(No.4): 230-8.

Silverstein J, Maclaren N, Riley W, Spillar R, Radjenovic D, Johnson S. (1988). Immunosuppression with azathioprine and prednisone in recent-onset insulin-dependent diabetes mellitus. *New England Journal of Medicine.* Vol.319(No.10): 599-604.

Simon G, Parker M, Ramiya V, Wasserfall C, Huang Y, Bresson D, Schwartz RF, Campbell-Thompson M, Tenace L, Brusko T, Xue S, Scaria A, Lukason M, Eisenbeis S, Williams J, Clare-Salzler M, Schatz D, Kaplan B, Von Herrath M, Womer K, Atkinson MA. (2008). Murine antithymocyte globulin therapy alters disease progression in NOD mice by a time-dependent induction of immunoregulation. *Diabetes.* Vol.57(No.2): 405-14.

Sizonenko SV, Halban PA. (1991). Differential rates of conversion of rat proinsulins I and II. Evidence for slow cleavage at the B-chain/C-peptide junction of proinsulin II. Biochemical Journal. Vol.278(Pt 3): 621-5.

Skyler JS, Krischer JP, Wolfsdorf J, Cowie C, Palmer JP, Greenbaum C, Cuthbertson D, Rafkin-Mervis LE, Chase HP, Leschek E. (2005). Effects of oral insulin in relatives of patients with type 1 diabetes: The Diabetes Prevention Trial--Type 1. *Diabetes Care.* Vol.28(No.5): 1068-76.

Skyler JS; Type 1 Diabetes TrialNet Study Group. (2008). Update on worldwide efforts to prevent type 1 diabetes. *Annals of the New York Academy of Sciences.* Vol.1150: 190-6.

Stadinski BD, Delong T, Reisdorph N, Reisdorph R, Powell RL, Armstrong M, Piganelli JD, Barbour G, Bradley B, Crawford F, Marrack P, Mahata SK, Kappler JW, Haskins K. (2010). Chromogranin A is an autoantigen in type 1 diabetes. *Nature Immunology.* Vol.11(No.3): 225-31.

Stiller CR, Dupré J, Gent M, Jenner MR, Keown PA, Laupacis A, Martell R, Rodger NW, von Graffenried B, Wolfe BM. (1984). Effects of cyclosporine immunosuppression in insulin-dependent diabetes mellitus of recent onset. *Science.* Vol.223(No.4643): 1362-7.

Solvason N, Lou YP, Peters W, Evans E, Martinez J, Ramirez U, Ocampo A, Yun R, Ahmad S, Liu E, Yu L, Eisenbarth G, Leviten M, Steinman L, Garren H. (2008). Improved efficacy of a tolerizing DNA vaccine for reversal of hyperglycemia through enhancement of gene expression and localization to intracellular sites. *Journal of Immunology.* Vol.181(No.12): 8298-307.

Sutherland DE, Gruessner RW, Dunn DL, Matas AJ, Humar A, Kandaswamy R, Mauer SM, Kennedy WR, Goetz FC, Robertson RP, Gruessner AC, Najarian JS. (2001). Lessons learned from more than 1,000 pancreas transplants at a single institution. *Annals of Surgical Innovation and Research.* Vol.233(No.4): 463-501.

Tang Q, Bluestone JA. (2006). Regulatory T-cell physiology and application to treat autoimmunity. *Immunological Reviews.* Vol.212: 217-37.

Tang Q, Bluestone JA. (2008). The Foxp3+ regulatory T cell: a jack of all trades, master of regulation. *Nature Immunology.* Vol.9(No.3): 239-44.

Thomas HE, Irawaty W, Darwiche R, Brodnicki TC, Santamaria P, Allison J, Kay TW. (2004). IL-1 receptor deficiency slows progression to diabetes in the NOD mouse. *Diabetes.* Vol.53(No.1): 113-21.

Tian J, Clare-Salzler M, Herschenfeld A, Middleton B, Newman D, Mueller R, Arita S, Evans C, Atkinson MA, Mullen Y, Sarvetnick N, Tobin AJ, Lehmann PV, Kaufman DL. (1996). Modulating autoimmune responses to GAD inhibits disease progression and prolongs islet graft survival in diabetes-prone mice. *Nature Medicine.* Vol.2(No.12): 1348-53.

Tisch R, Liblau RS, Yang XD, Liblau P, McDevitt HO. (1998). Induction of GAD65-specific regulatory T-cells inhibits ongoing autoimmune diabetes in nonobese diabetic mice. *Diabetes.* Vol.47(No.6): 894-9.

Tisch R, Yang XD, Liblau RS, McDevitt HO. (1994). Administering glutamic acid decarboxylase to NOD mice prevents diabetes. *Journal of Autoimmunity.* Vol.7(No.6): 845-50.

Tisch R, Yang XD, Singer SM, Liblau RS, Fugger L, McDevitt HO. (1993). Immune response to glutamic acid decarboxylase correlates with insulitis in non-obese diabetic mice. *Nature.* Vol.366(No.6450): 72-5.

Tisch R, Wang B, Weaver DJ, Liu B, Bui T, Arthos J, Serreze DV. (2001). Antigen-specific mediated suppression of beta cell autoimmunity by plasmid DNA vaccination. *Journal of Immunology.* Vol.166(No.3): 2122-32.

Tritt M, Sgouroudis E, d'Hennezel E, Albanese A, Piccirillo CA. (2008). Functional waning of naturally occurring CD4+ regulatory T-cells contributes to the onset of autoimmune diabetes. *Diabetes.* Vol.57(No.1):113-23.

Tsai S, Shameli A, Yamanouchi J, Clemente-Casares X, Wang J, Serra P, Yang Y, Medarova Z, Moore A, Santamaria P. (2010). Reversal of autoimmunity by boosting memory-like autoregulatory T cells. *Immunity.* Vol.23;32(No.4): 568-80.

Vague P, Vialettes B, Lassmann-Vague V, Vallo JJ. (1987). Nicotinamide may extend remission phase in insulin-dependent diabetes. *Lancet.* Vol.329(No.8533): 619-20.

Valle A, Jofra T, Stabilini A, Atkinson M, Roncarolo MG, Battaglia M. (2009). Rapamycin prevents and breaks the anti-CD3-induced tolerance in NOD mice. *Diabetes.*

Waid DM, Vaitaitis GM, Wagner DH Jr. (2004). Peripheral CD4loCD40+ auto-aggressive T cell expansion during insulin-dependent diabetes mellitus. *European Journal of Immunology.* Vol.34(No.5): 1488-97.

Walter M, Kaupper T, Adler K, Foersch J, Bonifacio E, Ziegler AG. (2010). No effect of the 1alpha, 25-dihydroxyvitamin D3 on beta-cell residual function and insulin requirement in adults with new-onset type 1 diabetes. *Diabetes Care.* Vol.33(No.7): 1443-8.

Weaver DJ Jr, Liu B, Tisch R. (2001). Plasmid DNAs encoding insulin and glutamic acid decarboxylase 65 have distinct effects on the progression of autoimmune diabetes in nonobese diabetic mice. *Journal of Immunology.* Vol.167(No.1): 586-92.

Wenzlau JM, Juhl K, Yu L, Moua O, Sarkar SA, Gottlieb P, Rewers M, Eisenbarth GS, Jensen J, Davidson HW, Hutton JC. (2007). The cation efflux transporter ZnT8 (Slc30A8) is a major autoantigen in human type 1 diabetes. *Proceedings of the National Academy of Sciences of the USA*. Vol.104(No.43): 17040-5.

Wolfe T, Bot A, Hughes A, Möhrle U, Rodrigo E, Jaume JC, Baekkeskov S, von Herrath M. (2002). Endogenous expression levels of autoantigens influence success or failure of DNA immunizations to prevent type 1 diabetes: addition of IL-4 increases safety. *European Journal of Immunology*. Vol.32(No.1): 113-21.

Xiu Y, Wong CP, Bouaziz JD, Hamaguchi Y, Wang Y, Pop SM, Tisch RM, Tedder TF. (2008). B lymphocyte depletion by CD20 monoclonal antibody prevents diabetes in nonobese diabetic mice despite isotype-specific differences in Fc gamma R effector functions. *Journal of Immunology*. Vol.180(No.5): 2863-75.

You S, Candon S, Kuhn C, Bach JF, Chatenoud L. (2008). CD3 antibodies as unique tools to restore self-tolerance in established autoimmunity their mode of action and clinical application in type 1 diabetes. *Advances in Immunology*. Vol.100: 13-37.

Zanin-Zhorov A, Tal G, Shivtiel S, Cohen M, Lapidot T, Nussbaum G, Margalit R, Cohen IR, Lider O. (2005). Heat shock protein 60 activates cytokine-associated negative regulator suppressor of cytokine signaling 3 in T cells: effects on signaling, chemotaxis, and inflammation. *Journal of Immunology*. Vol.175(No.1): 276-85.

Zhang L, Nakayama M, Eisenbarth GS. (2008). Insulin as an autoantigen in NOD/human diabetes. *Current Opinion in Immunology*. Vol.20(No.1): 111-8.

Zhang W, Jin H, Hu Y, Yu Y, Li X, Ding Z, Kang Y, Wang B. (2010). Protective response against type 1 diabetes in nonobese diabetic mice after coimmunization with insulin and DNA encoding proinsulin. *Hum Gene Therapy*. Vol.21(No.2): 171-8.

Zheng XX, Steele AW, Hancock WW, Kawamoto K, Li XC, Nickerson PW, Li Y, Tian Y, Strom TB. (1999). IL-2 receptor-targeted cytolytic IL-2/Fc fusion protein treatment blocks diabetogenic autoimmunity in nonobese diabetic mice. *Journal of Immunology*. Vol.163(No.7): 4041-8.

17

Type 1 Diabetes Immunotherapy - Successes, Failures and Promises

Brett E. Phillips and Nick Giannoukakis
Children's Hospital of Pittsburgh of UPMC
United States of America

1. Introduction

Type 1 diabetes is an autoimmune disease that usually strikes during adolescence resulting in uncontrolled blood glucose levels. Auto-reactive T-cells target the insulin producing beta cells of the pancreas resulting in their destruction. The only treatment currently available is lifelong administration of insulin to bring blood glucose levels back under control. The identification of insulin and its mass production were the first major success in the treatment of the disease. Building on the work of others, Frederick Banting and Charles Best demonstrated the ability of insulin to maintain normoglycemia in pancreatectomized dogs in 1921 (Banting; Best; Collip, et al., 1922) and with the help of Eli Lilly the mass production of insulin was under way by 1922 for clinical use. Prior to this the disease was fatal by 3 years. No less than 4 Nobel prizes have been rewarded over the years for research on insulin's indentification, sequence, structure, and the production of recombinant human insulin.

Despite the success of insulin therapy, it is now obvious that even rigorous control of blood glucose with insulin injections only delays, but does not prevent the development of diabetic complications (The DCCT Research Group, 1993). Diabetic complications, which include cardiovascular disease, diabetic retinopathy, kidney failure, and neuropathy, account for significant diabetes-related patient morbidity and mortality. Islet transplantation has been attempted to restore the normal release patterns of insulin, but sufficient source donors are limiting, the possibility of lifelong anti-rejection drugs may prove worse than diabetes, and the autoimmune process that destroyed the original beta cells are still active (Huurman; Hilbrands; Pinkse, et al., 2008, Marzorati; Pileggi&Ricordi, 2007, Roelen; Huurman; Hilbrands, et al., 2009, Van Belle&von Herrath, 2008). Therefore therapeutics that modify the immune response and restore normal immune function are necessary to improve the outcomes of patients with type 1 diabetes. Little has changed in the primary treatment of type 1 diabetes over the last 90 years, but immunotherapy techniques hold the promise of finding a true cure.

2. Immunotherapy - small windows of opportunity

Immunotherapy techniques have the potential to restore the proper immune system balance preventing further beta cell death and increasing insulin production with the subsiding of beta cell inflammation (Dib&Gomes, 2009, Mortensen; Hougaard; Swift, et al., 2009, Papoz; Lenegre; Hors, et al., 1990). A favorable window of opportunity must be selected for immunotherapy techniques to have the greatest impact, especially since patients may have lost as much as 80% of their beta cell mass by the time of clinical diagnosis of type 1 diabetes(Bresson&von Herrath, 2007). Late treatment after further cell loss may not allow for sustainable insulin production levels to maintain euglycemia and therefore would only be a benefit if used in combination with regenerative medicine or beta cell replacement. For this reason, the effective window of opportunity must be explored for each proposed immunotherapy.

2.1 Disease prediction failure

Preservation of beta cell mass sufficient to meet the patients' insulin needs is the target goal of immunotherapy. The chances of successful treatment increase with a greater beta cell preservation and allows a buffer against possible future relapses. Since disease onset rapidly reduces the beta cell population, early detection of the disease or even pre-clinical detection would greatly enhance patient outcomes. Along these lines, efforts have been made to identify predictive biomarkers for type 1 diabetes. These markers include genetic susceptibility loci, autoantibodies, and the population size of regulatory immune cells. With a sufficient understanding of how these factors change at disease onset and over the course of the disease, we could some day even preemptively treat healthy patients that are at significant risk to develop type 1 diabetes.

The human genome has been mined for susceptibility genes that will affect the probability of developing type 1 diabetes. In animal models this is a lengthy process in controlled inter-breeding of two mouse strains. Mice within each strain are genetically identical. By breeding a diabetes-prone mouse strain with a normal mouse strain, the offspring contain one set of chromosomes from each strain. Continued breeding of these offspring over several generations to the normal mouse strain results in a number of new mouse lines that are mostly normal, but contain different fragments of DNA from the diabetes-prone animals. The percentage of animals in each new strain that develop diabetes can then be compared to which DNA fragments they received to identify possible susceptibility genes. For humans, DNA sequence variations are compared in families with a known history of type 1 diabetes. Four genetic regions have been linked to the disease thus far among different populations and they are the HLA locus, Insulin, cytotoxic T lymphocyte antigen-4 (CTLA-4), and phosphatase non-receptor type 22 (PTPN22).

In retrospect, it is not surprising that insulin is one of the identified susceptibility genes for type 1 diabetes. The human insulin 5' promoter region exhibits variability in DNA sequence length depending on the number of a variable number of tandom repeats (VTNR) variation it contains. These variants are named VTNR1, VTNR2, and VTNR3, which are arranged in lengths of increasing order. VTNR1 class alleles are associated with diabetes susceptibility and reduced insulin expression in the thymus (Kantarova&Buc, 2007, Maier&Wicker, 2005). Insulin production in the thymus is closely linked to the expression of the Autoimmune Regulator (AIRE) transcription factor whose role is to participate in the transactivation of a wide range of self-antigens necessary for T-cell negative selection (Anderson; Venanzi; Chen, et al., 2005). The consensus model posits that low levels of thymic insulin facilitates the escape of insulin-reactive thymocytes which enter the periphery and at some point later in life are activated to recognize beta cell insulin (Liston; Lesage; Wilson, et al., 2003). Recent work has demonstrated that AIRE can bind the VTNR1 class allele promoter with a marked reduction in insulin mRNA production(Cai; Zhang; Breslin, et al., 2011). Indeed AIRE disruption leads to a number of other autoimmune diseases.

The strongest genetic linkage to diabetes lies on chromosome 6 (6p21.3) where HLA (MHC in mouse) genes are located (Kantarova&Buc, 2007, Maier&Wicker, 2005). The HLA system encodes a number of highly-polymorphic cell surface proteins that present self and processed antigens to T-cells. HLA class I molecules are expressed on most cells in the body and identify the cell as "self" or part of the body. HLA class II molecules are used to display foreign antigens captured by antigen presenting cells (APC) of the immune system such as dendritic cells (DC). Interactions between DC's HLA class II molecules and T-cell's T-cell Receptor (TCR) activate T-cells to proliferate and to target cells expressing those specific targets. The highest HLA risk is conferred by the DR and DQ alleles. This risk accounts for 40% of the genetic risk for type 1 diabetes (Kantarova&Buc, 2007).

Two additional susceptibility loci are associated with regulation of T-cell activation. CTLA-4 is a protein that is expressed on the surface of activated T-cells. For T-cells to become fully activated, co-stimulatory molecules on DC's interact with the T-cell after initial HLA class II and TCR interaction, and can result in pro-inflammatory cytokine release from the dendritic cells (Bluestone, 1996, Clarkson&Sayegh, 2005, Kishimoto; Dong&Sayegh, 2000, Lenschow; Walunas&Bluestone, 1996, Sayegh&Turka, 1995). CTLA-4 can directly interact with co-stimulatory molecules CD80 and CD86 reducing IL-2 receptor activation and IL-2 production (Kantarova&Buc, 2007). IL-2 is a strong pro-inflammatory cytokine involved in growth and survival for T-cells which undergo apoptosis if IL-2 is removed. T regulatory (Treg) cells characterized as CD4+ CD25+ can also negatively regulate T-cell activation and require CTLA-4 to elicit some of its regulatory actions (Kantarova&Buc, 2007, Maier&Wicker, 2005). Inactive splice variants of CTLA-4 have been detected in mice, but have yet to be identified in human disease (Maier&Wicker, 2005). Disregulated and hypersensitive T-cell populations can develop with genetic modifications to the PTPN22 gene. It's gene product, lymphoid protein tyrosine kinase (LYP), is active at the cell membrane and improper localization results in T-cell defects (Kantarova&Buc, 2007, Maier&Wicker, 2005). Other autoimmune diseases such rheumatoid arthiritis, systemic lupus, and Graves disease have been similarly linked to HLA class II, CTLA-4, and PTPN22 genes and establish a connection between these genes and immune system dysregulation (Jones; Fugger; Strominger, et al., 2006, Kantarova&Buc, 2007, Maier&Wicker, 2005). Further research is still needed to use this information to develop a predictive test that can be used in a wide segment of the population.

2.2 Auto-antibodies and early disease detection failure

Type 1 diabetes is associated wtih the production of a number of auto-antibodies that bind to a number of self-antigens. Among these are antibodies recognising islet cell antigens of a general nature (ICA), glutamic acid decarboxylase (GAD), islet cell antigen 512 (IA-2) and insulin (IAA) (Isermann; Ritzel; Zorn, et al., 2007). Unfortunately the predictive value of these antibodies cannot reach a level permissive for preemptive clinical intervention. The percentage of diabetic patients that have IA-2 and IAA is reduced as the age of disease onset increases making it challenging to use these criteria as airtight predicitive markers (Isermann; Ritzel; Zorn, et al., 2007) (Bingley; Bonifacio; Williams, et al., 1997, Verge; Howard; Rowley, et al., 1994). Measurement variations between testing labs is still a major concern (Schlosser; Mueller; Torn, et al., 2010), especially in the case of ICA testing where results are dependent on the experience of the operator (Isermann; Ritzel; Zorn, et al., 2007). A single positive auto-antibody titer is also not sufficient to predict the development of diabetes, only 30% of those patients develop diabetes over the course of 15 years (Verge; Gianani; Kawasaki, et al., 1996).

The current methods cannot accurately predict diabetes development and thus, it is difficult to accept these markers to drive an intervention prior to clinical disease onset. In general, any predictive markers must have a low margin of error and high prediction certainty to justify treating healthy patients for diseases they don't yet have. Additionally it is highly unlikely the entire population will receive the proper diagnostic pre-screening tests to identify all potential type 1 diabetes patients. For these reasons, immunotherapeutics have been focused on diabetes reversal in new onset patients during their "honeymoon" period where blood glucose is elevated but they still have beta cell mass.

3. Immunotherapy treatments - bench and bedside

Immunotherapy defines a broad range of strategies to inhibit autoimmune processes with the intended outcome the long-term restoration of normal immune system function. The most direct approach is to induce the elimination or the silencing of immune cells responsible for the autoimmunity. Other approaches attempt to restore self-antigen tolerance by providing large amounts of self-antigen, or self-antigen decoys to minimize the interaction between HLA and the peptides. Cell based therapies are also underway that introduce modified immune cells to abrogate autoimmune processes. The current clinical status of these methods and others will be covered here in an overview.

3.1 Targeted cell ablation

The beta cells of the pancreas are directly destroyed by activated auto-reactive T-cells making these T-cells an attractive therapeutic target. The two antibodies that have been developed to target T-cells for elimination are specific for CD3 and CD4. These surface proteins are abundant on cytotoxic T-cells, but unfortunately in the case of CD4, can also be found on anti-inflammatory Treg cells characterized as CD4+ CD25+. While treatment with anti-CD4 antibodies did reverse new onset diabetes in the Non-Obese Diabetic (NOD) mouse model, Treg populations were not positively effected and systemic immunosuppression occurred (Makhlouf; Grey; Dong, et al., 2004). The anti-CD3 antibody was also able to reverse new onset diabetes in the NOD mouse model but without these complications (Chatenoud; Primo&Bach, 1997, Chatenoud; Thervet; Primo, et al., 1994). The anti-CD3 antibody treatment elevated Treg cell populations in mouse (Belghith; Bluestone; Barriot, et al., 2003) and then in humans (Bisikirska; Colgan; Luban, et al., 2005, Chatenoud, 2010). These promising data were used to translate the CD3 antibody into expanded phase II and III trials. Cytokine production profiles also were shifted with a reduction in IL-2 and an increase in IL-10 permissive for a more anti-inflammatory state (Herold; Burton; Francois, et al., 2003). Despite the apparent trend towards a more balanced pro-/anti- inflammatory state, non-specific T-cell activation was observed (Chatenoud, 2010). Nevertheless, despite almost a decade of testing, Phase III trials were recently stopped by MacroGenics and Lilly since insulin requirements and Hemogoblin A1C levels remained unaffected after 1 year of drug treatment http://www.bizjournals.com/washington/quick_news/2010/10/macrogenics-lilly-abandon-diabetes-drug.html; AND http://www.inpharm.com/news/150858/gsk-tolerx-otelixizumab-phase-iii-failure

Autoantibody production occurs in a number of autoimmune diseases and contributes to ongoing pathogenesis. Under normal conditions, B cells generate antibodies to allow the body to quickly recognize and clear antigens it has encountered in the past. This system is particularly dangerous when auto-anitbodies are generated because it establishes an ongoing and self-sustaining immune reaction in the host. For this reason the anti-CD20 antibody Rituximab was developed to deplete B cell populations and their ability to produce antibodies. Rituximab was initially approved for the treatment of Non-Hodgkin's Lymphoma (McLaughlin; White; Grillo-Lopez, et al., 1998, Scott, 1998) and later rheumatoid arthritis (Edwards; Szczepanski; Szechinski, et al., 2004). Numerous clinical trials are now underway for the treatment of other autoimmune diseases (Reis; Athanazio; Lima, et al., 2009, Suzuki; Nagasawa; Kameda, et al., 2009) (Hauser; Waubant; Arnold, et al., 2008) including type 1 diabetes due to favorable pre-clinical NOD mouse data (Hu; Rodriguez-Pinto; Du, et al., 2007, Xiu; Wong; Bouaziz, et al., 2008). The Phase II trial results did show a trend towards increased beta cell mass preservation, but the treated group did not have significantly different C-peptide levels and were all still insulin dependent during the course of the trial (Pescovitz; Greenbaum; Krause-Steinrauf, et al., 2009). At this time cell ablation strategies have not been effective in the treatment of type 1 diabetes and confer numerous side effects.

3.2 Competitive and non-competitive tolerance induction

T-cells are educated in the thymus to learn the difference between "self" and foreign antigens and under normal conditions self reactive T-cells are destroyed. This process breaks down with type 1 diabetes and other autoimmune diseases resulting in autoreactive T-cells that attacks the host's body. In some instances this may be due to decreased insulin expression in the thymus, which is believed to be the reason why insulin promoter variations lead to genetic susceptibility(Cai; Zhang; Breslin, et al., 2011). This has lead to the idea that increasing a patient's exposure to self-antigens may allow the T-cells to be properly educated. Clinical trials are currently underway where patients are given insulin through oral (2009, Skyler; Krischer; Wolfsdorf, et al., 2005) or nasal (Harrison; Dempsey-Collier; Kramer, et al., 1996, Harrison; Honeyman; Steele, et al., 2004) routes of delivery. At least one study using oral insulin delivery, ORALE, failed to show any preservation in beta cell function (Chaillous; Lefevre; Thivolet, et al., 2000). Similarly, synthetic peptides are under development that have greater stability and can be delivered by injection. Both heat shock protein 60 (HSP60) (Atkinson&Maclaren, 1994, Delovitch&Singh, 1997, Durinovic-Bello, 1998, Wicker; Todd&Peterson, 1995) and GAD65 (Agardh; Cilio; Lethagen, et al., 2005, Hinke, 2008, Ludvigsson, 2010) are diabetes auto-antigens being considered as treatment. DeveloGen Inc has manufactured DiaPep277 which shares sequence homology with amino acids 437-460 of HSP60. To increase peptide stability, two single amino acid changes were made at the 6th and 11th position changing cysteine to valine (Raz; Avron; Tamir, et al., 2007, Raz; Elias; Avron, et al., 2001). Early trials have showed a trend in preserved C-peptide levels(Schloot; Meierhoff; Lengyel, et al., 2007). Additionally, increases in anti-inflammatory cytokine IL-10 and T-helper 2 cells (Th2) were observed in ongoing phase II clinical trials(Huurman; van der Meide; Duinkerken, et al., 2008). Likewise the GAD65 peptide Diamyd has conferred increased levels of anti-inflammatory cytokines and the Treg transcription factor marker forkhead box protein (FOXP3) in clinical trials (Agardh; Cilio; Lethagen, et al., 2005, Hinke, 2008, Ludvigsson, 2010). Phase III trials are still ongoing for Diamyd (Ludvigsson, 2010). The clinical outcomes of insulin requirements or restoration of euglycemia have yet to be addressed, but at the very least these studies hold promise at delaying disease onset.

Altered peptide ligands (APL) offer a similar antigen based strategy but their mechanism of action appears to involve competition for the natural antigen at the TCR. The T-cell's TCR have highly variable structures that allow for conformations that can identify all the possible antigens the body has previous been exposed to, in the context of presentation by HLA class I and II. Each individual T-cell has only one TCR confirmation capable of recognizing a single specific antigen. The TCR is targeted to a short amino acid sequence found in the antigen, with important specific primary and secondary sites needed for T-cell activation(Sloan-Lancaster&Allen, 1996). Modification to the amino acid sequence at the primary site allows the TCR to bind the antigen but maintains the specific T-cell subset in an inactive state(Sloan-Lancaster&Allen, 1996). This phenomenon has been exploited for beta cell reactive T-cells, most notably with Neurocrine Biosciences NBI-6024 APL (Nicholson&Kuchroo, 1997, Sloan-Lancaster&Allen, 1996) (Alleva; Gaur; Jin, et al., 2002). NBI-6024 is an insulin APL that covers amino acid region 9-23, the primary TRC recognition site for insulin(Alleva; Crowe; Jin, et al., 2001, Alleva; Gaur; Jin, et al., 2002, Wong; Karttunen; Dumont, et al., 1999). Positions 16 and 19 are modified to alanine. Initial studies in the NOD mouse model demonstrated increased anti-inflammmatory Th2 cells and their production of IL-4 and IL-10(Alleva; Gaur; Jin, et al., 2002, Alleva; Maki; Putnam, et al., 2006). Administration into the NOD mouse strain delayed the onset and reduced the incidence of diabetes development (Alleva; Gaur; Jin, et al., 2002). Unfortunately phase I and II clinical trials were unable to demonstrate preserved beta cell mass resulting in the cessation of testing(Alleva; Maki; Putnam, et al., 2006, Walter; Philotheou; Bonnici, et al., 2009).

A serious hurdle to tolerance induction using peptide antigens may be the sheer number of auto-antigens detected by the immune system. While a single target may exist at disease onset, continued inflammation in the beta cells leads to the development of additional self-antigen targets. Therefore early detection of pre-clinical diabetes might be required for this approach to prevent diabetes. Additionally a single universal disease-initiating auto-antigen would have to be identified, or if this does not exist, a means of screening for which autoantigens are present at clinical onset in order to select an agent that would eliminate those specific T-cells.

3.3 Cell based therapeutics

Cell based therapeutics use natural or modified immune cells transplanted into a host in an attempt to restore the balance of pro- and anti-inflammatory cells. The majority of cell-based research to date has focused on DC's, the regulators of the immune system(Shortman&Naik, 2007). In 2010 the FDA approved the first DC based approach for the treatment of prostate cancer which has been recently accepted for coverage by medicare(Perrone, 2011). That approach is focused on hyperstimulating patient DC *ex vivo* with prostate cancer antigens, while applications for type 1 diabetes have focused on dampening the immune response. Under normal conditions the DC migrate through the body sampling the environment around them. DC then present the self-antigens to naïve T-cells promoting and maintaining self-tolerance(Kurts; Cannarile; Klebba, et al., 2001, Kurts; Carbone; Barnden, et al., 1997, Lutz&Schuler, 2002, Randolph, 2001, Shortman&Naik, 2007, Vlad; Cortesini&Suciu-Foca, 2005). If instead, a foreign antigen is detected, the DC undergo a series of maturation steps that increase surface levels of HLA class II complex and co-stimulatory molecules which in turn facilitate T-cell activation(Mellman&Steinman, 2001). T-cell hypo-responsiveness to self and foreign antigens has been clearly demonstrated in a number of models when costimulatory molecule interaction between DC and T-cells is inhibited (Bluestone, 1996, Clarkson&Sayegh, 2005, Hackstein; Morelli&Thomson, 2001, Kishimoto; Dong&Sayegh, 2000, Lenschow; Herold; Rhee, et al., 1996, Morelli&Thomson, 2003, Sayegh&Turka, 1995, Steinman, 2003, Steinman; Inaba; Turley, et al., 1999). This aspect of DC makes it an ideal target for autoimmune disease therapy in order to maintain auto-reactive T-cell populations silent or hyporesponsive.

DC based therapies have been successful in the treatment of type 1 diabetes in the NOD mouse model. NFkappaB decoys have been employed to prevent DC maturation preventing co-stimulatory molecule expression and reducing the incidence of diabetes development(Ma; Qian; Liang, et al., 2003). Administration of DC treated ex vivo with antisense oligonucleotides (AS-ODN) targeting the co-stimulatory molecules CD40, CD80, and CD86 similarly prevent diabetes development and could reverse new-onset diabetes in NOD mice(Harnaha; Machen; Wright, et al., 2006, Machen; Harnaha; Lakomy, et al., 2004, Phillips, B.; Nylander; Harnaha, et al., 2008). The effects of the treatment extended beyond cyto-toxic T-cell hyporesponsiveness and include the augmentation of anti-inflammatory Treg (Harnaha; Machen; Wright, et al., 2006, Machen; Harnaha; Lakomy, et al., 2004, Phillips, B.; Nylander; Harnaha, et al., 2008). Both methods are based on harvesting DC's from the mouse and then modifying *ex vivo* before being reintroduced back into the mouse. In essence, co-stimulation deficient DC are phenotypically idnetical to immature DC which promote T-cell hyporesponsiveness and an overall state of tolerance. Stabilization of DC in an immature state has been a popular method of promoting auto- and allo-antigen tolerance in a variety of models (Beissert; Schwarz&Schwarz, 2006, Chen, 2006, Enk, 2006, Harnaha; Machen; Wright, et al., 2006, Huber&Schramm, 2006, Hugues; Boissonnas; Amigorena, et al., 2006, Lohr; Knoechel&Abbas, 2006, Ma; Qian; Liang, et al., 2003, Machen; Harnaha; Lakomy, et al., 2004, Marguti; Yamamoto; da Costa, et al., 2009, Nouri-Shirazi&Thomson, 2006, Phillips, B.; Nylander; Harnaha, et al., 2008, Roncarolo; Gregori; Battaglia, et al., 2006, Shevach; DiPaolo; Andersson, et al., 2006, Tang&Bluestone, 2006, Tarbell; Yamazaki; Olson, et al., 2004, Verhagen; Blaser; Akdis, et al., 2006, Yamazaki; Iyoda; Tarbell, et al., 2003, Zhang; Yi; Xia, et al., 2006). Recently, a phase I trial of AS-ODN treated DC's was completed in our center in established type 1 diabetic patients.

Immunotherapeutic treatments often track Treg frequency as an indicator of increased regulation of the immune system and overall tolerance. Methods have been developed to induce Treg differentiation and expand existing Treg populations so sufficient Treg cells could be generated to directly use as a therapeutic (Apetoh; Quintana; Pot, et al., 2010, Gandhi; Kumar; Burns, et al., 2010). Initial studies in the NOD mouse model have also demonstrated the importance of Treg functions in controlling the autoimmune process and role in new onset diabetes reversal(Godebu; Summers-Torres; Lin, et al., 2008, Luo; Tarbell; Yang, et al., 2007, Tang; Henriksen; Bi, et al., 2004, Weber; Harbertson; Godebu, et al., 2006). Regulation afforded by Treg extends beyond single auto-antigens making it an attractive choice in light of antigen spreading effects seen with type 1 diabetes (Luo; Tarbell; Yang, et al., 2007, Tarbell; Yamazaki; Olson, et al., 2004). Given these factors it seems likely that at Treg cell-based therapeutic will be developed.

3.4 Polymer drug delivery

Polymers are typically immunologically and biologically inert molecules that can be used for drug delievery. DNA oligonuceotides, proteins, or antibodies are examples of biologically active compounds that can be conjugated to or carried by polymers(Phillips, B.E.&Giannoukakis, 2010). AS-ODN targeting the co-stimulatory molecules CD40, CD80, and CD86 have been used to treat DC *ex vivo* for administration to diabetic animals(Harnaha; Machen; Wright, et al., 2006, Machen; Harnaha; Lakomy, et al., 2004, Phillips, B.; Nylander; Harnaha, et al., 2008). These same AS-ODN molecules have been formulated into polymer microsphere particles consisting of polyethylene glycol (PEG), polyvinyl pyrrolidone (PVP), and poly-L-lysine-hydrobromide. Administration of these drug carrying microspheres results in similar reversal of new onset diabetes in the NOD mouse model(Phillips, B.; Nylander; Harnaha, et al., 2008). This technique is able to function because DC constantly sample their surrounding environment picking up these AS-ODN containing microspheres. Microsphere administration is promising in that it is far less invasive and costly than harvesting, treating, and re-introducing cells back into a patient. Also given the limited window of treatment for immunotherapeutics, they can be an off the shelf drug that can be immediately administered to newly diagnosed patients.

4. Conclusion

Immunotherapies are immerging for the treatment of type 1 diabetes. For the first time treatments are focusing on preserving beta cell mass and restoring proper function of the immune system instead of just maintaining blood glucose levels. Independence from insulin treatment could remove concerns of patient compliance in blood glucose monitoring and diabetic complications that occur even with intensive insulin therapy. The technology promises much in improvements in patient health, but has a number of hurdles it must first overcome. The current window of treatment is still very small using these techniques. Treatment must begin within months of diabetes onset to preserve the largest number of beta cells as possible. Unfortunately at this time an effective means of identifying individuals prone to develop diabetes has not been fully developed. Concerns also exist about the ethics of treating patients for a disease they may never develop even if at high genetic risk. The predictive value of any such method would need a high level of confidence and be inexpensive enough to adopt for universal screening. Falling short in either category will result in continued disease detection after disease onset. For these reasons, it seems likely that therapeutics will continue to be designed for new onset treatment unless paired with a cell replacement strategy.

Extensive basic and clinical testing is still required to determine patient outcome. Tolerance induction treatments have reached phase III clinical testing, but they have not examined the restoration of euglycemia and insulin independence. The general trend for these studies is they may delay disease onset. While this is not a cure, it can still be important considering the early age onset of the disease. Patient compliance in blood glucose monitoring is not ideal even in adults so delaying onset in children may help them to reach a more mature age to improve self-monitoring. Diabetic complications are also a function of disease maintenance and length. Even rigorous insulin therapy does not prevent complications, so in well-maintained patients a delay in onset could facilitate a delay in complications onset. Antibody based approaches of cell depletion have had mixed results. Anti-CD3 drugs for T-cell ablation confer extensive side effects and recently failed phase III clinical trials. Other antobody appraoches like Rituximab still have not shown unequivocal effectiveness in preserving residual beta cell function. Last, are the cell-based treatments which are the most and least advanced of the techniques. DC based treatments have already been approved for use in cancer patients with minimal side effects, but are just completing phase I clinical trials for the treatment of diabetes. *In vivo* cell modification may prove even less invasive and costly, but have yet to reach trials. The future of any treatment will require additional observation as relapse is possible over the lifetime of the patient, but there is promise in the fact that the field is finally moving beyond simple blood glucose control and trying to cure the underlying autoimmune pathology of type 1 diabetes.

5. References

Agardh, C.D.; Cilio, C.M.; Lethagen, A.; Lynch, K.; Leslie, R.D.; Palmer, M.; Harris, R.A.; Robertson, J.A.&Lernmark, A., (2005). Clinical evidence for the safety of GAD65 immunomodulation in adult-onset autoimmune diabetes. J Diabetes Complications, Vol.19, No. 4, pp. 238-246, ISSN 1056-8727

Alleva, D.G.; Crowe, P.D.; Jin, L.; Kwok, W.W.; Ling, N.; Gottschalk, M.; Conlon, P.J.; Gottlieb, P.A.; Putnam, A.L.&Gaur, A., (2001). A disease-associated cellular immune response in type 1 diabetics to an immunodominant epitope of insulin. J Clin Invest, Vol.107, No. 2, pp. 173-180, ISSN 0021-9738

Alleva, D.G.; Gaur, A.; Jin, L.; Wegmann, D.; Gottlieb, P.A.; Pahuja, A.; Johnson, E.B.; Motheral, T.; Putnam, A.; Crowe, P.D.; Ling, N.; Boehme, S.A.&Conlon, P.J., (2002). Immunological characterization and therapeutic activity of an altered-peptide ligand, NBI-6024, based on the immunodominant type 1 diabetes autoantigen insulin B-chain (9-23) peptide. Diabetes, Vol.51, No. 7, pp. 2126-2134, ISSN 0012-1797

Alleva, D.G.; Maki, R.A.; Putnam, A.L.; Robinson, J.M.; Kipnes, M.S.; Dandona, P.; Marks, J.B.; Simmons, D.L.; Greenbaum, C.J.; Jimenez, R.G.; Conlon, P.J.&Gottlieb, P.A., (2006). Immunomodulation in type 1 diabetes by NBI-6024, an altered peptide ligand of the insulin B epitope. Scand J Immunol, Vol.63, No. 1, pp. 59-69, ISSN 0300-9475

Anderson, M.S.; Venanzi, E.S.; Chen, Z.; Berzins, S.P.; Benoist, C.&Mathis, D., (2005). The cellular mechanism of Aire control of T cell tolerance. Immunity, Vol.23, No. 2, pp. 227-239, ISSN 1074-7613

Apetoh, L.; Quintana, F.J.; Pot, C.; Joller, N.; Xiao, S.; Kumar, D.; Burns, E.J.; Sherr, D.H.; Weiner, H.L.&Kuchroo, V.K., (2010). The aryl hydrocarbon receptor interacts with c-Maf to promote the differentiation of type 1 regulatory T cells induced by IL-27. Nat Immunol, Vol.11, No. 9, pp. 854-861, ISSN 1529-2916

Atkinson, M.A.&Maclaren, N.K., (1994). The pathogenesis of insulin-dependent diabetes mellitus. N Engl J Med, Vol.331, No. 21, pp. 1428-1436, ISSN 0028-4793

Banting, F.G.; Best, C.H.; Collip, J.B.; Campbell, W.R.&Fletcher, A.A., (1922). Pancreatic Extracts in the Treatment of Diabetes Mellitus. Can Med Assoc J, Vol.12, No. 3, pp. 141-146, ISSN 0008-4409

Beissert, S.; Schwarz, A.&Schwarz, T., (2006). Regulatory T cells. J Invest Dermatol, Vol.126, No. 1, pp. 15-24, ISSN 0022-202X

Belghith, M.; Bluestone, J.A.; Barriot, S.; Megret, J.; Bach, J.F.&Chatenoud, L., (2003). TGF-beta-dependent mechanisms mediate restoration of self-tolerance induced by antibodies to CD3 in overt autoimmune diabetes. Nat Med, Vol.9, No. 9, pp. 1202-1208, ISSN 1078-8956

Bingley, P.J.; Bonifacio, E.; Williams, A.J.; Genovese, S.; Bottazzo, G.F.&Gale, E.A., (1997). Prediction of IDDM in the general population: strategies based on combinations of autoantibody markers. Diabetes, Vol.46, No. 11, pp. 1701-1710, ISSN 0012-1797

Bisikirska, B.; Colgan, J.; Luban, J.; Bluestone, J.A.&Herold, K.C., (2005). TCR stimulation with modified anti-CD3 mAb expands CD8+ T cell population and induces CD8+CD25+ Tregs. J Clin Invest, Vol.115, No. 10, pp. 2904-2913, ISSN 0021-9738

Bluestone, J.A., (1996). Costimulation and its role in organ transplantation. Clin Transplant, Vol.10, No. 1 Pt 2, pp. 104-109, ISSN 0902-0063

Bresson, D.&von Herrath, M., (2007). Moving towards efficient therapies in type 1 diabetes: to combine or not to combine? Autoimmun Rev, Vol.6, No. 5, pp. 315-322, ISSN 1568-9972

Cai, C.Q.; Zhang, T.; Breslin, M.B.; Giraud, M.&Lan, M.S., (2011). Both polymorphic variable number of tandem repeats and autoimmune regulator modulate differential expression of insulin in human thymic epithelial cells. Diabetes, Vol.60, No. 1, pp. 336-344, ISSN 1939-327X

Chaillous, L.; Lefevre, H.; Thivolet, C.; Boitard, C.; Lahlou, N.; Atlan-Gepner, C.; Bouhanick, B.; Mogenet, A.; Nicolino, M.; Carel, J.C.; Lecomte, P.; Marechaud, R.; Bougneres, P.; Charbonnel, B.&Sai, P., (2000). Oral insulin administration and residual beta-cell function in recent-onset type 1 diabetes: a multicentre randomised controlled trial. Diabete Insuline Orale group. Lancet, Vol.356, No. 9229, pp. 545-549, ISSN 0140-6736

Chatenoud, L., (2010). Immune therapy for type 1 diabetes mellitus-what is unique about anti-CD3 antibodies? Nat Rev Endocrinol, Vol.6, No. 3, pp. 149-157, ISSN 1759-5037

Chatenoud, L.; Primo, J.&Bach, J.F., (1997). CD3 antibody-induced dominant self tolerance in overtly diabetic NOD mice. J Immunol, Vol.158, No. 6, pp. 2947-2954, ISSN 0022-1767

Chatenoud, L.; Thervet, E.; Primo, J.&Bach, J.F., (1994). Anti-CD3 antibody induces long-term remission of overt autoimmunity in nonobese diabetic mice. Proc Natl Acad Sci U S A, Vol.91, No. 1, pp. 123-127, ISSN 0027-8424

Chen, W., (2006). Dendritic cells and (CD4+)CD25+ T regulatory cells: crosstalk between two professionals in immunity versus tolerance. Front Biosci, Vol.11, No. pp. 1360-1370, ISSN 1093-4715

Clarkson, M.R.&Sayegh, M.H., (2005). T-cell costimulatory pathways in allograft rejection and tolerance. Transplantation, Vol.80, No. 5, pp. 555-563, ISSN 0041-1337

Delovitch, T.L.&Singh, B., (1997). The nonobese diabetic mouse as a model of autoimmune diabetes: immune dysregulation gets the NOD. Immunity, Vol.7, No. 6, pp. 727-738, ISSN 1074-7613

Dib, S.A.&Gomes, M.B., (2009). Etiopathogenesis of type 1 diabetes mellitus: prognostic factors for the evolution of residual beta cell function. Diabetol Metab Syndr, Vol.1, No. 1, pp. 25, ISSN 1758-5996

Durinovic-Bello, I., (1998). Autoimmune diabetes: the role of T cells, MHC molecules and autoantigens. Autoimmunity, Vol.27, No. 3, pp. 159-177, ISSN 0891-6934

Edwards, J.C.; Szczepanski, L.; Szechinski, J.; Filipowicz-Sosnowska, A.; Emery, P.; Close, D.R.; Stevens, R.M.&Shaw, T., (2004). Efficacy of B-cell-targeted therapy with rituximab in patients with rheumatoid arthritis. N Engl J Med, Vol.350, No. 25, pp. 2572-2581, ISSN 1533-4406

Eising, S.; Nilsson, A.; Carstensen, B.; Hougaard, D.M.; Norgaard-Pedersen, B.; Nerup, J.; Lernmark, A.&Pociot, F., (2011). Danish children born with glutamic acid decarboxylase-65 and islet antigen-2 autoantibodies at birth had an increased risk to develop type 1 diabetes. Eur J Endocrinol, Vol.164, No. 2, pp. 247-252, ISSN 1479-683X

Enk, A.H., (2006). DCs and cytokines cooperate for the induction of tregs. Ernst Schering Res Found Workshop, No. 56, pp. 97-106, ISSN 0947-6075

Gandhi, R.; Kumar, D.; Burns, E.J.; Nadeau, M.; Dake, B.; Laroni, A.; Kozoriz, D.; Weiner, H.L.&Quintana, F.J., (2010). Activation of the aryl hydrocarbon receptor induces human type 1 regulatory T cell-like and Foxp3(+) regulatory T cells. Nat Immunol, Vol.11, No. 9, pp. 846-853, ISSN 1529-2916

Godebu, E.; Summers-Torres, D.; Lin, M.M.; Baaten, B.J.&Bradley, L.M., (2008). Polyclonal adaptive regulatory CD4 cells that can reverse type I diabetes become oligoclonal long-term protective memory cells. J Immunol, Vol.181, No. 3, pp. 1798-1805, ISSN 1550-6606

Hackstein, H.; Morelli, A.E.&Thomson, A.W., (2001). Designer dendritic cells for tolerance induction: guided not misguided missiles. Trends Immunol, Vol.22, No. 8, pp. 437-442, ISSN 1471-4906

Harnaha, J.; Machen, J.; Wright, M.; Lakomy, R.; Styche, A.; Trucco, M.; Makaroun, S.&Giannoukakis, N., (2006). Interleukin-7 is a survival factor for CD4+ CD25+ T-cells and is expressed by diabetes-suppressive dendritic cells. Diabetes, Vol.55, No. 1, pp. 158-170, ISSN 0012-1797

Harrison, L.C.; Dempsey-Collier, M.; Kramer, D.R.&Takahashi, K., (1996). Aerosol insulin induces regulatory CD8 gamma delta T cells that prevent murine insulin-dependent diabetes. J Exp Med, Vol.184, No. 6, pp. 2167-2174, ISSN 0022-1007

Harrison, L.C.; Honeyman, M.C.; Steele, C.E.; Stone, N.L.; Sarugeri, E.; Bonifacio, E.; Couper, J.J.&Colman, P.G., (2004). Pancreatic beta-cell function and immune responses to insulin after administration of intranasal insulin to humans at risk for type 1 diabetes. Diabetes Care, Vol.27, No. 10, pp. 2348-2355, ISSN 0149-5992

Hauser, S.L.; Waubant, E.; Arnold, D.L.; Vollmer, T.; Antel, J.; Fox, R.J.; Bar-Or, A.; Panzara, M.; Sarkar, N.; Agarwal, S.; Langer-Gould, A.&Smith, C.H., (2008). B-cell depletion with rituximab in relapsing-remitting multiple sclerosis. N Engl J Med, Vol.358, No. 7, pp. 676-688, ISSN 1533-4406

Herold, K.C.; Burton, J.B.; Francois, F.; Poumian-Ruiz, E.; Glandt, M.&Bluestone, J.A., (2003). Activation of human T cells by FcR nonbinding anti-CD3 mAb, hOKT3gamma1(Ala-Ala). J Clin Invest, Vol.111, No. 3, pp. 409-418, ISSN 0021-9738

Hinke, S.A., (2008). Diamyd, an alum-formulated recombinant human GAD65 for the prevention of autoimmune diabetes. Curr Opin Mol Ther, Vol.10, No. 5, pp. 516-525, ISSN 1464-8431

Hu, C.Y.; Rodriguez-Pinto, D.; Du, W.; Ahuja, A.; Henegariu, O.; Wong, F.S.; Shlomchik, M.J.&Wen, L., (2007). Treatment with CD20-specific antibody prevents and reverses autoimmune diabetes in mice. J Clin Invest, Vol.117, No. 12, pp. 3857-3867, ISSN 0021-9738

Huber, S.&Schramm, C., (2006). TGF-beta and CD4+CD25+ regulatory T cells. Front Biosci, Vol.11, No. pp. 1014-1023, ISSN 1093-4715

Hugues, S.; Boissonnas, A.; Amigorena, S.&Fetler, L., (2006). The dynamics of dendritic cell-T cell interactions in priming and tolerance. Curr Opin Immunol, Vol.18, No. 4, pp. 491-495, ISSN 0952-7915

Huurman, V.A.; Hilbrands, R.; Pinkse, G.G.; Gillard, P.; Duinkerken, G.; van de Linde, P.; van der Meer-Prins, P.M.; Versteeg-van der Voort Maarschalk, M.F.; Verbeeck, K.; Alizadeh, B.Z.; Mathieu, C.; Gorus, F.K.; Roelen, D.L.; Claas, F.H.; Keymeulen, B.; Pipeleers, D.G.&Roep, B.O., (2008). Cellular islet autoimmunity associates with clinical outcome of islet cell transplantation. PLoS One, Vol.3, No. 6, pp. e2435, ISSN 1932-6203

Huurman, V.A.; van der Meide, P.E.; Duinkerken, G.; Willemen, S.; Cohen, I.R.; Elias, D.&Roep, B.O., (2008). Immunological efficacy of heat shock protein 60 peptide DiaPep277 therapy in clinical type I diabetes. Clin Exp Immunol, Vol.152, No. 3, pp. 488-497, ISSN 1365-2249

Isermann, B.; Ritzel, R.; Zorn, M.; Schilling, T.&Nawroth, P.P., (2007). Autoantibodies in diabetes mellitus: current utility and perspectives. Exp Clin Endocrinol Diabetes, Vol.115, No. 8, pp. 483-490, ISSN 0947-7349

Jones, E.Y.; Fugger, L.; Strominger, J.L.&Siebold, C., (2006). MHC class II proteins and disease: a structural perspective. Nat Rev Immunol, Vol.6, No. 4, pp. 271-282, ISSN 1474-1733

Kantarova, D.&Buc, M., (2007). Genetic susceptibility to type 1 diabetes mellitus in humans. Physiol Res, Vol.56, No. 3, pp. 255-266, ISSN 0862-8408

Kishimoto, K.; Dong, V.M.&Sayegh, M.H., (2000). The role of costimulatory molecules as targets for new immunosuppressives in transplantation. Curr Opin Urol, Vol.10, No. 2, pp. 57-62, ISSN 0963-0643

Kurts, C.; Cannarile, M.; Klebba, I.&Brocker, T., (2001). Dendritic cells are sufficient to cross-present self-antigens to CD8 T cells in vivo. J Immunol, Vol.166, No. 3, pp. 1439-1442, ISSN 0022-1767

Kurts, C.; Carbone, F.R.; Barnden, M.; Blanas, E.; Allison, J.; Heath, W.R.&Miller, J.F., (1997). CD4+ T cell help impairs CD8+ T cell deletion induced by cross-presentation of self-antigens and favors autoimmunity. J Exp Med, Vol.186, No. 12, pp. 2057-2062, ISSN 0022-1007

Lenschow, D.J.; Herold, K.C.; Rhee, L.; Patel, B.; Koons, A.; Qin, H.Y.; Fuchs, E.; Singh, B.; Thompson, C.B.&Bluestone, J.A., (1996). CD28/B7 regulation of Th1 and Th2 subsets in the development of autoimmune diabetes. Immunity, Vol.5, No. 3, pp. 285-293, ISSN 1074-7613

Lenschow, D.J.; Walunas, T.L.&Bluestone, J.A., (1996). CD28/B7 system of T cell costimulation. Annu Rev Immunol, Vol.14, No. pp. 233-258, ISSN 0732-0582

Liston, A.; Lesage, S.; Wilson, J.; Peltonen, L.&Goodnow, C.C., (2003). Aire regulates negative selection of organ-specific T cells. Nat Immunol, Vol.4, No. 4, pp. 350-354, ISSN 1529-2908

Lohr, J.; Knoechel, B.&Abbas, A.K., (2006). Regulatory T cells in the periphery. Immunol Rev, Vol.212, No. pp. 149-162, ISSN 0105-2896

Ludvigsson, J., (2010). GAD-alum (Diamyd)--a new concept for preservation of residual insulin secretion. Expert Opin Biol Ther, Vol.10, No. 5, pp. 787-799, ISSN 1744-7682

Luo, X.; Tarbell, K.V.; Yang, H.; Pothoven, K.; Bailey, S.L.; Ding, R.; Steinman, R.M.&Suthanthiran, M., (2007). Dendritic cells with TGF-beta1 differentiate naive

CD4+CD25- T cells into islet-protective Foxp3+ regulatory T cells. Proc Natl Acad Sci U S A, Vol.104, No. 8, pp. 2821-2826, ISSN 0027-8424

Lutz, M.B.&Schuler, G., (2002). Immature, semi-mature and fully mature dendritic cells: which signals induce tolerance or immunity? Trends Immunol, Vol.23, No. 9, pp. 445-449, ISSN 1471-4906

Ma, L.; Qian, S.; Liang, X.; Wang, L.; Woodward, J.E.; Giannoukakis, N.; Robbins, P.D.; Bertera, S.; Trucco, M.; Fung, J.J.&Lu, L., (2003). Prevention of diabetes in NOD mice by administration of dendritic cells deficient in nuclear transcription factor-kappaB activity. Diabetes, Vol.52, No. 8, pp. 1976-1985, ISSN 0012-1797

Machen, J.; Harnaha, J.; Lakomy, R.; Styche, A.; Trucco, M.&Giannoukakis, N., (2004). Antisense oligonucleotides down-regulating costimulation confer diabetes-preventive properties to nonobese diabetic mouse dendritic cells. J Immunol, Vol.173, No. 7, pp. 4331-4341, ISSN 0022-1767

Maier, L.M.&Wicker, L.S., (2005). Genetic susceptibility to type 1 diabetes. Curr Opin Immunol, Vol.17, No. 6, pp. 601-608, ISSN 0952-7915

Makhlouf, L.; Grey, S.T.; Dong, V.; Csizmadia, E.; Arvelo, M.B.; Auchincloss, H., Jr.; Ferran, C.&Sayegh, M.H., (2004). Depleting anti-CD4 monoclonal antibody cures new-onset diabetes, prevents recurrent autoimmune diabetes, and delays allograft rejection in nonobese diabetic mice. Transplantation, Vol.77, No. 7, pp. 990-997, ISSN 0041-1337

Marguti, I.; Yamamoto, G.L.; da Costa, T.B.; Rizzo, L.V.&de Moraes, L.V., (2009). Expansion of CD4+ CD25+ Foxp3+ T cells by bone marrow-derived dendritic cells. Immunology, Vol.127, No. 1, pp. 50-61, ISSN 1365-2567

Marzorati, S.; Pileggi, A.&Ricordi, C., (2007). Allogeneic islet transplantation. Expert Opin Biol Ther, Vol.7, No. 11, pp. 1627-1645, ISSN 1744-7682

Maziarz, M.; Janer, M.; Roach, J.C.; Hagopian, W.; Palmer, J.P.; Deutsch, K.; Sanjeevi, C.B.; Kockum, I.; Breslow, N.&Lernmark, A., (2010). The association between the PTPN22 1858C>T variant and type 1 diabetes depends on HLA risk and GAD65 autoantibodies. Genes Immun, Vol.11, No. 5, pp. 406-415, ISSN 1476-5470

McLaughlin, P.; White, C.A.; Grillo-Lopez, A.J.&Maloney, D.G., (1998). Clinical status and optimal use of rituximab for B-cell lymphomas. Oncology (Williston Park), Vol.12, No. 12, pp. 1763-1769; discussion 1769-1770, 1775-1767, ISSN 0890-9091

Mellman, I.&Steinman, R.M., (2001). Dendritic cells: specialized and regulated antigen processing machines. Cell, Vol.106, No. 3, pp. 255-258, ISSN 0092-8674

Morelli, A.E.&Thomson, A.W., (2003). Dendritic cells: regulators of alloimmunity and opportunities for tolerance induction. Immunol Rev, Vol.196, No. pp. 125-146, ISSN 0105-2896

Mortensen, H.B.; Hougaard, P.; Swift, P.; Hansen, L.; Holl, R.W.; Hoey, H.; Bjoerndalen, H.; de Beaufort, C.; Chiarelli, F.; Danne, T.; Schoenle, E.J.&Aman, J., (2009). New definition for the partial remission period in children and adolescents with type 1 diabetes. Diabetes Care, Vol.32, No. 8, pp. 1384-1390, ISSN 1935-5548

Nicholson, L.B.&Kuchroo, V.K., (1997). T cell recognition of self and altered self antigens. Crit Rev Immunol, Vol.17, No. 5-6, pp. 449-462, ISSN 1040-8401

Nouri-Shirazi, M.&Thomson, A.W., (2006). Dendritic cells as promoters of transplant tolerance. Expert Opin Biol Ther, Vol.6, No. 4, pp. 325-339, ISSN 1744-7682

Papoz, L.; Lenegre, F.; Hors, J.; Assan, R.; Vague, P.; Tchobroutsky, G.; Passa, P.; Charbonnel, B.; Mirouze, J.; Feutren, G.&et al., (1990). Probability of remission in individual in early adult insulin dependent diabetic patients. Results from the Cyclosporine Diabetes French Study Group. Diabete Metab, Vol.16, No. 4, pp. 303-310, ISSN 0338-1684

Pescovitz, M.D.; Greenbaum, C.J.; Krause-Steinrauf, H.; Becker, D.J.; Gitelman, S.E.; Goland, R.; Gottlieb, P.A.; Marks, J.B.; McGee, P.F.; Moran, A.M.; Raskin, P.; Rodriguez, H.; Schatz, D.A.; Wherrett, D.; Wilson, D.M.; Lachin, J.M.&Skyler, J.S., (2009). Rituximab, B-lymphocyte depletion, and preservation of beta-cell function. N Engl J Med, Vol.361, No. 22, pp. 2143-2152, ISSN 1533-4406

Phillips, B.; Nylander, K.; Harnaha, J.; Machen, J.; Lakomy, R.; Styche, A.; Gillis, K.; Brown, L.; Lafreniere, D.; Gallo, M.; Knox, J.; Hogeland, K.; Trucco, M.&Giannoukakis, N., (2008). A microsphere-based vaccine prevents and reverses new-onset autoimmune diabetes. Diabetes, Vol.57, No. 6, pp. 1544-1555, ISSN 1939-327X

Phillips, B.E.&Giannoukakis, N., (2010). Drug delivery technologies for autoimmune disease. Expert Opin Drug Deliv, Vol.7, No. 11, pp. 1279-1289, ISSN 1744-7593

Randolph, G.J., (2001). Dendritic cell migration to lymph nodes: cytokines, chemokines, and lipid mediators. Semin Immunol, Vol.13, No. 5, pp. 267-274, ISSN 1044-5323

Raz, I.; Avron, A.; Tamir, M.; Metzger, M.; Symer, L.; Eldor, R.; Cohen, I.R.&Elias, D., (2007). Treatment of new-onset type 1 diabetes with peptide DiaPep277 is safe and associated with preserved beta-cell function: extension of a randomized, double-blind, phase II trial. Diabetes Metab Res Rev, Vol.23, No. 4, pp. 292-298, ISSN 1520-7552

Raz, I.; Elias, D.; Avron, A.; Tamir, M.; Metzger, M.&Cohen, I.R., (2001). Beta-cell function in new-onset type 1 diabetes and immunomodulation with a heat-shock protein peptide (DiaPep277): a randomised, double-blind, phase II trial. Lancet, Vol.358, No. 9295, pp. 1749-1753, ISSN 0140-6736

Reis, E.A.; Athanazio, D.A.; Lima, I.; Oliveira e Silva, N.; Andrade, J.C.; Jesus, R.N.; Barbosa, L.M.; Reis, M.G.&Santiago, M.B., (2009). NK and NKT cell dynamics after rituximab therapy for systemic lupus erythematosus and rheumatoid arthritis. Rheumatol Int, Vol.29, No. 4, pp. 469-475, ISSN 1437-160X

Roelen, D.L.; Huurman, V.A.; Hilbrands, R.; Gillard, P.; Duinkerken, G.; van der Meer-Prins, P.W.; Versteeg-van der Voort Maarschalk, M.F.; Mathieu, C.; Keymeulen, B.; Pipeleers, D.G.; Roep, B.O.&Claas, F.H., (2009). Relevance of cytotoxic alloreactivity under different immunosuppressive regimens in clinical islet cell transplantation. Clin Exp Immunol, Vol.156, No. 1, pp. 141-148, ISSN 1365-2249

Roncarolo, M.G.; Gregori, S.; Battaglia, M.; Bacchetta, R.; Fleischhauer, K.&Levings, M.K., (2006). Interleukin-10-secreting type 1 regulatory T cells in rodents and humans. Immunol Rev, Vol.212, No. pp. 28-50, ISSN 0105-2896

Sayegh, M.H.&Turka, L.A., (1995). T cell costimulatory pathways: promising novel targets for immunosuppression and tolerance induction. J Am Soc Nephrol, Vol.6, No. 4, pp. 1143-1150, ISSN 1046-6673

Schloot, N.C.; Meierhoff, G.; Lengyel, C.; Vandorfi, G.; Takacs, J.; Panczel, P.; Barkai, L.; Madacsy, L.; Oroszlan, T.; Kovacs, P.; Suto, G.; Battelino, T.; Hosszufalusi, N.&Jermendy, G., (2007). Effect of heat shock protein peptide DiaPep277 on beta-cell function in paediatric and adult patients with recent-onset diabetes mellitus type 1: two prospective, randomized, double-blind phase II trials. Diabetes Metab Res Rev, Vol.23, No. 4, pp. 276-285, ISSN 1520-7552

Schlosser, M.; Mueller, P.W.; Torn, C.; Bonifacio, E.&Bingley, P.J., (2010). Diabetes Antibody Standardization Program: evaluation of assays for insulin autoantibodies. Diabetologia, Vol.53, No. 12, pp. 2611-2620, ISSN 1432-0428

Scott, S.D., (1998). Rituximab: a new therapeutic monoclonal antibody for non-Hodgkin's lymphoma. Cancer Pract, Vol.6, No. 3, pp. 195-197, ISSN 1065-4704

Shevach, E.M.; DiPaolo, R.A.; Andersson, J.; Zhao, D.M.; Stephens, G.L.&Thornton, A.M., (2006). The lifestyle of naturally occurring CD4+ CD25+ Foxp3+ regulatory T cells. Immunol Rev, Vol.212, No. pp. 60-73, ISSN 0105-2896

Shortman, K.&Naik, S.H., (2007). Steady-state and inflammatory dendritic-cell development. Nat Rev Immunol, Vol.7, No. 1, pp. 19-30, ISSN 1474-1733

Skyler, J.S.; Krischer, J.P.; Wolfsdorf, J.; Cowie, C.; Palmer, J.P.; Greenbaum, C.; Cuthbertson, D.; Rafkin-Mervis, L.E.; Chase, H.P.&Leschek, E., (2005). Effects of oral insulin in relatives of patients with type 1 diabetes: The Diabetes Prevention Trial--Type 1. Diabetes Care, Vol.28, No. 5, pp. 1068-1076, ISSN 0149-5992

Sloan-Lancaster, J.&Allen, P.M., (1996). Altered peptide ligand-induced partial T cell activation: molecular mechanisms and role in T cell biology. Annu Rev Immunol, Vol.14, No. pp. 1-27, ISSN 0732-0582

Steinman, R.M., (2003). The control of immunity and tolerance by dendritic cell. Pathol Biol (Paris), Vol.51, No. 2, pp. 59-60, ISSN 0369-8114

Steinman, R.M.; Inaba, K.; Turley, S.; Pierre, P.&Mellman, I., (1999). Antigen capture, processing, and presentation by dendritic cells: recent cell biological studies. Hum Immunol, Vol.60, No. 7, pp. 562-567, ISSN 0198-8859

Suzuki, K.; Nagasawa, H.; Kameda, H.; Amano, K.; Kondo, T.; Itoyama, S.; Tanaka, Y.&Takeuchi, T., (2009). Severe acute thrombotic exacerbation in two cases with anti-phospholipid syndrome after retreatment with rituximab in phase I/II clinical trial for refractory systemic lupus erythematosus. Rheumatology (Oxford), Vol.48, No. 2, pp. 198-199, ISSN 1462-0332

Tang, Q.&Bluestone, J.A., (2006). Regulatory T-cell physiology and application to treat autoimmunity. Immunol Rev, Vol.212, No. pp. 217-237, ISSN 0105-2896

Tang, Q.; Henriksen, K.J.; Bi, M.; Finger, E.B.; Szot, G.; Ye, J.; Masteller, E.L.; McDevitt, H.; Bonyhadi, M.&Bluestone, J.A., (2004). In vitro-expanded antigen-specific regulatory T cells suppress autoimmune diabetes. J Exp Med, Vol.199, No. 11, pp. 1455-1465, ISSN 0022-1007

Tarbell, K.V.; Yamazaki, S.; Olson, K.; Toy, P.&Steinman, R.M., (2004). CD25+ CD4+ T cells, expanded with dendritic cells presenting a single autoantigenic peptide, suppress autoimmune diabetes. J Exp Med, Vol.199, No. 11, pp. 1467-1477, ISSN 0022-1007

The DCCT Research Group, The Diabetes Control and Complications Trial (DCCT) (1993). The effect of intensive treatment of diabetes on the development and progression of long-term complications in insulin-dependent diabetes mellitus. The Diabetes Control and Complications Trial Research Group. N Engl J Med, Vol.329, No. 14, pp. 977-986, ISSN 0028-4793

Van Belle, T.&von Herrath, M., (2008). Immunosuppression in islet transplantation. J Clin Invest, Vol.118, No. 5, pp. 1625-1628, ISSN 0021-9738

Verge, C.F.; Gianani, R.; Kawasaki, E.; Yu, L.; Pietropaolo, M.; Jackson, R.A.; Chase, H.P.&Eisenbarth, G.S., (1996). Prediction of type I diabetes in first-degree relatives using a combination of insulin, GAD, and ICA512bdc/IA-2 autoantibodies. Diabetes, Vol.45, No. 7, pp. 926-933, ISSN 0012-1797

Verge, C.F.; Howard, N.J.; Rowley, M.J.; Mackay, I.R.; Zimmet, P.Z.; Egan, M.; Hulinska, H.; Hulinsky, I.; Silvestrini, R.A.; Kamath, S.&et al., (1994). Anti-glutamate decarboxylase and other antibodies at the onset of childhood IDDM: a population-based study. Diabetologia, Vol.37, No. 11, pp. 1113-1120, ISSN 0012-186X

Verhagen, J.; Blaser, K.; Akdis, C.A.&Akdis, M., (2006). Mechanisms of allergen-specific immunotherapy: T-regulatory cells and more. Immunol Allergy Clin North Am, Vol.26, No. 2, pp. 207-231, vi, ISSN 0889-8561

Vlad, G.; Cortesini, R.&Suciu-Foca, N., (2005). License to heal: bidirectional interaction of antigen-specific regulatory T cells and tolerogenic APC. J Immunol, Vol.174, No. 10, pp. 5907-5914, ISSN 0022-1767

Walter, M.; Philotheou, A.; Bonnici, F.; Ziegler, A.G.&Jimenez, R., (2009). No effect of the altered peptide ligand NBI-6024 on beta-cell residual function and insulin needs in new-onset type 1 diabetes. Diabetes Care, Vol.32, No. 11, pp. 2036-2040, ISSN 1935-5548

Weber, S.E.; Harbertson, J.; Godebu, E.; Mros, G.A.; Padrick, R.C.; Carson, B.D.; Ziegler, S.F.&Bradley, L.M., (2006). Adaptive islet-specific regulatory CD4 T cells control autoimmune diabetes and mediate the disappearance of pathogenic Th1 cells in vivo. J Immunol, Vol.176, No. 8, pp. 4730-4739, ISSN 0022-1767

Wicker, L.S.; Todd, J.A.&Peterson, L.B., (1995). Genetic control of autoimmune diabetes in the NOD mouse. Annu Rev Immunol, Vol.13, No. pp. 179-200, ISSN 0732-0582

Wong, F.S.; Karttunen, J.; Dumont, C.; Wen, L.; Visintin, I.; Pilip, I.M.; Shastri, N.; Pamer, E.G.&Janeway, C.A., Jr., (1999). Identification of an MHC class I-restricted autoantigen in type 1 diabetes by screening an organ-specific cDNA library. Nat Med, Vol.5, No. 9, pp. 1026-1031, ISSN 1078-8956

Xiu, Y.; Wong, C.P.; Bouaziz, J.D.; Hamaguchi, Y.; Wang, Y.; Pop, S.M.; Tisch, R.M.&Tedder, T.F., (2008). B lymphocyte depletion by CD20 monoclonal antibody prevents diabetes in nonobese diabetic mice despite isotype-specific differences in Fc gamma R effector functions. J Immunol, Vol.180, No. 5, pp. 2863-2875, ISSN 0022-1767

Yamazaki, S.; Iyoda, T.; Tarbell, K.; Olson, K.; Velinzon, K.; Inaba, K.&Steinman, R.M., (2003). Direct expansion of functional CD25+ CD4+ regulatory T cells by antigen-processing dendritic cells. J Exp Med, Vol.198, No. 2, pp. 235-247, ISSN 0022-1007

Zhang, L.; Yi, H.; Xia, X.P.&Zhao, Y., (2006). Transforming growth factor-beta: an important role in CD4+CD25+ regulatory T cells and immune tolerance. Autoimmunity, Vol.39, No. 4, pp. 269-276, ISSN 0891-6934

18

Immunotherapy for Type 1 Diabetes - Necessity, Challenges and Unconventional Opportunities

Rachel Gutfreund and Abdel Rahim A. Hamad
Department of Pathology; Johns Hopkins University School of Medicine, Baltimore, USA

1. Introduction

Type 1 diabetes (T1D) is the leading autoimmune disease of childhood. In this review / prospective, we discuss (1) why there is an urgent need of an immunotherapy for T1D despite success of insulin therapy in improving quality of life of patients and (2) why the limited efficacy of current therapies in phase I/II clinical trials has necessitated a quest for new approaches. In addition, we offer novel views on the potentials of targeting the Fas death pathway as an unconventional therapeutic approach for T1D that is unlikely to cause immune suppression.

2. Why immunotherapy for T1D?

Type 1 diabetes (TID), also known as insulin dependent diabetes, is a chronic progressively worsening autoimmune disease that occurs early in life and is the leading autoimmune disease of childhood (Bluestone et al.). In genetically susceptible individuals, autoimmune T-cells infiltrate pancreatic islets where they proliferate and destroy insulin-producing beta cells, resulting in insulin deficiency and impaired blood glucose homeostasis manifested as hyperglycemia. Hyperglycemia causes many serious complications including renal failure, proliferative retinopathy/blindness, peripheral neuropathy, and vascular disease. Therefore, all T1D patients need to take exogenous insulin on a daily basis to keep the blood glucose level within a physiologic range. Since insulin is not a cure for the disease, patients must take it throughout life, a routine that requires significant dedication and time from patients and parents in case of children. In addition, patients need to observe a strict diet, check their blood sugar levels on a regular basis, and adjust the insulin dose accordingly. Even with tight glucose control, patients eventually develop a multitude of life threatening vascular and neurologic complications as mentioned above. Thus, although insulin therapy is currently the best available option to manage T1D, it remains a palliative measure and a cure for the disease remains an urgent goal. Consequently, intensive efforts are being directed towards developing an immunotherapy for the disease. These efforts are facilitated by the significant advances made in understanding the disease pathogenesis that resulted in uncovering a multitude of potentially therapeutic targets to control the diabetogenic T cells that drive the disease process.

3. High standard for T1D immunotherapy

The goal of immunotherapy, in general, is to thwart the unwanted immune cells that precipitate and drive the autoimmune response that impairs or destroys the target organ; the pancreas in the case of T1D. Studies in animal models have identified the T cell as the key mediator of the autoimmune responses that destroy insulin-producing beta cells in pancreata of T1D (Anderson and Bluestone, 2005). Therefore, many recent and current T1D immunotherapies are aimed at the T cell. Significant advances have been made in identifying and characterizing molecules and mediators, including cytokines, which regulate T cell activation, trafficking, and effector functions. These advances offer potential targets that can be modulated using recombinant ligands or specific antibodies to suppress or eliminate autoreactive T cells. These molecules and mediators, however, are used primarily by protective T cells to defend individuals from infections. Therefore, while theoretically many approaches can be used to successfully prevent or arrest the autoimmune response by targeting diabetogenic T cells; most of these approaches lack specificity and carry the inherent risk of paralyzing the whole T cell repertoire, resulting in systemic immune suppression. The difficulty is, therefore, lies in finding means to specifically target and safely suppress and/or eliminate autoreactive T cells without damaging protective T cells and causing immunosuppression.

The risk of immune suppression is an accepted trade-off in life threatening autoimmune diseases such as multiple sclerosis, but not for T1D patients. There is an exceptionally high safety standard for immunotherapy for T1D patients. A primary reason for this is the effectiveness of insulin therapy in allowing T1D patients to maintain a significantly good quality of life for a long time. Secondly, most T1D patients are young people with their productive years of life ahead of them. Therefore, the benefits of a successful immunotherapy for T1D must supersede those of the insulin therapy. It must be a cure and not an alternative palliative measure, and must carry minimal risk of causing immunosuppression. The side effects should be tolerable. In summary, although T1D is usually associated with devastating long-term complications, it is currently fairly manageable by the insulin therapy and thus benefits of any appealing immunotherapy should far exceed those of the insulin therapy. In other words, as a gold standard, immunotherapy for T1D must provide a cure for T1D: freedom from insulin usage, and negligible risk of immunosuppression.

4. Limited efficacy of clinically tested T1D immunotherapies generates new challenges

The non-obese diabetic (NOD) mouse is the widely-used animal model to study the pathogenesis of T1D. T1D disease development in these mice shares many properties with T1D disease development in humans (Anderson and Bluestone, 2005) and many key insights into the etiology and pathogenesis of the disease have been initially discovered in NOD mice (Anderson and Bluestone, 2005), resulting in a wide range of potential therapeutic targets, a number of which have been tested in clinical trials. These agents can generally be divided into two categories: nonspecific and antigen specific modulators. Among the promising non-specific modulators are anti-CD3 mAb and more recently, anti-CD20 therapy that modulate and temporally delete T and B cells, respectively. Among antigen specific therapies, attention is focused on GAD65 and insulin therapies. Because both non-specific and antigen specific therapies can potentially cause serious side effects depending on the dosage and frequency of administration, therapeutic regimens are carefully calculated.

Therapeutic trials of two humanized Fc-engineered monoclonal anti-CD3 antibodies called teplizumab (Herold et al., 2005; Herold et al., 2002) and otelixizumab (Bolt et al., 1993; Keymeulen et al., 2005) showed initial promising results. Short term treatment of recently-diagnosed T1D patients demonstrated a significant reduction in the loss of beta-cell function for at least two years. These subjects showed no evidence of long term immune suppression and experienced improvement in hemoglobin A1c levels and insulin usage. Although anti-CD3 mAb treatment was generally well-tolerated due to the largely-eliminated T cell activation-associated cytokine storm with the development of a non-Fc binding anti-CD3 mAb, some subjects experienced flu-like side effects in the first days and weeks after treatment that were attributed to cytokine release. Symptoms were severe enough to cause 10% of subjects to discontinue treatment. In the European trial, some subjects experienced transient reactivation of Epstein-Barr virus, however, these EBV copies returned to normal pre-treatment levels within 3 weeks in all cases (Keymeulen et al.).

A humanized CD20 mAb called Rituximab, which was initially approved to treat lymphomas, has also advanced to T1D clinical trials. A recent randomized, double-blind trial of Rituximab on newly-diagnosed T1D patients showed promise (Pescovitz et al., 2009). Three months after treatment, Rituximab-treated subjects had significantly lower hemoblogin A1c levels, reduced insulin use, and improved beta-cell function compared to placebo. Rituximab patients, however, experienced a decline in beta-cell function that paralleled those of placebo-treated subjects at months 3-12 of the study. Despite this, Rituximab patients showed overall improvement in the previously described clinical parameters at 1 year compared to placebo-treated subjects.

Antigen specific immunization with beta cell autoantigens (Insulin and GAD65) also made it to clinical trials. Glutamate Decarboxylase 65 (GAD65) is secreted by all endocrine islet cells and is thought to be one of the earliest autoantibody targets during the initiation of T1D (Kaufman et al., 1993; Tisch et al., 1993). The antigenic region of the GAD protein is initially a small region consisting of two adjacent peptides. T cell autoimmunity eventually spreads intermolecularly to additional GAD determinants and then to other beta-cell antigens, resulting in a diverse population of autoreactive T cells. Elimination of the anti-GAD T cell response halts the spread of autoimmunity to other beta-cell antigens and disease progression. Based on success in animal studies (Tian et al., 1996), two clinical trials using alum-formulated human recombinant GAD65 have shown encouraging results. Agardh et al. (2005) conducted a Phase II study to evaluate dosage and safety in adults (Agardh et al., 2005). No adverse effects of treatment were identified and both fasting and stimulated c-peptide levels were increased from baseline in the group receiving 20 μg compared to placebo at 24 weeks. A different trial conducted by Ludvigsson et al., (2011) on recent onset adolescents showed longer preservation of both fasting and stimulated C-peptide levels in GAD-treated subjects as compared to placebo. This study also demonstrated that improvement in clinical parameters after GAD treatment was most pronounced in patients with <6 months disease duration at baseline.

Much attention has been given to insulin and its immunogenic epitopes as inducers of immune tolerance in pre-T1D and newly diagnosed T1D patients. Insulin and proinsulin are thought to be some of the primary autoantigens targeted by the immune system during T1D initiation (Nakayama et al., 2005; Narendran et al., 2003). Mucosal exposure to insulin was shown to impart a T_{reg}-associated delay in disease onset and a reduction in incidence of T1D in NOD mice (Harrison and Hafler, 2000). Due to the largely successful outcomes of laboratory studies, oral and nasal insulin treatment progressed to clinical trials to explore treatment of both prediabetic and recent onset patients. A trial conducted by Harrison et al. (2004) recruited subjects who had antibodies to at least one islet antigen (Harrison et al., 2004). The trial demonstrated that nasally-administered insulin therapy did not result in adverse side effects or accelerated destruction of beta-cells. Subjects also experienced a decrease in T cell response to insulin and increase in antibody which were consistent with mucosal insulin tolerance.

Other trials, however, have indicated that insulin-treated prediabetic subjects were no less likely to develop T1D or experience a delay in T1D onset than their placebo-treated counterparts and that insulin therapy could possibly cause accelerated beta-cell destruction (Skyler et al., 2005; Sosenko et al., 2006).

While assessment of the results of clinical trials has demonstrated feasibility, evaluation of efficacy produced the conclusion that none of the agents currently under clinical investigation hold the key for the cure as a sole therapy. Since escalating dose is not an option because of the serious side effects of these agents, combination therapy strategies are currently being evaluated (Skyler and Ricordi; von Herrath). A prime example combines an antigen-specific therapy with a broad spectrum immunosuppressive drug. Nasally-introduced proinsulin II peptide in combination with anti-CD3 mAb was shown to significantly increase T_{reg} induction in 2 mouse models (Bresson et al., 2006). In contrast, neither therapy alone could achieve operational antigen-specific T_{reg} induction late in diabetogenesis. It is suggested by the authors of this study that the induction of proinsulin-specific T_{reg} cells was made possible by the transient decrease in autoreactive T cells via anti-CD3 mAb, allowing for the modulation of APCs in the PLNs. The hope is to increase the efficacy through synergistic or additive effects of agents that target different pathways. In addition, significant efforts are also being directed towards identifying new, non-suppressive therapeutic agents. In summary, as only few of the diverse immunomodulating agents that have so far been examined in clinical trials show promise, efforts are being directed towards identifying new therapeutic agents and assessing efficacy of combination therapy.

5. The Fas pathway as a counter-intuitive therapeutic target for T1D

For obvious reasons, the focus of immunotherapy for T1D has been on T cells, antigen presenting cells (APC), and molecules that control T cell activation. As noted above, the intimate roles for these cells and molecules in regulating host response to infections has limited the degree to which their activity can be modulated to treat or prevent T1D without causing immune suppression to infections. In this regard, The Fas pathway represents a unique molecule that is not essential for host immune response yet plays a critical role in regulating pathogenesis of autoimmune diabetes in the NOD mouse.

5.1 The Fas pathway regulates T cell homeostasis

The Fas pathway is the prototypical apoptosis pathway that mediates contraction and death of activated T cells (Hamad; Lenardo et al., 1999; Pinkoski and Green, 1999; Takahashi et al., 1994; Watanabe-Fukunaga et al., 1992). It is an extrinsic signaling pathway that initiates apoptosis, or programmed cell death. The Fas receptor (also known as Apo-1 or CD95) is a transmembrane protein member of the tumor necrosis factor (TNF) receptor superfamily (Strasser et al., 2009). It contains a "death domain" of approximately 80 amino acids in its cytoplasmic region that is essential for apoptotic signal transduction (Lenardo, 1996). Binding of FasL to its receptor results in the formation of a death-inducing signaling complex (DISC) composed of Fas-associated death domain protein (FADD) and caspase 8. The Fas-DISC complex allows for autocatalytic activation of procaspase 8. In type 1 cells, processed caspase-8 directly activates caspase 3 and other caspases which cleave cell substrates and initiate apoptosis. In type 2 cells, less DISC is formed, thus the apoptotic signal must by amplified via a positive feedback loop that involves the release of mitochondrial pro-apoptotic factors.

Increasing evidence indicates that the Fas pathway is critical for elimination of chronically-activated T cells, especially an abnormal subset of double negative (DN) alpha/beta T cells from secondary lymphoid organs (Hamad; Stranges et al., 2007). Spontaneous loss-of-function mutation in either Fas (lpr mutation) or FasL (gld mutation) impairs Fas-mediated apoptosis and animals bearing these mutations develop an age-dependent lymphoproliferation in which DN T cells predominate (Takahashi et al., 1994; Watanabe-Fukunaga et al., 1992). In humans, defects in the Fas pathway cause an autoimmune lymphoproliferative syndrome (ALPS) that is similar to the disease in mutant mice (Fischer et al., 1995).

5.2 Fas/FasL interaction controls a main pathogenic mechanism in insulitis development

Despite the lymphoproliferation, NOD mice (the widely used model for T1D) bearing homozygous gld or lpr mutations become completely resistant to autoimmune diabetes and several other organ-specific autoimmune diseases (Chervonsky et al., 1997; Hamad; Kim et al., 2000; Mohamood et al., 2007; Thomas et al., 1999; Waldner et al., 1997) (Nakayama et al., 2002). The diabetogenic process is arrested at a pre-insulitis stage by the lpr or gld mutation (Chervonsky et al., 1997; Mohamood et al., 2007; Su et al., 2000). This finding established the Fas/FasL interaction as a pivotal pathogenic mechanism that regulates insulitis development.

FasL is not required for the normal immune response. Therefore, it has been puzzling that NOD mice bearing homozygous lpr or gld mutations become resistant to autoimmune diabetes. The disease process is arrested at a pre-insulitis stage in mutant NOD mice and the mice never develop overt disease. Initially, it was thought that the protection is due to an essential role of Fas/FasL interactions in mediating death of the insulin-producing beta cells; a mechanism which, if true, would be extremely useful for engineering disease-resistant islets (Chervonsky et al., 1997). Specific deletion of the Fas molecule on pancreatic islets, however, did not spare beta cells from autoimmune attack and destruction or mice from developing overt disease (Allison and Strasser, 1998; Apostolou et al., 2003; Kim et al., 1999; Savinov et al., 2003). In the absence of a plausible alternative explanation of how inhibition of the Fas pathway prevents autoimmune diabetes and the tight association of the protection with lymphoaccumulation of DN T cells, interest in the therapeutic value of targeting the Fas pathway simply faded away.

5.3 Separation of lymphoproliferation from the protective effect of the gld mutation revitalizes interest in therapeutic potential of FasL

Unlike most effector molecules and cytokines that inhibit autoimmune processes, the Fas pathway is not needed for generation of adaptive immune responses and mice bearing spontaneous lpr or gld mutation remain immune competent. The main side effects of

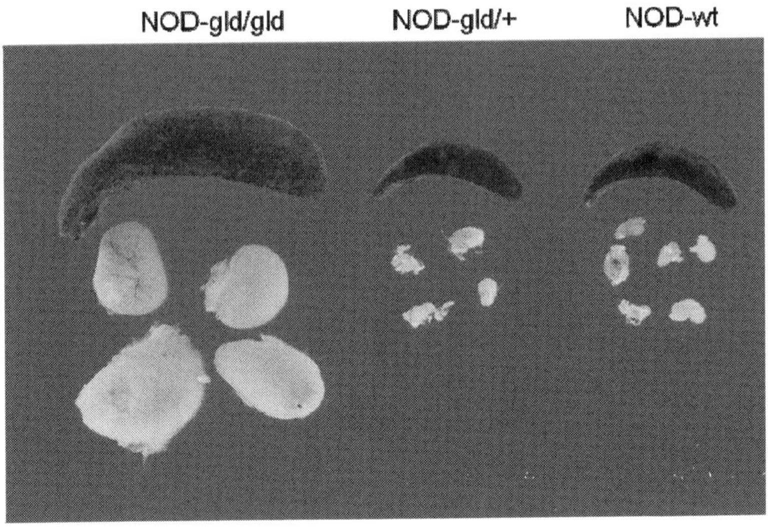

Fig. 1. Comparison of sizes of spleens and lymph nodes of 16-week-old NOD-gld/gld, NOD-gld/+, and NOD-wt mice. Adopted from ref. Mohamood et al. 2007 with copy right permission from Copyright © 201X, AMERICAN SOCIETY FOR INVESTIGATIVE PATHOLOGY. Published by ELSEVIER INC.

inactivating the Fas pathway are the age-dependent benign lymphoproliferation that occurs in some strains of mice together with lupus-like syndrome (Hamad; Mohamood et al., 2008; Nagata and Suda, 1995). It was believed that the lymphoproliferation and protection from autoimmune diabetes are tightly associated, leading to loss of interest in the therapeutic potential of targeting FasL. We therefore predicted that modulation of FasL to prevent autoimmune diabetes without causing lymphoproliferation will revitalize interest in assessing the therapeutic potential of targeting the Fas pathway: an approach that is unlikely to cause immune suppression. In support of this concept, studies by Su et al and our group showed that protection from autoimmune diabetes as a function of targeting FasL is indeed separable from the lymphoproliferation. NOD mice bearing heterozygote gld mutation (NOD-gld/+) develop no lymphoproliferation **(Figure 1)**, show mild or no insulitis **(Figure 2)**, completely protected from autoimmune diabetes **(Figure 3A)**, and show no sign of producing autoantibodies **(Figure 3B)**. We have not detected a single incidence of diabetes in NOD-gld/+ mice of various ages in our colony whereas NOD-wt littermates developed diabetes with a predicted incidence rate. Insulitis was also curtailed; the majority of NOD-gld/+ mice remained free of insulitis and fewer animals developed peri- or mild insulitis that did not progress to full destruction of islets and diabetes **(Fig. 2)**. NOD-gld/+ mice did not develop significant levels of anti-nuclear antibodies, whereas modest and infrequent anti-nuclear antibodies (ANA) were observed in NOD-gld/gld mice **(Fig. 3B)**. We concluded that complete inactivation of FasL was not essential for prevention of spontaneous diabetes in NOD mice and that partial blockade could be used to induce protection from autoimmune diabetes in wt mice without impairing T cell homeostasis.

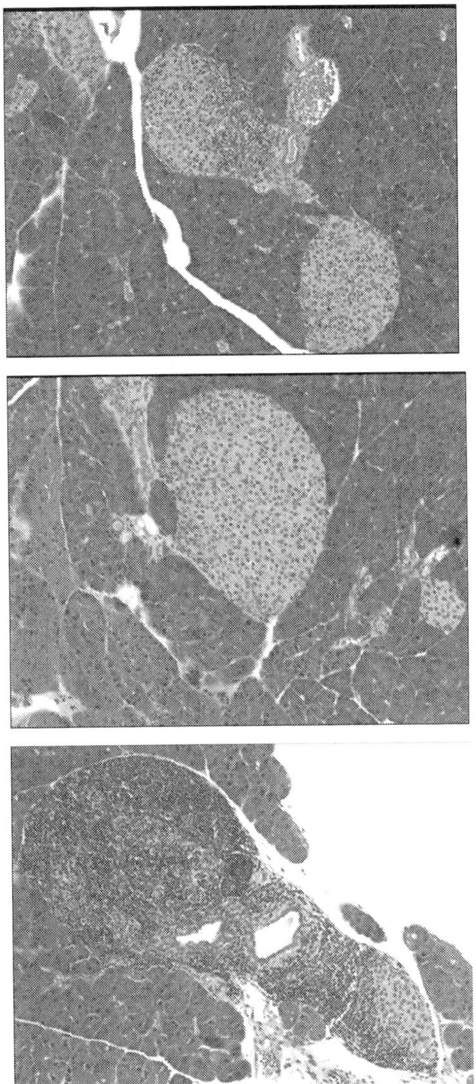

Fig. 2. NOD-gld/+ mice develop mild or no insulitis. Pancreata from 12-week-old NOD-wt, NOD-gld/+, or NOD-gld/gld mice were formalin-fixed, sectioned, H&E-stained, and compared with age-matched NOD-wt mice for insulitis. Three mice per group were examined. Top photo: NOD-gld/+ ; Middle photo: NOD-gld/gld , Bottom photo: NOD-WT Adopted from ref. Mohamood et al. 2007 with copy right permission from Copyright © 201X, AMERICAN SOCIETY FOR INVESTIGATIVE PATHOLOGY. Published by ELSEVIER INC.

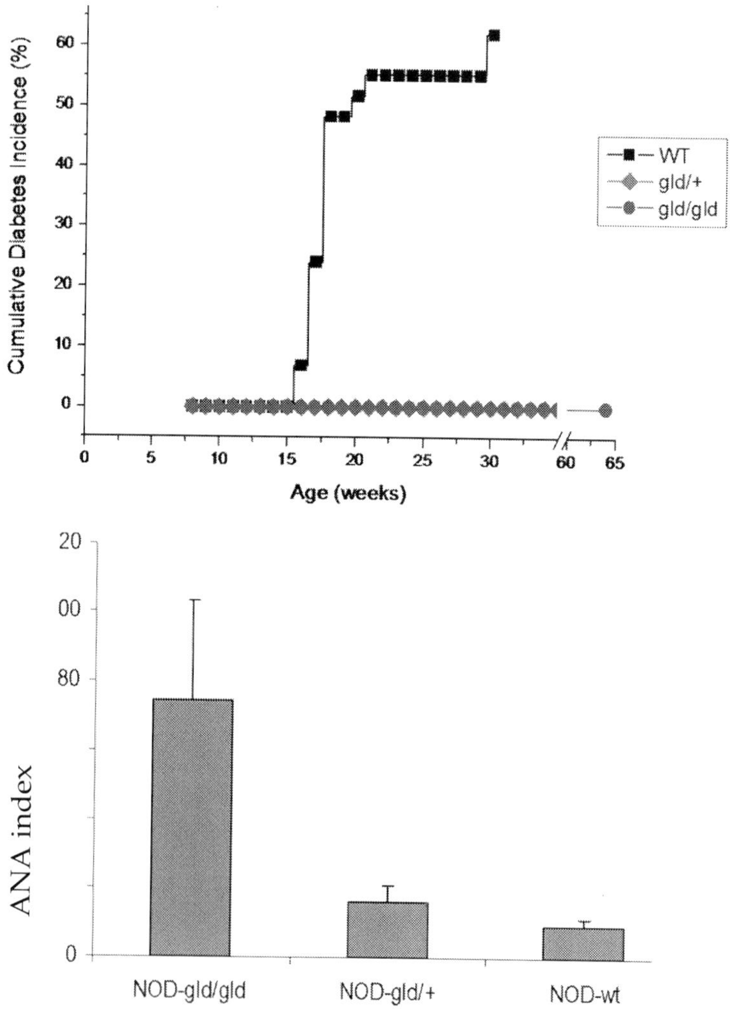

Fig. 3. *Top:* Cumulative diabetes incidence in NOD-gld/gld (n = 14), NOD-gld/+ (n = 35), and NOD-wt (n = 29) mice that were up to 65 weeks of age.
Bottom: Heterozygote gld mutation does not cause production of antinuclear antibodies (ANAs). ANAs in the sera from NOD-gld/gld, NOD-gld/+, and NOD-wt mice between the ages of 15 to 30 weeks (n = 6 per group). The concentration of ANAs in each sample is calculated as ANA index (AI), which is defined as the ratio of absorbance of the test sample and net absorbance of the negative (endpoint-cutoff) control. AI >22 is considered positive. Adopted from ref. Mohamood et al. 2007 with copy right permission from Copyright © 201X, AMERICAN SOCIETY FOR INVESTIGATIVE PATHOLOGY. Published by ELSEVIER INC.

FasL molecules randomly preassociate to form functional homotrimers that interact with corresponding Fas homotrimers (Orlinick et al., 1999; Schneider et al., 1997). In NOD mice bearing heterozygote gld mutation, about 85% of FasL homotrimers are inactive due to their incorporation of one or more gld molecules. Mechanistic analyses show that the remaining functional FasL homotrimers (~15%) suffice to maintain T cell homeostasis. Thus, it appears that more or less fully-functional FasL is required to drive the pathogenesis of autoimmune diabetes in NOD mice whereas partially functional FasL is sufficient to maintain immune homeostasis. The results offer the NOD-gld/+ mouse as a model to study the role of FasL in T cell tolerance without the complication caused by the massive DN T cell accumulation.

5.4 FasL-neutralizing antibody prevents diabetes in NOD-wt mice

Indeed, we found that brief antibody blockade of FasL using MFL4 neutralizing mAb (Kayagaki et al., 1997) prevents T1D in NOD mice without causing lymphoproliferation , thereby demonstrating the therapeutic potential of targeting FasL **(Figure 4)**. We treated prediabetic NOD female mice with MFL4 FasL-neutralizing antibody(Kayagaki et al., 1997) as described in Figure legend and monitored them for development of diabetes. Control NOD mice that were treated in parallel with hamster IgG developed diabetes with the normal incidence rate. In contrast, none of the mice in the treated group developed diabetes **(Fig.4, top)**. Analysis of pancreata from treated mice showed that blockade of FasL also prevented insulitis in the majority of the mice in the group although a few mice developed perinsulitis, whereas severe insulitis was observed in the control group (ref. (Mohamood et al., 2007) and data not shown). Furthermore, anti-FasL treatment was associated with only a small and transient increase in the frequency of DN T cells, which did not exceed 6% of T cells in any of the treated mice **(Fig. 4, bottom)**. As in NOD-gld/+ mice, protection from diabetes was not associated with systemic increase in the level of antinuclear antibodies [(ref. (Mohamood et al., 2007)]. Thus, it appears that there is a wide window for maneuvering to block most FasL activity to inhibit its pathogenic effect without interfering with T cell homeostasis. Together, these studies show the feasibility and suggest that FasL-based intervention may prove beneficial in the future to protect high-risk individuals from T1D. These findings revitalize interest in the therapeutic potentials of targeting FasL by showing that major side effects are avoidable by calibrating the dose.

5.5 Significance of targeting FasL

Developing an immunotherapy that would promote immune tolerance to beta cell autoantigens without generally weakening the immune system is the ultimate goal of researchers involved in studying T1D. Autoreactive T cells that cause T1D utilize more or less the same pathways for their activation, expansion, and differentiation as T cells that protect hosts from infections. Therefore, attempts to inactivate autoreactive T cells by targeting any of the large arrays of molecules along these pathways is inherently fraught with inactivating normal T cells required for fighting legitimate foreign pathogens. This fact imposes heavy restraints on therapeutic strategies targeting these pathways. To circumvent these restrains, scientists resort to using short courses and carefully calibrated doses of neutralizing reagents that undermine efficacy (Greenbaum and Atkinson; Skyler and Ricordi). Using combination therapy is another strategy that is being pursued to maximize additive effects of targeting more than one molecule (von Herrath). Another promising approach aims at expanding regulatory T cells specific for islet antigens that can be used to suppress autoreactive T cells.

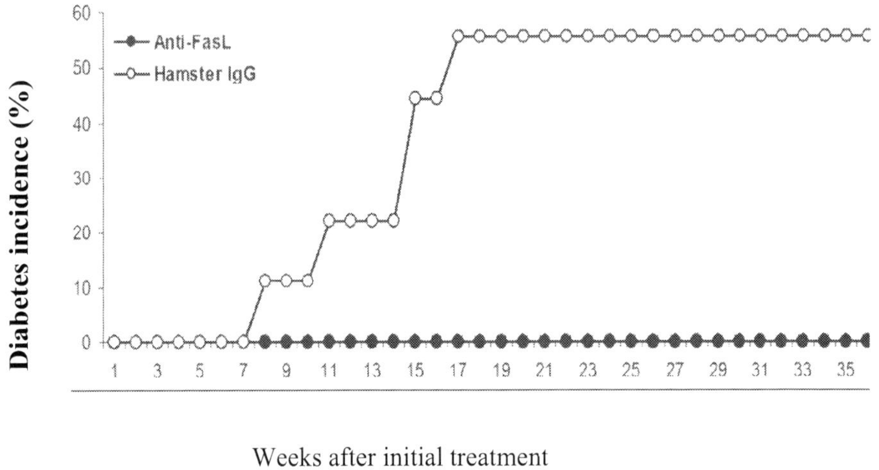

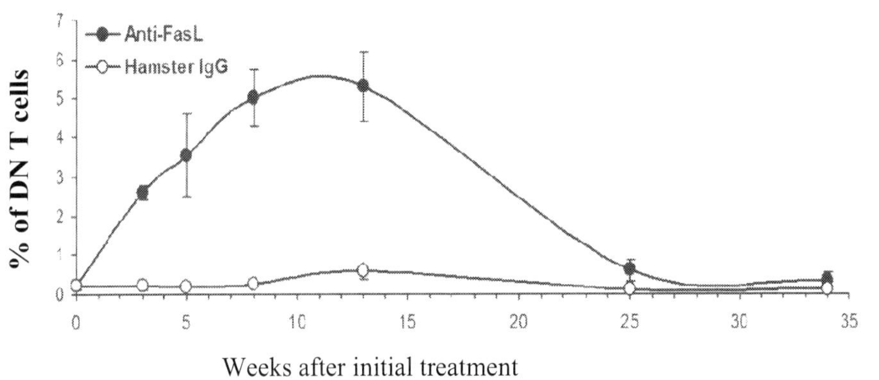

Fig. 4. *Top:* Diabetes incidence and blood glucose levels in mice treated with FasL-neutralizing antibody or hamster IgG control antibody.
Bottom: Blockade of FasL leads to mild and transient increase in the frequency of DN T cells in peripheral blood. Blood samples were collected and stained with TCR-, CD4-, and CD8-specific antibodies and analyzed by fluorescence-activated cell sorting. After gating on TCR^+ cells, the frequency of DN T cells was determined. Adopted from ref. Mohamood et al. 2007 with copy right permission from Copyright © 201X, AMERICAN SOCIETY FOR INVESTIGATIVE PATHOLOGY. Published by ELSEVIER INC.

The Fas pathway is unique in this regard and stands in a separate class: FasL is not essential for promoting normal immune response and hence immunosuppression is not a major concern in calibrated targeting of FasL (Hamad; Mohamood et al., 2008). In fact, there is a wide window for modulating FasL activity to suppress autoimmunity without disturbing immune homeostasis (Mohamood et al., 2008; Mohamood et al., 2007). Mechanistically, the long lasting tolerance to beta cell antigens mediated by FasL blockade is due to local immune modulation at the site of inflammation (Xiao et al., In press). It appears that regulatory cells play an important role in controlling diabetogenic T cells as transfer of splenocytes from NOD-gld/+ mice into NOD-scid mice results in diabetes development [ref. (Mohamood et al., 2007) and (Fig. 5)]. We envision that targeting Fas pathway could result in tissue specific tolerance without weakening the immune system.

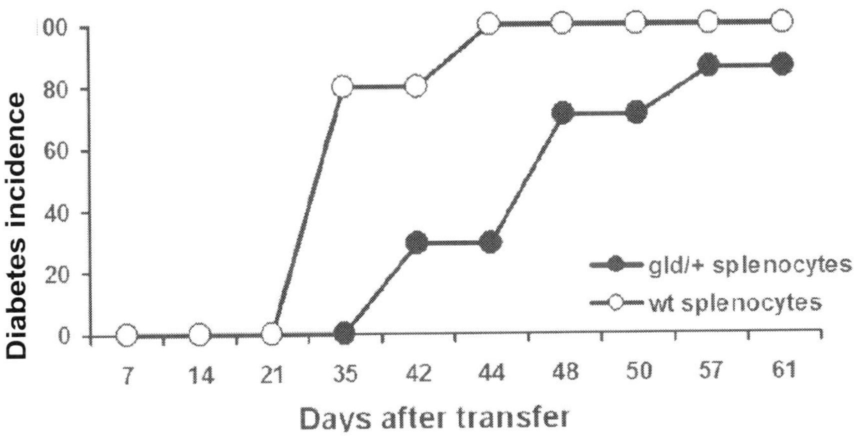

Fig. 5. **Disease-free NOD-gld/+ mice harbor diabetogenic lymphocytes that transfer diabetes to NOD-scid mice**. Diabetogenicity of 2 x10^7 splenocytes from diabetes-free NOD-gld/+ mice was tested in adoptive NOD-scid hosts after i.v. transfer and compared to that of equal number of splenocytes from age-matched NOD-wt mice (n = 7 per group). Blood glucose levels were monitored weekly to determine diabetes induction. Mice with two consecutive blood glucose levels of ≥250 mg/dL were considered diabetic. Results are from one of two similar experiments. Adopted from ref. Mohamood et al. 2007 with copy right permission from Copyright © 201X, AMERICAN SOCIETY FOR INVESTIGATIVE PATHOLOGY. Published by ELSEVIER INC.

5.6 What should be done to realize the therapeutic potentials of FasL?

Efforts will be directed towards mechanistic understanding of how inactivating FasL prevents T1D and assessing its preclinical ability to reverse new-onset disease in NOD mice. Also, attempts should be made to assess whether blockade of FasL synergizes with anti-CD3 or antigen specific therapy to produce a more effective and safer therapy. Thus, successful testing of the proposed idea is expected to provide convincing rationale for considering FasL as an immunotherapeutic target for T1D.

6. Conclusion

Type 1 diabetes (T1D) is the leading autoimmune disease of childhood. Long term complications association with the disease despite careful use of insulin therapy and restrict diet show the need of an immunotherapy for T1D. Assessment of the results of clinical trials has demonstrated feasibility, but evaluation of efficacy produced the conclusion that none of the agents currently under clinical investigation hold the key for the cure as a sole therapy. Our data and those published by others in the roles of FasL in pathogenesis of T1D offer novel views on the potentials of targeting the Fas death pathway as an unconventional therapeutic approach for T1D that is unlikely to cause immune suppression.

7. Acknowledgment

This work is supported by grants from the JDRF (1-2006-676), NIH grant 1R56AI083444-01A2, and American Heart Association (10Grant4200003). Also with support by P&F grant from the Baltimore Diabetes Research and Training Center Grant [P60DK079637]

8. References

Agardh, C.D., Cilio, C.M., Lethagen, A., Lynch, K., Leslie, R.D., Palmer, M., Harris, R.A., Robertson, J.A., and Lernmark, A. (2005). Clinical evidence for the safety of GAD65 immunomodulation in adult-onset autoimmune diabetes. J Diabetes Complications *19*, 238-246.

Allison, J., and Strasser, A. (1998). Mechanisms of beta cell death in diabetes: a minor role for CD95. Proc Natl Acad Sci U S A *95*, 13818-13822.

Anderson, M.S., and Bluestone, J.A. (2005). The NOD mouse: a model of immune dysregulation. Annu Rev Immunol *23*, 447-485.

Apostolou, I., Hao, Z., Rajewsky, K., and von Boehmer, H. (2003). Effective destruction of Fas-deficient insulin-producing beta cells in type 1 diabetes. J Exp Med *198*, 1103-1106.

Bluestone, J.A., Herold, K., and Eisenbarth, G. Genetics, pathogenesis and clinical interventions in type 1 diabetes. Nature *464*, 1293-1300.

Bolt, S., Routledge, E., Lloyd, I., Chatenoud, L., Pope, H., Gorman, S.D., Clark, M., and Waldmann, H. (1993). The generation of a humanized, non-mitogenic CD3 monoclonal antibody which retains in vitro immunosuppressive properties. Eur J Immunol *23*, 403-411.

Bresson, D., Togher, L., Rodrigo, E., Chen, Y., Bluestone, J.A., Herold, K.C., and von Herrath, M. (2006). Anti-CD3 and nasal proinsulin combination therapy enhances remission from recent-onset autoimmune diabetes by inducing Tregs. J Clin Invest *116*, 1371-1381.

Chervonsky, A.V., Wang, Y., Wong, F.S., Visintin, I., Flavell, R.A., Janeway, C.A., Jr., and Matis, L.A. (1997). The role of Fas in autoimmune diabetes. Cell *89*, 17-24.

Fischer, G., Rosenberg, F., Straus, S., Dale, L., Middelton, L., A., L., W., S., Lenardo, M., and J., P. (1995). Dominant interfering Fas gene mutations impair apoptosis in a human autoimmune lymphoproliferative syndrome. Cell *81*, 1935 - 1946.

Greenbaum, C., and Atkinson, M.A. Persistence is the twin sister of excellence: an important lesson for attempts to prevent and reverse type 1 diabetes. Diabetes *60*, 693-694.

Hamad, A.R. Analysis of gene profile, steady state proliferation and apoptosis of double-negative T cells in the periphery and gut epithelium provides new insights into the biological functions of the Fas pathway. Immunol Res *47*, 134-142.

Harrison, L.C., and Hafler, D.A. (2000). Antigen-specific therapy for autoimmune disease. Curr Opin Immunol *12*, 704-711.

Harrison, L.C., Honeyman, M.C., Steele, C.E., Stone, N.L., Sarugeri, E., Bonifacio, E., Couper, J.J., and Colman, P.G. (2004). Pancreatic beta-cell function and immune responses to insulin after administration of intranasal insulin to humans at risk for type 1 diabetes. Diabetes Care *27*, 2348-2355.

Herold, K.C., Gitelman, S.E., Masharani, U., Hagopian, W., Bisikirska, B., Donaldson, D., Rother, K., Diamond, B., Harlan, D.M., and Bluestone, J.A. (2005). A single course of anti-CD3 monoclonal antibody hOKT3gamma1(Ala-Ala) results in improvement in C-peptide responses and clinical parameters for at least 2 years after onset of type 1 diabetes. Diabetes *54*, 1763-1769.

Herold, K.C., Hagopian, W., Auger, J.A., Poumian-Ruiz, E., Taylor, L., Donaldson, D., Gitelman, S.E., Harlan, D.M., Xu, D., Zivin, R.A., and Bluestone, J.A. (2002). Anti-CD3 monoclonal antibody in new-onset type 1 diabetes mellitus. N Engl J Med *346*, 1692-1698.

Kaufman, D.L., Clare-Salzler, M., Tian, J., Forsthuber, T., Ting, G.S., Robinson, P., Atkinson, M.A., Sercarz, E.E., Tobin, A.J., and Lehmann, P.V. (1993). Spontaneous loss of T-cell tolerance to glutamic acid decarboxylase in murine insulin-dependent diabetes. Nature *366*, 69-72.

Kayagaki, N., Yamaguchi, N., Nagao, F., Matsuo, S., Maeda, H., Okumura, K., and Yagita, H. (1997). Polymorphism of murine Fas ligand that affects the biological activity. Proc Natl Acad Sci U S A *94*, 3914-3919.

Keymeulen, B., Candon, S., Fafi-Kremer, S., Ziegler, A., Leruez-Ville, M., Mathieu, C., Vandemeulebroucke, E., Walter, M., Crenier, L., Thervet, E., *et al.* Transient Epstein-Barr virus reactivation in CD3 monoclonal antibody-treated patients. Blood *115*, 1145-1155.

Keymeulen, B., Vandemeulebroucke, E., Ziegler, A.G., Mathieu, C., Kaufman, L., Hale, G., Gorus, F., Goldman, M., Walter, M., Candon, S., *et al.* (2005). Insulin needs after CD3-antibody therapy in new-onset type 1 diabetes. N Engl J Med *352*, 2598-2608.

Kim, S., Kim, K.A., Hwang, D.Y., Lee, T.H., Kayagaki, N., Yagita, H., and Lee, M.S. (2000). Inhibition of autoimmune diabetes by Fas ligand: the paradox is solved. J Immunol *164*, 2931-2936.

Kim, Y.H., Kim, S., Kim, K.A., Yagita, H., Kayagaki, N., Kim, K.W., and Lee, M.S. (1999). Apoptosis of pancreatic beta-cells detected in accelerated diabetes of NOD mice: no role of Fas-Fas ligand interaction in autoimmune diabetes. Eur J Immunol *29*, 455-465.

Lenardo, M., Chan, F., Hornug, F., McFarland, H., Siegel, R., Wang, J., and Zheng, L. (1999). Mature T lymphocytes apoptosis-immune regulation in a dynamic and unpredictable antigenic environment. Annu. rev. Immunol. *17*, 221-253.

Lenardo, M.J. (1996). Fas and the art of lymphocyte maintenance. JEM *183*, 721.

Mohamood, A.S., Bargatze, D., Xiao, Z., Jie, C., Yagita, H., Ruben, D., Watson, J., Chakravarti, S., Schneck, J.P., and Hamad, A.R. (2008). Fas-Mediated Apoptosis Regulates the Composition of Peripheral alphabeta T Cell Repertoire by Constitutively Purging Out Double Negative T Cells. PLoS ONE *3*, e3465.

Mohamood, A.S., Guler, M.L., Xiao, Z., Zheng, D., Hess, A., Wang, Y., Yagita, H., Schneck, J.P., and Hamad, A.R. (2007). Protection from autoimmune diabetes and T-cell lymphoproliferation induced by FasL mutation are differentially regulated and can be uncoupled pharmacologically. Am J Pathol *171*, 97-106.

Nagata, S., and Suda, T. (1995). Fas and Fas ligand:lpr and gld mutations. Immunol. Today *16*, 39-43.

Nakayama, M., Abiru, N., Moriyama, H., Babaya, N., Liu, E., Miao, D., Yu, L., Wegmann, D.R., Hutton, J.C., Elliott, J.F., and Eisenbarth, G.S. (2005). Prime role for an insulin epitope in the development of type 1 diabetes in NOD mice. Nature *435*, 220-223.

Nakayama, M., Nagata, M., Yasuda, H., Arisawa, K., Kotani, R., Yamada, K., Chowdhury, S.A., Chakrabarty, S., Jin, Z.Z., Yagita, H., *et al.* (2002). Fas/Fas ligand interactions play an essential role in the initiation of murine autoimmune diabetes. Diabetes *51*, 1391-1397.

Narendran, P., Mannering, S.I., and Harrison, L.C. (2003). Proinsulin-a pathogenic autoantigen in type 1 diabetes. Autoimmun Rev *2*, 204-210.

Orlinick, J.R., Vaishnaw, A.K., and Elkon, K.B. (1999). Structure and function of Fas/Fas ligand. Int Rev Immunol *18*, 293-308.

Pescovitz, M.D., Greenbaum, C.J., Krause-Steinrauf, H., Becker, D.J., Gitelman, S.E., Goland, R., Gottlieb, P.A., Marks, J.B., McGee, P.F., Moran, A.M., *et al.* (2009). Rituximab, B-lymphocyte depletion, and preservation of beta-cell function. N Engl J Med *361*, 2143-2152.

Pinkoski, M.J., and Green, D.R. (1999). Fas ligand, death gene. Cell Death Differ *6*, 1174-1181.

Savinov, A.Y., Tcherepanov, A., Green, E.A., Flavell, R.A., and Chervonsky, A.V. (2003). Contribution of Fas to diabetes development. Proc Natl Acad Sci U S A *100*, 628-632.

Schneider, P., Bodmer, J.L., Holler, N., Mattmann, C., Scuderi, P., Terskikh, A., Peitsch, M.C., and Tschopp, J. (1997). Characterization of Fas (Apo-1, CD95)-Fas ligand interaction. J Biol Chem *272*, 18827-18833.

Skyler, J.S., Krischer, J.P., Wolfsdorf, J., Cowie, C., Palmer, J.P., Greenbaum, C., Cuthbertson, D., Rafkin-Mervis, L.E., Chase, H.P., and Leschek, E. (2005). Effects of oral insulin in relatives of patients with type 1 diabetes: The Diabetes Prevention Trial--Type 1. Diabetes Care *28*, 1068-1076.

Skyler, J.S., and Ricordi, C. Stopping type 1 diabetes: attempts to prevent or cure type 1 diabetes in man. Diabetes *60*, 1-8.

Sosenko, J.M., Palmer, J.P., Greenbaum, C.J., Mahon, J., Cowie, C., Krischer, J.P., Chase, H.P., White, N.H., Buckingham, B., Herold, K.C., *et al.* (2006). Patterns of metabolic progression to type 1 diabetes in the Diabetes Prevention Trial-Type 1. Diabetes Care *29*, 643-649.

Stranges, P.B., Watson, J., Cooper, C.J., Choisy-Rossi, C.M., Stonebraker, A.C., Beighton, R.A., Hartig, H., Sundberg, J.P., Servick, S., Kaufmann, G., *et al.* (2007). Elimination of antigen-presenting cells and autoreactive T cells by fas contributes to prevention of autoimmunity. Immunity *26*, 629-641.

Strasser, A., Jost, P.J., and Nagata, S. (2009). The many roles of FAS receptor signaling in the immune system. Immunity *30*, 180-192.

Su, X., Hu, Q., Kristan, J.M., Costa, C., Shen, Y., Gero, D., Matis, L.A., and Wang, Y. (2000). Significant role for Fas in the pathogenesis of autoimmune diabetes. J Immunol *164*, 2523-2532.

Takahashi, T., Massato Tanaka, Camilynn I. Brannan, Nancy A. Jenkins, Neal G.Copeland, Takashi Suda, and Nagata, S. (1994). Generalized lymphoproliferative disease in mice caused by a point mutation in the Fas ligand. Cell *76*, 969-976.

Thomas, H.E., Darwiche, R., Corbett, J.A., and Kay, T.W. (1999). Evidence that beta cell death in the nonobese diabetic mouse is Fas independent. J Immunol *163*, 1562-1569.

Tian, J., Clare-Salzler, M., Herschenfeld, A., Middleton, B., Newman, D., Mueller, R., Arita, S., Evans, C., Atkinson, M.A., Mullen, Y., *et al.* (1996). Modulating autoimmune responses to GAD inhibits disease progression and prolongs islet graft survival in diabetes-prone mice. Nat Med *2*, 1348-1353.

Tisch, R., Yang, X.D., Singer, S.M., Liblau, R.S., Fugger, L., and McDevitt, H.O. (1993). Immune response to glutamic acid decarboxylase correlates with insulitis in non-obese diabetic mice. Nature *366*, 72-75.

von Herrath, M. Combination therapies for type 1 diabetes: why not now? Immunotherapy *2*, 289-291.

Waldner, H., Sobel, R.A., Howard, E., and Kuchroo, V.K. (1997). Fas- and FasL-deficient mice are resistant to induction of autoimmune encephalomyelitis. J Immunol *159*, 3100-3103.

Watanabe-Fukunaga, R., Brannan, C., Copeland, N., Jenkins, N., and Nagata, S. (1992). Lymphoproliferation disorder in mice explained by defects in Fas antigen that mediates apoptosis. Nature *356*, 314-317.

Xiao, X., Mohamood, A.S., Uddin, S., Gutfreund, R., Nakata, S., Marshall, A., Kimura, H., Caturegli, P., Womer, K.L., Huang, Y., *et al.* (In press). Inhibition of Fas ligand in NOD mice unmasks a protective role for IL-10 against insulitis development.

19

Autoantigen-Specific Immunotherapy

Shuhong Han[1], William Donelan, Westley Reeves[1] and Li-Jun Yang[2]

[1]Department of Medicine,

[2]Department of Pathology,

[1,2]Immunology, and Laboratory Medicine, University of Florida, Gainesville, Florida, USA

1. Introduction

The incidence of type 1 diabetes (T1D) is increasing dramatically and new treatment modalities are needed urgently. Arising from autoimmune destruction of the pancreatic β-cells, T1D manifests itself when less than 10-20% of functional β-cells remain in the islets and is characterized as a disorder of glucose regulation due to the insufficient production of insulin. Insulin is a hormone secreted by pancreatic islet β-cells and its main function is to move blood sugar into cells where it is stored and later used for energy. In T1D, the β-cells are destroyed by the patients' immune cells leading to limited or no insulin production. Without enough insulin, glucose accumulates in the bloodstream instead of entering the cells, causing symptoms of hyperglycemia. Chronic hyperglycemia can lead to many serious complications. Insulin replacement therapy is the current standard for treatment involving injection of recombinant insulin. Normal pancreatic insulin secretion is exquisitely sensitive to the minute-to-minute changes in blood glucose and glucose-stimulated insulin secretion (GSIS) and cannot be mimicked precisely by exogenous insulin injections. Thus, while insulin treatment successfully prolongs the life of affected individuals, it fails to prevent some of the serious complications of T1D that adversely affect quality of life and ultimately lead to significant morbidity and mortality. An alternative promising therapy is islet cell transplantation, but this suffers from several drawbacks including limited pancreatic islet tissue from cadaveric donors, the requirement for lifelong immunosuppression, and the increased risk of infection due to non-specific suppression of the immune system.

To cure T1D, researchers are pursuing combined immunological and biological strategies for restoring β-cell mass. Strategies for increasing β-cell mass include promoting endogenous pancreatic β-cell regeneration, reprogramming non-pancreatic cells into insulin-producing cells (IPCs), and generating unlimited autologous pancreatic β-cells from induced pluripotent stem (iPS) cells of the T1D patients. At the same time, there is considerable interest in approaches for modulating and suppressing autoimmunity to pancreatic β-cells and surrogates of IPCs. An individual's pancreatic β-cell mass is tightly regulated according to insulin demand, reflecting a balance between the rate of β-cell replication, regeneration/reprogramming, and the rate of β-cell apoptosis. Research efforts are focusing on how best to expand, reprogram, or generate β-cells or their surrogates from pancreatic stem/precursor cells, non-pancreatic adult/stem cells, or the iPS cells of T1D patients for β-cell replacement therapy. However, without preventing ongoing autoimmune destruction of β-cells, the regenerated, reprogrammed, or replaced β-cells or their surrogates may suffer the same fate as the endogenous pancreatic β-cells.

The loss of pancreatic β-cells in T1D is a T cell-mediated autoimmune process orchestrated by CD4+ and CD8+ T cells specific for β-cell antigens. Pathogenic diabetogenic T cells and autoantibodies to β-cell specific autoantigens have been found in T1D patients and non-obese diabetic (NOD) mice, a well-studied animal model of T1D. These T cells employ a variety of mechanisms to destroy β-cells. Moreover, genetic susceptibility factors for T1D mainly affect the ontogeny and survival of immune cell subsets at the level of the thymic selection and in the peripheral tolerance. T1D is an organ-specific autoimmune disease where the immune tolerance to the β-cells is broken and the immune system attacks and eliminates these β-cells. So, restoration of self-tolerance to β-cells and suppression of β-cell autoimmunity combined with increasing β-cell mass are the key components for β-cell replacement therapy.

Experimental evidence indicates that the immune system can be modulated and immune tolerance to β-cells can be restored in experimental animal models of T1D. Self-tolerance can be re-established centrally or peripherally by broad-based immunoregulatory strategies, including the inhibition or deletion of lymphocyte subsets and/or the use of agents proposed to induce or re-establish immune tolerance via activation of regulatory T (Treg) cells. An example is the use of nonmitogenic anti-CD3 or antithymocyte globulin. However, the induction of antigen-specific tolerance to β-cell antigens is a highly desirable objective because only the pathogenic autoreactive T cells are inactivated whereas the remainder of immune system remains unperturbed. Many autoantigens have been identified and implicated in relation to T1D. Well-established autoantigens include insulin (Palmer et al., 1983), glutamic acid decarboxylase 65 (GAD65) (Baekkeskov et al., 1990), insulinoma associated-2 antigen (IA-2) (Bonifacio et al., 1995), and heat shock protein (HSP) (Birk et al., 1996), as well as newly discovered β-cell-specific autoantigens zinc transporter-8 (ZnT8) (Wenzlau et al., 2007), pancreatic duodenal homeobox factor 1 (PDX1) (Li et al., 2010), and chromogranin A (CHGA) (Stadinski et al., 2010). These markers of T1D are useful for diagnosis as well as for prediction prior to disease onset and may prove useful for intervention by restoring immune tolerance[See table-1].

Antigen-specific immunoregulatory therapies are currently being evaluated for preventing and treating T1D and they include autoantigen therapy, dendritic cell (DC)-based strategies, and adoptive transfer of Treg cells. This chapter will review recent work on the antigen specific immunotherapy of T1D including strategies for tolerance induction.

2. The importance and feasibility of antigen specific immunotherapy

Nonspecific and specific approaches have been exploited by immunologists to control the autoimmune response in T1D. They include deleting pathogenic T cells and activating regulatory T cells to induce immune tolerance against β-cells. Non specific approaches included using immunosuppressive drugs such as steroids or cyclosporin A as well as some monoclonal or polyclonal antibodies. Polyclonal anti-lymphocyte antisera and anti-CD3 or anti-CD4 monoclonal antibodies have been used to cure early diabetic disease in murine models for T1D (Maki et al., 1992; Chatenoud et al., 1994; Makhlouf et al., 2004). Anti-lymphocyte antisera and anti-CD4 antibodies are strong immune suppressors and principally act on depleting the autoaggressive T cells. In contrast, anti-CD3 antibodies function as immune modulators (Chatenoud et al., 2007) since they can maintain long term

Autoantigen	Protein	Function	Antigen specific immunotherapy in humans
(Pre)(pro)insulin	Precursor and processed product	Hormone	??
GAD65	Gutamic acid decarboxylase - Mr 65,000 isoform	GABA producing enzyme	Alum-formulated GAD65 preserves beta-cell function
IA-2	Islet antigen-2	tyrosine phosphatase-like protein - unknown function	To be tested
ZnT8	Zn T8 transporter	One of several Zn transporters but specific to the beta cells	To be tested
PDX1	pancreatic and duodenal homeobox 1	a transcriptional activator of several genes, including insulin	To be tested
DiaPep277	HSP60	chaperone	DiaPep277 preserves beta cell function.

Table 1. Islet autoantigens in type 1 diabetes

immune tolerance through inducing adaptive Tregs, interfere with T cell activation, and induce anergy/apoptosis in activated cells. Based on results from the mouse model, the humanized anti-CD3 antibodies (teplizumab and otelixizumab) were explored in phase II trials. It was found that anti-CD3 antibody treatment could preserve endogenous insulin secretion and reduce HBA1c levels and insulin requirement in the treated group during a two year period in recent onset T1D. Recent follow-up studies indicate that the beneficial effects extend over a period of up to 5 years following a single treatment (Cernea et al., 2010). However, some patients develop "flu-like" symptoms due to significant cytokine release by antibody-bound T cells, and recurrent Epstein-Barr viral infections (Keymeulen et al., 2010). It is well known that steroid and and cyclosporin A therapy have very serious side effects. The common problem of antibody-based immunotherapies is that they can't discriminate between normal versus autoimmune effector T cells. The safety concerns and adverse effects of antigen nonspecific interventions, as well as the lack of permanent remission of disease with any agent tested to date have prompted interest in antigen specific interventions that might modulate the autoimmune aspect of the disease. Compared with nonspecific immune-approach, antigen-based immunotherapy allows selective targeting of disease-relevant T cells, while leaving the remainder of the immune system intact. Numerous studies have demonstrated that antigen specific immunotherapy can be highly effective in preventing and suppressing autoimmunity in rodent models of T1D and other autoimmune diseases (Harrison et al., 2000).

The concept of antigen-specific tolerance has been apparent for some years. The presence of self-reactive lymphocytes in the blood of healthy individuals (Burns et al., 1983) implies that self-antigen-specific regulatory mechanisms are physiological and prevent pathological autoimmunity. Antigen-specific tolerance operates directly on effector T cells (via apoptosis or anergy) and via Treg cells that secrete anti-inflammatory cytokines or compete with effector T cells at the level of the antigen presenting cell (APC). Many factors determine the induction of antigen specific tolerance including: 1) characters/properties of antigen, dose/concentration, physical form (soluble or aggregated, intact protein or peptide), chemical composition, affinity for MHC molecule, content of CD4+ and CD8+ T cell epitopes and 'immunodominance', purity and contaminants (e.g. endotoxin), and adjuvants; 2) route of administration; 3) level of co-stimulation; and 4) antigen-specific precursor cell frequency and duration of treatment (Harrison et al. 2000). High-dose soluble peptide or monomeric protein delivered by the intraperitoneal (i.p.), subcutaneous (s.c.), or intravenous (i.v.) route induces clonal deletion or clonal anergy (Liblau et al., 1997). Delivering antigen through mucosal routes, for example oral and naso-respiratory routes, could induce mucosal immune tolerance that suppresses subsequent systemic priming to the antigen (Faria et al., 1999). Oral tolerance means the specific suppression of immune responses to an antigen by prior administration of the antigen by the oral route. Oral tolerance is an active immunologic process that is mediated by more than one mechanism and is dose-dependent. Low doses have been shown to induce differentiation of regulatory T cells capable of downregulating T cells specific for distinct antigens within a given tissue. This phenomenon of bystander suppression in oral tolerance is associated with the induction of Th2 and TGF-β-secreting Tregs (Anderton et al., 1999) whereas higher doses favor the induction of clonal anergy or deletion (Chen et al., 1995).

T cells recognize antigen peptide via the T cell receptor (TCR) and produce a spectrum of responses that range from activation to anergy or cell death. In the late 1980s, peptides were modified to interfere with the MHC/peptide/TCR complex to prevent autoaggressive T cell activation (Adorini et al., 1988). Later on, this type of peptide was termed an altered peptide ligand (APL). In APLs, TCR contact residues in an immunodominant self-epitope are altered to impair the T cell strength of signal. So, APLs could induce anergy by engaging less than optimal numbers of TCRs. APLs have been applied therapeutically in animal models of autoimmune diseases and in the clinical trial (Harrison et al. 2000). One recent paper reported that proinsulin-derived APLs (prAPLs) modulate the cytokine signature of proinsulin-reactive T cells at a micromolar range by increasing anti-inflammatory cytokines, including TGF-β1 (van et al., 2010). The results suggest that APLs do not act as antagonists *in vivo* but mediate bystander suppression, probably by the generation of Treg cells.

Treg cells have an ability to regulate immune response by non specific bystander suppression in response to specific antigen that is recognized locally at the site of the lesion or in the draining lymph node. During the disease process of animal models and human T1D, T cell autoimmunity progressively spreads intra- and inter-molecularly among β-cell autoantigens such as insulin, GAD65, HSP, and IGRP (van Belle et al., 2011). Bystander suppression resolves the dilemma of multiple autoantigens in human autoimmune diseases by obviating the need to know if the antigen used to induce tolerance is the major or primary pathogenic autoantigen (Tang et al., 2008). Therefore, antigen-specific approaches use only one antigen to tolerize against multiple autoreactivities. In the long term, Treg cells create a regulatory environment by producing TGF-β and/or by substantially changing DC functions to promote new Treg cell production. These processes promote bystander suppression and are critical to the creation of infectious tolerance that can spread beyond the local tissue and exert long-lasting influence over the immune system. In contrast, tolerance-based on anergy or deletion is limited to each individual antigen.

Antigen-specific therapy is logically appealing and demonstrably effective in experimental autoimmune disease animal models. This proof-of-concept and its safety make it an attractive approach for treatment of human autoimmune disease including T1D.

3. Antigen specific immune tolerance induction strategies

Immunotherapy for T1D has been attempted at two main stages of the disease process - prior to clinical onset but after the appearance of islet autoantibodies (secondary prevention) and immediately after diagnosis (intervention) (Staeva-Vieira, T. et al. 2007) .

Prevention of T1D, meaning intervening early during the development of disease, holds greater promise for success because, in this stage, organ damage has not progressed very far and β-cells are still capable of self regeneration. Successful prevention of T1D depends on: 1) a good prediction/identification of at-risk individuals and 2) a safe intervention that causes no harm in those individuals who would have never developed T1D. In T1D, identifying the individuals at risk for developing disease can be obtained through screening islet autoantibodies, combined with genetic markers in the HLA region, and additional risk factors (Siljander et al., 2009). Moreover, metabolic assessments can also be included to identify late-stages of disease development, at which there is already some loss of glycemic control. Thus, it is now feasible to 'stage' individuals according to various modeled rates of progression to T1D (Staeva-Vieira et al., 2007). Currently, preventive trials for T1D include two main classes, antigen- or non-antigen-specific. Compared with a non-antigen specific-approach, an antigen-specific immune tolerance holds more promise and advantage. Many antigen-specific prevention trials have been conducted in recent years. Of note is the oral insulin trial used in relatives of T1D patients following screening of 103,391 first- and second-degree relatives of patients with T1D. Of them, 97,273 samples were analyzed for islet cell antibodies and 2,523 underwent genetic, immunological, and metabolic staging to quantify risk of developing T1D. This trial concluded that it is possible to identify individuals at high risk for T1D and enroll them in a large, multisite, randomized, and controlled clinical trial (Skyler et al., 2005).

Immune intervention for recent onset T1D aims to prevent or reverse the disease by blocking autoimmunity, thereby preserving/restoring β-cell mass and function and decreasing the likelihood of both hypoglycemia and long-term complications. It is a clinically feasible approach because potential subjects are readily identified and efficacy can be evaluated within a much shorter time frame. Currently, large quantities of evidence show that it is possible to reverse clinically established T1D. Firstly, evidence shows that loss of β-cells is a gradual process and that newly diagnosed patients still have 10-20% of functional β-cells remaining within the islets. Therefore, the reversal of hyperglycemia could be obtained through (1) promoting endogenous regeneration and replication of remaining β-cells, (2) reducing metabolic stress on the remaining β-cells, (In support, it is known that early and intensive insulin therapy in patients with recent onset T1D can clearly reduce the loss of remaining β-cell capacity (Shah et al., 1989).), (3) changing immune environment from producing proinflammatory (IFNγ) to anti-inflammatory (IL-10) cytokines (Alizadeh et al., 2006), and (4) suppressing recurrent β-cell autoimmunity. In support, it was found that anti-CD3 antibody could induce durable regression of recently diagnosed T1D in NOD mice by restoring self-tolerance following short-term treatment (Chatenoud 2003). According to this evidence, it is very clear that interventions in recent onset T1D have to be operational within a small and clearly defined window, which might also vary on an individual basis. In this stage patients still have sufficient remaining β-cell mass that can be assessed by C-peptide measurements (Staeva-Vieira, T. et al.2007). In order to maintain or restore critical mass of viable and functional β-cells in T1D patients for developing immune intervention, many approached are being explored. They include (1) stimulation of β-cell regeneration/proliferation in vivo through hormone and growth factor treatment, (2) direct conversion by in vivo reprogramming of adult pancreatic exocrine cells to transform into β-cells, (3) isolation and in vitro differentiation of pancreatic progenitors, embryonic stem cells, or extrapancreatic adult stem cells, and (4) induction of iPS cells from adult-differentiated cells through targeted reprogramming with soluble factors (5) islet transplantation (Guo T et al. 2009). As soon as these approaches for increasing viable and functional β-cells become readily available, immune intervention will be feasible for recent onset T1D patients and even for late stage patients.

4. Antigen-specific immunotherapy approaches

4.1 Autoantigen therapy

Antigens may behave as immunogens that provoke an adaptive immune response or as tolerogens that induce a state of specific immunological unresponsiveness (immune tolerance) to subsequent challenging doses of the antigen. Several factors determine the immunogenic versus tolerogenic capacity of an antigen, including its molecular form, the nature of APCs, the dose, the route of administration and local response environment (Anderton et al., 1999). Many attempts have been made to induce or restore tolerance in T1D by the use of candidate autoantigens.

Insulin

Insulin and proinsulin molecules have been identified to play a primary role in the initiation of the autoimmune process that ultimately leads to destruction of β-cells and onset of clinical T1D for both humans and the NOD mouse. Insulin autoantibodies usually precede the development of T1D and can be utilized to assist in disease prediction. Transplanted T cell clones recognizing insulin, both CD4+ and CD8+, can transfer disease to young mice or immunodeficient animals. Specific insulin peptides reacting with these clones have been identified (Gottlieb et al., 2002). Based on knowledge about insulin immunity in T1D, insulin specific tolerance induction approaches for prevention and immune intervention have been explored in T1D animal models and patients[See table-2].

Group	Antigen	Route	Protection from diabetes	Reference
BB rat (DP, DR)	Insulin, high dose continuous	Subcutaneously	Yes	41,42
BB rat (DP, DR)	Insulin	Oral	No	42
NOD mouse	Insulin	Subcutanously	Yes	22
NOD mouse	B chain	Subcutanously	Yes	44
NOD mouse	B9-23	Subcutanously	Yes	26,27
NOD mouse	B9-23	Intranasally	Yes	23,26,27
NOD mouse	B10-24	Intranasally	Yes	45
NOD mouse	Proinsulin	DNA	Yes	51
LCMV mouse	Insulin B chain	Oral DNA	Yes	47-49
PVG RT1u Rat	B1-18	Intrathymic	Yes	50
Human, new onsets	Insulin	Oral	No	56
Human, high risk prediabetic	Insulin, low dose continous	Subcutaneous	No	55
Human, new onset disbetes	APL of B9-23	Subcutanous	?	38
Human, medium-risk prediabetic	Insulin	Oral	?	55

Reference: Gottlieb PA, Eisenbarth GS. Insulin-specific tolerance in diabetes. Clin Immunol. 2002, 102(1):2-11

Table 2. Insulin Immunotherapy of Type 1 Diabetes [Gottlieb PA, 2002-p2]

In NOD mice, reports demonstrated that delivery of insulin (intravenously, subcutaneously, orally, or intranasally), proinsulin, or insulin peptides could delay the onset and reduce the incidence of T1D (Chatenoud 2010). Further study investigating the protection mechanism indicated that administration of insulin could induce active tolerance against T1D (Aspord et al., 2002). Insulin-derived mutated proinsulin peptide B24-C36 was shown to induce anti-diabetogenic regulatory T cells that block the adoptive transfer of T1D and protect the NOD mice from T1D (Fierabracci 2011).

Based on the success in animal models, clinical trials of oral or nasal insulin have been conducted in humans. These trials can be divided into prevention trials and intervention trials. One human prevention trial has included a double-blinded crossover safety study conducted in 38 individuals with antibodies to one or more islet antigens (insulin, GAD65, or IA-2) and the results showed intranasal insulin does not accelerate loss of β-cell function in individuals at risk for T1D and induces immune changes consistent with mucosal tolerance to insulin (Harrison et al., 2004). This is the first report that showed intranasal insulin was immunotherapeutic and retarded progression to clinical T1D. However, another double blind prevention trial with nasal insulin obtained contradictory findings. In this trial, 224 infants and 40 siblings positive for two or more autoantibodies received short-acting human insulin or placebo once a day intranasally. Median duration of the intervention was 1.8 years. The results showed that, in children with HLA-conferred susceptibility to T1D, administration of nasal insulin immediately following detection of autoantibodies could not be shown to prevent or delay T1D. The prevention efficacy of oral insulin was also tested in 388 prediabetic patients who were first- and second-degree relatives of T1D patients and were also classified as having increased risk for developing T1D by genetic, immunological, and metabolic staging (Skyler et al., 2005; Sosenko et al., 2006). It was concluded that oral insulin did not delay or prevent T1D. However, according to subgroup analysis, it appeared that there might be a potential benefit in T1D prevention in those subjects with higher autoantibody levels. Reasons for failure may include insufficient dosing as well as the fact that by the time an individual is identified with autoantibodies, the disease process is well established and difficult to reverse. Moreover, the dose, frequency of mucosal antigen administration, and timing of antigen delivery are critical determinants of tolerance induction and subsequent suppression of T cell mediated autoimmune disease.

Intervention trials were also performed in patients with recent onset T1D with insulin. In one trial, 52 adults with recent onset T1D were given nasal insulin. It was found that nasal insulin did not retard loss of residual β-cell function, but the evidence showed that it could induce immune tolerance to insulin and it provided a rationale for its application to prevent T1D in at-risk individuals (Fourlanos et al., 2011). Two studies including about 100 patients each tested the use of oral insulin at a limited dose range and they didn't observe clinical efficacy (Chaillous et al., 2000; Pozzilli et al., 2000). A large phase II clinical trial with NBI 6,024 (an altered peptide ligand of the 9–23 insulin B chain peptide) showed there is no efficacy of APL treatment in patients at the stage of overt disease (Walter et al., 2009). It did not cause significant changes in insulin requirement, metabolic control, hypoglycemic and hyperglycemic events, autoantibody concentrations, or CD4+ and CD8+ T cell numbers. The lack of response may reflect a fundamental defect in the proposed mechanism of action or inadequacy of exposure (dose), frequency, or timing of injected peptide.

GAD65

GAD65 is one of the major T1D-related autoantigens recognized by self-reactive T cells. T cells specific for GAD65 are among the first to enter inflamed pancreatic islets and may be important for the initiation of autoimmunity (Kaufman et al., 1993). Moreover, GAD65 is also an early target of autoantibodies during the initiation of T1D. Immune therapies targeting GAD65 have been tested in both animal models and in human T1D patients [See table-3].

Group	Antigen	Route	Protection from diabetes	Reference
NOD mice	GAD65	Intraperitoneally	Yes	Peterson 1994 and 1997
BB rats	GAD65	IV	No	Pleau 1995
NOD mice	GAD65 peptide	Nasal	Yes	Wang 2009
NOD mice	GAD65 peptides	Intranasal	Yes	Tian 1996
NOD mice, diabetic	GAD65	IV	Yes	Tisch 1998
NOD mice	DNA	Intramuscular	Yes	Tisch 2001
NOD mice	rVV-GAD65	Intraperitoneally	Yes	Jun 2002
NOD mice, diabetic	DNA	Intramuscular	Yes	Goudy 2008
Human, onset diabetes	GAD-alum (Diamyd)	Subcutaneously	Yes	Agardh 2005
Human, onset diabetes	GAD-alum (Diamyd)	Subcutaneously	Yes	Ludvigsson 2011 and 2008

Table 3. GAD65 Immunotherapy of Type 1 Diabetes

In NOD mice, administration of GAD65 can prevent and block autoimmune destruction of pancreatic β-cells and subsequent need for exogenous insulin replacement. It was found that oral administration of a fusion protein composed of cholera toxin B subunit (CTB) and GAD65 peptide could significantly reduce pancreatic islet inflammation and delay the development of T1D through generating regulatory T cells and induction of immunological tolerance (Gong et al., 2010). Intravenous injections of GAD during the later stages of disease still effectively blocked disease progression in prediabetic mice and protected syngeneic islet graft survival in diabetic NOD mice (Tian et al., 1996). The identification of CD4+ Treg cells in GAD-treated mice suggests a major role for bystander suppression in the induction of tolerance by treatment with this autoantigen (Tisch et al., 1998).

Based on the above convincing data from NOD mice, autoantigen immunotherapy with GAD65 was tried in human. GAD-Alum (Diamyd Therapeutics) is an adjuvant-formulated vaccine incorporating recombinant human GAD65 which is the specific isoform of GAD expressed in human pancreatic β-cells and a major antigen targeted by autoreactive T lymphocytes in T1D. It was shown to be safe and to preserve residual insulin secretion in patients with late onset T1D of adulthood (Agardh et al., 2005). A subsequent phase II trial in recent onset T1D showed significant preservation of residual insulin secretion and a GAD-specific immune response, both humoral and cell mediated immune response (Agardh et al., 2009). Moreover, Alum-formulated GAD65 has been given subcutaneously in two injections with one month apart to recent onset T1D patients with positive GAD65 autoantibodies. The injections were found to preserve residual β-cell function without treatment related serious adverse events (Agardh et al., 2005). Further study showed that two injections of GAD-Alum to children and adolescents with T1D could induce GAD specific CD4+CD25high forkhead box P3 (Foxp3)+ regulatory T cells and secretion of Th2 and regulatory cytokines (Hjorth et al., 2011). These data support a long-lasting immunomodulatory effect of GAD-Alum treatment. Follow-up after 5 years completed in

2008 still show a significantly beneficial effect of the Diamyd (Morales et al., 2011). According to these promising clinical data, Phase III studies in children with recent onset T1D are ongoing along with a study (DIAPREV-IT) aimed at testing whether Diamyd® may prevent the clinical onset of T1D in non-diabetic children with GAD65 autoantibodies and at least one more islet autoantibody (Larsson et al., 2011). Also, Diamyd Medical is currently conducting two clinical Phase III studies on T1D: one in Europe and one in the United States. Here, the formulation is crucial to Dyamid's GAD drug because *1)* adjuvant reduces the required quantity of antigen by maximizing its immunogenicity and *2)* aluminum salts preferentially induce a humoral rather than cellular immune response. Immune readouts show an increase in FoxP3 and transforming growth factor-β in cells from GAD-Alum-treated patients compared with placebo after 15 months (Ludvigsson 2009). In summary, GAD 65 vaccination has shown encouraging results with preservation of residual insulin secretion in 10- to 18-year-old type 1 diabetic patients with recent onset. In patients with short T1D duration, the effect was quite pronounced. These effects were reached with a very well tolerated treatment. Future studies will show if the good effect seen so far can be confirmed. There is a hope that GAD vaccination will cause remission or even cure and prevention of T1D seem to be a realistic possibility (Morales et al., 2011).

DiaPep277

HSP60 is a ubiquitous protein that is part of a highly conserved family of intracellular chaperones and is also located in the mitochondria and mature insulin-secretory granules of pancreatic β-cells with an important regulatory role in the innate immune system and considered an important autoantigen in T1D (Birk et al., 1996). Although HSP60 autoantibodies are not yet considered a diagnostic tool for T1D, the evidence suggests this autoantigen may be important in disease development. Therefore, vaccine strategies that are based on HSP60 as a T1D autoantigen have been tested in mouse models and human T1D patients [See table-4].

Group	Antigen	Route	Protection from diabetes	Reference
NOD mice, prediabetic and diabetic	DiaPep277	Subcutaneous	Yes	Elias 1995 and 1997
STZ-C57BL/KsJ diabetes mice model	DiaPep277	Subcutanous	Yes	Elias 1996
NOD mice, prediabetic	DiaPep277	Intraperitoneally	Yes	Elias 1991
NOD mice, prediabetic	DiaPep277	Trans inoculations	Yes	Jin 2008
BB-DP rats, Prediabetic	DiaPep277	Oral	Yes	Brugman 2004
NOD mice, Prediabetic	Pep277	Nasal	Yes	Liang 2010
NOD mice, , prediabetic and diabetic	Pep 277	several	No	Bowman 2002
Human, on-set	DiaPep277	Subcutaneous	Yes	Raz 2001 and 2007
Human, on-set	DiaPep277	Subcutaneous	Yes	Huurman 2008 and 2007
Human, paediatric on-set	DiaPep277	Subcutaneous	?	Schloot 2007
Human, on-set	DiaPep277	Subcutaneous	?	Schloot 2007
Children, on-set	DiaPep277	Subcutaneous	No	Lazer 2007

Table 4. DiaPep277 Immunotherapy of Type 1 Diabetes

DiaPep277 is a 24 amino acid synthetic peptide derived from the C 31 terminus of the human HSP60. Compared with HSP60, DiaPep277 activates T cell TLR2 receptors but has no effect on macrophage TLR4 receptors. So, DiaPep277 only mediated anti-inflammatory effect on T cells and lacked pro-inflammatory effect on innate immune cells. In NOD mice, nasal administration of a diabetogenic peptide Pep277 showed significant anti-inflammatory immune response (Liang et al., 2010). Moreover, neonatal oral administration of DiaPep277 combined with hydrolysed casein diet could protect against T1D in BB-DP rats. All the results showed that DiaPep277 could significantly prevent T1D development and arrest the progression of insulitis in mice that have already become hyperglycemic (Fierabracci 2011). These promising experimental results led to clinical trials with DiaPep277. It was found that DiaPep277 treatment for patients with recent onset T1D could prevent further β-cell loss (Raz et al., 2001; Raz et al., 2007). Specific intervention with DiaPep277 re-establishes the balance in the immune system by enhancing the Th2-type cytokine production and inducing a strong signal for the development of Th2 cells. Phase II clinical trials in adult subjects with T1D have shown suggestive evidence of better preservation of C-peptide and cessation of destruction of β-cells with DiaPep277 (Raz et al., 2001). Moreover, the adult trials showed significantly better preservation of insulin synthesis as measured by C-peptide production in the treated groups compared with placebo, but this effect was not seen in the pediatric trial. Similar results were observed in one other trial performed in pediatric patients (Schloot et al., 2007). Diapep277 was more pronounced in patients with a high β-cell reserve at the start of the treatment. The phase III study has began in 40 medical centers worldwide and the results are expected in 2011 (Eldor et al., 2009). If DiaPep277 proves to be efficacious, it will cause a paradigm shift in the treatment of T1D from treating the subsequent insulin deficiency to addressing the initial autoimmune process that is at the core of the disease (Eldor et al., 2009).

In summary, efficacy of autoantigen therapy has been disappointing. Based on preclinical models, several factors are emerging as critical in determining the outcome of Autoantigen immunization most notably dose, route, adjuvant, and frequency of administration. Studies have shown that too frequent antigen administrations, as well as very high dosages, do not result in optimal induction of immune regulation and tolerance (Peakman M et al. 2010). Another challenge for developing effective autoantigen therapy is to know the role that β-cell autoantigens play in islet inflammation and restoration of immunological tolerance, for example, how DCs recognize autoantigens and how autoantigen exposed DCs guide T cell development into immunosuppressive or autoreactive T cell subsets. The other important questions that need to be answered include precisely which autoantigen epitopes should be targeted and whether the use of a single antigen is sufficient in order to induce immune tolerance and stop an ongoing T cell response to multiple autoantigens. Moreover, only blood samples are readily available from patients to evaluate efficiency of antigen immunotherapy. The question is if peripheral T cell populations reflect the T cell population infiltrating the target organ. Another important concern is if immune deviation and functional dominance of regulatory responses are reflected by changes in peripheral antigen-specific T cells. More-sensitive assays are necessary to develop to evaluate the impact of immunotherapy on disease progression through analysis of peripheral cells. All these issues need to be addressed by performing autoantigen specific immunotherapy studies in future clinical trials.

4.2 Dendritic cell (DC)-based immunotherapy

4.2.1 Brief overview of DC biology

Dendritic cells (DCs) are a special subset of leukocytes able to alert the immune system of the presence of infections and are responsible for the activation and the control of adaptive immune responses. There is also mounting evidence that DCs establish and maintain immunological tolerance. Indeed, DCs can prevent, inhibit, or modulate T cell mediated effector responses through a variety of mechanisms including T cell anergy, T cell deletion, immune deviation (i.e. polarization of T cell cytokine profiles), and the expansion or induction of Tregs. The induction/expansion of FoxP3+ Tregs is one of the major mechanisms by which DCs maintain immune tolerance (Steinman et al., 2003).

DCs are a heterogeneous mix of the distinct leukocyte subsets that have different functions and homing patterns. In humans, there are two major and intrinsically different subpopulations of DCs: myeloid DCs (myDCs) and plasmacytoid DCs (pDCs). These two DC subsets recognize different microbial pathogens by expressing distinct repertoires of toll-like receptors (TLR) and induce different types of innate and adaptive immune responses depending on environmental factors. Much evidence supports the presence of DCs with tolerogenic properties in both myDCs and pDC subsets (Gregori 2010). Both myDC and pDCs develop from hematopoietic bone marrow progenitor cells that turn into DC precursors (pre-pDCs) upon encounter of Flt3-ligand (Flt-3L). Pre-DCs migrate from the bone marrow to the bloodstream where they circulate as immature DCs characterized by low expression of HLA class II and co-stimulatory molecules, high endocytic activity, and low T cell activation potential. Immature myDCs and pDCs encounter pathogens and become activated mature DCs to prime CD4+ and CD8+ T cells (Liu et al., 2010). In addition to their potential to become activated DCs, immature myDCs and pDCs in the steady state are also critically involved in homeostasis and in promoting and maintaining peripheral tolerance, primarily via the induction of CD4+ Tregs. Of note, the DCs with tolerogenic function not only comprise immature DCs, but also include other DCs covering a spectrum of different maturation states. The induced CD4+ Tregs include the naturally occurring Tregs (nTregs) and the adaptive Tregs. Thymic-derived nTregs are defined by the constitutive high expression of FoxP3 (Sakaguchi et al., 2010). Adaptive Tregs composed of different Treg subsets are generated in the periphery in tolerogenic microenvironments and suppress T cell responses via immunomodulatory cytokines. The best characterized are the IL-10-producing type 1 regulatory T (Treg1) cells that depend on IL-10 for their generation and functions (Allan et al., 2008).

According to current understanding of DC development, protocols have been set up for *in vitro* propagation of large numbers of activated and tolerogenic DCs using defined growth factors as well as biological, genetic, and pharmacological modifications (Morelli et al., 2007). Depending on the agent used for tolerogenic DC induction, the resulting DCs are equipped with defined tolerogenic molecules which determine their ability to promote different subsets of Treg cells. Tolerogenic DCs secreting high levels of IL-10 in the absence of IL-12 are primarily involved in the induction of adaptive IL-10-producing Treg1 cells. FoxP3-inducer DCs express low levels of co-stimulatory molecules and express indoleamine 2,3-dioxygenase which allows them to secrete TGF-β and retinoic acid and to promote FoxP3+ Treg cells (Gregori 2010). According to these prerequisites, it can be postulated that depending on the type of Tregs required for promoting tolerance toward a given antigen, different protocols for *in vitro* generation of tolerogenic myDC with the desired phenotypic and functional characteristics could be designed. In general, tolerogenic potential of DCs were determined by low-expression of co-stimulatory molecules, microenvironmental factors (in particular, immunosuppressive cytokines), expression of death-inducing ligands, (in particular Fas ligand (FasL)), and inhibition of gene transcription regulatory proteins (e.g. NF-kB) (Morelli et al., 2007). The development of culture methods for generating large numbers of DCs that can be pharmacologically or biologically manipulated opens important new perspectives for the development of DC-based cell therapy protocols.

4.2.2 DC-based therapeutic approach

DCs are critical for both preventing and perpetuating autoimmunity, reflecting their dual roles in regulating the immune system, i.e., maintenance of T cell tolerance and induction of pro-inflammatory immune responses. The defects in immune regulation by DCs may play a central role in T1D (Anderson et al., 2005). In T1D, abnormalities in DC phenotype and function in both NOD mice and humans may result in the skewing response toward pathogenic Th1 cells (Feili-Hariri et al., 2006). The purpose of using tolerogenic DC therapy for T1D is to re-balance dysregulated immune responses that have already been ongoing for some time. A number of studies have shown that therapy with various forms of DCs can protect mice from T1D development. For example, DCs generated from the bone marrow of NOD mice by culturing DCs in granulocyte-macrophage colony-stimulating factor (GM-CSF), IL-4, and fetal bovine serum (FBS) could prevent T1D in some recipients when administered to young (5-week-old) NOD mice (Feili-Hariri et al., 1999). Transfer of DCs *ex vivo* stimulated with IFN-γ down-modulates T1D in NOD mice (Shinomiya et al., 1999). However, one study showed that only DCs from pancreatic lymph nodes (panLNs), but not DCs from other anatomical sites, could protect from disease, presumably because panLN-derived DCs would present β-cell-derived antigens after adoptive transfer (Clare-Salzler et al., 1992). This study indicated that autoantigen exposed DCs have better protection effects.

4.2.2.1 Exposure of therapeutic DCs to antigen *ex vivo*

The original observation that DCs from the panLNs could prevent T1D when transferred to NOD mice, while those from other sites could not, suggests the potential importance of the incorporation of β-cell antigens into DC-based therapeutics for this disease (Mukherjee et al. 2010). The von Herrath group explored this approach in a rat model (Haase et al., 2005). They utilized the rat insulin promoter (RIP)-LCMV model of T1D in which disease is induced upon LCMV infection. BM-DCs were generated and pulsed with a viral peptide recognized by CD8+ T cells. It was found that the antigen pulsed DCs have stronger ability to inhibit development of T1D than the unpulsed DCs. This study suggests that disease relevant antigen exposed tolerogenic DCs have therapeutic benefit for T1D. Next, autoantigen pulsed DCs were explored for treating T1D in NOD mice. It was found that adoptive transfer of insulin peptide- pulsed, immature DCs could protect NOD mice from T1D whereas unpulsed DCs had no effect on T1D development (Haase et al., 2010). In another study, immature DCs derived from BM were pulsed with antigen-specific apoptotic bodies from the β-cell line NIT-1 cells and the administration of these cells to NOD could decrease T1D incidence significantly and correlated positively with insulitis reduction (Marin-Gallen et al., 2010). All these results show that DC therapy is capable of preventing T1D in an antigen-specific manner in animal model and DCs expressing disease-associated antigens constitutes a promising strategy to prevent T1D. The mechanism for preventing and delaying development of T1D with autoantigen exposed DCs is inducing expansion of regulatory T cells (Cheatem et al., 2009).

4.2.2.2 Targeting of antigens to DCs *in vivo*

Loading antigen ex vivo to DCs is challenging and faces many problems including labor-intensive procedure for each patient, high cost, and limited DC number (Tacken et al., 2007). Thus, many studies have begun to explore the utility of *in vivo* delivery of β-cell antigens to DCs for the prevention and treatment of T1D.

Many receptors used in targeting DC studies belong to the C-type lectin receptor (CLR) family, a family of calcium-dependent lectins that share primary structural homology in their carbohydrate recognition domain (CRD). Through their CRD, the CLRs bind to specific self or non-self sugar residues. Many of these lectins were shown to be associated with antigen uptake by DCs.Approaches to targeting CLRs fall into two categories: based on the binding of natural receptor ligands and exploited antibodies against the receptor. CD205 belongs to type I CLR family and study indicated that it is a suitable target for in vivo antigen-targeting studies. CD205 recycles through late endosomal or lysosomal compartments and mediates antigen presentation. (Tacken et al. 2007).

Much evidence shows that DEC-205 is involved in antigen processing and presentation. In mice, DEC205 expression is relatively DC restricted: it is highly expressed by mature DCs (mDCs), thymic epithelium, at low levels by B cells, and at very low levels by T cells and granulocytes. Therefore, DEC205 is an excellent target to study *in vivo* DC targeting. The therapeutic potential of DEC-205-mediated antigen delivery has begun to be explored in mouse models of T1D (Mukhopadhaya et al., 2008; Bruder et al., 2005). In Mukhopadhaya A et al's study, autoantigen peptide-linked anti-DEC-205 could lead to deletion of autoreactive CD8+ T cells even in the context of ongoing autoimmunity in NOD mice and induce subsequent immune tolerance to β-cells. This study provides support for the development of DC targeting of self antigens for treatment of chronic T cell-mediated autoimmune diseases. Bruder D et al. utilized the INS-HA/TCR-HA transgenic mouse model for T1D. It was found that T1D was prevented in most animals when treated with HA peptide linked anti-DEC-205. Further analysis showed that these HA-specific CD4+ T cells from anti-DEC-HA-treated mice exhibited increased expression of FoxP3, cytotoxic T-lymphocyte-associated antigen-4, and the immunosuppressive cytokines interleukin-10 and TGF-β. The findings indicate that targeting of the HA antigen to immature DCs in vivo leads to a relative increase of antigen-specific $FoxP3^+$ regulatory T cells that suppress the development of T1D. Another recent related study showed that targeting a mimotope peptide to the endocytic receptor DEC-205 on DCs in NOD mice induces efficient conversion of pancreatic β-cell-reactive BDC2.5 CD4+ T cells into long-lived FoxP3+ Treg cells (Petzold et al., 2010). These results suggest that promoting antigen-specific Treg cells in vivo might be a feasible approach in T1D with DC in vivo targeting.

4.2.3 Future challenges for DC based approaches

4.2.3.1 Challenge for exposure of DCs to antigen *ex vivo*

Adoptive cellular therapy with tolerogenic DCs has potential applications not only in human autoimmune diseases but also for allogeneic tissue transplantation and hypersensitivity. One big challenge is to generate tolerogenic DCs with a stable phenotype which are resistant to maturation mediated by pro-inflammatory mediators.

Currently, DCs for clinical use are generated from peripheral blood monocytes of the patients. However, the number of monocytes obtained from the patients is limited and the potential of monocytes to differentiate into DCs varies depending on the blood donor. Thus, the issue of limited cells is a serious obstacle for DC therapy. ES cells and iPS cells have pluripotency and unlimited propagation capacity and may be an ideal cell source for DC-therapy. Several groups have developed methods to generate DCs from ES cells or iPS cells (Menendez et al., 2005).

Developing tolerogenic DC-based therapies also requires optimizing the following conditions. (1) To define the best source of DC precursors for the *in vitro* induction of tolerogenic DCs, i.e. peripheral blood monocytes *vs* bone marrow CD34+ cells. Studies performed in non-human primates indicate that bone marrow cells are a good source of tolerogenic DCs (Steinman et al., 2003). (2) To determine the disease stage, route of delivery, and dose (Lo J et al., 2006) of DC transfer. Because the autoimmune response leading to TID in humans takes place for several years before hyperglycemia develops, it may be important to determine a critical stage for initiation of DC-based therapy. The study from NOD mice indicates that prevention initialized at early stage has a positive effect. Future studies are needed to establish whether DC-based therapies block disease onset at advanced stages of islet destruction or even reverse acute onset T1D. For the route of DCs administration, until now, there is no solid evidence to show which administration route is the best. It was noted DCs have different migration in different administration route. For example, subcutaneous injected DCs home mainly to the draining lymph nodes whereas intravenous administration mainly goes to the spleen, lungs, and liver. Concerning the injection dose, the effect of the number per treatment has not been comparatively evaluated. Of note, the lifespan of DCs in vivo is limited to about 2-3 weeks. Therefore, it could be envisaged to perform repetitive injections unless a single injection would be sufficient to generate a microenvironment suitable for sustaining *de novo in vivo* induction of tolerogenic DCs (Morelli et al., 2007).

4.2.3.2 Challenge for targeting DC *in vivo*

When developing DEC-205-mediated therapeutic strategies for T1D, the choice of antigen is a major consideration. Until now, the antibody can be modified to include an antigen and it proves difficult to combine multiple antigens. As mentioned before, multiple antigens are targeted by T cells in both NOD mice and T1D patients (DiLorenzo et al., 2002). Particularly in humans, it is unclear which of these are the most 'important', i.e. critical for disease initiation and/or progression. However, accumulating evidence suggests that insulin and GAD65 are key targets of pathogenic T cells in T1D in both NOD mice and humans and that they may be candidates for targeting to DEC205 in T1D.

DCs have two functions, maintaining tolerance to self and inducing immunity. In the context of activation stimuli such as those found during inflammation, infection, or tissue destruction, DCs induce prolonged T cell activation and in steady state, they induce tolerance. This character of DCs was also shown in the Hawiger D study. It was found that HEL linked anti-DEC 205 could induce immune tolerance under physiological conditions but induce prolonged T cell activation and immunity against HEL when performed in conjunction with an agonistic anti-CD40 antibody. (Hawiger et al., 2001). It indicated antigen delivery to DCs in the context of an inflammatory environment may lead to exacerbation of a pathogenic autoimmune response rather than tolerance induction. So, when considering the translation of such a strategy to humans, the potential remedy should be considered. (Mukherjee et al. 2010)

Another potential concern is that CD205 expression in humans is less DC restricted than in mice, and targeting constructs might also be endocytosed by several other cell types for example B cells, T cells, monocytes, macrophages, and natural killer (NK) cells (Erbacher et al., 2009). It still needs to be confirmed if targeting these cells has any side effects. On the whole, many issues need to be resolved before translating DC based approaches into human T1D prevention and treatment.

4.3 Adoptive transfer of Tregs

4.3.1 Brief overview of Tregs

Tregs play a crucial role in the maintenance of immune homeostasis. The two best studied types of CD4+ regulatory T cells are the FoxP3+ Tregs and Th1 cells secreting IL-10. Large quantities of evidence show that CD4+ regulatory T cells play a protective role in autoimmune disease (Spoerl et al., 2011).

CD4+FoxP3+ Tregs account for approximately 5-10% of the total CD4+ T cells in the periphery, most prominently in the lymphoid organs such as the spleen and lymph nodes, with a small subset found in the non-lymphoid tissues. FoxP3+ Tregs suppress both innate and adaptive immune cells through several mechanisms and maintain tolerance and immune homeostasis. They exert suppression by cell contact-dependent mechanisms (for example, functional modulation by means of CD39, CD73, and LAG-3, or killing of APCs or responder T cells by means of granzyme and perforin) as well as mechanisms mediated by soluble factors (for example, secretion of immunosuppressive cytokines such as IL-10, TGF-β, IL-35, and galectin-1), or deprivation of cytokines (for example, IL-2) necessary for the expansion and/or survival of responder T cells (Zhang et al., 2009). Moreover, Tregs have two key characters that are very important for their translational application; (1) Bystander suppression: When Tregs are first activated through their respective TCRs to induce suppressive activity, but once activated, the cells are capable of suppressing responses in a non-specific manner. (2) Infectious tolerance: The transferred Tregs generate an immunoregulatory milieu that persists long after the removal of the eliciting cell population. This occurs as new regulatory cell populations are activated by antigen in the context of tolerogenic APCs and Tregs. These two characteristics allow Tregs of single or limited-antigen specificity to establish a broad and stable immunoregulatory effect and constitute the quintessential Treg phenotype (Brusko et al., 2008b). Phenotypically, CD4+FoxP3+ Tregs express multiple cell surface markers such as CD25, CTLA-4, GITR (glucocorticoid-induced tumor necrosis factor receptor), OX40, CD103, CD39, and CD73, many of which are also expressed by activated CD4+ T effector cells (Kang et al., 2007). Thus, these markers are not Treg specific.

CD4+FoxP3+ Tregs are not a uniform cell population, but consisted of those that developed in the thymus (nTregs) and those that are derived from T effector cells in the periphery (adaptive or induced Tregs, iTregs). nTregs are shown to arise as a committed lineage in the thymus and bear a diverse TCR repertoire against a broad range of self antigens. iTreg cells are induced under particular conditions of antigenic stimulation both in vitro and in vivo. Furthermore, iTregs are particularly unstable and tend to lose FoxP3 expression more easily than nTregs, which is likely related to epigenetic differences in the FoxP3 gene in both subsets. Indeed, certain non-coding regions in the FoxP3 gene in nTregs have been shown to be completely demethylated while such regions are often methylated in iTregs (Curotto de Lafaille et al., 2009). Such differences may be important in therapeutic manipulation of nTregs and iTregs (Spoerl et al., 2011).

Another important development about Tregs is that many protocols were developed for isolating and expanding nTregs for therapeutic applications from healthy individuals and patients (Brusko et al., 2008a). This provides important tools and principles for translating Treg therapies into clinical treatments for patients with T1D and other autoimmune disorders.

4.3.2 Tregs in the pathophysiology of T1D

A growing body of evidence suggests that an imbalance in the immune system plays a major role in the pathogenesis of autoimmune disease (Brusko et al., 2008b). Tregs play a major role in controlling the activity of self-aggressive T cells that were not deleted in the thymus and are one of the key factors for maintaining homeostatic balance in the immune system (Chatenoud et al., 2001). Defects in the number and function of Tregs and a resistance of effector T cells to Treg-mediated suppression could each contribute to failed T cell regulation. Each of these defects contributes to the development of autoimmune disease including T1D (Buckner 2010).

A role for nTreg cells in T1D is evident in individuals with IPEX, in which the absence of nTreg cells results in enhanced susceptibility to T1D. In NOD mice, reduced CD4+ Treg cell frequencies or function represent a primary predisposing factor to T1D (Sgouroudis et al., 2009). The adoptive transfer of Tregs could suppress disease through reducing effector Th1 T cells and macrophages and inhibiting effector T cell cytokine and chemokine production (Tonkin et al., 2009). However, Tritt M et al. have contradicting reports as they couldn't detect the defect of cellular frequency of FoxP3+ nTreg cells in the lymphoid tissues. However, the nTreg cell functional potency and intra-pancreatic proliferative potential declines with age, in turn augmenting diabetogenic responses and disease susceptibility (Tritt et al., 2008). On the whole, strong evidence shows that complete absence of Tregs precipitates T1D and the disease can be prevented by the adoptive transfer of additional Tregs (Sgouroudis et al., 2009).

Most studies investigating the role of Tregs in human T1D showed contradictory results in the peripheral blood frequency and suppression function of these cells between T1D and control subjects when the expression of transcription factor FoxP3 was used for their identification (Alonso et al., 2009). One reason is that FoxP3 is an unreliable marker for Tregs in humans, as it is also expressed in activated effector T cells. Moreover, unlike mice, the frequency of Tregs in islet couldn't be obtained from human. The results obtained from blood samples might not indicate the involvement of Tregs in the pathophysiology of T1D. Moreover, the method used to isolate Tregs may influence the degree of suppression observed in vitro. This effect may also account for some of the discrepancies in the reported functions of these cells in T1D (Brusko et al., 2008b). The above data from mice and human indicated central importance of Tregs in the pathogenesis and potentially the treatment of T1D.

4.3.3 Therapy of T1D with Tregs

In the mouse animal model, the adoptive transfer of CD4+ CD25+ Treg cells has been shown to protect from T1D (Salomon et al., 2000; Tonkin et al., 2008; Tonkin et al., 2009). According to published results, the adoptive Treg cells include polyspecific and autoantigen specific. Now the evidence is very clear that antigen-specific Tregs are more effective in several autoimmune syndromes when compared with polyclonal populations (Brusko et al., 2008b). According to a study by Wu AJ, polyspecific Tregs had to be transferred regularly (twice weekly) in high doses and mice developed T1D after Treg transfer had been stopped (Wu et al., 2002). This makes this approach difficult to be performed in human patients. The other concerns about polyspecific Tregs include the efficacy and safety of these Tregs related to their polyspecificity and a paucity of information about their stability, function, and fate in vivo. So, autoantigen-specific Tregs would have more advantages in terms of safety and efficacy because they could specifically recognize antigens from the target tissue to achieve tissue specific immunoregulation. Several studies already showed natural CD4+ CD25+ Tregs from the NOD mouse specific for an islet antigen were more protective than their polyspecific Tregs (Tang et al., 2004; Tarbell et al., 2004; Tarbell et al., 2007). Compared with poly specific Tregs, relatively small numbers of islet autoantigen-specific Tregs prevent T1D in NOD mice. Moreover, it was found that adoptive transfer of islet specific Tregs showed considerable efficacy in ameliorating ongoing T1D in NOD mice (Tarbell et al., 2007). Until now, not many treatments were shown to interfere with disease pathophysiology at later disease stages in the NOD mouse. Therefore, adoptive autoantigen specific regulatory T cells should have great potential therapeutic benefit in humans.

For developing adoptive autoantigen specific regulatory T cell therapy, in vitro expansion of this unique cell population becomes very important. Several research groups already developed the expansion protocol of autoantigen specific Tregs from peripheral blood in vitro (Dromey et al., 2011; Tang et al., 2004; Tarbell et al., 2004). Because proinsulin and GAD65 usually are targets of autoreactive T cells in human T1D (Harrison 2008). Tregs specific for these autoantigens are being attempted to expand in vitro and they will have potential application for adoptive immunotherapy of T1D.

4.3.4 Future challenges for Treg therapy

Translating Tregs into the clinical setting still faces several challenges. Firstly, until now, no unique cell surface markers were identified for human Tregs. Because activated effector T cells also express CD25, there exits high frequency of activated effector T cells contamination present in the CD4+ CD25+ fraction with present Treg isolating kits. So, for the isolation of human Tregs, the combination of the surface markers CD4+ CD25high CD127low results in a population which is enriched in Tregs with fewer recently activated effector T cells (Brusko et al., 2008b). Second, another major challenge in antigen-specific Treg therapy lies in the isolation of sufficient quantities of antigen-specific T cells. In order to obtain enough cell number for adoptive transfer, in vitro expansion of this population is necessary. Although several groups already developed protocols for expanding autoantigen specific Treg cells, the current technology may not provide a robust method for isolating and expanding a sufficient quantity of these cells for use in the clinic. The next most important factor will be the stability of the Treg differentiation phenotype. Recent animal studies provide evidence for functional heterogeneity and lineage plasticity within the Treg compartment (Addey et al., 2011). In the healthy immune system, the majority of natural Tregs are relatively stable, but the study showed that 10-15% of "stable" Treg cells were found to lose FoxP3 expression after adoptive transfer into lymphopenic hosts (Zhou et al., 2009). There are two fates for Tregs that lose FoxP3 in lymphopenic hosts: death or de-differentiation. One study showed that half of the Tregs transferred into lymphopenic hosts did not die but rather began producing IL-2 and IFNγ and became effector T cells with the same antigen specificity (Komatsu et al., 2009). These reverted autoreactive effector cells will aggravate the autoimmune damage.

The studies described above suggest a critical challenge in the transition of Treg-based cell therapies from animal studies to human clinical trials. Knowledge of the purity, stability, and phenotypic characteristics of cell therapy products will be essential prior to their introduction into patients.

5. The importance of combination therapy

After several attempts to develop potent immunotherapy to cure T1D, the results are disappointing. Because of the multifaceted nature of this disease, a monotherapy will not be sufficient to combat T1D. The best approach is to use a combination therapy. Two major goals have to be accomplished: (1) the rapid blockade of the immune system and dampening of any auto-reactive responses without strong side-effects and (2) the regeneration of a critical β-cell mass in order to maintain euglycemia without repetitive insulin injections (Bresson et al., 2007). Each of these goals can be achieved by different means, but the combination of different therapies is very necessary for successful prevention and treatment for T1D. It should be noted that the ideal combination therapy would utilize two or more agents whose mechanisms of action are complementary and that have already been demonstrated as safe T1D monotherapies in humans.

5.1 Combination of anti-CD3 Ab with antigen-specific approach

The first and key step for treatment of T1D is dampening the auto-reactive responses and maintaining permanent tolerance to islet cells. In order to obtain this goal, the combination of immunotherapy approaches including nonspecific immunoregulatory and antigen-specific tolerance strategies are necessary. It was found that efficacy of antigen-specific therapy can be greatly enhanced when combined with anti-CD3 in recent onset T1D. A previous study (Bresson et al., 2006) showed that combination treatment with anti-CD3 specific antibody and intranasal administration of proinsulin peptide can reverse recent onset T1D in murine T1D models with much higher efficacy than with monotherapy using anti-CD3 or antigen alone. Further in vivo analysis showed that expansion of insulin-specific CD25+Foxp3+ Tregs producing IL-10, TGF-β, and IL-4 was strongly enhanced. These cells could transfer dominant tolerance to immunocompetent recent onset T1D recipients and suppressed autoaggressive CD8 responses. Moreover, the combination using anti-CD3 antibody and GAD65-expressing plasmid was shown to reverse recent onset T1D in RIP-LCMV-GP mice models (Bresson et al., 2010). Thus, the efficacy of antigen-specific therapy to induce Tregs and long-term tolerance can be greatly enhanced by addition of anti-CD3 treatment. The potential reasons include: (1) It was found that Tregs were not able to suppress activated autoaggressive T cells within the islets and PLNs (Nagler-Anderson et al., 2004; Tarbell et al., 2004). That is the reason why antigen-specific therapies were only effective during the prediabetic phase in animal models. Anti-CD3 antibody could directly decrease numbers of autoaggressive T cells in mice as described in the study (Herold et al., 2002) and create a systemic immunomodulatory milieu to facilitate the islet antigen–specific induction of Tregs. (2) Anti-CD3 has been shown in some settings to directly promote the generation of Tregs. In NOD studies by Chatenoud and others, anti-CD3 increased the number of CD4+CD25+ cells as well as systemic TGF-β production, which was required for therapeutic efficacy (Chatenoud et al., 2007). According to these results, an ideal combination therapy will consist of an islet antigen-specific immune tolerance induction, such as autoantigen immunization, coupled with a systemic drug that dampens islet destructive immunity but does not affect Tregs. Anti-CD3 treatment is suggested as a good candidate for this. In summary, the combination therapies with anti-CD3 Ab and antigen specific tolerance induction constitutes a great hope towards the development of safer and more effective immuno-interventions and would be excellent candidates for clinical studies in humans.

5.2 Combination of immunotherapy and β-cell regeneration

Since β-cell mass decreases over time, patients with long-standing T1D are very likely to have lost most of their insulin producing cells. Thus, treatments that only target the autoreactive immune system would not obviate the need for insulin injections in these patients. So, improving β-cell function at the time of diagnosis is an important determinant of response to treatment with immune therapy, and therefore strategies that improve β-cell mass and/or function may have a positive effect on response to immune treatment. Much evidence showed that reduced β-cell mass can eventually be restored endogenously. It has been demonstrated that β-cells can replicate, differentiate, or transdifferentiate from various endocrine or non-endocrine cells. Specifically, certain peptides and growth factors such as gastrin and glucagon-like peptide 1 (GLP1) can increase β-cell mass and restore normoglycaemia in animal models of T1D in the absence of immunosuppressants (Suarez-Pinzon, WL et al. 2008). So, it is necessary and feasible to develop combination therapy including improving β-cell regeneration and immunotherapy. Sherry NA et al. reported the efficiency of such combination therapy. They found that treatment with glucagon-like peptide-1 receptor agonist enhances remission of T1D in NOD mice treated with anti-CD3 Ab by enhancing the recovery of the residual islets (Sherry et al., 2007). Also, it was demonstrated that exendin-4 synergistically augments the remission-inducing effect of anti-lymphocyte serum in NOD mice (Ogawa et al., 2004). These results suggested that this combinatorial approach may be useful in treatment of patients with recent onset T1D. Accordingly, a new phase II study about combination of regenerative agents (lansoprazole and sitagliptin) and Diamyd are recruiting patients. Currently, this is the only clinical trial combining a treatment to control the autoimmune attack with autoantigen vaccine and a treatment to help the body generate more insulin. It is believed that combinations like this represent a very promising approach to the future cure for T1D

6. Conclusion remark

Antigen specific tolerance induction is the targeted therapy for prevention or early reversal of T1D. Ideally the tolerance therapy would specifically target β-cell antigens and create a local tolerance environment for inhibiting ongoing autoimmune attack against β-cells and contributing to β-cell regeneration.

Development of safe and effective prevention of T1D is becoming a major worldwide public health goal. While many preventive modalities have succeeded in animal models of T1D, prevention of human T1D remains elusive. With further understanding of genetic and environmental factors that determine the relapsing-remitting course of β-cell destruction and autoimmune mechanisms of β-cell destruction, primary prevention with antigen specific immune tolerance induction will likely be the optimal approach for the prevention of T1D in high-risk groups.

As patients develop autoimmunity, β-cell function declines. At this stage, efficacy of antigen-specific therapies is limited. The experience accumulated from previous clinical trials indicated that combination therapies may enhance efficacy while lowering risk. It is likely that one day combination therapy including systemic immune modulators, antigen specific immune tolerance induction, and a compound with positive effects on β-cell proliferation will become the standard of care for newly diagnosed T1D.

7. References

Addey, C.; White, M.; Dou, L.; Coe, D.; Dyson, J., & Chai, J. G. (2011). Functional plasticity of antigen-specific regulatory T cells in context of tumor. *J Immunol* 186(8):4557-4564.

Adorini, L.; Muller, S.; Cardinaux, F.; Lehmann, P. V.; Falcioni, F., & Nagy, Z. A. (1988). In vivo competition between self peptides and foreign antigens in T-cell activation. *Nature* 334(6183):623-625.

Agardh, C. D.; Cilio, C. M.; Lethagen, A.; Lynch, K.; Leslie, R. D.; Palmer, M.; Harris, R. A.; Robertson, J. A., & Lernmark, A. (2005). Clinical evidence for the safety of GAD65 immunomodulation in adult-onset autoimmune diabetes. *J Diabetes Complications* 19(4):238-246.

Agardh, C. D.; Lynch, K. F.; Palmer, M.; Link, K., & Lernmark, A. (2009). GAD65 vaccination: 5 years of follow-up in a randomised dose-escalating study in adult-onset autoimmune diabetes. *Diabetologia* 52(7):1363-1368.

Alizadeh, B. Z.; Hanifi-Moghaddam, P.; Eerligh, P.; van der Slik, A. R.; Kolb, H.; Kharagjitsingh, A. V.; Pereira Arias, A. M.; Ronkainen, M.; Knip, M.; Bonfanti, R.; Bonifacio, E.; Devendra, D.; Wilkin, T.; Giphart, M. J.; Koeleman, B. P.; Nolsoe, R.; Mandrup, P. T.; Schloot, N. C., & Roep, B. O. (2006). Association of interferon-gamma and interleukin 10 genotypes and serum levels with partial clinical remission in type 1 diabetes. *Clin.Exp.Immunol* 145(3):480-484.

Allan, S. E.; Broady, R.; Gregori, S.; Himmel, M. E.; Locke, N.; Roncarolo, M. G.; Bacchetta, R., & Levings, M. K. (2008). CD4+ T-regulatory cells: toward therapy for human diseases. *Immunol Rev.* 223(391-421.

Alonso, N.; Soldevila, B.; Sanmarti, A.; Pujol-Borrell, R., & Martinez-Caceres, E. (2009). Regulatory T cells in diabetes and gastritis. *Autoimmun.Rev.* 8(8):659-662.

Anderson, M. S. & Bluestone, J. A. (2005). The NOD mouse: a model of immune dysregulation. *Annu.Rev.Immunol* 23(447-485.

Anderton, S.; Burkhart, C.; Metzler, B., & Wraith, D. (1999). Mechanisms of central and peripheral T-cell tolerance: lessons from experimental models of multiple sclerosis. *Immunol Rev.* 169(123-137.

Aspord, C. & Thivolet, C. (2002). Nasal administration of CTB-insulin induces active tolerance against autoimmune diabetes in non-obese diabetic (NOD) mice. *Clin.Exp.Immunol* 130(2):204-211.

Baekkeskov, S.; Aanstoot, H. J.; Christgau, S.; Reetz, A.; Solimena, M.; Cascalho, M.; Folli, F.; Richter-Olesen, H., & De, C. P. (1990). Identification of the 64K autoantigen in insulin-dependent diabetes as the GABA-synthesizing enzyme glutamic acid decarboxylase. *Nature* 347(6289):151-156.

Birk, O. S.; Elias, D.; Weiss, A. S.; Rosen, A.; van-der, Z. R.; Walker, M. D., & Cohen, I. R. (1996). NOD mouse diabetes: the ubiquitous mouse hsp60 is a beta-cell target antigen of autoimmune T cells. *J Autoimmun.* 9(2):159-166.

Bonifacio, E.; Lampasona, V.; Genovese, S.; Ferrari, M., & Bosi, E. (1995). Identification of protein tyrosine phosphatase-like IA2 (islet cell antigen 512) as the insulin-dependent diabetes-related 37/40K autoantigen and a target of islet-cell antibodies. *J Immunol* 155(11):5419-5426.

Bresson, D.; Fradkin, M.; Manenkova, Y.; Rottembourg, D., & von, H. M. (2010). Genetic-induced variations in the GAD65 T-cell repertoire governs efficacy of anti-CD3/GAD65 combination therapy in new-onset type 1 diabetes. *Mol.Ther.* 18(2):307-316.

Bresson, D.; Togher, L.; Rodrigo, E.; Chen, Y.; Bluestone, J. A.; Herold, K. C., & von, H. M. (2006). Anti-CD3 and nasal proinsulin combination therapy enhances remission from recent-onset autoimmune diabetes by inducing Tregs. *J Clin.Invest* 116(5):1371-1381.

Bresson, D. & von, H. M. (2007). Moving towards efficient therapies in type 1 diabetes: to combine or not to combine? *Autoimmun.Rev.* 6(5):315-322.

Bruder, D.; Westendorf, A. M.; Hansen, W.; Prettin, S.; Gruber, A. D.; Qian, Y.; von, B. H.; Mahnke, K., & Buer, J. (2005). On the edge of autoimmunity: T-cell stimulation by steady-state dendritic cells prevents autoimmune diabetes. *Diabetes* 54(12):3395-3401.

Brusko, T. & Bluestone, J. (2008a). Clinical application of regulatory T cells for treatment of type 1 diabetes and transplantation. *Eur.J Immunol* 38(4):931-934.

Brusko, T. M.; Putnam, A. L., & Bluestone, J. A. (2008b). Human regulatory T cells: role in autoimmune disease and therapeutic opportunities. *Immunol Rev.* 223(371-390.

Buckner, J. H. (2010). Mechanisms of impaired regulation by CD4(+)CD25(+)FOXP3(+) regulatory T cells in human autoimmune diseases. *Nat Rev.Immunol* 10(12):849-859.

Burns, J.; Rosenzweig, A.; Zweiman, B., & Lisak, R. P. (1983). Isolation of myelin basic protein-reactive T-cell lines from normal human blood. *Cell Immunol* 81(2):435-440.

Cernea, S.; Dobreanu, M., & Raz, I. (2010). Prevention of type 1 diabetes: today and tomorrow. *Diabetes Metab Res.Rev.* 26(8):602-605.

Chaillous, L.; Lefevre, H.; Thivolet, C.; Boitard, C.; Lahlou, N.; tlan-Gepner, C.; Bouhanick, B.; Mogenet, A.; Nicolino, M.; Carel, J. C.; Lecomte, P.; Marechaud, R.; Bougneres, P.; Charbonnel, B., & Sai, P. (2000). Oral insulin administration and residual beta-cell function in recent-onset type 1 diabetes: a multicentre randomised controlled trial. Diabete Insuline Orale group. *Lancet* 356(9229):545-549.

Chatenoud, L. (2003). CD3-specific antibody-induced active tolerance: from bench to bedside. *Nat Rev.Immunol* 3(2):123-132.

Chatenoud, L. (2010). Immune therapy for type 1 diabetes mellitus-what is unique about anti-CD3 antibodies? *Nat Rev.Endocrinol.* 6(3):149-157.

Chatenoud, L. & Bluestone, J. A. (2007). CD3-specific antibodies: a portal to the treatment of autoimmunity. *Nat Rev.Immunol* 7(8):622-632.

Chatenoud, L.; Salomon, B., & Bluestone, J. A. (2001). Suppressor T cells--they're back and critical for regulation of autoimmunity! *Immunol Rev.* 182(149-163.

Chatenoud, L.; Thervet, E.; Primo, J., & Bach, J. F. (1994). Anti-CD3 antibody induces long-term remission of overt autoimmunity in nonobese diabetic mice. *Proc.Natl.Acad.Sci.U.S.A* 91(1):123-127.

Cheatem, D.; Ganesh, B. B.; Gangi, E.; Vasu, C., & Prabhakar, B. S. (2009). Modulation of dendritic cells using granulocyte-macrophage colony-stimulating factor (GM-CSF) delays type 1 diabetes by enhancing CD4+CD25+ regulatory T cell function. *Clin.Immunol* 131(2):260-270.

Chen, Y.; Inobe, J.; Marks, R.; Gonnella, P.; Kuchroo, V. K., & Weiner, H. L. (1995). Peripheral deletion of antigen-reactive T cells in oral tolerance. *Nature* 376(6536):177-180.

Clare-Salzler, M. J.; Brooks, J.; Chai, A.; Van, H. K., & Anderson, C. (1992). Prevention of diabetes in nonobese diabetic mice by dendritic cell transfer. *J Clin.Invest* 90(3):741-748.

Curotto de Lafaille, M. A. & Lafaille, J. J. (2009). Natural and adaptive foxp3+ regulatory T cells: more of the same or a division of labor? *Immunity* 30(5):626-635.

DiLorenzo, T. P.; Lieberman, S. M.; Takaki, T.; Honda, S.; Chapman, H. D.; Santamaria, P.; Serreze, D. V., & Nathenson, S. G. (2002). During the early prediabetic period in NOD mice, the pathogenic CD8(+) T-cell population comprises multiple antigenic specificities. *Clin.Immunol* 105(3):332-341.

Dromey, J. A.; Lee, B. H.; Yu, H.; Young, H. E.; Thearle, D. J.; Jensen, K. P.; Mannering, S. I., & Harrison, L. C. (2011). Generation and expansion of regulatory human CD4(+) T-cell clones specific for pancreatic islet autoantigens. *J Autoimmun.* 36(1):47-55.

Eldor, R.; Kassem, S., & Raz, I. (2009). Immune modulation in type 1 diabetes mellitus using DiaPep277: a short review and update of recent clinical trial results. *Diabetes Metab Res.Rev.* 25(4):316-320.

Faria, A. M. & Weiner, H. L. (1999). Oral tolerance: mechanisms and therapeutic applications. *Adv.Immunol* 73(153-264.

Feili-Hariri, M.; Dong, X.; Alber, S. M.; Watkins, S. C.; Salter, R. D., & Morel, P. A. (1999). Immunotherapy of NOD mice with bone marrow-derived dendritic cells. *Diabetes* 48(12):2300-2308.

Feili-Hariri, M.; Flores, R. R.; Vasquez, A. C., & Morel, P. A. (2006). Dendritic cell immunotherapy for autoimmune diabetes. *Immunol Res.* 36(1-3):167-173.

Fierabracci, A. (2011). Peptide immunotherapies in Type 1 diabetes: lessons from animal models. *Curr.Med Chem.* 18(4):577-586.

Fourlanos, S.; Perry, C.; Gellert, S. A.; Martinuzzi, E.; Mallone, R.; Butler, J.; Colman, P. G., & Harrison, L. C. (2011). Evidence that nasal insulin induces immune tolerance to insulin in adults with autoimmune diabetes. *Diabetes* 60(4):1237-1245.

Gong, Z.; Pan, L.; Le, Y.; Liu, Q.; Zhou, M.; Xing, W.; Zhuo, R.; Wang, S., & Guo, J. (2010). Glutamic acid decarboxylase epitope protects against autoimmune diabetes through activation of Th2 immune response and induction of possible regulatory mechanism. *Vaccine* 28(24):4052-4058.

Gottlieb, P. A. & Eisenbarth, G. S. (2002). Insulin-specific tolerance in diabetes. *Clin.Immunol* 102(1):2-11.

Gregori, S. (2010). Dendritic cells in networks of immunological tolerance. *Tissue Antigens* 77(2):89-99.

Guo T and Hebrok M (2009). Stem cells to pancreatic beta-cells: new sources for diabetes cell therapy. *Endocr Rev.* 30(3):14-227

Haase, C.; Ejrnaes, M.; Juedes, A. E.; Wolfe, T.; Markholst, H., & von Herrath, M. G. (2005). Immunomodulatory dendritic cells require autologous serum to circumvent nonspecific immunosuppressive activity in vivo. *Blood* 106(13):4225-4233.

Haase, C.; Yu, L.; Eisenbarth, G., & Markholst, H. (2010). Antigen-dependent immunotherapy of non-obese diabetic mice with immature dendritic cells. *Clin.Exp.Immunol* 160(3):331-339.

Harrison, L. C. (2008). Vaccination against self to prevent autoimmune disease: the type 1 diabetes model. *Immunol Cell Biol.* 86(2):139-145.

Harrison, L. C. & Hafler, D. A. (2000). Antigen-specific therapy for autoimmune disease. *Curr.Opin.Immunol* 12(6):704-711.

Harrison, L. C.; Honeyman, M. C.; Steele, C. E.; Stone, N. L.; Sarugeri, E.; Bonifacio, E.; Couper, J. J., & Colman, P. G. (2004). Pancreatic beta-cell function and immune responses to insulin after administration of intranasal insulin to humans at risk for type 1 diabetes. *Diabetes Care* 27(10):2348-2355.

Hawiger, D.; Inaba, K.; Dorsett, Y.; Guo, M.; Mahnke, K.; Rivera, M.; Ravetch, J. V.; Steinman, R. M., & Nussenzweig, M. C. (2001). Dendritic cells induce peripheral T cell unresponsiveness under steady state conditions in vivo. *J Exp.Med* 194(6):769-779.

Herold, K. C.; Hagopian, W.; Auger, J. A.; Poumian-Ruiz, E.; Taylor, L.; Donaldson, D.; Gitelman, S. E.; Harlan, D. M.; Xu, D.; Zivin, R. A., & Bluestone, J. A. (2002). Anti-CD3 monoclonal antibody in new-onset type 1 diabetes mellitus. *N.Engl.J Med* 346(22):1692-1698.

Hjorth, M.; Axelsson, S.; Ryden, A.; Faresjo, M.; Ludvigsson, J., & Casas, R. (2011). GAD-alum treatment induces GAD65-specific CD4+CD25highFOXP3+ cells in type 1 diabetic patients. *Clin.Immunol* 138(1):117-126.

Lo J, Clare-Salzler MJ (2006) Dendritic cell subsets and type I diabetes: focus upon DC-based therapy. *Autoimmun Rev.* 5(6):419-423.

Kang, S. M.; Tang, Q., & Bluestone, J. A. (2007). CD4+CD25+ regulatory T cells in transplantation: progress, challenges and prospects. *Am.J Transplant.* 7(6):1457-1463.

Kaufman, D. L.; Clare-Salzler, M.; Tian, J.; Forsthuber, T.; Ting, G. S.; Robinson, P.; Atkinson, M. A.; Sercarz, E. E.; Tobin, A. J., & Lehmann, P. V. (1993). Spontaneous loss of T-cell tolerance to glutamic acid decarboxylase in murine insulin-dependent diabetes. *Nature* 366(6450):69-72.

Keymeulen, B.; Candon, S.; Fafi-Kremer, S.; Ziegler, A.; Leruez-Ville, M.; Mathieu, C.; Vandemeulebroucke, E.; Walter, M.; Crenier, L.; Thervet, E.; Legendre, C.; Pierard, D.; Hale, G.; Waldmann, H.; Bach, J. F.; Seigneurin, J. M.; Pipeleers, D., & Chatenoud, L. (2010). Transient Epstein-Barr virus reactivation in CD3 monoclonal antibody-treated patients. *Blood* 115(6):1145-1155.

Komatsu, N.; Mariotti-Ferrandiz, M. E.; Wang, Y.; Malissen, B.; Waldmann, H., & Hori, S. (2009). Heterogeneity of natural Foxp3+ T cells: a committed regulatory T-cell lineage and an uncommitted minor population retaining plasticity. *Proc.Natl.Acad.Sci.U.S.A* 106(6):1903-1908.

Larsson, H. E. & Lernmark, A. (2011). Does immune-tolerance treatment with Alum-formulated GAD65 protect insulin-production in the pancreatic islet ss cells? *Hum.Vaccin.* 7(1):

Li, S. W.; Koya, V.; Li, Y.; Donelan, W.; Lin, P.; Reeves, W. H., & Yang, L. J. (2010). Pancreatic duodenal homeobox 1 protein is a novel beta-cell-specific autoantigen for type I diabetes. *Lab Invest* 90(1):31-39.

Liang, J.; Aihua, Z.; Yu, W.; Yong, L., & Jingjing, L. (2010). HSP65 serves as an immunogenic carrier for a diabetogenic peptide P277 inducing anti-inflammatory immune response in NOD mice by nasal administration. *Vaccine* 28(19):3312-3317.

Liblau, R.; Tisch, R.; Bercovici, N., & McDevitt, H. O. (1997). Systemic antigen in the treatment of T-cell-mediated autoimmune diseases. *Immunol Today* 18(12):599-604.

Liu, K. & Nussenzweig, M. C. (2010). Origin and development of dendritic cells. *Immunol Rev.* 234(1):45-54.

Ludvigsson, J. (2009). Therapy with GAD in diabetes. *Diabetes Metab Res.Rev.* 25(4):307-315.

Makhlouf, L.; Grey, S. T.; Dong, V.; Csizmadia, E.; Arvelo, M. B.; Auchincloss, H., Jr.; Ferran, C., & Sayegh, M. H. (2004). Depleting anti-CD4 monoclonal antibody cures new-onset diabetes, prevents recurrent autoimmune diabetes, and delays allograft rejection in nonobese diabetic mice. *Transplantation* 77(7):990-997.

Maki, T.; Ichikawa, T.; Blanco, R., & Porter, J. (1992). Long-term abrogation of autoimmune diabetes in nonobese diabetic mice by immunotherapy with anti-lymphocyte serum. *Proc.Natl.Acad.Sci.U.S.A* 89(8):3434-3438.

Marin-Gallen, S.; Clemente-Casares, X.; Planas, R.; Pujol-Autonell, I.; Carrascal, J.; Carrillo, J.; Ampudia, R.; Verdaguer, J.; Pujol-Borrell, R.; Borras, F. E., & Vives-Pi, M. (2010). Dendritic cells pulsed with antigen-specific apoptotic bodies prevent experimental type 1 diabetes. *Clin.Exp.Immunol* 160(2):207-214.

Menendez, P.; Bueno, C.; Wang, L., & Bhatia, M. (2005). Human embryonic stem cells: potential tool for achieving immunotolerance? *Stem Cell Rev.* 1(2):151-158.

Morales, A. E. & Thrailkill, K. M. (2011). GAD-alum immunotherapy in Type 1 diabetes mellitus. *Immunotherapy.* 3(3):323-332.

Morelli, A. E. & Thomson, A. W. (2007). Tolerogenic dendritic cells and the quest for transplant tolerance. *Nat Rev.Immunol* 7(8):610-621.

Mukherjee G, Dilorenzo TP (2010) The immunotherapeutic potential of dendritic cells in type 1 diabetes. *Clin Exp Immunol.* 161(2):197-207.

Mukhopadhaya, A.; Hanafusa, T.; Jarchum, I.; Chen, Y. G.; Iwai, Y.; Serreze, D. V.; Steinman, R. M.; Tarbell, K. V., & DiLorenzo, T. P. (2008). Selective delivery of beta cell antigen to dendritic cells in vivo leads to deletion and tolerance of autoreactive CD8+ T cells in NOD mice. *Proc.Natl.Acad.Sci.U.S.A* 105(17):6374-6379.

Nagler-Anderson, C.; Bhan, A. K.; Podolsky, D. K., & Terhorst, C. (2004). Control freaks: immune regulatory cells. *Nat Immunol* 5(2):119-122.

Ogawa, N.; List, J. F.; Habener, J. F., & Maki, T. (2004). Cure of overt diabetes in NOD mice by transient treatment with anti-lymphocyte serum and exendin-4. *Diabetes* 53(7):1700-1705.

Palmer, J. P.; Asplin, C. M.; Clemons, P.; Lyen, K.; Tatpati, O.; Raghu, P. K., & Paquette, T. L. (1983). Insulin antibodies in insulin-dependent diabetics before insulin treatment. *Science* 222(4630):1337-1339.

Peakman M and von Herrath M (2010). Antigen-specific immunotherapy for type 1 diabetes: maximizing the potential. *Diabetes*.59(9):2087-2093

Petzold, C.; Riewaldt, J.; Koenig, T.; Schallenberg, S., & Kretschmer, K. (2010). Dendritic cell-targeted pancreatic beta-cell antigen leads to conversion of self-reactive CD4(+) T cells into regulatory T cells and promotes immunotolerance in NOD mice. *Rev.Diabet.Stud.* 7(1):47-61.

Pozzilli, P.; Pitocco, D.; Visalli, N.; Cavallo, M. G.; Buzzetti, R.; Crino, A.; Spera, S.; Suraci, C.; Multari, G.; Cervoni, M.; Manca Bitti, M. L.; Matteoli, M. C.; Marietti, G.; Ferrazzoli, F.; Cassone Faldetta, M. R.; Giordano, C.; Sbriglia, M.; Sarugeri, E., & Ghirlanda, G. (2000). No effect of oral insulin on residual beta-cell function in recent-onset type I diabetes (the IMDIAB VII). IMDIAB Group. *Diabetologia* 43(8):1000-1004.

Raz, I.; Avron, A.; Tamir, M.; Metzger, M.; Symer, L.; Eldor, R.; Cohen, I. R., & Elias, D. (2007). Treatment of new-onset type 1 diabetes with peptide DiaPep277 is safe and associated with preserved beta-cell function: extension of a randomized, double-blind, phase II trial. *Diabetes Metab Res.Rev.* 23(4):292-298.

Raz, I.; Elias, D.; Avron, A.; Tamir, M.; Metzger, M., & Cohen, I. R. (2001). Beta-cell function in new-onset type 1 diabetes and immunomodulation with a heat-shock protein peptide (DiaPep277): a randomised, double-blind, phase II trial. *Lancet* 358(9295):1749-1753.

Sakaguchi, S.; Miyara, M.; Costantino, C. M., & Hafler, D. A. (2010). FOXP3+ regulatory T cells in the human immune system. *Nat Rev.Immunol* 10(7):490-500.

Salomon, B.; Lenschow, D. J.; Rhee, L.; Ashourian, N.; Singh, B.; Sharpe, A., & Bluestone, J. A. (2000). B7/CD28 costimulation is essential for the homeostasis of the CD4+CD25+ immunoregulatory T cells that control autoimmune diabetes. *Immunity* 12(4):431-440.

Schloot, N. C.; Meierhoff, G.; Lengyel, C.; Vandorfi, G.; Takacs, J.; Panczel, P.; Barkai, L.; Madacsy, L.; Oroszlan, T.; Kovacs, P.; Suto, G.; Battelino, T.; Hosszufalusi, N., & Jermendy, G. (2007). Effect of heat shock protein peptide DiaPep277 on beta-cell function in paediatric and adult patients with recent-onset diabetes mellitus type 1: two prospective, randomized, double-blind phase II trials. *Diabetes Metab Res.Rev.* 23(4):276-285.

Sgouroudis, E. & Piccirillo, C. A. (2009). Control of type 1 diabetes by CD4+Foxp3+ regulatory T cells: lessons from mouse models and implications for human disease. *Diabetes Metab Res.Rev.* 25(3):208-218.

Shah, S. C.; Malone, J. I., & Simpson, N. E. (1989). A randomized trial of intensive insulin therapy in newly diagnosed insulin-dependent diabetes mellitus. *N.Engl.J Med* 320(9):550-554.

Sherry, N. A.; Chen, W.; Kushner, J. A.; Glandt, M.; Tang, Q.; Tsai, S.; Santamaria, P.; Bluestone, J. A.; Brillantes, A. M., & Herold, K. C. (2007). Exendin-4 improves reversal of diabetes in NOD mice treated with anti-CD3 monoclonal antibody by enhancing recovery of beta-cells. *Endocrinology* 148(11):5136-5144.

Shinomiya, M.; Fazle Akbar, S. M.; Shinomiya, H., & Onji, M. (1999). Transfer of dendritic cells (DC) ex vivo stimulated with interferon-gamma (IFN-gamma) down-modulates autoimmune diabetes in non-obese diabetic (NOD) mice. *Clin.Exp.Immunol* 117(1):38-43.

Siljander, H. T.; Simell, S.; Hekkala, A.; Lahde, J.; Simell, T.; Vahasalo, P.; Veijola, R.; Ilonen, J.; Simell, O., & Knip, M. (2009). Predictive characteristics of diabetes-associated autoantibodies among children with HLA-conferred disease susceptibility in the general population. *Diabetes* 58(12):2835-2842.

Skyler, J. S.; Krischer, J. P.; Wolfsdorf, J.; Cowie, C.; Palmer, J. P.; Greenbaum, C.; Cuthbertson, D.; Rafkin-Mervis, L. E.; Chase, H. P., & Leschek, E. (2005). Effects of oral insulin in relatives of patients with type 1 diabetes: The Diabetes Prevention Trial--Type 1. *Diabetes Care* 28(5):1068-1076.

Sloan-Lancaster, J. & Allen, P. M. (1996). Altered peptide ligand-induced partial T cell activation: molecular mechanisms and role in T cell biology. *Annu.Rev.Immunol* 14(1-27.

Sosenko, J. M.; Palmer, J. P.; Greenbaum, C. J.; Mahon, J.; Cowie, C.; Krischer, J. P.; Chase, H. P.; White, N. H.; Buckingham, B.; Herold, K. C.; Cuthbertson, D., & Skyler, J. S. (2006). Patterns of metabolic progression to type 1 diabetes in the Diabetes Prevention Trial-Type 1. *Diabetes Care* 29(3):643-649.

Spoerl, S. & Li, X. C. (2011). Regulatory T cells and the quest for transplant tolerance. *Discov.Med* 11(56):25-34.

Stadinski, B. D.; Delong, T.; Reisdorph, N.; Reisdorph, R.; Powell, R. L.; Armstrong, M.; Piganelli, J. D.; Barbour, G.; Bradley, B.; Crawford, F.; Marrack, P.; Mahata, S. K.; Kappler, J. W., & Haskins, K. (2010). Chromogranin A is an autoantigen in type 1 diabetes. *Nat Immunol* 11(3):225-231.

Staeva-Vieira, T.; Peakman, M., & von, H. M. (2007). Translational mini-review series on type 1 diabetes: Immune-based therapeutic approaches for type 1 diabetes. *Clin.Exp.Immunol* 148(1):17-31.

Steinman, R. M.; Hawiger, D., & Nussenzweig, M. C. (2003). Tolerogenic dendritic cells. *Annu.Rev.Immunol* 21(685-711.

Suarez-Pinzon WL, Power RF, Yan Y et al. (2008).Combination therapy with glucagon-like peptide-1 and gastrin restores normoglycemia in diabetic NOD mice. *Diabetes.* 57(12):3281-3288.

Tacken, P. J.; de, V., I; Torensma, R., & Figdor, C. G. (2007). Dendritic-cell immunotherapy: from ex vivo loading to in vivo targeting. *Nat Rev.Immunol* 7(10):790-802.

Tang, Q. & Bluestone, J. A. (2008). The Foxp3+ regulatory T cell: a jack of all trades, master of regulation. *Nat Immunol* 9(3):239-244.

Tang, Q.; Henriksen, K. J.; Bi, M.; Finger, E. B.; Szot, G.; Ye, J.; Masteller, E. L.; McDevitt, H.; Bonyhadi, M., & Bluestone, J. A. (2004). In vitro-expanded antigen-specific regulatory T cells suppress autoimmune diabetes. *J Exp.Med* 199(11):1455-1465.

Tarbell, K. V.; Petit, L.; Zuo, X.; Toy, P.; Luo, X.; Mqadmi, A.; Yang, H.; Suthanthiran, M.; Mojsov, S., & Steinman, R. M. (2007). Dendritic cell-expanded, islet-specific CD4+ CD25+ CD62L+ regulatory T cells restore normoglycemia in diabetic NOD mice. *J Exp.Med* 204(1):191-201.

Tarbell, K. V.; Yamazaki, S.; Olson, K.; Toy, P., & Steinman, R. M. (2004). CD25+ CD4+ T cells, expanded with dendritic cells presenting a single autoantigenic peptide, suppress autoimmune diabetes. *J Exp.Med* 199(11):1467-1477.

Tian, J.; Clare-Salzler, M.; Herschenfeld, A.; Middleton, B.; Newman, D.; Mueller, R.; Arita, S.; Evans, C.; Atkinson, M. A.; Mullen, Y.; Sarvetnick, N.; Tobin, A. J.; Lehmann, P. V., & Kaufman, D. L. (1996). Modulating autoimmune responses to GAD inhibits disease progression and prolongs islet graft survival in diabetes-prone mice. *Nat Med* 2(12):1348-1353.

Tisch, R.; Liblau, R. S.; Yang, X. D.; Liblau, P., & McDevitt, H. O. (1998). Induction of GAD65-specific regulatory T-cells inhibits ongoing autoimmune diabetes in nonobese diabetic mice. *Diabetes* 47(6):894-899.

Tonkin, D. R. & Haskins, K. (2009). Regulatory T cells enter the pancreas during suppression of type 1 diabetes and inhibit effector T cells and macrophages in a TGF-beta-dependent manner. *Eur.J Immunol* 39(5):1313-1322.

Tonkin, D. R.; He, J.; Barbour, G., & Haskins, K. (2008). Regulatory T cells prevent transfer of type 1 diabetes in NOD mice only when their antigen is present in vivo. *J Immunol* 181(7):4516-4522.

Tritt, M.; Sgouroudis, E.; d'Hennezel, E.; Albanese, A., & Piccirillo, C. A. (2008). Functional waning of naturally occurring CD4+ regulatory T-cells contributes to the onset of autoimmune diabetes. *Diabetes* 57(1):113-123.

van Belle, T. L.; Coppieters, K. T., & von Herrath, M. G. (2011). Type 1 diabetes: etiology, immunology, and therapeutic strategies. *Physiol Rev.* 91(1):79-118.

van, A. D.; Kalbacher, H.; Palesch, D.; Zou, F.; Spyrantis, A.; Rosinger, S.; Boehm, B. O., & Burster, T. (2010). A proinsulin 74-90-derived protease-resistant, altered peptide ligand increases TGF-beta 1 secretion in PBMC from patients with type 1 diabetes mellitus. *J Leukoc.Biol.* 87(5):943-948.

Walter, M.; Philotheou, A.; Bonnici, F.; Ziegler, A. G., & Jimenez, R. (2009). No effect of the altered peptide ligand NBI-6024 on beta-cell residual function and insulin needs in new-onset type 1 diabetes. *Diabetes Care* 32(11):2036-2040.

Wenzlau, J. M.; Juhl, K.; Yu, L.; Moua, O.; Sarkar, S. A.; Gottlieb, P.; Rewers, M.; Eisenbarth, G. S.; Jensen, J.; Davidson, H. W., & Hutton, J. C. (2007). The cation efflux transporter ZnT8 (Slc30A8) is a major autoantigen in human type 1 diabetes. *Proc.Natl.Acad.Sci.U.S.A* 104(43):17040-17045.

Wu, A. J.; Hua, H.; Munson, S. H., & McDevitt, H. O. (2002). Tumor necrosis factor-alpha regulation of CD4+CD25+ T cell levels in NOD mice. *Proc.Natl.Acad.Sci.U.S.A* 99(19):12287-12292.

Zhang, G. Y.; Hu, M.; Wang, Y. M., & Alexander, S. I. (2009). Foxp3 as a marker of tolerance induction versus rejection. *Curr.Opin.Organ Transplant.* 14(1):40-45.

Zhou, X.; Bailey-Bucktrout, S.; Jeker, L. T., & Bluestone, J. A. (2009). Plasticity of CD4(+) FoxP3(+) T cells. *Curr.Opin.Immunol* 21(3):281-285.

20

Multi-Component Vaccines for Suppression of Type 1 Diabetes

William H.R. Langridge and Oludare J. Odumosu
Loma Linda University School of Medicine, Center for Health Disparities and Molecular Medicine, Loma Linda, U.S.A.

1. Introduction

Many individual therapeutic strategies involving oral delivery of diabetes autoantigens such as insulin and GAD have been shown to provide partial short term suppression of organ specific type 1 diabetes autoimmunity (Weiner et al. 1991; Zhang et al. 1991; Nakayama et al. 2005). However, few individual therapies have been able to demonstrate effective, safe and persistent protection against type 1 diabetes onset or progression (Hutchings and Cooke 1998). More recently, combinatorial therapeutic strategies that incorporate immunostimulatory molecules such as the cholera toxin B subunit (CTB), linked to a diabetes autoantigen (eg. insulin or GAD), were shown to substantially enhance immune suppression of juvenile (Type 1) diabetes autoimmunity to provide more effective, safe and sustainable disease prevention (Arakawa et al. 1998; Denes et al. 2006). Combinatorial vaccines involving oral delivery of the cholera toxin B subunit (CTB) linked to pancreatic autoantigens such as proinsulin and GAD delivered together were shown to provide additive enhancement of autoantigen mediated suppression of diabetes insulitis and hyperglycemia in contrast to inoculation of prediabetic mice with CTB::GAD or CTB::proinsulin alone (Arakawa, Chong, and Langridge 1998). Most recently, combinatorial DNA vaccination experiments including genes encoding CTB::GAD together with the immunosuppressive cytokine IL-10 were shown to completely suppress type 1 diabetes onset in non-obese prediabetic (NOD) mice (Denes et al. 2010). Thus, it is now clear that combinatorial vaccination strategies have the ability to completely prevent diabetes onset in genetically susceptible mammals.

However, to harness and transfer this promising combinatorial vaccination strategy for effective and safe clinical therapy in type 1 diabetes patients, cellular and molecular mechanisms underlying multi-component vaccine stimulation of immunological tolerance must be defined. Initial steps required to attain this goal, will involve identification of mechanisms responsible for vaccine interactions with cells of the innate immune system i.e., dendritic cells (DCs), involved in the initial processing vaccine autoantigens.

In order to understand how multi-component vaccines may function to prevent the development of chronic islet inflammation (insulitis) progressing to high blood sugar (hyperglycemia), it will be important to understand the nature of immune responses underlying type 1 diabetes disease onset. To accomplish this goal, hypotheses must be tested that suggest how adjuvant-autoantigen fusion proteins may enhance immunotolerance e.g.

through initial activation of sensor cells of the innate immune system predominantly immature dendritic cells (iDC). Of importance will be to determine how DCs process adjuvant-autoantigen fusion proteins, and how these processing reactions result in the initiation of immuno-reactive or immuno-suppressive T cell populations responsible for inhibiting the development of autoreactive effector T cell responses? Throughout the development of this review, we will examine the role of protein adjuvants such as CTB in combination with autoantgens and anti-inflammatory cytokines that can act in concert to stimulate proliferation and activation of regulatory T cell subsets potentially key players in the inhibition of DC maturation and stimulation of T cell morphogenesis into autoreactive T cells. To rescue the large numbers of existing diabetes patients in which diabetes has progressed to a hyperglycemic state, it will be important to understand mechanisms responsible for diabetes development and how combinatorial vaccines may interact with cells of the immune system to suppress diabetes progression. An improved understanding of these mechanisms will establish a basis for development of safer, more effective and durable vaccine strategies for prevention of diabetes onset and for improvement of combinatorial therapeutic strategies for restoration of immunological homeostasis and ultimately restoration of euglycemia in type 1 diabetes patients.

2. Type 1 diabetes results from genetic predisposition and a breakdown in the mechanisms responsible for immunological tolerance

In juvenile diabetes mellitus, (type 1 diabetes), insulin-producing beta cells in the pancreatic Islets of Langerhans are attacked and destroyed by aberrant immune responses to insulin and progressively to other islet beta cell products. Diabetic patients that have progressed to hyperglycemia must regularly inject insulin multiple times a day, or risk diabetic shock, coma and death. Regulation of immunological homeostasis, among the approximate 10^{14} commensal microorganisms living on the 10^{13} cells of the human body's mucosae requires a delicate balance of activation and suppression of immunity, (Lodinova-Zadnikova et al. 2004). The first step in disruption of homeostasis leading to islet-cell mortality is initiated by events that trigger maturation of antigen-presenting cells (APCs), largely dendritic cells (DC), responsible for inducing the morphogenesis of autoreactive CD8+, CD4+ T cells and B cells, which results in the production of anti-beta cell antibodies (Atkinson et al. 1994; Han et al. 2005; Tisch and McDevitt 1996). The continuous loss of islet β-cell function results in a progressive deficiency of insulin production leading to a gradual elevation of blood sugar levels (hyperglycemia), that triggers an increase in cellular oxidative stress leading to chronic inflammation and an associated risk for secondary neural and circulatory pathological complications that include amputation, blindness, kidney failure, heart attack and stroke (Libby et al. 2005; Shen and Bornfeldt 2007). Diabetes hyperglycemia represents the end stage of an immunological process that develops over months in mice to years in humans (Vendrame, Zappaterreno, and Dotta 2004). While most type 1 diabetes (T1D) cases develop in pre-adolescence, late onset diabetes (LADA), may appear generally from 40-60 yr of age and is often confused with type 2 diabetes. The progression of diabetes symptoms may be responsible for 10-15% of diabetes related heart disease mortality especially in low income socio-economic groups which are at greatest risk for diabetes related health disparities in the U.S (Kobayashi et al. 2006; Maioli, Puddu, and Pes 2006). Diagnosis and treatment of hyperglycemia is poor, as islet β-cell destruction is completely asymptomatic until more than half of the approximately 1×10^6 pancreatic islets have been destroyed or inactivated (Tang et al. 2006). Approximately 3 million Americans, or about 15-20% of citizens currently afflicted with all forms of diabetes, suffer from type 1 diabetes and > 13,000 children are diagnosed with type 1 diabetes in the U.S. annually - (about 35 children / day), (International 2005). Alarmingly, type 1 diabetes in pre-adolescent children is increasing at about 0.3-0.5% annually, (Gale 2002; International 2005). Familial inheritance studies show that genetic predisposition factors (genotype DRB1*0301/04, DQB1*0201/0302), play a significant role in T1D development (Rewers et al. 1996). At least 15 genetic loci have been linked to T1D in the non-obese diabetic (NOD) mouse, a relevant mammalian T1D model (Makino et al. 1980). In humans, genetic risk factors were identified in the leukocyte antigen (HLA) complex on chromosome 6, CTLA-4 gene polymorphisms on chromosome 2, and in the insulin gene variable number tandem repeat region on chromosome 11 (Onengut-Gumuscu and Concannon 2002). Since Type 1 diabetes ranges from 23 - 53% among monozygotic twins, genetic risk factors are insufficient to account for disease occurrence (Tatersall R. B. 1972).

Environmental factors, including virus infection and dietary components are considered to modify diabetes susceptibility (Jun and Yoon 2001; Akerblom HK 2002). Cytotoxic CD8+ T cells were shown to be involved in diabetes initiation and progression(Walter and Santamaria 2005). Further, recruitment of naïve diabetogenic β-cell-reactive CTLs to the pancreatic islets were shown to require β-cell-reactive CD4+ Th1 cells(Delovitch and Singh 1997). Following $CD4^{+}$ Th cell infiltration of pancreatic islets in NOD mice, autoreactive Th1 lymphocytes were shown to secrete inflammatory cytokines IFN-γ and IL-2 that stimulate macrophage and CTL secretion of oxidative compounds and inflammatory cytokines that induce chronic pancreatic inflammation (insulitis), ultimately responsible for apoptosis of islet insulin-producing β-cells(Romagnani 1998). Diabetes onset is not always marked by circulating auto-Ab to β-cell autoantigens and a variety of immune cells including B cells, dendritic cells, macrophages and natural killer (NK) cells have been shown to be involved in diabetes pathogenesis(Yoon, Jun, and Santamaria 1998; Dai, Carayanniotis, and Sercarz 2005; Tian et al. 2006; Silveira and Grey 2006; Cardell 2006). A recently identified rat diabetes model was shown to be quantitatively up-regulated from 2.0 -100% diabetes by antibody depletion of regulatory T cells suggesting a significant role for regulatory T cells in diabetes suppression(Mordes et al. 2005). Thus, dendritic cell, autoreactive T cell, T regulatory cell and B cell pathways may all interact to establish or break immunological homeostasis(Mostarica-Stojkovic 2005).

2.1 Diabetes autoantigen therapy can restore immunological tolerance

While, deletion of autoreactive T cells is generally achieved in the thymus (central tolerance), a few autoreactive T lymphocytes escape deletion and appear in the periphery(Song et al. 2004). Interestingly, autoreactive T cell clones specific for self-proteins were shown to arise spontaneously from normal peripheral blood mononuclear cells in healthy people (Wucherpfennig et al. 1994). Thus, autoimmunity may have the opportunity to exist to some degree in everyone. Insulin was shown to be an early major diabetes autoantigen(Palmer et al. 1983; Jaeckel, Lipes, and von Boehmer 2004; Jaeckel et al. 2003; Kent et al. 2005). The insulin leader, A, B and C protein chains all were shown to contain CD4+ and CD8+ immunodominant T cell epitopes (Di Lorenzo, Peakman, and Roep 2007). Progressive islet β-cell destruction was shown to lead to the appearance of additional β-cell autoantigens (Ag spreading), a factor that exacerbates β-cell destruction(Baekkeskov et al.

1990). Immunotherapy with major β-cell antigens such as insulin, glutamate decarboxylase (GAD), or heat shock protein (hsp60), was shown to delay or even prevent the onset of type 1 diabetes, providing a potentially useful therapeutic approach to treatment of T cell-mediated autoimmunity(Elliott et al. 1994; Tisch and McDevitt 1996). Oral inoculation with small amounts of islet autoantigens was shown to induce self-tolerance through IL-4 and Stat 6 activation of $CD4^+$ Th2 and Th3 regulatory T cells that down-modulate autoreactive effector T cell inflammation at close proximity e.g., "bystander suppression", (Hommann et al. 2001; Weiner 2001). Protection against T1D was shown to be associated with Th3 regulatory lymphocyte secretion of TGF-β in prediabetic NOD mice gavaged with insulin, (Zhang et al. 1991). Further, oral auto-Ag inoculation generated partial diabetes suppression in patients (Millington, Mowat, and Garside 2004; Chaillous et al. 2000). In several related Th1 cell mediated autoimmune diseases, collagen-induced arthritis (Thompson and Staines 1986) and encephalomyelitis (Higgins and Weiner 1988) disease suppression was observed after prolonged feeding of small amounts of specific auto-Ags. The induction of multiple sclerosis in animals was not only halted but reversed by feeding small amounts of myelin basic protein suggesting that this type of oral auto-Ag therapy can suppress and even aid in recovery from autoimmunity (Bitar and Whitacre 1988).

2.2 Cholera toxin B subunit (CTB), enhances autoantigen mediated immunotolerance

Immunotherapy with adjuvants such as Complete Freund's Adjuvant (CFA) co-injected intradermally with insulin, or inoculation with CTB-insulin B chain polypeptide fusion proteins significantly suppressed diabetes early onset demonstrating the usefulness of immunostimulatory molecules in diabetes suppression (Hutchings and Cooke 1998). Additional studies in BB rats suggest that CFA may mediate diabetes suppression through induction of regulatory T cells (Qin et al. 1993). Thus, a number of biological mechanisms may contribute to suppression of autoimmunity. Cholera toxin (CTX), from *Vibrio cholerae* contains a toxic ADP-ribosyltransferase A subunit (CTA1), linked by a small helical (A2) peptide to a pentamer of non-toxic carrier B subunits (CTB), (Eriksson and Holmgren 2002). CTX induces DC maturation and migration to the Peyer's patches while the CTB subunit was shown to inhibit DC maturation and to bind GM1-ganglioside, a receptor found on most epidermal cells, thereby providing an efficient transmucosal carrier for autoantigen induction of peripheral tolerance (Shreedhar, Kelsall, and Neutra 2003; Lycke 2004; Sun, Holmgren, and Czerkinsky 1994). Oral delivery of CTB was shown to directly stimulate DC induction of T cell IL-4 secretion and to exert a variety of distinct anti-inflammatory effects resulting in immunological suppression (Holmgren et al. 1994; Li and Fox 1996; Holmgren and Czerkinsky 2005). Oral delivery of CTB conjugated to specific autoantigens was shown to protect mice against several Th1 cell mediated autoimmune diseases including autoimmune encephalomyelitis (Sun et al. 1996; Sun et al. 2000), autoimmune chondritis (Kim et al. 2001) and uveitis (Phipps et al. 2003). Further, CTB-insulin conjugates were shown to suppress diabetes in NOD mice (Bergerot et al. 1997; Arakawa, Chong, and Langridge 1998), a result associated with reduced IFN-γ production and Tr1 regulatory T cell migration into pancreatic islets (Aspord et al. 2002; Roncarolo et al. 2001). Further, linkage of CTB to insulin generated up to a 10,000-fold reduction in autoantigen required for immuno-tolerization (Bergerot et al. 1997; Arakawa et al. 1998; George-Chandy et al. 2001). Thus, current evidence suggests that mechanisms responsible for CTB modulated immune suppression may include inhibition of DC maturation by suppressing the expression of surface co-stimulatory molecules resulting in the increased secretion of IL-10 and a concurrent suppression of IL-12, inhibition of autoreactive T cell development and/or stimulation of Th2 and regulatory T cell proliferation and activation (Marinaro et al. 1995; Lavelle et al. 2003; Odumosu et al. 2010).

2.3 Dendritic cells can initiate immunological tolerance

Dendritic cells may play a primary role in antigen priming of naïve T helper cells (Th0) and modulation of their development into autoreactive Th1 or immunosuppressive Th2 lymphocytes important for maintenance of immunological homeostasis (Pulendran et al. 1999; Pulendran et al. 2001; Itano et al. 2003).

Immuno-cytochemical analyses showed that oral inoculation of autoantigens results in their uptake from M cells in the intestinal mucosa into peripheral (lamina propria) DCs via several routes that may influence the nature of the immune response (Yoon and Jun 2005).

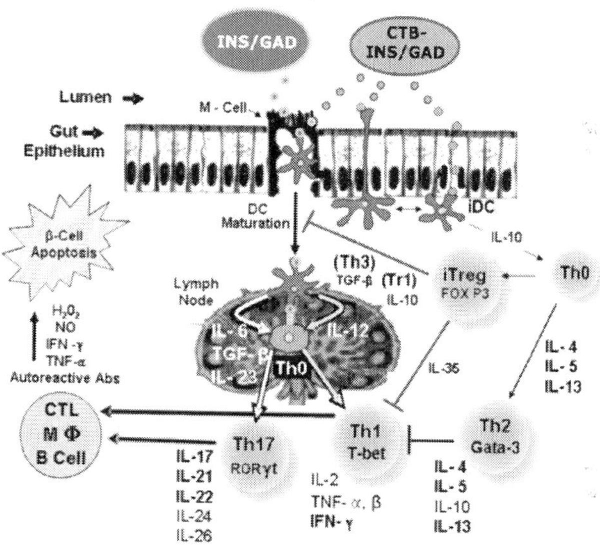

Fig. 1. Adjuvant-autoantigen fusion protein suppression of autoimmunity. Immature dendritic cells (iDC) take up CTB:GAD/Insulin autoantigen fusion proteins through the intestinal epithelium. Low levels of oral delivered auto-Ags stimulate DC secretion of anti-inflammatory cytokines IL-10 and IL-4 which guide cognate naïve Th0 lymphocyte development of into immunosuppressive Th2 and iTreg lymphocyte phenotypes (Iwasaki and Kelsall 2000; Afzali et al. 2007).

Autoantigens may be taken up and processed by immature, partially activated semi-mature or mature DC subsets (Lutz and Schuler 2002). These DCs may remain in the periphery or migrate to lymph nodes, where they present antigen peptides on MHCII receptors, synthesize co-stimulatory molecules and in the absence of additional cytokine production, may induce the morphogenesis of Ag-specific IL-10 producing CD4+CD25+ T regulatory (Tr1) cells (Enk 2005) **Figure 1.** Co-stimulation appears to be less or absent for tolerogenic responses, thus, interactions between autoantigens, DCs and T cells in the gut associated lymphoid tissues may result in tolerogenic outcomes following autoAg presentation (Lycke 2004). Peyer's patches DCs that synthesize IL-10 were shown to down-regulate Th1 cell mediated autoimmunity (Steinbrink et al. 1997). Immature or peripheral DCs (iDCs), that had low expression of co-stimulatory molecules, secreted cytokine IL-10, remained in the periphery and were shown to induce Th2 lymphocyte mediated immunological tolerance (Rissoan et al. 1999; Liu et al. 2001; Li et al. 2006). Further studies showed that a major function of peripheral iDCs was maintenance of self-tolerance (Wilson, El-Sukkari, and Villadangos 2004; Steinman and Pope 2002). In alternative, experiments, adding IL-12 to iDCs induced Th1 cell morphogenesis and accelerated type 1 diabetes in NOD mice (Trembleau et al. 1995). In response to microbial antigens, DCs may secrete inflammatory cytokines IL-6 and IL-23 that stimulate naïve Th0 cell development into IL-17 inflammatory cytokine secreting Th17 effector T cells (Figure 1). Th17 cells have been implicated in the induction of organ-specific autoimmune arthritis, multiple sclerosis, psoriasis, and inflammatory bowel disease as well as type 1 diabetes (Cua et al. 2003; Langrish et al. 2005; Duerr et al. 2006; Murphy et al. 2003; Nakae et al. 2003; Zheng et al. 2007; Mensah-Brown, Shahin, Al-Shamisi et al. 2006; Mensah-Brown, Shahin, Al-Shamsi et al. 2006). Together, the experimental evidence suggests development of type 1 diabetes may be under DC control (Shinomiya et al. 1999). However, there is some debate about the role of Th17 cells in diabetogenesis suggesting that Th17 cells are not important in the disease process but rather are plastic cell that become become Th1(Bending et al. 2009).

2.4 CTB enhances immune tolerance by upregulating DC tolerogenic toll-like receptors

Dendritic cells, macrophages, and granulocytes derived from hematopoietic stem cells provide the first line of defense against infectious pathogens attacking mucosal surfaces. Thus, DCs (found in most abundance in the mucosae and skin), must recognize pathogen antigens, autoantigens and innocuous antigens in order to maintain immunological homeostasis. To accomplish this task, DCs bind small conserved pathogen antigen segments; pathogen associated molecular patterns (PAMPS), to their trans-membrane toll-like receptor (TLR) domains, (Takeda, Kaisho, and Akira 2003; Wen et al. 2004). Different PAMPS stimulate specific TLRs that activate one of several DC signal transduction pathways leading to synthesis of transcriptional regulators e.g., NFkB. These transcriptional activators switch on genes encoding specific cytokines, costimulatory molecules and chemokines that enable DCs to direct naïve cognate Th0 cell development into (1) immunoreactive Th1 lymphocytes, (2) immunosuppressive Th2 effector cell and (3) T regulatory cell subsets (Kaisho and Akira 2002). Autoreactive T cells involved in experimental autoimmune encephalomyelitis (EAE) and other chronic inflammatory autoimmune diseases are considered to follow TLR defined pathways of DC processing and auto-Ag presentation triggered by environment signals (Haverkos et al. 2003; Bach 2005). Recently, examination of TLR2 and TLR4 expression in monocytes from T1D patients showed that TLR2 and TLR4 surface expression and mRNAs were significantly increased in T1D monocytes in comparison with the controls (Devaraj et al. 2007). Further, downstream targets of TLRs, NFKb, MyD88, Trif and pIRAK, were also significantly upregulated. Antigen ligation to TLR2 is generally known to induce a Th2 immunosuppressive cytokine profile (Ferwerda et al. 2005). Whether CTB binds and activates TLR2 or TLR4 is presently

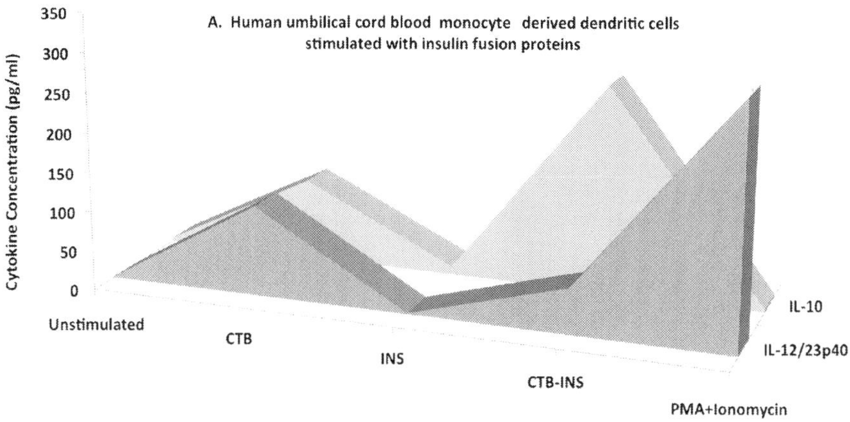

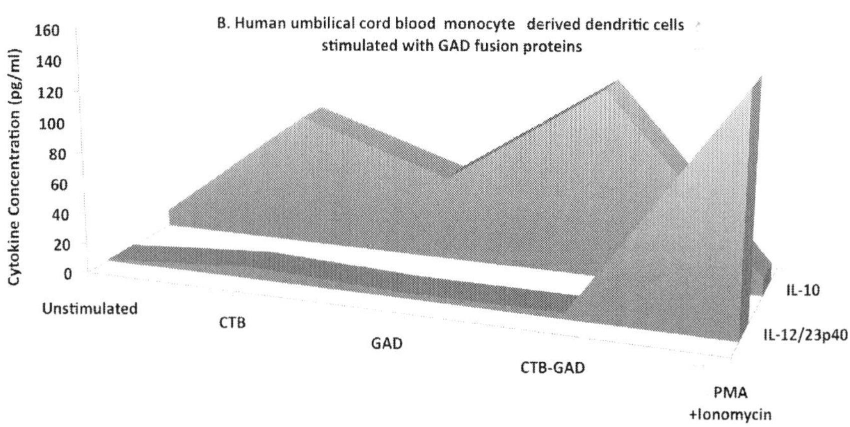

Fig. 2. Measurement of anti-inflammatory cytokine IL-10 and inflammatory cytokine IL-12/23p40 subunit levels by Cytometric Bead Array flow cytometry, from cell supernatants removed from iDCs inoculated with CTB-insulin (CTB::INS) fusion protein, (Panel A) or CTB::GAD fusion protein (Panel B). For each treatment the concentration of IL-10 and IL-12/23p40 subunit was normalized to standard IL-10 and IL-12/23p40 cytokine curve and given in pg/ml. The data represent the Mean and SE (*P<0.001) of repeated independent experiments in comparison with the control sample.

unknown. However, the structurally similar *E. coli* AB enterotoxin B subunit (LTB) was shown to stimulate TLR2, resulting in regulatory T cell proliferation which ultimately lead to inhibition of iDC maturation, IL-10 secretion and induction of immunosuppressive Th2 lymphocyte development (Hajishengallis et al. 2005; Sutmuller et al. 2006). Examination of CTB mediated suppression of DC maturation suggests that TLR2 may be selectively upregulated (Odumosu et al. 2010). The observed selectivity may be due to TLR2 dependent hydrophobic interactions for ligand binding as previously observed for the E. coli enterotoxin B subunit LTBIIb (Seong and Matzinger 2004; Okusawa et al. 2004). Alternatively, multiple bacterial products including lipo-polysaccharide (LPS), were shown to undergo DC processing independently of TLR signaling, via stimulation of the pannexin - 1 hemi-channel protein–cryopyrin receptor pathway (Kanneganti et al. 2007) Thus, in addition to immunosuppressive TLR receptor binding, alternative signaling pathways could be involved in iDC processing of CTB-INS fusion protein potentially favoring CTB induced DC synthesis of IL-10 leading to induction of Th0 -> Th2 cell morphogenesis and suppression of autoreactive Th1 lymphocyte development (**Figure 2**).

2.5 Regulatory T cells inhibit dendritic cell maturation

The suppression of autoreactive T cells is essential for establishment of peripheral tolerance and maintenance of immunological homeostasis, (Vigouroux et al. 2004; Stassen et al. 2004). Natural CD4+CD25+ regulatory T cells (nTregs) of thymus origin, have a high avidity for self-antigens and were shown to link central tolerance to induction of regulatory functions in the periphery (Sakaguchi et al. 1995; Sakaguchi and Sakaguchi 2005; Sakaguchi 2005; Taams and Akbar 2005; Bresson et al. 2006). Natural Treg immunosuppressive functions are antigen independent and are largely under control of the forkhead box p3 transcription factor FOXP3 (Fontenot, Gavin and Rudensky 2003; Hori, Nomura and Sakaguchi 2003). While nTregs inhibit DC maturation in an antigen independent manner, they were also shown to be important for down-regulating Th1 cell mediated autoimmunity in thyroiditis, diabetes, encephalomyelitis, and oophoritis (Tarbell et al. 2004). Further, the glucocorticoid-induced tumor necrosis factor receptor (GITR), cytotoxic T-lymphocyte antigen 4 (CTLA-4), and LAG-3 surface markers were identified on antigen-activated nTregs (Nocentini and Riccardi 2005; Huang et al. 2004; Oderup et al. 2006). Further evidence supporting Treg suppression of autoimmunity, mutations in the mouse *foxp3* gene resulted in development of systemic autoimmunity, characterized by inflammatory lymphocyte infiltration and destruction of tissues by autoreactive T-cells, leading to spontaneous development of a number of Th1 cell mediated autoimmune diseases including type 1 diabetes (Hori and Sakaguchi 2004; Ehrenstein et al. 2004; Lindley et al. 2005; Viglietta et al. 2004).

Incubation of DCs with nTregs increased IL-10 secretion and reduced CD40, CD80/86 co-stimulatory molecule expression reinforcing the hypothesis that nTregs modulate autoimmunity through suppression of DC immunostimulatory functions (Veldhoen et al. 2006; Misra et al. 2004; Yang et al. 2006). Recent experiments clearly show that Tregs interact with antigen-bearing DCs to prevent naïve autoreactive CD4+CD25-- effector Th0 cell priming (Tang et al. 2006). Adoptive transfer experiments further confirmed nTreg-DC interaction was essential for autoreactive Th1 cell inhibition (Tarbell et al. 2004; Kelsen et al. 2006). Regulation of DC processing of autoantigens, in the absence of sufficient nTregs, requires additional regulatory T cell induction from the CD4+ CD25-- T cell population(Bluestone and Abbas 2003; Filippi, Bresson, and von Herrath 2005) . Two human CD4+CD25+ nTreg subsets were shown to convey immuno-suppressive capabilities to $CD4^+$ CD25-- T cells. Natural Tregs expressing $\alpha 4\beta 7$ integrin induced IL-10 secreting Tr1-like suppressor T cells, while nTregs expressing $\alpha 4\beta 1$ integrin induced TGF-β secreting Th3-like suppressor T cells (Stassen et al. 2004). Secreted TGF-β1 was shown to suppress DC activation during maturation (Rastellini et al. 1995; Yamaguchi et al. 1997; King et al. 1998).

Further, TGF-β1 inhibited DC expression of chemokine receptor CCR7, responsible for DC migration to lymph nodes (MartIn-Fontecha et al. 2003). Secretion of IL-10 by Tr1 iTregs inhibited DC maturation by blocking IL-12 synthesis and skewing Th1/Th2 polarity toward Th2 cells *in vivo* by inhibiting both Th1 cell proliferation and monocyte secretion of IFN-γ, TNF-β and IL-2 cytokines (De Smedt et al. 1997; Sela 2006). DCs were shown to expand and differentiate Foxp3+CD25+CD4+ Tregs from Foxp3–CD25–CD4+ thymocytes with specificity for self-antigens presented by thymic medullary DCs maturing in response to thymic stromal lymphopoietin (Watanabe et al. 2005). In vivo, repeated injection of preprocessed peptides (Apostolou and von Boehmer 2004) or the targeting of intact antigens to immature DCs (Kretschmer et al. 2005) convert antigen-specific Foxp3–CD25–CD4+ T cells to Foxp3+CD25+CD4+ Tregs bearing the same TCR. DCs also induce other regulatory populations, such as IL-10-producing Tr1 (Levings et al. 2005; Akbari, DeKruyff, and Umetsu 2001; Akbari et al. 2002; Stock et al. 2004) and IL-10-producing regulatory DCs (Kojo et al. 2005). Diabetes-susceptible NOD mice appear to generate normal numbers of Foxp3 T-cells over their lifetimes (Tritt et al. 2008). However, Piccirillo and his colleagues at McGill University showed that T-cell functional potency declined with age, leaving potential autoimmune responses in the pancreas unchecked. These authors suggest that certain genetic predispositions, coupled with the possible contribution of external environmental factors or infections, could potentially alter regulatory T-cell function in susceptible individuals and trigger a full-scale diabetic autoimmune reaction in the pancreas (Tritt et al. 2008).

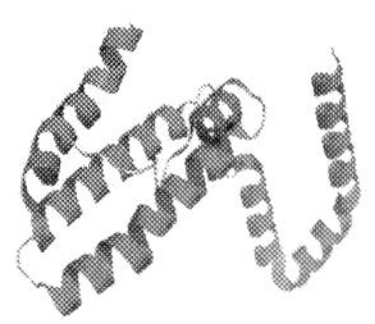

Ribon
diagram of
Human IL-10

2.6 Immunosuppressive properties of anti-inflammatory cytokine IL-10

Human IL-10 is a homodimeric anti-inflammatory cytokine protein (molecular structure at left), with a subunit length of 160 amino acids and 73 percent amino acid homology with its murine orthologue(Yoon et al. 2006; Moore et al. 1990). Mouse knockout studies showed that IL-10 down-regulates autoimmunity in the intestinal tract and is active in suppression of Crohn's disease (Minderhoud, Samsom, and Oldenburg 2007, 2007). In confirmation, the inability to clear persistent viral infections was shown to result from T-cell inactivation generated by APC up-regulation of anti-inflammatory IL-10 biosynthesis (Seyfert-Margolis et al. 2006). Thus, suppression of inflammatory responses mediated by DC up-regulation of IL-10 may play a significant role in virus-mediated suppression of type 1 diabetes in NOD mice and BB rats (Tracy and Drescher 2007; Schwimmbeck, Dyrberg, and Oldstone 1988). Alternative mechanisms that may play a role in cytokine enhancement of immune suppression include IL-10 blockage of NF-kappa B activity and regulation of the JAK-STAT signaling pathway (Donnelly, Dickensheets, and Finbloom 1999; Leceta et al. 2000).

A regulatory role for autocrine IL-10 has been described for APCs such as monocytes, macrophages and dendritic cells (de Waal Malefyt et al. 1991; Sica et al. 2000). Autocrine production of IL-10 by immature DCs, was shown to inhibit production and release of pro-inflammatory cytokines (IL-12, TNF-α, IL-6, LTB4, NO, PGE2), and to suppress Th1 lymphocyte activity by down-regulation of costimulatory molecule expression on the APC surface (Harizi and Gualde 2006; Grutz 2005; Moore et al. 1993). Through inhibition of these endogenous pro-inflammatory mediators, IL-10 has demonstrated a central role in down-regulating DC mediated inflammatory responses and maintenance of DCs in an immature state (Harizi and Gualde 2006).

In paracrine fashion, IL-10 synthesized by DCs can regulate immune responses by altering the function of different adjacent cell types. In several studies IL-10 secreted by iDCs stimulated morphogenesis of cognate Th0 cell development into immunosuppressive Th2 lymphocytes, or into suppressor CD4+ regulatory T cells (Stassen, Schmitt, and Jonuleit 2004; Romagnani et al. 1998). In addition, IL-10 was shown to increase effector functions of CD8+ T cells (Groux et al. 1999). In addition, IL-10 may be crucial for controlling chronic inflammatory responses *in vivo*. Inhibition of LPS-induced CD40 signaling by IL-10 suppressed multiple sclerosis and rheumatoid arthritis, confirming the value of IL-10 as a therapeutic for autoimmunity (Qin et al. 2006). Further, IL-10 was shown to play a role in partial suppression of type 1 diabetes (Slavin, Maron, and Weiner 2001; Battaglia et al. 2006; Goudy et al. 2001; Goudy et al. 2003). Thus, through activation of several biological mechanisms, IL-10 may provide significant enhancement to CTB-diabetes autoantigen mediated immune suppression.

2.7 Virus vaccine delivery does not inhibit immunotolerance

In addition to its function as a vehicle for subunit vaccine delivery, vaccinia virus was shown to stimulate production of anti-inflammatory cytokines IL-10 and TGF-β in skin epithelial cells(Liu et al. 2005). As these cytokines are known to inhibit inflammation and Th1 responses, vaccinia demonstrates properties known to suppress inflammation. Further, vaccinia virus expressing the pancreatic islet auto-Ag glutamic acid decarboxylase (GAD) was shown to be 90% effective in prevention of diabetes in NOD mice (Jun, Khil, and Yoon 2002; Jun et al. 2002). (1) Vaccinia multiplies in the cytoplasm, excluding genetic modification of infected cells (Moss 1996). (2) All human cell types tested produce viral infection with high efficiency. Viral or foreign proteins are synthesized and undergo appropriate post-translational modification (Moss 1991). (3) Multiple autoantigen genes (up to 25 kb), can be tolerated in dispensable regions of the vaccinia genome without impacting virus growth. (4) Because recombinant vaccinia virus proteins expressed in mammalian cells are properly folded, processed and transported normally, they can be used to induce or bind antibodies that recognize conformational epitopes (Otteken, Earl, and Moss 1996). (5) The safety of a live attenuated VV vaccine was clearly shown in a major smallpox eradication program (Moss 1991). (6) Patients injected with an attenuated VV strain expressing cytokines showed no evidence of systemic virus spread, organ dysfunction or other major hematological or biochemical changes (Robinson, Cornelius et al. 1998; Robinson, Mukherjee et al. 1998; Mastrangelo et al. 1999). (7) Construction of safer, hyper-attenuated replication-deficient and –competent strains of vaccinia is underway (Denes et al. 2006), which could be used for treatment of diabetes. Recent experiments in our laboratory showed that vaccinia virus delivered CTB-INS autoantigens suppress type 1 diabetes insulitis and hyperglycemia in NOD mice (Denes, Fodor and Langridge 2010). Of specific relevance to this proposal, addition of vaccinia as an alternate CTB-INS delivery vehicle will permit priming and boosting CTB-INS immunosuppressive responses without the possibility for generation of immunity to the vector, which could potentially ameliorate immunological tolerization to the autoantigen and degrade the contribution of the adjuvant to enhanced immunosuppression. Further, delivery of subunit vaccines, which are often lacking in immunogenicity may benefit from increased immunostimulation provided by heterologous prime/boost inoculation regimes. Vaccinia prime, plant boost strategies may provide an increased level of immunosuppression.

2.8 Plants block type 1 diabetes onset and act as production and delivery vehicles for diabetes vaccines.

The B subunit of the AB toxin isolated from the castor oil plant *Ricinus communis,* when linked as a fusion protein at the C-terminus of proinsulin and expressed in potato plants, was shown to significantly suppress the onset of type 1 diabetes (Carter et al. 2010; Carter et. al. 2006). Because food plants are generally devoid of pathogen associated molecular patterns (PAMPs), they are well tolerated by the inate and adaptive arms of the immune system. Their ease of genome manipulation via genetic engineering techniques, their ability to correctly modify recombinant proteins while retaining biological activity and their simplicity for oral vaccine administration makes them ideal production and delivery vehicles for mucosal vaccination (Fuchs and Gonsalves 2007; Horn, Woodard, and Howard 2004; Streatfield 2006). Further, the federal government has confirmed the safety of transgenic plants for human consumption as no human toxicity has been detected since their first appearance two decades ago (Konig et al. 2004; Flachowsky, Chesson, and Aulrich 2005). Having completed phase 3 trials, several plant synthesized pharmaceuticals have already emerged into the marketplace (Horn, Woodard, and Howard 2004). In contrast to injected vaccines that stimulate only IgG antibody production, plant based vaccines stimulate both IgA and IgG antibody biosynthesis, protecting mucosal epithelia as well as blood perfused tissues. Further, plants do not become infected with animal pathogens, and since they are delivered by the digestive tract, they eliminate needle based injuries and cross infection. In terms of stimulating immunity, heterologous plant prime-boost vaccination regimes were shown to generate high levels of antibody protection in mice (Webster et al. 2006). Important to this review, plant vaccines have also been shown to suppress autoimmune diseases (Arakawa, Chong, and Langridge 1998; von Herrath and Whitton 2000). The addition of immunomodulators to autoantigens in prime-boost regimens was shown to significantly enhance immunological suppression of autoimmunity and allergy (Ulmer, Wahren, and Liu 2006, 2006). Alternatively, virus delivered CTB::INS and CTB::GAD fusion genes expressed in primate and human cells were shown to partially suppress insulitis and hyperglycemia in NOD mice providing the option for development of virus prime-plant boost strategies for enhanced suppression of autoimmunity (Denes et al. 2005; Denes et al. 2006). Thus, in addition to providing nutrition, transgenic plant tissues can provide proteins that both suppress diabetes autoimmunity and serve as production and delivery vehicles for multi-component vaccines that can suppress autoimmunity.

3. Conclusions

A variety of bacterial and plant enterotoxin B subunit immunomodulatory molecules linked to diabetes autoantigens were shown to safely generate substantial increases in immunological tolerance in vaccinated prediabetic mice. Additional evidence from NOD mouse vaccination experiments showed that this multifactorial vaccination strategy in combination with the anti-inflammatory cytokine IL-10 is both effective and safe for durable suppression of chronic insulitis responsible for type 1 diabetes onset. Recent *ex vivo* monocyte derived DC - CTB::autoantigen fusion protein inoculation experiments showed that enhancement of immunological tolerance correlated with vaccine suppression of DC biosynthesis of co-stimulatory factors CD86, CD83 and CD80. In addition, vaccine inoculated DCs were shown to further suppress diabetes autoimmunity by down-regulating inflammatory cytokine IL-12 and IL-6 secretion and up-regulating secretion of the anti-inflammatory cytokine IL-10. In future experiments, incubation of adjuvant-autoantigen inoculated DCs with naïve Th0 lymphocytes will determine the degree to which CTB-autoantigen fusion proteins can stimulate naïve Th0 lymphocyte development into anti-inflammatory Th2 or regulatory T cells. Further, these experiments may also establish whether CTB adjuvant-autoantigen fusion proteins suppress diabetes autoimmunity by enhancing DC inhibition of autoreactive Th1 or Th17 lymphocyte development.

4. References

Afzali, B., G. Lombardi, R. I. Lechler, and G. M. Lord. 2007. The role of T helper 17 (Th17) and regulatory T cells (Treg) in human organ transplantation and autoimmune disease. *Clin Exp Immunol* 148 (1):32-46.

Akbari, O., R. H. DeKruyff, and D. T. Umetsu. 2001. Pulmonary dendritic cells producing IL-10 mediate tolerance induced by respiratory exposure to antigen. *Nat Immunol* 2 (8):725-31.

Akbari, O., G. J. Freeman, E. H. Meyer, E. A. Greenfield, T. T. Chang, A. H. Sharpe, G. Berry, R. H. DeKruyff, and D. T. Umetsu. 2002. Antigen-specific regulatory T cells develop via the ICOS-ICOS-ligand pathway and inhibit allergen-induced airway hyperreactivity. *Nat Med* 8 (9):1024-32.

Akerblom HK, Vaarala O, Hyoty H, Ilonen J, Knip M. . 2002. Environmental factors in the etiology of type 1 diabetes. *Am J Med Genet.* 115 (1):18-29.

Apostolou, I., and H. von Boehmer. 2004. In vivo instruction of suppressor commitment in naive T cells. *J Exp Med* 199 (10):1401-8.

Arakawa, T., D. K. Chong, and W. H. Langridge. 1998. Efficacy of a food plant-based oral cholera toxin B subunit vaccine. *Nat Biotechnol* 16 (3):292-7.

Arakawa, T., J. Yu, D. K. Chong, J. Hough, P. C. Engen, and W. H. Langridge. 1998. A plant-based cholera toxin B subunit-insulin fusion protein protects against the development of autoimmune diabetes. *Nat Biotechnol* 16 (10):934-8.

Aspord, C., C. Czerkinsky, A. Durand, A. Stefanutti, and C. Thivolet. 2002. alpha4 integrins and L-selectin differently orchestrate T-cell activity during diabetes prevention following oral administration of CTB-insulin. *J Autoimmun* 19 (4):223-32.

Atkinson, M. A., M. A. Bowman, L. Campbell, B. L. Darrow, D. L. Kaufman, and N. K. Maclaren. 1994. Cellular immunity to a determinant common to glutamate decarboxylase and coxsackie virus in insulin-dependent diabetes. *J Clin Invest* 94 (5):2125-9.

Bach, J. F. 2005. A Toll-like trigger for autoimmune disease. *Nat Med* 11 (2):120-1.

Baekkeskov, S., H. J. Aanstoot, S. Christgau, A. Reetz, M. Solimena, M. Cascalho, F. Folli, H. Richter-Olesen, and P. De Camilli. 1990. Identification of the 64K autoantigen in insulin-dependent diabetes as the GABA-synthesizing enzyme glutamic acid decarboxylase. *Nature* 347 (6289):151-6.

Battaglia, M., A. Stabilini, E. Draghici, B. Migliavacca, S. Gregori, E. Bonifacio, and M. G. Roncarolo. 2006. Induction of tolerance in type 1 diabetes via both CD4+CD25+ T regulatory cells and T regulatory type 1 cells. *Diabetes* 55 (6):1571-80.

Bending, D., H. De La Pena, M. Veldhoen, J. M. Phillips, C. Uyttenhove, B. Stockinger, and A. Cooke. 2009. Highly purified Th17 cells from BDC2.5NOD mice convert into Th1-like cells in NOD/SCID recipient mice. *J Clin Invest* 119 (3):565-72.

Bergerot, I., C. Ploix, J. Petersen, V. Moulin, C. Rask, N. Fabien, M. Lindblad, A. Mayer, C. Czerkinsky, J. Holmgren, and C. Thivolet. 1997. A cholera toxoid-insulin conjugate as an oral vaccine against spontaneous autoimmune diabetes. *Proc Natl Acad Sci U S A* 94 (9):4610-4.

Bitar, D. M., and C. C. Whitacre. 1988. Suppression of experimental autoimmune encephalomyelitis by the oral administration of myelin basic protein. *Cell Immunol* 112 (2):364-70.

Bluestone, J. A., and A. K. Abbas. 2003. Natural versus adaptive regulatory T cells. *Nat Rev Immunol* 3 (3):253-7.

Bresson, D., L. Togher, E. Rodrigo, Y. Chen, J. A. Bluestone, K. C. Herold, and M. von Herrath. 2006. Anti-CD3 and nasal proinsulin combination therapy enhances remission from recent-onset autoimmune diabetes by inducing Tregs. *J Clin Invest* 116 (5):1371-81.

Cardell, S. L. 2006. The natural killer T lymphocyte: a player in the complex regulation of autoimmune diabetes in non-obese diabetic mice. *Clin Exp Immunol* 143 (2):194-202.

Chaillous, L., H. Lefevre, C. Thivolet, C. Boitard, N. Lahlou, C. Atlan-Gepner, B. Bouhanick, A. Mogenet, M. Nicolino, J. C. Carel, P. Lecomte, R. Marechaud, P. Bougneres, B. Charbonnel, and P. Sai. 2000. Oral insulin administration and residual beta-cell function in recent-onset type 1 diabetes: a multicentre randomised controlled trial. Diabete Insuline Orale group. *Lancet* 356 (9229):545-9.

Cua, D. J., J. Sherlock, Y. Chen, C. A. Murphy, B. Joyce, B. Seymour, L. Lucian, W. To, S. Kwan, T. Churakova, S. Zurawski, M. Wiekowski, S. A. Lira, D. Gorman, R. A. Kastelein, and J. D. Sedgwick. 2003. Interleukin-23 rather than interleukin-12 is the critical cytokine for autoimmune inflammation of the brain. *Nature* 421 (6924):744-8.

Dai, Y. D., G. Carayanniotis, and E. Sercarz. 2005. Antigen processing by autoreactive B cells promotes determinant spreading. *Cell Mol Immunol* 2 (3):169-75.

De Smedt, T., M. Van Mechelen, G. De Becker, J. Urbain, O. Leo, and M. Moser. 1997. Effect of interleukin-10 on dendritic cell maturation and function. *Eur J Immunol* 27 (5):1229-35.

de Waal Malefyt, R., J. Abrams, B. Bennett, C. G. Figdor, and J. E. de Vries. 1991. Interleukin 10(IL-10) inhibits cytokine synthesis by human monocytes: an autoregulatory role of IL-10 produced by monocytes. *J Exp Med* 174 (5):1209-20.

Delovitch, T. L., and B. Singh. 1997. The nonobese diabetic mouse as a model of autoimmune diabetes: immune dysregulation gets the NOD. *Immunity* 7 (6):727-38.

Denes, B., I. Fodor, and W. H. Langridge. 2010. Autoantigens plus interleukin-10 suppress diabetes autoimmunity. *Diabetes Technol Ther* 12 (8):649-61.

Denes, B., V. Krausova, N. Fodor, T. Timiryasova, D. Henderson, J. Hough, J. Yu, I. Fodor, and W. H. Langridge. 2005. Protection of NOD mice from type 1 diabetes after oral inoculation with vaccinia viruses expressing adjuvanted islet autoantigens. *J Immunother* 28 (5):438-48.

Denes, B., J. Yu, N. Fodor, Z. Takatsy, I. Fodor, and W. H. Langridge. 2006. Suppression of hyperglycemia in NOD mice after inoculation with recombinant vaccinia viruses. *Mol Biotechnol* 34 (3):317-27.

Devaraj, S., A. T. Cheung, I. Jialal, S. C. Griffen, D. Nguyen, N. Glaser, and T. Aoki. 2007. Evidence of increased inflammation and microcirculatory abnormalities in patients with type 1 diabetes and their role in microvascular complications. *Diabetes* 56 (11):2790-6.

Di Lorenzo, T. P., M. Peakman, and B. O. Roep. 2007. Translational mini-review series on type 1 diabetes: Systematic analysis of T cell epitopes in autoimmune diabetes. *Clin Exp Immunol* 148 (1):1-16.

Donnelly, R. P., H. Dickensheets, and D. S. Finbloom. 1999. The interleukin-10 signal transduction pathway and regulation of gene expression in mononuclear phagocytes. *J Interferon Cytokine Res* 19 (6):563-73.

Duerr, R. H., K. D. Taylor, S. R. Brant, J. D. Rioux, M. S. Silverberg, M. J. Daly, A. H. Steinhart, C. Abraham, M. Regueiro, A. Griffiths, T. Dassopoulos, A. Bitton, H. Yang, S. Targan, L. W. Datta, E. O. Kistner, L. P. Schumm, A. T. Lee, P. K. Gregersen, M. M. Barmada, J. I. Rotter, D. L. Nicolae, and J. H. Cho. 2006. A genome-wide association study identifies IL23R as an inflammatory bowel disease gene. *Science* 314 (5804):1461-3.

Ehrenstein, M. R., J. G. Evans, A. Singh, S. Moore, G. Warnes, D. A. Isenberg, and C. Mauri. 2004. Compromised function of regulatory T cells in rheumatoid arthritis and reversal by anti-TNFalpha therapy. *J Exp Med* 200 (3):277-85.

Elliott, J. F., H. Y. Qin, S. Bhatti, D. K. Smith, R. K. Singh, T. Dillon, J. Lauzon, and B. Singh. 1994. Immunization with the larger isoform of mouse glutamic acid decarboxylase (GAD67) prevents autoimmune diabetes in NOD mice. *Diabetes* 43 (12):1494-9.

Enk, A. H. 2005. Dendritic cells in tolerance induction. *Immunol Lett* 99 (1):8-11.

Eriksson, K., and J. Holmgren. 2002. Recent advances in mucosal vaccines and adjuvants. *Curr Opin Immunol* 14 (5):666-72.

Ferwerda, G., S. E. Girardin, B. J. Kullberg, L. Le Bourhis, D. J. de Jong, D. M. Langenberg, R. van Crevel, G. J. Adema, T. H. Ottenhoff, J. W. Van der Meer, and M. G. Netea. 2005. NOD2 and toll-like receptors are nonredundant recognition systems of Mycobacterium tuberculosis. *PLoS Pathog* 1 (3):279-85.

Filippi, C., D. Bresson, and M. von Herrath. 2005. Antigen-specific induction of regulatory T cells for type 1 diabetes therapy. *Int Rev Immunol* 24 (5-6):341-60.

Flachowsky, G., A. Chesson, and K. Aulrich. 2005. Animal nutrition with feeds from genetically modified plants. *Arch Anim Nutr* 59 (1):1-40.

Fontenot, J. D., M. A. Gavin, and A. Y. Rudensky. 2003. Foxp3 programs the development and function of CD4+CD25+ regulatory T cells. *Nat Immunol* 4 (4):330-6.

Fuchs, M., and D. Gonsalves. 2007. Safety of virus-resistant transgenic plants two decades after their introduction: lessons from realistic field risk assessment studies. *Annu Rev Phytopathol* 45:173-202.

Gale, E. A. 2002. The rise of childhood type 1 diabetes in the 20th century. *Diabetes* 51 (12):3353-61.

George-Chandy, A., K. Eriksson, M. Lebens, I. Nordstrom, E. Schon, and J. Holmgren. 2001. Cholera toxin B subunit as a carrier molecule promotes antigen presentation and increases CD40 and CD86 expression on antigen-presenting cells. *Infect Immun* 69 (9):5716-25.

Goudy, K. S., B. R. Burkhardt, C. Wasserfall, S. Song, M. L. Campbell-Thompson, T. Brusko, M. A. Powers, M. J. Clare-Salzler, E. S. Sobel, T. M. Ellis, T. R. Flotte, and M. A. Atkinson. 2003. Systemic overexpression of IL-10 induces CD4+CD25+ cell populations in vivo and ameliorates type 1 diabetes in nonobese diabetic mice in a dose-dependent fashion. *J Immunol* 171 (5):2270-8.

Goudy, K., S. Song, C. Wasserfall, Y. C. Zhang, M. Kapturczak, A. Muir, M. Powers, M. Scott-Jorgensen, M. Campbell-Thompson, J. M. Crawford, T. M. Ellis, T. R. Flotte, and M. A. Atkinson. 2001. Adeno-associated virus vector-mediated IL-10 gene delivery prevents type 1 diabetes in NOD mice. *Proc Natl Acad Sci U S A* 98 (24):13913-8.

Groux, H., F. Cottrez, M. Rouleau, S. Mauze, S. Antonenko, S. Hurst, T. McNeil, M. Bigler, M. G. Roncarolo, and R. L. Coffman. 1999. A transgenic model to analyze the immunoregulatory role of IL-10 secreted by antigen-presenting cells. *J Immunol* 162 (3):1723-9.

Grutz, G. 2005. New insights into the molecular mechanism of interleukin-10-mediated immunosuppression. *J Leukoc Biol* 77 (1):3-15.

Hajishengallis, G., S. Arce, C. M. Gockel, T. D. Connell, and M. W. Russell. 2005. Immunomodulation with enterotoxins for the generation of secretory immunity or tolerance: applications for oral infections. *J Dent Res* 84 (12):1104-16.

Han, B., P. Serra, J. Yamanouchi, A. Amrani, J. F. Elliott, P. Dickie, T. P. Dilorenzo, and P. Santamaria. 2005. Developmental control of CD8 T cell-avidity maturation in autoimmune diabetes. *J Clin Invest* 115 (7):1879-87.

Harizi, H., and N. Gualde. 2006. Pivotal role of PGE2 and IL-10 in the cross-regulation of dendritic cell-derived inflammatory mediators. *Cell Mol Immunol* 3 (4):271-7.

Haverkos, H. W., N. Battula, D. P. Drotman, and O. M. Rennert. 2003. Enteroviruses and type 1 diabetes mellitus. *Biomed Pharmacother* 57 (9):379-85.

Higgins, P. J., and H. L. Weiner. 1988. Suppression of experimental autoimmune encephalomyelitis by oral administration of myelin basic protein and its fragments. *J Immunol* 140 (2):440-5.

Holmgren, J., and C. Czerkinsky. 2005. Mucosal immunity and vaccines. *Nat Med* 11 (4 Suppl):S45-53.

Holmgren, J., C. Czerkinsky, N. Lycke, and A. M. Svennerholm. 1994. Strategies for the induction of immune responses at mucosal surfaces making use of cholera toxin B subunit as immunogen, carrier, and adjuvant. *Am J Trop Med Hyg* 50 (5 Suppl):42-54.

Hommann, M., U. Schotte, K. K. Richter, U. Moller, R. Basciani, and J. Scheele. 2001. [HELLP Syndrome as an indication for liver transplantation]. *Gynakol Geburtshilfliche Rundsch* 41 (1):8-11.

Hori, S., T. Nomura, and S. Sakaguchi. 2003. Control of regulatory T cell development by the transcription factor Foxp3. *Science* 299 (5609):1057-61.

Hori, S., and S. Sakaguchi. 2004. Foxp3: a critical regulator of the development and function of regulatory T cells. *Microbes Infect* 6 (8):745-51.

Horn, M. E., S. L. Woodard, and J. A. Howard. 2004. Plant molecular farming: systems and products. *Plant Cell Rep* 22 (10):711-20.

Huang, J. B., Y. Takeda, Y. Araki, F. Sendo, and H. R. Petty. 2004. Molecular proximity of complement receptor type 3 (CR3) and the glycosylphosphatidylinositol-linked protein GPI-80 on neutrophils: effects of cell adherence, exogenous saccharides, and lipid raft disrupting agents. *Mol Immunol* 40 (17):1249-56.

Hutchings, P., and A. Cooke. 1998. Protection from insulin dependent diabetes mellitus afforded by insulin antigens in incomplete Freund's adjuvant depends on route of administration. *J Autoimmun* 11 (2):127-30.

International, Juvenile Diabetes Research Foundation, ed. 2005. *KRC Research for JDRF*. New York.

Itano, A. A., S. J. McSorley, R. L. Reinhardt, B. D. Ehst, E. Ingulli, A. Y. Rudensky, and M. K. Jenkins. 2003. Distinct dendritic cell populations sequentially present antigen to CD4 T cells and stimulate different aspects of cell-mediated immunity. *Immunity* 19 (1):47-57.

Iwasaki, A., and B. L. Kelsall. 2000. Localization of distinct Peyer's patch dendritic cell subsets and their recruitment by chemokines macrophage inflammatory protein (MIP)-3alpha, MIP-3beta, and secondary lymphoid organ chemokine. *J Exp Med* 191 (8):1381-94.

Jaeckel, E., L. Klein, N. Martin-Orozco, and H. von Boehmer. 2003. Normal incidence of diabetes in NOD mice tolerant to glutamic acid decarboxylase. *J Exp Med* 197 (12):1635-44.

Jaeckel, E., M. A. Lipes, and H. von Boehmer. 2004. Recessive tolerance to preproinsulin 2 reduces but does not abolish type 1 diabetes. *Nat Immunol* 5 (10):1028-35.

Jun, H. S., Y. H. Chung, J. Han, A. Kim, S. S. Yoo, R. S. Sherwin, and J. W. Yoon. 2002. Prevention of autoimmune diabetes by immunogene therapy using recombinant vaccinia virus expressing glutamic acid decarboxylase. *Diabetologia* 45 (5):668-76.

Jun, H. S., L. Y. Khil, and J. W. Yoon. 2002. Role of glutamic acid decarboxylase in the pathogenesis of type 1 diabetes. *Cell Mol Life Sci* 59 (11):1892-901.

Jun, H. S., and J. W. Yoon. 2001. The role of viruses in type I diabetes: two distinct cellular and molecular pathogenic mechanisms of virus-induced diabetes in animals. *Diabetologia* 44 (3):271-85.

Kaisho, T., and S. Akira. 2002. Toll-like receptors as adjuvant receptors. *Biochim Biophys Acta* 1589 (1):1-13.

Kanneganti, T. D., M. Lamkanfi, Y. G. Kim, G. Chen, J. H. Park, L. Franchi, P. Vandenabeele, and G. Nunez. 2007. Pannexin-1-mediated recognition of bacterial molecules activates the cryopyrin inflammasome independent of Toll-like receptor signaling. *Immunity* 26 (4):433-43.

Kelsen, J., C. L. Hvas, J. Agnholt, and J. F. Dahlerup. 2006. [CD4 + CD25 + regulatory T cells and their importance to human illnesses]. *Ugeskr Laeger* 168 (1):32-7.

Kent, S. C., Y. Chen, L. Bregoli, S. M. Clemmings, N. S. Kenyon, C. Ricordi, B. J. Hering, and D. A. Hafler. 2005. Expanded T cells from pancreatic lymph nodes of type 1 diabetic subjects recognize an insulin epitope. *Nature* 435 (7039):224-8.

Kim, J. J., J. S. Yang, L. K. Nottingham, W. Tang, K. Dang, K. H. Manson, M. S. Wyand, D. M. Wilson, and D. B. Weiner. 2001. Induction of immune responses and safety profiles in rhesus macaques immunized with a DNA vaccine expressing human prostate specific antigen. *Oncogene* 20 (33):4497-506.

King, C., J. Davies, R. Mueller, M. S. Lee, T. Krahl, B. Yeung, E. O'Connor, and N. Sarvetnick. 1998. TGF-beta1 alters APC preference, polarizing islet antigen responses toward a Th2 phenotype. *Immunity* 8 (5):601-13.

Kobayashi, T., S. Tanaka, N. Harii, K. Aida, H. Shimura, M. Ohmori, M. Kanesige, A. Shimada, and T. Maruyama. 2006. Immunopathological and genetic features in slowly progressive insulin-dependent diabetes mellitus and latent autoimmune diabetes in adults. *Ann N Y Acad Sci* 1079:60-6.

Kojo, S., K. Seino, M. Harada, H. Watarai, H. Wakao, T. Uchida, T. Nakayama, and M. Taniguchi. 2005. Induction of regulatory properties in dendritic cells by Valpha14 NKT cells. *J Immunol* 175 (6):3648-55.

Konig, A., A. Cockburn, R. W. Crevel, E. Debruyne, R. Grafstroem, U. Hammerling, I. Kimber, I. Knudsen, H. A. Kuiper, A. A. Peijnenburg, A. H. Penninks, M. Poulsen, M. Schauzu, and J. M. Wal. 2004. Assessment of the safety of foods derived from genetically modified (GM) crops. *Food Chem Toxicol* 42 (7):1047-88.

Kretschmer, K., I. Apostolou, D. Hawiger, K. Khazaie, M. C. Nussenzweig, and H. von Boehmer. 2005. Inducing and expanding regulatory T cell populations by foreign antigen. *Nat Immunol* 6 (12):1219-27.

Langrish, C. L., Y. Chen, W. M. Blumenschein, J. Mattson, B. Basham, J. D. Sedgwick, T. McClanahan, R. A. Kastelein, and D. J. Cua. 2005. IL-23 drives a pathogenic T cell population that induces autoimmune inflammation. *J Exp Med* 201 (2):233-40.

Lavelle, E. C., E. McNeela, M. E. Armstrong, O. Leavy, S. C. Higgins, and K. H. Mills. 2003. Cholera toxin promotes the induction of regulatory T cells specific for bystander antigens by modulating dendritic cell activation. *J Immunol* 171 (5):2384-92.

Leceta, J., R. P. Gomariz, C. Martinez, C. Abad, D. Ganea, and M. Delgado. 2000. Receptors and transcriptional factors involved in the anti-inflammatory activity of VIP and PACAP. *Ann N Y Acad Sci* 921:92-102.

Levings, M. K., S. Gregori, E. Tresoldi, S. Cazzaniga, C. Bonini, and M. G. Roncarolo. 2005. Differentiation of Tr1 cells by immature dendritic cells requires IL-10 but not CD25+CD4+ Tr cells. *Blood* 105 (3):1162-9.

Li, T. K., and B. S. Fox. 1996. Cholera toxin B subunit binding to an antigen-presenting cell directly co-stimulates cytokine production from a T cell clone. *Int Immunol* 8 (12):1849-56.

Li, Y. Y., Y. Yang, M. Bao, C. K. Edwards, 3rd, and J. R. Parnes. 2006. Mouse splenic B lymphocyte activation using different activation stimuli induces in vitro splicing of tumor necrosis factor-alpha nuclear pre-mRNA. *Mol Immunol* 43 (6):613-22.

Libby, P., D. M. Nathan, K. Abraham, J. D. Brunzell, J. E. Fradkin, S. M. Haffner, W. Hsueh, M. Rewers, B. T. Roberts, P. J. Savage, S. Skarlatos, M. Wassef, and C. Rabadan-Diehl. 2005. Report of the National Heart, Lung, and Blood Institute-National Institute of Diabetes and Digestive and Kidney Diseases Working Group on Cardiovascular Complications of Type 1 Diabetes Mellitus. *Circulation* 111 (25):3489-93.

Lindley, S., C. M. Dayan, A. Bishop, B. O. Roep, M. Peakman, and T. I. Tree. 2005. Defective suppressor function in CD4(+)CD25(+) T-cells from patients with type 1 diabetes. *Diabetes* 54 (1):92-9.

Liu, L., Z. Xu, R. C. Fuhlbrigge, V. Pena-Cruz, J. Lieberman, and T. S. Kupper. 2005. Vaccinia virus induces strong immunoregulatory cytokine production in healthy human epidermal keratinocytes: a novel strategy for immune evasion. *J Virol* 79 (12):7363-70.

Liu, Z., K. Geboes, P. Hellings, P. Maerten, H. Heremans, P. Vandenberghe, L. Boon, P. van Kooten, P. Rutgeerts, and J. L. Ceuppens. 2001. B7 interactions with CD28 and CTLA-4 control tolerance or induction of mucosal inflammation in chronic experimental colitis. *J Immunol* 167 (3):1830-8.

Lodinova-Zadnikova, R., L. Prokesova, H. Tlaskalova, I. Kocourkova, J. Zizka, and Z. Stranak. 2004. [Influence of oral colonization with probiotic E. coli strain after birth on frequency of recurrent infections, allergy and development of some immunologic parameters. Long-term studies]. *Ceska Gynekol* 69 Suppl 1:91-7.

Lutz, M. B., and G. Schuler. 2002. Immature, semi-mature and fully mature dendritic cells: which signals induce tolerance or immunity? *Trends Immunol* 23 (9):445-9.

Lycke, N. 2004. ADP-ribosylating bacterial enzymes for the targeted control of mucosal tolerance and immunity. *Ann N Y Acad Sci* 1029:193-208.

Maioli, M., L. Puddu, and G. M. Pes. 2006. [Latent autoimmune diabetes in adults]. *Clin Ter* 157 (1):69-78.

Makino, S., K. Kunimoto, Y. Muraoka, Y. Mizushima, K. Katagiri, and Y. Tochino. 1980. Breeding of a non-obese, diabetic strain of mice. *Jikken Dobutsu* 29 (1):1-13.

Marinaro, M., H. F. Staats, T. Hiroi, R. J. Jackson, M. Coste, P. N. Boyaka, N. Okahashi, M. Yamamoto, H. Kiyono, H. Bluethmann, K. Fujihashi, and J. R. McGhee. 1995. Mucosal adjuvant effect of cholera toxin in mice results from induction of T helper 2 (Th2) cells and IL-4. *J Immunol* 155 (10):4621-9.

MartIn-Fontecha, A., S. Sebastiani, U. E. Hopken, M. Uguccioni, M. Lipp, A. Lanzavecchia, and F. Sallusto. 2003. Regulation of dendritic cell migration to the draining lymph node: impact on T lymphocyte traffic and priming. *J Exp Med* 198 (4):615-21.

Mastrangelo, M. J., H. C. Maguire, Jr., L. C. Eisenlohr, C. E. Laughlin, C. E. Monken, P. A. McCue, A. J. Kovatich, and E. C. Lattime. 1999. Intratumoral recombinant GM-CSF-encoding virus as gene therapy in patients with cutaneous melanoma. *Cancer Gene Ther* 6 (5):409-22.

Mensah-Brown, E. P., A. Shahin, M. Al-Shamisi, X. Wei, and M. L. Lukic. 2006. IL-23 leads to diabetes induction after subdiabetogenic treatment with multiple low doses of streptozotocin. *Eur J Immunol* 36 (1):216-23.

Mensah-Brown, E. P., A. Shahin, M. Al-Shamsi, and M. L. Lukic. 2006. New members of the interleukin-12 family of cytokines: IL-23 and IL-27 modulate autoimmune diabetes. *Ann N Y Acad Sci* 1079:157-60.

Millington, O. R., A. M. Mowat, and P. Garside. 2004. Induction of bystander suppression by feeding antigen occurs despite normal clonal expansion of the bystander T cell population. *J Immunol* 173 (10):6059-64.

Minderhoud, I. M., M. Samsom, and B. Oldenburg. 2007. Crohn's disease, fatigue, and infliximab: is there a role for cytokines in the pathogenesis of fatigue? *World J Gastroenterol* 13 (14):2089-93.

———. 2007. What predicts mucosal inflammation in Crohn's disease patients? *Inflamm Bowel Dis* 13 (12):1567-72.

Misra, N., J. Bayry, S. Lacroix-Desmazes, M. D. Kazatchkine, and S. V. Kaveri. 2004. Cutting edge: human CD4+CD25+ T cells restrain the maturation and antigen-presenting function of dendritic cells. *J Immunol* 172 (8):4676-80.

Moore, K. W., A. O'Garra, R. de Waal Malefyt, P. Vieira, and T. R. Mosmann. 1993. Interleukin-10. *Annu Rev Immunol* 11:165-90.

Moore, K. W., P. Vieira, D. F. Fiorentino, M. L. Trounstine, T. A. Khan, and T. R. Mosmann. 1990. Homology of cytokine synthesis inhibitory factor (IL-10) to the Epstein-Barr virus gene BCRFI. *Science* 248 (4960):1230-4.

Mordes, J. P., D. L. Guberski, J. H. Leif, B. A. Woda, J. F. Flanagan, D. L. Greiner, E. H. Kislauskis, and R. S. Tirabassi. 2005. LEW.1WR1 rats develop autoimmune diabetes spontaneously and in response to environmental perturbation. *Diabetes* 54 (9):2727-33.

Moss, B. 1991. Vaccinia virus: a tool for research and vaccine development. *Science* 252 (5013):1662-7.

———. 1996. Genetically engineered poxviruses for recombinant gene expression, vaccination, and safety. *Proc Natl Acad Sci U S A* 93 (21):11341-8.

Mostarica-Stojkovic, M. 2005. [Mechanisms of the induction of autoimmunity]. *Srp Arh Celok Lek* 133 Suppl 1:9-15.

Murphy, C. A., C. L. Langrish, Y. Chen, W. Blumenschein, T. McClanahan, R. A. Kastelein, J. D. Sedgwick, and D. J. Cua. 2003. Divergent pro- and antiinflammatory roles for IL-23 and IL-12 in joint autoimmune inflammation. *J Exp Med* 198 (12):1951-7.

Nakae, S., A. Nambu, K. Sudo, and Y. Iwakura. 2003. Suppression of immune induction of collagen-induced arthritis in IL-17-deficient mice. *J Immunol* 171 (11):6173-7.

Nakayama, M., N. Abiru, H. Moriyama, N. Babaya, E. Liu, D. Miao, L. Yu, D. R. Wegmann, J. C. Hutton, J. F. Elliott, and G. S. Eisenbarth. 2005. Prime role for an insulin epitope in the development of type 1 diabetes in NOD mice. *Nature* 435 (7039):220-3.

Nocentini, G., and C. Riccardi. 2005. GITR: a multifaceted regulator of immunity belonging to the tumor necrosis factor receptor superfamily. *Eur J Immunol* 35 (4):1016-22.

Oderup, C., L. Cederbom, A. Makowska, C. M. Cilio, and F. Ivars. 2006. Cytotoxic T lymphocyte antigen-4-dependent down-modulation of costimulatory molecules on dendritic cells in CD4+ CD25+ regulatory T-cell-mediated suppression. *Immunology* 118 (2):240-9.

Odumosu, O., K. Payne, I. Baez, J. Jutzy, N. Wall, and W. Langridge. 2010. Suppression of dendritic cell activation by diabetes autoantigens linked to the cholera toxin B subunit. *Immunobiology.*

Okusawa, T., M. Fujita, J. Nakamura, T. Into, M. Yasuda, A. Yoshimura, Y. Hara, A. Hasebe, D. T. Golenbock, M. Morita, Y. Kuroki, T. Ogawa, and K. Shibata. 2004. Relationship between structures and biological activities of mycoplasmal diacylated lipopeptides and their recognition by toll-like receptors 2 and 6. *Infect Immun* 72 (3):1657-65.

Onengut-Gumuscu, S., and P. Concannon. 2002. Mapping genes for autoimmunity in humans: type 1 diabetes as a model. *Immunol Rev* 190:182-94.

Otteken, A., P. L. Earl, and B. Moss. 1996. Folding, assembly, and intracellular trafficking of the human immunodeficiency virus type 1 envelope glycoprotein analyzed with monoclonal antibodies recognizing maturational intermediates. *J Virol* 70 (6):3407-15.

Palmer, J. P., C. M. Asplin, P. Clemons, K. Lyen, O. Tatpati, P. K. Raghu, and T. L. Paquette. 1983. Insulin antibodies in insulin-dependent diabetics before insulin treatment. *Science* 222 (4630):1337-9.

Phipps, P. A., M. R. Stanford, J. B. Sun, B. G. Xiao, J. Holmgren, T. Shinnick, A. Hasan, Y. Mizushima, and T. Lehner. 2003. Prevention of mucosally induced uveitis with a HSP60-derived peptide linked to cholera toxin B subunit. *Eur J Immunol* 33 (1):224-32.

Pulendran, B., P. Kumar, C. W. Cutler, M. Mohamadzadeh, T. Van Dyke, and J. Banchereau. 2001. Lipopolysaccharides from distinct pathogens induce different classes of immune responses in vivo. *J Immunol* 167 (9):5067-76.

Pulendran, B., J. L. Smith, G. Caspary, K. Brasel, D. Pettit, E. Maraskovsky, and C. R. Maliszewski. 1999. Distinct dendritic cell subsets differentially regulate the class of immune response in vivo. *Proc Natl Acad Sci U S A* 96 (3):1036-41.

Qin, H., C. A. Wilson, K. L. Roberts, B. J. Baker, X. Zhao, and E. N. Benveniste. 2006. IL-10 inhibits lipopolysaccharide-induced CD40 gene expression through induction of suppressor of cytokine signaling-3. *J Immunol* 177 (11):7761-71.

Qin, H. Y., M. W. Sadelain, C. Hitchon, J. Lauzon, and B. Singh. 1993. Complete Freund's adjuvant-induced T cells prevent the development and adoptive transfer of diabetes in nonobese diabetic mice. *J Immunol* 150 (5):2072-80.

Rastellini, C., L. Lu, C. Ricordi, T. E. Starzl, A. S. Rao, and A. W. Thomson. 1995. Granulocyte/macrophage colony-stimulating factor-stimulated hepatic dendritic cell progenitors prolong pancreatic islet allograft survival. *Transplantation* 60 (11):1366-70.

Rewers, M., J. M. Norris, G. S. Eisenbarth, H. A. Erlich, B. Beaty, G. Klingensmith, M. Hoffman, L. Yu, T. L. Bugawan, A. Blair, R. F. Hamman, M. Groshek, and R. S. McDuffie, Jr. 1996. Beta-cell autoantibodies in infants and toddlers without IDDM relatives: diabetes autoimmunity study in the young (DAISY). *J Autoimmun* 9 (3):405-10.

Rissoan, M. C., V. Soumelis, N. Kadowaki, G. Grouard, F. Briere, R. de Waal Malefyt, and Y. J. Liu. 1999. Reciprocal control of T helper cell and dendritic cell differentiation. *Science* 283 (5405):1183-6.

Robinson, B. W., S. A. Mukherjee, A. Davidson, S. Morey, A. W. Musk, I. Ramshaw, D. Smith, R. Lake, T. Haenel, M. Garlepp, J. Marley, C. Leong, I. Caminschi, and B. Scott. 1998. Cytokine gene therapy or infusion as treatment for solid human cancer. *J Immunother* 21 (3):211-7.

Robinson, C. P., J. Cornelius, D. E. Bounous, H. Yamamoto, M. G. Humphreys-Beher, and A. B. Peck. 1998. Characterization of the changing lymphocyte populations and cytokine expression in the exocrine tissues of autoimmune NOD mice. *Autoimmunity* 27 (1):29-44.

Romagnani, S. 1998. The Th1/Th2 paradigm and allergic disorders. *Allergy* 53 (46 Suppl):12-5.

Romagnani, S., M. Kapsenberg, A. Radbruch, and L. Adorini. 1998. Th1 and Th2 cells. *Res Immunol* 149 (9):871-3.

Roncarolo, M. G., R. Bacchetta, C. Bordignon, S. Narula, and M. K. Levings. 2001. Type 1 T regulatory cells. *Immunol Rev* 182:68-79.

Sakaguchi, S. 2005. Naturally arising Foxp3-expressing CD25+CD4+ regulatory T cells in immunological tolerance to self and non-self. *Nat Immunol* 6 (4):345-52.

Sakaguchi, S., and N. Sakaguchi. 2005. Regulatory T cells in immunologic self-tolerance and autoimmune disease. *Int Rev Immunol* 24 (3-4):211-26.

Sakaguchi, S., N. Sakaguchi, M. Asano, M. Itoh, and M. Toda. 1995. Immunologic self-tolerance maintained by activated T cells expressing IL-2 receptor alpha-chains (CD25). Breakdown of a single mechanism of self-tolerance causes various autoimmune diseases. *J Immunol* 155 (3):1151-64.

Schwimmbeck, P. L., T. Dyrberg, and M. B. Oldstone. 1988. Abrogation of diabetes in BB rats by acute virus infection. Association of viral-lymphocyte interactions. *J Immunol* 140 (10):3394-400.

Sela, M. 2006. Immunomodulatory vaccines against autoimmune diseases. *Rejuvenation Res* 9 (1):126-33.

Seong, S. Y., and P. Matzinger. 2004. Hydrophobicity: an ancient damage-associated molecular pattern that initiates innate immune responses. *Nat Rev Immunol* 4 (6):469-78.

Seyfert-Margolis, V., T. D. Gisler, A. L. Asare, R. S. Wang, H. M. Dosch, B. Brooks-Worrell, G. S. Eisenbarth, J. P. Palmer, C. J. Greenbaum, S. E. Gitelman, G. T. Nepom, J. A. Bluestone, and K. C. Herold. 2006. Analysis of T-cell assays to measure autoimmune responses in subjects with type 1 diabetes: results of a blinded controlled study. *Diabetes* 55 (9):2588-94.

Shen, X., and K. E. Bornfeldt. 2007. Mouse models for studies of cardiovascular complications of type 1 diabetes. *Ann N Y Acad Sci* 1103:202-17.

Shinomiya, M., S. M. Fazle Akbar, H. Shinomiya, and M. Onji. 1999. Transfer of dendritic cells (DC) ex vivo stimulated with interferon-gamma (IFN-gamma) down-modulates autoimmune diabetes in non-obese diabetic (NOD) mice. *Clin Exp Immunol* 117 (1):38-43.

Shreedhar, V. K., B. L. Kelsall, and M. R. Neutra. 2003. Cholera toxin induces migration of dendritic cells from the subepithelial dome region to T- and B-cell areas of Peyer's patches. *Infect Immun* 71 (1):504-9.

Sica, A., A. Saccani, B. Bottazzi, N. Polentarutti, A. Vecchi, J. van Damme, and A. Mantovani. 2000. Autocrine production of IL-10 mediates defective IL-12 production and NF-kappa B activation in tumor-associated macrophages. *J Immunol* 164 (2):762-7.

Silveira, P. A., and S. T. Grey. 2006. B cells in the spotlight: innocent bystanders or major players in the pathogenesis of type 1 diabetes. *Trends Endocrinol Metab* 17 (4):128-35.

Slavin, A. J., R. Maron, and H. L. Weiner. 2001. Mucosal administration of IL-10 enhances oral tolerance in autoimmune encephalomyelitis and diabetes. *Int Immunol* 13 (6):825-33.

Song, F., I. E. Gienapp, T. Shawler, Z. Guan, and C. C. Whitacre. 2004. The thymus plays a role in oral tolerance induction in experimental autoimmune encephalomyelitis. *Ann N Y Acad Sci* 1029:402-4.

Stassen, M., S. Fondel, T. Bopp, C. Richter, C. Muller, J. Kubach, C. Becker, J. Knop, A. H. Enk, S. Schmitt, E. Schmitt, and H. Jonuleit. 2004. Human CD25+ regulatory T cells: two subsets defined by the integrins alpha 4 beta 7 or alpha 4 beta 1 confer distinct suppressive properties upon CD4+ T helper cells. *Eur J Immunol* 34 (5):1303-11.

Stassen, M., E. Schmitt, and H. Jonuleit. 2004. Human CD(4+)CD(25+) regulatory T cells and infectious tolerance. *Transplantation* 77 (1 Suppl):S23-5.

Steinbrink, K., M. Wolfl, H. Jonuleit, J. Knop, and A. H. Enk. 1997. Induction of tolerance by IL-10-treated dendritic cells. *J Immunol* 159 (10):4772-80.

Steinman, R. M., and M. Pope. 2002. Exploiting dendritic cells to improve vaccine efficacy. *J Clin Invest* 109 (12):1519-26.

Stock, P., O. Akbari, G. Berry, G. J. Freeman, R. H. Dekruyff, and D. T. Umetsu. 2004. Induction of T helper type 1-like regulatory cells that express Foxp3 and protect against airway hyper-reactivity. *Nat Immunol* 5 (11):1149-56.

Streatfield, S. J. 2006. Mucosal immunization using recombinant plant-based oral vaccines. *Methods* 38 (2):150-7.

Sun, J. B., J. Holmgren, and C. Czerkinsky. 1994. Cholera toxin B subunit: an efficient transmucosal carrier-delivery system for induction of peripheral immunological tolerance. *Proc Natl Acad Sci U S A* 91 (23):10795-9.

Sun, J. B., C. Rask, T. Olsson, J. Holmgren, and C. Czerkinsky. 1996. Treatment of experimental autoimmune encephalomyelitis by feeding myelin basic protein conjugated to cholera toxin B subunit. *Proc Natl Acad Sci U S A* 93 (14):7196-201.

Sun, J. B., B. G. Xiao, M. Lindblad, B. L. Li, H. Link, C. Czerkinsky, and J. Holmgren. 2000. Oral administration of cholera toxin B subunit conjugated to myelin basic protein protects against experimental autoimmune encephalomyelitis by inducing transforming growth factor-beta-secreting cells and suppressing chemokine expression. *Int Immunol* 12 (10):1449-57.

Sutmuller, R. P., M. E. Morgan, M. G. Netea, O. Grauer, and G. J. Adema. 2006. Toll-like receptors on regulatory T cells: expanding immune regulation. *Trends Immunol* 27 (8):387-93.

Taams, L. S., and A. N. Akbar. 2005. Peripheral generation and function of CD4+CD25+ regulatory T cells. *Curr Top Microbiol Immunol* 293:115-31.

Takeda, K., T. Kaisho, and S. Akira. 2003. Toll-like receptors. *Annu Rev Immunol* 21:335-76.

Tang, Q., J. Y. Adams, A. J. Tooley, M. Bi, B. T. Fife, P. Serra, P. Santamaria, R. M. Locksley, M. F. Krummel, and J. A. Bluestone. 2006. Visualizing regulatory T cell control of autoimmune responses in nonobese diabetic mice. *Nat Immunol* 7 (1):83-92.

Tarbell, K. V., S. Yamazaki, K. Olson, P. Toy, and R. M. Steinman. 2004. CD25+ CD4+ T cells, expanded with dendritic cells presenting a single autoantigenic peptide, suppress autoimmune diabetes. *J Exp Med* 199 (11):1467-77.

Tatersall R. B., and Pyke, D.A. . 1972. Diabetes in identical twins. *Lancet* 2 (7787):1120-1125.

Thompson, H. S., and N. A. Staines. 1986. Gastric administration of type II collagen delays the onset and severity of collagen-induced arthritis in rats. *Clin Exp Immunol* 64 (3):581-6.

Tian, J., D. Zekzer, Y. Lu, H. Dang, and D. L. Kaufman. 2006. B cells are crucial for determinant spreading of T cell autoimmunity among beta cell antigens in diabetes-prone nonobese diabetic mice. *J Immunol* 176 (4):2654-61.

Tisch, R., and H. McDevitt. 1996. Insulin-dependent diabetes mellitus. *Cell* 85 (3):291-7.

Tracy, S., and K. M. Drescher. 2007. Coxsackievirus infections and NOD mice: relevant models of protection from, and induction of, type 1 diabetes. *Ann N Y Acad Sci* 1103:143-51.

Trembleau, S., T. Germann, M. K. Gately, and L. Adorini. 1995. The role of IL-12 in the induction of organ-specific autoimmune diseases. *Immunol Today* 16 (8):383-6.

Tritt, M., E. Sgouroudis, E. d'Hennezel, A. Albanese, and C. A. Piccirillo. 2008. Functional waning of naturally occurring CD4+ regulatory T-cells contributes to the onset of autoimmune diabetes. *Diabetes* 57 (1):113-23.

Ulmer, J. B., B. Wahren, and M. A. Liu. 2006. DNA vaccines: recent technological and clinical advances. *Discov Med* 6 (33):109-12.

———. 2006. Gene-based vaccines: recent technical and clinical advances. *Trends Mol Med* 12 (5):216-22.

Veldhoen, M., R. J. Hocking, C. J. Atkins, R. M. Locksley, and B. Stockinger. 2006. TGFbeta in the context of an inflammatory cytokine milieu supports de novo differentiation of IL-17-producing T cells. *Immunity* 24 (2):179-89.

Vendrame, F., A. Zappaterreno, and F. Dotta. 2004. Markers of beta cell function in type 1 diabetes mellitus. *Minerva Med* 95 (2):79-84.

Viglietta, V., C. Baecher-Allan, H. L. Weiner, and D. A. Hafler. 2004. Loss of functional suppression by CD4+CD25+ regulatory T cells in patients with multiple sclerosis. *J Exp Med* 199 (7):971-9.

Vigouroux, S., E. Yvon, E. Biagi, and M. K. Brenner. 2004. Antigen-induced regulatory T cells. *Blood* 104 (1):26-33.

von Herrath, M. G., and J. L. Whitton. 2000. DNA vaccination to treat autoimmune diabetes. *Ann Med* 32 (5):285-92.

Walter, U., and P. Santamaria. 2005. CD8+ T cells in autoimmunity. *Curr Opin Immunol* 17 (6):624-31.

Watanabe, N., Y. H. Wang, H. K. Lee, T. Ito, W. Cao, and Y. J. Liu. 2005. Hassall's corpuscles instruct dendritic cells to induce CD4+CD25+ regulatory T cells in human thymus. *Nature* 436 (7054):1181-5.

Webster, D. E., S. D. Smith, R. J. Pickering, R. A. Strugnell, I. B. Dry, and S. L. Wesselingh. 2006. Measles virus hemagglutinin protein expressed in transgenic lettuce induces neutralising antibodies in mice following mucosal vaccination. *Vaccine* 24 (17):3538-44.

Weiner, H. L. 2001. Induction and mechanism of action of transforming growth factor-beta-secreting Th3 regulatory cells. *Immunol Rev* 182:207-14.

Weiner, H. L., Z. J. Zhang, S. J. Khoury, A. Miller, A. al-Sabbagh, S. A. Brod, O. Lider, P. Higgins, R. Sobel, R. B. Nussenblatt, and et al. 1991. Antigen-driven peripheral immune tolerance. Suppression of organ-specific autoimmune diseases by oral administration of autoantigens. *Ann N Y Acad Sci* 636:227-32.

Wen, L., J. Peng, Z. Li, and F. S. Wong. 2004. The effect of innate immunity on autoimmune diabetes and the expression of Toll-like receptors on pancreatic islets. *J Immunol* 172 (5):3173-80.

Wilson, N. S., D. El-Sukkari, and J. A. Villadangos. 2004. Dendritic cells constitutively present self antigens in their immature state in vivo and regulate antigen presentation by controlling the rates of MHC class II synthesis and endocytosis. *Blood* 103 (6):2187-95.

Wucherpfennig, K. W., J. Zhang, C. Witek, M. Matsui, Y. Modabber, K. Ota, and D. A. Hafler. 1994. Clonal expansion and persistence of human T cells specific for an immunodominant myelin basic protein peptide. *J Immunol* 152 (11):5581-92.

Yamaguchi, Y., H. Tsumura, M. Miwa, and K. Inaba. 1997. Contrasting effects of TGF-beta 1 and TNF-alpha on the development of dendritic cells from progenitors in mouse bone marrow. *Stem Cells* 15 (2):144-53.

Yang, S., W. Li, W. Liu, C. Gao, B. Zhou, S. Li, Y. Li, and Y. Kong. 2006. IL-10 gene modified dendritic cells induced antigen-specific tolerance in experimental autoimmune myocarditis. *Clin Immunol* 121 (1):63-73.

Yoon, J. W., and H. S. Jun. 2005. Autoimmune destruction of pancreatic beta cells. *Am J Ther* 12 (6):580-91.

Yoon, J. W., H. S. Jun, and P. Santamaria. 1998. Cellular and molecular mechanisms for the initiation and progression of beta cell destruction resulting from the collaboration between macrophages and T cells. *Autoimmunity* 27 (2):109-22.

Yoon, S. I., N. J. Logsdon, F. Sheikh, R. P. Donnelly, and M. R. Walter. 2006. Conformational changes mediate interleukin-10 receptor 2 (IL-10R2) binding to IL-10 and assembly of the signaling complex. *J Biol Chem* 281 (46):35088-96.

Zhang, Z. J., L. Davidson, G. Eisenbarth, and H. L. Weiner. 1991. Suppression of diabetes in nonobese diabetic mice by oral administration of porcine insulin. *Proc Natl Acad Sci U S A* 88 (22):10252-6.

Zheng, Y., D. M. Danilenko, P. Valdez, I. Kasman, J. Eastham-Anderson, J. Wu, and W. Ouyang. 2007. Interleukin-22, a T(H)17 cytokine, mediates IL-23-induced dermal inflammation and acanthosis. *Nature* 445 (7128):648-51.

Part 7

Beta Cell Replacement

21

Porcine Islet Xenotransplantation for the Treatment of Type 1 Diabetes

Dana Mihalicz, Ray V. Rajotte and Gina R. Rayat
University of Alberta
Canada

1. Introduction

Type 1 diabetes is a disease that typically occurs in childhood and adolescence and has been estimated to account for 5% to 10% of all diagnosed cases of diabetes. It is caused by the destruction of beta cells in the islets of pancreas resulting in insulin deficiency that eventually leads to high glucose levels in the blood. If not properly treated, this condition can lead to long-term secondary complications of diabetes such as kidney disease, heart disease, and blindness. Individuals with type 1 diabetes require insulin injections for survival, but insulin injection never achieves perfect regulation of glucose in the blood and secondary complications of diabetes still develop. An attractive alternative treatment for type 1 diabetes is the replacement of islets by transplantation. Islet transplantation offers a physiological means of delivering insulin thus has the potential to control better the levels of glucose in the blood. With an islet transplant, the beta cells that have been destroyed are replaced by new beta cells in the islets, which are able to sense the changes in blood glucose levels.

The very first attempts at islet transplantation occurred prior to the discovery of insulin in 1922 (Banting & Best, 1922) when Von Mering and Minkowski demonstrated in 1889 that the pancreas was responsible for the regulation of blood glucose as removal of the pancreas made the dogs diabetic (von Mering, 1889). Minkowski subsequently attempted to reverse diabetes in the diabetic dogs by auto-transplanting fragments of pancreas under the skin but his attempt failed (Minkowski, 1892). Subsequent advances in rodent models established the foundation for techniques used in current day islet transplantation. In 1989, the Islet Transplant Group at the University of Alberta carried out Canada's first islet transplant (Warnock et al., 1989). Long-term insulin independence was achieved when a combination of freshly isolated and cryopreserved islets were used (Warnock et al., 1992). Up to 1999, of the 267 islet allografts transplanted worldwide, only 12.4% have resulted in insulin independence for periods of more than 1 week, and only 8.2% have done so for periods of more than 1 year (Brendel et al., 1999). Despite these sobering long-term results, compared with intensive exogenous insulin therapy, islet transplantation provided superior metabolic control, prevented hypoglycemic events and held the potential to decrease secondary complications of diabetes (Alejandro et al., 1997) - a substantial impetus to encourage continued support of the field. Islet transplantation, however, faces a number of challenges, including a shortage of suitable human donors for transplantation and the required long-term use of harmful immunosuppressive drugs in order to prevent rejection of the graft. For these reasons, islet transplantation is currently reserved for patients with brittle diabetes. However, as improved anti-rejection regimens are being developed, islet transplantation is becoming a viable option for more patients with type 1 diabetes. This only serves to widen the gap between the supply and demand of islets for transplantation. A potential strategy to overcome this challenge is the transplantation of xenogeneic tissue, or tissue from a different species, as an alternative source of islets. The first recorded attempt at using xenotransplantation to treat type 1 diabetes was performed by Watson-Williams and Harsant in 1893, when they treated a young boy in diabetic ketoacidosis by implanting fragments of a sheep's pancreas subcutaneously. Although there was a temporary improvement in the young boy's glycosuria, he ultimately died shortly thereafter (Williams, 1894). Since this time a number of xenogeneic sources of insulin producing cells have been explored including porcine (Korbutt et al., 1996), bovine (Marchetti et al., 1995), rabbit (Lacy et al., 1989) and fish Brockman bodies (Wright et al., 1992). Arguably, the most attractive alternative source of islets for human transplantation are porcine islets (Figure 1).

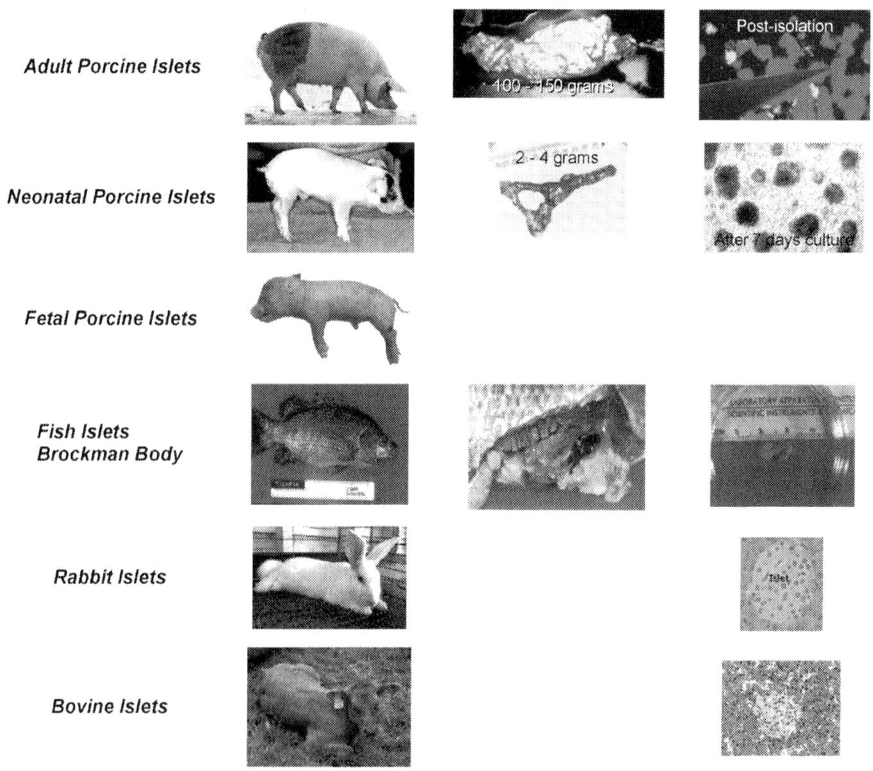

Fig. 1. Xenogeneic sources of insulin producing tissue. Each of these sources have been examined, however, the most promising source for clinical islet transplantation is porcine islets.

2. Porcine islets as a potential solution to the shortage of human islets

Pigs have been the focus of islet xenotransplantation for a number of reasons - they are inexpensive, readily available, breed quickly and produce large litters. Their islets display many morphologic and structural similarities to human islets, and respond to glucose levels in the same physiologic range (Cardona et al., 2007). Porcine insulin differs from human insulin by only one amino acid, and as such has been used clinically to treat patients with type 1 diabetes for many years (Dufrane & Gianello, 2009). Pig donors have many advantages with respect to transplantation: i) they are not exposed to compromising conditions such as comorbidity, brain death and cold ischemic injury as many deceased human donors are; ii) they may be housed in pathogen-free facilities which may allow for an on-demand source of islets with limited risk of pathogen transmission; iii) they may be genetically modified in order to change the expression of proteins, which may ultimately allow for the procurement of less immunogenic tissue (Hering & Walawalker, 2009; Ricordi et al., 1990; Korbutt et al., 1996).

2.1 The optimal age of the donor pig

Three main age groups of donor pigs have been investigated to date - adult, fetal, and neonatal - however, the optimal age is still being debated. Adult pigs are a potential source of tissue, as the isolated islets function well both *in vitro* and *in vivo* immediately upon isolation, and the yield is substantial. Ricordi et al. demonstrated that approximately 255,000 islets could be isolated per adult pig pancreas, using a technique modified from the human islet isolation procedure. The final preparation was 85-90% pure and reversed hyperglycemia in nude mice (Ricordi et al., 1990). Adult pig islets, however, do have their disadvantages. They are difficult to isolate and maintain in culture, are fragile, and are more susceptible to ischemic and hypoxic damage than neonatal porcine islets. In addition, they lack growth potential (Smith & Mandel, 2000), which limits their ability to recover from any damage upon transplantation. Adult islets may also be relatively more immunogenic upon transplantation, which may only increase the need for immunosuppression (Bloch et al., 1999). In order to be suitable for clinical transplantation, the pigs must be maintained in a pathogen-free environment until they are of an appropriate age for donation. This can be very costly and logistically very difficult, which can limit the applicability of adult pigs as islet donors.

The processing of fetal pig pancreata yield porcine fetal islet-like clusters (FICC), an immature group of cells that is capable of producing insulin. In 1988, a simplified procedure for the procurement of FICC was developed by Korsgren et al., which is a simple procedure that does not require the ductal infusion of collagenase or ficoll gradient separation of islets that is seen in adult islet isolation. Media changes every second day purifies the islets, but the functional ability of the FICC is still poor due to their immaturity. They can be maintained in culture for up to 30 days, and are capable of proliferating, however, *in vivo* reversal of hyperglycemia in animals can take months (Korsgren et al., 1991). In addition, the yield of FICC per pancreas is low, and an estimated 100 porcine donors would be necessary to transplant one 70-kg patient (Korsgren et al., 1991).

A functionally mature islet source with the isolation ease seen in fetal pig donors can be found in neonatal porcine donors. Korbutt et al. developed a protocol in 1996 for the isolation of neonatal porcine islets (NPI), which is easy to perform, with a consistent yield of approximately 50,000 islets per pancreas. The preparation consists of 35% fully differentiated islets, and approximately 57% endocrine precursor cells (Korbutt et al., 1996). These precursor cells allow the islets to differentiate and divide in the post-transplantation period (Binett et al., 2001; Hering & Walawalker, 2009; Korbutt et al., 1996; Rayat et al., 1999). NPI have been shown to reverse diabetes in both small and large animal models, including non-human primate (NHP) models, after a delay of up to 8 weeks due to their immaturity (Arefanian et al., 2007; Arefanian et al., 2010; Cardona et al., 2006; Kobayashi et al., 2005; Korbutt et al., 1996; Rayat & Gill, 2005; Ramji et al., 2010). They are also believed to be more resistant to hypoxic injury and less immunogenic than adult islets (Bloch et al., 1999). In addition, neonatal pigs require fewer facilities and resources in order to house them compared with adult pigs.

There are two major disadvantages of using NPI as a source for transplantation. First, a yield of 50,000 NPI per pancreas translates to the need for approximately 70 donor piglets per patient, which is much greater than adult pig donors (Korbutt et al., 1996). Second, NPI express antigens on their surface that can predispose the tissue to rejection upon transplantation. Although the most studied of these antigens is galactose α(1,3) galactose (Gal), it is not likely the only xeno-antigen responsible for rejection (Rayat et al., 1998).

A concern regarding the use of porcine tissue in humans is the possible transmission of xenosis, in particular, the transmission of porcine endogenous retrovirus (PERV). PERV is present in all pigs, as is a retrovirus encoded in their germline, and is therefore a potential source of xenosis. To date, however, there has been no evidence of transmission of this virus to humans or non-human primates (Cardona et al., 2007; Hering et al., 2006; Rood et al., 2007; Valdes-Gonzales et al., 2005).

2.2 Immunological responses to porcine islets

After the transplantation of xenogeneic tissue, there are 3 major pathways of rejection that can destroy the graft in a rapid manner - the innate immune system, hyperacute rejection mediated by pre-formed natural antibodies and complement, and acute cell mediated rejection.

2.2.1 Innate immune system – instant blood mediated inflammatory reaction (IBMIR)

The innate immune system in the form of IBMIR is the major pathway of the first mechanism of graft loss. When islets are injected into the portal vein of the recipient, there are a number of factors that activate both the coagulation cascade and platelets (van der Windt et al., 2007). The intrinsic pathway of coagulation is activated due to the remnants of collagen in the graft, which is not normally in contact with blood. In addition, tissue factor (TF), which is expressed on both α and β cells, as well as on contaminating ductal structures, activates the extrinsic pathway of coagulation. Due to molecular incompatibilities between the xenogeneic tissue and the recipient, normal feedback mechanisms, such as porcine membrane TF pathway inhibitor, which limit coagulation, do not occur (van der Windt et al., 2007). Platelets are also activated through the presence of thrombin, collagen, and von Willebrand factor bound collagen. These pathways lead to thrombus formation and subsequent ischemia and necrosis of the graft. The complement system is also activated and this is followed by infiltration of $CD11^+$ polymorphonuclear cells and macrophages, which lead to enzymatic digestion and phagocytosis of the islets, as well as the release of cytokines that can induce apoptosis (Nilsson, 2008; Van der Windt et al., 2007). As a result, significant tissue damage occurs, and often the majority of the graft is destroyed within 24 hrs. The damaged islets expel their insulin, and animals are at risk of becoming hypoglycemic. Although it has been demonstrated in primate models that insulin independence can be achieved even after such a significant loss of tissue, this is likely because a very large islet mass was transplanted initially. IBMIR is not limited to xenotransplantation, but the reaction is often more pronounced in this circumstance (van der Windt et al., 2007). Many strategies are being developed to attenuate this destructive reaction, including the addition of heparin in the islet preparation as seen in current clinical practice (Cabric et al., 2007), the administration of low-molecular weight dextran sulphate, and various other compounds (Johansson et al., 2006; van der Windt et al., 2007).

2.2.2 Hyperacute rejection

Natural pre-formed antibodies can lead to a dramatic reaction and loss of the graft. In solid organ transplantation, discordant grafts are rejected due to antibodies to carbohydrate moieties, in particular the Gal antigen. The Gal epitope, which is the result of the enzyme α1,3-galactosyltransferase catalyzing the transfer of an α-galactosyl residue to a terminal β-galactose, is present on all cell surface glycoproteins and glycolipids of all mammals except humans, apes, and Old World Monkeys (Galili & Swanson, 1991). These animals develop antibodies due to exposure to the epitope through enteric bacteria and other pathogens. Due to this humoral response, solid organ xenografts can exhibit significant destruction, and IgG deposits are associated with the grafts by 12 hours post-transplantation. By 2 days, there is significant IgM and C3, C5, and C9 complement depositions within 2 days of transplantation.

Porcine islet grafts, however, seem to evade the hyperacute response that solid organ xenografts experience. The typical antibody and complement deposition that is seen in solid organ grafts is not observed when porcine islets are transplanted into non-human primates (Hering et al., 2006). In addition, the use of α1,3-galactosyltransferase gene-knockout (GT-KO) pigs as donors has not yet proved to reduce the post-transplant graft loss as compared to wild-type pigs (Rood et al., 2007). Only approximately 5% of adult pig islets express Gal on their surface, whereas approximately 20% of NPI express it (Rayat et al., 2003). During both *in vitro* and *in vivo* maturation models of NPI, the expression of Gal is shown to reduce significantly as the precursor cells evolve into mature β cells (Rayat et al., 2003). Regardless, it has been demonstrated that NPI expressing and not expressing Gal can be susceptible to hyperacute rejection *in vitro*, suggesting that Gal is not the only xenoantigen responsible for this phenomenon (Rayat et al., 1998). Islet xenografts are also mainly revascularized by recipient endothelial cells (Nyqyist et al., 2005). It is for these reasons the natural pre-formed anti-Gal antibodies are not considered a major factor in the loss of islet graft tissue in the early post-transplant period (Cardona et al., 2006; Hering et al., 2006; Hering & Walawalker, 2009).

2.2.3 Cell mediated rejection

Likely the most important mechanism of rejection of porcine xenografts is via T-cell mediated processes. In rodent models, acute cellular rejection appears to be mediated predominately by CD4$^+$ T-cells, as CD8 knockout but not CD4 knockout mice, reject their xenografts. In addition, due to the degree of phylogenic disparity between mice and the donor pig, the bias would be against direct recognition by CD8$^+$ T cells. The signals required for direct T cell activation may not occur because of incompatibilities of molecular interactions between the pig antigen presenting cells (APCs) and the mouse T cells (Rayat et al., 2003; Koulmanda et al., 2004). In genetically modified mice, which are MHC II deficient and therefore lack an indirect response, the rejection of fetal porcine islet xenografts is delayed. The depletion of $CD4^+$ T cells further prolongs graft survival in these mice; however rejection is not completely prevented. This suggests that a direct response must occur by some mechanism upon T cell recovery in order for an immune response to occur (Koulmanda et al., 2004). However, in NHP and human models, the direct presentation route may be more significant, as it has been demonstrated that both $CD4^+$ and $CD8^+$ human T-cells can respond to porcine APCs (Yamada et al., 1995).

The likely mechanism is the processing of porcine antigens by recipient APCs and presentation to recipient $CD4^+$ T cells, which can then activate the pathways necessary to destroy the xenograft. In acute cellular rejection, macrophages, eosinophils, and T cells infiltrate the xenograft and reach a maximum infiltrate within 4-6 days (Smith & Mandel, 2000). $CD8^+$ T cells likely contribute to this rejection as well, although the mechanism of their involvement is not clear. Their activation may be through either donor presentation (direct) or cross-presentation by the host APCs (Rayat & Gill, 2003).

2.2.4 Autoimmune recognition

Type 1 diabetes is an autoimmune disorder, and as such, the prevention of the preceding mechanisms of rejection is not relevant if the xenogeneic tissue is recognized by the preexisting autoimmune repertoire. At present, the evidence suggests that this repertoire may be partially species specific, therefore the xenogeneic tissue may escape the effects of the autoreactivity; however the extent of this specificity is yet to be determined. If donor tissue shares epitopes with the target of the autoimmune cells and antibodies, they too may be targeted and destroyed by the native disease process.

The animal model that has been developed to investigate this is the non-obese diabetic (NOD) mouse. These mice spontaneously begin to develop diabetes after 12 weeks, and 90% of female mice will be fully diabetic by 30 weeks. The mechanism of diabetes development is similar to that which is found in human type 1 diabetes patients, where autoreactive T cells infiltrate the islets and specifically attack the β cells (Anderson & Bluestone, 2005). Strategies that have been shown to be effective in chemically induced diabetic mice have not been effective in NOD mice (Arefanian et al., 2007; Koulmanda et al., 2003). For example in our experience, the short-term administration of 2 monoclonal antibodies targeted against T cell activation failed to promote survival of NPI xenografts in NOD mice despite being highly effective in B6 mice. Graft survival in the NOD mice required the administration of an additional monoclonal antibody against $CD4^+$ T cells (Arefanian et al., 2007). Koulmanda et al. have also demonstrated that the depletion of $CD4^+$ T cells in NOD mice allowed for the prolonged survival of adult porcine islet xenografts. Interestingly, no further survival benefit was found when $CD8^+$ T cells were also depleted. However, further results have demonstrated that autoimmunity may not be the reason for the difficulty in inducing tolerance in NOD mice. When the NOD mice were treated with streptozotocin (STZ) prior to the onset of diabetes, autoimmunity was avoided, as subsequent islet isografts were not rejected as they are in spontaneously diabetic NOD mice. The prolongation of adult porcine islet survival was virtually identical in both the spontaneously diabetic and STZ treated NOD mice, supporting the idea that recurrent autoimmunity does not substantially contribute to the rejection of islet xenografts (Koulmanda et al., 2003).

3. Current tolerance induction strategies

In order for T cell activation to occur, and therefore for an immune response to an antigen to occur, it must first receive two signals. The first is engagement of the antigen-specific T cell receptor and the second is a non-antigen-specific co-stimulatory signal, which is provided by an active APC. Both the direct and indirect pathways of antigen presentation, as seen primarily in NHP and rodents respectively, require this co-stimulatory interaction in order to activate T cells. It therefore seems intuitive that interference with these interactions would lead to tolerance to the foreign antigens, specifically the porcine islets. Monoclonal antibodies provide this interference and have the ability to provide long-term graft protection with only a short course of treatment, thus negating the requirement of continuous immunosuppression.

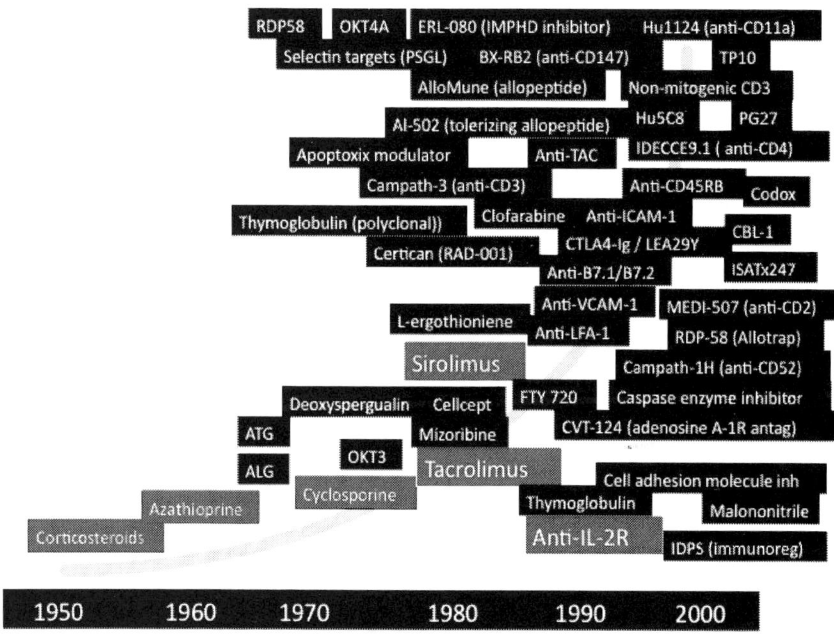

Fig. 2. The multiple strategies used over time to attempt to prevent the rejection of islet transplants.

3.1 Biologic agents - monoclonal antibodies

3.1.1 Anti-LFA-1 monoclonal antibody (mAb)

Leukocyte function antigen-1 (LFA-1) is an important adhesion molecules expressed on a variety of cells including macrophages, monocytes, and NK cells, but is most heavily expressed on T and B cells. This molecule interacts with intercellular adhesion molecules-1 (ICAM-1), which is present on vascular endothelium, lymphocytes, and macrophages. The interaction of these two molecules provides a number of functions which include: *i)* facilitating the migration of lymphocytes to the site of inflammation; *ii)* strengthening the binding of T cells to antigen presenting cells; *iii)* providing signals necessary for the activation of T cells; and *iv)* further activating APCs to secrete cytokines and recruit other cells (Dougherty & Hogg, 1987). Due to the number and significance of these functions, interfering with this interaction can therefore lead to tolerance, which can be achieved by an anti-LFA-1 mAb.

The administration of this mAb has been shown to be effective in a number of allograft models, including cardiac, renal, and islet graft models (Nicolls et al., 2000; Poston et al., 2000; Vincenti et al., 2007). Clinically, the humanized form, Efalizumab, has been used to treat another autoimmune disorder, plaque psoriasis, with few acute side effects (Lebwohl et al., 2003). There have been 2 trials to date in clinical islet allotransplantation that have reported its efficacy (Posselt et al., 2010; Turgeon et al., 2010). In one trial, all 8 patients who received an islet transplant and were treated with an Efalizumab-based regimen achieved insulin independence; 4 of these patients achieved independence after a single islet transplant (Posselt et al, 2010). In the second study, the 4 patients that were treated with an Efalizumab based regimen achieved insulin independence after a single islet transplant (Turgeon et al., 2010). Efalizumab was ultimately removed from the market in 2009 due to 4 cases of progressive multifocal leukoencephalopathy (PML), however, none of the recipients in either of these studies demonstrated evidence of this disease (Posselt et al., 2010; Turgeon et al., 2010). In fact, these 4 cases arose from over 40,000 patients who had been treated with the medication for greater than 4 years (Turgeon et al., 2010). Although the risk-benefit profile of this medication is unfavorable for the treatment of a relatively minor condition such as psoriasis, it is perhaps better than that of the traditional immunosuppressive agents currently being used in clinical transplantation. It is therefore still being investigated as a possible agent to prevent graft rejection.

With respect to xenotransplantation, the anti-LFA-1 mAb has been shown to be effective both *in vitro* and *in vivo* (Rayat & Gill, 2005; Tredget et al., 2008). In a concordant rat to mouse model, the administration of this mAb prevented islet graft rejection in 27 of 28 mice from up to 100 days (Tredget et al., 2008). In a discordant NPI to mouse model, only 7/15 mice achieved normoglycemia with the short-term administration of anti-LFA-1 mAb, and only 6/15 maintained long-term graft survival (Rayat & Gill, 2005). Anti-LFA-1 mAb has also been shown to improve the function of adult porcine islets in mice when added to a CTLA4Ig and anti-CD154 mAb regimen (Kumagai-Braesch et al., 2007). Collectively, these studies show us that the anti-LFA-1 mAb can be efficacious in preventing islet allograft rejection, and is very promising in the prevention of xenograft rejection, however monotherapy with this medication is not sufficient.

3.1.2 Anti-CD154 mAb

CD154 is a costimulatory molecule that is a member of the Tumor Necrosis Factor (TNF) family that is predominately present on T cells. It binds with CD40 on the surface of APCs and the interaction of these molecules is thought to be critical to the maturation of APCs, the promotion of antigen presentation, and the priming and proliferation of both cytotoxic and helper T cells (Seijkens et al., 2010). In NHP models of islet allotransplantation, the administration of the humanized form of anti-CD154 mAb (hu5c8) has demonstrated significant efficacy in preventing rejection (Kenyon et al., 1999a, 1999b). In three of three baboons who received islet allografts and were treated with short-term anti-CD154 mAb, delayed rejection of their grafts was observed. This rejection was reversed by the readministration of the mAb (Kenyon et al., 1999a). In rhesus macaques, six of six recipients of islet allografts and anti-CD154 mAb induction therapy plus monthly maintenance therapy achieved and maintained insulin independence for >100 days, with no evidence of rejection in 5 of the 6 animals (Kenyon et al., 1999b). Thus in allotransplantation, the benefits of the anti-CD154 mAb are clear.

In NPI xenograft models, the administration of anti-CD154 mAb (MR-1) as a monotherapy has yielded only modest results, with approximately 40% of diabetic mice achieving normoglycemia (Rayat & Gill, 2005). However, combination therapy of anti-LFA-1 and anti-CD154 mAbs has improved survival of porcine islet xenografts. In mice transplanted with NPI, short-term treatment with both anti-LFA-1 and anti-CD154 mAbs allowed 100% of the mice to demonstrate long-term survival of the grafts (>100 days) with only 10% rejecting prior to 300 days post-transplant (Arefanian et al., 2010). These results are substantial and clearly demonstrate that simultaneous interference of adhesion and costimulatory pathways can lead to islet xenograft tolerance. Pre-clinical models with the transplantation of either NPI or adult porcine islets have demonstrated that the humanized form of anti-CD154 mAb (H106, ABI793) is very effective when combined to existing regimens, such as basiliximab, sirolimus, and FTY720 or belatacept (Cardona et al., 2006; Cardona et al., 2007; Hering et al., 2006).

The unfortunate side effect of the humanized form of anti-CD154 mAb is that it has been shown to increase the incidence of thrombo-embolic events in both human and non-human primates (Kawai et al., 2000). The administration of heparin concomitantly with the mAb did decrease this incidence, however it remains above the acceptable limit for clinical use (Kawai et al., 2000). Non-human primate models also suggest that the administration of aspirin during the treatment with anti-CD154 mAb therapy could greatly reduce the incidence of these events (van der Windt, et al., 2009). Investigation is currently underway to search for compounds that can interfere with the CD154/CD40 interaction on the surface of T cells and APCs, respectively without the increase in thrombotic events. There is promise in the use of small inhibitory molecules which have demonstrated their ability to bind to CD154 *in vitro* and effectively block its binding to CD40 (Buchwald et al., 2009; Margolles-Clark et al., 2009; Margolles-Clark et al., 2010). These small inhibitory molecules have been identified as a number of organic dyes, including Direct Red 80 (DR80) and Mordant Brown 1 (MB1), compounds traditionally used in textile industry. They have been found to bind to CD154 and block its interaction with CD40 in a dose dependent manner, with a much higher affinity than that of the anti-CD154 mAb itself. This inhibitory effect does translate to the inhibition of B and T cell proliferation *in vitro* (Buchwald et al., 2009; Margolles-Clark et al., 2009; Margolles-Clark et al., 2010; Mihalicz et al, 2011). Preliminary *in vivo* studies have demonstrated no effect as monotherapy in the prevention of NPI xenograft rejection in mice. In combination with anti-LFA-1 mAb, however, DR80 allowed 6 of 10 mice to achieve long-term normoglycemia after transplantation of NPI. However, the compounds used in this experiment are impure with the commercially available products containing only 25-40% dye content. The rate of mice maintaining normoglycemia with this regimen is expected to improve as purification of these dyes is perfected. With less impurities, there is a greater proportion of the injected compound that is biologically active, and likely less toxicity (Mihalicz et al., 2011).

3.2 Co-Transplantation with Sertoli cells

A number of anatomical immunoprivileged sites have been identified that provide immune protection to local tissues via a variety of mechanisms. These include the testes, anterior chamber of the eye, the brain, and the placenta (Cobbold et al., 2006), and transplanted tissue in these sites have extended survival when compared with conventional sites (Streillein, 1995). (Figure 3). The testes are of particular interest, as they seem to not only prevent inflammatory reactions and therefore bystander damage, but they also contain Sertoli cells that have a number of roles. They support the germ cells that are developing within the testes and protect them from being eliminated by the immune system. They are believed to confer this immune privilege through the release of local factors that inhibit the immune response, such as TGF-β, clusterin, serine protease inhibitors, and Fas ligand, which induces apoptosis of activated T cells (De Cesaros et al., 1992). It is possible that the co-transplantation of Sertoli cells with porcine islets could protect the graft from rejection via the same physiologic factors that protect the germ cells *in vivo*. When NPI were transplanted with Sertoli cells under the kidney capsules of rats, 66% were able to survive for >90 days with only a single injection of antilymphocyte serum (Dufour et al., 2003). Unfortunately subsequent studies have failed to support these findings. Studies with non-human primates examined the co-transplantation of NPI with neonatal porcine Sertoli cells in a number of anatomical sites including the omental pouch, kidney, pancreas, and liver. After 2 months, no insulin positive cells could be seen on immunohistochemistry, concluding that the Sertoli cells had limited ability to protect the graft (Wang et al., 2005). A controversial clinical study performed in Mexico, although deemed unjustifiable at that time by the International Xenotransplant Association ethics committee (Sykes et al., 2006), demonstrated prolonged survival of NPI xenografts when transplanted with Sertoli cells in a steel wire mesh device (Valdes-Gonzalez et al. 2005). Half of the 12 adolescent recipients showed greatly reduced insulin requirements at one year post-transplantation.

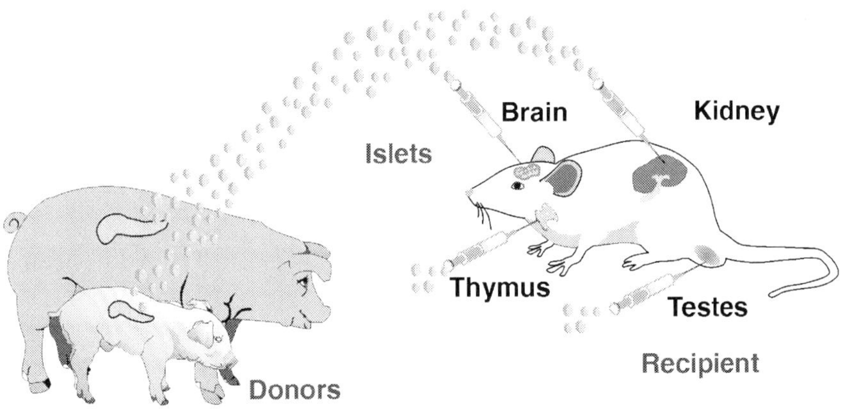

Fig. 3. Immunoprivileged sites that may be capable of conferring protection to transplanted islet xenografts.

The co-culture of Sertoli cells and islets prior to transplantation may confer additional benefits. When co-cultured with islets, Sertoli cells have been shown to facilitate maturation, expansion, and functioning of islets. It is possible that the Sertoli cells provide similar trophic support and nutrients to the islets as they do to germ cells in the native testes through secretion of various factors. In a study by Basta et al, neonatal porcine pancreatic endocrine precursor cells were cultured with Sertoli cells conditioned media, and subsequently showed enhanced differentiation into insulin secreting endocrine cells (Basta et al.,2004). This suggests that a secreted substance is inducing these changes and is particularly exciting in the transplantation of NPI, which contain a high proportion of these endocrine precursor cells and may be influenced by these factors in a way that adult porcine islets could not.

The addition of biologic therapy to this strategy of co-transplantation has been shown to increase its efficacy. In a recent study by our group, we confirmed that the co-transplantation of NPI and Sertoli cells in mice was not sufficient to prevent rejection. However, when anti-LFA-1, anti-CD154, or anti-CD45RB monotherapy was added, NPI graft survival increased beyond that of either treatment alone. For example, 7/7 mice who were transplanted with NPI and Sertoli cells, and were treated with a short course of anti-LFA-1 mAb achieved long-term graft survival >100 days. This is in comparison with 3/7 mice, which were transplanted with NPI alone and treated with anti-LFA-1 mAb, and 0/8 mice who were transplanted with NPI and Sertoli cells but received no mAb therapy. It appears as though the synergistic effect of the immunological protection of the Sertoli cells with the inhibition of immune cell activation by the mAb therapy is able to promote long-term porcine islet xenograft survival (Ramji et al., 2010).

Although the results of the preceding studies are exciting, there is still much to be examined in order to properly bring this to clinical studies. The mechanism of this protection is as of yet unknown, and the consequences of transplanting Sertoli cells into humans, particularly female patients, is to be determined.

3.3 Microencapsulation of NPI

Immunoisolation is another strategy to protect islets from rejection, by in a sense "hiding the islets from the recipients' immune system. By providing either a micro or macro barrier around the tissue, the ideal immunoisolation device will allow for the free passage of glucose, insulin, waste and nutrients, but excluding the passage of immune cells and antibodies responsible for the rejection process. A number of devices have been studied including cellulose membranes (Risbud & Bhondem, 2001), chitosan-polyvinyl pyrrolidone hydrogels (Risbud et al., 2000), and even steel wire meshes (Valdes-Gonzales et al., 2005). (Figure 4). Perhaps the most studied, and most promising, device for immunoisolation are alginate microcapsules.

The presence of an alginate capsule can protect the NPI from destruction by human antibody and complement *in vitro* (Rayat et al., 2000). In addition, when cultured in the presence of autologous pig serum, the microencapsulated NPI mature quickly, and are able to reverse hyperglycemia in diabetic mice at a more rapid rate than non-encapsulated NPI (Rayat et al., 2000). The proposed mechanism is by providing an extracellular support matrix to the NPI, and a possible barrier to the action of $CD4^+$ T cells. While some groups have reported that microencapsulated porcine islets can survive after xenotransplantation without the use of immunosuppressive medications (Duvivier-Kali et al., 2004; Sun et al., 1996), there is further evidence that microencapsulation alone is likely not sufficient to prevent rejection (Kobayashi et al., 2005, 2008). When microencapsulated NPI are transplanted into immune competent mice without the use of immunosuppressive medications, a progressive amount of $CD4^+$ T cells, macrophages, and B cells are seen on the surface of the capsule over time. At no time points are immune cells seen within the capsule, however, there is evidence that complement (C3 and C4) and anti-porcine IgG antibody are able to traverse the barrier. This antigen-specific response suggests that xenoantigens are

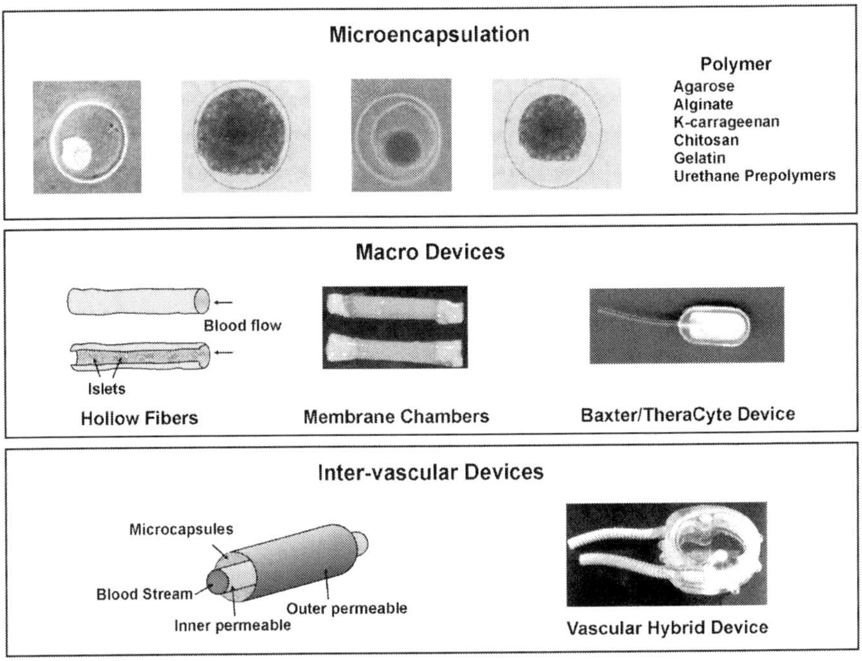

Fig. 4. Various immunoisolation devices examined for the transplantation of islets in an effort to evade the host immune system.

likely shed from the capsule which can then interact with the recipient APCs, leading to an indirect immune response. This immune response is sufficient to kill the NPI, as none of the transplanted B6 mice achieved normoglycemia, and by day 50 post-transplantation, nearly half of the cells in the NPI were non-viable (Kobayashi et al., 2005). The *in vivo* maturation of microencapsulated NPI in immunodeficient mice did improve the survival of the grafts in subsequent transplantation into immune competent mice. This seems to be due to the maturation of intact NPI and a decrease in their immunogenicity (Kobayashi et al., 2008).

Microencapsulated islet graft survival can be prolonged when the combination of anti-LFA-1 and anti-CD154 mAbs are also administered *in vivo*. In one study, all mice that were transplanted with microencapsulated NPI and treated with these mAbs achieved normoglycemia, with >50% maintaining normoglycemia for over 100 days. This is in contrast to only 1/20 untreated mice achieving normoglycemia. The therapy appears to prevent a humoral response, which may be the result of an altered indirect antigen response. It also prevented the migration of immune cells to the microencapsulated islets possibly through interfering with the secretion of chemokines, cell motility, and ultimately T cell activation (Kobayashi et al., 2005).

Although it seems clear that microencapsulation alone is likely not sufficient to prevent the xenorejection of NPI, when combined with other strategies such as the *in vivo* maturation of NPI and the administration of mAb therapy, it does provide some beneficial effects. Microencapsulation remains a promising strategy in providing protection to NPI and warrants further investigation. In fact, a recent study by Dufrane et al. demonstrated survival of microencapsulated adult porcine islets for 6 months post-transplantation without immunosuppression under the kidney capsule in non-diabetic primates (Dufrane et al., 2006). This same group later showed that macroencapsulated porcine islets in a monolayer cellular device can reverse diabetes in NHP for up to 6 months post-transplantation in the absence of immunosuppression (Dufrane et al., 2010). These studies established that both micro- and macroencapsulated porcine islets are able to function long-term in stringent xenogeneic models. The challenge will be to provide the appropriate additional support, possibly in the form of the aforementioned monoclonal antibodies, in order to carry survival of the islets past the 6 month mark.

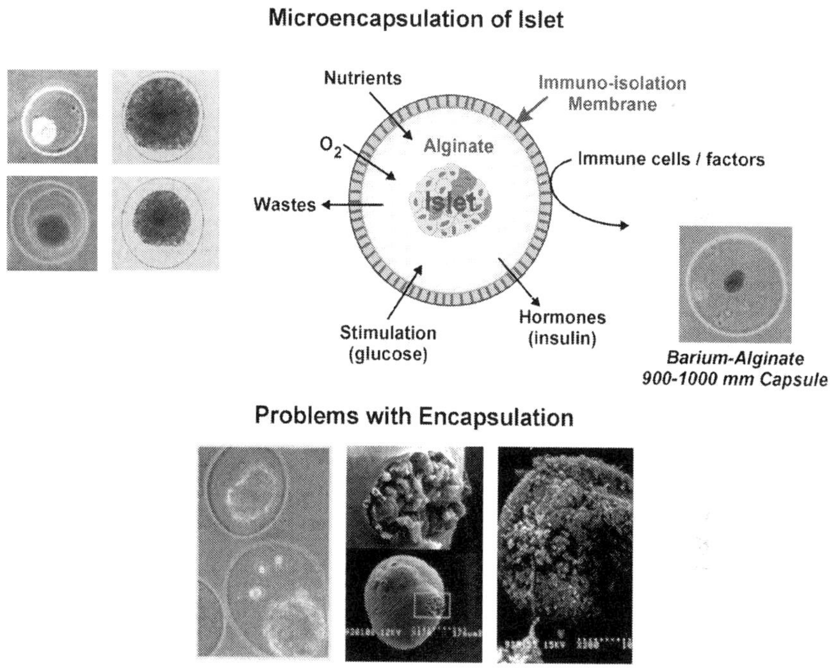

Fig. 5. Microencapsulation of islets for transplantation. The capsule allows for the passage of insulin and wastes out of the islets cells, while nutrients, including glucose are able to enter the islets. Immune cells, however, are not able to pass through the barrier, potentially protecting the islets from rejection. Problems with microencapsulation include protrusion of islets which could cause rupture of the capsule attracting the immune cells leading to graft failure.

4. Future prospects for tolerance induction

The future of tolerance induction in porcine islet xenotransplantation may in the use of genetically modified pig donors such as human CD46 (hCD46) transgenic pigs (van der

Windt et al., 2009), N-acetylglucosaminyltransferase-III (GnT-III) transgenic pigs (Komoda et al., 2005), and alpha 1,3-galactosyltransferase knock-out (GT-KO) pigs (Casu et al., 2010). GnT-III transgenic pigs have been shown to have significantly down-regulated xenoantigens, both Gal and non-Gal, due to a mechanism that is not fully understood. Cynomolgus monkeys were transplanted with these islets under their kidney capsule showed slightly longer survival than wild-type pig islets in the absence of immune suppression, although these results were not significant, and question regarding the usefulness of these donors has arisen (Komoda et al., 2005). GT-KO pigs lack the enzyme alpha 1,3-galactosyltransferase, therefore the donor tissue lacks the xenoantigen Gal (Casu et al., 2005). This mutation has been shown to have minimal effect on glucose metabolism in the donor pig (Casu et al., 2005), however has shown little in the way of advantage in terms of transplant rejection in preliminary animal models (Bottino et al., 2007).

The hCD46 transgene has been introduced into porcine donors in an attempt to circumvent the IBMIR reaction. CD46 is a human complement regulatory protein, and as such is believed to assist in the avoidance of complement mediated early destruction of islets upon portal infusion. In a preclinical model using Cynomolgus monkeys, the hCD46 transgenic pigs did allow for a significantly longer period of insulin independence, even up to one year post-transplantation, as compared to wild-type pig donors, who only maintained normoglycemia up to 36 days. In addition, both sets of islets were bound with anti-pig antibodies, however, only wild-type pig islets were bound with complement. Despite this fact, early graft loss was detected in both groups, as evidenced by a release of C-peptide and hypoglycemia in the recipient (van der Windt et al., 2009). The numbers of recipients in this study was small, however the results are perhaps the most promising of any of the studies involving transgenic pigs to date.

Another future prospect for the induction of tolerance is the creation of mixed hematopoetic chimerism. Creation of this chimeric state can occur after hematopoietic stem cell transplantation, or bone marrow transplantation, which can effectively induce tolerance to the subsequent islet graft. This is done by establishing "self" tolerance to the islet graft by the donor immune cells. This has been performed in both allotransplantation and rat to mouse xenotransplantation, leading to graft acceptance and ultimately normoglycemia in the host animals. This strategy has also been shown to reduce the number of allogeneic islets required to achieve normoglycemia in NOD mice (Zhang et al., 2010). In xenotransplantation, the simultaneous or subsequent transplantation of rat bone marrow and islets to chemically-induced diabetic mice resulted in the grafts being permanently accepted and allowed the recipients to achieve normoglycemia (Zeng et al., 1992; Li et al., 1994).

The practicality of chimerism for tolerance induction in NPI transplantation is in question, however, as multiple neonatal donors will be required for one human recipient. This would require a large amount of bone marrow transplantations which may not be feasible, as there may be a limit to the number of bone marrow strains that can repopulate an animal (Chester et al., 1989). In addition the engraftment of the bone marrow tissue itself currently requires an immunosuppressive regimen, trading one potentially harmful regimen for another.

5. Cultural views of porcine islet xenotransplantation

Additional barriers to the clinical use of islet xenotransplantation as a treatment for type 1 diabetes are the ethical and cultural issues surrounding it. A number of surveys have examined public opinion on this issue, dating back to the mid 1980's (Hagelin, 2004). Although often flawed and biased, review of these articles reveals that there is not overwhelming support for xenotransplantation, with acceptance rates of 40-50%, which can increase to 70-80% in the case of patients who may directly benefit from xenotransplantation (Deschamps et al., 2000; Hagelin, 2004; Persson et al., 2003). However, the proportion of people directly opposing it appears to be decreasing over time (Hagelin, 2004). Some studies identified factors such as a lower level of education, an older population, female gender, and being very religious as factors that decreased the likelihood of supporting xenotransplantation (Hagelin, 2004; Rios et al., 2010). In a study of Latin American health care workers, the acceptance of xenotransplantation was influenced by their specific job in the field, specifically physicians being more supportive of the idea (77%) compared with auxiliary staff being less supportive (40%) (Rios et al., 2010).

Specific to islet xenotransplantation, a recent survey of Latin-American diabetic patients revealed 79% indicated acceptance of porcine islet xenotransplantation. Seventy-five percent indicated they would accept the porcine tissue even if it only reduced their insulin requirements, temporarily prevented the progression of secondary complications, or needed to be repeated every six months. Interestingly, 40% indicated that they believe living with porcine cells could cause them psychological distress (Abalovich et al., 2010). This is in contrast to a French study from 5 years previous, where it was found that the proportion of individuals with type 1 diabetes willing to accept a transplant was much lower. Before the risks of the procedure were explained, 52% said they would agree to islet xenotransplantation. After it was explained that xenotransplantation may require more intense immunosuppression than conventional allotransplantation, leaving the patient more vulnerable to infections and malignancies, 70.5% refused. Patients also stated that insulin independence was their greatest priority, taking precedence over a reduction in complications or an increased life expectancy, therefore if this is not achieved, they were not willing to accept the risks of the procedure. Other reasons for refusal were cited as the risk of disease transmission and other risks that may not be yet identified (Deschamps et al., 2005). Although these are reasonable concerns, as the strategies to overcome these barriers are developed, it is possible these issues will be addressed by the time islet xenotransplantation becomes a viable clinical option. Therefore, although in some regions the acceptance of islet xenotransplantation may currently be limited, it is still prudent to continue the research in this area to develop a safe and acceptable treatment regimen.

6. Conclusions

Type 1 diabetes is a debilitating and costly disease, but the use of islet transplantation can reduce the burden on both the patient and the healthcare system. Due to a shortage of donor tissue, xenogeneic tissues, in particular porcine islets, are being investigated as a source of insulin producing cells. The main challenge in using these tissues is to provide a means to evade the host immune system in order to maintain a viable and functioning graft. Many methods are under investigation in order to induce tolerance, many with promising results. Due to the redundancy within the highly sophisticated immune system, the likely solution will be a combination of these strategies, which will allow us to circumvent these immune mechanisms from more than one angle at a time.

7. Acknowledgements

The authors would like to acknowledge our funding sources including the Juvenile Diabetes Research Foundation, Canadian Diabetes Association, Edmonton Civic Employees Charitable Assistance Fund, Canadian Institutes for Health Research, Muttart Diabetes Research and Training Centre, University Hospital Foundation, Stollery Children's Hospital Foundation, the MacLachlan Fund, the Diabetes Association (Brooks and District), the Alberta Diabetes Foundation, and the Alberta Diabetes Institute. We would also like to thank Dawne Colwell for her assistance with the figures.

8. References

Abalovich, A., Wechsler, C., & Bervottini, M. (2010). Pig islet xenotransplantation acceptance in a Latin-American diabetic population. *Xenotransplantation,* Vol. 17, pp. (263-266), ISSN 1399-3089

Alejandro, R., Lehmann, R., Ricordi, C., Kenyon, NS., Angelico, MC., Burke, G., Esquenazi, V., Nery, J., Betancourt, AE., Kong, SS., Miller, J. & Mintz, DH. (1997). Long-term function (6 years) of islet allografts in type 1 diabetes. *Diabetes,* Vol. 46, pp. (1983-1989), ISSN 0012-1797

Anderson, MS. & Bluestone, JA. (2005). The NOD mouse: A model of immune dysregulation. *Annual Review of Immunology,* Vol. 23, pp. (447-485), ISSN 0732-0582

Arefanian, H., Tredget, EB., Rajotte, RV., Korbutt, GS., Gill, RG. & Rayat GR. (2007). Combination of anti-CD4 with anti-LFA-1 and anti-CD154 monoclonal antibodies promotes long-term survival and function of neonatal porcine islet xenografts in spontaneously diabetic NOD mice. *Cell Transplantation,* Vol. 16, pp. (787-798), ISSN 0963-6897

Arefanian, H., Tredget, EB., Rajotte, RV., Gill, RG., Korbutt, GS. & Rayat, GR. (2010). Short-term administrations of a combination of anti-LFA-1 and anti-CD154 monoclonal antibodies induce tolerance to neonatal porcine islet xenografts in mice. *Diabetes,* Vol. 59, pp. (958-966), ISSN 0012-1797

Banting, FG. & Best, CH. (1922). The internal secretion of the pancreas. *Journal of Laboratory and Clinical Medicine,* Vol. 7, pp. (256-271), ISSN 0022-2143

Basta, G., Racanicchi, L., Mancuso, F., Guido, L., Luca, G., Macchiarulo, G., Brunetti, P., & Calafiore, R. (2004). Transdifferentiation molecular pathways of neonatal pig pancreatic duct cells into endocrine cell phenotypes. *Transplantation Proceedings,* Vol. 36, pp. (2857-2863), ISSN 0041-1345

Beckwith, J., Nyman, JA., Flanagan, B., Schrover, R., & Schuurman, H-J. (2010). A health-economic analysis of porcine islet xenotransplantation. *Xenotransplantation.* Vol. 17, pp. (233-242), ISSN 1399-3089

Binett, TM., Dufour, JM., & Korbutt, GS. (2001). In vitro maturation of neonatal porcine islets: a novel model for the study of islet development and xenotransplantation. *Annals of the New York Academy of Sciences,* Vol. 944, pp. (47-61), ISSN 0077-8923

Bloch, K., Assa, S., Lazard, D., Abramov, N., Shalitin S., Weintrob, N., Josefsberg, Z., Rapoport, M., & Vardi, P. (1999). Neonatal pig islets induce a lower T-cell response than adult pig islets in IDDM patients. *Transplantation*, Vol. 67, Issue 5, pp. (748-752), ISSN 0931-0509

Bottino, R., Balamurugan, AN., Smetanka, C., Bertera, S., He, J., Rood, PPM, Cooper, DKC., & Trucco., M. (2007). Isolation outcome and functional characteristics of young and adult pig pancreatic islets for transplantation studies. *Xenotransplantation*, Vol. 14, pp. (74-82), ISSN 1399-3089

Brendel, M., Hering, B., Schultz, A., & Bretzel, R. (1999). International Islet Transplant Registry Report. Giessen, Germany: University of Giessen, pp. (1-20)

Buchwald, P., Margolles-Clark, E., Kenyon, NS., & Ricordi, C. (2010). Organic dyes as small molecule protein-protein interaction inhibitors of the CD40-CD154 costimulatory interaction. *Journal of Molecular Recognition*. Vol. 23, No. 1, pp. (65-73), ISSN 0952-3499

Cabric, S., Sanchez, J., Lundgren, T., Foss, A., Felldin, M., Källen, R., Salmela, K., Tibell, A., Tufveson, G., Larsson, R., Korsgren, O., & Nilsson, B. (2007). Islet surface heparinization prevents the instant blood-mediated inflammatory reaction in islet transplantation. *Diabetes*, Vol. 56, No. 8, pp. (2008-2015), ISSN 0012-1797

Cardona, K., Korbutt, GS., Milas, Z., Lyon, J., Cano, J., Jiang, W., Bello-Laborn, H., Hacquoil, B., Strobert, E., Gangappa, S., Weber, CJ., Pearson, TC., Rajotte, RV., & Larsen, CP. (2006). Long-term survival of neonatal porcine islets in nonhuman primates by targeting costimulation pathways. *Nature Medicine*, Vol. 12, No. 3, pp. (304-306), ISSN 1078-8956

Cardona, K., Milas, Z., Strobert, E., Cano, K., Jiang, W., Safely, SA., Gangappa, S., Hering, BJ., Weber, CJ., Pearson, TC., & Larsen, CP. (2007). Engraftment of adult porcine islet xenografts in diabetic nonhuman primates through targeting of costimulation pathways. *American Journal of Transplantation*, Vol. 7, No. 10, pp. (2260-2268), ISSN 1600-6135

Casu, A., Echeverri, GJ., van der Windt, DJ., He, J., Ekser, B., Ball, S., Ayares, D., & Cooper, DKC. (2010). Insulin secretion and glucose metabolism in alpha 1,3-galactosyltransferase knock-out pigs compared to wild-type pigs. *Xenotransplantation*, Vol. 17, pp. (131-139), ISSN 1399-3089

Chester, CH., Sykes, M., & Sachs, DH. (1989). Multiple mixed chimeras: reconstitution of lethally irradiated mice with syngeneic plus allogeneic bone marrow from multiple strains. *Research in Immunology*, Vol. 140, No. 5-6, pp. (503-516), ISSN 0923-2494

Cobbold, SP., Adams, E., Graca, L., Daley, S., Yates, S., Paterson, A., Robertson, NJ., Nolan, KF, Fairchild, PJ., & Waldmann, H. (2006). Immune privilege induced by regulatory T cells in transplantation tolerance. *Immunology Review*, Vol. 213, pp. (239-255), ISSN 1077-5552

De Cesaris, P., Filippini, A., Cervelli, C., Riccioli, A., Muci, S., Starace, G., Stefanini, M., & Ziparo, E. (1992). Immunosuppressive molecules produced by Sertoli cells cultured in vitro: biological effects on lymphocytes. *Biochemical and Biophysical Research Communications*, Vol. 186, No. 3, pp. (1639-1646), ISSN 1090-2104

Deschamps, J-Y, Chaillous, L., Gouin E., & Saï, P. (2000). Acceptability of pig xenografts by patients with type 1 diabetes and the general population. *Diabetes Care*, Vol. 23, pp. (412-414), ISSN 0149-5992

Deschamps, J-Y., Roux, FA., Gouin, E., & Saï, P. (2005). Reluctance of French patients with type 1 diabetes to undergo pig pancreatic islet xenotransplantation. *Xenotransplantation,* Vol. 12, pp. (175-180), ISSN 1399-3089

Dougherty, GJ. & Hogg, N. (1987). The role of monocyte lymphocyte function-associated antigen 1 (LFA-1) in accessory cell function. *European Journal of Immunology,* Vol. 17, pp. (943-947), ISSN 0014-2980

Dufour, JM., Rajotte, RV., Kin, T., & Korbutt, GS. (2003). Immunoprotection of rat islet xenografts by cotransplantation with Sertoli cells and a single injection of antilymphocyte serum. *Transplantation,* Vol. 75, No. 9, pp. (1594-1596), ISSN 0931-0509

Dufrane, D., & Gianello, P. (2009). Pig islets for clinical islet transplantation. *Current Opinion in Nephrology and Hypertension,* Vol. 18, No. 6, pp. (495-500), ISSN 1062-4821

Dufrane, D., Goebbels RM., Saliez, A., Guiot, Y., & Gianello, P. (2006). Six month survival of microencapsulated pig islets and alginate biocompatibility in primates: Proof of concept. *Xenotransplantation,* Vol. 81, pp. (1345-1353), ISSN 1399-3089

Dufrane, D., Goebbels, RM, & Gianello, P. (2010). Alginate macroencapsulation of pig islets allows correction of streptozotocin-induced diabetes in primates up to 6 months without immunosuppression. *Transplantation,* Vol. 90, pp. (1054-1062), ISSN 0931-0509

Ferguson, J. & Scothorne, RJ. (1977). Extended survival of pancreatic islet allografts in the testis of guinea pigs. *Journal of Anatomy,* Vol. 124, pp. (1-8), ISSN 0021-8782

Galili, U. & Swanson, K. (1991). Gene sequences suggest inactivation of α-1-3-galactosyltransferase in catarrhines after the divergence of apes from monkeys. *Proceedings of the National Academy of Sciences USA,*Vol. 8, No. 16, pp. (7401-7404), ISSN 0027-8424

Hagelin J. (2004). Public opinion surveys about xenotransplantation. *Xenotransplantation,* Vol. 11, No. 6, pp. (551-558), ISSN 1399-3089

Han, J., Le, H., Kwon, H., Shin, S., Yoon, J., & Jun, H. (2007). Engineered enteroendocrine cells secrete insulin in response to glucose and reverse hyperglycemia in diabetic mice. *Molecular Therapy,* Vol. 15, No. 6, pp. (1195-1202), ISSN 1525-0016

Hering, BJ., Wijkstom, M., Graham, ML., Hardstedt, M., Aasheim, TC., Jie, T., Ansite, JD., Nakano, M., Cheng, J., Moran, K., Christians, U., Finnegan, C., Mills, CD., Sutherland, DE., Bansal-Pakala, P., Murtaugh, MP., Kirchof, N., & Schuurman, HJ. (2006). Prolonged diabetes reversal after intraportal xenotransplantation of wild-type porcine islets in immunosuppressed nonhuman primates. *Nature Medicine,* Vol. 12, No. 3, pp. (301-303), ISSN 1078-8956

Hering, BJ. & Walawalkar, N. (2009). Pig-to-nonhuman primate islet xenotransplantation. *Transplant Immunology,* Vol. 21, No. 2, pp. (81-86), ISSN 0966-3274

Isaac, JR., Skinner, S., Elliot, R., Salto-Tellez, M., Garkavenko, O., Khoo, A., Lee, KO., Caine, R., & Wang, DZ. (2005). Transplantation of neonatal porcine islets and Sertoli cells into non-immunosuppressed nonhuman primates. *Transplant Proceedings,* Vol. 37, No. 1, pp. (487-488), ISSN 0041-1345

Johansson, H., Goto, M., Dufrane, D., Siegbahn, A., Elgue, G., Gianello, P., Korsgren, O., & Nilsson, B. (2006). Low molecular weight dextran sulfate: a strong candidate drug to block IBMIR in clinical islet transplantation. *American Journal of Transplantation*, Vol. 6, No. 2, pp. (305-312), ISSN 1600-6135

Kasper, DL. & Harrison, TR. (2005). Harrison's principles of internal medicine (McGraw-Hill, Medical Pub. Division, New York)

Kawai, T., Andrews, D., Colvin, RB., Sachs, DH., & Cosimi, AB. (2000). Thromboembolic complications after treatment with monoclonal antibody against CD40 ligand. *Nature Medicine*, Vol. 6, No. 2, pp. (114), ISSN 1078-8956

Kenyon, NS., Chatzipetrou, M., Masetti, M., Ranuncoli, A., Oliveria, M., Wagner, JL., Kirk, AD., Harlan, DM., Burkly, LC., & Ricordi, C. (1999). Long-term survival and function of intrahepatic islet allografts in rhesus monkeys treated with humanized anti-CD154. *Proceedings of the National Academy of Sciences USA*, Vol. 96, pp. (8132-8137), ISSN 0027-8424

Kenyon, NS., Fernandez, LA., Lehmann, R., Masetti, M., Ranuncoli, A., Chatzipetrou, M., Iaria, G., Han, D., Wagner, JL., Ruiz, P., Berho, M., Inverardi, L., Alejandro, R., Mintz, DH., Kirk, AD., Harlan, DM., Burkly, LC., & Ricordi, C. (1999). Long-term survival and function of intrahepatic islet allografts in baboons treated with humanized anti-CD154. *Diabetes*, Vol. 48, pp. (1-9), ISSN 0012-1797

Kobayashi, T., Harb, G., & Rayat, GR. (2005). Prolonged survival of microencapsulated neonatal porcine islets in mice treated with a combination of anti-CD154 and anti-LFA-1 monoclonal antibodies. *Transplantation*, Vol. 80, No. 6, pp. (821-827), ISSN 0931-0509

Kobayashi, T., Harb, G., Rajotte, RV., Korbutt, GS., Mallett, AG., Arefanian, H., Mok, D., & Rayat, GR. (2006). Immune mechanisms associated with the rejection of encapsulated neonatal porcine islet xenografts. *Xenotransplantation*, Vol. 13, No. 6, pp. 547-559, ISSN 1399-3089

Kobayashi, T., Arefanian, H., Harb, G., Tredget, EB., Rajotte, RV., Korbutt, GS., & Rayat, GR. (2008). Prolonged survival of microencapsulated neonatal porcine islet xenografts in immune-competent mice without antirejection therapy. *Cell Transplantation*, Vol. 17, No. 10-11, pp. (1243-1256), ISSN 0963-6897

Komoda, H., Miyagawa, S., Omori, T., Takahagi, Y., Murakami, H., Shigehisa, T., Ito, T., Matsuda, H., & Shirakura, R. (2005). Survival of adult islet grafts from transgenic pigs with N-acetylglucosaminyltransferase-III (GnT-III) in cynomolgus monkeys. *Xenotransplantation*, Vol. 12, pp. (209-216), ISSN 1399-3089

Korbutt, GS., Elliott, JF., Ao, Z., Smith, DK., Warnock, GL., & Rajotte, RV. (1996). Large scale isolation, growth, and function of porcine neonatal islet cells. *Journal of Clinical Investigation*, Vol. 97, No. 9, pp. (2119-2129), ISSN 0021-9738

Korsgren, O., Jansson, L., Eizirik, D., & Andersson, A. (1991). Functional and morphological differentiation of fetal porcine islet-like clusters after transplantation into nude mice. *Diabetologia*, Vol. 34, No. 6, pp. (379-386), ISSN 0012-186X

Koulmanda, M., Qipo, A., Smith, RN., & Auchincloss, H Jr. (2003). Pig islet xenografts are resistant to autoimmune destruction by NOD recipients after anti-CD4 treatment. *Xenotransplantation*, Vol. 10, No. 2, pp. (178-184), ISSN

Koulmanda, M., Laufer, TM., Auchincoss, H Jr., & Smith, RN. (2004). Prolonged survival of fetal pig islet xenografts in mice lacking the capacity for an indirect response. *Xenotransplantation*, Vol. 11, No. 6, pp. (525-530), ISSN 1399-3089

Kumagai-Braesch, M., Ekberg, H., Wang, F., Österholm, C., Ehrnfelt, C., Sharma, A., Lindeborg, E., Holgersson, J., & Corbascio, M. (2007). Anti-LFA-1 improves pig islet xenograft function in diabetic mice when long-term acceptance is induced by CTLA4Ig/Anti-CD40L. *Transplantation*, Vol. 83, pp. (1259-1267), ISSN 1534-0608

Lacy, PE., Ricordi, C., & Finke, EH. (1989). Effect of transplantation site and alpha L3T4 treatment on survival of rat, hamster, and rabbit islet xenografts in mice. *Transplantation*, Vol. 47, No. 5, pp. (761-766), ISSN 1534-0608

Lebwohl, M., Tyring, Sk., Hamilton, TK., Toth, D., Glazer, S., Tawfik, NH., Walicke, P., Dummer, W., Wang, X., Garovoy, MR., & Pariser, D: Efalizumab Study Group. (2003). A novel targeted T-cell modulator, efalizumab, for plaque psoriasis. *New England Journal of Medicine*, Vol. 349, pp. (2004-2013), ISSN 0028-4793

Marchetti, P., Giannarelli, R., Cosmi, S., Masiello, P., Coppelli, A., Viacava, P., & Navalesi, R. (1995). Massive isolation, morphological and functional characterization, and xenotransplantation of bovine pancreatic islets. *Diabetes*, Vol. 44, pp. (375-381), ISSN 0012-1797

Margolles-Clark, E., Umland, O., Kenyon, NS., Ricordi, C., & Buchwald, P. (2009). Small-molecule co-stimulatory blockade: organic dye inhibitors of the CD40-CD154 interaction. *Journal of Molecular Medicine*, Vol. 87, No. 11, pp. (1133-1143), ISSN 0946-2716

Margolles-Clark, E., Kenyon, NS., Ricordi, C., & Buchwald, P. (2010). Effective and specific inhibition of the CD40-CD154 co-stimulatory interaction by a napthalenesulphonic acid derivative. *Chemical Biology and Drug Design*, Vol. 76, No. 4, pp. (305-313), ISSN 1747-0277

Mihalicz, D., Bayrack, K., Alavi, F., Le, C., Buchwald, P., Williams, D., Rajotte RV., & Rayat, GR. (2011) The potential of novel organic dyes to prevent the rejection of porcine islets in mice. (Abstract) Canadian Society of Transplantation, 2011 Annual Scientific Meeting (Mont-Tremblant, Quebec, Canada, March 2-5, 2011)

Minkowski, O. (1894). Weitere Mitteilungen uber den diabetes mellitus nach extirpation des pancreas. *British Medical Journal*, Vol. 2, pp. (1303-1304), ISSN 0959-8138

Mirabet, M., Barrabes, JA., Quiroga, A. & Garcia-Dorado, D. (2008). Platelet pro-aggregatory effects of CD40L monoclonal antibody. *Molecular Immunology*, Vol. 45, No. 4, pp. (937-944), ISSN 0161-5890

Moberg L. (2005). The role of the innate immunity in islet transplantation. *Upsala Journal of Medical Sciences*, Vol. 110, pp. (17-55), ISSN 0300-9734

Muller, YD., Golshayan, D., Ehirchiou, D., Wekerle, T., Seebach, JD., & Buhler, LH. (2009). T regulatory cells in xenotransplantation. *Xenotransplantation*, Vol. 16, No. 3, pp. (121-128), ISSN 1399-3089

Nicolls, MR., Coulombe, M., Yang, H., Bolwerk, A. & Gill, RG. (2000). Anti-LFA-1 therapy induces long-term islet allograft acceptance in the absence of IFN-γ or IL-4. *The Journal of Immunology*, Vol. 164, pp. (3627-3634), ISSN 0022-1767

Nilsson, B. (2008). The instant blood-mediated inflammatory reaction in xenogeneic islet transplantation. *Xenotransplantation,* Vol. 15, No. 2, pp. (96-98), ISSN 1399-3089

Nyqvist, D., Koehler, M., Wahlstedt, H., & Berggren, PO. (2005). Donor islet endothelial cells participate in formation of functional vessels within pancreatic islet grafts. *Diabetes,* Vol. 54, No. 8, pp. (2287-2293), ISSN 0012-1797

Persson, MO., Persson, NH., Ranstam, J., & Hermerén, G. (2003). Xenotransplantation public opinion perceptions: rather cells than organs. *Xenotransplantation,* Vol. 10, pp. (72-79), ISSN 1399-3089

Posselt, AM., Bellin, MD., Tavakol, M., Szot, GL., Frassetto, LA., Masharani, U., Kerlan, RK., Fong, L., Vincenti, FG., Hering, BJ., Bluestone, JA., & Stock, PG. (2010). Islet transplantation in type 1 diabetics using an immunosuppressive protocol based on the anti-LFA-1 antibody Efalizumab. *American Journal of Transplantation,* Vol. 10, No. 8, pp. (1870-1880), ISSN 1600-6135

Poston, RS., Robbins, RC., Chan, B., Simms, P., Presta, L., Jardieu, P., & Morris, RE. (2000). Effects of humanized monoclonal antibody to rhesus CD11a in rhesus monkey cardiac allograft recipients. *Transplantation,* Vol. 69, No. 10, pp. (2005-2013), ISSN 0963-6897

Ramji, Q., Arefanian, H., Rajotte, RV., & Rayat, GR. (2010). Short-term administration of a monoclonal antibody therapy is effective in preventing islet xenograft rejection when islets are co-transplanted with Sertoli cells. (Abstract) 10th Annual Rachmiel Levine Symposium for Diabetes and Obesity (Las Vegas, Nevada, USA, March 14-17, 2010)

Rayat, GR., Rajotte, RV., Elliott, JF., & Korbutt, GS. (1998). Expression of Galα(1,3)Gal on neonatal porcine islet beta cells and susceptibility to human-complement lysis. *Diabetes,* Vol. 47, pp. (1406-1411), ISSN 0012-1797

Rayat, GR., Rajotte, RV., & Korbutt, GS. (1999). Potential application of neonatal porcine islets as treatment for type 1 diabetes: A review. *Annals of the New York Academy of Sciences,* Vol. 875, pp. (175-188), ISSN 0077-8923

Rayat, GR., Rajotte, RV., Ao, Z., & Korbutt, GS. (2000). Microencapsulation of neonatal porcine islets: protection from human antibody/complement-mediated cytolysis in vitro and long-term reversal of diabetes in nude mice. *Transplantation,* Vol. 69, No. 6, pp. (1084-1090), ISSN 0963-6897

Rayat ,GR., Rajotte, RV., Hering, BJ., Binette, TM., & Korbutt, GS. (2003). In vitro and in vivo expression of Galα(1,3)Gal on porcine islet cells is age-dependent. *Journal of Endocrinology,* Vol. 177, pp. (127-135), ISSN 0022-0795

Rayat, GR. & Gill, RG. (2003). Pancreatic islet xenotransplantation: Barriers and prospects. *Transplantation,* Vol. 3, No. 4, pp. (336-343), ISSN 0963-6897

Rayat, GR., Johnson, ZA., Beilke, JN., Korbutt, GS., Rajotte, RV., & Gill, RG. (2003). The degree of phylogenetic disparity of islet grafts dictates the reliance on indirect CD4 T-cell antigen recognition for rejection. *Diabetes,* Vol. 52, No. 6, pp. (1433-1440), ISSN 0012-1797

Rayat, GR. & Gill, RG. (2005). Indefinite survival of neonatal porcine islet xenografts by simultaneous targeting of LFA-1 and CD-154 or CD45RB. *Diabetes,* Vol. 54, No. 2, pp. (443-451), ISSN 0012-1797

Ricordi, C., Socci, C., Davalli, AM., Staudacher, C., Baro, P., Vertova, A., Sassi, I., Gavazzi, F., Pozza, G., & Di Carlo, V. (1990). Isolation of the elusive pig islet. *Surgery*, Vol. 107, No. 6, pp. (688-694), ISSN 1530-0358

Ríos, A., Martìnez-Alarcón, MA., Ayala-García, MJ., Sebastián, A., Abdo-Cuza, A., López-Navas, A., López-López, A., Ramírez, EJ., Muñoz, G., Camacho, A., Suárez-López, J., Castellanos, R., Rodríguez, JS., Martínez, MA., Nieto, A., Ramis, G., Ramírez, P., & Parrilla, P. (2010). Level of acceptance of a clinical solid organ xenotransplantation program among personnel in organ transplant-related services in Spanish, Mexican, and Cuban hospital centers. *Transplantation Proceedings,* Vol. 42, pp. (222-227), ISSN 0041-1345

Risbund, MV., Hardikar, A., & Bhonde, R. (2000). Chitosan-polyvinyl pyrrolidone hydrogels as candidate for islet immunoisolation: in vitro biocompatibility studies. *Cell Transplantation,* Vol. 9, No.1, pp. (25-31), ISSN 0963-6897

Risbund, MV. & Bhonde, RR. (2001). Suitability of cellulose molecular dialysis membrane for bioartificial pancreas: in vitro biocompatibility studies. *Journal of Biomedical Materials Research,* Vol. 54, No. 3, pp. (436-444), ISSN 1552-4965

Rood, PP., Bottino, R., Balamurugan, AN., Smetanka, C., Ayares, D., Groth, CC., Murase, N., Cooper, DKC. & Trucco, M. (2007). Reduction of early graft loss after intraportal porcine islet transplantation in monkeys. *Transplantation,* Vol. 83, No. 2, pp. (202-210), ISSN 0963-6897

Seijkens, T., Engel, D., Tjwa, M., & Lutgens, E. (2010). The role of CD154 in hematopoietic development. *Journal of Thrombosis and Haemostasis,* Vol. 104, No. 4, pp. 693-701, ISSN 1538-7933

Smith, RM. & Mandel, TE. (2000). Pancreatic islet xenotransplantation: the potential for tolerance induction. *Immunology Today*, Vol. 21, No. 1, pp. (42-47), ISSN 0167-4919

Streilein, JW. (1995). Unraveling immune privilege. *Science,* Vol. 270, pp. (1158-1159), ISSN 0036-8075

Sykes M, Cozzi, E., d'Apice, A., Pierson, R., O'Connell, P., Cowan, P., Dorling, A., Hering, B., Leventhal, J., Rees, M., & Sandrin, M. (2006). Clinical trial of islet xenotransplantation in Mexico. *Xenotransplantation*, Vol. 13, No. 5, pp. (371-372), ISSN 1399-3089

Sun, Y., Ma, X., Zhou, D., Vacek, I., & Sun, A. (1996). Normalization of diabetes in spontaneously diabetic cynomolgus monkeys by xenografts of microencapsulated porcine islets without immunosuppression. *Journal of Clinical Investigation,* Vol. 98, No. 6, pp. (1417-1422), ISSN 0021-9738

Tredget, EB., Arefanian, H., Gill, RG., Rajotte, RV., & Rayat, GR. (2008). Monotherapy with anti-LFA-1 monoclonal antibody promotes long-term survival of rat islet xenografts. *Cell Transplantation*, Vol. 17, No. 6, pp. (599-608), ISSN 0963-6897

Turgeon, NA., Avila, JG., Cano, JA., Hutchinson, JJ., Badell, IR., Page, AJ., Adams, AB., Sears, MH., Bowen, PH., Kirk, AD., Pearson, TC., & Larsen, CP. (2010). Experience with a novel Efalizumab-based immunosuppressive regimen to facilitate single donor islet cell transplantation. *American Journal of Transplantation,* Vol. 10, pp. (2082-2091), ISSN 1600-6135

Valdes-Gonzales, RA., Dorantes LM, Garibay, GN., Bracho-Blanchet, E., Mendez, AJ, Davila-Perez, R., Elliott, RB., Teran, L. & White, DJG. (2005). Xenotransplantation of porcine neonatal islets of Langerhans and Sertoli cells: a 4-year study. *European Journal of Endocrinology*, Vol. 153, No. 3, pp. (419-427), ISSN 0804-4643

Van der Windt, DJ., Bottino, R., Casu, A., Campanile, N., & Cooper, DKC. (2007). Rapid loss of intraportally transplanted islets: an overview of pathophysiology and preventive strategies. *Xenotransplantation,* Vol. 14, No. 4, pp. (288-297), ISSN 1399-3089

Van der Windt, DJ., Bottino, R., Casu, A., Campanile, N., Smetanka, C., He, J., Murase, N., Hara, H., Ball, S., Loveland, BE., Ayares, D., Lakkis, FG., Cooper, DKC., & Trucco, M. (2009). Long-term controlled normoglycemia in diabetic non-human primates after transplantation with hCD46 transgenic porcine islets. *American Journal of Transplantation,* Vol. 9, pp. (2716-2726), ISSN 1600-6135

Vincenti, F., Mendez, R., Pescovitz, M., Rajagopalan, PR., Wilkinson, AH., Butt, K., Laskow, D., Slakey, DP., Lorber MI., Garg, JP., & Garovoy, M. (2007). A phase I/II randomized open-label multicenter trial of efalizumab, a humanized anti-CD11a, anti-LFA-1 in renal transplantation. *American Journal of Transplantation,* Vol. 7, No. 7, pp. (1770-1777), ISSN 1600-6135

Von Mering J, MO. (1889). *Archives of Experimental Pathology and Pharmakology,* Vol. 26, pp. 371 , ISSN 0365-2009

Wang, DZ., Skinner, S., Elliot, R., Escobar, L., Salto-Tellez, M., Garkavenko, O., Khoo, A., Lee, KO., Calne, R., & Isaac, JR. (2005). Xenotransplantation of neonatal porcine islets and Sertoli cells into immunosuppressed streptozotocin-induced diabetic rats. *Transplantation Proceedings*, Vol. 37, No. 1, pp. (470-471), ISSN 0041-1345

Warnock, GL., Kneteman, NM., Ryan, EA., Evans, MG., Seelis, REA., Halloran, PF., Rabinovitch, A., & Rajotte, RV. (1989). Continued function of pancreatic islets after transplantation in type 1 diabetics. *The Lancet*, Vol. 334, No. 8662, pp. (570-572), ISSN 0140-6736

Warnock, GL., Kneteman, NM., Ryan, EA., Rabinovitch, A., & Rajotte, RV. (1992). Long-term follow-up after transplantation of insulin-producing pancreatic islets into patients with type 1 (insulin-dependent) diabetes mellitus. *Diabetologia*, Vol. 35, No. 1, pp. (89-95), ISSN 0012-186X

Williams, P. (1894). Notes on diabetes treated with extract and by grafts of sheep's pancreas. *British Medical Journal,* Vol. 2, pp. (1303- 1304), ISSN 0959-8138

Wright, JR., Polvi, S., & MacLean, S. (1992). Experimental transplantation with principal islets of teleost fish (Brockman bodies). Long-term function of tilapia islet tissue in diabetic nude mice. *Diabetes*, Vol. 41, No. 12, pp. (1528-1532), ISSN 0012-1797

Yamanda, K., Sachs, DH., & DerSimonian, H. (1995). Human anti-porcine xenogeneic T cell response. Evidence for allelic specificity of mixed leukocyte reaction and for both direct and indirect pathways of recognition. *Journal of Immunology*, Vol. 155, pp. (5249-5256), ISSN 0022-1767

Zeng, Y., Ildstad, ST., Wren, SM., Rilo, HLR., Bereiter, DR., Carroll, PB., Tzakis, AG., Starzl, TE. & Ricordi, C. (1992). Long-term survival of donor-specific pancreatic islet xenografts in fully xenogeneic chimeras. *Transplantation Proceedings,* Vol. 24, No. 3, pp. (985), ISSN 0041-1345

Zhang, C., Wang, M., Rcine, JJ., Liu, H., Lin, C., Nair, I., Lau, J., Cao, Y., Todorov, I., Atkinson, M., & Zeng, D. (2010). Induction of chimerism permits low-dose islet grafts in the liver or pancreas to reverse refractory autoimmune diabetes. *Diabetes*, Vol. 59, pp. (2228-2236), ISSN 0012-1797

Beta Cell Replacement Therapy

Jeffrey A. SoRelle and Bashoo Naziruddin
Institute of Biomedical Studies, Baylor University, Waco, Texas
and Baylor University Medical Center, Dallas, Texas
United States of America

1. Introduction

Type 1 Diabetes mellitus (T1D) is an autoimmune disorder caused by destruction of pancreatic beta cells which produce insulin. Current estimates have shown that T1D affects about 0.4 to 0.8% of the population worldwide accounting for 5-10% of all diabetes cases (Stock and Bluestone, 2004). It is seen as an increasing health hazard. For T1D, exogenous insulin administration is the most widely used treatment. However, this treatment has several limitations including development of secondary health complications over time. There are several approaches already in practice to replace the damaged beta cells in T1D. They include whole organ pancreas or isolated islet cell transplantation. Several novel approaches are currently in development such as expansion of adult beta cells and stem/progenitor cells which can be transformed into beta cells. This review summarizes recent progress made in beta cell replacement therapy for T1D. Diabetes mellitus has been known for thousands of years. Diabetes comes from an ancient Greek word coined by Arataeus of Cappadocia, and mellitus from the Latin word honey associated with sweet urine. (Medvei, 1993).

The pathogenesis of T1D has been attributed to an autoimmune response. Currently the mechanism that triggers this disease is still unknown, but it seems to be a combination of environmental and genetic factors. T-cells in the host's body become sensitized to protein that naturally occurs in the beta cells of the pancreas and the immune system begins to mount a specific attack leading to destruction of the islets of Langerhans. Several candidate proteins have been identified including GAD65, insulin, and ZnT8 (Harlan et al., 2009, Shapiro et al., 2003). Reducing the autoimmune effect in beta cell replacement is very important, but before moving onto the strategies for beta cell replacement therapy it is important to describe the standard therapy for T1D and how it falls short of providing for all the needs of diabetic patients.

Exogenous insulin therapy continues to be the leading therapy for T1D today, but there are several complications associated with it. However, even intensive monitoring of blood glucose and injection of insulin is not enough to halt the secondary complications of diabetes (Harlan et al., 2009). Diabetes mellitus can decrease patients' lifespan, especially in severe cases. Lowered blood sugar levels, which can result if too much insulin is administered, can also lead to a hypoglycemic episode (Cooke and Plotnick, 2008). These episodes are typified by ketoacidosis, where in an effort to find energy, the body burns fatty acids leading to the production of acidic ketones that can be detected by an alcoholic smell on the breath. Hypoglycemic episodes can lead to coma and even death, and is considered the most severe side effect of diabetes. Secondary complications such as blindness, peripheral neuropathy, and cardiovascular complications result from destruction of microvasculature. Additionally, the quality of life is lower even for patients with well regulated blood sugar.

There are several methods both clinical and experimental that are being developed to provide optimal beta cell replacement. The first type that was developed and successfully applied to the clinical setting was that of whole organ pancreas transplant (WOP). Next, in an effort to transplant only the insulin secreting portion of the pancreas, islet transplantation was explored and has been applied through several clinical trials. Efforts have been made to improve this technique by perfecting the techniques of islet isolation and immunosuppression; immunoisolation and xenotransplantation are also being explored. However, even if all donor human pancreases were effectively used, they would be insufficient to treat every patient eligible for transplant. This emphasizes the importance of current studies into beta cell regeneration from many sources including embryonic stem cells, and pancreatic ductal and acinar cells.

2. Pancreas transplantation

Transplantation of whole allogenic pancreas is an established procedure. The first clinical transplant of a whole vascularized pancreas was at the University of Minnesota in 1966. Initial results showed very poor graft survival rates; less than 5% of grafts survived after six months. Important advances were made in surgical technique and post-transplant monitoring. Because the pancreas is a very large, immunogenic organ, large doses of immunosuppressants are required to prevent rejection. Immunosuppression protocols had to be adjusted to prevent graft rejection while not being so strong as to damage the beta cells. However, the addition of mycophenolate mofetil and tacrolimus to regimens suppressing the immune system dramatically increased the success of whole pancreas transplant from 20% to 80% survival after one year. One important stepping stone in anti-rejection therapy was the elimination of steroids. The addition of sirolimus, an immunosuppressant lacking nephrotoxic or beta cell toxic properties, along with an antilymphocyte antibody induction allowed the discontinuation of steroids from maintenance therapy. This immune therapy led to a low rejection rate of pancreas. Three year survival rate, defined as insulin independence, is around 80% according to the International Pancreas Transplant Registry (Gruessner, 2001).

Transplanting a whole pancreas simultaneously or after a kidney transplant has provided significant improvement in patients. Since diabetes affects the function of the renal system, many patients will have a history of dialysis. Such an issue would call for a kidney transplant, and since this would already require a surgical procedure and immunosuppression, adding a pancreas transplant in a simultaneous fashion could prove beneficial (Humar et al., 2000). In fact, the development of secondary complications is attenuated by an allogenic pancreas transplant. Further, the progression of nephropathy is decreased from diabetic effects with the simultaneous transplant of a pancreas and kidney. There also appears to be improvements to the quality of life and in the damage to the peripheral nerve system (Venstrom et al., 2003).

Although transplant of whole allogenic pancreases offers the above advantages, it comes with the serious complications associated with surgery. A study by the Univeristy of Pennsylvania (Frank et al., 2004) compared 30 whole pancreas and 27 isolated islet transplants. This investigation showed that 7 patients (23%) required post-transplant surgery while only 1 islet recipient (7%) needed surgery. There was a significant difference in the number of patients requiring blood transfusions post-transplant from whole pancreas (43%) versus islet transplant (7%). The main reason that would account for the differences in surgical complications can be attributed to the invasiveness of the whole pancreas transplant versus the relatively non-invasive islet transplant, which is performed by percutaneous puncture and infusion into the portal vein of the liver. Thus long hospital stays are required of whole pancreas transplant cases whereas islet transplantation is an outpatient procedure leading to a lower estimated cost. Despite the lower surgical risk and cost of islet transplantation it has not yet achieved the duration or rate of graft success found in whole pancreas transplantation.

An issue for beta cell replacement is the low number of donors compared to the number of eligible recipients (Matsumoto et al., 2006). In the United States, there are an estimated 7,000 available donor pancreases, but the number of pancreases available for clinical transplant are much lower due to many exclusion criteria. For whole organ transplant, young donors (<50 years old), with low BMI are preferred. Although the islets received from young donors are suggested to display greater functionality, it is very difficult to effectively isolate a sufficient number of islets for transplant from these donors. Also, obese donor pancreases are associated with higher surgical complication rates. Conversely, isolations from pancreata from older, obese (BMI>30) donors produce higher yields of islets that are still functional and qualify for clinical transplant. Thus islet transplant has the ability to utilize marginally acceptable pancreases for clinical transplant, increasing the ability to perform beta cell replacement. These non-overlapping criteria for whole organ and islet isolation reinforce the notion that these two treatments are not competitive, but rather complementary.

The important advances and improvements of whole organ pancreas transplant over the past two decades have given significant momentum to this method of beta cell replacement in patients with life-threatening diabetes. Although the one year rejection rate is higher at 8% for solitary pancreas transplant in preuremic patients than the rejection rate of 2% seen in persons receiving simultaneous pancreas and kidney transplants, the increased success of the procedure still warrants its application (Gruessner, 2001). However, this treatment is still limited to patients with brittle diabetes experiencing uncontrolled blood glucose levels and hypoglycemic unawareness despite intensive insulin therapy. The risk of morbidity, the need to open the abdominal cavity during surgery, and the strong immunosuppressive regimen required for solid organ transplant substantiates a long, hard look at alternative methods of beta cell replacement.

3. Islet cell transplantation

The transplantation of pancreatic islets of Langerhans is an exciting alternative, because it reduces the surgical risk of complication by being less invasive (Frank et al., 2004). Furthermore, transplanting only the functional, insulin secreting portion of the pancreas reduces the risk of activating the exocrine, digestive portion of the pancreas, which could lead to deterioration of endocrine function.

Islet transplantation also provides several other exciting possibilities. One such possibility is the ability to manipulate islets prior to implantation to protect them from the immune system or to attach biologically active molecules that could aid in engraftment. Beta cell regeneration by embryonic or adult stem cells also provides the possibility of a large population of renewable insulin secreting cells, but the risk of neoplasm formation still remains a potential issue (Borowiak & Melton, 2009; Ricordi & Edlund, 2008). Xenogenic, porcine islets could also fill the gap between beta cell supply and demand (Hering & Walawalkar, 2009). Each of these methods contains complicating factors that do not allow current application to the clinical setting, but recent advances have put them closer in reach than ever before.

A comparison of the historical progress of whole organ transplant to that of islet transplantation would provide an objective basis to evaluate the progress of islet transplantation. Although whole organ treatment achieved high levels of graft survival in the years 1994-1997, the islet survival rate at five years has reached around fifty percent in 2010-2011, comparable to the level of whole pancreas graft success (Rickels et al, 2011). From this perspective, islet transplantation is not inferior to pancreas organ transplantation, though it may not have reached its full potential yet.

In the past decade since the publication of the Edmonton Protocol (Shapiro et al., 2000), there have been many advances in the field of islet transplantation, primarily in the area of islet isolation technique and immunosuppression therapy. Breakthroughs have been made in the area of pancreas procurement and preservation with study into ductal preservation, the two layer method, and the type of preservation solution used. Furthermore, there has been much progress in the islet isolation process by bringing standards up to cGMP qualifications, optimization of collagenase enzymes, and using iodixanol for continuous density gradient purification (Matsumoto et al., 2009). With the introduction of thymoglobulin at induction phase and the combination of prograf and mycophenolate mofitil as maintenance immunosuppressive agents, the islet transplant survival rate has significantly improved recently.

3.1 Pancreas preservation and islet isolation

The islet isolation process is fundamental to islet transplantation. The main stages in isolation are pancreas procurement and preservation, digestion of the organ, and purification of the islets. First, the pancreas is obtained from the organ procurement organization, prepared with certain preservation solutions and injections as described later. Upon arrival at the isolation facility, the pancreas is disinfected and injected with a digestion enzyme that degrades the pancreas and releases islets. Lastly, the mixture of pancreatic tissue is centrifuged with a density gradient to separate the endocrine tissue from the exocrine tissue. Within each of these procedures are detailed methodologies that have been explored to improve both islet yield and function.

3.1.1 cGMP facility

One major requirement for islet cell preparations and isolations is that it should be performed under current good manufacturing practices (cGMP). An important requirement of cGMP facilities is the validation and sterilization of all equipment (Garfinkel et al., 2004). Although initially assumed to increase the cost of establishing an islet isolation program, the guidelines of cGMP ensure the efforts of improving safety of islet preparations. Documentation of errors, corrective measures, and preventative actions minimize costs and provides the ability to critically evaluate the impact of certain actions. Validation of instruments prevents false bias readings, and validation of processes indicates whether assumptions about the production are correct or not (Yamamoto et al., 2009).

Documentation not only proves the correctness of the manufacturing, but also provides data for scientific reports. However, some of these requirements still can create a large amount of work.

3.1.2 Pancreas preservation

In the area of organ preservation, damage due to low oxygenation and warm ischemia are important hurdles to overcome. Warm ischemia is the time between the cessation of a heart beat in a donor's body and when cold preservation solutions can be injected. Ischemia is the loss of blood circulation to an organ that consequently causes a lack of oxygen, glucose, and other helpful molecules in the blood. In general, warm ischemia times greater than fifteen minutes cause pancreases to be of marginal quality and times exceeding thirty minutes usually disqualifies the organ for transplantation. Significant amounts of damage are incurred to the pancreas and islets during warm ischemia time, but cold ischemia time should also be limited as much as possible. Cold ischemia time is incurred during procurement and transportation of the organ, and should be lower than twelve hours. In addition to ischemic injury, there is also the danger of hypoxic damage from low oxygenation conditions (Sawada et al., 2003). Following procurement, donor pancreases were initially preserved in University of Wisconsin solution (UW) or Histidine-Tryptophan-Ketoglutarate solution (HTK). Although these solutions are standard for tissue preservation of other organs, other preservation methods were attempted to improve the results of islet isolation. The two layer method and ductal preservation have emerged as two techniques that preserve the pancreas while leading to increased islet yield and quality from isolation.

The advent of perfluorocarbon as an excellent oxygen carrier led to significant improvements in reducing hypoxic damage. Perfluorocarbon (PFC) is a hydrocarbon derived chemical where all of the hydrogens of a carbon chain are replaced by fluorine atoms. The uniform covering of fluorines prevents polarization of the electron clouds, which explains the low van der Waals forces and non-polar nature of the molecule (Lamal, 2004). The property of PFC that makes it particularly attractive as an organ preservation and oxygenation solution is the capacity to dissolve large amounts of oxygen. This high dissolving power of PFC combined with a low oxygen binding constant, due to low intermolecular forces, allows PFC to release oxygen more effectively than hemoglobin (F2 Chemicals Ltd., 2003).

The Two-Layer Method (TLM) involves placing PFC, which is almost twice as dense as water, beneath the UW/HTK solution and oxygenating the solution before adding a procured pancreas. The addition of a water based preservation solution above the PFC solution prevented the loss of dissolved oxygen (Matsumoto & Kuroda, 2002). The distinction between the static and original TLM is that the original method provides continuous oxygen supplied to the PFC, while static method precharges the PFC with oxygen before the organ is added. Cold ischemia time for human pancreata can be extended up to thirteen hours using TLM. Islet yield, viability, and functionality were significantly improved by both two-layer methods compared to UW solution alone. The human islet isolations with the two layer methods yielded about twice as many islets (2,659 ± 549 IEQ/g in the static TLM, 2,244 ± 557 IEQ/g in the original TLM) compared to the UW method (1,293 ± 451 IEQ/g). This study showed that the islet yield, viability, and *in-vitro* function were significantly improved by both TLM approaches with similar results. Since the static

TLM is easier and yields comparable results as the original method it has subsequently attained widespread use in clinical studies. In contrast, a larger study comparing the effectiveness of TLM vs preservation in UW solution alone reported no significant advantage in using TLM method (Caballero-Corbalan et al., 2007)

Although this TLM is effective at oxygenating the pancreas, the organ is still a thick tissue with inner, non-accessed parts being exposed to a higher risk of damage. It has been hypothesized that the ductal system is thus especially susceptible to cold ischemic injury. This could result in the inability to properly perfuse collagenase (an essential reagent discussed later) by intraductal distention. By injecting cold preservation solution in the opposite direction through the main pancreatic duct, a majority of the inner spaces of the pancreas can be reached, preserving a greater number of islets for isolation, and allowing greater distention of the organ during collagenase injection (Matsumoto et al., 2002). Functionality results for islets isolated from pancreata receiving ductal injections of cold preservation solution were evaluated by an *in-vivo* assay, insulin secretion, and by viability testing. Ductal preservation significantly reduced the number of nonviable cells from around sixty percent to lower than twenty percent. Using this method, the insulin secretion ability of islets was also improved. The best determinant of islet quality is the *in-vivo* assay, which involves the transplantation of isolated islets under the kidney capsule of a diabetic nude mouse. This further confirmed that islets not preserved with ductal injection could not cure diabetic mice in any of the cases, whereas islets from pancreata perfused with UW solution showed a similar curative rate compared to islets from a fresh pancreas (Sawada et al., 2003).

Protecting the pancreas from ischemic damage between procurement and processing is an important aspect of islet isolation. Although islets only constitute about 2-5% of the total pancreatic mass, they use over 10% of the organ's blood supply. Therefore, sufficient oxygenation is important for islet function. Previous studies performed have demonstrated the ability of the two layer method and ductal preservation to yield higher numbers of improved quality islets.

3.1.3 Collagenase

Pancreas digestion is performed by injection of collagenase enzyme that cleaves the basic connective tissue. Successful human islet isolations hinge upon the quality of the collagenase used, which is the blade that cuts islets from the pancreas providing isolated islets. The types of collagenase traditionally used are derived from *Clostridium histolyticum* (Linetsky et al., 1997). Liberase HI is a blend of purified collagenases and protease that showed significantly higher islet yields when compared to crude collagenase extracts (Linetsky et al., 1997, Olack et al., 1999). Liberase HI provided the advantage of not only higher islet yields compared to crude collagenase, but also a reduction in contaminating enzymes and endotoxin. Despite these advantages, Liberase HI appeared to have inconsistencies between lots, and exhibited poor storage stability (Barnett et al., 2005). This enzyme blend further fell out of favor, because animal products such as bovine brain extract were used in the manufacturing process (Shimoda et al., 2010). Many centers turned to NB-1 collagenase products (SERVA/Nordmark) in order to avoid the potential safety risks (Bucher et al., 2005, Shimoda et al., 2010). Results from many centers that used this enzyme are mixed in terms of generating islet yields and quality similar to those achieved by Liberase HI (Barnett et al., 2005; Yamamoto, 2007).

To show the further usefulness of an optimal collagenase, human pancreas isolations were performed by Balamurugan et al., (2010) with collagenase from VitaCyte (n=28) and Serva/Nordmark (n=30). The results of these isolations show that VIzyme produced significantly higher yields of islets. The final islet equivalent (IEQ) per gram of pancreas for VitaCyte enzyme versus Serva's enzyme was 414,700±175,900 versus 213,400±152,400 with a p value of 0.002. Islet equivalent (IEQ) is the standard unit of measurement of islets and corresponds to a round islet with a diameter of 150 micrometers. From these isolation results, six clinical islet transplantations were performed. Two patients received islets isolated from Serva's NB-1; one patient achieved normoglycemia for over 700 days and the other had evidence of graft failure on day 84. Of four patients transplanted with islets isolated using collagenase from VitaCyte, three were insulin independent for more than 350 days. Although this clinical data is not conclusive, it does demonstrate that the utilization of VIzyme in islet isolation may prove beneficial to increasing islet yields. Further independent studies are warranted to validate such claims.

3.1.4 Purification

The final stage in the islet isolation process is purification to separate functional islets, from the contaminating acinar cells. The positive aspect of this process is a higher purity of islets to transplant; also the packed cell volume will be lower, decreasing the risk of an embolism or other risks associated with the islet infusion process.

This separation process takes advantage of the different densities of acinar and islet cells, with acinar tissue being more dense than islets. However, one disadvantage is that the islet post-purification recovery is mostly decreased. The traditional gold standard for this process was the use of Ficoll, a heavy, multi-branched sugar that readily dissolves in water, based density gradient combined with semiautomated centrifugation with a COBE-2991 cell processor to achieve optimal results (Matsumoto et al., 2006). The centrifugation process can be mechanically stressful and damaging to islets; further the exposure to enzyme and endotoxin in the isolation can lead to apoptosis, inflammation, and attack by the immune system post-transplant. An alternative density solution, iodixanol, is a neutral iso-osmotic contrast solution used clinically in the imaging field. Iodixanol's effect on the purification was studied along with the production of pro-inflammatory cytokines after islet isolation (Mita et al., 2010). Islets purified by iodixanol-based gradients yielded significantly lower levels of cytokines and chemokines when compared to Ficoll-based gradient solutions. The inflammatory molecules that were downregulated include interleukin-1 beta (IL-1β), tumor necrosis factor-alpha (TNF-α), interferon-gamma (IFN-γ), IL-6, IL-8, macrophage inflammatory protein 1beta(MIP-1β), and monocyte chemoattractant-1 (MCP-1). These cytokines are known to not only be pro-inflammatory, but some are also associated with apoptosis and necrosis. These results provide compelling data that iodixanol has a protective effect on islet preparations when used in density gradient purifications. Furthermore, Hering et al. (2005) have reported that islet preparations purified using iodixanol-based gradients were able to cure eight patients with a single transplantation.

In the Edmonton protocol (2000), islets were transplanted immediately after isolation, without a period of culturing. Although this may cause attrition of islets, some argue that the culture period allows damaged ineffective islets to die off while permitting enough time for functional testing of islets prior to transplantation. Further, the culturing period could be used to pretreat the recipient or the islets themselves.

The culture of islets up to 48 hours pre-transplant has gained some popularity for several reasons. This culture time allows depletion of apoptotic islets and testing for sterility, microbiology, viability, and *in vitro* glucose stimulated insulin secretion response. The patient does not have to be rushed into a radiology suite to receive the infusion, but this time could allow for the start of an immune cell depleting induction therapy.

Thus, the advances made in the area of islet isolation have been substantial over the past decade. The standardization to cGMP facilities, preservation with the two layer method and ductal injection method have all improved the preparative conditions for conducting an isolation. The optimization of the collagenase solution continues to improve islet yields after pancreatic digestion. By currently using iodixanol based density gradient solutions, the risk of apoptotic islet damage both after isolation and after transplantation has been reduced by the lowering of inflammatory cytokines. These improvements have led to higher yields and islets with greater functionality, which provides transplant recipients a greater chance at achieving insulin independence.

3.2 Advances in immunosuppression to prevent islet graft rejection

Although it is difficult to obtain islet preparations of an adequate quantity and quality for transplantation, it is also very difficult to protect and maintain the allogenic islet function after transplantation. There are several aspects of the immune system that prevent the long term survival of islet cells. The first reaction encountered by islets is the instant blood mediated inflammatory response (IBMIR), primarily mediated by the innate immune system which leads to islet destruction (Bennett et al., 1999). Islets surviving this initial, short term inflammatory response are later subjected to targeting of autoimmune and alloimmune responses. The alloimmune response is primarily directed against mismatched HLA. The autoimmune response which already exists in type 1 diabetic recipients, being the source of the pathogenesis of the disease and is specifically reactive to beta cell markers such as glutamic acid decarboxylase (GAD65) and islet cell antigen (ICA) (Shapiro et al., 2003). Immunosuppressive regimens for islet cell transplant recipients must counter these aspects of the whole immune response for improved graft survival.

Immunosuppression after islet transplantation is comprised of two phases namely induction and maintenance therapies. The induction phase is characterized by anti-inflammatory drugs and monoclonal or polyclonal antibodies that deplete immune cells (anti-CD3 and anti-thymocyte globulin) or prevent T-cell activation (anti-IL-2 receptor) (Stock & Bluestone, 2004; Matsumoto et al., 2011). The maintenance drug regimen is focused on suppression of T-cells by various strategies including calcineurin inhibitors such as tacrolimus, and cyclosporine. Other drugs such as mycophenolate mofetil (MMF) have also been used with good outcomes.

In the early days of islet transplantation, drugs administered to counter the immune system were found to be toxic to islet cells (Stock & Bluestone, 2004). Beta cells naturally have lower levels of anti-oxidant enzymes, which put them at an increased risk. Further, the hepatic graft site puts islets in contact with blood that has higher concentrations of the immunosuppressive drugs, increasing any negative side effects. The advent of the Edmonton protocol demonstrated successful islet transplantations, with a part of the accomplishment being attributed to minimizing calcineurin inhibitors and a steroid-free induction process.

3.2.1 Induction therapy

The first stage of treatment for islet transplantation is the induction therapy that attempts to reduce the inflammatory effects of the short term immune system. It has been estimated that during the initial phase after transplant, as much as 50 to 60% of the islets graft is lost due to IBMIR (Bennett, 1999). Within as little as five minutes, natural IgG and IgM lead to complement activation starts to attack it by creating perforin complexes that lead to cell lysis (Tiernberg, 2008). Another significant physiological change involved in IBMIR is the dramatic, rapid increase in cytokine levels such as IL-2, TNF-α, IL-1β, and IFN-γ. Due to diabetogenic effects glucocorticoids are avoided in the immunosuppressive regimens turning to newer alternatives (Shapiro et al., 2000). An alternative to steroids is daclizumab, a humanized monoclonal antibody with specific affinity to the IL-2 receptor. This receptor on T-cells is responsible for the main activation pathway, which triggers an immune response against beta cells.

Thymoglobulin has become a popular agent for the reduction in host T-cells (Finke, 2009). This thymoglobulin is a polycolonal antibody that targets T-cells, thus depleting the cells required to mount a specific response to islets even before they enter the body.

Another T-cell depleting agent used for induction therapy is alemtuzumab (Maggliocca, 2006). Alemtuzumab is a monoclonal antibody against CD52, which is a marker of mature lymphocytes. One specific complication is that it increases the chance of infections while also increasing the possibility of reactivation of cytomegalovirus.

Another target of induction therapy includes the proinflammatory cytokine response. Our group and others have shown that IL-1β plays an important role in the onset of T1D. Additionally TNF-α blockage was shown to significantly improve the clinical outcome of patients based on the collaborative islet transplant registry (CITR) database (CITR Report 2009). To abrogate the inflammatory effects of these cytokines a combined treatment of eternacept and anakinra was used for induction therapy (Matsumoto, 2011). Etanercept is a TNF-α inhibitor, acting as a decoy receptor and blocking the true effect of TNF. Anakinra is an IL-1 receptor antagonist blocking the activity of IL-1β. This anti-inflammatory response was combined with thymoglobulin for the induction therapy. All patients undergoing this therapy were able to achieve insulin independence following a single islet infusion. Gene microarray analysis was performed on blood samples taken within the first week post-transplant. The results of the gene microarray demonstrated that genes related to cytotoxic T cells were repressed; however, there was upregulation seen in inflammation and neutrophil related genes. This suggests that there may be alternative inflammatory cytokines and agents that may be relevant to the immediate immune reaction.

3.2.2 Inhibition of NF-kB to prevent inflammation

Instead of trying to target all of the extracellular agents that might cause an inflammatory reaction, an effort was made to find and inhibit a downstream signaling protein that is activated by pro-inflammatory cytokines. Nuclear factor kappa-light-chain-enhancer of activated B-cells (NF-κB) is a protein that regulates transcription of several sequences of DNA and is activated through a canonical pathway by inflammatory cytokines (Hawiger, 2001). This led us to believe that inhibition of NF-κB would inhibit the collective effects of circulating cytokines.

An inhibitor of NF-κB activation was found in traditional eastern medicine from the plant *Withania somnifera* extract called Withaferin A, WA (Kaileh et al., 2007). Withaferin A is a steroidal lactone that prevents the phosphorylation and subsequent degradation of inhibitor of kappaB (IkB), which sequesters NF-κB in the cytoplasm. Studies by Peng et al. (2010) showed that RNA transcripts of inflammatory cytokines and chemokines such as IP-10 (CXCL10), RANTES (CCL5), MIP-1 (CCL4), and MCP-1 (CCL-2) were upregulated in human islets in the presence of cytokines. However, WA was able to inhibit this effect. WA was not shown to decrease islet viability or functionality, while simultaneously inhibiting the inflammatory response. This result demonstrates that careful regulation of NF-κB can have a beneficial effect for islet transplantation by preventing the effects of cytokine induced damage.

Another NF-κB inhibitor was found to improve intraportal islet transplantation by IKK-β inhibition (Chen et al., 2011). This study showed higher retention of insulin independence in a xenogenic model when a proprietary NF- κB inhibitor drug was injected once, thirty minutes before the transplantation. The primary anticipated effect of NF- κB inhibition is on the IMBIR reaction which is more easily studied in a syngenic model, where the only source of graft failure is IBMIR rather than a specific adaptive immune response.

3.2.3 Maintenance therapy

The purpose of the maintenance therapy is to suppress the specific alloimmune and autoimmune responses mediated by T and B lymphocytes. The drugs typically used for this purpose include Prograf, Rapamycin, MMF, and blockers of co-stimulation. Several combinations of these therapeutic agents have been attempted in clinical islet transplantations to increase the longevity of the graft while minimizing the beta cell toxicity and patient related adverse events.

The types of immunosuppression traditionally used for transplantation are the calcineurin inhibitors tacrolimus and cyclosporine, but often these agents were associated with toxic effects for beta cells (Drachenberg, 1999). Tacrolimus is an immunosuppressant that was found to inhibit NF-AT activation. The original molecule was found in the fermentation of a soil sample containing the bacterium *Streptomyces tsukobensis* (Pritchard, 2005). Tacrolimus inhibits the activation of NF-AT and its translocation to the nucleus by forming a complex with the immunophilin FKBP12 to inhibit the activation of calcineurin and subsequent T-cell activation (Liu, 1991). This action also leads to the arrest of the cell cycle, preventing it from moving from the G_0 stage to the G_1 stage; thus cellular proliferation is prevented. Cyclosporin acts in a similar way as tacrolimus, binding to cyclophilin to prevent calcineurin mediated dephosphorylation of NF-AT; however tacrolimus exhibits greater potency with fewer harmful side effects compared to cyclosporine.

Although the calcineurin inhibitors have been effective at inhibiting rejection in solid organ transplant, they have also been associated with the onset of diabetes mellitus. This is a serious implication for a transplantation procedure trying to prevent this very condition. This side effect was histologically analyzed in solid pancreas transplants for patients receiving either tacrolimus or cyclosporine in a randomized fashion (Drachenberg, 1999). Sectioned biopsy samples from 1 to 8 months post-transplant revealed cytoplasmic swelling, vacuolization, apoptosis and irregular insulin staining of islets for patients receiving both drugs. Although islet cell damage was more frequent for patients receiving tacrolimus versus cyclosporine (10/13 versus 5/13 respectively), it was not significantly different. Since tacrolimus is more effective with less side effects, it is used more often. But as this study shows it should be administered in low doses to prevent beta cell toxicity.

Reference	# of Patients	Insulin Independence (%)	Long Term Follow Up	Immunosuppression
Shapiro et al., 2000	8	100%	18% at 5yrs	Daclizumab (Dac), Rapamycin (Rap), Tacrolimus (Tac)
Noguchi et al., 2005	5	60%	NA	Basiliximab, Rap, Tac
Ryan et al., 2005	65	90%	70% at 1yr 10% at 5yrs	Dac, Rap, Tac
Toso et al., 2006	8	100%	71% at 1 & 2 yrs	Dac, Rap, Tac
Vantyghem et al., 2009	5	60%	20% After 1yr	ATG, Rap/ Tac
	14	100%	71% at 1 yr 57% at ~3yr	Dac, Rap, Tac
Froud et al., 2008	3	66%	66% After 2 yr	Alemtuzumab, Rap/Tac (3 mo.), then Rap/MMF
Matsumoto et al., 2010	3	100%	53±7 days	ATG, Tac, MMF, Enteracept, Anakinra
Posselt et al., 2010	3	100%	40±4 days	Dac, Rap, Tac, Enteracept
	8	100%	75% at 1 yr* 38% at 2yrs*	ATG, Efalizumab, Rap, MMF
Shapiro et al., 2010	12	100%	83% at 3yrs	Alemtuzumab, Tac, MMF
Hering et al., 2011	16	88%	38%	Dac, Rap/ Tac
	8	100%	63% at 1 yr	ATG, Dac, Enteracept, MMF, Rap, Tac

*These numbers are limited, because the drug being tested, Efalizumab, was withdrawn from the market during treatment.

Table 1. Summary of Clinical Islet Transplantation Outcome.

Rapamycin (sirolimus) has a different mechanism of action and side effects compared to the calcineurin inhibitors (Pritchard, 2005). Although rapamycin binds to FKBP12 in a similar mechanism like tacrolimus, it does not inhibit calcineurin, rather the complex inhibits mTOR (mammalian Target Of Rapamycin). This inhibits the second phase of T-cell activation, whereas tacrolimus and cyclosporine inhibit the first phase. So rapamycin also inhibits signal transduction leading to IL-2 production and clonal proliferation, and since it affects a different part of T-cell activation it can be used synergistically with calcineurin inhibitors. One of the side effects associated with this drug is oral ulcers that make ingestion of food difficult. Rapamycin is thus a potential alternative or adjunct to calcineurin inhibitor mediated T-cell inhibition.

Another widely used immunosuppressant is mycophenolate mofetil, MMF, which prevents B and T-cell proliferation (Ransom, 1995). This is the first of two enzymes responsible for the production of guanosine monophosphate from inosine monophosphate; lymphocytes are particularly dependent on this pathway for the subsequent synthesis of GDP, GTP, and dGTP. The reduction of GTP and dGTP levels in lymphycytes results in a decreased ability to perform DNA synthesis and GTP dependent metabolism. Some of the adverse events associated with this drug include nausea, infections, leucopenia, and anemia. This alternative mechanism of specific immune system suppression has led to the widespread use of MMF in combination with tacrolimus or sirolimus. One such study was performed recently by Shapiro et al. in 2010 by combining MMF with tacrolimus for maintenance with alemtuzumab induction. This study was compared to the original Edmonton protocol which used daclizumab for induction and a combination of tacrolimus and sirolimus as seen in Table 1. It was hypothesized that MMF would be better tolerated than high dose sirolimus. Of the 12 patients with completed islet infusions, 83% (10/12) are still insulin independent at 36 months, whereas two patient's grafts failed after removing immunosuppressants due to infections. The mechanism underlying this tolerance seemed to be linked to a unique donor specific IL-10 regulated immune response, leading to improved insulin independence rates.

There have also been several antibody mediated approaches to preventing T-cell activation by blocking costimulation. This approach enabled a calcineurin inhibitor and gluococorticoid free immunosuppression regimen; the antibody used was efalizumab (anti-LFA 1 antibody) (Posselt et al., 2010). These antibodies were used as supplements to sirolimus/MMF maintenance therapy. The result was that 5/5 of patients receiving eflizumab achieved insulin independence with several maintaining graft function for over a year. Unfortunately, this therapy cannot be continued, because efalizumab was withdrawn from the market by the FDA in mid 2009 (Posselt et al., 2009). Despite the progress made, any use of immunosuppressants will slow the widespread applicability of islet transplantation, since the cost benefit analysis of immunosuppression must be compared to insulin therapy alone.

3.3 Xenogenic porcine islets for transplantation

Even if all pancreatic islet cell transplantations became successful and only required one pancreas to achieve insulin independence, there would still be an insufficient number of pancreata to treat all type 1 diabetic patients. There are approximately 7,000 pancreases available for donation in the United States per year, but diabetes milletus affects as many as 3 million people in the United States and as many as 16 million people worldwide. This shortage in human islet cells from organ donor sources has led to a search for alternative sources (Hering & Walawalkar, 2009). One source that has been identified is porcine islets, which secrete physiologically functional insulin but can be highly immunogenic to humans and carry a risk of cross-species infection by pig endogenous retroviruses.

A particular surface epitope that has led to increased xenoreactivity is galactose-α1,3-galactose (Rayat et al., 1998; Korbutt et al., 1997). Through genetic engineering of pig herds, a knockout animal which lacks this epitope has been successfully bred (Puga Yung et al., 2009). However kidney transplantation results using this animal have shown only modest gains.

Another fear of porcine islet transplantation is that pig endogenous retrovirus (PERV) could be transmitted from the porcine islets transplanted into the human recipient. Although pigs can be bred in pathogen-free facilities that shields them from contracting microbes that can be transmitted, PERV is integrated into the genome and the risk of infection cannot be so easily removed. When recipients are immunosuppressed, porcine cytomegalovirus or pig lymphotrophic herpes virus are common infections that can be activated under immunosuppression. There have been conflicting reports of PERV manifesting in non-obese diabetic mice transplanted with pig islets. For humans, sensitive detection techniques such as quantitative polymerase chain reaction or immunoblotting assays for PERV proteins. With respect to clinical trials of xenotransplantation, there is little evidence of transmission of xenogenic endogenous virus transmission (Elliott et al., 2005; Garkavenko et al., 2011).

Porcine islets have even been used in two clinical trials of islet transplantation, one in Mexico (Valdes-Gonzales et al., 2005) and one in New Zealand (Garkavenko et al., 2011). The Mexico trial involved transplantation of collagen generating devices embedded with islet and sertoli cells into twelve juvenile type 1 diabetic patients. The purpose of the sertolli cells was to prevent the action of the immune system. This procedure did not produce long term insulin independence, but glycemic control was improved along with positive porcine C-peptide in patient urine during long term follow-up.

A second noteworthy clinical trial is being performed in New Zealand using alginate encapsulated neonatal porcine islets transplanted into the peritoneal cavity of type 1 diabetic patients. The pigs used were raised in pathogen-free facilities with a donor herd free from conventional pathogens and non-transmittable PERV. This unique lack of exposure to viruses is a characteristic of these pigs which were raised on the island of New Zealand with limited exposure to foreign diseases. In terms of xenogenic related infection, zoonosis has been rigorously monitored with no evidence of cross-species infection. Again, no patients became insulin independent, but there was a significant reduction in hypoglycemic unawareness episodes. This encapsulation method demonstrates the usefulness of immunoisolation in islet transplantation (Elliott RB, 2011).

Porcine islets have been used to explore alternative transplant sites, since blood in the portal vein of the liver often contains higher concentrations of immunosuppressants and other toxins, while containing low concentrations of oxygen. Areas of porcine islet transplantation into non-human primates include intraperitoneum, renal subcapsule, subcutaneous, the omentum pouch, and the mesentery (Hering & Walawalkar, 2009). The efficacy of each transplant site is difficult to determine as various immunosuppressive therapies were used in addition to encapsulation and the use of a subcutaneous mono-layer device. These large animal studies have shown some success demonstrating the ability in some cases to create insulin independence with immunosuppressants. Finally, genetic modification of donor pigs permits the upregulation of certain genes that would have cytoprotective or immunomodulatory effects to improve engraftment and reduce the effect of the immune response.

3.4 Islet Immunoisolation

The leading strategy to reduce or eliminate the most risky aspect of islet transplantation, namely immunosuppression drugs, is immunoisolation. To protect islets from the recognition of the immune system, two strategies have been used, specifically encapsulation and surface modification (Wilson & Chaikof, 2007) as shown in Figure 1. Encapsulation involves, as its name suggests, enclosing an islet in a capsule that is impermeable to the immune system. These capsules are typically composed of agarose or poly(vinyl alcohol) alginate. The capsules must have defined pore sizes that allow the influx of glucose as well as the secretion of insulin, while simultaneously preventing intrusion by complement or antibodies. These modifications also allow drug delivery by covalent attachment of antithrombogenic or immunosuppressive agents, which would be applicable to both human allotransplantation or xenotransplantation.

3.4.1 Encapsulation

The encapsulation method is limited by bioincompatibility and biodegradation of the materials in addition to hypoxic damage to the islets (Lee & Byun, 2010). Further there is the practical limitation of size; the typical islet diameter of 150 μm is often increased by as much as 5 fold, leading to a volume increase greater than 100 fold. Since more than 500,000 islet equivalents are now required to cure diabetes (~10mL islet pellet volume), that volume would be increased to over 1 liter with encapsulated islets. This would exclude transplantation into the portal vein of the liver, because this volume of islets would significantly increase the risk of portal vein thrombosis and other bleeding complications. Thus, alternative sites of injection such as subcutaneous, intraperitoneal, or intramuscular have to be validated. However, this technique still would have the issue of incomplete encapsulation or variable number of islets entrapped.

3.4.2 Surface modification

An alternative to macroencapsulation is surface modification, which uses the islet surface as the scaffolding upon which to build protective barriers. One such surface modification method is conformal coating, which uses derivatives of the molecule diacrylate (Cruise et al., 1999) Conformal coating uses the islet surface to deposit or chemically grow a protective barrier without as large of a size increase; the final diameter is only increased by 30 to 50μm in human and porcine islets.

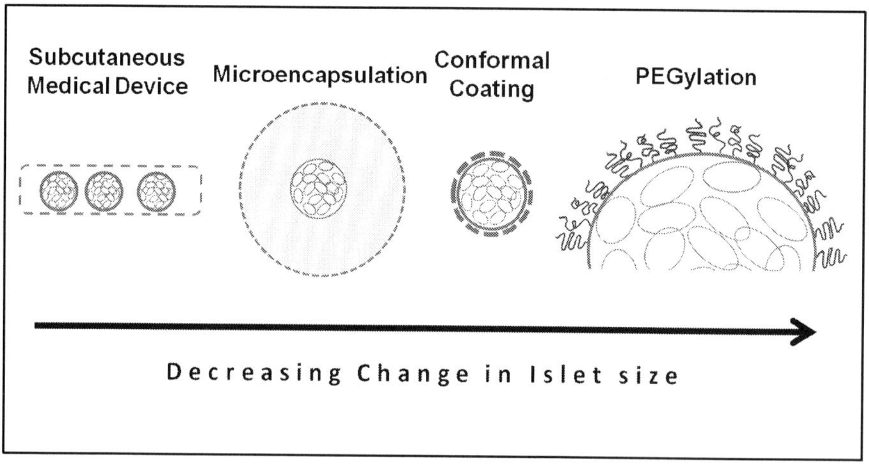

Fig. 1. Immunoisolation methods for islets from largest size to smallest increase in size.

Another study demonstrated the use of proteins as a protective barrier by reacting a disuccinimidyl bifunctional poly-ethylene glycol (PEG) molecule on one side with the islet surface and the other side to albumin (Xie et al., 2005). Another method of surface modification is PEGylation, which attaches long chains of PEG, a hydrophilic, biologically inert, flexible polymer chain. This method of surface modification has been applied previously to the immunoisolation of red blood cells to mask the ABO surface antigens from host antibodies (Scott et al., 1997; Murad et al., 1999). These experiments show that surface PEGylation of islets can be accomplished successfully without loss in viability or functionality. One of the main advantages of PEGylation to islets is that there is no significant size increase like that associated with macroencapsulation. There is only a microscopic increase in size, because the PEG conjugated islets (PEGylated islets) are modified at the molecular level. The traditional and most widely used PEGylation technique applied uses a succinimidyl functionalized PEG (N-hydroxysuccinimide, NHS), which reacts to surface amine groups on the islet surface (Lee et al., 2007). However, there are several other surface moieties that can be targeted by chemical modification. There have been studies that investigate PEGylation by targeting the lipid membrane (Teramura et al., 2007), and surface sugars (Wilson et al., 2010). This same study also analyzed optimization of surface modification by varying reaction time and concentration of the functionalized PEG; the new oxidative method was even combined with the traditional NHS method. However there remain more surface modification targets available such as disulfide bridges; even photochemical techniques that have been applied to protein linkage of tissue (Zhang et al., 2004). Another poorly studied aspect of islet surface modification is in relation to the longevity of the modification methods. The islet surface is a dynamic environment, with constant turnover and regeneration of the cell membrane. Almost all of the PEGylation techniques mentioned only look at the uniformity and quantity of the PEG immediately after modification. If PEG is supposed to protect islets from the immune system, it should be robust and remain for a long time in order to protect islets from T-cell mediated rejection. Biologically active agents that have been attached to islet surfaces include heparin, activated protein C, urokinase, or thrombomodulin (Cabric et al., 2007; Contreras et al., 2004; Teramura & Iwata, 2008; Stabler et al., 2007). Development of a standardized analytic method that determines PEG density/ islet (size adjusted) and uniformity over a long time period would provide the ability to compare surface modification chemistries and optimize PEGylation reactions.

4. Beta cell regeneration

Development of type 1 diabetes is a consequence of loss of functional beta cell mass. Hence the objective of many therapeutic approaches to treat T1D is to restore beta cell mass sufficient to maintain normoglycemia. Results from the clinical islet transplantation trials have reinforced this concept. In a healthy individual, the beta cells lost are constantly replenished by beta cell neogenesis through mechanisms which are not clearly understood. Beta cell mass is maintained and regulated in response to pharmacological and nutritional stimuli which include glucose, insulin, epidermal growth factor (EGF), gastrin and glucagon like peptide (GLP-1). Physiological stimuli such as pregnancy, obesity and pancreatic tissue damage also significantly regulate beta cell mass. Beta cell development in pancreas is regulated by the hierarchical expression of a specific complement of transcription factor proteins (Edlund H, 1998). Originating from cells expressing homeodomain transcription factor PDX1 (pancreatic/duodenal homeobox 1) and repressing sonic hedgehog, both endocrine and exocrine cells of the adult pancreas arise from endodermal cells expressing PDX1 and Ptfla. Fibroblast growth factor family of proteins stimulate the proliferation of progenitor cells in addition to specific stimuli from mesenchymal cells. Formation of beta cells is further driven by the transient expression of Pax4 in ngn 3-expressing cells. Beta cell expansion begins when transcription factor complement being driven by PDX1, Pax6, Nkx2.2 and Nkx6.1 (Edlund H, 1998).

In the adult pancreas, beta cell replication is a key phenomenon for the emergence of neogenic beta cells, however, the rates of beta cells replication is extremely low. The origin of neogenic beta cells is unclear. Several possibilities including differentiation of pancreatic stem cells or ductal or acinar cells are proposed. The plasticity of adult pancreatic cells is thought to play an important role in the neogenesis of beta cells. Attempts to transdifferentiate liver cells or intestinal K cells in insulin producing beta cells have also been reported through coordinated alteration in gene expression and cellular phenotype (Campbell and Macfarlane, 2007). A number of hormones and growth factors have been shown to stimulate renewal of beta cells which include GLP1 analog, EGF and gastrin. GLP1 is an incretin hormone produced by L-cells of the intestine. GLP-1 augments insulin secretion (Melloul et al, 2002). GLP-1 binds to specific GLP-1 receptor and activates intracellular signaling events involving protein kinase A and changes in cyclic AMP levels. GLP-1 released from the intestinal L-cells is rapidly degraded by the dipeptidase enzyme DPPIV. Inhibitors of DPPIV are now increasingly used to control glucose levels in type 2 diabetic patients. GLP-1 has also been shown to increase PDX1 gene expression in ductal cells during the regeneration of pancreas (Sharma et al., 1999). A similar line of action has been proposed for thiazolidinediones in the enhancement of neogenic beta cell function through activation of nuclear receptor peroxisome proliferator activator gamma (PPAR) (Richardson et al., 2006)

5. Stem cells

Stem cells have the potential to undergo symmetric cell divisions as well as asymmetric cell divisions for lineage commitment such as differentiation into insulin-producing cells. Stem cells may offer an important and unlimited source for beta cell replacement. Stem cells can be broadly classified as embryonic (ESC) or adult (ASC) stem cells. ESCs are isolated from the blastocyst which is formed during embryonic development while ASCs are detected within tissues (Fuchs et al., 2004). Both cell types are capable of commitment to specific cell lineages. ESCs exhibit greater plasticity (pluripotency) in terms of differentiation into almost any cell type, however, ASCs are limited in their commitment to repertoire of cell types (multipotency).

ESCs offer a potential source for beta cell neogenesis. However, it is difficult to maintain human ESCs in an undifferentiated state under *in vitro* culture conditions. The molecular mechanisms that derive ESCs into insulin producing are not clearly defined yet; however, nutrients, oxygen and other growth factors have been shown to play a critical role (Smith, 1991). Only a small percentage (<2%) of ESCs have been shown to spontaneously differentiate into insulin producing cells, thus limiting their clinical application. Several cell culture strategies have been proposed to increase the percentage of insulin producing cells from ESCs. Unfortunately the amount insulin obtained with these strategies is extremely low when compared to insulin content of the beta cells of pancreas (Roche and Soria, 2006). Despite their limited capacity for proliferation ASCs offer the advantage of immune compatibility in the development of beta cell replacement therapies. However, ASCs may still be targeted by the autoimmune response. ASCs isolated from pancreatic tissue have been shown to differentiate *in vitro* into islet-like structures (Bonner-Weir et al., 2000; Ramiya et al., 2000) lending support to the notion that ductal cells may serve as islet progenitors. Culture of ductal cells isolated from human pancreas under specific conditions resulted in islet-like clusters that exhibited islet-specific hormones and transcription factors. Further, these islet-like clusters showed increased insulin response to glucose challenge. In contrast, Dor et al., (2004) have proposed that beta cell neogenesis in adult pancreas is solely derived from replication of pre-existing beta cells and not from stem cell precursors. Thus identification of true islet progenitors and the mechanisms that differentiate stem cells into normal insulin producing beta cells are still under progress.

In summary, great strides have been made in development of a physiological treatment for insulin-dependent diabetes. Four broad types of approaches as shown in figure 2 are currently being pursued to find a cure for this increasing health hazard. While some of these approaches have progressed well enough to find clinical application, others are lagging behind due to technological deficiencies. Transplantation of allogenic pancreas organ or

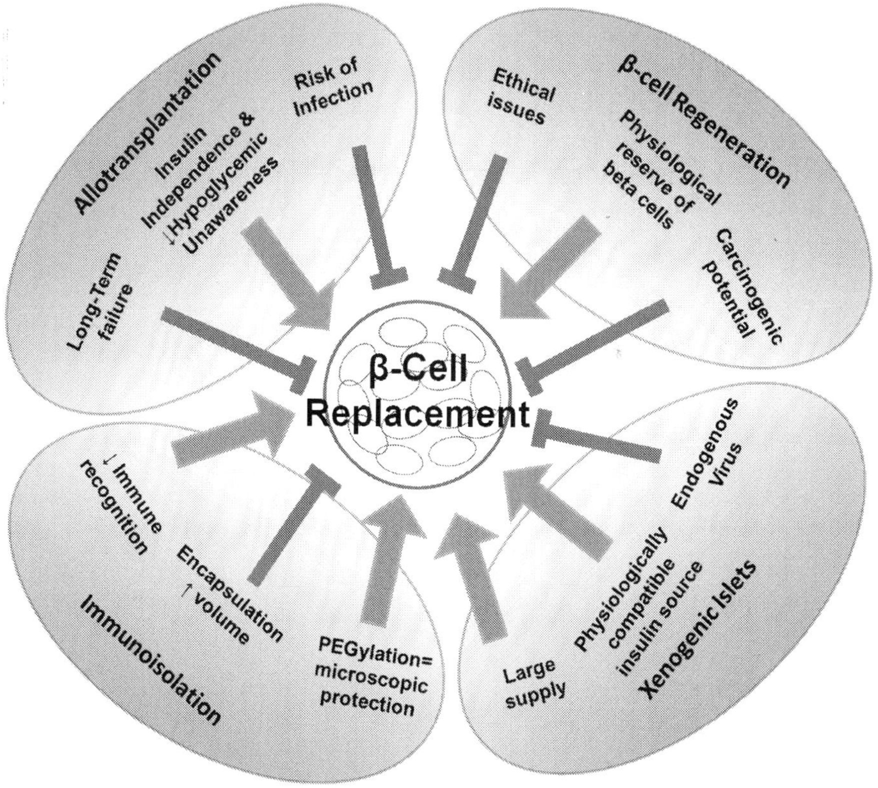

Fig. 2. Opportunities and Challenges to beta cell replacement therapies. Green colored arrows indicate opportunities and the red colored hammer indicates challenges.

isolated pancreatic islets have shown the most progress in terms of clinical application and are currently limited by the lack of suitable organ supply and islet-friendly immunosuppression. Transplantation of pig islets could overcome the hurdle of donor organ shortage, but the safety and efficacy of such xenotransplantation remains to be determined. Immune isolation of allogenic and xenogenic islets will significantly prolong the survival of transplanted islets and also prevent the harmful effects of host immune response. Optimization of encapsulation technologies to support islet cell function in the long term is not fully developed yet. Replacement of beta cells derived from alternative sources such as stem cells has the potential to offer unlimited supply of beta cells and is currently receiving greater attention from the research community.

6. Conclusion

Incidence of diabetes is increasing at an alarming rate in different populations all over the world. Diagnosis of T1D is also following this increasing trend, constituting 5-10% of the total diabetes cases. Exogenous insulin therapy is proving to be adequate for majority of T1D patients; however, for "brittle" T1D patients control of blood glucose levels is very difficult using this treatment. Transplantation of whole organ pancreas is an established procedure to restore beta cell mass to attain normoglycemia. Transplantation of isolated islets has seen a tremendous growth in the past decade in terms of the number of transplant recipients, improvement in the islet isolation methodologies and post-transplant graft survival and function. Due to limited supply of qualified pancreata for transplantation, other approaches to replace beta cells are gaining attention. Pig islets are an attractive option in terms of abundant supply and physiological similarity of insulin despite the possible risk of infection. Beta cell replacement using regeneration of stem cells or other cell types have shown promising results, however, are too far away from clinical application. Importantly, immune isolation of transplanted islets or beta cells using macro- or micro-encapsulation technology may significantly improve the current outcomes of cell-based therapy.

7. Acknowledgement

This work was supported by a grant (#5-2010-668) from the Juvenile Diabetes Research Foundation (to B.N.) and by the Baylor Health Care System. JAS is supported by a fellowship from Baylor University Institute of Biomedical Studies, Waco, Texas. The authors thank Ana Rahman and Yoshiko Tamura for their help in preparation of the manuscript.

8. References

Balamurugan AN, Breite AG, Anazawa T, Loganathan G, Wilhelm JJ, Papas KK, et al. Successful human islet isolation and transplantation indicating the importance of class 1 collagenase and collagen degradation activity assay. *Transplantation*, Vol. 89, No.8, (April 2010), pp. 954-961

Barnett MJ, Zhai X, LeGatt DF, Cheng SB, Shapiro AMJ, Lakey JRT. Quantitative assessment of collagenase blends for human islet isolation. *Transplantation*, Vol. 80, No. 6 (September 2005), pp. 723-728

Bennet W, Sundberg B, Groth CG, Brendel MD, Brandhorst D, Brandhorst H, et al. Incompatibility between human blood and isolated islets of Langerhans: a finding with implications for clinical intraportal islet transplantation? *Diabetes*, Vol. 48, No. 10, (October, 1999), pp. 1907-1914

Bonner-Weir S, Taneja M, Weir GC et al., In vitro cultivation of human islets from expanded ductal tissue. *Proc Natl Acad Sci USA*, Vol. 97, No. 14, (July 2000), pp.7999-8004.

Borowiak M, Melton DA. How to make [beta] cells? *Current Opinion in Cell Biology*, Vol. 21, No. 6, (December 2009), pp.727-732

Bucher P, Mathe Z, Morel P, Bosco D, Andres A, Kurfuest M, et al. Assessment of a novel two-component enzyme preparation for human islet isolation and transplantation. *Transplantation*, Vol. 79, No. 1, (January 2005), pp. 91-97

Cabric S, Sanchez J, Lundgren T, Foss A, Felldin M, Källen R, et al. Islet Surface Heparinization Prevents the Instant Blood-Mediated Inflammatory Reaction in Islet Transplantation. *Diabetes*, Vol. 56, No. 8, (August 2007), pp. 2008 -2015

Caballero-Corbalan J, Eich T, Lundgren T, Foss A, Felldin M, Kallen R, Salmela K, et al. No beneficial effect of two-layer storage compared with UW-storage on human islet isolation and transplantation. *Transplantation*, Vol. 84, No. 7, (October 2007), pp. 864-9

Cambell SC, Macfarlane W. Approaches to beta-cell regeneration and neogenesis. In: Islet Transplantation and Beta Cell Replacement Therapy. (Eds) A.M. James Shapiro and James A. M. Shaw, (2007), pp. 293-309

Chen C, Moreno R, Samikannu B, Bretzel RG, Schmitz ML, Linn T. Improved intraportal islet transplantation outcome by systemic IKK-beta inhibition: NF-κB activity in pancreatic islets depends on oxygen availability. *Am. J. Transpl*ant, Vol.11, No.2, (February 2011), pp. 215-224

CITR report, Collaborative Islet Transplant Registry Sixth Annual Report, (2009) www.citregistry.org

Cruise GM, Hegre OD, Lamberti FV, Hager SR, Hill R, Scharp DS, et al. In vitro and in vivo performance of porcine islets encapsulated in interfacially photopolymerized poly (ethylene glycol) diacrylate membranes. *Cell Transplant*, Vol. 8, No. 3, (June 1999), pp. 293-306

Cooke DW PL, Plotnick L. Type 1 diabetes mellitus in pediatrics. *Pediatr Rev*, Vol. 29, No. 11, (November 2008), pp. 374–84

Dor Y, Brown J, Martinez OI, Melton DA. Adult pancreatic beta cells are formed by self-duplication rather than stem-cell differentiation, *Nature*, (May 2004), 6;429(6987):41-46

Drachenberg CB, Klassen DK, Weir MR, Wiland A, Fink JC, Bartlett ST, et al. Islet cell damage associated with tacrolimus and cyclosporine: morphological features in pancreas allograft biopsies and clinical correlation. *Transplantation*. Vol. 68, No. 3, (August, 1999), pp. 396-402

Elliott RB; on behalf of Living Cell Technologies. Toward xenotransplantation of pig islets in the clinic, *Curr Opin Organ Transplant*, (April 2011), 16(2):195-200

Finke J, Bethge WA, Schmoor C, Ottinger HD, Stelljes M, Zander AR, et al. Standard graft-versus-host disease prophylaxis with or without anti-T-cell globulin in haematopoietic cell transplantation from matched unrelated donors: a randomised, open-label, multicentre phase 3 trial. *The Lancet Oncology*, Vol. 10, No. 9, (September 2009), pp. 855-864

Fuchs E, Tumbar T, Guasch G. Socializing with the neighbors: Stem cells and their niche. *Cell*, (March 2004), 116:639-648

Garfinkel MR, Connors M, Ostrega D, Jarosz J, Philipson L, Millis JM. Islet isolation under cGMP conditions: replacing the coil. *Transplantation Proceedings*, Vol. 36, No.4, (May 2004), pp. 1031-1033

Garkavenko O, Durbin K, Tan P, Elliott R. Islets transplantation: New Zealand experience. *Xenotransplantation*, Vol. 18, No. 1, (January 2011), pp. 60-60

Gruessner AC, Sutherland DE. Analysis of United States (US) and non-US pancreas transplants reported to the United network for organ sharing (UNOS) and the international pancreas transplant registry (IPTR) as of October 2001. *Clin Transpl*, (October 2001), pp. 41-72

Hawiger J. Innate Immunity and Inflammation: A Transcriptional Paradigm. *IR*, Vol. 23, No. 2-3, (2001), pp. 99-110

Hering BJ, Kandaswamy R, Ansite JD, Eckman PM, Nakano M, Sawada T, et al. Single-donor, marginal-dose islet transplantation in patients with type 1 diabetes. *JAMA*, Vol. 293, No. 7, (February 2005), pp. 830-835

Hering BJ, Walawalkar N. Pig-to-nonhuman primate islet xenotransplantation. *Transpl. Immunol*, Vol. 21, No. 2, (June 2009), pp. 81-86

Humar A, Kandaswamy R, Granger D, Gruessner RW, Gruessner AC, Sutherland DER. Decreased Surgical Risks of Pancreas Transplantation in the Modern Era. *Ann Surg*, Vol. 231, No, 2, (Februaryruary 2000), pp. 269-275

Kaileh M, Vanden Berghe W, Heyerick A, Horion J, Piette J, Libert C, et al. Withaferin a strongly elicits IkappaB kinase beta hyperphosphorylation concomitant with potent inhibition of its kinase activity. *J. Biol. Chem*, Vol. 282, No. 7, (February 2007), pp. 4253-4264

Lee DY, Byun Y. Pancreatic islet PEGylation as an immunological polymeric restraint. *Biotechnol Bioproc E*, Vol. 15, No. 1, (2010), pp. 76-85

Lemal David M. Perspective on fluorocarbon chemistry. *J. Org. Chem*, Vol. 69, No. 1, (January 2004), pp. 1–11

Linetsky E, Bottino R, Lehmann R, Alejanuarydro R, Inverardi L, Ricordi C. Improved human islet isolation using a new enzyme blend, liberase. *Diabetes*, Vol. 46, No. 7, (July 1997), pp. 1120-1123

Liu J, Farmer JD Jr, Lane WS, Friedman J, Weissman I, Schreiber SL. Calcineurin is a common target of cyclophilin-cyclosporin A and FKBP-FK506 complexes. *Cell*, Vol. 66, No. 4, (August 1991), pp. 807-815

Magliocca JF, Knechtle SJ. The evolving role of alemtuzumab (Campath-1H) for immunosuppressive therapy in organ transplantation. *Transplant International*, Vol. 19, No. 9, (September 2006), pp. 705-714

Matsumoto S, Kuroda Y. Perfluorocarbon for organ preservation before transplantation. *Transplantation*, Vol. 74, No. 12, (December 2002), pp. 1804-1809

Matsumoto S, Noguichi H, Shimoda M, Ikemoto T, Naziruddin B, Jackson A, et al. Seven Consecutive Successful Clinical Islet Isolations With Pancreatic Ductal Injection. *Cell Transplant*, Vol. 19, No. 3, (2010), pp. 291-297

Matsumoto S, Rigley TH, Qualley SA, Kuroda Y, Reems JA, Stevens RB. Efficacy of the oxygen-charged static two-layer method for short-term pancreas preservation and islet isolation from nonhuman primate and human pancreata. *Cell Transplant*, Vol. 11, No. 8, (2002), pp. 769-777

Matsumoto S, Takita M, Chaussabel D, Noguchi H, Shimoda M, Sugimoto K, Itoh T, Chujo D, SoRelle JA, Onaca N, Naziruddin B, Levy MF. Improving Efficacy of Clinical Islet Transplantation with Iodixanol Based Islet Purification, Thymoglobulin Induction and Blockage of IL-1-beta and TNF-alpha. *Cell Transplant*, (Epub, March 8, 2011)

Mccarthy R, Spurlin B, Wright M, Breite A, Sturdevant L, Dwulet C, et al. Development and Characterization of a Collagen Degradation Assay to Assess Purified Collagenase Used in Islet Isolation. *Transplantation Proceedings*, Vol. 40, No. 2, (2008), pp. 339-342

McCarthy RC, Spurlin B, Wright MJ, Breite AG, Sturdevant LK, Dwulet CS, et al. Development and characterization of a collagen degradation assay to assess purified collagenase used in islet isolation. *Transplant. Proc*, Vol. 40, No. 2, (March 2008), pp. 339-342

Melloul D, Marshak S, Cerasi E. Regulation of insulin gene transcription. *Diabetologia*, (2002) 45:309-326

Mita A, Ricordi C, Messinger S, Miki A, Misawa R, Barker S, et al. Antiproinflammatory effects of iodixanol (OptiPrep)-based density gradient purification on human islet preparations. *Cell Transplant*, Vol. 19, No. 12, (2010), pp. 1537-1546

Murad KL, Mahany KL, Brugnara C, Kuypers FA, Eaton JW, Scott MD. Structural and Functional Consequences of Antigenic Modulation of Red Blood Cells With Methoxypoly(Ethylene Glycol). *Blood*, Vol. 93, No. 6, (March 1999), pp. 2121 -2127

Olack BJ, Swanson CJ, Howard TK, Mohanakumar T. Improved method for the isolation and purification of human islets of langerhans using Liberase enzyme blend. *Hum. Immunol*, Vol. 60, No. 12, (December 1999), pp. 1303-1309

Posselt AM, Szot G, Frassetto L, Masharani U, Tavakol M, Vincenti F, et al. Islet Allograft Survival in Type 1 Diabetic Patients Using Calcineurin Inhibitor-Free Protocols Based on T-Cell Adhesion or Costimulation Blockade: 2566. *Transplantation*, Vol.90, (2010)

Pritchard DI. Sourcing a chemical succession for cyclosporin from parasites and human pathogens. *Drug Discov. Today*, Vol. 10, No. 10, (May 2005), pp. 688-691

Puga Yung G, Schneider MK, Seebach JD. Immune responses to alpha 1,3 galactosyltransferase knockout pigs. *Curr Opin Organ Transplant.*, Vol. 14, No. 2, (2009), pp. 154-160

Ramiya VK, Maraist M, Arfors KE, Schatz DA, Peck AB et al., Reversal of insulin-dependent diabetes using islets generated in vitro from pancreatic stem cells. *Nat Med*, (2000), 6:278-282

Ransom JT. Mechanism of action of mycophenolate mofetil. *Ther Drug Monit*, Vol. 17, No. 6, (December 1995), pp. 681-684

Rayat GR, Rajotte RV, Elliott JF, Korbutt GS. Expression of Gal alpha(1,3)gal on neonatal porcine islet beta-cells and susceptibility to human antibody/complement lysis. *Diabetes*, Vol. 47, No. 9, (1998), pp. 1406 -1411

Rickels M, Barton FB, Alejandro R, Pattou F, Berney T, Senior P et al. Factors of islet transplant success: Results from the Collaborative Islet Transplant Registry 1999-2010. *Rev Diabetic Stud*, Vol. 8, No. 1, (2011), pp.101

Ricordi C, Edlund H. Toward a renewable source of pancreatic [beta]-cells. *Nat Biotech*, Vol. 26, No. 4, (April 2008), pp. 397-398

Richardson H, Campbell SC, Smith SA, Macfarlane WM. Effects of rosiglitazone and metformin on pancreatic beta-cell gene expression. *Diabetologia*, (2006), 4:685-696

Roche E, Soria B. Stem cell approaches for beta-cell replacement. In: Islet Transplantation and Beta Cell Replacement Therapy. (Eds.) A.M. James Shapiro and James A. M. Shaw, (2007), pp:311-325

Sawada T, Matsumoto I, Nakano M, Kirchhof N, Sutherland DER, Hering BJ. Improved islet yield and function with ductal injection of University of Wisconsin solution before pancreas preservation. *Transplantation*, Vol. 75, No. 12, (June 2003), pp. 1965-1969

Scott MD, Murad KL, Koumpouras F, Talbot M, Eaton JW. Chemical camouflage of antigenic determinants: Stealth erythrocytes. *Proc Natl Acad Sci U S A*, Vol. 94, No. 14, (July 1997), pp. 7566-7571

Shapiro AM, Lakey JR, Ryan EA, Korbutt GS, Toth E, Warnock GL, et al. Islet transplantation in seven patients with type 1 diabetes mellitus using a glucocorticoid-free immunosuppressive regimen. *N. Engl. J. Med*, Vol. 343, No. 4, (2000 July), pp. 230-238

Shapiro AMJ, Nanji SA, Lakey JRT. Clinical islet transplant: current and future directions towards tolerance. *Immunological Reviews*, Vol. 196, No. 1, (December 2003), pp. 219-236

Shapiro AMJ, Toso C, Koh A, Calne SR, Kin T, O'Gorman D, et al. Alemtuzumab Induction and Tac/Mmf Maintenance Substantially Improves Long Term Insulin Independence Rates After Clinical Islet Transplantation, and Strongly Suppresses Both Auto and Alloreactivity. *Transplantation*, Vol. 90, (2010), Abstract 2026

Sharma A, Zangen DH, Reitz P et al. The homeodomain protein IDX-1 increases after an early burst of proliferation during pancreatic regeneration. *Diabetes*, (1999), 48:507-513

Shimoda M, Noguchi H, Naziruddin B, Fujita Y, Chujo D, Takita M, et al. Assessment of human islet isolation with four different collagenases. *Transplant. Proc*, Vol. 42, No. 6, (August 2010), pp. 2049-2051

Smith AG. Culture and differentiation of embryonic stem cells. *J Tissue Cult Meth.* (1991), Vol. 19, pp. 1341-1343

Stabler CL, Sun X-L, Cui W, Wilson JT, Haller CA, Chaikof EL. Surface re-engineering of pancreatic islets with recombinant azido-thrombomodulin. Bioconjug. Chem, Vol. 18, No. 6 (November 2007), pp. 1713-1715

Stock PG, Bluestone JA. Beta-Cell Replacement for Type I Diabetes. *Annu. Rev. Med*, Vol. 55, No. 1, (2004), pp. 133-156

Sutherland DER, Gores PF, Farney AC, Wahoff DC, Matas AJ, Dunn DL, et al. Evolution of kidney, pancreas, and islet transplantation for patients with diabetes at the University of Minnesota. *The American Journal of Surgery*, Vol. 166, No. 5, (November 1993), pp. 456-491

Takemoto N, Teramura Y, Iwata H. Islet Surface Modification with Urokinase through DNA Hybridization. *Bioconjug Chem*, (Epub, March 22, 2011)

Teramura Y, Iwata H. Islets Surface Modification Prevents Blood-Mediated Inflammatory Responses. *Bioconjugate Chemistry*, Vol. 19, No. 7, (July 2008), pp. 1389-1395

Teramura Y, Kaneda Y, Iwata H. Islet-encapsulation in ultra-thin layer-by-layer membranes of poly(vinyl alcohol) anchored to poly(ethylene glycol)-lipids in the cell membrane. *Biomaterials*, Vol. 28, No. 32. (November 2007), pp. 4818-4825

Tjernberg J, Ekdahl KN, Lambris JD, Korsgren O, Nilsson B. Acute antibody-mediated complement activation mediates lysis of pancreatic islets cells and may cause tissue loss in clinical islet transplantation. *Transplantation*, Vol. 85, No. 8, (April 2008), pp. 1193-1199

Valdes-Gonzalez RA, Dorantes LM, Garibay GN, Bracho-Blanchet E, Mendez AJ, Davila-Perez R, et al. Xenotransplantation of porcine neonatal islets of Langerhans and Sertoli cells: a 4-year study. *Eur J Endocrinol*, Vol. 153, No. 3, (September 2005), pp. 419-427

Venstrom JM, McBride MA, Rother KI, Hirshberg B, Orchard TJ, Harlan DM. Survival After Pancreas Transplantation in Patients With Diabetes and Preserved Kidney Function. *JAMA*, Vol. 290, No. 21, (December 2003), pp. 2817 -2823

Vézina C, Kudelski A, Sehgal SN. Rapamycin (AY-22,989), a new antifungal antibiotic. I. Taxonomy of the producing streptomycete and isolation of the active principle. *J. Antibiot*, Vol. 28, No. 10, (October 1975), pp. 721-726

Wilson JT, Chaikof EL. Challenges and emerging technologies in the immunoisolation of cells and tissues. *Advanced Drug Delivery Reviews*, Vol. 60, No. 2, (January 2008), pp. 124-145

Wilson JT, Haller CA, Qu Z, Cui W, Urlam MK, Chaikof EL. Biomolecular surface engineeng of pancreatic islets with thrombomodulin. *Acta Biomaterialia*, Vol. 6, No. 6, (June 2010), pp. 1895-1903

Xie D, Smyth CA, Eckstein C, Bilbao G, Mays J, Eckhoff DE, et al. Cytoprotection of PEG-modified adult porcine pancreatic islets for improved xenotransplantation. *Biomaterials*, Vol. 26, No. 4, (February 2005), pp. 403-412

Yamamoto T, Horiguchi A, Ito M, Nagata H, Ichii H, Ricordi C, et al. Quality control for clinical islet transplantation: organ procurement and preservation, the islet processing facility, isolation, and potency tests. *J Hepatobiliary Pancreat Surg*, Vol 16, No. 2, (2009), pp. 131-136

Yamamoto T, Ricordi C, Messinger S, Sakuma Y, Miki A, Rodriguez R, et al. Deterioration and Variability of Highly Purified Collagenase Blends Used in Clinical Islet Isolation. *Transplantation*, Vol 84, No. 8, (2007), pp. 997-1002

Yun Lee D, Hee Nam J, Byun Y. Functional and histological evaluation of transplanted pancreatic islets immunoprotected by PEGylation and cyclosporine for 1 year. *Biomaterials*, Vol. 28, No. 11, (April 2007), pp. 1957-1966

Zhang JR, Woods RJ, Brown PB, Mowery RA, Kane RR. Photochemical tissue bonding using monomeric 4-amino-1,8 naphthalimides. *J Biomed. Op*, Vol. 9, No. 5, (September 2004), pp. 1089-92

Part 8

Genetics

23

Genetics of Type 1 Diabetes

Tatijana Zemunik and Vesna Boraska
*University of Split School of Medicine,
Split,
Croatia*

1. Introduction

Type 1 diabetes (T1D) is an autoimmune disease characterized by immune destruction of insulin-producing pancreatic β cells. This leads to dysfunctional regulation of blood glucose levels in T1D patients. The destruction of β cells of Langerhans islets is caused by infiltration of dendritic cells, macrophages and T lymphocytes. The destruction of β cells starts with an autoimmune process that is followed by massive destruction of β cells later on. Autoantibodies against T1D-specific antigens are present in serum and can be detected in the early stage of the disease (Ounisis-Benkalha & Polychronakos, 2008). There are several main types of T1D autoantibodies: islet antibodies, antibodies to insulin (IAA), glutamic acid decarboxilase (GADA) and tyrosine phosphatise IA-2. In the last few years antibodies to zinc transporter (ZnT8) have been added to this group (Mehers & Gillespie, 2008). It is generally accepted that T1D occurs as a result of genetic and environmental factors when presence of many alleles combined with effects of numerous environmental factors lead to disease development (Pociot et al., 2010). Research of T1D genetic basis and environmental factors has increased dramatically in the last two decades. Today it is considered that beside *HLA* region on chromosome 6q21 that contributes approximately with 40% to T1D development, more than 50 non-*HLA* genes significantly increase the risk of T1D occurrence (MacFarlane et al., 2009, Ziegler et al., 2010; Concannon et al., 2010). The final aim of genetic research is integration with clinical practice, which is expected once the main understanding of genetic etiology of T1D is achieved. Translation to clinics includes development of genetic-based diagnostic tests, population screening methods and prevention strategies, and finally, development of new treatments and therapies (Manolio et al., 2009).

2. Genetic studies

There are two main approaches in dissecting T1D genetic background: linkage analysis and association analysis (Figure 1). Linkage analysis is based on simple Mendelian inheritance and it uses affected relatives (typically siblings) to identify regions on chromosomes that are shared more frequently than expected by chance. Since affected siblings are relatively rare in T1D, linkage studies have been performed in somewhat unique subgroup of families with T1D (Concannon et al., 2009). In general, samples are genotyped for a modestly dense panel of markers, typically microsatellites, to search for linked alleles i.e. alleles that are inherited together. Regions in the genome with accumulating evidence of linkage are further fine mapped, which means that additional markers are typed in the same chromosomal region,

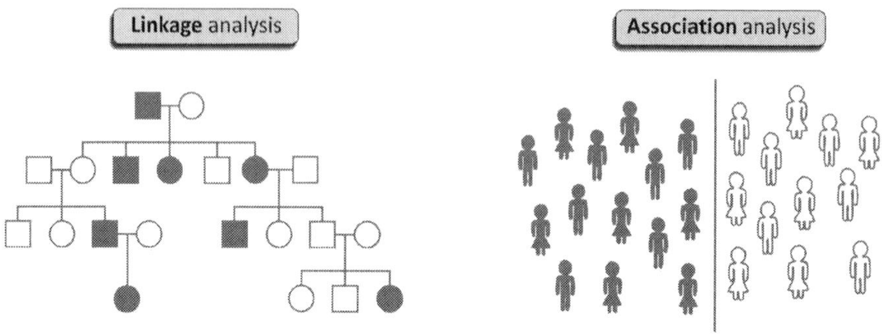

Fig. 1. Linkage analysis tests for the co-segregation of alleles within family members whereas association analysis searches for the difference in allele frequency between unrelated groups of affected and unaffected individuals or within families. Adapted from Concannon et al., 2009.

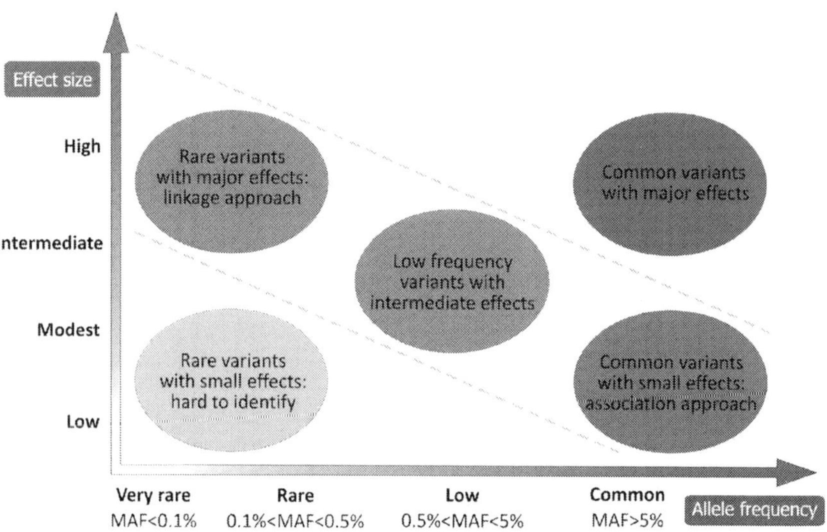

Fig. 2. Relation of risk allele frequencies, effect sizes (odds ratios) and feasibility of identifying risk variants by common genetic tests. Generally, linkage studies are better in indentifying low-frequency alleles with larger effect sizes, whereas association studies are more effective in identifying common variants with small to moderate effects. Adapted from McCarthy et al., 2008 & Manolio et. al., 2009.

in order to narrow down regions associated with disease. Linkage analyses are most effective in identifying rare alleles with large effect sizes (Figure 2) (Concannon et al., 2009). On the other hand, common alleles with modest and small effect sizes can be identified through association analysis. Association studies test for association of genotyped marker (typically single nucleotide polymorphism, SNP) with the disease of interest in a case-control or family-based sample. These studies rely on the assumption that investigated allele is associated with disease if it differs in frequency between two investigated groups of individuals. Tested polymorphism is usually not the causative one but it will show an association if it is in linkage disequilibrium (LD) with an unknown causative, risk or protective, variant. Human genome is divided into regions of high and low LD, and if allele resides in the region of high LD that means that many SNPs from the same region will be inherited together and therefore reflect one another. This means that genotyping of only limited, but carefully selected, set of SNPs can actually capture a majority of information within tested gene region (Lander, 2011).

For the last decade the most common design of association analysis used to be candidate gene approach that searches for differences in allele frequencies in specifically selected genes between affected and healthy groups of individuals or affected subjects and their parents. There are few general limits of candidate gene studies that include modest sample sizes, limited number of investigated variants, the fact that selection of genes/variants is often based on inadequate understanding of biological pathways and, most importantly, observed associations are usually difficult to replicate (Manolio et al., 2009). However, just few years ago a complete dominance in association analyses design was taken by genome-wide association studies (GWAS) approach. These are hypothesis free studies that usually test between 300,000 up to 1 million directly genotyped SNPs that capture substantial proportion of common genetic variation of the genome (McCarthy et al. 2008). The methodology behind the GWAS is the same as in any association study and that is to map susceptibility variants through identification of associations between allele (genotype) frequency and disease status (McCarthy et al. 2008). The development of both, high-throughput genotyping platforms and a catalogue of human variation by International HapMap Project (http://hapmap.ncbi.nlm.nih.gov/) and The 1000 Genomes project (http://www.1000genomes.org/) have made possible high utilization of GWAS. In addition, development of imputation methods that infer missing genetic variants enabled inclusion and comparison of different GWAS in large-scale meta-analysis framework (Marchini & Howie, 2010). Also, huge collaborative international projects such as The Type 1 Diabetes Genetics Consortium (T1DGC) (https://www.t1dgc.org/home.cfm) have put efforts to collect and systemise data from several thousand T1D affected and healthy individuals worldwide in order to identify genes contributing to an individual's risk for T1D susceptibility. Overall, the combination of linkage, association and large-scale GWAS approaches provided evidence of genetic contribution of many common and rare alleles with wide range of effect sizes to the T1D development.

2.1 Linkage analysis approach

Genetic linkage studies have shown the biggest success in discovering genetic loci underlying monogenic disorders where risk factors, even rare in frequency, have large effects and often lead to change in amino acid sequence (Smith & Newton-Cheh 2009). In complex diseases, such as T1D, situation is less straightforward since there are loci of small, modest and large effect sizes contributing to the disease (Concannon et al., 2009; Kere, 2010).

Several linkage analyses of T1D provided evidence for linkage between the *HLA* region on chromosome 6p21 and T1D. There were also other non-*HLA* loci findings but these were not consistently replicated among studies, mostly because of limited sample sizes. T1DGC conducted linkage meta-analysis of most of T1D genome-wide linkage studies and showed strong evidence of linkage with *HLA* class II genes encoding *HLA-DR* and *HLA-DQ*. In addition, this study demonstrated supporting evidence of linkage of additional genes within *HLA* region and small number of other regions in the genome (Concannon et al., 2009).

2.2 Association analysis approach

2.2.1 Case–control design

Case-control design is one of the most common association study designs. Case-control study compares two groups of individuals, one with the disease (cases) and the other without disease (controls). It is assumed that cases have higher prevalence of susceptibility alleles for disease of interest than controls and that susceptibility alleles can be detected through direct comparison of allele frequencies between two groups (McCarthy et al. 2008). A lot of attention is given to case ascertainment to minimize phenotypic heterogeneity. In addition, study power can be improved by selection of cases, for example to those with the extremes of phenotypes (McCarthy et al. 2008). Since it is observed that incident rates of T1D highly increase in the very young group of children, an early age of disease onset could be an example of extreme T1D phenotype and enrichment of those cases in the sample set is likely to improve power (McCarthy et al. 2008; Maahs et al. 2010).

In genetic epidemiological studies a lot of attention is given to control selection. Controls are matched with cases by ethnicity to avoid problems of population stratification that may result with spurious associations (false positives). This means that controls are selected from the same population, preferably from the same region, as cases (Zondervan & Cardon 2007). Nowadays, with the genome-wide data, it is possible to estimate the level of relatedness among individuals and, also, the matching of cases and controls by ancestry (Anderson et al. 2010). Principal component analysis is one of the most common methods that enables clustering of individuals by ancestry (Figure 3). To further reduce stratification within the sample set, controls can also be matched to cases by age, sex and environmental factors. Usually, association analyses are adjusted for covariates with strong impact on phenotype to reduce non-genetic contribution to phenotype variation (Smith & Newton-Cheh 2009).

2.2.2 Family-based design

Family-based association studies, most commonly in the form of parent–offspring trios, use another analytical approach to test for association. To make assumptions on association with the disease these studies examine the transmission of alleles from heterozygous parents to affected offspring that is observed more frequently than expected by chance (Smith & Newton-Cheh 2009). Since these studies are conducted within families they offer a protection from population stratification but they also rely on informative parent–offspring trios which usually reduce the effective sample size, thus power as well (McCarthy et al. 2008; Smith & Newton-Cheh 2009). Family-based studies are particularly useful in finding variants underlying relatively rare phenotypes that segregate within families. Also, these studies have advantages when age of disease onset is low, as in the case of T1D, because it enables easier collection of many family members (Smith & Newton-Cheh 2009).

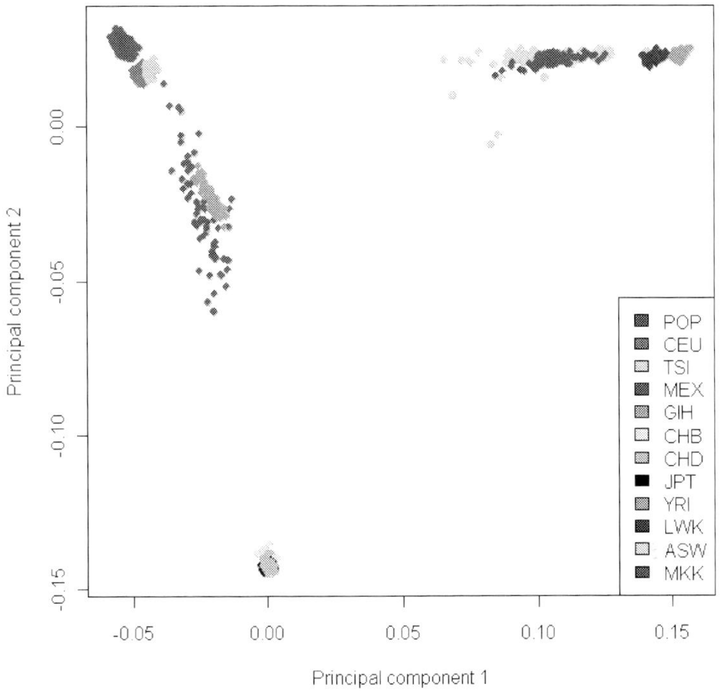

Fig. 3. Principal component analysis of samples deriving from population of interest (POP) and 11 HapMap phase II populations (CEU - Utah residents with Northern and Western European ancestry from the CEPH collection; TSI - Toscans in Italy; MEX - Mexican ancestry in Los Angeles; GIH - Gujarati Indians in Houston; CHB - Han Chinese in Beijing, China; CHD - Chinese in Metropolitan Denver; JPT - Japanese in Tokyo, YRI - Yoruba in Ibadan, Nigeria; LWK - Luhya in Webuye, Kenya; ASW - African ancestry in Southwest USA; MKK - Maasai in Kinyawa, Kenya)

2.2.3 Genome-wide association studies (GWAS) and meta-analyses

Rationale underlying GWAS is the 'common disease, common variant' hypothesis. It is believed that both, common and rare variants, contribute to complex disease risk. However, GWAS are generally powered only to detect association of common variants (allelic variants present in more than 5% of the population) with modest to large effect sizes (Manolio et al., 2009). GWAS are not designed to identify multiple rare mutations within a gene (Kere, 2010).

Because of the modest sample sizes individual GWAS have limited power to detect all associations underlying complex diseases. Increase in sample size achieved by combination of statistical evidence of individual studies through meta-analysis approach can improve study power and raise a discovery of susceptibility loci. Nowdays, a majority of new genetic findings underlying complex traits are found through meta-analysis approach. Since different studies differ in design, sample collection, genotyping platform and analysis methodology, one of the most important prerequisites for meta-analysis is capability to uniform study results. Most genotyping platforms have different representation of genetic markers and harmonisation of studies through expansion of SNP coverage can be achieved by imputation processes. Imputation infers and fills in missing genotypes on the basis of HapMap, the 1000 Genomes or other reference panels to allow different studies to analyse the same set of common SNPs (de Bakker et al., 2010). The biggest meta-analysis for T1D combined results from two studies and included total of 7,514 cases and 9,045 reference samples. This study identified another 18 regions associated with T1D that suggested novel candidate genes such as *IL10, IL19, IL20, GLIS3, CD69* and *IL27* (Barrett et al., 2009).

2.3 Other types of genetic research

There are many other types of genetic research that contribute to understanding of complex disease mechanisms. Many of these studies use knowledge on susceptible genetic variation accumulated through linkage and association studies. Identified variants are usually additionally analysed for gene-gene and gene-environment interactions. Also, it is well known that genes interact through complex molecular networks and integrating the prior knowledge of biological pathways of genes of interest may increase a chance to find genes involved in disease development. These pathway-based analyses use different software packages that search through variety of web-based databases and take into account the existing data on biological pathways of investigated genes (Wang et al., 2010). Cross-disorder overlap is another search that looks for evidence of potential overlapping regions of the genome affecting various different diseases, such as T1D and other autoimmune traits (Eyre et al. 2010). All these supplementary analyses help in elucidating genetic contribution in complex disease development.

There are functional studies that also use data derived from genetic analyses. Most commonly performed ones are gene expression analyses that may investigate susceptible genes/gene variants in different tissues or investigate them under different environmental stimuli. Combining the information on gene expression profiles and alternate splicing sites across a range of human tissues together with genetic mapping for the same samples will be valuable in deciphering the roles of genetic variants (McCarthy et al., 2008). Genetical genomics analysis also offers new means in understanding the genetic architecture of gene expression (Cui et al., 2010)

2.4 Finding the missing heritability

GWAS have identified more than 50 genetic variants associated with T1D. However, just like in most other complex traits, associated variants explain only a small proportion of heritability of T1D ($\lambda s \sim 5$, whereas it is estimated to be 15) and have rather small effect on disease risk (Clayton, 2009). The remaining missing heritability can be explained in several different ways such as an influence of much larger number of common variants of smaller effect sizes that still need to be identified, an influence of rare variants of modest and small effect sizes that have not yet been discovered because of their underrepresentation in the current genotyping platforms and because of underpowered sample sizes, an influence of structural variants that are also poorly captured by existing platforms and generally low power to detect gene-gene and gene-environment interactions (Manolio et al., 2009). Sample size is generally one of the major limiting factors for discovery of common alleles with small effect sizes. Augmenting the number of investigated individuals through meta-analysis approach to more than tens of thousands of individuals is another way for discovery of new genetic loci (Lander, 2011). On the other hand sequencing is the best way for discovering rare and structural variants such as copy number variants, inversions, translocations, microsatellite repeat expansions, insertions of new sequence and complex rearrangements (Manolio et al., 2009). Because of immense decrease in price, sequencing is becoming a common practice and next generation sequencing (exon or whole-genome sequencing) might provide many clues for missing heritability. The 1000 Genomes Project (http://www.1000genomes.org/) aims to provide a complete catalogue of human genome sequence variation and the pilot phase of the project already identified around 15 million SNPs, 1 million short insertions and deletions and 20,000 structural variants (The 1000 Genomes Project Consortium et al., 2010). Most of these variants were previously unknown and will provide a foundation for future genetic research of human diseases, including T1D. Also, sequencing of individuals with extreme phenotypes, for example individuals with the extreme age of T1D diagnosis, might provide important findings because it is thought that they carry more deleterious, loss-of-function mutations (Romeo et al., 2007).

It is also thought that some of the missing heritability might be discovered by conducting studies in populations of non European ancestry. Most genetic studies have been limited to European populations even it is known that genetic variation is highest in the populations of recent African ancestry. These studies might prove useful in detecting rare variants associations and narrowing down associated regions due to smaller LD windows (International HapMap Consortium et al., 2007). Family studies and isolated populations are another sample sets that might help in identifying missing heritability due to their enrichment of unique genetic variants (Sabatti et al., 2009).

2.5 Prevention, diagnostics and clinical application of genetic findings

Genetic research of complex diseases aims to improve understanding of biological and physiological pathways involved in disease etiology. The main goal is integration of newly accumulated knowledge with clinical practice by development of more effective means of diagnosis, prevention, treatment and response to therapies. Identification of predictive variants for considerable proportion of disease, even with identification of many other risk variants with smaller effect sizes, is very challenging (Manolio et al., 2009). The biggest influence for T1D development is carried by *HLA* loci and it is shown that only few *HLA* SNPs capture most of the heritability of T1D risk that is attributable to *HLA* associations (Clayton, 2009). There is substantial genetic risk to T1D that can be attributable to yet undiscovered loci and it is assumed that the majority of these loci will have smaller effects than those loci which have already been discovered (Clayton, 2009). So far, genetic prediction for T1D is modest and it is still not reaching criteria required for a targeted disease prevention strategy (Clayton, 2009). However, it is believed that a small proportion of population at the highest risk will be identifiable and the development of diagnostic and targeted prevention strategies for those individuals will be feasible. These diagnostic and interventional strategies will require more accurate genetic prediction and it is necessary that they are developed through ethical, safe, effective and individualized approach (Manolio et al., 2009; Clayton, 2009). One of suggested ways to discover individuals at risk is through population screening which means genotyping specific genetic variants, whole-genome typing and whole-genome sequencing of entire population (Manolio et al., 2009; Pharoah et al., 2008). Figure 4 shows the ways of translation of genetic findings into clinical practice and disease management.

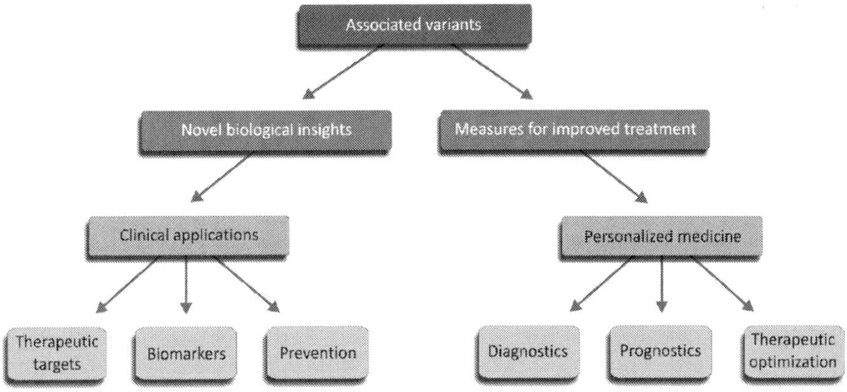

Fig. 4. Translation of genetic information into clinical practice. Adapted from McCarthy et al. 2008.

3. Genetic background of T1D

3.1 Rare monogenetic forms of T1D

Very rare form of autoimmune diabetes is monogenetic diabetes, which means that it is caused by mutation of a single gene. In such cases, diabetes occurs as part of multiple set of autoimmune diseases. One of them is known as the immune dysregulation, polyendocrinopathy, enteropathy, X-linked (IPEX) syndrome in which a function of regulatory T cells is impaired (van Belle et al., 2011). It occurs as a result of mutations of *FOXP3*, the master gene for normal functioning of regulatory T cells (Wang et al., 2010). About 80% of children with IPEX syndrome develop autoimmune diabetes at an early age (van Belle et al., 2011). Another example of multiple autoimmune disease is autoimmune polyendocrine syndrome type 1 (APS-1) or autoimmune polyendocrinopathy-candidiasis-ectodermal dystrophy (APECED) (van Belle et al., 2011). The main cause of APECED development is mutations in the autoimmune regulator (AIRE) protein (Villaseñor et al. 2005). Lack of AIRE protein decreases the expression of insulin and other peripheral molecules in the thymus. This allows effector T cells escape to the periphery and prevent their negative selection in the thymus through apoptosis (Liston et al., 2004). About 20% of APS1 or APECED patients develop T1D (van Belle et al., 2011). Although the number of patients with this monogenic form of T1D is almost negligible, these findings indicate the high impact of immune status on the disease occurrence (van Belle et al., 2011).

3.2 Family history of T1D

Over 85% of T1D patients do not have positive family history of T1D, however there is a 6% of disease clustering among siblings. Siblings have 15 times greater chance of developing T1D in comparison with the general population which gives strong evidence of the genetic background of this disease. The pattern of inheritance seems very complicated, and disease development further depends on the triggers from the environment. Long-term monitoring showed that the concordance rate of inheritance is greater than 50% in monozygous twins, while it is 6-10% in dizygous twins, which is similar to that of siblings. Interestingly, the siblings who share both identical haplotypes of *DR3/DR4 HLA* class II region, which shows highest susceptibility to T1D, have a higher risk of disease development than those who share only one or no haplotypes of that region. (Steck & Rewers 2011).

3.3 *HLA*

First and consistent evidence of *HLA* gene contribution to the disease was provided by linkage analyses and further confirmed by association analyses. *HLA* genes contribute with approximately 40% of genetic risk to T1D development (MacFarlane et al., 2009). The proteins encoded by *HLA* genes are cell-surface proteins grouped in class I (A, B and C) and class II (DP, DQ and DR) of *HLA* region on chromosome 6p21 (Figure 5). Both groups of proteins are essential in self and non-self immune recognition. The proteins encoded by the *HLA* class I genes are single chain proteins that present intracellular antigen to CD8+ T killer cells while proteins encoded by *HLA* class II are built of two chains and present extracellular antigen to CD4+ T helper cells (Ounisis-Benkalha & Polychronakos, 2008). It is considered today that the *HLA* region class II has the strongest input in the development of T1D, which has been deeply investigated in the past several decades (van Belle et al., 2011). *HLA DR4* and *DR3* class II haplotypes are of particular importance in the T1D development. Even greater risk of T1D development have individuals with genetic combinations of two susceptible alleles, *DR3/DR4*. *HLA* region on chromosome 6p21.3 comprises more than 200

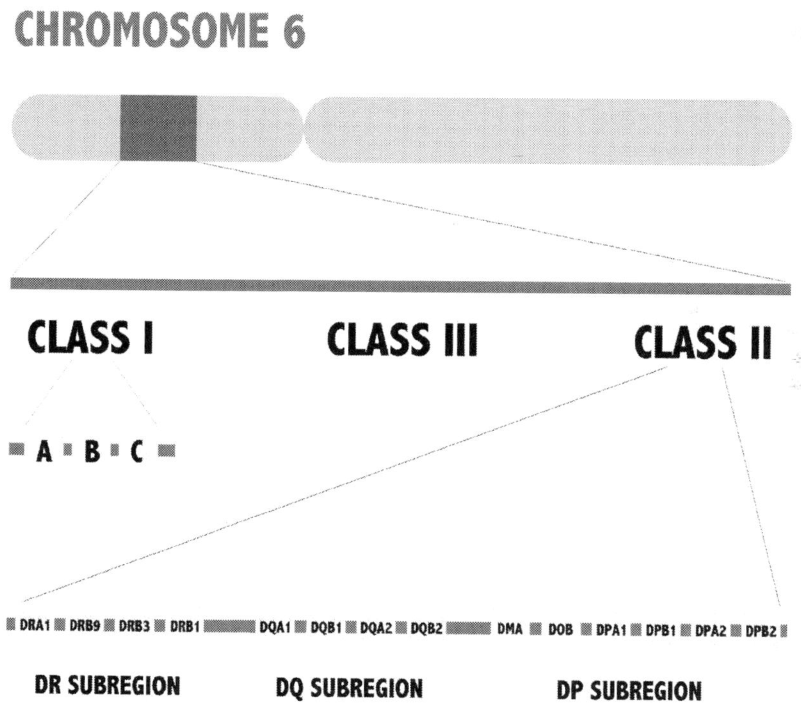

Fig. 5. *HLA* region on hromosome 6p21.3. Adapted from Mehers & Gillespie, 2008.

genes that are in high LD. Therefore, it is difficult to determine which gene gives the observed effect. It is considered that haplotypes of high risk for T1D are *DRB1*0401-DQA1*0301-DQB1*0302* and *DRB1*0301-DQA1*0501-DQB1*0201*(Mehers & Gillespie, 2008; Skrodeniene et al., 2010). Antigen-presenting cells (APC) carry HLA class II molecules that bind key T1D autoantigens such as preproinsulin, insulinoma associated antigen 2, glutamic acid decarboxilase (GAD) and zinc transporter (ZnT8) and present them to thymocites in the thymus. Strongly self-reactive thymocites die by apoptosis, negative selection that eliminates 98% of thymocytes. Only 2% of thymocytes that have low affinity migrate as mature T cells in the periphery where they develop into $CD4^+$ and $CD8^+$ T cells. $CD4^+$ T cells are helper cells to $CD8^+$ T killer cells in the processes of destruction of pancreatic islet β cells (Figure 6). It is believed that the most important autoantigen in the onset of T1D is preproinsulin, whose N-terminal signal peptide and the peptidase cleavage site is recognised by $CD8^+$ T killer cells. The proteins encoded by *HLA* class I, *HLA-A* and *HLA-B* exert smaller effects in the pathogenesis of T1D. Proteins encoded by class I *HLA* genes are expressed on nucleated cells, often in the pancreatic insulin-producing β cells. These proteins present antigens directly to the $CD8^+$ T killer cells (Figure 6) (Ounisis-Benkalha & Polychronakos, 2008; Todd, 2010; Pociot et al., 2010; Blueston et al., 2010; van Belle et al., 2011). However, it was observed that some *HLA* haplotype combinations have protective association with T1D. It is believed that haplotype *DR15-DQ6*, which was found in about 20% of the general population and even less than 1% of patients with T1D has protective effect (Ounisis-Benkalha & Polychronakos, 2008).

3.4 Other non-*HLA* pathways

Linkage analyses additionally pointed to linkage of some non-*HLA* loci but without consistent replication. Candidate-gene association studies have further confirmed *HLA* loci as the major T1D genetic factors but also identified four other T1D susceptibility loci: gene for insulin (*INS*), cytotoxic T-lymphocyte-associated protein 4 (*CTLA4*), protein tyrosine phosphatise, non-receptor type 22 (lymphoid) (*PTPN22*) and interleukin 2 receptor, alpha (*IL2RA*) (Bell et al., 1984; Nisticò et al., 1996; Bottini et al., 2004; Lowe et al., 2007).

The first strong non-*HLA* association with T1D was shown with polymorphisms within the *INS* gene (Bell et al., 1984). Variable number of tandem repeats (VNTR) composed of 14-15 bp tandem repeat sequence (ACAGGGGTGTGGGG) is located 596 bp upstream of the *INS* gene on chromosome 11p15 and regulates gene transcription (Ounissi-Benkalha & Polychronakos, 2008). Alleles of this region are divided into three classes with respect to the number of consecutive VNTRs: class I VNTR alleles (short, 26-63 repeats), class II VNTR alleles (63-140 repeats) and class III VNTR alleles (long, 141-209) (Durinovic-Bello et al., 2010). They correlate with *INS* mRNA production in pancreas and thymus. Class I alleles of the *INS* VNTR increase the risk of T1D and have been associated with high mRNA levels in pancreas and low levels in thymus. Class III alleles are associated with 20% lower mRNA than class I in pancreas but two to three times higher mRNA levels in thymus and therefore are considered to be protective. It seems that high levels of proinsuline in the thymus may stimulate negative selection (dying by apoptosis) of insulin specific T-lymphocits crucial in the pathogenesis of T1D. On the other hand it is believed that lower levels of proinsuline in thymus affect the positive selection of T cells in the thymus, migration of $CD4^+$ proinsulin specific T cells in the periphery, that increase risk to T1D. In that way, the genetically regulated selection mechanisms affect the selection of autoreactive cells in the immune response to autoantigenes (Todd, 2010; Pociot et al., 2010; Ounissi-Benkalha & Polychronakos, 2008).

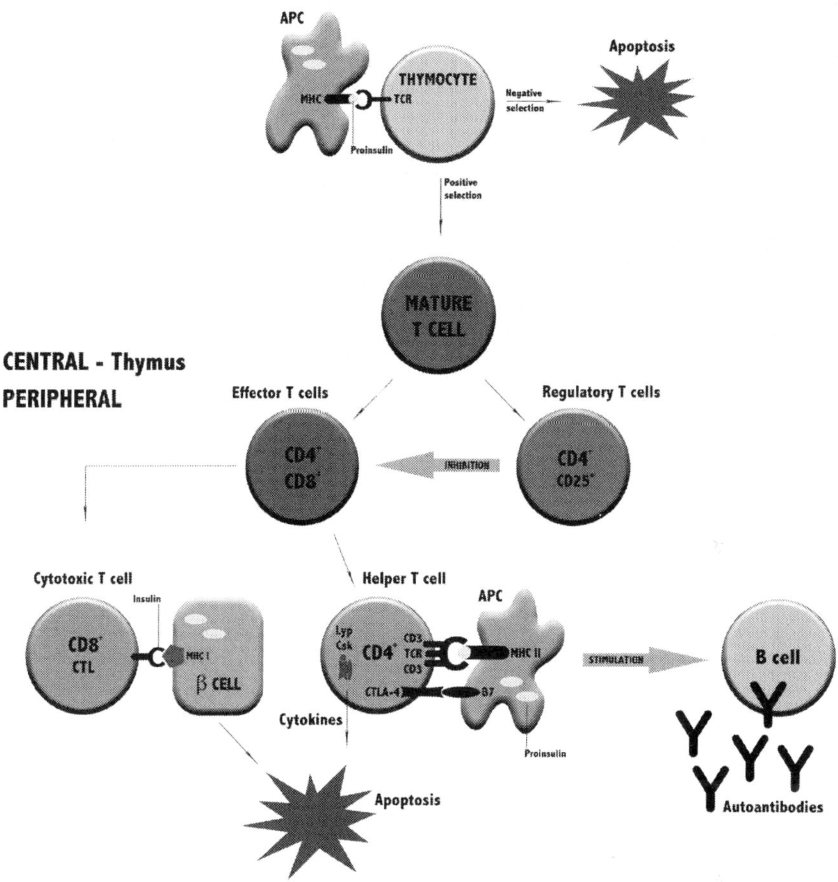

Fig. 6. The development of an autoimmune reaction in T1D. Adapted from Ounisis-Benkalha & Polychronakos, 2008.

In 1996 *CTLA4* gene located on chromosome 2q33 was confirmed as another T1D susceptibility gene (Nistico L et al., 1996.). CTLA4 protein is a co-stimulatory receptor on the cell surface of CD4+ T cells. It binds B7 ligands of APCs that activate main component of the co-receptor, CD28. In the same time intracellular part of the CTLA4 interact with intracellular domain of CD3 receptor and start phosphorylation of the several downstream target molecules. Consequently, this leads to activation of T cells after their binding to HLA molecules on APCs (Figure 6) (Ounissi-Benkalha & Polychronakos, 2008). Reduction of the CTLA4 protein in CD4+ T cells increases susceptibility to T1D (Todd, 2010; Pociot et al., 2010). The A49G polymorphism in exone 1 causes substitution of an alanine with a threonine in the signal sequence of CTLA4 protein that leads to incorrect glycosylation of mutant protein and reduction of its expression on T-cell surface. Conversely, C318T polymorphism of the *CTLA4* promoter gene region causes higher promoter activity and increases the amount of CTL4 protein on the T cell surface. Therefore, it can be considered as protective polymorphism of this gene (Ounissi-Benkalha & Polychronakos, 2008).

More recently in 2004, *PTPN22* gene located on chromosome 1q13 that encodes lymphoid tyrosine phosphatase was recognized as further T1D susceptibility gene (Bottini et al., 2004). Lymphoid tyrosine phosphatise "Lip" inhibits T cell receptor (TCR) signal transduction and causes inhibition of $CD4^+$ T-cell activation (Figure 6). The Lyp inhibitory function is enhanced by its interaction with C-terminal Src tyrosine kinase (Csk). T1D is associated with a polymorphism at position 1858 by replacing the C to T, which leads to the substitution of arginine to tryptophan at position 620 of Lyp protein (R620W) (Ounissi-Benkalha & Polychronakos, 2008; Mehers & Gillespie, 2008; Todd, 2010; Pociot et al., 2010). The Lyp interaction with tyrosine kinase Csk occurs just in the 620 region. A 620W allele interacts less strongly with Csk than 620R allele. A 620W homozygous shows increased inhibition of TCR signalling, reduces $CD4^+$ T cell activation thus resulting in increased autoimmunity (Todd, 2010; Pociot et al., 2010; Ziegler et al., 2010).

Another strongly associated gene, *IL2RA* located on chromosome 10p15 that encodes alpha chain (CD25) molecules of IL-2 receptor has been reported as T1D associated gene (Vella et al. 2005). The CD25 is responsible for binding of IL-2 and proliferation of regulatory T cell and consequently, it affects their function in inhibition of effector T cells and autoimmune disease (Figure 6). T1D-predisponding alleles of *IL2RA* gene correlate with lower amounts of CD25 on the surface of the regulatory T cells which are suppressors of autoreactivity and that can be important in regulation of T-cell proliferation by an immunogenic stimulus (Ounissi-Benkalha & Polychronakos, 2008; Mehers & Gillespie, 2008; Todd, 2010; Pociot et al., 2010).

Since 2001 a significant number of GWA studies have been reported. Data from The International Type 1 Diabetes Genetics Consortium (T1DGC) collected through multiple genome-wide association studies are available to the scientific community by request. Recently, GWAS and large scale meta-analyses identified more than 40 loci that affect the risk of developing T1D (Table 1.) (Barrett et al., 2009, Pociot et al., 2010). The analysis included 7.514 cases and 9.045 control samples. Fifteen of these regions have been previously reported as regions associated with T1D susceptibility. Eighteen additional regions showed significant association with T1D and several of them contain new candidate genes of possible relevance to T1D (*IL10, IL19, IL20, GLIS3, CD69* and *IL27*) (Pociot et al., 2010). Most of the listed genes mediate the immune response, some exert their functions in the process of destruction of pancreatic β cells and some have a dual role (Pociot et al., 2010). A list of SNPs and genes associated with T1D is presented in Table 1.

SNP	Chromosome	OR minor allele	Gene of interest
rs2476601	1p13.2	2.05	PTPN22
rs2269241	1p31.3	1.10	PGM1
rs2816316	1q31.2	0.89	RGS1
rs3024505	1q32.1	0.84	IL10 (CNTN2)
rs1534422	2p25.1	1.08	(gene desert)

SNP	Chromosome	OR minor allele	Gene of interest
rs917997	2q12.1	0.83	IL18RAP
rs1990760	2q24.2	0.86	IFIH1
rs3087243	2q33.2	0.88	CTLA4
rs11711054	3p21.31	0.85	CCR5
rs10517086	4p15.2	1.09	(gene desert)
rs4505848	4q27	1.13	IL2
rs6897932	5q13.2	0.89	IL7R
rs9268645	6p21.32	6.8	MHC
rs11755527	6q15	1.13	BACH2
rs9388489	6q22.32	1.17	C6orf173
rs2327832	6q23.3	0.90	TNFAIP3
rs1738074	6q25.3	0.92	TAGAP
rs7804356	7p15.2	0.88	SKAP2
rs4948088	7p12.1	0.77	COBL
rs7020673	9p24.2	0.88	GLIS3
rs12251307	10p15.1	1.61	IL2RA
rs11258747	10p15.1	0.84	PRKCQ
rs10509540	10q23.31	0.75	RNLS
rs7111341	11p15.5	2.38	INS (TH)
rs4763879	12p13	1.09	CD69
rs2292239	12q13.2	1.31	ERBB3
rs1678536	12q13.3.		Multiple (MMP19-LOCx-GSTPP)
rs3184504	12q24.12	1.28	SH2B3
rs1465788	14q24.1	0.86	C14orf181
rs4900384	14q32.2	1.09	(0; gene desert)
rs3825932	15q25.1	0.86	CTSH
rs12708716	16p13.13	0.81	CLEC16A
rs12444268	16p12.3	1.10	UMOD
rs4788084	16p11.2	0.86	IL27 (NUPR1)
rs7202877	16q23.1	1.28	CTRB1
rs16956936	17p13.1	0.92	DNAH2
rs2290400	17q12	0.87	ORMDL3 (GSDML3)
rs7221109	17q21.2	0.95	SMARCE1
rs1893217	18p11.21	1.28	PTPN2
rs763361	18q22.2	1.16	CD226
rs425105	19q13.32	0.86	PRKD2
rs2281808	20p13	0.90	SIRPG
rs11203203	21q22.3	1.13	UBASH3A
rs5753037	22q12.2	1.10	LOC729980/HORMAD2
rs229541	22q13.1	1.12	C1QTNF6
rs2664170	Xq28	1.16	GAB3

Table 1. SNPs associated with T1D according to Pociot et al. 2010 & Barret et al 2008.

Additional functional studies provided evidence of causality of several genes within established loci, such as several cytokines and their receptors (*IL10, IL2, IL27, IL7R, CCR5, SH2B3, IL18RAP*), immunomodulatory molecules (*IFIH1, TLR7-TLR8, TAGAP)* and other types of proteins (*PTPN2, GLIS3*). However, for the majority of associated regions the most likely causal gene still needs to be identified (Todd, 2010). *IFIH1* gene on chromosome 2q24.2 encodes intracellular pathogen receptor, MDA5, responsible for binding of viral RNA. This binding stimulates the production of type 1 interferon that could enhance cytotoxic activity of T cells on pancreatic β cells. *TLR7-TLR8* genes on chromosome Xp22.2 also encode intracellular receptors for viral RNA. This may explain induction of autoimmune destruction of β cells by numerous viral infections that may raise type 1 interferon levels (Todd, 2010; Pociot et al., 2010; Concannon et al., 2010). *GLIS3* acts as both transcriptional activator and repressor and is specifically involved in the development of pancreatic β cells. Mutations in this gene have been associated with a rare syndrome of neonatal diabetes and congenital hypothyroidism (Grant SF et al., 2009). It is the only gene that shows overlap between T1D and T2D that may be due to its function in the development and/or function of β cells (Todd, 2010).

There are more than 300 candidate genes that are in LD with T1D associated genetic regions. Also, it has been shown that at least 10 T1D associated regions do not contain a functional candidate gene which suggests that distant, long-range gene regulation might underly some of the observed associations. The main focus of current research is to identify causal risk genes and to understand how they influence the disease (Todd, 2010; Pociot et al., 2010). T1DGC is involved in the research of many autoimmune diseases since it is believed that many of them share common genetic background. A genotyping assay called ImmunoChip, that includes ~200 000 SNPs that are expected to be involved or were previously associated with immune reactions, was developed in order to disentangle the genetic background of various autoimmune diseases including T1D (Pociot et al., 2010).

3.5 Genetic markers in prediction and prevention of T1D

Recently, several population studies attempted to stratify children at birth according to their predisposition for T1D development by examining their *HLA* genotypes and insulin gene polymorphisms. Denver, Germany and Finland studies showed that children with the high risk *HLA* genotypes or polymorphisms within the insulin gene have about 50% higher risk of developing T1D-specific antibodies by the age of 5 (Barker et al., 2004, Walter et al., 2003, Hummel et al, 2004, Steck & Rewers, 2011). Assessment of risk can be extended by including other polymorphisms of susceptible genes for T1D development as well as family history of diabetes (Steck & Rewers, 2011). The application of preventive therapy would be focused on those individuals who have the highest genetic predisposition for the T1D development. Animal model of mucosal administration of insulin in the prevention of autoimmune diabetes has proven to be safe. Mucosal administration of insulin as a self-antigen stimulates a protective immune response that has the potential to affect the destructive immune response that would otherwise follow. Low doses of autoantigenes induce regulatory T cells that release inhibitory cytokines, while high doses destroy autoreactive effector T cells. Pre-POINT (Primary Oral Insulin) Trial in siblings with the high genetic risk for T1D, involving several European populations, Canada and USA, plans to investigate such treatment. Children aged 18 months and 7 years with a family history and genetic predisposition to T1D will be enrolled in the study. Conduction of study is planned in two steps: –step one -

genetic screening and determination of serum antibodies: step two - recruitment of selected children and treatment (test of four doses of insulin). As the effect depends on the dose and route at which insulin is administred in primary mucosal insulin therapy, goal of this study is to find a safe dose (applied orally or intranasal) that will induce an immune response to insulin. Pre-POINT studies should continue with POINT study with the determinate set dose. The main objective of this study is to determine whether the use of oral insulin can prevent or delay the onset of T1D in individuals with high genetic risk (Steck & Rewers, 2011, Achenbac et al, 2008).

4. Epigenetics

There is a significant increase in the incidence of T1D in the last 50 years that is mainly explained by changes in the environment. It is believed that environmental factors can affect epigenetic mechanisms of candidate genes expression and development of T1D. Epigenetic mechanisms encouraged with environmental factors can cause identical genotypes to exhibit different phenotypes. The proposed environmental factors that can trigger an autoimmune process involve nutrition and viruses. Nutrients that may trigger epigenetic mechanisms are considered to be substances that provide a methyl group (methionine, choline) or cofactors (folic acid, vitamin B12 and pyridoxal phosphate) required for DNA and histone methylation (Hewagama & Richardson, 2009). Actually, there are three ways in which phenotype can be altered by epigenetic modifications of gene expression: methylation of DNA, histone modification or activation of micro-RNA. It is well known that silencing of gene expression can be achieved by methylation of cytosine in CpG dinucleotides. Acetylation, methylation, phosphorilation and ubiquitination of histones modify the chromatin conformation, which can stimulate or silent gene expression. MicroRNAs bind to mRNA causing degradation before the translation in protein. These mechanisms that alter gene expression may influence development and function of immune system, as well as development, function and recovery of pancreatic β cells. Differentiation of T-helper cells is regulated by a complex epigenetic control. Critical epigenetic process in T-helper cells differentiation is DNA methylation, which can affect the expression of specific cytokines (interferons, interleukins) and encourage autoreactivity. Development, function and regeneration of pancreatic β cells largely depend on the genetic profile that will be expressed. Progressive decline of pancreatic β cells in type 1 and type 2 diabetes is strongly associated with the expression of genes responsible for the development and function of β cells. It is shown that the activity of the insulin gene is dependent on mechanisms of histone acetylation and methylation. It was also shown that the blood glucose concentration can affect the activity of enzymes that regulate the methylation process, but this seems to be associated with type 2 diabetes (MacFarlane et al., 2009).

5. Environment

Numerous environmental factors are implicated in T1D disease development in genetically susceptible individuals. Many of these factors act in uterine life, infancy and early childhood and are namely associated with viral infections and diet (Norris, 2010; Roivainen & Klingel, 2010).

Viral infections are considered to be the major environmental factors predisposing to T1D. Rotaviruses, adenoviruses, retroviruses, reoviruses, cytomegalovirus, Epstein-Barr virus, mumps virus and rubella virus are the ones that have been implicated in T1D pathogenesis but the most risk ones are human enteroviral (HEV) intestinal infections. Coxsackievirus and echovirus serotypes of HEV infections, are highly cytolitic and can cause β cell cytolysis and activate innate and adaptive immune system but can also activate autoreactive T cells (Roivainen & Klingel, 2010). A recent study examined autoimmune microbiome for T1D and came out with conclusion that microbiomes of healthy children differ to those of children that develop T1D later in their lives. This means that microbiome could be used as bacterial marker for the early T1D diagnosis. Also, the "healthy" microbiome could be used in the prevention of T1D development in children at genetically high risk of developing disease (Giongo et al. 2011).

The maternal diet during pregnancy, such as vegetable and vitamin D consumption, and wheat, cow's milk and omega-3 fatty acids early exposures in life are speculated to have a role in the aetiology of the disease. Introduction of cow's milk and meat prior 6 months of age have shown to have risk effects. Likewise, cereal, gluten or wheat antigens may cause an aberrant response in developing immune system. Some other factors may have protective effects against T1D development, such as early introduction of vegetable oil and high omega-3 fatty acid intake (Norris, 2010). Huge international collaborative effort, The Environmental Determinants of Diabetes in the Young (TEDDY) (http://teddy.epi.usf.edu/), was developed with the aim of identifying environmental factors that modify risk for T1D (TEDDY, 2008).

It is generally considered that environmental and behavioural factors have stronger effects on disease development than genetic loci itself, but it is very hard to accurately identify and measure them. The largest effects are expected from gene and environment interaction in individuals that are genetically at high-risk for disease development (Clayton, 2009).

6. Conclusion

The main genetic predisposition for developing T1D comes from the HLA region. There are currently identified additional ~50 non-HLA loci that predispose to risk of T1D. It is expected that the remaining T1D susceptible loci will be explained by additional common and rare genetic variants, structural polymorphisms, gene-gene and gene-environment interactions and epigenetic events. A role of associated genes and their protein products in disease aetiology is under intense investigation but the candidacy of many loci implicate to the combined effect of adaptive and innate immune action in insulin-producing β cell destruction. Further genetic studies performed on much bigger datasets comprising tens of thousands of individuals, detailed genetic mapping, genotype-phenotype correlation studies and other functional studies will be crucial in deciphering a complete genetic architecture of T1D and understanding the disease mechanisms. The main goal of genetic research is to link research findings with advances in therapy such as screening of individuals and implementation of preventive measures to those with high genetic predisposition to T1D and development of new, more efficient treatments and therapies. Detection of major pathways in the development of T1D opens up new therapeutic targets, development of more efficient treatments and individual approaches to patients.

7. Acknowledgement

We would like to thank Marina Pehlić, MD and Ante Kokan for their help in preparation of figures.

8. References

1000 Genomes Project Consortium, Durbin, R.M., Abecasis, G.R., Altshuler, D.L., Auton, A., Brooks, L.D., Durbin, R.M., Gibbs, R.A., Hurles, M.E. & McVean, G.A. (2010). A map of human genome variation from population-scale sequencing. *Nature*, Vol.467, No.7319, (Oct 2010), pp.1061-1073, ISSN 0028-0836

Achenbach P, Barker J, Bonifacio E; Pre-POINT Study Group. (2008). Modulating the natural history of type 1 diabetes in children at high genetic risk by mucosal insulin immunization. *Current diabetes reports*, Vol.8, No.2, (Apr 2008), pp.87-93, ISSN 1534-4827

Anderson, C.A., Pettersson, F.H., Clarke, G.M., Cardon, L.R., Morris, A.P., Zondervan, K.T. (2010). Data quality control in genetic case-control association studies. *Nature Protocols*, Vol.5, No.9, (Sep 2010), pp.1564-1573, ISSN 1754-2189

de Bakker, P.I., Neale, B.M., Daly, M.J. (2010). Meta-analysis of genome-wide association studies. *Cold Spring Harbor Protocols*, Vol.6, (Jun 2010), pdb.top81, ISSN 1559-6095

Barker, J.M., Goehrig, S.H., Barriga, K., Hoffman, M., Slover, R., Eisenbarth, G.S., Norris, J.M., Klingensmith, G.J., Rewers, M, DAISY study. (2004). Clinical characteristics of children diagnosed with type 1 diabetes through intensive screening and follow-up. *Diabetes Care*, Vol.27, No.6, (Jun 2004), pp.1399-404, ISSN 0149-5992

Barrett, J.C., Clayton, D.G., Concannon, P., Akolkar, B., Cooper, J.D., Erlich, H.A., Julier, C., Morahan, G., Nerup, J., Nierras, C., Plagnol, V., Pociot, F., Schuilenburg, H., Smyth, D.J., Stevens, H., Todd, J.A., Walker, N.M. & Rich, S.S. (2009). Type 1 Diabetes Genetics Consortium. Genome-wide association study and meta-analysis find that over 40 loci affect risk of type 1 diabetes. *Nature Genetics*, Vol.41, No.6, (Jan 2009), pp.703-707, ISSN 1061-4036

Bell, G.I., Horita, S. & Karam, J,H. (1984). A polymorphic locus near the human insulin gene is associated with insulin-dependent diabetes mellitus. *Diabetes*, Vol.33, No.2, (Feb 1984), pp.176-183, ISSN 0012-1797

van Belle, T.L., Coppieters, K.T., von Herrath, M.G. (2011). Type 1 diabetes: etiology, immunology, and therapeutic strategies. *Physiological reviews*, Vol. 91, No.1, (Jan 2011), pp. 79-118. ISSN 0031-9333

Bluestone, J.A., Herold, K. & Eisenbarth, G. (2010). Genetics, pathogenesis and clinical interventions in type 1 diabetes. *Nature*, Vol.464, No.7293, (Apr 2010), pp.1293-1300, ISSN 0028-0836

Bottini, N., Musumeci, L., Alonso, A., Rahmouni, S., Nika, K., Rostamkhani, M., MacMurray, J., Meloni, G.F., Lucarelli, P., Pellecchia, M., Eisenbarth, G.S., Comings, D. & Mustelin, T. (2004). A functional variant of lymphoid tyrosine phosphatase is associated with type I diabetes. *Nature Genetics*, Vol.36, No.4, (Apr 2004), pp.337-338, ISSN 1061-4036

Clayton, D.G. (2009). Prediction and interaction in complex disease genetics: experience in type 1 diabetes. *PLoS Genetics*, Vol.5, No.7, (Jul 2009), e1000540, ISSN 1553-7390

Concannon, P., Rich, S.S. & Nepom, G.T. (2009). Genetics of type 1A diabetes. *The New England Journal of Medicine*, Vol.360, No.16, (Apr 2009), pp.1646-1654, ISSN 0028-4793

Cui, Y., Li, G., Li, S. & Wu, R. (2010). Designs for linkage analysis and association studies of complex diseases. *Methods in Molecular Biology*, Vol.620, Part.2, pp.219-242, ISSN 1064-3745

Durinovic-Belló, I., Wu, R.P., Gersuk, V.H., Sanda, S., Shilling, H.G., Nepom, G.T. (2010). Insulin gene VNTR genotype associates with frequency and phenotype of the autoimmune response to proinsulin. *Genes and immunity*, Vol.11, No.2, (Mar 2010), pp.188-93, ISSN 1466-4879

Eyre, S., Hinks, A., Bowes, J., Flynn, E., Martin, P., Wilson, A.G., Morgan, A.W., Emery, P., Steer, S., Hocking, L.J., Reid, D.M., Harrison, P., Wordsworth, P., Yorkshire Early Arthritis Consortium, Biologics in RA Control Consortium, Thomson, W., Worthington, J., Barton, A. (2010). Overlapping genetic susceptibility variants between three autoimmune disorders: rheumatoid arthritis, type 1 diabetes and coeliac disease. *Arthritis Research & Therapy*, Vol.12, No.5, (2010), R175, ISSN 1478-6354

Giongo, A., Gano, K.A., Crabb, D.B., Mukherjee, N., Novelo, L.L., Casella, G., Drew, J.C., Ilonen, J., Knip, M., Hyöty, H., Veijola, R., Simell, T., Simell, O., Neu, J., Wasserfall, C.H., Schatz, D., Atkinson, M.A., Triplett, E.W. (2011). Toward defining the autoimmune microbiome for type 1 diabetes. *Multidisciplinary Journal of Microbial Ecology*, Vol.5, No.1, (Jan 2011), pp. 82-91, ISSN 1751-7362

Grant, S.F., Qu, H.Q., Bradfield, J.P., Marchand, L., Kim, C.E., Glessner, J.T., Grabs, R., Taback, S.P., Frackelton, E.C., Eckert, A.W., Annaiah, K., Lawson, M.L., Otieno, F.G., Santa, E., Shaner, J.L., Smith, R.M., Skraban, R., Imielinski, M., Chiavacci, R.M., Grundmeier. R.W., Stanley, C.A., Kirsch, S.E., Waggott, D., Paterson, A.D., Monos, D.S., DCCT/EDIC Research Group, Polychronakos, C., Hakonarson, H. (2009). Follow-up analysis of genome-wide association data identifies novel loci for type 1 diabetes. *Diabetes*, Vol.58, No.1, (Jan 2009), pp.:290-5, 0012-1797

Hewagama, A., Richardson, B. (2009). The genetics and epigenetics of autoimmune diseases. *Journal of autoimmunity*. Vol. 3, No.1, (Aug 2009), pp.3-11, ISSN 0896-8411

Hummel, M., Bonifacio, E., Schmid, S., Walter, M., Knopff, A., Ziegler, A.G. (2004). Brief communication: early appearance of islet autoantibodies predicts childhood type 1 diabetes in offspring of diabetic parents. *Annals of internal medicine*, Vol.140, No.11, (Jun 2004), pp.82-6, ISSN 0003-4819

International HapMap Consortium, Frazer, K.A., Ballinger, D.G. et al. (2007). A second generation human haplotype map of over 3.1 million SNPs. *Nature*, Vol.18, No.449, (Oct 2007), pp.851-861, 0028-0836

Kere, J. (2010). Genetics of complex disorders. *Biochemical and Biophysical Research Communications*. Vol.21, No.396, (May 2010), pp.143-6, ISSN 0006-291X

Lander, E.S. (2011). Initial impact of the sequencing of the human genome. *Nature*, Vol.470, No.7333, (Feb 2011), pp.187-197, ISSN 0028-0836

Liston, A., Gray, D.H., Lesage, S., Fletcher, A.L., Wilson, J., Webster, K.E., Scott, H.S., Boyd, R.L., Peltonen, L., Goodnow, C.C. (2004). Gene dosage--limiting role of Aire in thymic expression, clonal deletion, and organ-specific autoimmunity. *The Journal of experimental medicine*. Vol.18, No.8, (Oct. 2004), pp.1015-26, ISSN 0022-1007

Lowe, C.E., Cooper, J.D., Brusko, T., Walker, N.M., Smyth, D.J., Bailey, R., Bourget, K., Plagnol, V., Field, S., Atkinson, M., Clayton, D.G., Wicker, L.S. & Todd, J.A. (2007). Large-scale genetic fine mapping and genotype-phenotype associations implicate polymorphism in the IL2RA region in type 1 diabetes. *Nature Genetics*, Vol.39, No.9, (Sep 2007), pp.1074-1082, ISSN 1061-4036

Maahs, D.M., West, N.A., Lawrence, J.M., Mayer-Davis, E.J. (2010). Epidemiology of type 1 diabetes. *Endocrinology and Metabolism Clinics of North America*, Vol.39, No.3, (Sep 2010), pp.481-497, ISSN 0889-8529

MacFarlane, A.J., Strom, A. & Scott, F.W. (2009). Epigenetics: deciphering how environmental factors may modify autoimmune type 1 diabetes. *Mammalian Genome*, Vol.20, No.9-10, (Sep-Oct 2009), pp.624-632, ISSN 0938-8990

Manolio, T.A., Collins, F.S., Cox, N.J., Goldstein, D.B., Hindorff, L.A., Hunter, D.J., McCarthy, M.I., Ramos, E.M., Cardon, L.R., Chakravarti, A., Cho, J.H., Guttmacher, A.E., Kong, A., Kruglyak, L., Mardis, E., Rotimi, C.N., Slatkin, M., Valle, D., Whittemore, A.S., Boehnke, M., Clark, A.G., Eichler, E.E., Gibson, G., Haines, J.L., Mackay, T.F., McCarroll, S.A. & Visscher, P.M. (2009). Finding the missing heritability of complex diseases. *Nature*, Vol.461, No.7265, (Oct 2009), pp.747-753, ISSN 0028-0836

Marchini, J. & Howie, B. (2010). Genotype imputation for genome-wide association studies. *Nature Reviews Genetics*, Vol.11, No.7, (Jun 2010), pp.499-511, ISSN 1471-0056

McCarthy, M.I., Abecasis, G.R., Cardon, L.R., Goldstein, D.B., Little, J., Ioannidis, J.P. & Hirschhorn, J.N. (2008). Genome-wide association studies for complex traits: consensus, uncertainty and challenges. *Nature Reviews Genetics*, Vol.9, No.5, (May 2008), pp.356-369, ISSN 1471-0056

Mehers, K.L., Gillespie, K.M. (2008). The genetic basis for type 1 diabetes. *British medical bulletin*, Vol.88, No.1, (2008), 115-29, ISSN 0007-1420

Nisticò, L., Buzzetti, R., Pritchard, L.E., Van der Auwera, B., Giovannini, C., Bosi, E., Larrad, M.T., Rios, M.S., Chow, C.C., Cockram, C.S., Jacobs, K., Mijovic, C., Bain, S.C., Barnett, A.H., Vandewalle, C.L., Schuit, F., Gorus, F.K., Tosi, R., Pozzilli, P. & Todd, J.A. (1996). The CTLA-4 gene region of chromosome 2q33 is linked to, and associated with, type 1 diabetes. Belgian Diabetes Registry. *Human Molecular Genetics*, Vol.5, No.7, (Jul 1996), pp.1075-1080, ISSN 0964-6906

Norris, J.M. (2010). Infant and childhood diet and type 1 diabetes risk: recent advances and prospects. *Current diabetes reports*, Vol.10, No.5, (Oct 2010), pp.345-349, ISSN 1534-4827

Ounissi-Benkalha, H., Polychronakos, C. (2008). The molecular genetics of type 1 diabetes: new genes and emerging mechanisms. *Trends in molecular medicine*, Vol.14, No.6, (Jun 2008), pp.268-75, ISSN 1471-4914

Pharoah, P.D., Antoniou, A.C., Easton, D.F., Ponder, B.A. (2008). Polygenes, risk prediction, and targeted prevention of breast cancer. *New England Journal of Medicine*, Vol.358, No.26, (Jun 2008), pp.2796-2803, ISSN 0028-4793

Pociot, F., Akolkar, B., Concannon, P., Erlich, H.A., Julier, C., Morahan, G., Nierras, C.R., Todd, J.A., Rich, S.S. & Nerup, J. (2010). Genetics of type 1 diabetes: what's next? *Journal of Diabetes*, Vol.59, No.7, (Jul 2010), pp.1561-1571, ISSN 1753-0407

Roivainen, M. & Klingel K. (2010). Virus infections and type 1 diabetes risk. *Current diabetes reports*, Vol.10, No.5, (Oct 2010), pp.350-356, ISSN 1534-4827

Romeo, S., Pennacchio, L.A., Fu, Y., Boerwinkle, E., Tybjaerg-Hansen, A., Hobbs, H.H. & Cohen, J.C. (2007). Population-based resequencing of ANGPTL4 uncovers variations that reduce triglycerides and increase HDL. *Nature Genetics*, Vol. 9, No.4, (Apr 2007), pp.513-516, ISSN 1061-4036

Sabatti, C., Service, S.K. Hartikainen, A.L., Pouta, A. Ripatti, S., Brodsky, J., Jones, C.G., Zaitlen, N.A., Varilo, T., Kaakinen, M., Sovio, U., Ruokonen, A., Laitinen, J., Jakkula, E., Coin,

L., Hoggart, C., Collins, A., Turunen, H., Gabriel, S., Elliot, P., McCarthy, M.I., Daly, M.J., Järvelin, M.R., Freimer, N.B. & Peltonen, L. (2009). Genome-wide association analysis of metabolic traits in a birth cohort from a founder population. *Nature Genetics,* Vol.41, No.1, (Jan 2009), pp. 35-46, ISSN 1061-4036

Skrodenienė, E., Marčiulionytė, D., Padaiga, Z., Jašinskienė, E., Sadauskaitė-Kuehne, V., Sanjeevi, C.B., Ludvigsson, J. (2010). HLA class II alleles and haplotypes in Lithuanian children with type 1 diabetes and healthy children (HLA and type 1 diabetes). *Medicina (Kaunas),* Vol.46, No.8, (2010), pp. 505-10, ISSN 1010-660X

Smith, J.G., Newton-Cheh, C. (2009). Genome-wide association study in humans. *Methods in Molecular Biology,* Vol.573, (2009), pp.231-258, ISSN 1064-3745

Smyth, D.J., Cooper, J.D., Bailey, R., Field, S., Burren, O., Smink, L.J., Guja, C., Ionescu-Tirgoviste, C., Widmer, B., Dunger, D.B., Savage, D.A., Walker, N.M., Clayton, D.G. & Todd, J.A. (2006). A genome-wide association study of nonsynonymous SNPs identifies a type 1 diabetes locus in the interferon-induced helicase (IFIH1) region. *Nature Genetics,* Vol.38, No.6, (Jun 2006), pp.617–619, ISSN 1061-4036

Steck AK, Rewers MJ. (2011). Genetics of type 1 diabetes. *Clinical chemistry,* Vol.57, No.2, (Feb 2011), pp.176-85, ISSN 0009-9147

TEDDY Study Group. (2008). The Environmental Determinants of Diabetes in the Young (TEDDY) Study. *Annals of the New York Academy of Sciences,* Vol.150, No.1150, (Dec 2008), 1-13, ISSN 0077-8923

Todd, J.A. Etiology of type 1 diabetes. (2010). *Immunity,* Vol.32, No.4, (Apr 2010), pp457-467, ISSN 1074-7613

Vella, A., Cooper, J.D., Lowe, C.E., Walker, N., Nutland, S., Widmer, B., Jones, R., Ring, S.M., McArdle, W., Pembrey, M.E., Strachan, D.P., Dunger, D.B., Twells, R.C., Clayton, D.G., Todd, J.A. (2005). Localization of a type 1 diabetes locus in the IL2RA/CD25 region by use of tag single-nucleotide polymorphisms. *The American Journal of Human Genetics,* Vol.76, No.5, (Maj 2005), pp.773–779, ISSN 0002-9297

Villaseñor, J., Benoist, C., Mathis, D. (2005). AIRE and APECED: molecular insights into an autoimmune disease. *Immunological reviews.* Vol.204, (Apr 2005), pp.156-64, ISSN 0105-2896.

Ziegler, A.G. & Nepom, G.T. (2010). Prediction and pathogenesis in type 1 diabetes. *Immunity,* Vol.32, No.4, (Apr 2010), pp.468-478, ISSN 1074-7613

Zondervan, K.T., Cardon, L.R. (2007). Designing candidate gene and genome-wide case-control association studies. *Nature Protocols,* Vol.2, No.10, (Oct 2007), pp.92-2501, ISSN 1754-2189

Walter, M., Albert, E., Conrad, M., Keller, E., Hummel, M., Ferber, K., Barratt, B.J., Todd, J.A., Ziegler, A.G., Bonifacio, E. (2003). IDDM2/insulin VNTR modifies risk conferred by IDDM1/HLA for development of Type 1 diabetes and associated autoimmunity. *Diabetologia,* Vol.46, No.5, (May 2003), pp.712-20, ISSN 0012-186X

Wang, J., Li, X., Jia, Z., Tian, Y., Yu, J., Bao, L., Wu, Y., Ni, B. (2010). Reduced FOXP3 expression causes IPEX syndrome onset: An implication from an IPEX patient and his disease-free twin brother. *Clinical Immunology,* Vol.137, No.1, (Oct 2010),pp. 178-80, ISSN 1744-666X

Wang, K., Li, M., Hakonarson, H. (2010). Analysing biological pathways in genome-wide association studies. *Nature Reviews Genetics,* Vol.11, No.12, (Dec 2010), pp.843-854, ISSN 1471-0056

24

The Genetics of Type 1 Diabetes

Kathleen M. Gillespie
University of Bristol
UK

1. Introduction

Type 1 diabetes (T1D) is an autoimmune disease caused by the destruction of insulin producing beta-cells in the pancreas. Individuals with T1D cannot survive without insulin replacement, and despite daily insulin treatment remain at risk of complications including nephropathy, retinopathy and coronary heart disease. Although commonly associated with onset in childhood and adolescence with a peak age at diagnosis of 12 years, many cases of T1D are diagnosed in adulthood. Epidemiological studies show that the incidence of T1D is unequally distributed in the world's population, with a high incidence rate in Caucasians (40/100 000/year in Finland) and an extremely low rate among Asian and South American populations (0.1/100 000/year) (Karvonen et al., 2000). T1D is increasingly considered a disease of "westernization" or affluence associated with improved hygiene, healthcare and living standards. The incidence of the condition has been increasing rapidly in recent decades for unknown reasons: the current rate of increase is 3% per year worldwide and it has been predicted that the incidence will be 40% higher by 2010 compared to 1998 (Onkamo et al., 1999). More recent predictions show that if present trends continue, doubling of new cases of type 1 diabetes in European children younger than 5 years will occur between 2005 and 2020, and prevalent cases younger than 15 years will rise by 70% (Patterson et al., 2009).

T1D is generally diagnosed on clinical grounds but can be confirmed by the presence of circulating antibodies in the blood (Baekkeskov et al., 1982). These antibodies are markers of ongoing autoimmune destruction (Bottatzo et al., 1985) and the best characterized are specific to the islet proteins insulin (Palmer et al., 1983), glutamic acid decarboxylase (GAD) (Baekkeskov et al., 1990), IA-2 (Christie et al., 1994) and the zinc transporter ZnT8 (Wenzlau et al., 2007, 2008). The autoimmune process begins very early in life: studies of neonatal diabetes suggest that most cases of diabetes diagnosed before 6 months are unlikely to be autoimmune, but those diagnosed after the age of 6 months have the genetic characteristics of T1D (Edghill et al., 2006) while islet autoantibodies are detectable by 5 years of age in most future T1D cases (Bonifacio et al., 2004); in many by 2 years of age (Zeigler et al., 1999), and antibodies to insulin (generally the first to appear) have been detected as early as 6 to 12 months of age (Roll et al., 1996).

T1D can be predicted accurately by the detection of multiple islet autoantibodies and their characteristics (Bingley et al. 1997; Achenbach et al., 2004a, 2004b). Trials of agents to prevent T1D however require identification of those at risk of T1D very early in life before the autoimmune process has been initiated. This is only possible by estimation of genetic risk.

2. The role of genes in susceptibility to T1D

Type 1 diabetes develops through the interaction of complex genetic and environmental influences. There are several lines of evidence indicating a strong genetic component causing susceptibility to the disease. Twin studies provide one line of evidence.

2.1 Twin studies

Concordance rates between monozygotic twins has been estimated at 30-50% compared to 10% in dizygotic twins (Olmos et al., 1988; Kaprio et al., 1992; Verge et al., 1995; Hyttinen et al., 2003) indicating that genetic mechanisms are involved but are not solely responsible for disease pathogenesis. While concordance rates do increase over the period of observation the window of greatest risk appears to be within 3 years of diagnosis of the index twin (Redondo et al. 2001). Familial clustering of type 1 diabetes provides further evidence for the role genes in T1D. The risk of developing type 1 diabetes for any individual is 0.4% (population frequency). However the risk to a sibling of someone already affected is 6%. This produces a sibling risk/population prevalence ratio (λ) of 15 (Risch et al., 1988) strongly suggesting a genetic component.

2.2 Genetic methodologies

Unraveling of genetic mechanisms underlying a complex multifactorial disease involving genetic and environmental determinants such as T1D is challenging and has been ongoing since the 1970s. Indeed studies of T1D lead the way for other complex diseases. Initially simple case control comparisons of the allele frequencies of candidate genes were used. Then, in the 1990s, linkage studies were used which search for the co-transmission in T1D families of a DNA marker with the disease. The marker locus itself usually is not directly involved in the disease process, but if it lies close to a locus that is, a disease associated allele will be observed more often in individuals with disease. This lead to the identification of more genetic loci associated with T1D but was hampered by the requirement for increased statistical power from larger patient populations.

The most recent, and successful methodologies however are genome wide association studies (GWAS). These studies have taken advantage of 1) collections of large cohorts of individuals (several thousand) with well classified disease and a similar number of matched healthy controls 2) a detailed map of the most common genetic variants in the human genome, single nucleotide polymorphisms (SNPs) and the completion of the HAPMAP (*www.hapmap.org/*) project which showed that not all genome wide SNPs need to be analysed to generate the maximum dataset and finally 3) improved methodologies for high throughput SNP genotyping.

Interestingly, all three methodologies identified the human leucocyte antigen (HLA) region (also known as the major histocompatibility complex(MHC)) on the short arm of chromosome 6 as the predominant genetic susceptibility factor for T1D. The HLA is crucial to immune recognition of self and non-self peptides. There are 3 classes of HLA molecules- I, II, III. Class I and II are distinct structural entities. Although there are multiple class I and II genes, all the gene products have similar overall structure. Class III is a diverse collection of more than 20 genes including those encoding complement proteins. The structure of the MHC gene cluster is shown on Figure 1.

Class I MHC molecules are found on all nucleated cells and present peptides to cytotoxic T cells. Class II MHC molecules are found on certain immune cells, chiefly macrophages, B

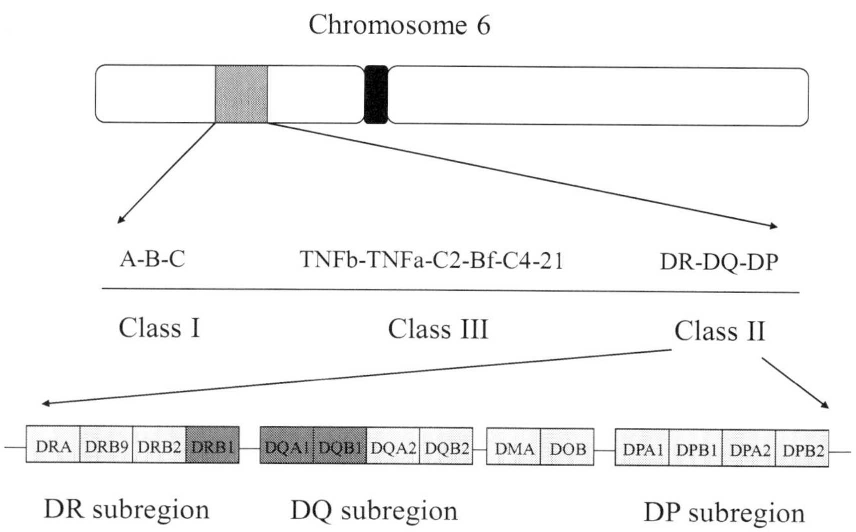

Fig. 1. The HLA region on chromosome 6 (from Mehers and Gillespie 2008). The T1D associated haplotypes are DRB1*03-DQB1*02 and DRB1*04-DQB1*0302

cells and dendritic cells, collectively known as professional antigen-presenting cells (APCs). The Class II MHC molecules on APCs present peptides to helper T cells, which stimulate an immune reaction as shown schematically on figure 2. It therefore intuitive that autoimmune diseases such as type 1 diabetes, caused by the erroneous recognition of pancreatic proteins as foreign, might involve HLA variants.

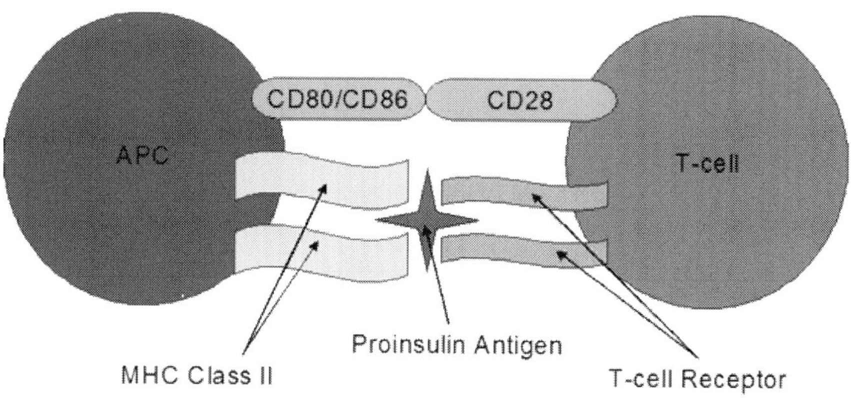

Fig. 2. A simplified schematic diagram of a proinsulin peptide being presented to a CD4 helper T cell by MHC Class II on an antigen presenting cells (from Mehers and Gillespie, 2008)

3. The HLA in susceptibility to T1D

In the early 1970s, Singal and colleagues, Nerup and colleagues and Cudworth and colleagues all independently showed show that HLA class 1 alleles B8 and B15 were more prevalent in individuals with T1D compared to healthy individuals who lacked these antigens (Singal and Blajchman, 1973; Nerup et al., 1974; Cudworth and Woodrow, 1975). It later became clear that it was HLA class II rather than HLA class I that had the closest association with T1D. In 1987 it was shown that HLA class II DQB1 plays important role in susceptibility and resistance to T1D susceptibility (Todd et al., 1987) and in 1988, Thomson and colleagues analysed 180 Caucasoid families with at least 2 affected children and showed that there was an increase in DRB1*03/DRB1*04 genotypes in T1D patients, compared to healthy controls. They identified HLA class II DRB1*03 as the recessive allele and DRB1*04 as dominant and that the heterozygous effect of the two susceptible alleles together, produced a higher risk genotype with a synergistic effect (Thomson et al., 1988). They also demonstrated that DRB1*02 conferred a protective role in T1D susceptibility. It is now common for HLA susceptibility to T1D to be discussed in terms of HLA DRB1 (DR) and DQB1 (DQ). 90% of childhood cases have at least one of the risk haplotypes DRB1*04-DRB1*0302 (DR4-DQ8) or DRB*03-DQB1*0201 (DR3-DQ2) while the frequency of the highest risk combined genotype DRB1*04-DRB1*0302 (DR4-DQ8) and DRB*03-DQB1*0201 (DR3-DQ2) is present in almost half of children diagnosed under the age of 5 years (Cailliat

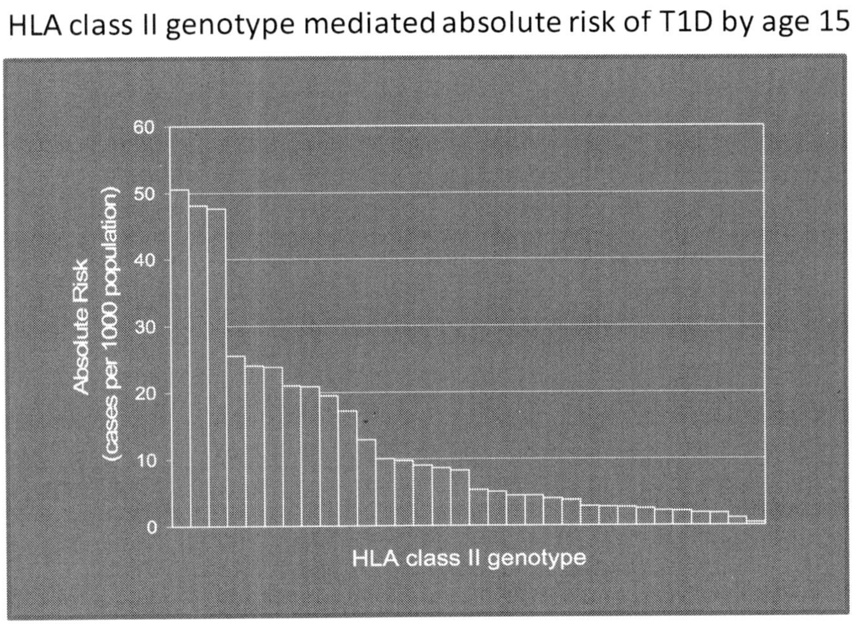

Fig. 3. Absolute risks associated with HLA class II genotypes for diagnosis of type 1 diabetes. The highest risk is associated with the genotype DRB1*03-DQB1*02/DRB1*04-DQB1*0302

Zucman et al., 1995, Gillespie et al., 2002). HLA class II haplotypes have been ranked in a risk hierarchy for T1D as shown in figure 3 (Lambert et al. 2004). Individuals with the highest risk genotype DRB1*03-DQB1*0201/DRB1*0401-DQB1*0302 have a 5% absolute risk of getting diabetes by the age of 15 years while DRB1*15-DQB1*0602 is protective (Thomson et al., 1988; Lambert et al., 2004; Pugliese et al., 1995). This haplotype is present only in about 1% of T1D cases but approximately 20% of the general population.

As the function of class II alleles is to present antigen or peptides to T cells in order to activate them, the ability of some alleles to contribute to susceptibility and others to protection is most likely to be effects on this activation pathway. Most studies have focused on the effects of different alleles on peptide binding, as it is in the peptide-binding groove where most of the HLA polymorphism is located. An early hypothesis focused on residue 57 in DQB alleles (Todd et al., 1987). All DQB1 alleles with an aspartic acid at residue 57 confer neutral to protective effects and the DQB1 alleles with alanine (*0201 and *0302) confer strong susceptibility in all ethnic groups. However this alone cannot explain all the observed associations with DQB1 alleles (Nepom et al, 1987).

A HLA class II gene which is clearly of importance in susceptibility to T1D but to a lesser extent than HLA DR and DQ is HLA DPBI. Studies have consistently shown that the DPB1*0301 allele is susceptible while the *0402 allele is protective and that these effects are independent of other HLA class II modulators (Noble et al., 2003; Cruz et al., 2004).

Intriguingly an "extreme" risk haplotype for T1D has been reported (Aly et al., 2006): siblings who share both extended high risk HLA DR3 and DR4 haplotypes identical by descent with the affected proband were shown to have a 55% risk of diabetes by the age of 12 years compared with a 7% risk of diabetes by age 12 in siblings not sharing both IBD haplotypes. These data suggest the presence of an important, and as yet recognized, modulator of risk within the HLA.

In the half century since HLA mediated susceptibility to type 1 diabetes was initially described, the HLA has consistently been replicated as the major determinant of genetic susceptibility with estimates suggesting that this gene family is responsible for 50% of susceptibility. Recent fine mapping of 8 megabases of the extended MHC region by genome wide association strategies have confirmed that the major susceptibility and resistance loci for T1D are within the HLA class II region (Nejentsev et al., 2007; Howson et al., 2009).

HLA susceptibility to T1D is dynamic

Intriguingly as the incidence of type 1 diabetes has been increasing, the frequency of HLA class II susceptibility genotypes in affected individuals has decreased (Herrman et al., 2003, Gillespie et al., 2004, Fourlanos et al., 2008). The frequency of individuals with the highest risk genotype DRB1*03-DQB1*0201/DRB1*0401-DQB1*0302 has been decreasing over the last half century while the frequency of those with the intermediate genotypes (carrying only one of the haplotypes DRB1*03-DQB1*0201 or DRB1*0401-DQB1*0302) has increased (figure 4). This was demonstrated by comparing HLA class II gene frequencies between a current T1D cohort, the Bart's Oxford (BOX) cohort and a cohort diagnosed before 1950 known as the Golden Years cohort. As the gene pool cannot change over this time frame, it appears that increasing environmental pressure is precipitating disease in individuals with less genetic susceptibility thus contributing to the ongoing increasing numbers of children developing T1D. This dynamic in assessment of genetic risk for T1D will create difficulties for therapeutic trials where accurate assessment of risk is crucial.

3.1 The role of HLA class I genes

As indicated above HLA class II genes do not account for all of the HLA-associated contribution with type 1 diabetes. The original serological associations between the HLA and type 1 diabetes were with class I B alleles. It is increasingly clear that although the predominant effect of the HLA on susceptibility is mediated through HLA class II, these effects are modulated by HLA class 1 alleles. In a Finnish study of extended haplotypes it was shown that the A2, Cw1, B56, DR4, DQ8 haplotype was present in 5.5% of individuals with diabetes compared with 1.1% of controls and has the highest risk for type 1 diabetes (Tienari et al., 1992). In Finns, the Cw1, B56, DR4, DQ8 haplotype is conserved and is only associated with four HLA-A alleles. Only the A2 allele is associated with diabetes suggesting that, at least on this haplotype, the class I region contributes to susceptibility.

The effect of class I alleles was also studied in non-DR3/non-DR4 or low genetic risk individuals with T1D (Fennessy et al. 1994) who were more likely to possess two of the HLA-A alleles associated with increased disease susceptibility. The haplotypes most frequently found in type 1 diabetes were the HLA-A alleles A28, A24, A3, A2 and A1. This group went on to show elevated risks for class I alleles B13, A24 and B62 in 801 newly diagnosed Finnish children (Langholz et al., 1995). In Japanese patients with type 1 diabetes, HLA-A24 is associated with rapid onset of the disease (Nakanishi et al., 1993) and may influence age of onset and disease progression. A study of 222 diabetic multiplex families from the Human Biological Data Interchange also showed the A*2402 allele has a significant effect on the age of onset distribution of DR-DQ haplotypes occurring at a higher frequency in those individuals diagnosed younger (Valdes et al 1999) while the A*0101 was associated with older age of onset.

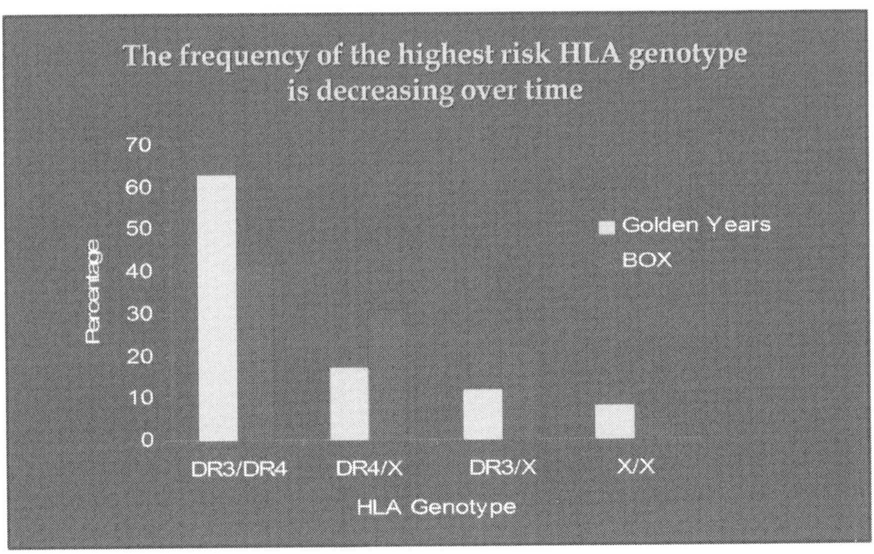

Fig. 4. The highest risk HLA DR3/DR4 genotypes is less frequent in a current T1D population (BOX) than in a population of individuals who developed T1D half a century earlier (adapted from Gillespie et al. Lancet 2004)

More recent studies by Nejentsev et al. in 2007 showed that after taking into account the effects of HLA class II, all remaining HLA effects on susceptibility to T1D are attributable to genes in HLA A and B. Most important was HLA B*39 as a susceptibility factor while the A*02 allele increases risk in individuals with the highest risk class II genotype. In the same way that HLA class II molecules present peptide to CD4 cells, HLA class I molecules present peptides to cytotoxic CD8+ T cells, increasingly accepted as the central cell in immune infiltration in human T1D pancreas and in the non-obese diabetic (NOD) mouse (discussed in section 7).

4. Non HLA genes in susceptibility to T1D

4.1 Insulin gene

In the early 1980s, a second genetic locus, the insulin gene, linked with susceptibility to T1D was identified (Bell et al., 1984). The Insulin gene (INS) on chromosome 11p15 encompasses 1430 base pairs (bp) and results in the translation of preproinsulin, the presursor of mature insulin. Preproinsulin is processed to proinsulin by removal of the signal peptide and then to mature biologically active insulin by removal of the C-peptide. It is increasingly clear that insulin is the primary autoantigen in T1D. A variable number tandem repeat (VNTR) region consisting of a 14 to 15 bp consensus sequence upstream of the INS gene, in the INS promoter, is comprised of three classes of alleles: there is a higher frequency of class I alleles with shorter repeat sequences in individuals with T1D (Bennett et al. 1995) while individuals with longer class III alleles are relatively protected from T1D. The VNTR regulates transcription rates of insulin and its precursors. Class I and Class III alleles differentially affect transcription of insulin in the thymus and pancreas (Vafiadis et al., 1997; Pugliese et al, 1997). Class III alleles result in 20% increased INS transcription in the thymus. This potentially results in more efficient negative selection of insulin reactive T cells and less susceptibility to T1D compared to class I alleles providing an attractive model for the role of the insulin gene in susceptibility to T1D but this hypothesis remains to be experimentally demonstrated.

4.2 CTLA-4

In 1996, the cytotoxic T-lymphocyte antigen-4 (CTLA-4) gene encoded on chromosome 2q33 was identified as a further T1D susceptibility gene (Nistico et al., 1996). CTLA-4 is a surface molecule found on activated T cells which produces a negative signal by inhibiting the T cell receptor signaling complex ligand interactions (blocks binding of CD80 and CD86) (Figure 2). Two major splice forms exist - encoding membrane bound and soluble forms. When CTLA-4 is knocked out, lymphoproliferative disorders result (Waterhouse et al., 1995). An A49G polymorphism in exon 1 of CTLA-4 changes the amino acid sequence resulting in reduced cell surface expression (Anjos et al., 2002). It is thought that inherited changes in CTLA-4 gene expression can increase T cell self-reactivity and therefore play an important role in autoimmune diseases such as T1D (Ueda et al., 2003).

4.3 PTPN22

More recently in 2004, protein tyrosine phosphatase non-receptor 22 (PTPN22), a gene found on chromosome 1p13 which encodes lymphoid protein tyrosine phosphatase (LYP) was found to be associated with susceptibility to T1D. Protein tyrosine phosphatases such as LYP are responsible for preventing spontaneous T cell activation and they have the ability to prevent the response to antigen by dephosphorylating and inactivating T cell receptors. It has been demonstrated that a single nucleotide polymorphism (SNP) in the PTPN22 gene can lead to susceptibility to autoimmune diseases such as T1D because of a decrease in negative regulation of hyper-reactive T cells (Bottini et al., 2004). The first complete resequencing of the human PTPN22 gene was carried out in 2005 (Criswell et al., 2005). This sequence was further analysed for polymorphisms associated with T1D and a SNP at 1858bp in codon 620 was found. Two alleles referred to as 1858C and 1858T were identified and the 1858T variant was shown to occur more often in T1D populations: 30.6% of people with TID compared to 21.3% healthy controls are heterozygous for the polymorphism p = 0.0006 (Bottini et al., 2006). LYP is expressed in other cells in addition to T cells including natural killer (NK) cells, B cells, macrophages and dendritic cells (DCs) and so could very well also have an effect on the function of several immune cells.

4.4 IL2RA/CD25

In 2005, the interleukin 2 receptor alpha (IL2RA) region on chromosome 10p15 was found to be associated with T1D (Vella et al., 2005). IL2RA encodes the α-chain of the IL-2 receptor complex (also referred to as CD25) which is responsible for binding IL-2, a key player in the proliferation of regulatory T cells. IL2R has also been associated with T1D in the non-obese diabetic (NOD) mouse (Wicker et al., 2005). Two IL-2R SNPs associated with the increased risk of T1D have been reported (Qu et al., 2007) with ss52580101 the most closely associated (Lowe et al., 2007). A recent study measuring expression of IL-2R in individuals homozygous for susceptible and protective SNPs associated with T1D demonstrated that on stimulation, higher percentages of CD69+ CD4+ memory T cells secreted IL-2 from individuals with the protective SNP compared to individuals with the susceptible SNP (Dendrou et al., 2009). More recently susceptibility genotypes were found to be associated with lower levels of soluble IL2Ralpha (sIL2Ra) ((Lowe et al. 2007, Maier et al. 2009) and *in vitro* stimulation of peripheral blood mononuclear cells from individuals with T1D results in lower levels compared to healthy controls (Giordano et al. 1989).

5. Genome wide association studies

In recent years methodologies to identify susceptibility factors underlying complex disorders have improved by orders of magnitude. In particular the success of the HapMap project in identifying stretches of linkage disequilibrium decreasing the number of SNPs requiring genotyping combined with increased capacity for high throughput SNP analysis has resulted in a genetic revolution. In 2007, results of the first genome-wide association studies in seven different complex diseases was published by the Wellcome Trust Case Control Consortium (2007). Later in 2007, a further genome wide association scan was carried out and confirmed the additional associations of 12q24, 12q13, 16p13 and 18p11 with T1D (Todd et al., 2007). More recently the Type 1 Genetics Consortium (TIDGC) has published over 40 genetic loci associated with T1D (Barrett et al., 2009). A selection of the best characterized are shown on Figure 5. The genes detailed above all remain associated with T1D and most of the newly identified susceptibility genes can be positioned on immune activation pathways while some loci have yet to have the disease associated gene identified. Despite the overwhelming success of GWAS in identifying susceptibility genes for common diseases using hypothesis-free methodologies the effects of the identified genes on improved genetic risk assessments have been minimal. This is because most of the newly identified loci make only a minimal contribution to risk with odds ratios (OR) in the range of 1.2-1.3 compared to 7 for the HLA locus (Figure 6). An OR of 1 indicates that risk is equal in healthy controls and individuals with disease. This has become known as the missing heritability and indicates, not surprisingly, that mechanisms other than common variants contribute to susceptibility to T1D. Candidates for such effects are rare variants as well as epigenetic modifications which cannot be detected by GWAS. Nevertheless the new loci identified by GWAS have informed ongoing functional studies and confirmed some interesting mechanistic loci such as IFIH1.

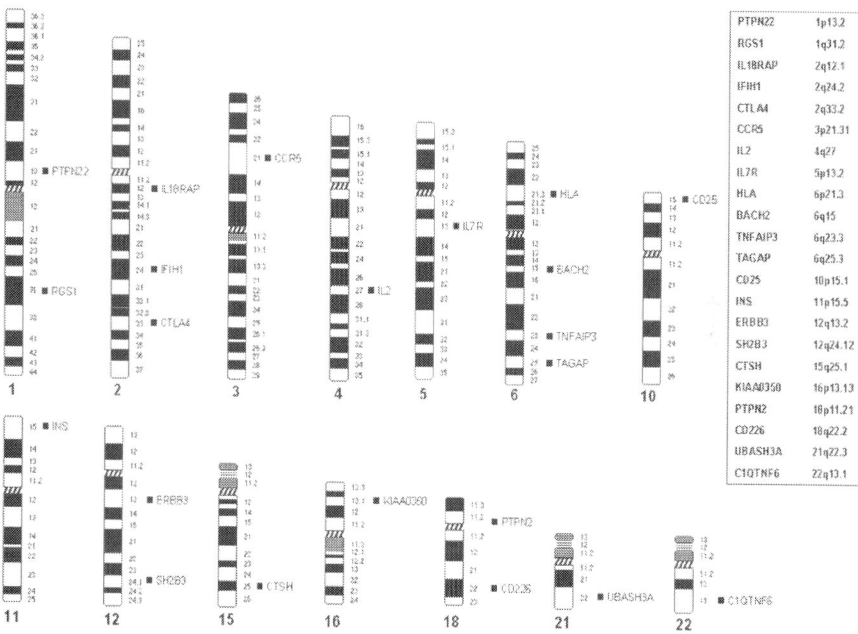

Fig. 5. Chromos omal localisation of selected T1D associated loci (adapted from Ye et al. 2010)

6. Genetic susceptibility to Type 1 diabetes in the post-GWAS era

6.1 IFIH1

In 2006, interferon induced with helicase C domain 1 (IFIH1) also known as MDA-5 on chromosome 2q24.3 was found to be strongly associated with T1D (Smyth et al., 2006) Later, in 2008, a follow up study on IFIH1 was carried out, confirming the strongest association to be with SNP rs1990760 (Qu et al., 2008). IFIH1 is particularly interesting because unlike the T1D susceptibility genes discussed so far, it is not involved in T cell activation but contributes to innate immune responses by releasing the cytokine interferon-gamma (IFN-γ) and inducing apoptosis of cells infected by picorna viruses of which enteroviruses such as coxsackie B4 which have been identified histologically in T1D pancreas (Dotta et al., 2007). This molecule may therefore provide molecular insights into the hypothesis that viral infection contributes to susceptibility to T1D as alterations in IFIH1

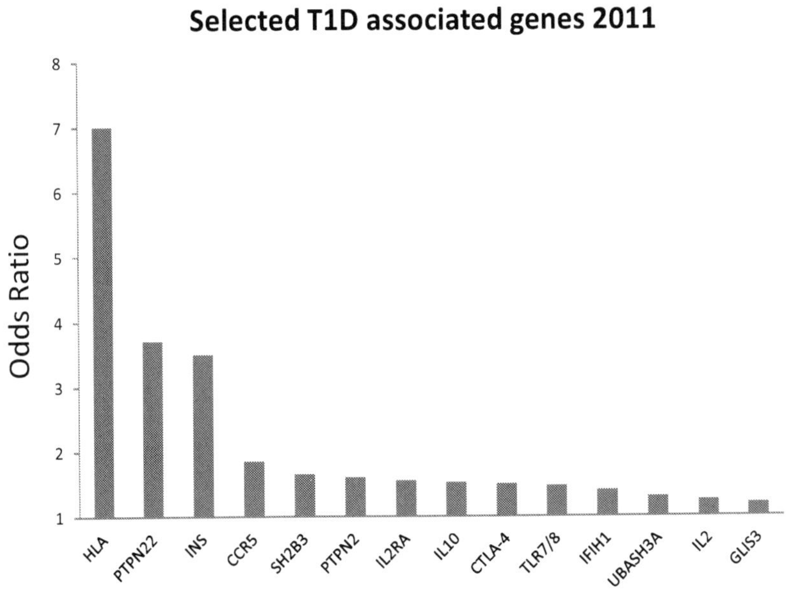

Fig. 6. The relative effect of selected T1D associated genes on susceptibility to T1D (adapted from Todd 2010)

activity could interfere with detection and clearance of virus. PBMC expression levels of IFIH1 have been reported to be higher in individuals with susceptibility genotypes (Liu et al. 2009). Recent resequencing of the IFIH1 gene identified four rare variants associated with T1D protection, which are predicted to play a role in altering the expression and structure of IFIH1 (Nejentsev et al., 2009).

6.2 TLR 7 and 8

The Toll-like receptor (TLR) family which plays a fundamental role in pathogen recognition and activation of innate immunity. TLRs are highly conserved and recognize pathogen-associated molecular patterns (PAMPs) that are expressed on infectious agents. Toll like receptors (TLR) 7 and 8 are located closely together on the X chromosome have recently been associated with T1D (Todd, 2010). TLR7 recognises single stranded RNA in endosomes, which is a common feature of viral genomes which are internalised by macrophages. Like IFIH1, the association of T1D with these receptors strengthens arguments for the involvement of viruses in the pathogenesis of disease.

6.3 CCR5

CCR5 is a chemokine receptor on the surface of several cells of the immune system including macrophages, NKT cells, CD4+ T cells and CD8+ T cells. It has been mapped to the short arm of chromosome 3 within the chemokine receptor gene cluster. Recent studies established that this gene comprises three exons spanning a region of about 6 kb. A 32bp insertion/deletion polymorphism exon 3 changes the open reading frame of CCR5 and results in a nonfunctional protein. This polymorphism is present only in 1% of the population but deletion homozygotes are protected against HIV-1 infection (Alexander et al., 2000) as well as T1D, rheumatoid arthritis and celiac disease (Smyth et al., 2008).

6.4 UBASH3A

A chromosome 21q22.3 T1D-associated locus (rs876498) has been identified (Concannon et al. 2008) and replicated (Grant et al., 2009). The only gene in the corresponding region of linkage disequilibrium is the Ubiquitin associated and SH3 domain containing A (UBASH3A) gene which comprises 15 exons, spans 40kb, and has been shown to be expressed in spleen, bone marrow and peripheral blood lymphocytes (Wattenhoffer et al., 2009). UBASH3A suppresses T cell receptor signalling (figure 7) and may therefore provide a candidate for the increased frequency of autoimmune disease in Down syndrome (Gillespie et al., 2006).

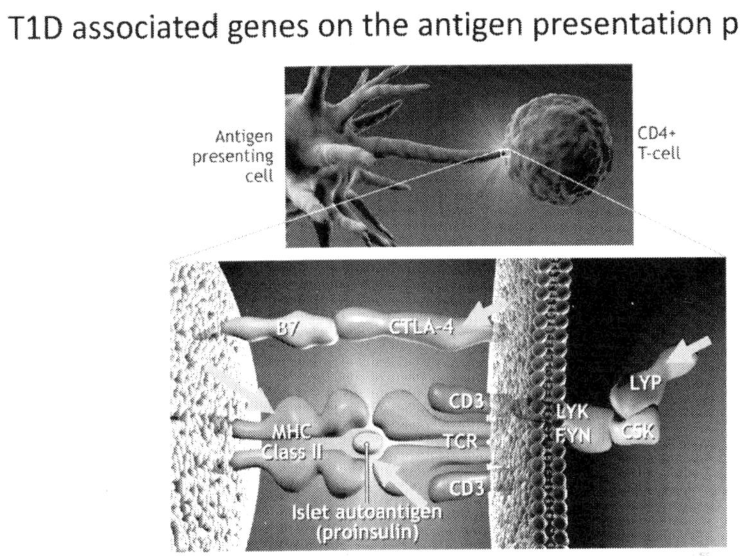

Fig. 7. Many of the T1D associated genes can be mapped onto this antigen presentation pathway when proinsulin peptide is presented to a CD4 helper T cell through the T cell receptor (TCR) this activating Lyp coded for by PTPN22 as well as PTPN2, IL2, IL2RA and UBASH3A and several others (adapted from Gillespie, 2006)

6.5 NK receptor/HLA class 1 interactions

Natural killer (NK) cells represent the first line of defence against viral infection. NK cell infiltrates have been identified in pancreas from individuals with type 1 diabetes (T1D) (Dotta et al. 2008) and increased NK cell activity has been reported in the periphery of individuals with T1D (Herold et al 1984, Nair et al 1986)]. NK cells act by either activating or inhibiting cytolysis and their activity is controlled by the balance of inhibitory and activating receptors on the cell surface. One set of human NK cell receptors are the killer immunoglobulin-like receptor (KIR) gene family on chromosome 19 [10] which consists of

16 genes; each is either inhibitory or activating in function and is polymorphic both in terms of gene content and allelic variation. Genome wide association studies of KIR in T1D are not yet available because this region of chromosome 19 does not have a high coverage SNP map but results from genetic studies of KIR in T1D increasingly show an association between T1D and the activating receptor KIR2DS2 (and its ligand, HLA C group 1). Van der Slik et al. (2003) analysed the KIR gene family and respective HLA class I ligands in 149 children diagnosed with diabetes under the age of 14 in a Dutch population and Shastry et al. (2008) carried out a similar analysis in 98 patients diagnosed with T1D under the age of 18 years compared to 70 healthy controls in a Latvian population. In addition Ramos-Lopez et al. (2009) showed, in a combined German/Belgian study of 1124 patients with T1D compared to 716 healthy controls, that a single nucleotide polymorphism (rs2756923) in exon 8 of the inhibitory gene KIR2DL2 was associated with T1D. More recent data show that activating combinations of KIR/HLA genes are more frequent in young T1D children diagnosed in the first 5 years of life suggesting that NK cell responses to viral infection are altered in this group (Mehers et al., submitted).

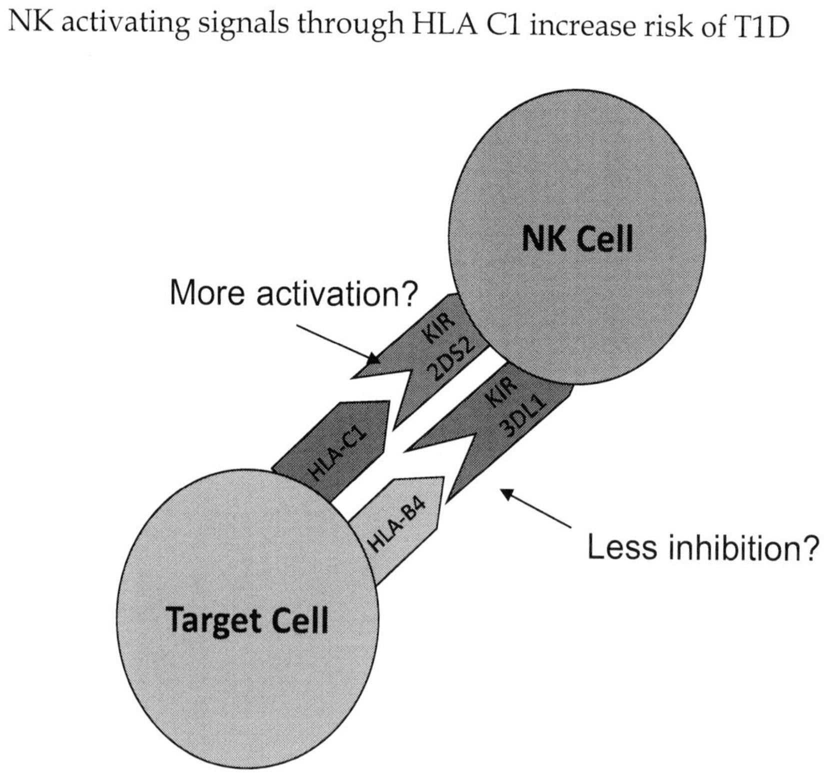

Fig. 8. Individuals with T1D more frequently express genetic combinations of NK cell activation

7. The NOD model of T1D

NOD mice, a commonly used mouse model for T1D, were generated following an experiment by Makino and colleagues in 1980 (Makino et al., 1980) where out-bred brother x sister Swiss mice were repetitively mated in order to produce a strain in which all mice developed cataracts. Mice without cataracts were found to have high blood glucose levels and were selectively bred in order to produce a mouse model strain of spontaneous diabetes development. These mice develop an autoimmune type of diabetes where pancreatic β-cells are damaged and destroyed by mononuclear cells infiltrating into the islets of langerhans (Fujino-Kurihara et al., 1985). The incidence of autoimmune diabetes in the female NOD mice varies in different colonies but generally is 60-80% and 20-30% in males (Kikutani and Makino, 1992; Atkinson and Leiter, 1999). This is in contrast to human T1D where males and females are equally affected early in life but the incidence is higher in males from adolescence onwards (Weets et al., 2001, Gale and Gillespie., 2002). Disease onset in the NOD usually occurs between 12-14 weeks in female mice and slightly later in males (Kikutani and Makino, 1992).

NOD mice are very sensitive to changes in their environment and geographical location. It has been demonstrated that changes in either of these circumstances results in a different rate of spontaneous diabetes development (Oldstone, 1988). Diabetes onset in NOD mice is prevented by administration of Complete Freund's Adjuvant (CFA), bacteria, parasites and the housing of the mice in dirty conditions, as well as many other treatments (Oldstone, 1990; Oldstone et al., 1990; Sobel et al., 1998b; Zaccone et al., 2004).

Multiple loci are involved in genetic susceptibility to autoimmune diabetes in the NOD mouse, as in humans. H-2g7, a mouse MHC haplotype, is the major genetic contributor to T1D genetic susceptibility (Kikutani and Makino, 1992; Atkinson and Leiter, 1999). Experiments investigating the MHC in the NOD mouse indicate that the MHC in mice is essential but not sufficient for β-cell destruction and development of diabetes in NOD mice (Kikutani and Makino, 1992) suggesting that, as in human T1D, other loci are important. It is increasingly clear that some susceptibility loci in humans and the NOD mouse are the same and this allows detailed functional analysis of genetic determinants of disease.

Regions of genetic association in the NOD mouse have been designated Idd numbers - for instance the MHC association is referred to as Idd1 while ctla4 is Idd5.1. As well as the membrane bound and soluble forms of ctla4 found in humans mice have a third form lacking a binding domain. Protection from diabetes can be mediated by over-expression of this mouse specific isoform. The IL2 signaling pathway, specifically IL2 (Lyons et al. 2000) has also been associated with diabetes in the NOD mouse (Idd3).

8. Common mechanisms of autoimmunity

More than 50 genome wide association studies have now been published and their power to identify complex gene networks that link biological pathways is increasingly clear and particularly so for autoimmunity. When data from several different forms of autoimmunity including rheumatoid arthritis, celiac disease, autoimmune thyroid disease, multiple sclerosis and type 1 diabetes are compared, common autoimmune pathways, including the HLA and genes such as PTPN22 that that regulateT cell activation have become apparent. This may offer the potential for flexible therapy in the future.

9. Other genetic mechanisms underlying susceptibility to T1D

9.1 Gender and Type 1 diabetes

Unlike most other autoimmune diseases where risk is greatest in females, type I diabetes is the only major organ-specific autoimmune disorder not to show a strong female bias with risk equal between males and females in childhood. Risk in males increases in adolescence and remains higher than females thereafter. The effects of hormonal changes on risk are unknown but effects on insulin resistance could be important. Furthermore, fathers with Type I diabetes are more likely than affected mothers to transmit the condition to their offspring (Warram et al. 1988) and this observation have never been explained. Women of childbearing age are therefore less likely to develop type I diabetes, and - should this occur - are less likely to transmit it to their offspring. Parent of origin effects, precipitated by epigenetic changes to DNA are worthy of investigation.

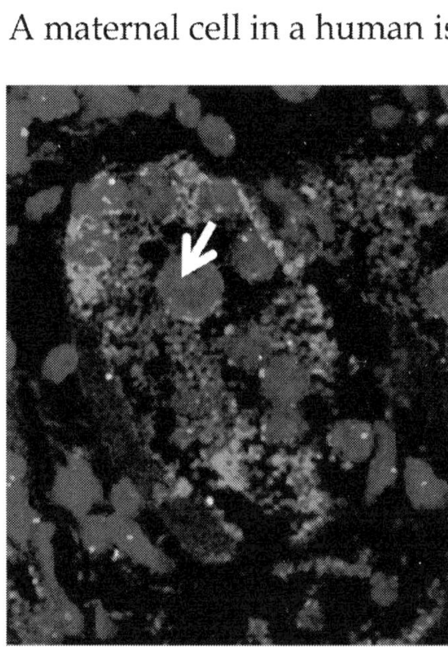

Fig. 9. A female nucleus (two red X chromosomes) in autopsy male pancreas tissue. The Y chromosme is represented as a light green dot and nuclei are stained blue with dapi. Insulin is stained green with fitc. Showing that this maternal cell lies within an islet. Adabted from van Zyl et al. 2010

9.2 Microchimerism

Some genetic mechanisms such as rare variants cannot be identified by GWAS and will be defined by high throughput next generation sequencing protocols as they increasingly become available. Other mechanisms that require further investigation are DNA methylation and other epigenetic changes to DNA that could increase risk of future type 1 diabetes. Further, over the last decade there have been several reports of associations between maternal cells, which are known to persist in her progeny for several decades (Maloney et al. 1998). Maternal DNA is often detected by testing for the presence of the non-inherited maternal allele (NIMA) and increased levels of maternal DNA or cells have been associated with several different autoimmune diseases (reviewed by Nelson 2008). One study of 464 T1D families by Pani et al. (2002) showed that the non-transmitted HLA DR3-DQ2 and DR4-DQ8 were more frequent in mothers than in fathers of all non- DQ2/DQ8 heterozygous diabetic offspring, as well as in offspring not carrying any HLA high-risk allele. In patients with either risk allele alone, more maternal than paternal non-transmitted risk alleles complemented the constellation to DQ2/DQ8. This suggested that the non-inherited maternal allele was contributing to T1D susceptibility. This observation however could not be replicated in two other studies (Lambert et al. 2003, Herrman et al. 2003). Several years later, using a more sensitive quantitative PCR for the NIMA, Nelson et al (2007) showed that NIMA levels were increased in children with T1D compared to unaffected siblings and healthy controls. Intriguingly using fluorescence in situ hybridization (FISH) for the X and Y chromosomes, this study also showed evidence for the presence of maternal cells in autopsy pancreatic islets of individuals with T1D and healthy controls, although the frequency of maternal cells was higher.

This increased frequency of maternal cells in autopsy T1D was confirmed in a follow up study (van Zyl et al. 2010). The role of these cells in T1D is, as yet, unclear. If they are functioning beta cells could represent the target of the immune response or alternatively could be immune effector cells. Further studies are required in this new area of biology.

10. Conclusions

Type 1 diabetes is a disease of major personal, medical and financial significance. The recent rapid increased in the frequency of the disease, especially in those diagnosed under the age of 5 years is alarming. Thirty years of research have demonstrated the importance of underlying genetic susceptibility. Major improvements in identifying the genetic determinants of complex disease have resulted in an explosion of information on the genetic pathways contributing to autoimmune diabetes. While these genetic determinants have not enhanced assessment of genetic risk for participation in intervention trials (HLA mediated risk remains the most robust means of estimating genetic risk), they have identified immune and biochemical pathways that may potentially be targeted therapeutically in the future.

11. References

Achenbach P, Koczwara K, Knopff A, Naserke H, Ziegler AG, Bonifacio E. (2004) Mature high-affinity immune responses to (pro)insulin anticipate the autoimmune cascade that leads to type 1 diabetes. *J Clin Invest* 114:589- 597.

Achenbach P, Warncke K, Reiter J, et al. (2004) Stratification of type 1 diabetes risk on the basis of islet autoantibody characteristics. *Diabetes* 53:384-392.

Alexander L, Weiskopf E, Greenough TC, Gaddis NC, Auerbach MR, Malim MH, O'Brien SJ, Walker BD, Sullivan JL, Desrosiers RC. (2000) Unusual polymorphisms in human immunodeficiency virus type 1 associated with nonprogressive infection. *J Virol.* 74:4361-76.

Aly TA, Baschal EE, Jahromi MM, et al. (2008) Analysis of single nucleotide polymorphisms identifies major type 1A diabetes locus telomeric of the major histocompatibility complex. *Diabetes* 57:770-776.

Aly TA, Ide A, Jahromi MM, et al. (2006) Extreme genetic risk for type 1A diabetes. *Proc Natl Acad Sci USA* 103:14074- 14079.

Anjos S, Nguyen A, Ounissi-Benkalha H, Tessier MC, Polychronakos C. (2002) A common autoimmunity predisposing Signal peptide variant of the cytotoxic T-lymphocyte antigen 4 results in inefficient glycosylation of the susceptibility allele. *J Biol Chem.* 277:46478-86.

Atkinson MA, Leiter EH. (1999) The NOD mouse model of type 1 diabetes: as good as it gets? *Nat Med.* 5:601-4.

Awata T, Kuzuya T, Matsuda A, Iwamoto Y, Kanazawa Y, Okuyama M et al. High frequency of aspartic acid at position 57 of the HLA-DQ □-chain in Japanese IDD patients and non-diabetic subjects. *Diabetes* 1990; 39:266-269.

Baekkeskov S, Aanstoot HJ, Christgau S, et al. (1990) Identification of the 64K autoantigen in insulin-dependent diabetes as the GABA-synthesizing enzyme glutamic acid decarboxylase. *Nature* 347:151-156.

Baekkeskov S, Nielsen JH, Marner B, Bilde T, Ludvigsson J, Lernmark A. (1982) Autoantibodies in newly diagnosed diabetic children immunoprecipitate human pancreatic islet cell proteins. *Nature* 298:167-169.

Bailey R, Cooper JD, Zeitels L, et al. (2007) Association of the vitamin D metabolism gene CYP27B1 with type 1 diabetes. *Diabetes* 56:2616-2621.

Barker JM, Barriga KJ, Yu L, et al. (2004) Prediction of autoantibody positivity and progression to type 1 diabetes: Diabetes Autoimmunity Study in the Young (DAISY). *J Clin Endocrinol Metab* 89:3896-3902.

Barrett JC, Clayton DG, Concannon P, Akolkar B, Cooper JD, Erlich HA, Julier C, Morahan G, Nerup J, Nierras C, Plagnol V, Pociot F, Schuilenburg H, Smyth DJ, Stevens H, Todd JA, Walker NM, Rich SS; Type 1 Diabetes Genetics Consortium. (2009) Genome-wide association study and meta-analysis find that over 40 loci affect risk of type 1 diabetes. *Nat Genet.* 41:703-7.

Bell GI, Horita S, Karam JH. (1984). A polymorphic locus near the human insulin gene is associated with insulin- dependent diabetes mellitus. *Diabetes* 33:176-183.

Bennett ST, Lucassen AM, Gough SC, et al. (1995) Susceptibility to human type 1 diabetes at IDDM2 is determined by tandem repeat variation at the insulin gene minisatellite locus. *Nat Genet* 9:284-292.

Bingley PJ, Bonifacio E, Williams AJ, Genovese S, Bottazzo GF, Gale EA. (1997) Prediction of IDDM in the general population: strategies based on combinations of autoantibody markers. *Diabetes* 46:1701-1710.

Bonifacio E, Hummel M, Walter M, Schmid S, Ziegler AG. (2004) IDDM1 and multiple family history of type 1 diabetes combine to identify neonates at high risk for type 1 diabetes. *Diabetes Care* 27:2695-2700.

Bottazzo GF, Dean BM, McNally JM, MacKay EH, Swift PG, Gamble DR. (1985) In situ characterization of autoimmune phenomena and expression of HLA molecules in the pancreas in diabetic insulitis. *N Engl J Med* 313:353- 360.

Bottini N, Musumeci L, Alonso A, et al. (2004) A functional variant of lymphoid tyrosine phosphatase is associated with type I diabetes. *Nat Genet* 36:337-338.

Bottini N, Vang T, Cucca F, Mustelin T. (2006) Role of PTPN22 in type 1 diabetes and other autoimmune diseases. *Semin Immunol* 18:207-213.

Caillat-Zucman S, Garchon HJ, Timsit J, Assan R, Boitard C, Djilali-Saiah I, Bougnères P, Bach JF. (1992) Age-dependent HLA genetic heterogeneity of type 1 insulin-dependent diabetes mellitus. *J Clin Invest.* 90:2242-50.

Christie MR, Genovese S, Cassidy D, Bosi E, Brown TJ, Lai M, Bonifacio E, Bottazzo GF. (1994) Antibodies to islet 37k antigen,but not to glutamate decarboxylase, discriminate rapid progression to IDDM in endocrine autoimmunity. *Diabetes* 43:1254-9.

Concannon P, Gogolin-Ewens KJ, Hinds DA, et al. (1998) A second-generation screen of the human genome for susceptibility to insulin-dependent diabetes mellitus. *Nat Genet* 19:292-296.

Concannon P, Onengut-Gumuscu S, Todd JA, Smyth DJ, Pociot F, Bergholdt R, Akolkar B, Erlich HA, Hilner JE, Julier C,

Morahan G, Nerup J, Nierras CR, Chen WM, Rich SS, Type 1 Diabetes Genetics Consortium. (2008) A human type 1 diabetes susceptibility locus maps to chromosome 21q22.3. *Diabetes* 57:2858-61,

Cox NJ, Wapelhorst B, Morrison VA, et al. P. (2001) Seven regions of the genome show evidence of linkage to type 1 diabetes in a consensus analysis of 767 multiplex families. *Am J Hum Genet* 69:820-830.

Criswell LA, Pfeiffer KA, Lum RF, Gonzales B, Novitzke J, Kern M, Moser KL, Begovich AB, Carlton VE, Li W, Lee AT, Ortmann W, Behrens TW, Gregersen PK. (2005) Analysis of families in the multiple autoimmune disease genetics consortium (MADGC) collection: the PTPN22 620W allele associates with multiple autoimmune phenotypes. *Am J Hum Genet.* 76:561-71.

Cruz TD, Valdes AM, Santiago A, et al. (2004) DPB1 alleles are associated with type 1 diabetes susceptibility in multiple ethnic groups. *Diabetes* 53:2158-2163.

Cucca F, Lampis R, Congia M, et al. (2001) A correlation between the relative predisposition of MHC class II alleles to type 1 diabetes and the structure of their proteins. *Hum Mol Genet* 10:2025-2037.

Cudworth AG, Woodrow JC. (1975) Evidence for HL-A-linked genes in 'juvenile' diabetes mellitus. *Br Med J* 1975;3:133- 135.

Davies JL, Kawaguchi Y, Bennett ST, et al. (1994) A genome-wide search for human type 1 diabetes susceptibility genes. *Nature* ;371:130-136.

Dendrou CA, Plagnol V, Fung E, Yang JH, Downes K, Cooper JD, Nutland S, Coleman G, Himsworth M, Hardy M, Burren O, Healy B, Walker NM, Koch K, Ouwehand WH, Bradley JR, Wareham NJ, Todd JA, Wicker LS. (2009) Cell-specific protein phenotypes for the autoimmune locus IL2RA using a genotype-selectable human bioresource. *Nat Genet.* 41:1011-5

Dotta F, Censini S, van Halteren AG, et al. (2007) Coxsackie B4 virus infection of beta cells and natural killer cell insulitis in recent-onset type 1 diabetic patients. *Proc Natl Acad Sci USA* 104:5115-5120.

Edghill EL, Dix RJ, Flanagan SE, et al. (2006) HLA genotyping supports a non-autoimmune etiology in patients diagnosed with diabetes under the age of 6 months. *Diabetes* 55:1895-1898.

Fennessy M, Metcalfe K, Hitman GA, Niven M, Biro PA, Tuomilehto J et al. (1995) A gene in the HLA class 1 region contributes to susceptibility to IDDM in the Finnish population. *Diabetologia* 37:937-944.

Fourlanos S, Varney MD, Tait BD, et al. (2008) The rising incidence of type 1 diabetes is accounted for by cases with lower-risk human leukocyte antigen genotypes. *Diabetes Care* 31:1546-1549.

Fujino-Kurihara H, Fujita H, Hakura A, Nonaka K, Tarui S. (1985) Morphological aspects on pancreatic islets of non- obese diabetic (NOD) mice. *Virchows Arch B Cell Pathol Incl Mol Pathol.* 1985 49:107-20.

Gale EA, Gillespie KM. (2001) Diabetes and gender. *Diabetologia.* 44:3-15.

Gale EA. (2002) The rise of childhood type 1 diabetes in the 20th century. *Diabetes* 51:3353-3361.

Gillespie KM, Gale EA, Bingley PJ. (2002) High familial risk and genetic susceptibility in early onset childhood diabetes. *Diabetes.* 51:210-4.

Gillespie KM, Dix RJ, Williams AJ, Newton R, Robinson ZF, Bingley PJ, Gale EA, Shield JP. (2006) Islet autoimmunity in children with Down's syndrome. *Diabetes.* 55:3185-8.

Gillespie KM, Bain SC, Barnett AH, et al. (2004) The rising incidence of childhood type 1 diabetes and reduced contribution of high-risk HLA haplotypes. *Lancet;* 364:1699-1700.

Giordano C, Pantò F, Caruso C, Modica MA, Zambito AM, Sapienza N, Amato MP, Galluzzo A. (1989) Interleukin 2 and soluble interleukin 2-receptor secretion defect in vitro in newly diagnosed type I diabetic patients. *Diabetes.* 38:310-5.

Grant SF, Qu HQ, Bradfield JP, Marchand L, Kim CE, Glessner JT, Grabs R, Taback SP, Frackelton EC, Eckert AW, Annaiah K, Lawson ML, Otieno FG, Santa E, Shaner JL, Smith RM, Skraban R, Imielinski M, Chiavacci RM, Grundmeier RW, Stanley CA, Kirsch SE, Waggott D, Paterson AD, Monos DS; DCCT/EDIC Research Group, Polychronakos C, Hakonarson H: (2009) Follow-up analysis of genome-wide association data identifies novel loci for type 1 diabetes. *Diabetes* 58:290-5

Hakonarson H, Grant SF, Bradfield JP, et al. (2007) A genome-wide association study identifies KIAA0350 as a type 1 diabetes gene. *Nature* 448:591-594.

Hashimoto L, Habita C, Beressi JP, et al. (1994) Genetic mapping of a susceptibility locus for insulin-dependent diabetes mellitus on chromosome 11q. *Nature* 371:161-164.

Hawkes CJ, Wasmeier C, Christie MR, Hutton JC. (1996) Identification of the 37 kDa antigen in IDDM as a tyrosine phosphatase-like protein (phogrin) related to IA-2. *Diabetes* 45:1187-1192.

Hermann R, Knip M, Veijola R, et al. (2003) Temporal changes in the frequencies of HLA genotypes in patients with Type 1 diabetes—indication of an increased environmental pressure? *Diabetologia* 46:420-425.

Hermann R, Veijola R, Sipilä I, Knip M, Akerblom HK, Simell O, Ilonen J. -to: Pani MA, Van Autreve J, Van Der Auwera BJ, Gorus FK, Badenhoop K (2002) Non-transmitted maternal HLA DQ2 or DQ8 alleles and risk of Type I diabetes in offspring: the importance of foetal or post partum exposure to diabetogenic molecules. *Diabetologia* 46:588-9

Herold KC, Huen A, Gould L, Traisman H, Rubenstein AH. (1984) Alterations in lymphocyte subpopulations in type 1 (insulin-dependent) diabetes mellitus:

exploration of possible mechanisms and relationships to autoimmune phenomena. *Diabetologia.* 27 Suppl:102-5.

Howson JM, Walker NM, Clayton D, Todd JA; Type 1 Diabetes Genetics Consortium. (2009) Confirmation of HLA class II independent type 1 diabetes associations in the major histocompatibility complex including HLA-B and HLA- A. *Diabetes Obes Metab.* 11 Suppl 1:31-45

Hyoty H. (2002) Enterovirus infections and type 1 diabetes. *Ann Med* 2002;34:138-147.

Hyttinen V, Kaprio J, Kinnunen L, Koskenvuo M, Tuomilehto J. (2003) Genetic liability of type 1 diabetes and the onset age among 22,650 young Finnish twin pairs: a nationwide follow-up study. *Diabetes* 52:1052-1055.

Kaprio J, Tuomilehto J, Koskenvuo M, Romanov K, Reunanen A, Eriksson J, Stengård J, Kesäniemi YA. (1992) Concordance for type 1 (insulin-dependent) and type 2 (non-insulin-dependent) diabetes mellitus in a population-based cohort of twins in Finland. *Diabetologia.* 35:1060-7.

Karvonen M, Viik-Kajander M, Moltchanova E, Libman I, LaPorte R, Tuomilehto J. (2000) Incidence of childhood type 1 diabetes worldwide. Diabetes Mondiale (DiaMond) Project Group. *Diabetes Care* 23:1516-26.

Kikutani H, Makino S. (1992) The murine autoimmune diabetes model: NOD and related strains. *Adv Immunol.* 51:285- 322.

Kukko M, Virtanen SM, Toivonen A, et al. (2004) Geographical variation in risk HLA-DQB1 genotypes for type 1 diabetes and signs of beta-cell autoimmunity in a high-incidence country. *Diabetes Care* 27:676-681.

Lambert AP, Gillespie KM, Thomson G, et al. (2004) Absolute risk of childhood-onset type 1 diabetes defined by human leukocyte antigen class II genotype: a population-based study in the United Kingdom. *J Clin Endocrinol Metab* 89:4037-4043.

Lambert AP, Gillespie KM, Bingley PJ, Gale EA. to: Pani MA, Van Autreve J, Van der Auwera BJ, Gorus FK, Badenhoop K. (2003) Non-transmitted maternal HLA DQ2 or DQ8 alleles and risk of Type 1 diabetes in offspring: the importance of foetal or post partum exposure to diabetogenic molecules *Diabetologia.* 46:590-1

Langholz B, Tuomilehto-Wolf E, Thomas DW, Pitkäniemi J, Tuomilehto J. Variation in HLA-associated risks of chilhood insulin-dependent diabetes in a Finnish population: I. Allele effects at A,B and DR loci. DiMe Study Group. Childhood Diabetes in Finland. *Genet Epidemiol* 1995; 12:441-453.

Lee C, Iafrate AJ, Brothman AR. (2007) Copy number variations and clinical cytogenetic diagnosis of constitutional disorders. *Nat Genet* 39:S48-S54.

Liu S, Wang H, Jin Y, Podolsky R, Reddy MV, Pedersen J, Bode B, Reed J, Steed D, Anderson S, Yang P, Muir A, Steed L, Hopkins D, Huang Y, Purohit S, Wang CY, Steck AK, Montemari A, Eisenbarth G, Rewers M, She JX. (2009) IFIH1 polymorphisms are significantly associated with type 1 diabetes and IFIH1 gene expression in peripheral blood mononuclear cells. *Hum Mol Genet.* 18:358-65.

Lowe CE, Cooper JD, Brusko T, et al. (2007) Large-scale genetic fine mapping and genotype-phenotype associations implicate polymorphism in the IL2RA region in type 1 diabetes. *Nat Genet* 39:1074-1082.

Lyons PA, Hancock WW, Denny P, Lord CJ, Hill NJ, Armitage N, Siegmund T, Todd JA, Phillips MS, Hess JF, Chen SL, Fischer PA, Peterson LB, Wicker LS. (2000) The

NOD Idd9 genetic interval influences the pathogenicity of insulitis and contains molecular variants of Cd30, Tnfr2, and Cd137. *Immunity* 13:107-15.

Maloney S, Smith A, Furst DE, Myerson D, Rupert K, Evans PC, Nelson JL. (1999) Microchimerism of maternal origin persists into adult life. *J Clin Invest.* 104:41-7.

Mathieu C, Laureys J, Sobis H, Vandeputte M, Waer M, Bouillon R. (1992) 1,25-dihydroxyvitamin D3 prevents insulitis in NOD mice. *Diabetes* 41:1491-1495.

Maier LM, Anderson DE, Severson CA, Baecher-Allan C, Healy B, Liu DV, Wittrup KD, De Jager PL, Hafler DA. (2009) Soluble IL-2RA levels in multiple sclerosis subjects and the effect of soluble IL-2RA on immune responses. *J Immunol.* 182:1541-7.

Makino S, Kunimoto K, Muraoka Y, Mizushima Y, Katagiri K, Tochino Y. (1980) Breeding of a non-obese, diabetic strain of mice. *Jikken Dobutsu.* 29:1-13.

Mein CA, Esposito L, Dunn MG, et al. (1998) A search for type 1 diabetes susceptibility genes in families from the United Kingdom. *Nat Genet* 19:297-300.

Modi WS, Lautenberger J, An P, et al. (2006) Genetic variation in the CCL18-CCL3-CCL4 chemokine gene cluster influences HIV type 1 transmission and AIDS disease progression. *Am J Hum Genet*;79:120-128.

Muller K, Bendtzen K. Inhibition of human T lymphocyte proliferation and cytokine production by 1,25- dihydroxyvitamin D3. (1992) Differential effects on CD45RA+ and CD45R0+ cells. *Autoimmunity* 14:37-43.

Nair MP, Lewis EW, Schwartz SA. (1986) Immunoregulatory dysfunctions in type I diabetes: natural and antibody- dependent cellular cytotoxic activities. *J Clin Immunol.* 6:363-72.

Nelson JL, Gillespie KM, Lambert NC, Stevens AM, Loubiere LS, Rutledge JC, Leisenring WM, Erickson TD, Yan Z, Mullarkey ME, Boespflug ND, Bingley PJ, Gale EA. (2007) Maternal microchimerism in peripheral blood in type 1 diabetes and pancreatic islet beta cell microchimerism. *Proc Natl Acad Sci U S A.* 104:1637-42.

Nakanishi K, Kobayishi T, Murase T, Nakatsuiji T, Inoko H, Tsuji K et al. (1993) Association of HLA-A24 with complete B cell destruction in IDDM. *Diabetes* 42:1086.

Näntö-Salonen K, Kupila A, Simell S, et al. (2008) Nasal insulin to prevent type 1 diabetes in children with HLA genotypes and autoantibodies conferring increased risk of disease: a double-blind, randomised controlled trial. *Lancet* 372:1746-1755.

Nejentsev S, Cooper JD, Godfrey L, et al. (2004) Analysis of the vitamin D receptor gene sequence variants in type 1 diabetes. *Diabetes* 53:2709-2712.

Nejentsev S, Howson JM, Walker NM, et al. (2007) Localization of type 1 diabetes susceptibility to the MHC class I genes HLA-B and HLA-A. *Nature* 450:887-892.

Nejentsev S, Reijonen H, Adojaan B, Kovalchuk L, Sochnevs A, Schwartz E et al. (1997) The effect of HLA-B allele on IDDM risk defined by DRB1*04 subtypes and DQB1*0302. *Diabetes* 46:1888-1892.

Nejentsev S, Walker N, Riches D, Egholm M, Todd JA. (2009) Rare variants of IFIH1, a gene implicated in antiviral responses protect against type 1 diabetes. *Science.* 324:387-9.

Nepom BS, Schwartz D, Palmer J, Nepom GT. (1987) Trans-complementation of HLA genes in IDDM. HLA-DQ alpha- and beta-chains produce hybrid molecules in DR3/4 heterozygotes. *Diabetes*; 36:114-117.

Nelson JL. Your cells are my cells. (2008) *Sci Am.* 298:64-71

Nerup J, Platz P, Andersen OO, et al. (1974) HL-A antigens and diabetes mellitus. *Lancet* 1974;2:864-866.

Nistico L, Buzzetti R, Pritchard LE, et al. (1996) The CTLA-4 gene region of chromosome 2q33 is linked to, and associated with type 1 diabetes. Belgian Diabetes Registry. *Hum Mol Genet* 5:1075-1080.

Noble JA, Valdes AM, Thomson G, Erlich HA. (2003) The HLA class II locus DPB1 can influence susceptibility to type 1 diabetes. *Diabetes.* 2000 Jan;49(1):121-5.

Olmos P, A'Hern R, Heaton DA, Millward BA, Risley D, Pyke DA, Leslie RD. (1988) The significance of the concordance rate for type 1 (insulin-dependent) diabetes in identical twins. *Diabetologia.* 31:747-50.

Onkamo P, Vaananen S, Karvonen M, Tuomilehto J. (1999) Worldwide increase in incidence of Type I diabetes—the analysis of the data on published incidence trends. *Diabetologia* 42:1395-1403.

Ounissi-Benkalha H, Polychronakos C. (2008) The molecular genetics of type 1 diabetes: new genes and emerging mechanisms. *Trends Mol Med* 14:268-275.

Palmer JP, Asplin CM, Clemons P, et al. (1983) Insulin antibodies in insulin-dependent diabetics before insulin treatment. *Science* 222:1337-1339.

Pani MA, Van Autreve J, Van der Auwera BJ, Gorus FK, Badenhoop K. (2002) Non-transmitted maternal HLA DQ2 or DQ8 alleles and risk of Type I diabetes in offspring: the importance of foetal or post partum exposure to diabetogenic molecules. *Diabetologia.* 45:1340-3.

Patterson CC, Dahlquist GG, Gyürüs E, Green A, Soltész G; EURODIAB Study Group. (2009) Incidence trends for childhood type 1 diabetes in Europe during 1989-2003 and predicted new cases 2005-20: a multicentre prospective registration study. *Lancet.* 373:2027-33

Pugliese A, Gianani R, Moromisato R, Awdeh ZL, Alper CA, Erlich HA, Jackson RA, Eisenbarth GS. (1995) HLA- DQB1*0602 is associated with dominant protection from diabetes even among islet cell antibody-positive first- degree relatives of patients with IDDM. *Diabetes.* 44:608-13.

Pugliese A, Zeller M, Fernandez A, et al. (1997) The insulin gene is transcribed in the human thymus and transcription levels correlated with allelic variation at the INS VNTR-IDDM2 susceptibility locus for type 1 diabetes. *Nat Genet* 15:293-297.

Oldstone MB. (1988) Prevention of type I diabetes in nonobese diabetic mice by virus infection. *Science.* 239:500-2.

Oldstone MB. Viruses as therapeutic agents. I. (1990) Treatment of nonobese insulin-dependent diabetes mice with virus prevents insulin-dependent diabetes mellitus while maintaining general immune competence. *J Exp Med.* Jun 1;171(6):2077-89.

Qu HQ, Marchand L, Grabs R, Polychronakos C. (2008) The association between the IFIH1 locus and type 1 diabetes. *Diabetologia* 51:473-475.

Qu HQ, Montpetit A, Ge B, Hudson TJ, Polychronakos C. (2007) Toward further mapping of the association between the IL2RA locus and type 1 diabetes. *Diabetes* 56:1174-1176.

Ramos-Lopez E, Scholten F, Aminkeng F, et al. (2009) Association of KIR2DL2 polymorphism rs2756923 with type 1 diabetes and preliminary evidence for lack of inhibition through HLA-C1 ligand binding. *Tissue Antigens* 73:599-603

Redondo MJ, Fain PR, Eisenbarth GS. (2001) Genetics of type 1A diabetes. *Recent Prog Horm Res* 56:69-89.

Risch N. (1987) Assessing the role of HLA-linked and unlinked determinants of disease. *Am J Hum Genet* 40:1-14.

Roll U, Christie MR, Fuchtenbusch M, Payton MA, Hawkes CJ, Ziegler AG. (1996) Perinatal autoimmunity in offspring of diabetic parents. The German Multicenter BABY-DIAB study: detection of humoral immune responses to islet antigens in early childhood. *Diabetes* 45:967-973.

Sabbah E, Kulmala P, Veijola R, et al. (1996) Glutamic acid decarboxylase antibodies in relation to other autoantibodies and genetic risk markers in children with newly diagnosed insulin-dependent diabetes. *J Clin Endocrinol Metab* 81:2455-2459.

Shastry A, Sedimbi SK, Rajalingam R, et al. (2008) Combination of KIR 2DL2 and HLA-C1 (Asn) confers susceptibility to type 1 diabetes in Latvians. *Int J Immunogenet* 35: 439-446

Singal DP, Blajchman MA. Histocompatibility (HL-A) antigens, lymphocytotoxic antibodies and tissue antibodies in patients with diabetes mellitus. *Diabetes* 1973;22:429-432.

Smyth DJ, Cooper JD, Bailey R, et al. (2006) A genome-wide association study of nonsynonymous SNPs identifies a type 1 diabetes locus in the interferon-induced helicase (IFIH1) region. *Nat Genet* 38:617-619.

Smyth DJ, Plagnol V, Walker NM, Cooper JD, Downes K, Yang JH, Howson JM, Stevens H, McManus R, Wijmenga C, Heap GA, Dubois PC, Clayton DG, Hunt KA, van Heel DA, Todd JA. (2008) Shared and distinct genetic variants in type 1 diabetes and celiac disease. *N Engl J Med*. 359:2767-77.

Sobel DO, Ahvazi B. (1998) Alpha-interferon inhibits the development of diabetes in NOD mice. *Diabetes*. 47:1867-72

Solimena M, Dirkx R Jr, Hermel JM, et al. (1996) ICA 512, an autoantigen of type I diabetes, is an intrinsic membrane protein of neurosecretory granules. *EMBO J*. 15:2102-2114.

The EURODIAB Substudy 2 Study Group. (1999) Vitamin D supplement in early childhood and risk for type I (insulin- dependent) diabetes mellitus. *Diabetologia* 42:51-54.

Thomson G, Robinson WP, Kuhner MK, et al. (1988) Genetic heterogeneity, modes of inheritance, and risk estimates for a joint study of Caucasians with insulin-dependent diabetes mellitus. *Am J Hum Genet* 43:799-816.

Thomson G. (1988) HLA disease associations: models for insulin dependent diabetes mellitus and the study of complex human genetic disorders. *Annu Rev Genet* 22:31-50.

Tienari PJ, Tuomilehto-Wolf E, Tuomilehto J, Peltonen L, The DIME Study Group. (1992) HLA haplotypes in Type 1 (insulin- dependent) diabetes mellitus: molecular analysis of the HLA-DQ locus. *Diabetologia* 35:254-260.

Todd JA. Etiology of type 1 diabetes. *Immunity*. 2010 32:457-67.

Todd JA, Bell JI, McDevitt HO. (1987) HLA-DQ beta gene contributes to susceptibility and resistance to insulin- dependent diabetes mellitus. *Nature* 329:599-604.

Todd JA, Walker NM, Cooper JD, et al. (2007) Robust associations of four new chromosome regions from genome-wide analyses of type 1 diabetes. *Nat Genet* 39:857-864.

Todd JA, Walker NM, Cooper JD, Smyth DJ, Downes K, Plagnol V, Bailey R, Nejentsev S, Field SF, Payne F, Lowe CE, Szeszko JS, Hafler JP, Zeitels L, Yang JH, Vella A, Nutland S, Stevens HE, Schuilenburg H, Coleman G, Maisuria M, Meadows W, Smink LJ, Healy B, Burren OS, Lam AA, Ovington NR, Allen J, Adlem E, Leung HT, Wallace C, Howson JM, Guja C, Ionescu-Tîrgovişte C; Genetics of Type 1 Diabetes in Finland, Simmonds MJ, Heward JM, Gough SC; Wellcome Trust Case Control Consortium, Dunger DB, Wicker LS, Clayton DG: (2007) Robust associations of four new chromosome regions from genome-wide analyses of type 1 diabetes. *Nat Genet* 39:857- 64,

Ueda H, Howson JM, Esposito L, et al. (2003) Association of the T-cell regulatory gene CTLA4 with susceptibility to autoimmune disease. *Nature* 423:506-511.

Vafiadis P, Bennett ST, Todd JA, et al. (1997) Insulin expression in human thymus is modulated by INS VNTR alleles at the IDDM2 locus. *Nat Genet*;15:289-292.

Valdes AM, Thomson G, Erlich H, Noble JA. (1999) Association between type 1 diabetes age of onset and HLA among sibling pairs. *Diabetes* 48:1658-1661.

Van der Auwera BJ, Schuit FC, Weets I, Ivens A, Van Autreve JE, Gorus FK. (2002) Relative and absolute HLA-DQA1- DQB1 linked risk for developing type I diabetes before 40 years of age in the Belgian population: implications for future prevention studies. *Hum Immunol* 63:40-50.

Van Zyl B, Planas R, Ye Y, Foulis A, de Krijger RR, Vives-Pi M, Gillespie KM. (2010) Why are levels of maternal microchimerism higher in type 1 diabetes pancreas? *Chimerism* 1(2):45-50.

Vella A, Cooper JD, Lowe CE, et al. (2005) Localization of a type 1 diabetes locus in the IL2RA/CD25 region by use of tag single-nucleotide polymorphisms. *Am J Hum Genet* 76:773-779.

Verge CF, Gianani R, Yu L, Pietropaolo M, Smith T, Jackson RA, Soeldner JS, Eisenbarth GS. (1995) Late progression to diabetes and evidence for chronic beta-cell autoimmunity in identical twins of patients with type I diabetes. *Diabetes* 44(10):1176-9.

Warram JH, Krolewski AS, Kahn CR. (1988) Determinants of IDDM and perinatal mortality in children of diabetic mothers. *Diabetes*;37:1328-1334.

Waterhouse P, Penninger JM, Timms E, Wakeham A, Shahinian A, Lee KP, Thompson CB, Griesser H, Mak TW.(1995) Lymphoproliferative disorders with early lethality in mice deficient in Ctla-4. *Science*. 270:985-8.

Wattenhofer M, Shibuya K, Kudoh J, Lyle R, Michaud J, Rossier C, Kawasaki K, Asakawa S, Minoshima S, Berry A, Bonne-Tamir B, Shimizu N, Antonarakis SE, Scott HS. (2001) Isolation and characterization of the UBASH3A gene on 21q22.3 encoding a potential nuclear protein with a novel combination of domains. *Hum Genet*. 108:140-7.

Weets I, Van Autreve J, Van der Auwera BJ, Schuit FC, Du Caju MV, Decochez K, De Leeuw IH, Keymeulen B, Mathieu C, Rottiers R, Dorchy H, Quartier E, Gorus FK; Belgian Diabetes Registry. (2001) Male-to-female excess in diabetes diagnosed in early adulthood is not specific for the immune-mediated form nor is it HLA-DQ restricted: possible relation to increased body mass index. *Diabetologia*. 44:40-7

Wellcome Trust Case Control Consortium. (2007) Genome-wide association study of 14,000 cases of seven common diseases and 3,000 shared controls. *Nature* 447:661-78.

Wenzlau JM, Juhl K, Yu L, et al. (2007) The cation efflux transporter ZnT8 (Slc30A8) is a major autoantigen in human type 1 diabetes. *Proc Natl Acad Sci USA* 104:17040-17045.

Wenzlau JM, Liu Y, Yu L, et al. (2008) A common nonsynonymous single nucleotide polymorphism in the SLC30A8 gene determines ZnT8 autoantibody specificity in type 1 diabetes. *Diabetes* 57:2693-2697.

Wicker LS, Clark J, Fraser HIG, et al. (2005) Type 1 diabetes genes and pathways shared by humans and NOD mice. *J Autoimmun* 25 Suppl: 29-33.

Williams AJ, Aitken RJ, Chandler MA, Gillespie KM, Lampasona V, Bingley PJ. (2008) Autoantibodies to islet antigen-2 are associated with HLA-DRB1*07 and DRB1*09 haplotypes as well as DRB1*04 at onset of type 1 diabetes: the possible role of HLA-DQA in autoimmunity to IA-2. *Diabetologia* 51:1444-1448.

Zaccone P, Raine T, Sidobre S, Kronenberg M, Mastroeni P, Cooke A. (2004) Salmonella typhimurium infection halts development of type 1 diabetes in NOD mice. *Eur J Immunol.* 34:3246-56.

Ziegler AG, Hummel M, Schenker M, Bonifacio E. (1999) Autoantibody appearance and risk for development of childhood diabetes in offspring of parents with type 1 diabetes: the 2-year analysis of the German BABYDIAB Study. *Diabetes* 1999;48:460-468.

25

Comparative Genetic Analysis of Type 1 Diabetes and Inflammatory Bowel Disease

Marina Bakay, Rahul Pandey and Hakon Hakonarson
Center for Applied Genomics, Children's Hospital of Philadelphia USA

1. Introduction

Genome-wide association studies (GWAS) have been fruitful in identifying common variants underlying many complex human diseases (McCarthy et al., 2008; Altshuler et al., 2008), with notable success especially in several autoimmune diseases (Lettre & Rioux 2008; Zhernakova et al., 2009). Hundreds of distinct genomic loci have been associated with various autoimmune diseases, including celiac disease (CeD), Crohn's disease (CD), ulcerative colitis (UC), multiple sclerosis (MS), rheumatoid arthritis (RA), systemic lupus erythematosus (SLE) and type 1 diabetes (T1D). Besides individual studies, recent meta-analysis of GWAS has also enabled the identification of dozens of susceptibility loci for T1D (Cooper et al., 2008; Barrett et al., 2009; Bradfield et al., 2011), CD (Barrett et al., 2009; Franke et al., 2010), and UC (McGovern et al., 2010; Anderson et al., 2011), since single studies are typically underpowered. Additionally, comparisons of susceptibility loci between different autoimmune diseases have revealed important insights into their common genetic architecture. For example, interleukin 23 receptor (IL23R) has been consistently implicated in multiple related autoimmune disorders including CD, UC, ankylosing spondylitis and psoriasis, suggesting that it may be a common susceptibility factor for the major seronegative diseases (Cargill et al., 2007; Duerr et al., 2006; Tremelling et al., 2007). Another study compared shared genetic risk factors for T1D and CeD and reported multiple identical risk alleles (Smyth et al., 2008), suggesting that common biologic mechanisms may be etiologic features of both diseases. Several similar studies that examined known CD susceptibility loci in GWAS for UC identified previously unreported susceptibility loci shared by these related disorders (Franke et al., 2008; Anderson et al., 2009; Anderson et al., 2011). Taken together, these studies suggest that examination of related autoimmune diseases can help reveal shared genetic pathways, and that evaluation of known susceptibility loci for one disease in GWAS for another disease may uncover novel disease-loci relationships. The GWAS approach has been made possible by the development of high-density genotyping arrays that leverage the knowledge generated from The International HapMap project (The International HapMap Project, 2003; International HapMap Consortium, 2005). As a consequence, it has been shown that the genome is laid out in discrete linkage disequilibrium (LD) blocks with limited haplotype diversity within each of these blocks. Therefore, a minimal set of SNPs can detect almost all common haplotypes present, thus improving genotyping accuracy and reducing cost. Genome-wide

genotyping with in excess of 500,000 SNPs can now be readily achieved to accurately tag the vast majority of the diversity in the genome (Steemers et al., 2006; Gunderson et al., 2005; Reich et al., 2005). GWAS has been enormously successful through large-scale studies of cohorts of patients and controls, providing compelling evidences for genetic variants involved in complex autoimmune diseases. A full catalog of these studies is now available at the NIH website: http://www.genome.gov/gwastudies (Hindorff et al., 2010). We are now in a rapid phase of data accumulation for many complex disorders, especially T1D and IBD. 57 loci have now been uncovered to date as being robustly associated with pathogenesis of T1D. The chronic IBDs have seen a great success as well. To date there are 99 IBD susceptibility loci: 71 associated with CD, 47 with UC, and 28 with both UC and CD.
In this review, we first provide a summary of these recent discoveries and then discuss the shared susceptibility loci implicated in T1D, UC and CD. Our study helps understanding the genetic architecture, including shared genetic pathways and risk factors with opposing effects for these related diseases. Data were obtained from two main sources: the National Human Genome Research Institute catalogue of published genome-wide association studies (http://www.genome.gov/gwastudies/; last accessed on 1 April 2011); and PubMed literature search.

2.1 Type 1 diabetes (T1D)

T1D results from autoimmune destruction of pancreatic beta cells, resulting in a lack of insulin production. Of all cases of diabetes, T1D represents approximately 10% and is most prevalent in populations of European ancestry, where there is ample evidence of increased annual incidence during the past five decades (Onkamo et al., 1999; EURODIAB ACE Study Group, 2000). T1D risk is strongly influenced by multiple genetic loci and poorly understood environmental factors.

2.1.1 A genetic component to type 1 diabetes

T1D is a complex trait that results from the interplay between environmental and genetic factors. Many evidences support a strong genetic component associated to T1D. The epidemiological data for geographic prevalence differences is one clear indicator, with populations of European ancestry having the highest presentation rate. T1D has high concordance among monozygotic twins (33 to 42%) (Redondo et al., 2001) and runs strongly in families, with the sibling risk being approximately 10 times greater than the general population (Clayton, 2009); this is in clear contrast to the "less genetic" type 2 diabetes (T2D), where the sibling risk ratio is relatively modest at 3.5 (Rich, 1990).

2.1.2 Before GWAS

Historically, prior to GWAS, only five loci have been fully established to be associated with T1D. It has been long established that approximately half of the genetic risk for T1D is conferred by the genomic region harboring the HLA class II genes (primarily HLA-DRB1, -DQA1 and -DQB1 genes), which encode the highly polymorphic antigen-presenting proteins. Recent fine mapping efforts of the MHC addressed why the class II genes HLA-DQB1 and HLA-DRB1 cannot completely explain the association between T1D and the MHC region (Nejentsev et al., 2007). It turned out that most of the remaining association that could be detected was due to signals in HLA-B and HLA-A, and that the existence of other major T1D genes in the extended MHC was unlikely. Other established loci prior to

GWAS are the genes encoding insulin (INS) (Bell et al., 1984; Bennett et al., 1995), cytotoxic T-lymphocyte-associated protein 4 (CTLA4) (Nistico et al., 1996; Anjos et al., 2004); protein tyrosine phosphatase, non-receptor type 22 (PTPN22) gene (Bottini et al., 2004; Smyth et al., 2004) and interleukin 2 receptor alpha (IL2RA) (Vella et al., 2005; Lowe et al., 2007). However, the majority of other reported associations in the pre-GWAS era have remained debatable (Guo et al., 2004; Mirel et al., 2002; Biason-Lauber et al., 2005), where an initial report of association does not hold up in subsequent replication attempts by other investigative groups, known as the "winner's curse" (Lohmueller et al., 2003).

2.1.3 GWAS of T1D

The advent of GWAS has changed the situation dramatically, provided pace and great benefit to the discovery of loci associated with T1D, increasing the number of associated regions by a factor of ten. An early genome-wide SNP genotyping approach, using only 6,500 nonsynonymous SNPs (Smyth et al., 2006), represented a precursor to the full GWAS approached soon after; however it did uncover a robust association to the interferon-induced with helicase C domain 1 (IFIH1) gene. IFIH1 exerts its influence through the apoptosis of virally infected cells in antiviral immune responses, which may in turn support the notion that there is a connection between viral infections and the pathogenesis of T1D (Knip et al., 2005). Of interest, subsequent re-sequencing revealed additional rarer, higher risk conferring variants residing within the exons of this gene (Nejentsev et al., 2009). The first full-scale GWAS for T1D came simultaneously from our group (Hakonarson et al., 2007) and the Wellcome Trust Case-Control Consortium (WTCCC, 2007). In our study we examined a large pediatric cohort of European descent using the Illumina HumanHap 550 BeadChip platform. The design involved 561 cases, 1,143 controls and 467 triads in the discovery stage followed by a replication effort in 939 nuclear families. In addition to finding the "usual" suspects, including an impressive 392 SNPs capturing the very strong association across the MHC, we identified significant association with variation at the KIAA0350 gene, which we replicated in an additional cohort. The WTCCC study investigated seven common complex diseases including T1D (WTCCC, 2007) by genotyping 2,000 cases and 3,000 controls with ~500,000 SNPs using the Affymetrix GeneChip and reported a number of novel T1D loci, including KIAA0350 genomic region. They confirmed these findings in a replication study in 4,000 cases and 5,000 controls plus nearly 3,000 T1D family trios that were reported in a companion paper that came out on the same day (Todd et al., 2007). In a separate replication effort we elected to fast-track 24 SNPs at 23 distinct loci that fell just below the bar for genome wide significance in our 2007 GWAS and established association to the 12q13 region, with a combined P-value of $9.13x10^{-10}$ (Hakonarson et al., 2008); this was the same locus as the one reported by the WTCCC and Todd et al., 2007. The 12q13 region harbors several genes, including ERBB3, RAB5B, SUOX, RPS26 and CDK2. Additional laboratory studies are needed to identify both the causative variant and the corresponding genes. The clarity of signals found in 2007-2009 T1D GWAS highlights the strength and consistency of GWAS approach in contrast to traditional candidate gene and family-based studies where the consensus amongst geneticist was weak (Lohmueller et al., 2003).

2.1.4 Meta-analyses of T1D GWAS datasets

To date, genome wide genotyping has been relatively expensive, and represents a large financial investment when leveraging large, well powered case-control cohorts. In order to get the most from such an endeavor, GWAS investigators have chosen to combine datasets from different investigative groups in order to carry out meta-analyses. We used this data-mining approach to determine additional novel loci associated with T1D (Grant et al., 2009) conferring increasingly modest risks in the region of 1.1 to 1.2. Through subsequent rounds of testing in an independent cohort of nuclear T1D families from Montreal, the Children's Hospital of Philadelphia and the Type 1 Diabetes Genetics Consortium (T1DGC), followed by the WTCCC dataset and the Diabetes Control and Complications Trial (DCCT)/Epidemiology of Diabetes Interventions and Complications (EDIC) study cohort, we observed convincing association with the genes encoding ubiquitin-associated and SH3 domain-containing protein A (UBASH3A) and BTB and broad complex-tramtrack-bric-a-brac (BTB) and cap 'n' collar (CNC) homology 2 (BACH2). In further support of our finding, the UBASH3A locus was subsequently implicated in T1D from a large linkage study using dense SNP genotyping data generated on affected sib pairs (Concannon et al., 2008).

A subsequent meta-analysis by Cooper and colleges (Cooper et al., 2008) using T1D datasets from the TCCC (Wellcome Trust Case Control Consortium, 2007) and the Genetics of Kidneys in Diabetes (GoKinD) study (Mueller et al., 2006; Manolio et al., 2007), confirmed association to the previously observed loci of PTPN22, CTLA4, MHC, IL2RA, 12q13, 12q24, CLEC16A and PTPN2 but yielded less evidence for the IFIH1 and INS loci without reporting new T1D loci reaching the threshold for genome wide significance. The SNPs with lowest nominal P-values were taken forward for further genotyping in an additional British cohort of approximately 6,000 cases, 7,000 controls and 2,800 families. As a result, the IL2-IL21 association strengthened further and they found strong evidence for the following loci: BACH2 (as we described previously (Grant et al., 2009)), a 10p15 region harboring the protein kinase C, theta gene (PRKCQ), a 15q24 region harboring nine genes including cathepsin H (CTSH) and a 22q13 region harboring the C1q and tumor necrosis factor related protein 6 (C1QTNF6) and somatostatin receptor 3 (SSTR3). Additional studies are required to elucidate the culprit genes and their mechanism at the 15q24 and 22q13 loci.

The meta-analysis reported by Barrett et al., 2009 uncovered in excess of forty loci, including 18 novel regions plus confirmed a number of loci uncovered through cross-disease comparisons (Smyth et al., 2008; Fung et al., 2009; Cooper et al., 2009). This study not only involved samples from WTCCC (WTCCC, 2007) and GoKinD study (Mueller et al., 2006) but also brought in a further large set of cases, controls and family sets from T1DGC. In addition to confirmation for already known loci they also reported association to 1q32.1 (which harbors the interleukin genes IL10, IL19 and IL20), Glis family zinc finger protein 3 (GLIS3) (first suggested by us (Grant et al., 2009), CD69 and IL27. These findings were further supported by our in silico replication efforts (Qu et al., 2010).

To identify additional genetic loci for T1D susceptibility, we examined associations in the largest meta-analysis to date between the disease and ~2.54 million SNPs in a combined cohort of 9,934 cases and 16,956 controls (Bradfield et al., 2011). Targeted follow-up of 53 SNPs in 1,120 affect trios uncovered three new loci associated with T1D that reached genome wide significance. The most significantly associated SNP (rs539514, $P = 5.66 \times 10^{-11}$) resided in an intronic region of the LMO7 (LIM domain only 7) gene on 13q22. The second most significantly associated SNP (rs478222, $P = 3.50 \times 10^{-9}$) resided in an intronic region of the EFR3B (protein EFR3 homolog B) gene on 2p23; however the region of linkage disequilibrium is approximately 800kb and harbors additional multiple genes, including NCOA1, C2orf79, CENPO, ADCY3, DNAJC27, POMC, and DNMT3A. The third most significantly associated SNP (rs924043, $P = 8.06 \times 10^{-9}$) lied in an intergenic region on 6q27, where the region of association is approximately 900kb and harbors multiple genes including WDR27, C6orf120, PHF10, TCTE3, C6orf208, LOC154449, DLL1, FAM120B, PSMB1, TBP and PCD2. These latest associated regions add to the growing repertoire of gene networks predisposing to T1D. Figure 1 summarizes the 57 coli reported to date.

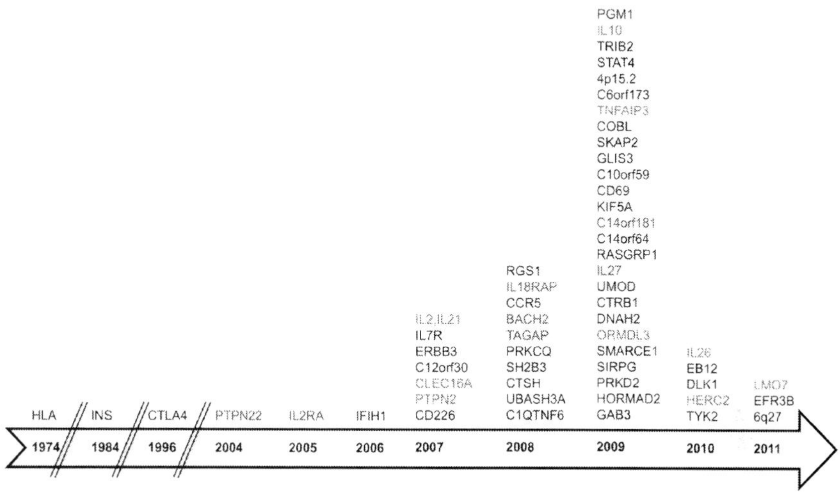

Fig. 1. The 57 type-1 diabetes loci described to date: a timeline. The loci in T1D are presented by the year they were first implicated in the disease. Those loci reported just as a chromosomal band are for those regions that are either gene deserts or harbor multiple genes from which not a single candidate gene has arisen. Green highlights genes common for T1D, CD & UC; Red-between T1D & UC; Blue-between T1D & CD.

2.2 Inflammatory bowel disease

The two IBD subtypes, Crohn's disease (CD) and ulcerative colitis (UC) collectively referred as Inflammatory bowel disease (IBD), common inflammatory disorders with complex etiology involving multiple genes and environmental factors, are characterized respectively by confluent inflammation of the colonic mucosa (UC) and discontinuous transmural intestinal inflammation (CD). IBD is thought to develop as a result of dysregulation of immune response to normal gut flora in a genetically susceptible host based on our current knowledge of clinical investigations, gene association studies and laboratory experiments. IBD impacts large number of people and is becoming more common in the rest of the world with adoption of Western lifestyle. The prevalence of CD and UC has increased significantly over the last decade with peak age of onset in the second to fourth decades of life (Lashner 1995). CD and UC are considered related disorders that have some shared and some distinct genetic susceptibility loci. IBD being highly heritable has a complex genetic basis as suggested by family, twin, and phenotype concordance studies. When compared to general population, familial aggregation studies have reported a greater relative risk for developing IBD among twins and first-degree relatives of affected individuals. Monozygotic twins compared to dizygotic twins have reported substantially higher disease concordance for both CD and UC (Thompson et al., 1996; Duerr, 2003; Halme et al., 2006)

It had proven difficult before the advent of GWA studies to isolate disease genes that confer susceptibility to CD and UC using classical candidate gene and linkage approaches, with two notable exceptions. 'Caspase recruitment domain family, member 15' (CARD15; also known as NOD2), the first and most widely replicated CD susceptibility gene was positionally cloned using linkage analysis in 2001 (Hugot et al., 2001; Hampe et al., 2001). Linkage studies approach also discovered CD risk haplotype spanning the organic cation transporter, SLC22A4, and other genes on chromosome 5q31 (IBD5) (Rioux et al., 2001; Peltekova et al., 2004). Due to extensive linkage disequilibrium (LD) in the region, the identity of the causative gene and associated variants has been debated (Duerr et al., 2006).

GWAS have yielded many positive associations within CD and UC and other autoimmune diseases. Duerr et al., 2006 reported the first GWA study of IBD and association between CD and variants in the interleukin 23 receptor (IL23R) on chromosome 1p31 in ileal CD cases of European ancestry.

Early-onset IBD demonstrates unique characteristics in clinical phenotype, severity, and familial clustering. Extensive anatomical involvement at presentation, with early disease progression is now clearly established as a feature of both childhoods CD (Vernier-Massouille et al., 2008) and UC (Van Limbergen et al., 2008a). Recent data suggest that stratifying subjects based upon age-of-onset may be effective in identifying genes contributing to IBD pathogenesis, and that individuals with early-onset disease may be more genetically enriched and thereby compensate for the relatively smaller pediatric cohorts (Kugathasan et al., 2008; Imielinski et al., 2009). Recent meta-analysis of published studies is another approach by which several common genetic factors can be identified. A handful of meta-analysis for common susceptibility loci between UC and CD have been performed most notably for NOD, PTPN22, ATG16L1, and IGRM (Barrett et al., 2008; McGovern et al., 2010; Franke et al., 2010; Anderson et al., 2011). GWAS studies to date, combining previously reported pediatric and adult onset IBD studies in a large meta-analysis, have confirmed 99 IBD susceptibility loci: 71 associated with CD, 47 with UC, and 28 with both UC and CD (Lees et al., 2011).

2.3 Comparisons between T1D and IBD

It is becoming apparent that there is cross-talk between genes influencing autoimmune diseases. For instance, it has been shown that the first T1D locus we reported, CLEC16A, has also yielded association to multiple sclerosis in a GWAS of that disease (De Jager et al., 2009) and that PTPN22 has been similarly implicated in Crohn's disease, rheumatoid arthritis, systemic lupus erythematosus and autoimmune thyroiditis (Hafler et al., 2007; Bottini et al., 2006). In addition, from our earlier comparative genetic analyses of inflammatory bowel disease and type 1 diabetes, we have intriguingly implicated multiple loci with opposite effects (Wang et al., 2010).

2.3.1 T1D and IBD (UC and CD) – common genes: IL10, IL2/IL21, ORMDL3, PTPN2, CLEC16A

IL10 (1q32)

The IL10 gene, located in chromosome 1, encodes Interleukin 10, which is an anti-inflammatory cytokine produced primarily by monocytes and lymphocytes. IL10 has pleiotropic effects in immunoregulation and inflammation. Franke et al., 2008 GWAS first reported SNP rs3024505 immediately flanking the IL10 gene in a region 1q32.1 associated

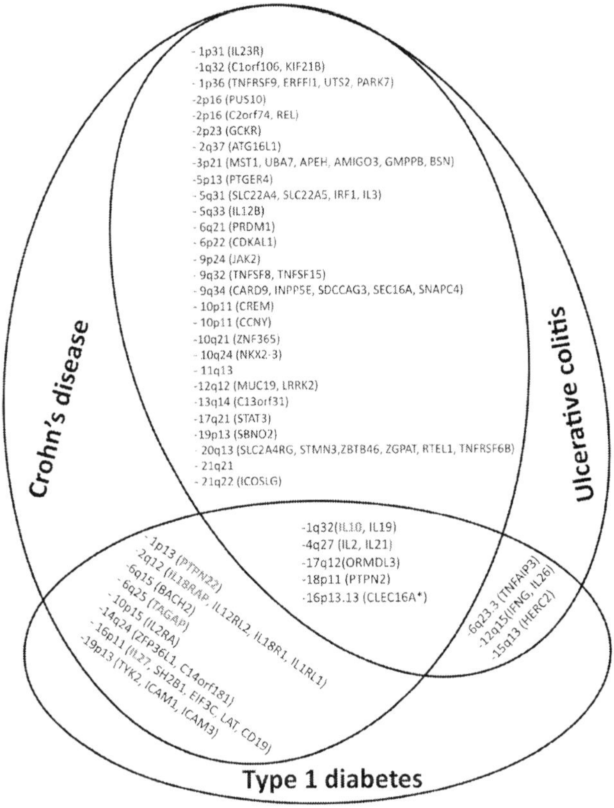

Fig. 2. Venn Diagram of known susceptibility loci that are shared by Crohn's disease, ulcerative colitis and type 1 diabetes. Red represents opposite direction for T1D and IBD: protection in one disease versus susceptibility in another.

with UC. Barrett et al., 2009 meta-analysis study revealed association with T1D. Study from our group (Wang et al., 2010) reported IL10 as novel association for CD with alleles having opposite direction of association between T1D and IBD (including both UC and CD) and the SNP rs3024505 confers protection to UC and CD. Later Franke et al., 2010 meta-analysis study of six Crohn's disease GWAS comprising of 6,333 affected individuals and 15,056 controls and followed up the top association signals in 15,694 cases, 14,026 controls and 414 parent-offspring trios confirmed the association.

IL2/IL21 (4q27)

The IL2 gene and IL21 gene are located on chromosome 4, encode Interleukin 2 and Interleukin 21, respectively. IL2 protein is a secreted cytokine important for the proliferation of T and B lymphocytes. IL2 signals through a receptor complex consisting of IL2 specific IL2 receptor alpha (CD25), IL2 receptor beta (CD122) and a common gamma chain shared by all members of this cytokine family. Binding activates the Ras/MAPK, JAK/Stat and PI

3-kinase/Akt signaling modules. Interleukin 21 is a cytokine with potent regulatory effects on cells of the immune system, including natural killer (NK) cells and cytotoxic T cells that can destroy virally infected or cancerous cells (Parrish-Novak et al., 2002).
GWAS provides evidences for 4q27 region association with a number of autoimmune phenotypes, type 1 diabetes and Graves' disease (GD) (Todd et al., 2007), systemic lupus erythematosus (SLE) (Sawalha et al., 2008), psoriatic arthritis (Liu et al., 2008) and juvenile idiopathic arthritis (Albers et al.,), ulcerative colitis (Festen et al., 2009), Crohn's disease (Marquez et al., 2009a), and celiac disease (Garner et al., 2009). This region contains four genes in strong linkage disequilibrium (LD): KIAA1109-TENR-IL2-IL21. KIAA1109 and ADAD1 (adenosine deaminase domain containing 1 protein with testis specific expression) genes have no known relationship to immune function, while IL2 and IL21 are both of interest, especially because IL2 is a risk gene for T1D in the non-obese diabetic mouse (Yamanouchi et al., 2007). The extensive linkage disequilibrium across the region is preventing fine-mapping efforts (Todd et al., 2007) suggesting resequencing followed by genotyping to identify all the variants with association in KIAA1109-TENR-IL2-IL21 region.

CLEC16A (16p13)

The CLEC16A gene, located on chromosome 16, encodes protein with unknown function. The exclusive expression specificity of CLEC16A in immune cells including dendritic cells, B lymphocytes and natural killer (NK) cells, all of which are pivotal in the pathogenesis of T1D (Poirot et al., 2004; Rodacki et al., 2007) indicates that the variant probably contributes to the disease by modulating immunity. Hakonarson et al., 2007 performed GWAS in a large pediatric cohort of European descent to identify new genetic factors that increase the risk of T1D and found that T1D was significantly associated with variation within a 233-kb linkage disequilibrium block on chromosome 16p13. Three common non-coding variants of the gene (rs2903692, rs725613 and rs17673553) in strong linkage disequilibrium reached genome-wide significance for association with T1D. A subsequent replication study in an independent cohort confirmed the association. There are no other genes in 16p13 region, making CLEC16A (also known as KIAA0350) a prime candidate for harboring the causative variant. We investigated the expression of KIAA0350 in four different NK cell lines and found higher expression in the NKL cell line; interestingly, this cell line is homozygous for allele A of rs2903692. WTCCC 2007 GWAS discovered KIAA0350 as T1D susceptibility locus. Several studies later confirmed the association with T1D (Todd et al., 2007; Cooper et al., 2008), pathogenesis of MS (De Jager et al., 2009) and Celiac disease (Dubois et al., 2010). Recent studies of the novel Drosophila gene, ema (endosomal maturation defective), orthologue of human CLEC16A, have defined roles for the protein in regulating endosomal trafficking (Kim et al., 2010). Such function suggests mechanisms by which CLEC16A may confer susceptibility to autoimmune disorders. In 2009, Marquez et al. concordantly with the already reported function of this locus in T1D and MS, showed the specific association of a CLEC16A/KIAA0350 polymorphism with a distinct group of NOD2-/CARD15 Crohn's disease patients. These new evidence argues in favor of the hypothesis that alterations in genetic factors involved in bacterial recognition through different pathways result in CD, which may allow more insight into processes critical to the pathogenesis of this IBD.

ORMDL3 (17p12)

The ORMDL3 gene, located on chromosome 17, encodes ORM1-like 3 protein of unknown function which is expressed heart, brain, lung liver and kidney. Common SNPs in the chromosome 17q12 region reported by GWAS is known to alter the risk for asthma and also linked with the expression level of the ORM1-like 3 (ORMDL3) gene (Moffat et al., 2007). SNP (rs7216389) was highlighted as the potential causal variant based on evolutionary conservation. Several studies have replicated this association for adult asthma in different ethnic groups (Sleiman et al., 2008; Madoreet et al., 2008; Galanter et al., 2008; Hirota et al., 2008). The rs7216389 SNP is found within a large linkage disequilibrium (LD) block that encompasses not only ORMDL3, but also gasdermin B (GSDMB), zona pellucida binding protein 2 (ZPBP2), and IKAROS family zinc finger 3 (Aiolos) (IKZF3) genes. Another variant (rs2872507) located within this same LD block has been associated with CD (Barrett et al., 2008 GWAS and Franke et al., 2010 meta-analysis), suggesting that the same polymorphism confers susceptibility to both CD and asthma. More recently, the same region was associated with the risk of type 1 diabetes (for SNP rs2290400) (Barrett et al., 2009) and UC (McGovern et al., 2010) for rs2305480. Further elucidation of the genetic mechanisms of transcriptional control of the ORMDL3 genomic region may potentially shed light on the pathogenesis of multiple complex diseases.

PTPN2 (18p11)

The PTPN2 gene, located on chromosome 18, encodes a tyrosine-protein phosphatase nonreceptor type 2, a key negative regulator of inflammatory responses is expressed in cells of the immune system and islet β-cells. Recent studies point out the possible role of PTPN2 in preventing β-cell apoptosis (Moore et al., 2009).

WTCCC 2007 and Barret et al., 2008 identified PTPN2 as CD susceptibility gene. Franke et al., 2008 and Dubois et al., 2010 GWAS associated PTPN2 as previously unknown disease loci for UC. Hakonarson et al., 2007 and Todd et al., 2007 GWAS, Cooper et al., 2008 and Barrett et al., 2009 meta-analysis associated PTPN2 as T1D susceptibility gene. Feston et al., 2011 meta-analysis identified PTPN2 as shared risk loci for Crohn's disease and celiac disease. Of special interest to CD, PTPN2 regulates intestinal epithelial barrier function, thus identifying a novel link between disease associated gene and a key patho-physiological event in CD (Scharl et al., 2009). SNP rs1893217(C), an autoimmune associated variant in PTPN2, reveals an impairment of IL2R signaling in CD4+ T cells (Long et al., 2011). Scharl et al., 2011 demonstrated that PTPN2 is activated by TNF-α and regulates TNF-α-induced MAPK signaling and on a functional level, loss of PTPN2 is associated with increased expression and secretion of proinflammatory mediators in the intestinal epithelium, a potential role for PTPN2 in the pathogenesis of CD.

2.3.2 Type 1 diabetes and Crohn's disease – common genes: PTPN22, IL18RAP, BACH2, TAGAP, IL2RA, IL27, TYK2, MTMR3)

PTPN22 (1p13)

The PTPN22 gene, located in chromosome 1, encodes tyrosine-protein phosphatase nonreceptor type 22, a lymphoid-specific phosphatase, an important downregulator of T cell activation. It is mainly expressed in T cells, B cells, NK cells, macrophages, monocytes, and dendritic cells. Initially PTPN22 polymorphism (C1858T) was associated and originally described in T1D patients (Bottini et al., 2004). This was consistently replicated in independent population's studies (Smyth et al., 2004; Santiago et al., 2007). Later the same polymorphism was associated with several autoimmune disorders, including rheumatoid arthritis (Begovich et al., 2004; Orozco et al., 2005), systemic lupus eritematosus (Orozco et al., 2005), Wegener's granulomatosis (Jagiello et al., 2005) and myasthenia gravis (Vandiedonck et al., 2006). C1858T polymorphism is a non-synonymous SNP with a substitution of arginine for tryptophan in the encoded protein (R620W). Functional studies in mice revealed that LYP (the mouse ortholog of PTPN22) has an increased phosphatase activity in presence of 1858T allele. The 620W autoimmune risk allele behaves as a gain-of-function mutation and results in a phosphatase with higher catalytic activity and more potent negative regulation of T-cell activation (Vang et al., 2005). By contrast, knockout mice have increased T-cell activation and an increased production of antibodies (Hasegawa et al., 2004).

PTPN22 was the first and most convincing example of common susceptibility genes underlying diverse autoimmune phenotypes. First GWAS for T1D reported PTPN22 as a susceptibility locus (Todd et al., 2007; Hakonarson et al., 2007). Later PTPN22 was associated with RA (Plenge et al., 2007, Stahl et al., 2010), Crohn's disease (Barrett et al., 2008), Graves' disease, Hashimoto thyroiditis, myasthenia gravis, systemic sclerosis, generalized vitiligo (Jin et al., 2010). For T1D and RA the 620W allele confers almost two-fold risk for the disease, with 3-4 odds rations for homozygous patients, making PTPN22 second in importance locus (after MHC), in terms of association strength, for these two diseases (Gregerson & Olsson, 2009). Barrett et al., 2008 was first to report "intriguing contrasts between genetic susceptibility to CD and other complex disorders". They found that the same coding variant (620W) that is a risk factor for T1D and RA provides protection from CD. Our group in latest GWAS confirmed both the association for T1D and CD as well as protection for CD (Wang et al., 2010). In summary, the minor allele of PTPN22 variant 620W predisposes a person to many immune-mediated diseases but is protective for Crohn's disease (Barrett et al., 2008; Wang et al., 2010).

IL18RAP (2q12)

The IL18RAP gene, located on chromosome 2, encodes Interleukin 18 receptor accessory protein. IL18RAP is strongly expressed in unstimulated T cells and NK cells (Su et al., 2004). The coexpression of IL18R1 and L18RAP is required for the activation of NF-κB and MAPK8 (JNK) in response to IL18.

IL18RAP is a long confirmed locus for type 1 diabetes. Smyth et al., 2008 genotyped DNA samples from 8064 T1D patients, 9339 control subjects, and 2828 families for eight loci previously known risk loci of celiac disease and reported association of IL18RAP and TAGAP genes with T1D ($P<1.00\times10^{-4}$) and showed that the minor alleles of the SNP rs917997-A for IL18RAP gene confers protection in T1D. Zhernakova et al., 2008 demonstrated strong association of rs917997 SNP for CD. The rs917997 genotype strongly correlates with lower IL18RAP expression in individuals homozygous for the risk allele, which may lead to differential IL18-mediated innate immune responses to infection (Zhernakova et al., 2010). In recent GWAS we confirmed IL18RAP region as T1D and CD loci and reported an opposite direction of association for the same allele residing in IL18RAP gene (rs917997) for T1D and CD (Wang et al., 2010). Meta-analysis studies by Franke et al., 2010 confirmed ones again IL18RAP as CD locus. Festen et al., 2011 meta-analysis study reported allele rs6708413-G residing in IL18RAP as a shared risk locus for CD and Celiac disease, validating previously identified associations.

BACH2 (6q15)

The BACH2 gene 'BTB and CNC homology 1, basic leucine zipper transcription factor 2', located on chromosome 6, encodes a protein which functions as a transcription repressor (Oyake et al., 1996). It possesses BTB/POZ domain and bZip domain. Bach2 forms heterodimers with the small Maf proteins (MafK, MafG and MafF) through the leucine zipper and then binds to the Maf-recognition elements (MARE). BACH2 is abundantly expressed in both B cells and neurons (Hoshino & Igarashi, 2002).

GWAS provided convincing associations of BACH2 with T1D in unrelated data sets (Grant et al., 2009; Cooper et al., 2008; Barrett et al., 2009). A second-generation GWAS of 4,533 celiac disease cases and 10,750 controls revealed rs10806425-A allele as a risk factor for celiac disease (Dubois et al., 2010). Meta analysis confirmed BACH2 as a susceptibility gene for both Celiac disease and CD, with rs1847472-G being a common risk allele (Franke et al., 2010).

TAGAP (6q25)

The TAGAP gene, located on chromosome 6, encodes T-cell activation RhoGTPase-activating protein, associated with multiple autoimmune diseases: T1D, CD, Celiac disease, and RA. With less known role in immune function, it has been found to be co-regulated with IL2 and is expected to play a role in T cell activation (Mao et al., 2004; Chang & Hsiao, 2005).

Smyth et al., 2008 first reported association of TAGAP with T1D ($P<1.00\times10^{-4}$). Recent genotyping study using the Sequenom MassArray platform reported TAGAP (rs182429) as an overlapping genetic susceptibility variant between three autoimmune disorders: RA, T1D and coeliac disease (Eyre et al., 2010). Franke et al., 2010 meta-analysis reported TAGAP association with CD, which was confirmed in another meta-analysis as common allele between CD and CelD (Festen et al., 2011). Interestingly, the TAGAP minor allele confers protection against RA (Eyre et al., 2010), similar to previous reports of T1D (Smyth et al., 2008) but contrasting in CD (Franke et al., 2010; Festen et al., 2011) and celiac disease (Smyth et al., 2008) in which the minor allele is associated with risk.

IL2RA (10p15)

The IL2RA gene, located on chromosome 10, encodes α subunit of the IL2 receptor complex, thus mediating IL2 signaling in host defense and regulating response to autoantigens by Tregs. The imbalance between Th1 and Th2 cytokines plays a crucial role in the regulation of the immune response and in the pathogenesis of autoimmune diseases (Cantagrel et al., 1999; Sartor, 1994). Thus, the genes encoding Th1 and Th2 cytokines and their receptors might be considered good candidates to modify the risk of these diseases.

IL2RA was associated with T1D even before advent of GWAS (Vella et al., 2005). Several GWAS consistently confirmed the association with (WTCCC 2007; Cooper et al., 2008; Barrett et al., 2009). IL2RA was also implicated in MS (Hafler et al., 2007; De Jager et al., 2009), RA (Stahl et al., 2010). Most recently meta-analysis confirmed the association with Crohn's disease (Franke et al., 2010).

ZFP36L1 (14q24)

14q24 is common susceptibility locus shared between T1D and CD. Barrett at al., 2009 meta-analysis first reported rs1465788-G (14q24.1) to be a risk allele for type 1 diabetes; with two genes to be present at this LD region: C14orf181 and ZFP36L1. rs4899260-A in region 14q24.1 was found in GWAS to be a risk allele for Celiac (Dubois et al., 2010). Meta-analysis study associated rs4902642-G in the same region as a risk allele for CD (Franke et al., 2010).

The region contains C14orf181 and ZFP36L1 gene. ZFP36L1 gene is a functionally interesting candidate located on chromosome 14, encodes Zinc finger protein 36 C3H type-like 1, a modulator of mRNA stability.

IL27 (16p11)

The IL27 gene, located on chromosome 16, encodes Interleukin 27, a cytokine secreted by stimulated antigen-presenting cells. IL27 is a member of the same family as IL12 and IL23. Initially it was associated only with the differentiation of TH1 lymphocytes, enhancement of the cellular type immune response, and the reciprocal inhibition of TH2 humoral immune reactions (Lucas et al., 2003). Later it was shown to play an important role in regulating the activity of B & T lymphocytes as well as NK cells (Larousserie et al., 2006). It could be important to pathogenesis of autoimmune diseases, that IL27 promotes cell-mediated immune reactions and limits inflammatory reactions (Jankowski et al., 2010). GWAS revealed association of IL27 with T1D (Barrett et al., 2009) and early onset IBD (Imielinski et al., 2009). In recent GWAS we confirmed IL27 (SNP rs4788084) as T1D locus and reported a new association with Crohn's disease. We also showed that T1D risk allele residing at the IL27 loci protects against CD (Wang et al., 2010). Recent meta-analysis of six CD GWAS confirmed IL27 as susceptibility locus for CD (Franke et al., 2010).

TYK2 (19p13)

The TYK2 gene, located on chromosome 19, encodes tyrosine kinase 2, a member of the JAK-signal transduction family. It is involved in cytokine signaling by IFN-γ, IL12 and IL23 and affects Th1 and Th17 lineage development. TYK2 also plays an important role in TLR-mediated responses in dendritic cells, including IL12 and IL23 production, and TYK2 mutations predispose to opportunistic infection (Ghoreschi et al., 2009). Initially, TYK2 gene has been associated with SLE (Suarez-Gestal et al., 2009) and MS (Mero et al., 2010). Only meta-analysis provided enough power to support at genome-wide significance for TYK2 associations with T1D (Wallace et al., 2010) and CD (Franke et al., 2010).

2.3.3 Type 1 diabetes and ulcerative colitis – common genes: TNFAIP3, IL26, HERC2

TNFAIP3 (6q23)

The TNFAIP3 gene, located on chromosome 6, encodes tumor necrosis factor, alpha-induced protein 3. This protein is a key regulator of NF-κB signaling pathway, modulates cell activation, cytokine signaling and apoptosis (Beyaert et al., 2000). The first association between autoimmune disease and SNPs spanning TNFAIP3 was identified for RA (Plenge et al., 2007). Then TNFAIP3 region was reported as a novel susceptibility locus for SLE (Graham et al., 2008) in Europeans and later it was confirmed in Asian populations (Han et al., 2009; Shimane et al., 2010). Fung et al., 2009 GWAS reported an association with T1D for two statistically independent SNPs rs6920220 and rs1049919. More recently, we tested this T1D loci susceptibility (TNFAIP3) in GWAS and discovered that it confers UC risk (Wang et al., 2010). Dubois et al., 2010 in GWAS reported association with celiac disease. Anderson et al., 2011 meta-analysis confirmed the association of TNFAIP3 as UC risk loci.

IL26 (12q15)

The IL26 (Interleukin 26) gene is located on chromosome 12 between the genes for two other important class 2 cytokines, IFN-γ and IL22 (Wilson et al., 2007). IL26 is a 171-amino acid protein and shares sequence homology to interleukin 10. IL26 signals through a receptor complex comprising two distinct proteins called IL20 receptor 1 and IL10 receptor 2 (Sheikh et al., 2004). First time, rs2870946-G and rs1558744-A in region 12q15 were associated with UC (Silverberg et al., 2009). Meta-analysis study further confirmed the association of rs1558744-A with UC (McGovern et al., 2010). Later GWAS from our group reported new association of rs1558744 variant with T1D (Wang et al., 2010).

HERC2 (15q13)

The HERC2 gene, located on chromosome 15, encodes a novel ubiquitin ligase required for DSB-associated histone ubiquitylation. This gene belongs to the HERC gene family that encodes a group of unusually large proteins with multiple structural domains. The protein has a COOH-terminal HECT domain, a motif responsible for E3 ubiquitin ligase activity. It was recently shown that HERC2 is implicated in DNA damage repair functions (Bekker-Jensen et al., 2010). At first in a GWAS, rs916977 variant in HERC2 was identified and confirmed as susceptibility loci specific to ulcerative colitis (Franke et al., 2008). GWAS from our group later identified rs916977 variant as novel association with T1D (Wang et al., 2010).

2.3.4 Crohn's disease and Ulcerative colitis – 32 common loci

IL23R (1p31)

The interleukin-23 receptor (IL23R) gene is located on chromosome 1p31 encodes receptor protein for IL23. IL23R is highly expressed in dendritic cells. This protein associates constitutively with JAK2, and also binds to transcription activator STAT3 in a ligand-dependent manner. Duerr et al., 2006 GWAS first identified the IL23R gene as a CD susceptibility gene in North American population, which indicated that the rare IL23R SNP rs11209026 (p.Arg381Gln; c.1142G>A) was associated with strong protection against CD. Since then this association has been replicated in both CD (Umeno et al., 2011; Ferguson et al., 2010) and UC (Umeno et al., 2011; Anderson et al., 2011; WatermanM et al., 2010), and also in pediatric CD (Baldassano et al., 2007; Gazouli M et al., 2010), psoriasis (Bowes & Barton, 2010), and ankylosing spondylitis (Laukens et al., 2010) by several GWAS and meta-analysis studies. Of importance, is notably the presence of multiple associations within the IL23R gene to CD and UC to date, suggests rigorous involvement of IL-23 pathway in IBD pathogenesis. These broad range associations might be attributed to the effect of different causal variants on different haplotypes or biological differences in the function of IL-23 and IL-23R signaling in different diseases. Additional genetic, bioinformatic, and laboratory assessments of association signals supplemented by deep resequencing efforts are needed to define more clearly susceptibility genes and contributing susceptibility alleles, especially where the association signals span several candidate genes to identify rare variants contributing to IBD pathophysiology.

KIF21B (1q32)

KIF21B gene, located on chromosome 1 encodes for Kinesin member 21B protein. Kinesin family proteins are microtubule-dependent molecular motors involved in the intracellular motile process and organelle transport. KIF21B expression is detected in lungs, brain, testes and thymus (Harada et al., 2007). In the immune system, expression is highest in $CD4^+$ and $CD8^+$ T cells, CD56bright NK cells and B cells (T1Dbase, http:// www.t1dbase.org/). Of importance, the mouse homologue, Kif21b, is located in a region linked to susceptibility (Idd5.4a) for a mouse model for diabetes (Hunter et al., 2007). SNP rs11584383, located downstream of KIF21B was one among the 21 novel loci reported to be associated with CD in GWAS by Barrett et al., 2008. Several GWAS later identified KIF21B as ulcerative colitis susceptibility loci (Franke et al., 2008; Anderson et al., 2009; McGovern et al., 2010). Recent meta-analysis studies have confirmed and reported it as common susceptibility loci between CD and UC (Anderson et al., 2011 and Umeno et al., 2011).

TNFRSF9, ERFFI1, UTS2, PARK7 (1p36)

The region 1p36 recently shown to be associated with IBD contains several genes. Tumor necrosis factor receptor superfamily, member 9 (TNFRSF9), contributes to the clonal expansion, survival, and development of T cells. ERBB receptor feedback inhibitor 1 (ERFFI1) is negative regulator for several RGFR family members. Urotensin 2 (UTS) is a potent vasoconstrictive peptide that regulates both endothelium-dependent and independent vasodilation. Parkinson disease autosomal recessive early onset 7 (PARK7) is positive regulator of androgen receptor-dependent transcription. Dubois et al., 2010 GWAS reported association of TNFRSF9 and PARK 7 with UC in European population. Anderson et al., 2011 meta-analysis further confirmed the reported association of 1p36.23 region with UC.

PUS10 (2p16)

PUS10 gene, located on chromosome 2, encodes 'pseudouridylate synthase 10' which catalyzes pseudouridination of universally conserved Psi55 in tRNA. These enzymes act as RNA chaperones, facilitating the correct folding and assembly of tRNAs (McCleverty et al., 2007). Barrett et al., 2008 was first to report PUS10 as susceptibility loci for Crohn's disease through GWAS. Meta-analysis study identified as a risk locus in UC (McGovern et al., 2010) and CelD (Dubois et al., 2010) indicating that this locus is a shared risk locus. Recently Festen et al., in 2011, through a meta-analysis of GWAS data from CD and CelD as a single disease phenotype established PUS10, as shared risk loci of genome-wide significance, with p-value of $1.38X10^{-11}$ along-with IL18RAP, PTPN2 and TAGAP, as shared risk loci for Crohn's Disease and Celiac Disease. This meta-analysis approach provided the power, lacking in individual disease-specific GWAS datasets, to identify shared risk loci with small effects in each single disease.

REL (2p16)

The REL gene located on chromosome 2, encodes c-Rel, a transcription factor that is a member of the Rel/NFKB family, which also includes RELA, RELB, NF-κB1/p50, and NF-κB2/p52. All five NF-kB members share a highly conserved 300 amino acid long N-terminal Rel homology domain (RHD), responsible for DNA binding, dimerization, nuclear localization, and binding to the NFKB inhibitor. REL plays a critical role through the production of pro-inflammatory cytokines and coordinating the expression of genes that control immune response, anti-apoptotic molecules and cell cycle modulators (Chen et al., 2003; Hayden et al., 2006; Belguise & Sonenshein, 2007; Tian & Liou 2009). Several studies have reported the effect of c-Rel in relation to autoimmune diseases, ESL (Burgos et al., 2000) and IBD (Neurath et al., 1998, Visekruna et al., 2006). The REL locus is common to UC, CD and RA. Zhernakova et al., 2008 reported moderate association of REL polymorphisms to UC. In 2009 Trynka et al., discovered two new loci, REL and OLIG3/TNFAIP3 to be associated to coeliac disease. Gregersen et al., 2009 described the association of the intronic single nucleotide polymorphism (SNP) rs13031237G→T in the REL gene as a risk factor for RA in an expansion of previous genome-wide association studies. Varade et al., 2011 reported first association of REL gene polymorphism in SLE. Recent GWAS studies reported epistasis between CARD9 and Rel in ulcerative colitis (McGovern et al., 2010) and Crohn's disease (Dubois et al., 2010). Franke et al., 2010 meta-analysis further established the Rel association, increasing the number of CD susceptibility loci to 71.

GCKR (2q23)

GCKR gene located on chromosome 2 encodes, glucokinase (hexokinase 4) regulatory protein belonging to the GCKR subfamily. GCKR is implicated in metabolic traits such as triglyceride (Aulchenko et al., 2009), fasting glucose (Dupuis et al., 2010) and serum uric acid (Kolz et al., 2009). Franke et al., 2010 meta-analysis first reported the association of GCKR as Crohn's disease susceptibility loci. Meta analysis study published by Umeno et al., 2011 confirmed the association of GCKR never had been shown associated with UC in any single studies performed to date. However, there is little information how this gene affects the development of CD and UC. Functional analysis will provide further understanding of the common pathogenesis of CD and UC.

ATG16L1 (2q37)

ATG16L1 gene, located on chromosome 2, encodes the autophagy-related 16-like 1 protein involved in the formation of autophagosomes during autophagy. Hampe et al., 2007 GWAS first identified ATG16L1 as a susceptibility gene for CD and demonstrated the expression of mRNA and protein in the colon, small intestine, intestinal epithelial cells and leukocytes with no difference in protein expression in intestinal tissues between CD and healthy controls. In constrast, Lees et al., 2008 demonstrated down-regulated ATG16L1 mRNA in colonic CD biopsies compared with healthy controls in microarray dataset. Analysis further confirmed the marker, rs2241880, was an SNP that encodes a threonine to alanine substitution (T300A) at amino acid position 300 which was correlated with the incidence of CD in two German and one British studies (Rioux et al., 2007). Prescott et al., 2007 reported a non-synonymous SNP in ATG16L1 predisposes to ileal Crohn's disease independent of CARD15 and IBD5. Roberts et al., 2007 reported strong association of IL23R, R381Q and ATG16L1 T300A with CD in a study of New Zealand Caucasians with IBD. Glas et al., 2008 reported strong association of ATG16L1 gene variants rs2241879 and rs2241880 (T300A) to CD in German population. Weersma et al., 2009 confirmed the genetic association of ATG16L1 along-with multiple CD susceptibility loci in a large Dutch-Belgian cohort. In addition, a number of studies included child-onset IBD cases, the results of which were also confusing and conflicting. Baldassano et al., 2007 reported association of the T300A non-synonymous variant of the ATG16L1 gene with susceptibility to pediatric Crohn's disease. Subsequently Van Limbergen et al., 2008b, reported ATG16L1 gene influences susceptibility and disease location but not childhood onset in Crohn's disease in Northern Europe population. The study by Latiano et al., 2008 confirmed the association ATG16L1 with CD, in both adult and pediatric-onset subsets. A meta-analysis in Spanish population by Marquez et al., 2009a reported Thr300Ala polymorphism association with CD, regardless of the CARD15 or IL23R status, but not with UC. The meta-analysis by Cheng et al., 2010 reported ATG16L1 T300A polymorphism with susceptibility to both CD and UC. Recent study by Platinga et al., 2011 demonstrates that the genetic variant of human ATG16L1, which confers a higher risk for CD is associated with elevated production of pro-inflammatory cytokines after engagement of NOD2, thereby provide an explanation for the excessive inflammatory response observed in CD caused by microorganisms that reside in the gut. These findings implicate the role of autophagy and intestinal microbes in the pathogenesis of IBD, and demonstrate the need for further studies.

MST1, UBA7, APEH, AMIGO3, GMPPB, BSN (3p21)

Raelson et al., 2007 GWAS first reported association of 3p21 SNP rs11718165 with CD. GWAS undertaken by the WTCCC 2007 reported different SNP rs9858542 associated with CD in Spanish population. Several studies have reported association with UC also (Fisher et al., 2008, Franke et al., 2008, & Anderson et al., 2011 meta-analysis). Marquez et al., 2009c reported two SNPs significantly associated with CD. Beckly et al., 2008 demonstrated strong epistasis with known CD associated variants in CARD15. Latiano et al., 2010 confirmed the association of variants (BSN and MST1) at the 3p21 locus influence susceptibility and phenotype both in adults and early-onset patients with IBD. Morgan et al., 2010 replicated the reported association in the 3p21 region with CD in New Zealand population. Meta-analysis by Umeno et al., 2011 confirmed the association of BSN-MST as common susceptibility loci between UC and CD. Designated as IBD9, 3p21 potentially is an important IBD locus, previously identified by early genome-wide linkage and fine mapping studies. This region contains CD candidate genes like MST1, UBA7, APEH, AMIGO3, GMPPB, and BSN. MST1, macrophage stimulatory protein 1, is involved in inflammation and tissue remodeling for wound healing. Goyette et al., 2008 first identified a non-synonymous coding variant (rs3197999, R689C) in MST1 gene associated with both CD and UC. APEH encodes a serine peptidase with a functional role in the degradation of bacterial peptide break down products in the gut to prevent excessive immune response. Amphoterin-Induced Gene and ORF 3 (AMIGO3), member of the AMIGO family of type I transmembrane proteins are thought to play roles in neuronal axon tract development and cell adhesion. Ubiquitin-like modifier-activating enzyme 7 protein in humans is encoded by the UBA7 gene. GPX1 encodes the antioxidant, glutathione peroxidase isoform 1. The BSN (bassoon) gene encodes a protein known neurotransmitter released at central nervous system synapses. Recent GWAS have provided evidence for the involvement of 3p21 in the pathogenesis of IBD, although it remains unclear which is the causative SNP and/or gene.

PTGER4 (5p13)

Prostaglandin E receptor 4 protein encoded by PTGER4 gene located on chromosome 5 belongs to the G-protein coupled receptor family and is one of four receptors identified for prostaglandin E2 (PGE2) that can activate T-cell factor signaling, mediates PGE2 induced expression of early growth response 1 (EGR1), regulates the level and stability of cyclooxygenase-2 mRNA, and lead to the phosphorylation of glycogen synthase kinase-3. Libioulle et al., 2007 first described the localization of PTGER4 as novel major susceptibility locus for CD to gene desert on 5p13.1 by GWA in Belgian cohort. Kurz et al., 2006 previously reported PTGER4 as asthma susceptibility loci through fine mapping and positional candidate studies on chromosome 5p13. PTGER4 is a strong candidate susceptibility gene for CD as PTGER4 knock-out mice have increased susceptibility to dextran sodium induced colitis (Kabashima et al., 2002), further supported by the observation that the CD susceptibility allele at marker rs4495224 was associated with increased PTGER4 transcript levels in lymphoblastoid cell lines. The association of PTGER4 as susceptibility loci for Crohn's disease was further replicated through independent GWAS (Barrett et al., 2008; Franke et al., 2010).

SLC22A4/SLC22A5/IRF1/IL3 (5q31)

The candidate genes encompassed at locus 5q31.1 includes a cytokine gene cluster (IL5, IL4, IL13), interferon regulator factor 1(IRF1), SLC22A4 (solute carrier family 22 member 4) and SLC22A5 (solute carrier family 22 member 5). SLC22A5 and SLC22A4 are high affinity sodium-dependent uptake transporters that function in the transport of L-carnitine and elimination of cationic drugs in the intestine. The locus 5q31 known as IBD5 was first associated with CD in genome-wide linkage scan in Canadian families (Rioux et al., 2001). Two pediatric studies reported in white populations confirmed an association of the SLC22A variants with CD (Babusukumar et al., 2006; Russell et al., 2006). Studies have also demonstrated IBD5 epitasis with NOD2/CARD15 for both CD and UC (Giallourakis et al., 2003; McGovern et al., 2003). First GWAS WTCCC 2007, confirmed the association of this locus with CD, followed by Raelson et al., 2007, Hampe et al., 2007, Franke et al., 2007. Furthermore, a meta-analysis by Barrett et al., 2008 pointed out another SNP, rs2188962, as the strongest disease-associated variant within IBD5. Besides CD, the TC haplotype has also been suggested to confer risk for UC (Waller et al., 2006; Palmieri et al., 2006). Preliminary data have also implicated this region associated to type I diabetes (Santiago et al., 2006). Although many studies have associated the region of chromosome 5, which contains SLC22A4 and SLC22A5 with CD, some investigators are hesitant to identify the mutations in these genes as causative of CD because of the tight linkage disequilibrium that exists between multiple genes in this chromosomal region. Hradsky et al., 2010 study on IBD5 confirmed the association of the IBD5 risk haplotype and showed prominent role of the rs6596075 and IGR2063b_1 in the Czech population. Franke et al., 2010 meta-analysis further confirmed the association with CD.

IL12B (5q33)

IL12B encodes the p40 subunit of the heterodimeric cytokines interleukin IL12 and IL23 (Langrish et al., 2004) produced by monocytes and dendritic cells. Association with CD was previously reported (WTCCC 2007) but not confirmed. The key role of the IL12/IL23 pathway in chronic intestinal inflammation is supported by the association between IL23R and CD3 and strong functional evidence from mouse models of colitis (Uhlig et al., 2006; Yen et al., 2006). Later polymorphisms at IL12B have been associated with both CD (Parkes et al., 2007; Barrett et al., 2008; McGovern et al., 2010) and UC in several GWAS (Franke et al., 2008; Fisher et al., 2008). Anderson et al., 2011 meta-analysis further confirmed the association with CD and UC. This gene also has been implicated in T1D susceptibility with inconsistent results (Howson et al., 2009). Recently, Ferguson et al., 2010 reported differential effect of two IL12B (rs1363670 and rs6887695) variants in New Zealand population (carrying the rs1363670 C variant increased CD risk while carrying the rs6887695 C variant decreased CD risk). Recent meta-analysies by Anderson et al., 2011 & Umeno et al., 2011 further confirmed the association of JAK2 with both UC and CD.

PRDM1 (6q21)

PRDM1 encodes for PR domain containing 1, with ZNF domain (also known as BLIMP1) protein known to play important roles in the proliferation, survival and differentiation of B and T lymphocytes. BLIMP-1 acts as master transcriptional regulator of plasma cells and repressor of beta-interferon (β-IFN) gene expression. Anderson et al., 2011 meta-analysis first reported and Umeno et al., 2011 meta-analysis further confirmed the association of PRDM1 with ulcerative colitis and Crohn's disease.

CDKAL1 (6p22)

CDKAL1 gene encodes CDK5 regulatory subunit associated protein 1-like 1 with unknown function which belongs to methyl-thiotransferase family. Variants in the intronic block of CDKAL1 have been associated with Crohn's disease (Barrett et al., 2008 GWAS) and T2D

(Zeggini et al., 2008). CDKAL1 shows inconsistent replication in ulcerative colitis (McGovern et al., 2010 GWAS and Anderson et al., 2008 GWAS), this gene is also associated with psoriasis but does not exhibit genome-wide significance (Quaranta et al., 2009).

JAK2 (9p24)

Janus kinase 2 (JAK2) is another common member of the IL23 pathway genes conferring susceptibility to IBD. Barrett et al., 2008 meta-analysis of GWAS first reported the association of polymorphism in the JAK2 promoter region with CD. Later, several studies reported association with UC (Fisher et al., 2008; Franke et al., 2008; Asano et al., 2009; Festen et al., 2009). McGovern et al., 2010 confirmed strong association of SNP rs10974944 in the JAK2 locus with UC in Dutch opulation. Franke et al., 2010 meta-analysis confirmed association with CD. Recent meta-analysis by Anderson et al., 2011 & Umeno et al., 2011 further confirmed the association of JAK2 with both UC and CD. JAK2 gene locus is currently the subject of detailed re-sequencing efforts and functional studies to identify the causal variants.

TNFSF15 (9q32)

TNFSF15 (tumor necrosis factor ligand superfamily, member 15) was identified as the first CD-susceptibility gene through a genome-wide association screening of 72738 SNPs in Japanese population (Yamazaki et al., 2005). The association has been well replicated by several studies; study in a Korean cohort (Yang et al., 2008), an independent Japanese cohort (Kakuta et al., 2006) and a US cohort (Picornell et al., 2007) and meta-analyses of GWAS in European populations (Barrett et al., 2008) although the association was less significant in Europeans than in Japanese or Korean individuals. Yang et al., 2008 replicated findings from studies on Caucasian populations and established TNFSF15 as CD susceptibility genes on Korean patients. However, the reports of TNFSF15 association with UC in Caucasians have been inconsistent (Franke et al., 2008; Wang et al., 2010; Haritunians et al., 2010). In contrast to his own previous finding, Yang et al., 2011 reported no association between TNFSF15 and IL23R with UC in Koreans. However, TNFSF15 showed a marginal association with UC in male patients only.

CARD9 (9q34)

CARD9 gene located on 9q34.3 encodes caspase recruitment domain family, member 9 protein, an adaptor molecule of PRR signaling. CARD9 is essential in the process of stimulating the innate immune signaling by intracellular and extracellular pathogens thus is an attractive candidate gene for IBD association (Underhill & Shimada, 2007). Zhernakova et al., 2008 performed a comprehensive analysis of candidate genes from 85 genes in the innate-immunity molecular pathway, in a group of 1851 IBD patients and 1936 controls, and observed association of the CARD9 variant, located in extended haploblock on 9q34.3, predominantly with UC and confirmed replication in the WTCCC GWAS data set. Later Barrett et al., 2009 GWAS study of UC confirmed CARD9 susceptibility. In 2010 McGovern et al., reported epistasis between CARD9 and Rel in Ulcerative colitis. Franke et al., 2010 also confirmed the association of CARD9 in UC and IBD.

CREM (10p11)

The cyclic adenosine 5'-monophosphate responsive element modulator (CREM) protein in humans encoded by the CREM gene binds to the IL2 gene promoter and suppresses expression of this cytokine (Tenbrock et al., 2002), critical for the initiation and termination of the immune response and T cell development. Meta-analysis studies by McGovern et al., 2010 confirmed the association of CREM with UC. Anderson et al., 2011 meta-analysis reported association with UC and CD. Recent meta-analysis study by Umeno et al., 2011 confirmed the association of CREM with UC.

CCNY (10p11)

Cyclin Y (CCNY) belongs to family of highly conserved proteins that activate cyclin-dependent kinases (Cdks) to regulate the cell cycle, transcription, and other cellular processes. Cyclin Y has not been characterized in any model organism. Very less is known for the human ortholog, CCNY. Franke et al., 2008 GWAS first reported association of SNP located in an intron of CCNY with the two IBD sub-phenotypes, CD and UC. Weersma et al., 2009 confirmed the association of CCNY as CD susceptibility loci in Dutch-Belgian cohort; though it is not yet clear whether CCNY plays a direct role in these diseases. Later the association of CCNY with UC and CD was confirmed in independent GWAS (Wang et al., 2010 and Waterman et al., 2010) and meta-analysis study by Umeno et al., 2011. First mutant allele reported for a Y-type cyclin, a null for Drosophila CycY generated by Liu & Finley, 2010 will provide further insight for the role of this conserved protein in human diseases.

ZNF365 (10q21)

Rioux et al., 2007 reported the first CD association with rs224136, a SNP ~40kb downstream from Zinc finger 365 (ZNF365). GWAS performed in populations of Northern European descent by WTCCC, 2007 and Barett et al., 2008 GWAS further confirmed the CD susceptibility. Torkvist et al., 2010 reported ZNF365 in analysis of 39 CD risk loci in Swedish inflammatory bowel disease patients. Amre et al., 2010 reported ZNF365 as susceptibility loci for CD in Canadian children. ZNF365 exists as four known transcript variants with variable expression across the species (ZNF365 isoforms A-D; GenBank NM_014951, NM_199450, NM_199451 and NM_199452). Of interest, studies in human colorectal cell lines showing interaction with histone acetyltransferase p300 during butyrate activation of the cyclin-dependent kinase inhibitor, p21waf1, a protein with increased levels in colonic crypts of patients with ulcerative colitis (Hofseth et al., 2003) and mice demonstrating dextran sulfate sodium-induced colitis homozygous for ZNF148-delN, highlight role for ZNF148 in gastrointestinal homoeostasis (Law et al., 2006). Haritunians et al., 2011 reported association of variant in ZNF365 isoform-D with CD. This study also demonstrated expression of ZNF365D in intestinal resections from both CD subjects and controls, markedly reduced expression levels of ZNF365D in EpsteineBarr virus-transformed lymphoblastoid cell lines from CD subjects homozygous for the risk allele (Ala), association of ZNF365D rs7076156 genotype and altered expression of ZNF148 (transcription factor) known to be involved in gut homeostatsis. Umeno et al., 2011, meta- analysis study further confirmed the association of ZNF365 as common susceptibility loci for Chron's disease and ulcerative colitis.

NKX2-3 (10q24)

NK2 transcription factor related, locus 3 (NKX2-3) is a member of the NKX family of homeodomain-containing transcription factors encoded by NKX2-3 gene is implicated in many aspects of cell type specification and maintenance of differentiated tissue functions. The rs10883365 variant of NKX2-3 gene on chromosome 10q24.2 was first identified as a CD susceptibility gene in the WTCCC 2007 GWAS in Caucasian patients. Parkes et al., 2007 reported association of SNP rs10883365 (P_{comb}=3.7 × 10^{-10}), within the NKX2-3 gene loci contributing to CD. In addition, Fisher et al., 2008 reported a modest association ($P = 3.3 \times 10^{-4}$ in the UC panel and $P = 2.4 \times 10^{-6}$ using the expanded WTCCC control panel) between rs10883365 and UC in a non-synonymous SNP scan. Franke et al., 2008 GWAS reported NKX2-3 previously unknown disease loci for UC from studies of CD. Further confirmed association between CD and UC came from Barrett et al., 2008 and Franke et al., 2010 GWAS. Replication studies from Netherlands (Weersma et al., 2009) and Japan (Yamazaki et al., 2009) further confirmed the association with CD. Dutch study demonstrated that the association between the rs10883365 variant of NKX2-3 and CD was linked to smoking status, with the risk being more pronounced in active and passive smokers (Van der Heide et al., 2010). Recently, Meggyesi et al., 2010 confirmed that rs10883365 variant was associated with UC and CD susceptibility in the allelic and genotypic models with an OR of 1.53 and 1.24 respectively in Eastern European patients.

LRRK2-MUC19 (12q12)

Leucine-rich repeat kinase 2 (LRRK2), also known as dardarin, member of leucine-rich repeat kinase family is an enzyme, in humans is encoded by LRRK2 gene. The protein is mainly expressed in the cytoplasm of neurons, myeloid cells and monocytes and is thought to be involved in the process of autophagy. LRRK2 was initially identified as the defective gene at PARK8 susceptibilty locus responsible for autosomal Parkinson's disease (PD). The meta-analysis of GWAS by Barrett et al., 2008 identified LRRK2-MUC19 as CD susceptibility loci. Franke et al., 2010 GWAS further confirmed the association with CD. However, Phillips et al., 2010 haplotype-tagging study of germline variation of MUC19 in inflammatory bowel disease suggested that LRRK2 represents the susceptibility gene at this region. Recently, meta-analysis of published studies by Umeno et al., 2011, reported LRR2-MUC19 as common susceptibility loci for CD and UC. With no known physiological substrate the role of LRRK2 in cellular context remains poorly understood. Zhang et al., 2009, GWAS reported association of an SNP located upstream from the LRRK2 locus with a higher susceptibility to Mycobacterium leprae. The study also highlighted other genes already known to be associated with CD, such as NOD2, TNFS15, and C13ORF31, suggesting that the pathways involved in the control of M. leprae might be also involved in the susceptibility to CD. Gardet et al., 2010 reported that LRRK2 is an IFN-γ target gene with increased expression in intestinal tissues upon CD inflammation, suggesting involvement in signaling pathways relevant to CD. Another member, MUC19, along-with LRRK2 is an important player in the rapidly evolving story of IBD. MUC19 encodes a mucin involved in epithelial cell lining protection (Hollingsworth & Swanson, 2004). Of interest, Mucin proteins protect the intestinal epithelium from injury are further supported by the fact that mucin deficiency leads to intestinal inflammation in mouse models of colitis (Van der Sluis et al., 2006). Meta-analysis by Umeno et al., 2011 reported LRRK2-MUC19 as novel susceptibility loci for CD and UC.

C13orf31 (13q14)

C13orf31 gene encoding chromosome 13 open reading frame 31 was first associated with leprosy in GWAS (Zhang et al., 2009). Meta-analysis by Anderson et al., 2011 reported C13orf31 as newly confirmed UC risk loci. Meta-analysis by Umeno et al., 2011 reported it as common susceptibility loci for both CD and UC.

STAT3 (17q21)

STAT3 codes for a transcription factor that is involved in multiple pathways and functions, including Jak-STAT pathway, neuron axonal guidance, apoptosis, activation of immune responses, and Th17 cell differentiation (Egwuagu, 2009). SNP (rs744166) within the STAT3 gene was associated to MS. Interestingly, the A allele of rs744166 tagging the MS-protective haplotype is associated with Crohn disease (Barrett et al., 2008 GWAS) and mutations in STAT3 are known to cause hyperimmunoglobulin E recurrent infection syndrome (HIES) (Holland et al., 2007), a rare autosomal-dominant disorder characterized by elevated immunoglobulin E levels and inflammation implying that STAT3 represents a shared risk locus for at least two autoimmune diseases. STAT3 was reported as T1D susceptibility locus by Fung et al., 2009, but it was not confirmed by other GWAS and meta-analysis studies. Recent meta-analyses by Anderson et al., 2011 and Umeno et al., 2011 confirmed the association with UC and CD.

SBNO2 (19p13)

Strawberry notch homologue 2 (SBNO2) gene located on chromosome 19 encodes for large 170-kDa proteins containing canonical DExD/H helicase domains. SBNO2 is key component of the IL-10 mediated anti-inflammatory pathway (Kasmi et al., 2007). Recent meta-analysis by Umeno et al., 2011 identified SBNO2 as novel common susceptibility loci for CD and UC.

TNFRSF6B, STMN3, RTEL1, ARFRP1, ZGPAT, SLC2A4RG, ZBTB46 (20q13)

The 20q13 signal resides in a complex telomeric region of LD and harbors the genes for STMN3 (stathmin-like 3), RTEL1 (regulator of telomere elongation helicase 1), TNFRSF6B (tumor necrosis factor receptor superfamily member 6B), ARFRP1 (ADP-ribosylation factor related protein 1), ZGPAT (zinc finger CCCH-type with G patch domain), LIME1 (Lck interacting transmembrane adaptor 1), SLC2A4RG (solute carrier family 2 member 4 regulator) and ZBTB46 (zinc finger and BTB domain containing 46). These loci contribute to both CD and UC susceptibility. The protein product for TNFRSF6B acts as a decoy receptor (DCR3) in preventing FasL-induced cell death, and a resistance to FasL-dependent apoptosis. Kugathasan et al., 2008 GWAS in a cohort of 1011 individuals using stratification of IBD by age of onset and 4250 matched controls identified previously unreported susceptibility loci for pediatric-onset IBD at 20q13 and 21q22. On the basis of the differences in serum DCR3 concentration between individuals with IBD with and without the identified SNPs, and its known biologic function, this study highlights TNFRSF6B as the most plausible candidate within the 20q13 locus.

ICOSLG (21q22)

Inducible costimulator-ligand (ICOS-L) is a member of the B7 family of costimulatory ligands (Coyle & Gutierrez-Ramos, 2001), shares 19–20% sequence identity with CD80 and CD86. ICOS-L binds to ICOS, a T cell-specific costimulatory molecule homologous to CD28 and CTLA-4. ICOSLG is intimately involved in proliferation and differentiation of T lymphocytes (Ito et al., 2007). Barrett et al., 2008 GWAS study first confirmed the association of ICOSLG with CD. The locus on chromosome 21q22 harboring genes including inducible T cell costimulator (ICOSLG) along-with autoimmune regulator (AIRE) and periodic tryptophan protein 2 homologue (PWP2) has been shown to influence susceptibility to both adult and pediatric CD and ulcerative colitis (UC). Imielinski et al., 2009 reported ICOSLG among the common variants at five new loci associated with early-onset inflammatory bowel disease. Franke et al., 2010 meta-analysis study further confirmed association with CD. Coquerelle et al., 2009 demonstrated that the treatment of trinitrobenzene sulfonic acid-induced murine colitis was ameliorated by anti-CTLA-4 antibodies through the induction of $ICOS^{high}$ T regulatory cells. Sato et al., 2004 demonstrated high expression of ICOS in activated CD4+ LPMC of IBD patients contributing to the dysregulated immune responses in IBD suggesting a role for the ICOS-ICOSLG interaction in CD pathogenesis. Henderson et al., 2011 using a genome wide haplotype tagging approach in first family-based association analysis strategy reported that variation in ICOSLG influences CD susceptibility and demonstrated that the signal at the 21q22 locus is most likely to be due to germline variation at the 3 end begging for deep sequencing of the 3'UTR of the gene to identify causative variants.

3. Conclusions

This chapter gives an overview of comparative genetic analyses for type 1 diabetes and inflammatory bowel disease. Genome wide association studies have revolutionized the field of complex disease genetics. For the first time there is real consensus on the role of specific genetic factors underpinning common disorders. However, such genome wide scans can lack coverage in certain regions where it is difficult to genotype so it is possible that other loci with reasonable effect sizes remain to be uncovered.

It is clear that larger sample sizes and bigger meta-analyses of GWAS datasets will lead to the uncovering of further loci, albeit with lower and lower effect sizes. However it has been predicted that there are a myriad of rare variants (possibly with larger effects) contributing to disease that cannot be detected on current genotyping platforms. To uncover the remaining "missing heritability" in complex diseases like T1D and IBD (Manolio et al., 2009), investigators in the near future will need to work on large, high-throughput sequencing efforts involving thousands of DNA samples from affected subjects and a similar number of controls.

Novel genomic techniques, such as Next-Generation DNA Sequencing (NGS), have opened new avenues in the elucidation of genetic defects and had speeded up the identification of causative gene variants to systematically tackle previously intractable genetic disorders which would be missed by GWAS. NGS involves the use of three specific techniques: DNA capture of specific regions (usually GWAS guided) usually in the 1-10 megabase range; exomic sequencing (the sequence of all coding regions of the genome), with capture of about 50 megabases; and the sequencing of entire human genome (~3 billion base pairs), in affected and unaffected individuals. Recent studies have used this approach to identify mutations for Miller syndrome (Roach et al., 2010) and Charcot-Marie-Tooth disease (Lupski et al., 2010). Although powerful, NGS is still very expensive and time consuming. However in future, with drop in costs of whole genome sequencing, it will likely become the dominant method for identifying mutations.

Recent GWAS have showed cross-talk of genes and autoimmune diseases. We report 16 common loci between T1D and IBD, six with opposite effects. As predicted, the role of some of the overlapping genes is not always the same for T1D, UC and CD. Thus, to discover all common, opposing and different variants for autoimmune disorders sequencing is necessary.

4. Acknowledgment

This research was financially supported by grant from National Institute of Health (DP3 DK085708-01) and an Institute Development Award to the Center for Applied Genomics from the Children's Hospital of Philadelphia.

5. References

Albers, H.; Kurreeman, F.; Stoeken-Rijsbergen, G.; Brinkman D.; Kamphuis, S. & Schilham M. (2009). Association of the autoimmunity locus 4q27 with juvenile idiopathic arthritis. *Arthritis Rheum.*, Vol.60, No.3, (March 2009), pp. 901-904.

Altshuler, D.; Daly, M. & Lander, E. (2008). Genetic mapping in human disease. *Science*, Vol.322, No.5903, (November 2008), pp. 881-888.

Amre, D.; Mack, D.; Morgan, K.; Israel, D.; Deslandres, C. & Levy, E. (2010). Susceptibility loci reported in genome-wide association studies are associated with Crohn's disease in Canadian children. *Aliment Pharmacol Ther.*, Vol.31, No.11, (June 2010), pp. 1186-91.

Anderson, C.; Massey, D.; Barrett, J.; Prescott, N.; Tremelling, M. & Parkes, M. (2009). Investigation of Crohn's disease risk loci in ulcerative colitis further defines their molecular relationship. *Gastroenterology*, Vol.136, No.2, (February 2009), pp. 523-9.

Anderson, C.; Boucher, G.; Lees, C.; Franke, A.; D'Amato, M. & Rioux JD. (2011). Meta-analysis identifies 29 additional ulcerative colitis risk loci, increasing the number of confirmed associations to 47. *Nat Genet.*, Vol.43, No.3, (March 2011), pp. 246-52.

Anjos, S.; Tessier, M. & Polychronakos, C. (2004). Association of the cytotoxic T lymphocyte-associated antigen 4 gene with type 1 diabetes: evidence for independent effects of two polymorphisms on the same haplotype block. *J Clin Endocrinol Metab.*, Vol.89, No.12, (December 2004), pp. 6257-65.

Asano, K.; Matsushita, T.; Umeno, J.; Hosono, N.; Takahashi, A. & Kubo M. (2009). A genome-wide association study identifies three new susceptibility loci for ulcerative colitis in the Japanese population. *Nat Genet.*, Vol.41, No.12, (December 2009), pp. 1325-9.

Aulchenko, Y.; Ripatti, S.; Lindqvist, I.; Boomsma, D.; Heid, I. & ENGAGE Consortium. (2009). Loci influencing lipid levels and coronary heart disease risk in 16 European population cohorts. *Nat Genet.*, Vol.41, No.1, (January 2009), pp. 47-55.

Babusukumar, U.; Wang, T.; McGuire, E.; Broeckel, U. & Kugathasan, S. (2006). Contribution of OCTN variants within the IBD5 locus to pediatric onset Crohn's disease. *Am J Gastroenterol.*, Vol.101, No.6, (June 2006), pp. 1354-61.

Baldassano, R.; Bradfield, J.; Monos, D.; Kim, C.; Glessner, J. & Hakonarson, H. (2007). Association of the T300A non-synonymous variant of the ATG16L1 gene with susceptibility to paediatric Crohn's disease. *Gut*, Vol.56, No.8, (August 2007), pp. 1171-3.

Barrett, J.; Hansoul, S.; Nicolae, D.; Cho, J.; Duerr, R. & Daly, M. (2008). Genome-wide association defines more than 30 distinct susceptibility loci for Crohn's disease. *Nat Genet.*, Vol.40, No.8, (August 2008), pp. 955-62.

Barrett, J.; Clayton, D.; Concannon, P.; Akolkar, B.; Cooper, J. & Rich, S. (2009). Genome-wide association study and meta-analysis find that over 40 loci affect risk of type 1 diabetes. Type 1 Diabetes Genetics Consortium. *Nat Genet.*, Vol.41, No.6, (June 2009), pp. 703-7.

Beckly, J.; Hancock, L.; Geremia, A.; Cummings, J.; Morris, A. & Jewell, D. (2008). Two-stage candidate gene study of chromosome 3p demonstrates an association between nonsynonymous variants in the MST1R gene and Crohn's disease. *Inflamm Bowel Dis.*, Vol.14, No.4, (April 2008), pp. 500-7.

Begovich, A.; Carlton, V.; Honigberg, L.; Schrodi, S.; Chokkalingam, A. & Gregersen, P. (2004). A missense single-nucleotide polymorphism in a gene encoding a protein tyrosine phosphatase (PTPN22) is associated with rheumatoid arthritis. *Am J Hum Genet.*, Vol.75, No.2, (August 2004), pp. 330-7.

Bekker-Jensen, S.; Rendtlew Danielsen, J.; Fugger, K.; Gromova, I.; Nerstedt, A. & Mailand, N.(2010). HERC2 coordinates ubiquitin-dependent assembly of DNA repair factors on damaged chromosomes. *Nat Cell Biol.*, Vol.12, No.1, (January 2010), pp. 80-6.

Belguise, K. & Sonenshein, G. (2007). PKCtheta promotes c-Rel-driven mammary tumorigenesis in mice and humans by repressing estrogen receptor alpha synthesis. *J Clin Invest.*, Vol.117, No.12, (December 2007), pp. 4009-21.

Bell, G.; Horita, S. & Karam, J. (1984). A polymorphic locus near the human insulin gene is associated with insulin-dependent diabetes mellitus. *Diabetes,* Vol.33, No.2, (February 1984), pp. 176-83.

Bennett, S.; Lucassen, A.; Gough, S.; Powell, E.; Undlien, D. & Todd, J. (1995). Susceptibility to human type 1 diabetes at IDDM2 is determined by tandem repeat variation at the insulin gene minisatellite locus. *Nature genetics,* Vol.9, No.3, (March 1995), pp. 284-92.

Beyaert, R.; Heyninck, K. & Van Huffel, S. (2000). A20 and A20-binding proteins as cellular inhibitors of nuclear factor-kappa B-dependent gene expression and apoptosis. *Biochem Pharmacol.,* Vol.60, No.8, (October 2000), pp. 1143-51.

Biason-Lauber, A.; Boehm, B.; Lang-Muritano, M.; Gauthier, B.; Brun, T. & Schoenle, EJ. (2005). Association of childhood type 1 diabetes mellitus with a variant of PAX4: possible link to beta cell regenerative capacity. *Diabetologia,* Vol.48, No.5, (May 2005), pp. 900-5.

Bottini, N.; Musumeci, L.; Alonso, A.; Rahmouni, S.; Nika, K. & Mustelin, T. (2004). A functional variant of lymphoid tyrosine phosphatase is associated with type I diabetes. *Nat Genet.*, Vol.36, No.4, (April 2004), pp. 337-8.

Bottini, N.; Vang, T.; Cucca, F. & Mustelin, T. (2006). Role of PTPN22 in type 1 diabetes and other autoimmune diseases. *Semin Immunol.,* Vol.18, No.4, (August 2006), pp. 207-13.

Bowes, J. & Barton, A. (2010). The genetics of psoriatic arthritis: lessons from genome-wide association studies. *Discov Med.*, Vol.10, No.52, (September 2010), pp. 177-83.

Bradfield, J.; Qu, H.; Wang, K.; Zhang, H.; Sleiman, P. & Hakonarson, H. (2011). A genome-wide meta-analysis of six type 1 diabetes cohorts identifies multiple associated loci. *PLoS Genet. In press.*

Burgos, P.; Metz, C.; Bull, P.; Pincheira, R.; Massardo, L. & González, A. (2000). Increased expression of c-rel, from the NF-kappaB/Rel family, in T cells from patients with systemic lupus erythematosus. *J Rheumatol.,* Vol.27, No.1, (January 2000), pp. 116-27.

Cantagrel, A.; Navaux, F.; Loubet-Lescoulié, P.; Nourhashemi, F.; Enault, G. & Mazières, B. (1999). Interleukin-1beta, interleukin-1 receptor antagonist, interleukin-4, and interleukin-10 gene polymorphisms: relationship to occurrence and severity of rheumatoid arthritis. *Arthritis Rheum.*, Vol.42, No.6, (June 1999), pp. 1093-100.

Cargill, M.; Schrodi, S.; Chang, M.; Garcia, V.; Brandon, R. & Begovich, A. (2007). A large-scale genetic association study confirms IL12B and leads to the identification of

IL23R as psoriasis-risk genes. *Am J Hum Genet.*, Vol.80, No.2, (February 2007), pp. 273-90.

Chang, I. & Hsiao, H. (2005). Induction of RhoGAP and pathological changes characteristic of Alzheimer's disease by UAHFEMF discharge in rat brain. *Curr Alzheimer Res.*, 2005 Dec; Vol.2, No.5, (December 2005), pp. 559-69.

Chen, X.; Kandasamy, K. & Srivastava, R. (2003). Differential roles of RelA (p65) and c-Rel subunits of nuclear factor kappa B in tumor necrosis factor-related apoptosis-inducing ligand signaling. *Cancer Res.*, Vol.63, No.5, (March 2003), pp. 1059-66.

Cheng, J.; Ning, Y.; Zhang, W.; Lu, Z. & Lin, L. (2010). T300A polymorphism of ATG16L1 and susceptibility to inflammatory bowel diseases: a meta-analysis. *World J Gastroenterol.*, Vol.16, No.10, (March 2010), pp. 1258-66.

Clayton, D. (2009). Prediction and interaction in complex disease genetics: experience in type 1 diabetes. *PLoS Genet.*, Vol.5, No.7, (July 2009), e1000540.

Concannon, P.; Onengut-Gumuscu, S.; Todd, J.; Smyth, D.; Pociot, F. & Rich, S. (2008). Type 1 Diabetes Genetics Consortium. A human type 1 diabetes susceptibility locus maps to chromosome 21q22.3. *Diabetes*, Vol.57, No.10, (October 2008), pp. 2858-61.

Cooper, J.; Smyth, D.; Smiles, A.; Plagnol, V.; Walker, N. & Todd, J. (2008). Meta-analysis of genome-wide association study data identifies additional type 1 diabetes risk loci. *Nat Genet.*, Vol.40, No.12, (December 2008), pp. 1399-401.

Cooper, J.; Walker, N.; Healy, B.; Smyth, D.; Downes, K.; Todd, J. &Type I Diabetes Genetics Consortium. (2009). Analysis of 55 autoimmune disease and type II diabetes loci: further confirmation of chromosomes 4q27, 12q13.2 and 12q24.13 as type I diabetes loci, and support for a new locus, 12q13.3-q14.1. *Genes Immun.*, Vol.10, Suppl.1, (December 2009), S95-120.

Coquerelle, C.; Oldenhove, G.; Acolty, V.; Denoeud, J.; Vansanten, G. & Moser, M. (2009). Anti-CTLA-4 treatment induces IL-10-producing ICOS+ regulatory T cells displaying IDO-dependent anti-inflammatory properties in a mouse model of colitis. *Gut*, Vol.58, No.10, (October 2009), pp. 1363-73.

Coyle, A. & Gutierrez-Ramos, J. (2001). The expanding B7 superfamily: increasing complexity in costimulatory signals regulating T cell function. *Nat Immunol.*, Vol.2, No.3, (March 2001), pp. 203-9.

De Jager, P.; Jia, X.; Wang, J.; de Bakker, P.; Ottoboni, L. & Oksenberg, J. (2009). Meta-analysis of genome scans and replication identify CD6, IRF8 and TNFRSF1A as new multiple sclerosis susceptibility loci. *Nat Genet.*, Vol.41, No.7, (July 2009), pp. 776-82.

Dubois, P.; Trynka, G.; Franke, L.; Hunt, K.; Romanos, J. & van Heel, D. (2010). Multiple common variants for celiac disease influencing immune gene expression. *Nat Genet.*, Vol.42, No.4, (April 2010), pp. 295-302.

Duerr, R. (2003). Update on the genetics of inflammatory bowel disease. *J Clin Gastroenterol.*, Vol.37, No.5, (Nov-Dec 2003), pp. 358-67.

Duerr, R.; Taylor, K.; Brant, S.; Rioux, J.; Silverberg, M. & Cho, J. (2006). A genome-wide association study identifies IL23R as an inflammatory bowel disease gene. *Science*, Vol.314, No.5804, (December 2006), pp. 1461-3.

Dupuis, J.; Langenberg, C.; Prokopenko, I.; Saxena, R.; Soranzo, N. & Barroso, I. (2010). New genetic loci implicated in fasting glucose homeostasis and their impact on type 2 diabetes risk. *Nat Genet.*, Vol.42, No.2, (February 2010), pp. 105-16.

Egwuagu, C. (2009). STAT3 in CD4+ T helper cell differentiation and inflammatory diseases. *Cytokine,* Vol.47, No.3, (September 2009), pp. 149-56.

EURODIAB ACE Study Group. (2000). Variation and trends in incidence of childhood diabetes in Europe. *Lancet,* Vol.355, No.9207, (March 2000), pp. 873-6.

Eyre, S.; Hinks, A.; Bowes, J.; Flynn, E.; Martin, P. & Barton, A. (2010). Overlapping genetic susceptibility variants between three autoimmune disorders: rheumatoid arthritis, type 1 diabetes and coeliac disease. *Arthritis Res Ther.,* Vol.12, No.5, (September 2010), R175.

Ferguson, L.; Han, D.; Fraser, A.; Huebner, C.; Lam, W. & Morgan, A. (2010). IL23R and IL12B SNPs and Haplotypes Strongly Associate with Crohn's Disease Risk in a New Zealand Population. *Gastroenterol Res and Pract.,* Vol.2010, (December 2010).

Festen, E.; Goyette, P.; Scott, R.; Annese, V.; Zhernakova, A. & Rioux, J. (2009). Genetic variants in the region harbouring IL2/IL21 associated with ulcerative colitis. *Gut,* Vol.58, No.6, (June 2009), pp. 799-804.

Festen, E.; Goyette, P.; Green, T.; Boucher, G.; Beauchamp, C. & Lagacé, C. (2011). A meta-analysis of genome-wide association scans identifies IL18RAP, PTPN2, TAGAP, and PUS10 as shared risk loci for Crohn's disease and celiac disease. *PLoS Genet.,* Vol. 7, No.1, (January 2011), e1001283.

Fisher, S.; Tremelling, M.; Anderson, C.; Gwilliam, R.; Bumpstead, S. & Satsangi, J. (2008). Genetic determinants of ulcerative colitis include the ECM1 locus and five loci implicated in Crohn's disease. *Nat Genet.,* Vol.40, No.6, (June 2008), pp. 710-712.

Franke, A.; Hampe, J.; Rosenstiel, P.; Becker, C.; Wagner, F. & Schreiber, S. (2007). Systematic association mapping identifies NELL1 as a novel IBD disease gene. *PLoS One,* Vol.2, No.1, (August 2007), e691.

Franke, A.; Balschun, T.; Karlsen, T.; Hedderich, J.; May, S. & Schreiber, S. (2008). Replication of signals from recent studies of Crohn's disease identifies previously unknown disease loci for ulcerative colitis. *Nat Genet.,* Vol.40, No.6, (June 2008), pp. 713-5.

Franke, A.; McGovern, D.; Barrett, J.; Wang, K.; Radford-Smith, G. & Parkes, M. (2010). Genome-wide meta-analysis increases to 71 the number of confirmed Crohn's disease susceptibility loci. *Nat Genet.,* Vol.42, No.12, (December 2010), pp. 1118-25.

Fung, E.; Smyth, D.; Howson, J.; Cooper, J.; Walker, N. & Todd, J. (2009) Analysis of 17 autoimmune disease-associated variants in type 1 diabetes identifies 6q23/TNFAIP3 as a susceptibility locus. *Genes and immunity,* Vol.10, No.2, (March 2009), pp. 188-91.

Galanter, J.; Choudhry, S.; Eng, C.; Nazario, S.; Rodríguez-Santana, J. & Burchard, E. (2008). ORMDL3 gene is associated with asthma in three ethnically diverse populations. *Am J Respir Crit Care Med.,* Vol. 177, No.11, (June 2008), pp. 1194–1200.

Gardet, A.; Benita, Y.; Li, C.; Sands, B.; Ballester, I. & Podolsky, D. (2010). LRRK2 is involved in the IFN-gamma response and host response to pathogens. *J Immunol.,* Vol.185, No.9, (November 2010), pp. 5577-85.

Garner, C.; Murray, J.; Ding, Y.; Tien, Z.; van Heel, D. & Neuhausen, S. (2009). Replication of celiac disease UK genome-wide association study results in a US population. *Hum Mol Genet.,* 2009, Vol.18, No.21, (November 2009), pp. 4219-4225.

Gazouli, M.; Pachoula, I.; Panayotou, I.; Mantzaris, G.; Chrousos, G. & Roma-Giannikou, E. (2010). NOD2/CARD15, ATG16L1 and IL23R gene polymorphisms and childhood

-onset of Crohn's disease. *World J Gastroenterol.,* Vol.16, No.14, (April 2010), pp. 1753-8.

Ghoreschi, K.; Laurence, A. & O'Shea, J. (2009). Janus kinases in immune cell signaling. *Immunol. Rev.,* Vol. 228, No.1, (March 2009), pp. 273–287.

Giallourakis, C.; Stoll, M.; Miller, K.; Hampe, J.; Lander, E. & Rioux, J. (2003). IBD5 is a general risk factor for inflammatory bowel disease: replication of association with Crohn disease and identification of a novel association with ulcerative colitis. *Am J Hum Genet.,* Vol. 73, No.1, (July 2003), pp. 205-211.

Glas, J.; Konrad, A.; Schmechel, S.; Dambacher, J.; Seiderer, J. & Brand, S. (2008). The ATG16L1 gene variants rs2241879 and rs2241880 (T300A) are strongly associated with susceptibility to Crohn's disease in the German population. *Am J Gastroenterol.,* Vol.103, No.3, (March 2008), pp. 682-91.

Goyette, P.; Lefebvre, C.; Ng, A.; Brant, S.; Cho, J. & Rioux, J. (2008). Gene-centric association mapping of chromosome 3p implicates MST1 in IBD pathogenesis. *Mucosal Immunol.,* Vol.1, No.2, (March 2008), pp. 131-8.

Graham, R.; Cotsapas, C.; Davies, L.; Hackett, R.; Lessard, C. & Parkin, M. (2008). Genetic variants near TNFAIP3 on 6q23 are associated with systemic lupus erythematosus. *Nat Genet.,* Vol.40, No.9, (September 2008), pp. 1059-61.

Grant, S.; Qu, H.; Bradfield, J.; Marchand, L.; Kim, C. & Hakonarson, H. (2009). Follow-up analysis of genome-wide association data identifies novel loci for type 1 diabetes. *Diabetes,* Vol.58, No.1, (January 2009), pp. 290-5.

Gregersen, P.; Amos, C.; Lee, A.; Lu, Y.; Remmers, E. & Siminovitch, K. (2009). REL, encoding a member of the NF-kappaB family of transcription factors, is a newly defined risk locus for rheumatoid arthritis. *Nat Genet.,* Vol.41, No.7, (July 2009), pp. 820–3.

Gregersen, P. & Olsson, L. (2009). Recent advances in the genetics of autoimmune disease. *Annu Rev Immunol,* Vol.27, pp. 363-91

Gunderson, K.; Steemers, F.; Lee, G.; Mendoza, L. & Chee, M. (2005). A genome-wide scalable SNP genotyping assay using microarray technology. *Nature genetics,* Vol.37, No.5, (May 2005), pp. 549-54.

Guo, D.; Li, M.; Zhang, Y.; Yang, P.; Eckenrode, S. & Wang, C. (2004). A functional variant of SUMO4, a new I kappa B alpha modifier, is associated with type 1 diabetes. *Nature genetics,* Vol.36, No.8, (August 2004), pp. 837-41.

Hafler, D.; Compston, A.; Sawcer, S.; Lander, E.; Daly, M. & Hauser, S. (2007). Risk alleles for multiple sclerosis identified by a genomewide study. *The New England journal of medicine,* Vol.357, No.9, (August 2007), pp. 851-62.

Hakonarson, H.; Grant, S.; Bradfield, J.; Marchand, L.; Kim, C. & Polychronakos, C. (2007). A genome-wide association study identifies KIAA0350 as a type 1 diabetes gene. *Nature,* 2007 Aug 2; Vol.448, No.7153, (August 2007), pp. 591-4.

Hakonarson, H.; Qu, H.; Bradfield, J.; Marchand, L.; Kim, C. & Polychronakos, C. (2008). A novel susceptibility locus for type 1 diabetes on Chr12q13 identified by a genome-wide association study. *Diabetes,* Vol.57, No.4, (April 2008), pp. 1143-6.

Halme, L., Paavola-Sakki, P.; Turunen, U.; Lappalainen, M.; Farkkila, M. & Kontula, K. (2006). Family and twin studiesin inflammatory bowel disease. *World Journal of Gastroenterology,* Vol.12, No.23, (June 2006), pp. 3668–72.

Hampe, J.; Cuthbert, A.; Croucher, P.; Mirza, M.; Mascheretti, S. & Mathew, C. (2001). Association between insertion mutation in NOD2 gene and Crohn's disease in German and British populations. *Lancet,* Vol.357, No.9272, (June 2001), pp. 1925–8.

Hampe, J.; Franke, A.; Rosenstiel, P.; Till, A.; Teuber, M. & Schreiber, S. (2007). A genome-wide association scan of nonsynonymous SNPs identifies a susceptibility variant for Crohn disease in ATG16L1. *Nat Genet.,* Vol. 39, No.2, (February 2007), pp. 207-211.

Han, J.; Zheng, H.; Cui, Y.; Sun, L.; Ye, D. & Zhang, X. (2009). Genome-wide association study in a Chinese Han population identifies nine new susceptibility loci for systemic lupus erythematosus. *Nat. Genet.,* Vol.41, No.11, (November 2009), pp. 1234–1237.

Harada, M.; Ishihara, Y.; Itoh, K. & Yamanaka, R. (2007). Kinesin superfamily protein-derived peptides with the ability to induce glioma-reactive cytotoxic T lymphocytes in human leukocyte antigen-A24+ glioma patients. *Oncol Rep.,* Vol.17, No.3, (March 2007), pp. 629-36.

Haritunians, T.; Taylor, K.; Targan, S.; Dubinsky, M.; Ippoliti, A. & McGovern, D. (2010). Genetic predictors of medically refractory ulcerative colitis. *Inflamm Bowel Dis.,* Vol.16, No.11, (November 2010), pp. 1830-40.

Haritunians, T.; Jones, M.; McGovern, D.; Shih, D.; Barrett, R. & Taylor, K. (2011). Variants in ZNF365 isoform D are associated with Crohn's disease. *Gut,* (January 2011).

Hasegawa, K.; Martin, F.; Huang, G.; Tumas, D.; Diehl, L. & Chan, A. (2004). PEST domain-enriched tyrosine phosphatase (PEP) regulation of effector/memory T cells. *Science,* Vol.303, No.5658, (January 2004), pp. 685–89.

Hayden, M.; West, A. & Ghosh, S. (2006). NF-kappaB and the immune response. *Oncogene,* Vol.25, No.51, (October 2006), pp. 6758– 80.

Henderson, P.; van Limbergen, J.; Anderson, N.; Nimmo, E.; Russell, R.; Satsangi, J. & Wilson, D. (2011). Variation in ICOSLG influences Crohn's disease susceptibility. *Gut,* (February 2011).

Hindorff LA, Junkins HA, Mehta JP, et al. A catalog of published genome-wide association studies 2010. Available at: www.genome.gov/gwastudies.

Hirota, T.; Harada, M.; Sakashita, M.; Doi, S.; Miyatake, A. & Tamari, M. (2008). Genetic polymorphism regulating ORM1- like 3 (Saccharomyces cerevisiae) expression is associated with childhood atopic asthma in a Japanese population. *J. Allergy Clin. Immunol.,* Vol.121, No.3, (March 2008), pp. 769–770.

Hofseth, L.; Saito, S.; Hussain, S.; Espey, M.; Miranda, K. & Harris, C. (2003). Nitric oxide-induced cellular stress and p53 activation in chronic inflammation. *Proc Natl Acad Sci USA,* Vol.100, No.1, (January 2003), pp. 143-8.

Holland, S.; DeLeo, F.; Elloumi, H.; Hsu, A.; Uzel, G. & Grimbacher, B. (2007). STAT3 mutations in the hyper-IgE syndrome. *N. Engl. J. Med.,* Vol.357, No.16, (October 2007), pp. 1608–1619.

Hollingsworth, M. & Swanson, B. (2004). Mucins in cancer: protection and control of the cell surface. *Nat Rev Cancer,* Vol.4, No.1, (January 2004), pp. 45–60.

Hoshino, H. & Igarashi, K. (2002). Expression of the oxidative stress-regulated transcription factor bach2 in differentiating neuronal cells. *J Biochem.,* Vol.132, No.3, (September 2002), pp. 427-31.

Howson, J.; Walker, N.; Smyth, D.; Todd, J. & Type I Diabetes Genetics Consortium. (2009). Analysis of 19 genes for association with type I diabetes in the Type I Diabetes. *Genes Immun.*, Vol.10, Suppl.1, (December 2009), S74-84.

Hradsky, O.; Dusatkova, P.; Lenicek, M.; Bronsky, J.; Duricova, D. & Cinek, O. (2010). Two independent genetic factors responsible for the associations of the IBD5 locus with Crohn's disease in the Czech population. *Inflamm Bowel Dis.*, (November 2010).

Hugot, J.; Chamaillard, M.; Zouali, H.; Lesage, S.; Cézard, J. & Thomas, G. (2001). Association of NOD2 leucinerich repeat variants with susceptibility to Crohn's disease. *Nature,* Vol.411, No.6837, (May 2001), pp. 599–603.

Hunter, K.; Rainbow, D.; Plagnol, V.; Todd, J.; Peterson, L. & Wicker, L. (2007). Interactions between Idd5.1/Ctla4 and other type 1 diabetes genes. *J Immunol,* Vol.179, No.12, (December 2007), pp. 8341-9.

Imielinski, M.; Baldassano, R.; Griffiths, A.; Russell, R.; Annese, V. & Hakonarson, H. (2009). Common variants at five new loci associated with early-onset inflammatory bowel disease. *Nat Genet.*, Vol.41, No.12, (December 2009), pp. 1335-40.

Ito, T.; Yang, M.; Wang, Y.; Lande, R.; Gregorio, J. & Gilliet, M. (2007). Plasmacytoid dendritic cells prime IL-10-producing T regulatory cells by inducible costimulator ligand. *J Exp Med.*, Vol.204, No.1, (January 2007), pp. 105–15.

Jagiello, P.; Aries, P; Arning, L.; Wagenleiter, S.; Csernok, E. & Epplen J. (2005). The PTPN22 620W allele is a risk factor for Wegener's granulomatosis. *Arthritis Rheum.*, Vol.52, No.12, (December 2005), pp. 4039-4043.

Jankowski, M.; Kopiński, P. & Goc, A. (2010). Interleukin-27: biological properties and clinical application. *Arch Immunol Ther Exp (Warsz),* Vol.58, No.6, (December 2010), pp. 417-25.

Jin, Y.; Birlea, S.; Fain, P.; Gowan, K.; Riccardi, S. Bennett, D. (2010). Variant of TYR and autoimmunity susceptibility loci in generalized vitiligo. *N Engl J Med.*, Vol.362, No.18, (May 2010), pp. 1686-97.

Kabashima, K.; Saji, T.; Murata, T.; Nagamachi, M.; Matsuoka, T. & Narumiya, S. (2002). The prostaglandin receptor EP4 suppresses colitis, mucosal damage and CD4 cell activation in the gut. *J Clin Invest.*, Vol.109, No.7, (April 2002), pp. 883–893.

Kakuta, Y.; Kinouchi, Y.; Negoro, K.; Takahashi, S. & Shimosegawa, T. (2006). Association study of TNFSF15 polymorphisms in Japanese patients with inflammatory bowel disease. *Gut,* Vol.55, No.10, (October 2006), pp. 1527-8.

Kasmi, K.; Smith, A.; Williams, L.; Neale, G.; Panopoulos, A. & Murray, P. (2007). A transcriptional repressor and corepressor induced by the STAT3-regulated anti-inflammatory signaling pathway. *J Immunol.*, Vol.179, No.11, (December 2007), pp. 7215-9.

Kim, S.; Wairkar, Y.; Daniels, R. & DiAntonio, A. (2010). The novel endosomal membrane protein Ema interacts with the class C Vps-HOPS complex to promote endosomal maturation. *Cell Biol.*, Vol.188, No.5, (March 2010), pp. 717-34.

Knip, M.; Veijola, R.; Virtanen, S.; Hyoty, H.; Vaarala, O. & Akerblom, H. (2005). Environmental triggers and determinants of type 1 diabetes. *Diabetes,* Vol.54, Suppl.2, (December 2005), S125-36.

Kolz, M.; Johnson, T.; Sanna, S.; Teumer, A.; Vitart, V. & Gieger, C. (2009). Meta-analysis of 28,141 individuals identifies common variants within five new loci that influence uric acid concentrations. *PLoS Genet.*, Vol.5, No.6, (June 2009), e1000504.

Kugathasan, S.; Baldassano, R.; Bradfield, J.; Sleiman, P.; Imielinski, M. & Hakonarson, H. (2008). Loci on 20q13 and 21q22 are associated with pediatric-onset inflammatory bowel disease. *Nature Genetics,* Vol.40, No.10, (October 2008), pp. 1211–5.

Kurz, T.; Hoffjan, S.; Hayes, M.; Schneider, D.; Nicolae, R. & Ober, C. (2006). Fine mapping and positional candidate studies on chromosome 5p13 identify multiple asthma susceptibility loci. *J Allergy Clin Immunol.,* Vol.118, No.2, (August 2006), pp. 396-402.

Langrish, C.; McKenzie, B.; Wilson, N.; de Waal Malefyt, R.; Kastelein, R. & Cua, J. (2004). IL-12 and IL-23: master regulators of innate and adaptive immunity. *Immunol Rev.,* Vol.202, (December 2004), pp. 96–105.

Larousserie, F.; Charlot, P.; Bardel, E.; Froger, J.; Kastelein, R. & Devergne, O. (2006). Differential effects of IL-27 on human B cell subsets. *J Immunol.,* Vol.176, No.10, (May 2006), pp. 5890-7.

Lashner, B. (1995). Epidemiology of inflammatory bowel disease. *Gastroenterology Clinics of North America,* Vol.24, No.3, (September 1995), pp. 467–74.

Latiano, A.; Palmieri, O.; Corritore, G.; Valvano, M.; Bossa, F. & Annese, V. (2010). Variants at the 3p21 locus influence susceptibility and phenotype both in adults and early-onset patients with inflammatory bowel disease. *Inflamm Bowel Dis.,* Vol.16, No.7, (July 2010), pp. 1108-17.

Laukens, D.; Georges, M.; Libioulle, C.; Sandor, C.; Mni, M. & De Vos, M. (2010). Evidence for significant overlap between common risk variants for Crohn's disease and ankylosing spondylitis. *PLoS One,* Vol.5, No.11, (November 2010), e13795.

Law, D.; Labut, E. & Merchant, J. (2006). Intestinal overexpression of ZNF148 suppresses ApcMin/+ neoplasia. *Mamm Genome,* Vol.17, No.10, (October 2006), pp. 999-1004.

Lees, C.; Barrett, J.; Parkes, M. & Satsangi, J. (2011). New IBD genetics: common pathways with other diseases. *Gut,* (February 2011).

Lettre, G. & Rioux, J. (2008). Autoimmune diseases: insights from genome-wide association studies. *Hum. Mol. Genet.,* Vol.17, R.2, (October 2008), R116–21.

Libioulle, C.; Louis, E.; Hansoul, S.; Sandor, C.; Farnir, F. & Georges, M. (2007). Novel Crohn disease locus identified by genome-wide association maps to a gene desert on 5p13.1 and modulates expression of PTGER4. *PLoS Genet.,* Vol.3, No.4, (April 2007), e58.

Liu, D. & Finley, R. (2010). Cyclin Y is a novel conserved cyclin essential for development in Drosophila. *Genetics,* Vol.184, No.4, (April 2010), pp. 1025-35.

Liu, Y.; Helms, C.; Liao, W.; Zaba, L.; Duan, S. & Bowcock, A. (2008). A genome-wide association study of psoriasis and psoriatic arthritis identifies new disease loci. *PLoS Genet,* Vol.4, No.3, (March 2008), e1000041.

Lohmueller, K.; Pearce, C.; Pike, M.; Lander, E. & Hirschhorn, J. (2003). Meta-analysis of genetic association studies supports a contribution of common variants to susceptibility to common disease. *Nature genetics,* Vol.33, No.2, (February 2003), pp. 177-82.

Long., S.; Cerosaletti, K.; Wan, J.; Ho, J.; Tatum, M. & Buckner, J. (2011). An autoimmune-associated variant in PTPN2 reveals an impairment of IL-2R signaling in CD4(+) T cells. *Genes Immun.,* Vol.12, No.2, (March 2011), pp. 116-25.

Lowe, C.; Cooper, J.; Brusko, T.; Walker, N.; Smyth, D. & Todd JA. (2007). Large-scale genetic fine mapping and genotype-phenotype associations implicate polymorphism in the IL2RA region in type 1 diabetes. *Nat Genet.*, Vol.39, No.9, (September 2007), pp. 1074-82.

Lucas, S.; Ghilardi, N.; Li, J. & de Sauvage, F. (2003). IL-27 regulates IL-12 responsiveness of naive CD4+ T cells through Stat1-dependent and -independent mechanisms. *Proc. Natl Acad. Sci. USA,* Vol.100, No.25, (December 2003), pp. 15047–52.

Lupski, J.; Reid, J.; Gonzaga-Jauregui, C.; Rio Deiros, D.; Chen, D. & Gibbs, R. (2010). Whole-genome sequencing in a patient with Charcot-Marie-Tooth neuropathy. *N Engl J Med.*, Vol.362, No.13, (April 2010), pp. 1181–1191.

Madore, A.; Tremblay, K.; Hudson, T. & Laprise, C. (2008). Replication of an association between 17q21 SNP and asthma in a French-Canadian familial collection. *Hum. Genet.*, Vol.123, No.1, (February 2008), pp. 93–95.

Manolio, T.; Collins, F.; Cox, N.; Goldstein, D.; Hindorff, L. & Visscher, P. (2009). Finding the missing heritability of complex diseases. *Nature,* Vol.461, No.7265, (October 2009), pp. 747-53.

Manolio, T.; Rodriguez, L.; Brooks, L.; Abecasis, G.; Collaborative Association Study of Psoriasis & Collins, F. (2007). New models of collaboration in genome-wide association studies: the Genetic Association Information Network. *Nature genetics,* Vol.39, No.9, (September 2007), pp. 1045-51.

Mao, M.; Biery, M.; Kobayashi, S.; Ward, T.; Schimmack, G. & Linsley, P. (2004). T lymphocyte activation gene identification by coregulated expression on DNA microarrays. *Genomics,* Vol.83, No.6, (June 2004), pp. 989-99.

Márquez, A.; Orozco, G.; Martínez, A.; Palomino-Morales, R.; Fernández-Arquero, M. & Urcelay, E. (2009a). Novel association of the interleukin 2-interleukin 21 region with inflammatory bowel disease. *Am J Gastroenterol.*, Vol.104, No.8, (August 2009), pp. 1968-1975.

Márquez, A.; Varadé, J.; Robledo, G.; Martínez, A.; Mendoza, J.; & Urcelay, E. (2009b). Specific association of a CLEC16A/KIAA0350 polymorphism with NOD2/CARD15(-) Crohn's disease patients. *Eur J Hum Genet.*, Vol.17, No.10, (October 2009), pp.1304-8.

Marquez, A.; Cénit, M.; Núñez, C.; Mendoza, J.; Taxonera, C. & Bartolomé, M. (2009c). Effect of BSN-MST1 locus on inflammatory bowel disease and multiple sclerosis susceptibility. *Genes Immun.*, Vol.10, No.7, (October 2009), pp. 631-5.

McCarthy, M.; Abecasis, G.; Cardon, L.; Goldstein, D.; Little, J.; Ioannidis, J. & Hirschhorn, J. (2008). Genome-wide association studies for complex traits: consensus, uncertainty and challenges. *Nat. Rev. Genet,* Vol.9, No.5, (May 2008), pp. 356–369.

McCleverty, C.; Hornsby, M.; Spraggon, G. & Kreusch, A. (2007). Crystal structure of human Pus10, a novel pseudouridine synthase. *J Mol Biol.*, Vol.373, No.5, (November 2007), pp. 1243-54.

McGovern, D.; Van Heel, D.; Negoro, K.; Ahmad, T. & Jewell, D. (2003). Further evidence of IBD5/CARD15 (NOD2) epistasis in the susceptibility to ulcerative colitis. *Am J Hum Genet.*, Vol.73, No.6, (December 2003), pp. 1465-6.

McGovern, D.; Gardet, A.; Törkvist, L.; Goyette, P.; Essers, J. & Green, T. (2010). Genome-wide association identifies multiple ulcerative colitis susceptibility loci. *Nat Genet.*, Vol.42, No.4, (April 2010), pp. 332-7.

Meggyesi, N.; Kiss, L.; Koszarska, M.; Bortlik, M.; Duricova, D. & Lakatos, P. (2010). NKX2-3 and IRGM variants are associated with disease susceptibility to IBD in Eastern

European patients. *World J Gastroenterol.*, Vol.16, No.41, (November 2010), pp. 5233-40.

Mero, I.; Lorentzen, A.; Ban, M.; Smestad, C.; Celius, E. & Harbo, H. (2010). A rare variant of the TYK2 gene is confirmed to be associated with multiple sclerosis. *Eur J Hum Genet.*, Vol.18, No.4, (April 2010), pp. 502-4.

Mirel, D.; Valdes, A.; Lazzeroni, L.; Reynolds, R.; Erlich, H. & Noble, J. (2002). Association of IL4R haplotypes with type 1 diabetes. *Diabetes,* Vol.51, No.11, (November 2002), pp. 3336-41.

Moffatt, M.; Kabesch, M.; Liang, L.; Dixon, A.; Strachan, D. & Rietschel, E. (2007). Genetic variants regulating ORMDL3 expression contribute to the risk of childhood asthma. *Nature,* Vol.448, No.7152, (July 2007), pp. 470-3.

Moore, F.; Colli, M.; Cnop, M.; Esteve, M.; Cardozo, A. & Eizirik, D. (2009). PTPN2, a candidate gene for type 1 diabetes, modulates interferon-gamma-induced pancreatic beta-cell apoptosis. *Diabetes,* Vol.58, No.6, (June 2009), pp. 1283-1291.

Morgan, A.; Han, D.; Lam, W.; Fraser, A. & Ferguson L. (2010). Association analysis of 3p21 with Crohn's disease in a New Zealand population. *Hum Immunol.*, Vol.71, No.6, (June 2010), pp. 602-9.

Mueller, P.; Rogus, J.; Cleary, P.; Zhao, Y.; Smiles, A. & Warram, J. (2006). Genetics of Kidneys in Diabetes (GoKinD) study: a genetics collection available for identifying genetic susceptibility factors for diabetic nephropathy in type 1 diabetes. *J Am Soc Nephrol.*, Vol.17, No.7, (July 2006), pp. 1782-90.

Nejentsev, S.; Howson, J.; Walker, N.; Szeszko, J.; Field, S. & Wellcome Trust Case Control Consortium. (2007). Localization of type 1 diabetes susceptibility to the MHC class I genes HLA-B and HLA-A. *Nature,* Vol.450, No.7171, (December 2007), pp. 887-92.

Nejentsev, S.; Walker, N.; Riches, D.; Egholm, M. & Todd, J. (2009). Rare variants of IFIH1, a gene implicated in antiviral responses, protect against type 1 diabetes. *Science,* Vol.324, No.5925, (April 2009), pp. 387-9.

Neurath, M.; Fuss, I.; Schürmann, G.; Pettersson, S.; Arnold, K. & Büschenfelde, K. (1998). Cytokine gene transcription by NF-kappa B family members in patients with inflammatory bowel disease. *Ann NY Acad Sci.*, Vol. 859, (November 1998), pp. 149–59.

Nisticò, L.; Buzzetti, R.; Pritchard, L.; Van der Auwera, B.; Giovannini, C. & Todd, J. (1996). The CTLA-4 gene region of chromosome 2q33 is linked to, and associated with, type 1 diabetes. Belgian Diabetes Registry. *Human molecular genetics,* Vol.5, No.7, (July 1996), pp. 1075-80.

Onkamo, P.; Vaananen, S.; Karvonen, M. & Tuomilehto, J. (1999). Worldwide increase in incidence of Type I diabetes-the analysis of the data on published incidence trends. *Diabetologia,* Vol.42, No.12, (December 1999), pp. 1395-403.

Orozco, G.; Sánchez, E.; González-Gay, M.; López-Nevot, M.; Torres, B. & Martín, J. (2005). Association of a functional single-nucleotide polymorphism of PTPN22, encoding lymphoid protein phosphatase, with rheumatoid arthritis and systemic lupus erythematosus. *Arthritis Rheum.*, Vol.52, No.1, (January 2005), pp. 219-224.

Oyake, T.; Itoh, K.; Motohashi, H.; Hayashi, N.; Hoshino, H. & Igarashi, K. (1996). Bach proteins belong to a novel family of BTB-basic leucine zipper transcription factors that interact with MafK and regulate transcription through the NF-E2 site. *Mol. Cell Biol.*, Vol.16, No.1, (November 1996), pp. 6083–6095.

Palmieri, O.; Latiano, A.; Valvano, R.; D'Incà, R.; Vecchi, M. & Annese, V. (2006). Variants of OCTN1-2 cation transporter genes are associated with both Crohn's disease and ulcerative colitis. *Aliment Pharmacol Ther.*, Vol.23, No.4, (February 2006), pp. 497–506.

Parkes, M.; Barrett, J.; Prescott, N.; Tremelling, M.; Anderson, C. & Mathew, C. (2007). Sequence variants in the autophagy gene IRGM and multiple other replicating loci contribute to Crohn's disease susceptibility. *Nat Genet.*, Vol.39, No.7, (July 2007), pp. 830-2.

Parrish-Novak, J.; Foster, D.; Holly, R. & Clegg, C. (2002). Interleukin-21 and the IL-21 receptor: novel effectors of NK and T cell responses. *J. Leukoc. Biol.*, Vol.72, No.5, (November 2002), pp. 856–63.

Peltekova, V.; Wintle, R.; Rubin, L.; Amos, C.; Huang, Q. & Siminovitch, K. (2004). Functional variants of OCTN cation transporter genes are associated with Crohn disease. *Nat Genet.*, Vol.36, No.5, (May 2004), pp. 471-475

Phillips, A.; Nimmo, E.; Van Limbergen, J.; Drummond, H.; Smith, L. & Satsangi, J. (2010). Detailed haplotype-tagging study of germline variation of MUC19 in inflammatory bowel disease. *Inflam Bowel Dis.*, Vol.16, No.4, (April 2010), pp.557-8.

Picornell, Y.; Mei, L.; Taylor, K.; Yang, H.; Targan, S. & Rotter, J. (2007). TNFSF15 is an ethnic-specific IBD gene. *Inflamm Bowel Dis.*, Vol.13, No.11, (November 2007), pp. 1333-8.

Plantinga, T.; Crisan, T.; Oosting, M.; van de Veerdonk, F.; de Jong, D. & Netea, M. (2011). Crohn's disease-associated ATG16L1 polymorphism modulates pro-inflammatory cytokine responses selectively upon activation of NOD2. *Gut*, (March 2011).

Plenge, R.; Seielstad, M.; Padyukov, L.; Lee, A.; Remmers, E. & Li, W. (2007). TRAF1-C5 as a risk locus for rheumatoid arthritis-a genomewide study. *N Engl J Med.*, Vol.357, No.12, (September 2007), pp. 1199-209.

Poirot, L.; Benoist, C. & Mathis, D. (2004). Natural killer cells distinguish innocuous and destructive forms of pancreatic islet autoimmunity. *Proc. Natl Acad. Sci. USA*, Vol.101, No.21, (May 2004), pp. 8102–8107.

Prescott, N.; Fisher, S.; Franke, A.; Hampe, J.; Onnie, C. & Mathew, C. (2007). A nonsynonymous SNP in ATG16L1 predisposes to ileal Crohn's disease and is independent of CARD15 and IBD5. *Gastroenterology*, Vol.132, No.5, (May 2007), pp. 1665-71.

Qu, H.; Bradfield, J.; Li, Q.; Kim, C.; Frackelton, E.; Grant, S.; Hakonarson, H. & Polychronakos C. (2010). In silico replication of the genome-wide association results of the Type 1 Diabetes Genetics Consortium. *Hum mol genetics*, Vol.19, No.12, (June 2010), pp. 2534-8.

Quaranta, M.; Burden, A.; Griffiths, C.; Worthington, J.; Barker, J.; Trembath, R. & Capon, F. (2009). Differential contribution of CDKAL1 variants to psoriasis, Crohn's disease and type II diabetes. *Genes Immun*, Vol.10, No.7, (October 2009), pp. 654-8.

Raelson, J.; Little, R.; Ruether, A.; Fournier, H.; Paquin, B. & Schreiber, S. (2007). Genome-wide association study for Crohn's disease in the Quebec founder population identifies multiple validated disease loci. *Proc Natl Acad Sci USA*, Vol.104, No.37, (September 2007), pp. 14747–52.

Redondo, M.; Yu, L.; Hawa, M.; Mackenzie, T.; Pyke, D.; Eisenbarth, G. & Leslie, R. (2001). Heterogeneity of type I diabetes: analysis of monozygotic twins in Great Britain and the United States. *Diabetologia,* Vol.44, No.3, (March 2001), pp. 354-62.

Reich, D.; Patterson, N.; De Jager, P.; McDonald, G.; Waliszewska, A. & Hafler, D. (2005). A whole-genome admixture scan finds a candidate locus for multiple sclerosis susceptibility. *Nature genetics,* Vol.37, No.10, (October 2005), pp. 1113-8.

Rich, S. (1990). Mapping genes in diabetes. Genetic epidemiological perspective. *Diabetes,* Vol.39, No.11, (November 1990), pp. 1315-9.

Rioux, J.; Daly, M.; Silverberg, M.; Lindblad, K.; Steinhart, H. & Hudson, T. (2001). Genetic variation in the 5q31 cytokine gene cluster confers susceptibility to Crohn disease. *Nat Genet.,* Vol.29, No.2, (October 2001), pp. 223–228.

Rioux, J.; Xavier, R.; Taylor, K.; Silverberg, M.; Goyette, P. & Brant, S. (2007). Genome-wide association study identifies new susceptibility loci for Crohn disease and implicates autophagy in disease pathogenesis. *Nat Genet.,* Vol.39, No.5, (May 2007), pp. 596-604.

Roach, J.; Glusman, G.; Smit, A.; Huff, C.; Hubley, R. & Galas, D. (2010). Analysis of genetic inheritance in a family quartet by whole-genome sequencing. *Science,* Vol.328, No.5978, (April 2010), pp. 636 - 639.

Roberts, R.; Gearry, R.; Hollis-Moffatt, J.; Miller, A.; Reid, J. & Kennedy, M. (2007). IL23R R381Q and ATG16L1 T300A are strongly associated with Crohn's disease in a study of New Zealand Caucasians with inflammatory bowel disease. *Am J Gastroenterol.,* Vol.102, No.12, (December 2007), pp. 2754-61.

Rodacki, M.; Svoren, B.; Butty, V.; Besse, W.; Laffel, L.; Benoist, C. & Mathis, D. (2007). Altered natural killer cells in type 1 diabetic patients. *Diabetes,* Vol.56, No.1, (January 2007), pp. 177–185.

Russell, R.; Drummond, H.; Nimmo, E.; Anderson, N.; Noble, C. & Satsangi, J. (2006). Analysis of the influence of OCTN1/2 variants within the IBD5 locus on disease susceptibility and growth indices in early onset inflammatory bowel disease. *Gut,* Vol.55, No.8, (August 2006), pp. 1114-1123.

Santiago, J.; Martinez, A.; de la Calle, H.; Fernandez-Arquero, M.; Figueredo, M.; de la Concha, E. & Urcelay, E. (2006). Evidence for the association of the SLC22A4 and SLC22A5 genes with type 1 diabetes: a case control study. *BMC Med Genet.,* Vol.7, (June 2006), 54.

Santiago, J.; Martínez, A.; de la Calle, H.; Fernández-Arquero, M.; Figueredo, M.; de la Concha, E. & Urcelay, E. (2007). Susceptibility to type 1 diabetes conferred by the PTPN22 C1858T polymorphism in the Spanish population. *BMC Med Genet.,* Vol.8, (August 2007), 54.

Sartor, R. (1994). Cytokines in intestinal inflammation: pathophysiological and clinical considerations. *Gastroenterology,* Vol.106, No.2, (February 1994), pp. 533-539.

Sato, T.; Kanai, T.; Watanabe, M.; Sakuraba, A.; Okamoto, S. & Hibi, T. (2004). Hyperexpression of inducible costimulator and its contribution on lamina propria T cells in inflammatory bowel disease. *Gastroenterology,* Vol.126, No.3, (March 2004), pp. 829–39.

Sawalha, A.; Kaufman, K.; Kelly, J.; Adler, A.; Aberle, T. & Harley, J. (2008). Genetic association of interleukin-21 polymorphisms with systemic lupus erythematosus. *Ann Rheum Dis.,* 2008, Vol.67, No.4, (April 2008), pp. 458-461.

Scharl, M.; McCole, D.; Weber, A.; Vavricka, S.; Frei, P. & Rogler, G. (2011). Protein tyrosine phosphatase N2 regulates TNFα-induced signalling and cytokine secretion in human intestinal epithelial cells. *Gut,* Vol.60, No.2, (February 2011), pp. 189-97.

Scharl, M.; Paul, G.; Weber, A.; Jung, B.; Docherty, M. & McCole, D. (2009). Protection of epithelial barrier function by the Crohn's disease associated gene protein tyrosine phosphatase n2. *Gastroenterology,* Vol.137, No.6, (December 2009), pp.2030-40.

Sheikh, F.; Baurin, V.; Lewis-Antes, A.; Shah, N.; Smirnov, S. & Kotenko, S. (2004). Cutting edge: IL-26 signals through a novel receptor complex composed of IL-20 receptor 1 and IL-10 receptor 2. *J. Immunol.,* Vol.172, No.4, (February 2004), pp. 2006–10.

Shimane, K.; Kochi, Y.; Horita, T.; Ikari, K.; Amano, H. & Yamamoto, K. (2010). The association of a nonsynonymous single-nucleotide polymorphism in TNFAIP3 with systemic lupus erythematosus and rheumatoid arthritis in the Japanese population. *Arthritis Rheum.,* Vol.62, No.2, (February 2010), pp. 574–579.

Silverberg, M.; Cho, J.; Rioux, J.; McGovern, D.; Wu, J. & Duerr, R. (2009). Ulcerative colitis-risk loci on chromosomes 1p36 and 12q15 found by genome-wide association study. *Nat Genet.,* Vol.41, No.2, (February 2009), pp. 216-20.

Sleiman, P.; Annaiah, K.; Imielinski, M.; Bradfield, J.; Kim, C. & Hakonarson, H. (2008). ORMDL3 variants associated with asthma susceptibility in North Americans of European ancestry. *J Allergy Clin Immunol,* Vol.122, No.6, (December 2008), pp. 1225–7.

Smyth, D.; Cooper, J.; Collins, J.; Heward, J.; Franklyn, J. & Todd, J. (2004). Replication of an association between the lymphoid tyrosine phosphatase locus (LYP/PTPN22) with type 1 diabetes, and evidence for its role as a general autoimmunity locus. *Diabetes,* Vol.53, No.11, (November 2004), pp. 3020-3.

Smyth, D.; Cooper, J.; Bailey, R.; Field, S.; Burren, O. & Todd J. (2006). A genome-wide association study of nonsynonymous SNPs identifies a type 1 diabetes locus in the interferon-induced helicase (IFIH1) region. *Nature genetics,* Vol.38, No.6, (June 2006), pp. 617-9.

Smyth, D.; Plagnol, V.; Walker, N.; Cooper, J.; Downes, K. & Todd, J. (2008). Shared and distinct genetic variants in type 1 diabetes and celiac disease. *N Eng J of Med,* Vol.359, No.26, (December 2008), pp. 2767-77.

Stahl, E.; Raychaudhuri, S.; Remmers, E.; Xie, G.; Eyre, S. & Alfredsson, L. (2010). Genome-wide association study meta-analysis identifies seven new rheumatoid arthritis risk loci. *Nat Genet.,* Vol.42, No.6, (June 2010), pp. 508-14.

Steemers, F.; Chang, W.; Lee, G.; Barker, D.; Shen R. & Gunderson, K. (2006). Whole-genome genotyping with the single-base extension assay. *Nature methods,* Vol.3, No.1, (January 2006), pp. 31-3.

Su, A.; Wiltshire, T.; Batalov, S.; Lapp, H.; Ching, K. & Hogenesch, J. (2004). A gene atlas of the mouse and human protein-encoding transcriptomes. *Proc Natl Acad Sci USA,* Vol.101, No.6, (april 2004), pp. 6062–7.

Suarez-Gestal, M.; Calaza, M.; Endreffy, E.; Pullmann, R.; Ordi-Ros, J. & European Consortium of SLE DNA Collections. (2009). Replication of recently identified systemic lupus erythematosus genetic associations: a case-control study. *Arthritis Res. Ther.,* Vol.11, No.3, (May 2009), R69.

Tenbrock, K.; Juang, Y.; Gourley, M.; Nambiar, M. & Tsokos, G. (2002). Antisense cyclic adenosine 5'-monophosphate response element modulator up-regulates IL-2 in T cells from patients with systemic lupus erythematosus. *J Immunol.*, Vol.169, No.8, (October 2002), pp. 4147–4152.

The International HapMap Consortium (2003). The International HapMap Project. *Nature*, Vol.426, No.6968, (December 2003), pp. 789-96.

The International HapMap Consortium (2005). A haplotype map of the human genome. *Nature*, Vol.437, No.7063, (October 2005), pp. 1299-320.

Thompson, N.; Driscoll, R.; Pounder, R. & Wakefield, A. (1996). Genetics versus environment in inflammatory bowel disease: results of a British twin study. *BMJ*, Vol.312, No.7023, (January 1996), pp. 95–6.

Tian, W. & Liou, H. (2009). RNAi-mediated c-Rel silencing leads to apoptosis of B cell tumor cells and suppresses antigenic immune response in vivo. *PLoS One*, Vol.4, No.4, (April 2009), e5028.

Todd, J.; Walker, N.; Cooper, J.; Smyth, D.; Downes, K. & Clayton, D. (2007). Robust associations of four new chromosome regions from genome-wide analyses of type 1 diabetes. *Nature genetics*, Vol.39, No.7, (July 2007), pp. 857-64.

Torkvist, L.; Halfvarson, J.; Ong, R.; Lördal, M.; Sjöqvist, U. & Pettersson, S. (2010). Analysis of 39 Crohn's disease risk loci in Swedish inflammatory bowel disease patients. *Inflamm Bowel Dis.*, Vol.16, No.6, (June 2010), pp. 907-9.

Tremelling, M.; Cummings, F.; Fisher, S.; Mansfield, J.; Gwilliam, R. & Satsangi, J. (2007). IL23R variation determines susceptibility but not disease phenotype in inflammatory bowel disease. *Gastroenterology*, Vol.132, No.5, (May 2007), pp. 1657-64.

Trynka, G.; Zhernakova, A.; Romanos, J.; Franke, L.; Hunt, K. & Wijmenga, C. (2009). Coeliac disease-associated risk variants in TNFAIP3 and REL implicate altered NF-kappaB signalling. *Gut*, 2009; Vol.58, No.8, (August 2009), pp. 1078–83.

Uhlig, H.; McKenzie, B.; Hue, S.; Thompson, C.; Joyce-Shaikh, B. & Powrie, F. (2006). Differential activity of IL-12 and IL-23 in mucosal and systemic innate immune pathology. *Immunity*, Vol.25, No.2, (August 2006), pp. 309–18.

Umeno, J.; Asano, K.; Matsushita, T.; Matsumoto, T.; Kiyohara, Y. & Kubo, M. (2011). Meta-analysis of published studies identified eight additional common susceptibility loci for Crohn's disease and ulcerative colitis. *Inflamm Bowel Dis.*, (February 2011).

Underhill, D. & Shimada, T. (2007). A pair of 9s: It's in the CARDs. *Nat. Immunol.*, Vol.8, No.2, (February 2007), pp.122–124.

Van der Heide, F.; Nolte, I.; Kleibeuker, J.; Wijmenga, C.; Dijkstra, G. & Weersma RK. (2010). Differences in genetic background between active smokers, passive smokers, and non-smokers with Crohn's disease. *Am J Gastroenterol.*, Vol.105, No.5, (May 2010), pp. 1165-1172.

Van der Sluis, M.; De Koning, B.; De Bruijn, A.; Velcich, A.; Meijerink, J. & Einerhand, A. (2006). Muc2-deficient mice spontaneously develop colitis, indicating that MUC2 is critical for colonic protection. *Gastroenterology*, Vol.131, No.1, (July 2006), pp. 117–129.

Van Limbergen, J.; Russell, R.; Drummond, H.; Aldhous, M.; Round, N. & Wilson, D. (2008a). Definition of phenotypic characteristics of childhood-onset inflammatory bowel disease. *Gastroenterology*, Vol.135, No.4, (October 2008), pp. 1114–22.

Van Limbergen, J.; Russell, R.; Nimmo, E.; Drummond, H.; Smith, L. & Satsangi, J. (2008b). Autophagy gene ATG16L1 influences susceptibility and disease location but not childhood-onset in Crohn's disease in Northern Europe. *Inflamm Bowel Dis.*, Vol.14, No.3, (March 2008), pp. 338-46.

Vandiedonck, C.; Capdevielle, C.; Giraud, M.; Krumeich, S.; Jais, J. & Garchon, H. (2006). Association of the PTPN22*R620W polymorphism with autoimmune myasthenia gravis. *Ann Neurol.*, Vol.59, No.2, (February 2006), pp. 404-407.

Vang, T.; Congia, M.; Macis, M.; Musumeci, L.; Orrú, V. & Bottini, N. (2005). Autoimmune-associated lymphoid tyrosine phosphatase is a gain-of-function variant. *Nat Genet.*, Vol.37, No.12, (December 2005), pp. 1317-1319.

Varade, J.; Palomino-Morales, R.; Ortego-Centeno, N.; Díaz-Rubio, M.; Fernández-Gutiérrez, B. & Martín, J. (2011). Analysis of the REL polymorphism rs13031237 in autoimmune diseases. *Ann Rheum Dis.*, Vol.70, No.4, (April 2011), pp. 711-2.

Vella, A.; Cooper, J.; Lowe, C.; Walker, N.; Nutland, S. & Todd, J. (2005). Localization of a type 1 diabetes locus in the IL2RA/CD25 region by use of tag single-nucleotide polymorphisms. *Am J Hum Genet.*, Vol.76, No.5, (May 2005), pp. 773-9.

Vernier-Massouille, G.; Balde, M.; Salleron, J.; Turck, D.; Dupas, J. & Colombel, J. (2008). Natural history of pediatric Crohn's disease: a population-based cohort study. *Gastroenterology,* Vol.135, No.4, (October 2008), pp. 1106–13.

Visekruna, A.; Joeris, T.; Seidel, D.; Kroesen, A.; Loddenkemper, C. & Steinhoff, U. (2006). Proteasome-mediated degradation of IkappaBalpha and processing of p105 in Crohn disease and ulcerative colitis. *J Clin Invest.*, Vol.116, No.12, (December 2006), pp. 3195-203.

Wallace, C.; Smyth, D.; Maisuria-Armer, M.; Walker, N.; Todd, J. & Clayton, D. (2010). The imprinted DLK1-MEG3 gene region on chromosome 14q32.2 alters susceptibility to type 1 diabetes. *Nat Genet.*, Vol.42, No.1, (January 2010), pp. 68-71.

Waller, S.; Tremelling, M.; Bredin, F.; Godfrey, L.; Howson, J. & Parkes, M. (2006). Evidence for association of OCTN genes and IBD5 with ulcerative colitis. *Gut,* Vol.55, No.6, (June 2006), pp. 809-14.

Wang, K.; Baldassano, R.; Zhang, H.; Qu, H.; Imielinski, M& Hakonarson, H. (2010). Comparative genetic analysis of inflammatory bowel disease and type 1 diabetes implicates multiple loci with opposite effects. *Hum Mol Genet.*, Vol.19, No.10, (May 2010), pp. 2059-67.

Waterman, M.; Xu, W.; Stempak, J.; Milgrom, R.; Bernstein, C. & Silverberg, M. (2010). Distinct and overlapping genetic loci in crohn's disease and ulcerative colitis: Correlations with pathogenesis. *Inflamm Bowel Dis.*, (December 2010).

Weersma, R.; Stokkers, P.; Cleynen, I.; Wolfkamp, S.; Henckaerts, L. & Vermeire, S. (2009). Confirmation of multiple Crohn's disease susceptibility loci in a large Dutch-Belgian cohort. *Am J Gastroenterol.*, Vol.104, No.3, (March 2009), pp. 630-638.

Wellcome Trust Case Control Consortium; Australo-Anglo-American Spondylitis Consortium (TASC); Burton, P.; Clayton, D.; Cardon, L. & Brown, M. (2007). Association scan of 14,500 nonsynonymous SNPs in four diseases identifies autoimmunity variants. *Nat Genet.*, Vol.39, No.11, (November 2007), pp. 1329-37.

Wilson, N.; Boniface, K.; Chan, J.; McKenzie, B.; Blumenschein, W. & de Waal Malefyt, R. (2007). Development, cytokine profile and function of human interleukin 17-producing helper T cells. *Nat Immunol.*, Vol.8, No.9, (September 2007), pp.950-7.

Yamanouchi, J.; Rainbow, D.; Serra, P.; Howlett, S.; Hunter, K. & Santamaria, P. (2007). Interleukin-2 gene variation impairs regulatory T cell function and causes autoimmunity. *Nat. Genet.*, Vol.39, No.3, (March 2007), pp. 329–37.

Yamazaki, K.; McGovern, D.; Ragoussis, J.; Paolucci, M.; Butler, H. & Nakamura, Y. (2005). Single nucleotide polymorphisms in TNFSF15 confer susceptibility to Crohn's disease. *Hum Mol Genet.*, Vol.14, No.22, (November 2005), pp. 3499-506.

Yamazaki, K.; Takahashi, A.; Takazoe, M.; Kubo, M.; Onouchi, Y. & Hata, A. (2009). Positive association of genetic variants in the upstream region of NKX2-3 with Crohn's disease in Japanese patients. *Gut*, Vol.58, No.2, (February 2009), pp. 228-232.

Yang, S.; Lim, J.; Chang, H.; Lee, I.; Li, Y.; Liu, J. & Song, K. (2008). Association of TNFSF15 with Crohn's disease in Koreans. *Am J Gastroenterol.*, Vol.103, No.6, (June 2008), pp. 1437-42.

Yang, S.; Jung, Y.; Hong, M.; Kim, H.; Ye, B.; Lee, I. & Song, K. (2011). No association between TNFSF15 and IL23R with ulcerative colitis in Koreans. *J Hum Genet.*, Vol.56, No.3, (March 2011), pp. 200-4.

Yen, D.; Cheung, J.; Scheerens, H.; Poulet, F.; McClanahan, T. & Rennick, D. (2006). IL-23 is essential for T cell-mediated colitis and promotes inflammation via IL-17 and IL-6. *J Clin Invest*, Vol.116, No.5, (May 2006), pp. 1310–6.

Zeggini, E.; Scott, L.; Saxena, R.; Voight, B.; Marchini, J. & Altshuler, D. (2008). Meta-analysis of genome-wide association data and large-scale replication identifies additional susceptibility loci for type 2 diabetes. *Nat Genet.*, Vol.40, No.5, (May 2008), pp. 638-45.

Zhang, H.; Qiu, L.; Chen, Y.; Zhu, W.; Mao, C. & Shi, J. (2009). ATG16L1 T300A polymorphism and Crohn's disease susceptibility: evidence from 13,022 cases and 17,532 controls. *Hum Genet.*, Vol.125, No.5-6, (June 2009), p. 627-631.

Zhernakova, A.; Festen, E.; Franke, L.; Trynka, G.; van Diemen, C. & Weersma, R. (2008). Genetic analysis of innate immunity in Crohn's disease and ulcerative colitis identifies two susceptibility loci harboring CARD9 and IL18RAP. *Am. J. Hum. Genet.*, Vol.82, No.5, (May 2008), pp. 1202–1210.

Zhernakova, A.; van Diemen, C. & Wijmenga, C. (2009). Detecting shared pathogenesis from the shared genetics of immune-related diseases. *Nat Rev Genet.*, Vol.10, No.1, (January 2009), pp. 43-55.

Zhernakova, A.; Elbers, C.; Ferwerda, B.; Romanos, J.; Trynka, G. & Wijmenga. C. (2010). Evolutionary and Functional Analysis of Celiac Risk Loci Reveals SH2B3 as a Protective Factor against Bacterial Infection. *Am J Hum Genet.*, Vol.86, No.6, (June 2010), pp. 970-7.

26

Genetics of Type 1 Diabetes

Marie Cerna
Charles University in Prague
The Czech Republic

1. Introduction

Type 1 diabetes (T1D) is considered as a complex genetic trait: not only do multiple genetic loci contribute to susceptibility, but environmental factors also play a major role in determining risk. A large body of evidence indicates that inherited genetic factors influence both susceptibility and resistance to the disease. There is significant familial clustering of T1D with an average prevalence risk in siblings of 7% and in a child of diabetic of 6%, compared to 0.4% in the general population. The degree of clustering of disease in families can be estimated from the ration of the risk for siblings or a patient with the disease and the population prevalence of that disease. If this ratio (λs) is close to 1, there is no evidence for familial clustering. For T1D, **the degree of familial clustering λs is about 15 (6/0.4%)**, which means that if a family has a child with T1D, then the other siblings are at a 15 times greater risk of developing diabetes than a member of the general population.

Genetic susceptibility in family members is clearly dependent on the degree of genetic identity with the proband, and in fact the risk of T1D in families has a non-linear correlation with the number of alleles shared with the proband; the highest risk is observed in monozygotic twins (100% sharing), followed by first and second degree relatives (50% and 25 % sharing respectively). Study of monozygotic twins provides a good opportunity to examine the expression of a human trait in a fixed genetic background: the absolute risk of a monozygotic twin of an effected individual gives a direct estimate of penetrance of this trait for a given environment. Although increased concordance rate for T1D has been found in monozygotic twins compared to dizygotic ones, it only reaches 40-50% with long-term follow-up.

The genetics of T1D has a long history of studies evaluating candidate genes for association with disease status in either case-control or family-based studies. Four chromosomal regions have emerged with consistent and significant evidence of association with T1D across multiple studies. These are the major locus - the human leukocyte antigen (HLA) region - on chromosome 6p21, the protein tyrosine phosphatase non receptor 22 (PTPN22) gene on chromosome 1p13, the insulin (INS) gene region on chromosome 11p15 and the high-affinity alpha chain of IL-2 receptor (IL2RA) gene on chromosome 10p15.

2. Strategies for identifying disease predisposing genes

Until very recently, three basic approaches have been used to identify genetic variants that may contribute to any human phenotype, including autoimmune disorders (Gregersen & Olsson, 2009). These approaches are a) candidate gene association studies, b) linkage analysis in multiplex families, and c) genome-wide association studies/scans (GWAS).

Candidate gene studies have been a mainstay for human genetic studies for several decades, and they will continue to play an important role. However, early candidate gene case-control studies often suffered from insufficient statistical power owing to inadequate sample sizes and to a lack of appreciation for the importance of careful matching of cases and controls. The strong publication bias for initial positive findings has been clearly documented (Ioannidis et al., 2001), and reports of candidate gene associations should be viewed with caution until multiple replications have been carried out. Candidate gene studies are usually done to address a plausible hypothesis, but plausibility should not mitigate the requirement for robust and reproducible statistical evidence.

Genetic linkage analysis depends on the cosegregation of chromosomal regions with a phenotypic trait within families, as is typical for highly penetrant Mendelian disorders. For most common autoimmune diseases, familial aggregation is rather modest, and therefore linkage analysis has quite low statistical power to detect chromosomal regions with shared genetic risk within families. Nevertheless, linkage approaches have occasionally contributed significantly to the identification of new risk genes.

In the last four years, GWAS have dominated efforts in gene mapping for autoimmune diseases, and these studies have led to the majority of the new genetic associations discussed in this review. Like candidate gene studies, the analysis is based on association, but in the case of GWAS, no particular hypothesis is being addressed. Rather, hundreds of thousands of hypotheses are being addressed simultaneously, without regard to biologic plausibility. This is a purely discovery-driven approach to gene identification, free of the limitations imposed by a priori assumptions about which genes and pathways are likely to be involved in the disease under study. Despite early skepticism, GWAS has proved to be a remarkably effective method of gene discovery.

Although the initial sequence of the human genome was an important first step, it is really the International HapMap Project that has provided the basis for a rational approach to GWAS (Frazer et al., 2007). When considering single nucleotide polymorphisms (SNPs), any two unrelated individuals in the population differ by approximately 0.1% across the 3.2 billion base pairs of the genome, or approximately 3 million SNPs. By studying 90 individuals in families from three major racial groups (Caucasian, Asian, and African), the HapMap Project has cataloged the majority of the common SNPs (e.g., SNPs with minor allele frequencies of 5% or greater) in these populations.

An important result of the HapMap Project has been the realization that to define most of the common variations among individuals, it is not necessary to genotype all 3 million SNP differences among them, but only a subset of these, on the order of 300,000 to 500,000 SNPs. This is because SNP alleles are distributed non-randomly among individuals, forming blocks of linkage disequilibrium (LD) that may extend from thousands to many hundreds of thousands of base pairs. This results in a kind of bar code that can be used to define the common genetic variation across the genome of a given individual.

This pattern of common variation across genomes had led to the concept of tagging SNPs (Chapman et al., 2003). This involves the use of a single SNP to tag a block of LD formed by many other SNPs, thus allowing for the interrogation of a large section of the genome with a single marker. A large block of LD encompasses several genes. Thus, many SNPs in this region are likely to provide evidence of association for diseases that are associated with the certain marker. Conversely, any association observed with such a SNP may be due to causal variants in any of the genes in this LD block. Additional functional and biological evidence, that this gene is involved in autoimmunity, is necessary to prove that the gene is the relevant risk gene in this region or that the marker used to first detect the association is causative. Once a SNP association is observed and confirmed, much work remains to be done to establish which genetic variants in the region are actually responsible (e.g., causative) for the association.

Furthermore, because many GWAS employ 500,000 or more SNPs across the genome, each addressing a separate hypothesis, the statistical significance levels must be adjusted for multiple testing. An overall p value of $< 5 \times 10^{-7}$ is now widely accepted as compelling evidence of true association, although it is quite clear that lower degrees of statistical significance often reflect real associations. In any case, truly convincing association always requires multiple replications in independent data sets.

A major consideration for GWAS, as well as any case-control association study, is the issue of proper matching of cases and controls. The availability of genome-wide SNP data across many different populations has now permitted the use of so-called ancestry informative markers (AIMS) to match more precisely cases and controls for their ethnic background. This is quite straightforward for major racial groups, such as Asian, Caucasian, and African, but is more challenging within these groups (Seldin & Price, 2008). Polymorphisms in European Caucasian populations nicely illustrate this problem. The certain SNP displays a wide range of allele frequencies in the normal population, generally increasing in frequency going from southern to northern Europe. Therefore, if the cases and controls are taken from different European subpopulations, there is considerable risk of false positive (or negative) results. This phenomenon is generally referred to as population stratification. In the experience of many investigators, self-report by study participants is an unreliable indicator of ancestry, but in the context of GWAS, it is possible to correct for unknown population stratification using the entire set of SNP markers.

Most of the associations with autoimmunity involve the detection of odds ratios between 1 and 2, with many associations on the lower end of this range. The sample sizes required to generate statistical significance in the setting of GWAS ($p < 5 \times 10^{-7}$) can be very large, depending on the allele frequency in the population and the odds ratios to be detected. For risk ratios on the order of 2 or more, sample sizes of 1000 are generally adequate. However, for risk ratios in the range of 1.2-1.3, even sample sizes of three or four thousand may have low statistical power depending on marker allele frequency (Iles, 2008). This magnitude of a population sample is now considered a minimum for a thorough analysis in the setting of a GWAS, and truly comprehensive genetic studies will require considerably larger sample sizes to be studied in the future.

3. HLA genes

The best evidence for a genetic component in the susceptibility to T1D comes from studies of the HLA genes in both populations and families as well as from animal models. It has been estimated that HLA provides up to 40-50% of the familial clustering of T1D. The contribution of the HLA region is easily detectable in genome-wide linkage analyses, as indicated by a LOD score of 65.8.

The HLA (human leukocyte antigens) region is a cluster of genes located within the major histocompatibility complex (MHC) on chromosome 6p21.3 (Mungall et al., 2003). MHC is a region of 4 million base pairs, what is 0.1% of the human genome. It contains over 100 genes, which are characterized by high degree of allele polymorphism. The human MHC is divided into three regions: class I, class II, and class III. **HLA class I genes** are located telomeric in the complex. They have single polypeptide chain containing 3 domains associated with β_2-microglobuline. The class I genes classically are HLA-A, -B and -C molecules. They are expressed on the surface of almost all tissue cells and their function is to present peptide antigens to CD8+ cytotoxic T-cells. **HLA class II genes** are located at the centromeric end of MHC and occupy a region of 1 million base pairs. Class II molecules are heterodimeric proteins consisting of heavy α-chain and lighter β-chain. Molecules are expressed on antigen presenting cells (monocytes, macrophages, B lymphocytes, dendritic cells and activated T lymphocytes). The HLA class II genes are HLA-DR, -DQ and -DP molecules and their major function is to present peptide antigens to CD4+ T-cells. **The MHC class III region** contains many genes with varying functions. The most studied genes are tumour necrosis factor and lymphotoxin (TNFA and TNFB).

The state of the immune tolerance to self antigens is maintained by a complex network of T and B lymphocytes and their regulatory products. The mechanisms, by which this discrimination between 'self' and 'non-self' is established, involved central thymic tolerance and peripheral or post-thymic tolerance (Roitt, Brostoff, Male, 2002). **Central thymic tolerance to self antigens (autoantigens)** results from deletion of differentiating T-cells that express antigen-specific receptors with high binding affinity for the HLA-peptide complex, where peptide antigen belongs to intrathymic self peptide antigens (negative selection). Low-affinity self-reactive T-cells, and T-cells with receptors specific for the HLA-peptide complex, where peptide antigens are not represented intrathymically, mature and join the peripheral T-cell pool (positive selection). **Post-thymic tolerance to self antigens** has five main mechanisms. Self-reactive T-cells in the circulation may ignore self antigens, for example when the antigens are in tissues sequestered from the circulation. Their response to a self antigen may be suppressed if the antigen is present in a privileged site. Self-reactive cells may under certain conditions be deleted or rendered anergic and unable to respond. Finally a state of tolerance to self antigens can also be maintained by immune regulation.

B-cell deletion takes place in both bone marrow and peripheral lymphoid organs. Differentiating B-cells that express surface immunoglobulin receptors with high binding affinity for self-membrane-bound antigens will be deleted soon after their generation in the bone marrow. A high proportion of short-lived, low-avidity, autoreactive B-cells appear in peripheral lymphoid organs. These cells may be recruited to fight against infection. From this point of view towards the HLA molecules, the discovery of function of HLA-DO, that is mainly expressed in B-cells and involved in antigenic peptide binding to HLA class II molecules in the endocytic pathway, has triggered interesting hypothesis.

The pathway resulting in the antigen processing and presentation of peptides on HLA class II begins with the biosynthesis of the HLA class II α and ß chains in the endoplasmic reticulum, where they form a trimeric complex with a co-expressed protein called invariant chain. The invariant chain, which fills the peptide-binding groove of the HLA class II molecule, directs the HLA class II molecule first to the Golgi and secondly to a specialized MHC class II compartment in the endosomal/lysosomal pathway. Here, invariant chain is proteolytically degraded in a stepwise fashion until only a fragment remains bound to the HLA class II molecule, called the class II-associated invariant chain peptide (CLIP). The exchange of CLIP for the stably binding antigenic peptides in the compartment is catalyzed by a specialized lysosomal chaperone called HLA-DM. The HLA class II peptide complexes are then transported to the cell surface for recognition by the CD4+ T lymphocytes.

HLA-DO molecule, expressed in B-cells, associates with DM thereby markedly affecting DM function. DO forms a unique, cell type-specific modulator that masters the immune response induced by B-cells (van Ham et al., 2000). First, DO reduces class II-mediated antigen presentation as a whole, leading to a generalized diminished CD4+ response. Second, DO regulates the composition of the class II-mediated peptide repertoire that will determine the specificity of the B cell-induced immune response. Both modulatory actions of DO may increase the threshold for nonspecific CD4+ activation and may prevent autoimmune responses, both of which could be obvious evolutionary selection criteria. In this respect, it is interesting to note that DO-deficient mice have a normal functioning immune system, but show higher levels of serum immunoglobulins. This may indicate that the absence of DO leads to a more generalized immune activation.

An association between HLA and autoimmune diabetes mellitus has been recognized for more than 20 years. The initial associations were found with the HLA class I serologically-defined alleles B8 and B15. When the HLA-DR locus was defined, it was found that T1D associated more closely with the **DR4** and **DR3** serotypes than the linked B8 and B15. Later, it was determined that DR4 was a haplotype consisting of a family of distinct HLA-DR and -DQ molecules. This led to the conclusion that the DQB1 locus of HLA-DQ is highly associated with T1D. Recent technologies, which have allowed for genome-wide searches for linkage in humans to T1D, have verified that HLA is a gene locus involved in T1D and, in fact, HLA is the major locus. The strongest association within the HLA gene complex is to combinations of DQA1 and DQB1.

Many studies have verified that **DQB1*0302** is a strong susceptibility gene and that the heterozygous combination of DQA1*0301-DQB1*0302 on the HLA-DR4 haplotype and DQA1*0501-DQB1*0201 on the HLA-DR3 haplotype results in a synergistically increased risk of T1D (Table 1). DQA1*0301-DQB1*0302 is the most prevalent risk conferring haplotype in Caucasians detected in 74% of type 1 diabetes patients followed by DQA1*0501-DQB1*0201 detected in 52% of Caucasian patients (Sanjeevi et al., 1995).

DQB1*0201	-	DQA1*0501	-	DRB1*0301
DQB1*0302	-	DQA1*0301	-	DRB1*0401

Table 1. Predisposition HLA haplotypes in T1D (marker IDDM1 of 6p21.3 locus).

Also, there is agreement that **DQB1*0602** allele, linked with DR2, is a strong protective gene (Kockum et al., 1993). The protective effect of DQB1*0602 is dominant to the susceptibility effects of DQB1*0302-DQA1*0301 and DQB1*0201-DQA1*0501 (Pugliese et al, 1995). A single copy of this DQB1*0602 allele is adequate to confer significant negative association.

HLA-DQ genes are of primary importance but HLA-DR genes modify the risk conferred by HLA-DQ (Sanjeevi et al., 1996). The risk associated with an HLA genotype is defined by the particular combination of susceptible and protective alleles. The frequencies of predisposition alleles, DQB1*0302 and DQB1*0201, are usually increased, while frequency of protective DQB1*0602 allele is usually decreased.

The categorization of T1D as an autoimmune disease is not ambiguous, with the presence of the predisposing HLA class II haplotypes, DRB1*04-DQB1*0302 and DRB1*03, in at least 90% of cases and the presence of autoantibodies and, more recently, autoreactive, anti-islet antigen-specific T-cells in the circulation of prediabetic individuals and of newly diagnosed and established cases (Todd, 2010). Transgenic mouse modeling (Nakayama et al., 2005; Mellanby et al., 2008) has provided direct support that it is the peptide-binding activity of the HLA class II molecules in antigen-presenting cells (APCs) for T lymphocyte peptide recognition that is the main mechanism of action of the DR and DQ molecules in T1D etiology. This is by far the major determinant of disease in the genome (Cucca et al., 2001; Zhang et al., 2008). In humans (and mice), susceptibility and resistance to T1D has been mapped to particular polymorphic peptide-binding pockets of the DQ molecule, pocket 9, and of DR, pockets 1 and 4 (and their mouse orthologs, IA and IE, respectively) (Cucca et al., 2001; Suri et al., 2005). It remains a goal to identify molecules that modulate the function of these pockets and could be therapeutic.

Class II molecules in APCs bind peptides from the currently identified autoantigens, preproinsulin (PPI), insulinoma-associated antigen 2 (I-A2), glutamic acid decarboxylase (GAD), and zinc transporter (ZnT8), and present these to CD4+ T-cell antigen receptors (TCRs) in the thymus and in the periphery, for example, in pancreatic lymph nodes and within the islets themselves (von Herrath, 2009). CD4+ T-cells provide help to CD8+ cytotoxic T-cells, which are the widely accepted most important killer of human islet beta cells in T1D autoimmunity (Skowera et al., 2008; Willcox et al., 2009).

Recent fine mapping of the extended MHC region, 8 Mb of chromosome 6p21, which was made possible by the development of high-throughput, dense, and genome-wide SNP genotyping (GWAS), has confirmed that the major susceptibility, and resistance, to T1D does indeed map to the HLA class II region of the MHC (Nejentsev et al., 2007; Howson et al., 2009).

This long-awaited comprehensive genetic mapping also showed that T1D susceptibility is modified, however, by lesser but still important effects of the specific allotypes of the equally polymorphic HLA class I molecules, HLA-B and HLA-A (Nejentsev et al., 2007; Howson et al., 2009). These molecules present peptides to cytotoxic CD8+ T-cells and are expressed strongly in the pancreatic insulin-producing beta cells (von Herrath, 2009). These recent HLA class I associations with T1D and additional histological evidence (Willcox et al., 2009) help secure a central role for CD8+ T-cells and their helpers, CD4+ T-cells and APCs, in T1D etiology.

4. Non-HLA genes

This central role for APC-peptide-T-cell interaction in T1D is emphasized. However, the etiopatogenesis of disease is completely dependent not only on the environment, but also on the alleles of multiple genes across the genome (Wicker et al., 2005), which products are involved in following immunological reactions. The specific MHC/peptide-TCR interaction, although necessary, is not sufficient to fully activate the T-cell. A second signal is required; otherwise the T-cell will become unresponsive. This second signal, also referred to as co-stimulation, is of crucial importance. The most potent co-stimulatory molecules known are B7s, which are Ig superfamily molecules, including B7-1 (CD80) and B7-2 (CD86). B7s exist as homodimers on the cell surface. These proteins are constitutively expressed on dendritic cells, but can be upregulated on monocytes, B-cells and probably other APCs. They are the ligands for other Ig superfamily molecules, CD28 and its homologue CTLA-4 (CD152) - which is expressed after T-cell activation. CD28 is the main co-stimulatory ligand expressed on naïve T-cells. CD28 stimulation has been shown to prolong and augment the production of IL-2 and other cytokines, and is probably important in preventing the induction of tolerance. CTLA-4, the alternative ligand for B7, is an inhibitory receptor limiting T-cell activation, resulting in less IL-2 production. Thus CD28, constitutively expressed, initially interacts with B7, leading to T-cell activation, but once this has peaked, the upregulation of CTLA-4 with its higher affinity limits the degree of activation, as available B7 will interact with CTLA-4.

Apart from the cell-surface interactions, cytokines, acting locally, are also involved in T-cell activation. IL-2 is responsible for promoting cell division in a resting T-cell. Triggering of the TCR along with co-receptors results in IL-2 synthesis by the T-cell itself. This binds to low-affinity IL-2 receptors on the T-cell surface that consist of two chains, beta and gamma. TCR triggering also results in expression of the alpha-chain of the IL-2 receptor, which, in conjugation with the other two chains, results in a high-affinity receptor. The alpha chain together with the beta chain binds IL-2, while the gamma chain signals to the cell. There is a transient production of IL-2 for 1-2 days. Other cytokines may also contribute to T-cell proliferation, and their relative representation in microenvironment determines development of certain T-cell subtypes. It is assumed that impairment of the balance between Th1 and Treg cells participates in etiopatogenesis of autoimmune diabetes. The transient expression of the high affinity IL-2 receptor for about 1 week after stimulation of the T-cell, together with the induction of CTLA-4 helps limit T-cell division. (In the absence of positive signals, the T-cells will start to die by programmed cell death, apoptosis.)

Based upon current analyses of completed genome screens, these non-HLA region genes may contribute relatively smaller (but significant) increments in genetic risk on an individual basis (Invernizzi & Gershwin, 2009). For example, PTPN22, INS, and IL2RA loci, which are the only other generally accepted genetic contributors to T1D risk, have a relative risk 3.9, 3.5 and 2.5, respectively. Other locus-specific effects range from 1.1-1.9.

In T1D, there are currently identified 52 non-HLA regions. For 15 of them, the most likely causal gene in the locus was defined, as supported by current functional evidence (Todd, 2010). Summary of candidate causal genes is in the Table 2. They are listed according to decreased relative risk. Further, there are currently identified 423 genes in the immediate high-association interval and 790 genes in the > 1 Mb regions. In addition, there are 167 and 433 non-protein-coding sequences in these two categories of regions, and these could well have altered functions owing to genome polymorphism.

Perhaps the most replicated and broadly relevant of these associations is with the intracellular **protein tyrosine phosphatase non receptor 22 (PTPN22)**. The gene for PTPN22 is located on chromosome 1p13.2. The initial association of PTPN22 with T1D was reported by Bottini et al., 2004, who took a candidate gene approach and focused on a nonsynonymous amino acid polymorphism (R620W, substitution of tryptophan for arginine) that was judged likely to have functional correlates. This polymorphism corresponds to a single nucleotide substitution of thymin for cytosine at the position 1858 of DNA (C1858T). In an independent effort, Begowich et al., 2004, selected PTPN22 as part of a limited genome-wide screen of likely functional variants in several thousand candidate genes, informed in part by previous linkage results. This led to the association of PTPN22 with RA. Both associations have now been widely replicated, and the PTPN22 associations with these and several other autoimmune diseases are among the most robust in the literature. For RA and T1D the PTPN22 620W allele confers a nearly two-fold risk for disease, with odds ratios in the range of 3-4 for homozygous individuals. Thus, in terms of strength of association, PTPN22 is second in importance only to the HLA for these two diseases.

Name	Original designation	Chromosome localization	RR value	Function in immune system
PTPN22		1p13.2	3,9	TCR and BCR signaling
INS	IDDM2	11p15.5	3,5	Autoantigen
IL2RA	IDDM10	10p15.1	2,5	T-cell and Treg homeostasis
CCR5		3p21.31	1,9	Th1-cell signaling
SH2B3		12q24.12	1,7	Intracellular adaptor protein
PTPN2		18p11.21	1,7	Negative regulation of T-cells
IL10		1q32.1	1,5	Inhibition of Th1-cells
CTLA-4	IDDM12	2q33.2	1,5	T-cell costimulatory inhibition
TLR7/TLR8		Xp22.2	1,4	Receptors for viral RNAs
IFIH1		2q24.2	1,4	Receptor for viral RNAs
IL2		4q27	1,3	T-cell and Treg homeostasis
GLIS3		9p24.2	1,3	Autoantigen
IKZF1		7p12.2	1,2	Lymphopoiesis regulation
IL7RA		5p13.2	1,2	Memory T-cell homeostasis
TAGAP	IDDM5	6q25.3	1,2	T-cell activation
IL18RAP		2q12.1	1,2	IFN-gamma induction

CCR5 = cytokine-chemokine receptor 5
CTLA-4 = cytotoxic T lymphocyte antigen 4
GLIS3 = GLIS family zinc finger 3
IFIH1 = interferon induced with helicase C domain 1
IKZF1 = IKAROS family zinc finger 1
IL2 = interleukin 2
IL10 = interleukin 10
IL2RA = interleukin 2 receptor alpha
IL7R = interleukin 7 receptor
IL18RAP = interleukin 18 receptor accessory protein
INS = insulin
PTPN22 = protein tyrosine phosphatase, non-receptor type 22
PTPN2 = protein tyrosine phosphatase, non-receptor type 2
SH2B3 = intracellular adaptor protein with PH and SH2 domains
TAGAP = T-cell activation RhoGTPase activating protein
TLR = Toll-like receptor

Table 2. The most significant non-HLA predisposition markers with known function in T1D (listed according to decreased value of RR).

The patterns of association between the PTPN22 620W allele and autoimmunity are instructive on many levels. First, PTPN22 was among the first and most convincing demonstrations that common susceptibility genes underlie diverse autoimmune phenotypes. In addition to T1D and RA, PTPN22 is associated with Graves' disease (Velaga et al., 2004), Hashimoto thyroiditis (Criswell et al., 2005), myasthenia gravis (Vandiedonck et al., 2006), systemic sclerosis (Dieude et al., 2008), generalized vitiligo (LaBerge et al., 2008), Addison's disease (Skinningsrud et al., 2008), and alopecia areata (Betz et al., 2008). Associations with juvenile idiopathic arthritis (JIA) and SLE have generally been weaker than for RA and T1D. Strikingly, there is no evidence of association with multiple sclerosis, and the 620W allele actually appears to be protective for Crohn's disease (Barrett et al., 2008). These contrasting patterns of association are likely to reflect fundamental similarities and differences in the mechanisms underlying the pathogenesis of these disorders. In general, it appears that an important feature of the PTPN22-associated diseases is that they all have a prominent component of humoral autoimmunity.

Knockout animals for Lyp (also known as PEP, the mouse ortholog of PTPN22) exhibit enhanced T-cell activation in combination with an increased production of antibodies (Hasegawa et al., 2004). This is consistent with the ability of PTPN22 to dephosphorylate Lck at the activating phosphotyrosine 394, leading to persistent phosphorylation and Lck activation in knockout animals. Lck is the tyrosine kinase of the Src family associated with CD4 and CD8. Yet somewhat surprisingly, the consequence of the 620W risk allele in humans is apparently a lower degree of T cell activation - an increased threshold for T-cell receptor signaling (Vang et al., 2005; Rieck et al., 2007). One clear biochemical consequence of the 620W polymorphism is to reduce the binding of PTPN22 with the intracellular kinase Csk (Bottini et al., 2004; Begovich et al., 2004). Indeed, amino acid position 620 of PTPN22 is located within one of several SH3 binding sites in the PTPN22 molecule. An important role of Csk is to inhibit Lck activity by phosphorylation of amino acid 505 of the Lck molecule (Vang et al., 2008). Whether this particular activity is affected by the 620W polymorphism in PTPN22 is unclear. Bottini and coworkers have proposed a model for interactions among Lck, PTPN22, and Csk that may explain the elevation of thresholds for TCR signaling, with the overall implication that reduced, rather than elevated, T-cell triggering may be part of the phenotypic predisposition to autoimmunity. A similar tendency to increased thresholds for receptor triggering has also been reported in B-cells (Rieck et al., 2007).

A second intracellular **protein tyrosine phosphatase non receptor 2 (PTPN2)** encoded on chromosome 18p11.21 has also been associated with human autoimmunity; convincing associations have been reported for T1D (Todd et al., 2007) and Crohn's disease (Wellcome Trust Case Control Consortium, 2007; Barrett et al., 2008), with odds ratios in the range of 1.3. PTPN2 is ubiquitously expressed and is clearly involved in immune function. PTPN2-knockout animals exhibit a fatal inflammatory wasting syndrome (Pao et al., 2007), with accompanying abnormalities in multiple cell types. PTPN2 appears to have a negative regulatory role on IL-2R signaling in T-cells, consistent with the fact that Janus family kinases 1 and 3 (Jak1 and Jak3) are among its substrates (Simoncic et al., 2002).

The **insulin (INS)** gene is located on chromosome 11p15.5. The immune-mediated process leading to development of T1D is highly specific to pancreatic beta cells. The insulin gene, therefore, is a plausible candidate susceptibility locus since preproinsulin has emerged as the most important autoantigen in childhood-onset T1D (Skowera et al., 2008).

Mutations of INS cause a rare form of diabetes that is similar to MODY (Maturity Onset Diabetes in the Young). Other variations of the insulin gene (variable number tandem repeats and SNPs) play a role in susceptibility to T1D and T2D. The polymorphism in the insulin minisatellite or variable number of tandem repeats (INS VNTR) are associated with the risk of diabetes and influence thymic insulin messenger RNA (Bell et al., 1984; Bennett et al., 1995, 1996). It is located 596bp upstream of the insulin gene translation initiation site and it is composed of a variable number of tandem repeats of 14-15bp in length based on the consensus sequence 5`-ACAGGGGTGTGGGG-3` (Bell et al., 1982). There are three main types of INS VNTR defined by their size: class I (26-63 repeats), class II (approximately 80 repeats) and class III (140-200 repeats). Each of them can be further divided based on the number of repeats and sequence. In white European population the minisatellite displays a bimodal allele size distribution with class I alleles and class III alleles at frequencies of 70% and 30%. Class II alleles are rare in white European population. Allelic variation in size of the insulin VNTR correlates with the expression of insulin in the pancreas and thymus and with placental expression of insulin growth factor-2 gene (IGF-2), which is downstream from the insulin gene (Moore et al., 2001).

Homozygosity for class I alleles is generally associated with high risk for diabetes, whereas class III alleles confer dominant protection. Class III alleles are associated with higher expression of insulin messenger RNA within the thymus and insulin with thymic transcription activity correlate inversely with susceptibility to diabetes in humans (Pugliese et al., 1997; Vafiadis et al., 1997). These findings support hypothesis that genetically determined differences in the expression of self antigens in the thymus could influence susceptibility to autoimmunity. High concentration of thymic insulin might lead to negative selection (deletion) of autoreactive T-cells bearing a TCR that is directed against self antigens and thus to the development of tolerance.

The gene encoding the **high-affinity alpha chain of the three-chain IL-2 receptor (IL2RA, CD25)** on chromosome 10p15.1 is also strongly associated with T1D with evidence for at least two distinct causal variants (Dendrou et al., 2009). Correlations, first with soluble CD25 in serum and plasma (Lowe et al., 2007), and then with mRNA and with CD25 surface expression (Dendrou et al., 2009), indicate unequivocally that IL2RA is a causal gene in this chromosome region. T1D-predisposing alleles of SNPs in intron 1 and the 5′region of the gene lower transcription, which results in lower amounts of CD25 on the surface of memory CD4+ T-cells and also in number of CD25+ naive CD4+ T-cells. One of the notable results to come out of this large-scale clinical study was that the expression of CD25 on memory T-cells was highly repeatable within the same person across several months and, thus, strongly heritable, indicating that here is an immunophenotype that is hard-wired into the human genome. For the 1% of the British population that have the most protective IL2RA genotype and most CD25 on these memory cells, there is considerable protection from T1D. Memory CD4+ T-cells with more CD25 on their surface secrete more IL-2 on stimulation, and hence, it is possible that T-cells are a source for IL-2, which could promote Treg cell function. From the results in T1D for the IL-2 and IL2R genes (there is an evidence for the exon 1 common synonymous SNP of IL2 and the SNP of IL2RB associations with T1D), one can ask the question: with such fundamental molecules being altered in the immune system, both of which are essential for immune tolerance, why are several immune diseases not associated with these variants? Answer can be simple: The balance between the functions of T effector and Treg cells appears to be important in human T1D (Lawson et al., 2008; Long et al., 2009, 2010).

Moreover, the **cytokine-chemokine receptor 5 (CCR5)** gene on chromosome 3p21.31, which has a naturally occurring, albeit rare (1% in populations), functionally disruptive variant, delta32 (the 32 base pair deletion), is associated with protection from T1D, RA, and celiac disease (Smyth et al., 2008), indicating the importance of chemokines and T-cell trafficking in T1D.

An exciting example of the rapid gain in knowledge is the **intracellular adaptor protein with PH and SH2 domains (SH2B3)** gene on chromosome 12q24.12. This gene was first associated with T1D (Todd et al., 2007), in which a nonsynonymous SNP, corresponding to a nonsynonymous amino acid polymorphism (R262W, substitution of tryptophan for arginine), was the most associated marker. The 262W allele is the nonancestral allele altering the sequence of a predicted functional pleckstrin homology domain, suggestive that this could be a causal SNP and gene. Subsequently, the same variant was associated with celiac disease (Hunt et al., 2008) and, most recently, with platelet count and cardiovascular disease (Soranzo et al., 2009). The latter study also focused on the R262W polymorphism and showed that the 262W allele lies on a very long extended conserved haplotype for which they provided evidence for very recent selection in European populations, presumably to help provide resistance to a pathogen(s). SH2B3 encodes Lnk, an important negative regulator of cell-signalling events from a number of receptors, including the TCR and MPL, the latter of which is the receptor for thrombopoietin on platelets. In general, Lnk negatively regulates lymphopoiesis and early hematopoiesis. It functions in responses controlled by cell adhesion and in crosstalk between integrin- and cytokine-mediated signalling (Takaki, 2008). The lnk-deficiency results in enhanced production of B-cells, and expansion as well as enhanced function of hematopoietic stem cells. These facts support the hypothesis that SH2B3 is the disease-causal gene in this chromosomal region.

Another candidate gene for T1D and other autoimmune diseases is located on chromosome 2q33.2 and encodes the T-cell costimulatory receptor, **cytotoxic T lymphocyte antigen 4 (CTLA-4, CD152)**. In addition to T1D (Ueda et al., 2003), many human autoimmune diseases are associated with SNPs in the CTLA-4 gene, including Graves' disease (Ueda et al., 2003), RA (Plenge et al., 2005), SLE (Barreto et al., 2004), and celiac disease (Smyth et al., 2008). Mutations or polymorphisms leading to altered activity of CTLA-4 are believed to play an important role in the risk for developing autoimmunity (Maier & Hafler, 2009). The effect of CTLA-4 gene seems to be independent of the HLA alleles or the insulin VNTR risk genotype (van der Auwera et al., 1997). There is a microsatellite marker in the 3'UTR of the CTLA-4 sequence, and several point polymorphisms have been detected at CTLA-4. A large-scale fine mapping and sequencing study has previously pinpointed the causal variant for T1D and Graves' disease to a SNP called CT60, which is located in the 3' untranslated region (UTR) of CTLA-4 near the polyA site. Such large-scale fine mapping studies are warranted for all other autoimmune diseases that have previously associated with variants at CTLA-4. Interestingly, some evidence has also been produced to suggest that CTLA-4 polymorphisms may influence gene expression. CTLA-4 functions as a potent negative T-cell regulator. Deficiency of CTLA-4 in mice leads to a lymphoproliferative disorder, causing death within 4 weeks of birth. More recently, its protein product has been shown to have an essential and specific role in Treg cell function in mice (Wing et al., 2008). One outstanding question is the role and function of the isoform of CTLA-4 that is missing the transmembrane domain (encoded by exon 3), referred to as soluble CTLA-4, and which is presumed to be secreted. The genetic analyses and correlation of CTLA-4 gene haplotypes with messenger RNA levels suggest that it is a reduction in the amount of soluble CTLA-4 that is responsible for the increased susceptibility to T1D in T-cells, including Treg cells (Atabani et al., 2005). Ueda et al., 2003, suggested that the disease susceptible genotype at the CT60 SNP (the G allele) influences the relative splicing efficiency and production of soluble CTLA-4 (sCTLA-4) versus full-length CTLA-4 (flCTLA-4) mRNA. In fact, GG homozygote individuals at CT60 (disease susceptible genotype) had half the levels of sCTLA-4 when normalized to flCTLA-4 compared with AA homozygote individuals at CT60. Indeed, the 3' UTR of CTLA-4 has been shown to regulate the mRNA steady-state levels of CTLA-4 and sequences in the 3' UTR regulate CTLA-4 mRNA stability and in vitro translation efficiency (Malquori et al., 2008). Another study has shown that the relative responsiveness of naive (CD4+ $CD45RA^{high}$) versus memory (CD4+ $CD45RA^{low}$) T-cell subsets to TCR signaling was altered in healthy donors with the susceptible G allele compared to healthy donors with the protective A allele at CT60 (Maier et al., 2007). The CT60 SNP, in combination with autoantibody measurement, has also allowed the identification of a subgroup of T1D subjects; the presence of autoantibodies against thyroid peroxidases (TPOAb) not only increases risk of T1D, but also results in an earlier age of onset of disease. Individuals with the G allele or GG genotype exhibit an almost twofold increased risk of having both T1D and TPOAbs (Howson et al., 2007). It is of interest to note that the CTLA4 association at CT60 with RA is also enhanced in subjects with RA who are seropositive for anti-citrulline antibodies (Plenge et al., 2005).

CTLA-4 is also important in preventing autoimmunity in a major mouse model of T1D, the non-obese diabetic (NOD) mouse. In addition to the full-length and soluble isoforms, a ligand-independent form of CTLA-4 (liCTLA-4) was discovered in mouse (Wicker et al., 2004). The mRNA for liCTLA-4 lacks exon 2 and therefore encodes a molecule lacking the CD80/CD86 ligand binding domain. In the NOD mouse, it is the liCTLA-4 isoform that is differentially regulated by susceptible and protective CTLA-4 alleles. This genotype-dependent expression of the liCTLA-4 isoform is most likely because of a synonymous SNP in an exon splicing silencer motif located in exon 2. The liCTLA-4 isoform was shown to strongly inhibit T-cell responses by binding and dephosporylating the TCR chain and emerged as a more potent negative T-cell regulator than flCTLA-4 in terms of proliferation and cytokine secretion (Vijayakrishnan et al., 2004). As reduced expression of sCTLA-4 and liCTLA-4 isoforms is associated with increased disease susceptibility in humans and the NOD mouse model, respectively, and liCTLA-4 has been shown to be a potent inhibitor of T-cell activation and/or expansion, human sCTLA-4 may have a similar role. These data suggest that autoimmune-susceptible alleles may directly predispose to loss or reduced levels of self-tolerance.

Concerning virus participation in disease etiopatogenesis, encouraging candidates for T1D are the **toll like receptor 7 - toll like receptor 8 (TLR7-TLR8)** region of chromosome Xp22.2 that encodes intracellular receptors for viral RNAs and for DNA and RNA from apoptotic cells, and the **interferon induced with helicase C domain 1 (IFIH1)** gene on chromosome 2q24.2 that also encodes intracellular receptor known to recognise viral RNA and mediate the innate immune response. IFIH1 is also termed as melanoma differentiation-associated protein 5 (MDA5). IFIH1 is causal in T1D based on the protective associations of four rare variants, where the derived alleles are predicted to reduce gene expression or function (Nejentsev et al., 2009). Most intriguingly, among the viruses detected by IFIH1 are viruses from the picornavirus family, of which enterovirus is a member. Enteroviruses, of which coxsackie virus is a member, are one of the most common types of viruses reported to be associated with T1D (Dotta et al., 2007). Binding of viral RNA to IFIH1 triggers the production of the type 1 interferons (alpha and beta), which could, in a highly plausible scenario, enhance anti-beta cell CD8+ cytotoxic T lymphocyte activity in islets via HLA class I upregulation on beta cells, and direct effects on CD4+ and CD8+ T-cells (Devendra & Eisenbarth, 2004; Li et al., 2008; von Herrath, 2009). The genetic results suggest that a variety of virus infections could, via increased type 1 interferon levels, enhance susceptibility to autoimmune beta-cell destruction and T1D, provided that susceptibility alleles at other loci are present. Seasonal differences in viral infections, combined with other seasonal effects such as reduced vitamin D levels in more northern countries during the winter months (Hyppönen & Power, 2007; Svoren et al., 2009), could help explain the well-established seasonality of T1D diagnosis itself.

The gene encoding the **GLI-similar 3 (GLIS3) protein** on chromosome 9p24.2 is also associated with T1D. GLIS3 protein belongs to a subfamily of the Krüppel-like zinc finger transcription factors. GLIS3 plays a key role in pancreatic development, particularly in the generation of beta-cells and in the regulation of insulin gene expression. It could be an autoantigen in T1D for which polymorphism in or near the gene alters its expression in beta-cells, as found for insulin. Mutations in GLIS3 have been implicated in a syndrome characterized by neonatal diabetes and congenital hypothyroidism (Senée et al., 2006) and in some patients accompanied by polycystic kidney disease, glaucoma and liver fibrosis. In addition, the GLIS3 gene has been associated with fasting glucose levels and type 2 diabetes (T2D) susceptibility (Dupuis et al., 2010). Therefore, this would be the first convincing example of a gene predisposing to both T1D and T2D. Otherwise, T1D and T2D are genetically and, therefore, etiologically distinct (Rafiq et al., 2008; Raj et al., 2009).

The gene on chromosome 7p12.2 encoding the **IKAROS family zinc finger 1 (IKZF1) protein,** that is an essential regulator of lymphopoiesis and immune homeostasis, has been implicated in the development of childhood acute lymphoblastic leukemia. The major IKZF1 genotype conferring susceptibility to this leukemia has been shown to protect against T1D (Swalford et al., 2011). This finding strengthens the link between autoimmunity and lymphoid cancers.

The gene encoding the **T-cell activation RhoGTPase activating protein (TAGAP)** on chromosome 6q25.3 is associated not only with T1D, but also with RA, celiac and Crohn's diseases. The TAGAP minor allele confers protection against RA, similar to previous reports of T1D but contrasting with celiac and Crohn's diseases in which the minor allele is associated with risk (Eyre et al., 2010). TAGAP is transiently expressed in activated T-cells, suggesting that it may have a role in immune regulation.

Exploring the genetic overlap between related diseases may reveal key common autoimmunity-inflammatory pathways, and that further combinations of more disease-specific variation at HLA and non-HLA genes, in interaction with epigenetic and environmental factors, determine the final clinical outcomes (Table 3).

It is interesting to note that the shared genetic predisposition between T1D and celiac disease (Smyth et al., 2008) supports further evaluation of the hypothesis that gut microflora dysbalance and gluten consumption might be an environmental factor in T1D leading to the alteration of the function of the gut immune system and its relationship with the pancreatic immune system (Turley et al., 2005; Vaarala et al., 2008; Wen et al., 2008). Conversely, genes classified as autoimmunity genes, because they are associated with T1D, contribute to celiac disease. However, there are some causal alleles with the effects in the opposite direction and some distinct differences in genetic susceptibility between the two diseases. There is also a certain significant overlap between T1D and RA that is much greater than between celiac disease and RA (Eyre et al., 2010). These data suggest that a common etiology may exist between T1D and celiac disease, but a common pathogenesis may exist between T1D and RA.

Shared causal variants among autoimmune diseases could suggest therapeutic targets applicable to more than one disease. However, the susceptibility loci unique to a particular disease are also of interest; differences may reflect genuine specificity between the diseases and may influence what determines the particular autoimmune phenotype that may have also clinical application.

Locus	Other autoimmune diseases
HLA	almost all autoimmune diseases
PTPN22	RA, Graves' disease, Hashimoto thyroiditis, myasthenia gravis, systemic sclerosis, generalized vitiligo, Addison's disease, alopecia areata, *weak association with* JIA and SLE, *opposite effect (protection) in* Crohn's disease, *no association with* celiac disease and multiple sclerosis
IL2RA	multiple sclerosis, *but no association with* celiac disease
CCR5	RA, celiac disease
SH2B3	celiac disease
PTPN2	celiac disease, Crohn's disease
CTLA4	Graves' disease, RA, SLE, celiac disease, Crohn's disease
TLR7/TLR8	celiac disease
IL7RA	multiple sclerosis
TAGAP	RA, *opposite effect (predisposition) in* celiac disease, Crohn's disease
IL18RAP	*opposite effect (predisposition) in* celiac disease, Crohn's disease

JIA = juvenile idiopathic arthritis
RA = rheumatic arthritis
SLE = systemic lupus erythematosus

Table 3. Predisposition loci in T1D associated with other autoimmune diseases.

5. Epigenetics

The other area that is relevant is the role of epigenetics (Wang et al., 2009; MacFarlane et al., 2009; Javierre et al., 2010), which provides a molecular bridge between genes and environment (Waterland et al., 2006; MacFarlane et al., 2009). Stochastic early epigenetic imprinting that can alter gene expression as well as environmentally-induced epigenetic changes (Waterland et al., 2006; MacFarlane et al., 2009; Tobi et al., 2009), including the aging process itself (Rakyan et al., 2010), could help account for the discordance of monozygotic twins for disease (Kaminsky et al., 2009). Recently, the first parentally imprinted susceptibility region has been reported, involving the DLK1-MEG3 locus on chromosome 14q32, in which expression of the maternal haplotype of these genes is suppressed by epigenetic mechanisms such that the risk of T1D at this locus is transmitted from fathers only (Wallace et al., 2010). Therefore, going forward, it will be necessary to combine studies correlating disease-associated SNP alleles and haplotypes with gene expression and splicing, with measurement of their methylation status (Todd, 2010). T1D genes are already known to have differentially-methylated regions that affect their expression, namely INS, IL2, and IL10.

6. Acknowledgments

This survey was funded by the Research design of the Ministry of Education and Youth of Czech Republic: Identification code: MSM 0021620814: Prevention, diagnostics and therapy of diabetes mellitus, metabolic and endocrine damage of organism.

7. References

Atabani SF, Thio CL, Divanovic S et al. (2005). Association of CTLA4 polymorphism with regulatory T cell frequency. *European Journal of Immunology*, 35, 2157-2162.

Barreto M, Santos E, Ferreira R et al. (2004). Evidence for CTLA4 as a susceptibility gene for systemic lupus erythematosus. *European Journal of Human Genetics*, 12, 620-626.

Barrett JC, Hansoul S, Nicolae DL et al. (2008). Genome-wide association defines more than 30 distinct susceptibility loci for Crohn's disease. *Nature Genetics*, 40, 955-962.

Begovich AB, Carlton VE, Honigberg LA et al. (2004). A missense single-nucleotide polymorphism in a gene encoding a protein tyrosine phosphatase (PTPN22) is associated with rheumatoid arthritis. *American Journal of Human Genetics*, 75, 330-337.

Bell GI, Selby MJ, Rutter WJ (1982). The highly polymorphic region near the human insulin gene is composed of simple tandemly repeating sequences. *Nature*, 295, 31-35.

Bell GI, Horita S, Karam JH (1984). A polymorphic locus near the human insulin gene is associated with insulin-dependent diabetes mellitus. *Diabetes*, 33, 176-183.

Bennett ST, Lucassen AM, Gough SC et al. (1995). Susceptibility to human type 1 diabetes at IDDM2 is determined by tandem repeat variation at the insulin gene minisatellite locus. *Nature Genetics*, 9, 284-292.

Bennett ST, Wilson AJ, Cucca F et al. (1996). IDDM2-VNTR-encoded susceptibility to type 1 diabetes: dominant protection and parental transmission of alleles of the insulin gene-linked minisatellite locus. *Journal of Autoimmunity*, 9, 415-421.

Betz RC, Konig K, Flaquer A et al. (2008). The R620W polymorphism in PTPN22 confers general susceptibility for the development of alopecia areata. *British Journal of Dermatology*, 158, 389-391.

Bottini N, Musumeci L, Alonso A et al. (2004). A functional variant of lymphoid tyrosine phosphatase is associated with type I diabetes. *Nature Genetics*, 36, 337-338.

Chapman JM, Cooper JD, Todd JA et al. (2003). Detecting disease associations due to linkage disequilibrium using haplotype tags: a class of tests and the determinants of statistical power. *Human Heredity*, 56, 18-31.

Criswell LA, Pfeiffer KA, Lum RF et al. (2005). Analysis of families in the multiple autoimmune disease genetics consortium (MADGC) collection: the PTPN22 620W allele associates with multiple autoimmune phenotypes. *American Journal of Human Genetics*, 76, 561-571.

Cucca F, Lampis R, Congia M et al. (2001). A correlation between the relative predisposition of MHC class II alleles to type 1 diabetes and the structure of their proteins. *Human Molecular Genetics*, 10, 2025-2037.

Dendrou CA, Plagnoi V, Fung E et al. (2009). Cell-specific protein phenotypes for the autoimmune locus IL2RA using a genotype-selectable human bioresource. *Nature Genetics*, 41, 1011-1015.

Devendra D, Eisenbarth GS (2004). Interferon alpha – a potential link in the pathogenesis of viral-induced type 1 diabetes and autoimmunity. *Clinical Immunology*, 111, 225-233.

Dieude P, Guedj M, Wipff J et al. (2008). The PTPN22 620W allele confers susceptibility to systemic sclerosis: findings of a large case-control study of European Caucasians and a meta-analysis. *Arthritis and Rheumatism*, 58, 2183-2188.

Dotta F, Censini S, van Halteren AG et al. (2007). Coxsackie B4 virus infection of beta cells and natural killer cell insulitis in recent-onset type 1 diabetic patients. *Proceedings of the National Academy of Sciences of the U.S.A.*, 104, 5115-5120.

Downes K, Pekalski M, Angus KL et al. (2010). Reduced expression of IFIH1 is protective for type 1 diabetes. *PLoS ONE*, 5, e12646.

Dupuis J, Langenberg C, Prokopenko I et al. (2010). New genetic loci implicated in fasting glucose homeostasis and their impact on type 2 diabetes risk. *Nature Genetics*, 42, 105-116.

Eyre S, Hinks A, Bowes J et al. (2010). Overlapping genetic susceptibility variants between three autoimmune disorders: rheumatoid arthritis, type 1 diabetes and coeliac disease. *Arthritis Research & Therapy*, 12, R175.

Frazer KA, Ballinger DG, Cox DR et al. (2007). A second generation human haplotype map of over 3.1 million SNPs. *Nature*, 449, 851-861.

Gregersen PK, Olsson LM (2009). Recent advances in the genetics of autoimmune disease. *Annual Review of Immunology*, 27, 363-391.

Hasegawa K, Martin F, Huang G et al. (2004). PEST domain-enriched tyrosine phosphatase (PEP) regulation of effector/memory T cells. *Science*, 303, 685-689.

Howson JM, Dunger DB, Nutland S et al. (2007). A type 1 diabetes sub-group with a female bias is characterized by failure in tolerance to thyroid peroxidase at an early age and a strong association with the cytotoxic T-lymphocyte-associated antigen-4 gene. *Diabetologia*, 50, 741-746.

Howson JM, Walker NM, Clayton D et al. (2009). Confirmation of HLA class II independent type 1 diabetes associations in the major histocompatibility complex including HLA-B and HLA-A. *Diabetes, Obesity & Metabolism*, 11 (Suppl.1), 31-45.

Hunt KA, Zhernakova A, Turner G et al. (2008). Newly identified genetic risk variants for celiac disease related to the immune response. *Nature Genetics*, 40, 395-402.

Hyppőnen E, Power C (2007). Hypovitaminosis D in British adults at age 45y: Nationwide cohort study of dietary and lifestyle predictors. *American Journal of Clinical Nutrition*, 85, 860-868.

Iles MM (2008). What can genome-wide association studies tell us about the genetics of common disease? *PLoS Genet*, 4, e33.

Invernizzi P, Gershwin ME (2009). The genetics of human autoimmune disease. *Journal of Autoimmunity*, 33, 290-299.

Ioannidis JP, Ntzani EE, Trikalinos TA et al. (2001). Replication validity of genetic association studies. *Nature Genetics*, 29, 306-309.

Javierre BM, Fernandez AF, Richter J et al. (2010). Changes in the pattern of DNA methylation associate with twin discordance in systemic lupus erythematosus. *Genome Research*, 20, 170-179.

Kaminsky ZA, Tang T, Wang SC et al. (2009). DNA methylation profiles in monozygotic and dizygotic twins. *Nature Genetics*, 41, 240-245.

Kang HS, ZeRuth G, Lichti-Kaiser K et al. (2010). Gli-similar (Glis) Krüppel-like zinc finger proteins: insights into their physiological functions and critical roles in neonatal diabetes and cystic renal disease. *Histology and Histopathology*, 25, 1481-1496.

Kockum I, Wassmuth R, Holmberg E et al. (1993). HLA-DQ primarily confers protection and HLA-DR susceptibility in type I (insulin-dependent) diabetes studied in population-based affected families and controls. *American Journal of Human Genetics,* 53, 150-167.

LaBerge GS, Bennett DC, Fain PR et al. (2008). PTPN22 is genetically associated with risk of generalized vitiligo, but CTLA4 is not. *Journal of Investigative Dermatology,* 128, 1757-1762.

Lawson JM, Tremble J, Dayan C et al. (2008). Increased resistance to CD4+CD25hi regulatory T cell-mediated suppression in patients with type 1 diabetes. *Clinical and Experimental Immunology,* 154, 353-359.

Li Q, Xu B, Michie SA et al. (2008). Interferon-alpha initiates type 1 diabetes in nonobese diabetic mice. *Proceedings of the National Academy of Sciences of the U.S.A.,* 105, 12439-12444.

Long SA, Walker MR, Rieck M et al. (2009). Functional islet-specific Treg can be generated from CD4+CD25- T cells of healthy and type 1 diabetic subjects. *European Journal of Immunology,* 39, 612-620.

Long SA, Cerosaletti K, Bollyky PL et al. (2010). Defects in IL-2R signaling contribute to diminished maintenance of FOXP3 expression in CD4(+)CD25(+) regulatory T-cells of type 1 diabetic subjects. *Diabetes,* 59, 407-415.

Lowe CE, Cooper JD, Brusko T et al. (2007). Large-scale genetic fine mapping and genotype-phenotype associations implicate polymorphism in the IL2RA region in type 1 diabetes. *Nature Genetics,* 39, 1074-1082.

MacFarlane AJ, Strom A, Scott FW (2009). Epigenetics: Deciphering how environmental factors may modify autoimmune type 1 diabetes. *Mammalian Genome,* 20, 624-632.

Maier LM, Anderson DE, De Jager PL et al. (2007). Allelic variant in CTLA4 alters T cell phosphorylation patterns. *Proceedings of the National Academy of Sciences of the U.S.A.,* 104, 18607-18612.

Maier LM, Hafler DA (2009). Autoimmunity risk alleles in costimulation pathways. *Immunological Reviews,* 229, 322-336.

Malquori L, Carsetti L, Ruberti G (2008). The 3′ UTR of the human CTLA4 mRNA can regulate mRNA stability and translational efficiency. *Biochimica et Biophysica Acta,* 1779, 60-65.

Mellanby RJ, Phillips JM, Parish NM et al. (2008). Both central and peripheral tolerance mechanisms play roles in diabetes prevention in NOD-E transgenic mice. *Autoimmunity,* 41, 383-394.

Moore GE, Abu-Amero SN, Bell G et al. (2001). Evidence that insulin is imprinted in the human yolk sac. *Diabetes,* 50, 199-203.

Mungall AJ, Palmer SA, Sims SK et al. (2003). The DNA sequence and analysis of human chromosome 6. *Nature,* 425, 805-811.

Nakayama M, Abiru N, Moriyama H et al. (2005). Prime role for an insulin epitope in the development of type 1 diabetes in NOD mice. *Nature,* 435, 220-223.

Nejentsev S, Howson JM, Walker NM et al. (2007). Localization of type 1 diabetes susceptibility to the MHC class I genes HLA-B and HLA-A. *Nature,* 450, 887-892.

Nejentsev S, Walker N, Riches D et al. (2009). Rare variants of IFIH1, a gene implicated in antiviral responses, protect against type 1 diabetes. *Science,* 324, 387-389.

Pao LI, Badour K, Siminovitch KA et al. (2007). Nonreceptor protein-tyrosine phosphatases in immune cell signaling. *Annual Review of Immunology,* 25, 473-523.

Plenge RM, Padyukov L, Remmers EF et al. (2005). Replication of putative candidate-gene associations with rheumatoid arthritis in >4,000 samples from North America and Sweden: association of susceptibility with PTPN22, CTLA4, and PADI4. *American Journal of Human Genetics,* 77, 1044-1060.

Pugliese A, Gianani R, Moromisato R et al. (1995). HLA-DQB1*0602 is associated with dominant protection from diabetes even among islet cell antibody-positive first-degree relatives of patients with IDDM. *Diabetes,* 44, 608-613.

Pugliese A, Zeller M, Fernandez A et al. (1997). The insulin gene is transcribed in the human thymus and transcription levels correlated with allelic variation at the INS VNTR-IDDM2 susceptibility locus for type 1 diabetes. *Nature Genetics,* 15, 293-297.

Rafiq S, Melzer D, Weedon MN et al. (2008). Gene variants influencing measures of inflammation or predisposing to autoimmune and inflammatory diseases are not associated with the risk of type 2 diabetes. *Diabetologia,* 51, 2205-2213.

Raj SM, Howson JM, Walker NM et al. (2009). No association of multiple type 2 diabetes loci with type 1 diabetes. *Diabetologia,* 52, 2109-2116.

Rakyan VK, Down TA, Maslau S et al. (2010). Human aging-associated DNA hypermethylation occurs preferentially at bivalent chromatin domains. *Genome Research,* 20, 434-439.

Rieck M, Arechiga A, Onengut-Gumuscu S et al. (2007). Genetic variation in PTPN22 corresponds to altered function of T and B lymphocytes. *Journal of Immunology,* 179, 4704-4710.

Roitt I, Brostoff J, Male D (2002). *Immunology* (6th ed.). Mosby, an imprint of Elsevier Science Limited.

Sanjeevi CB, Landin-Olsson M, Kockum I et al. (1995). Several residues in the DQA1 and DQB1 chain are either positively or negatively associated with insulin-dependent diabetes mellitus. *Diabetes,* 44, S1-S241.

Sanjeevi CB, Falorni A, Kockum I et al. (1996). HLA and glutamic acid decarboxylase in human insulin-dependent diabetes mellitus. *Diabetic Medicine,* 13, 209-217.

Seldin MF, Price AL (2008). Application of ancestry informative markers to association studies in European Americans. *PLoS Genet,* 4, e5.

Senée V, Chelala C, Duchatelet S et al. (2006). Mutations in GLIS3 are responsible for a rare syndrome with neonatal diabetes mellitus and congenital hypothyroidism. *Nature Genetics,* 38, 682-687.

Simoncic PD, Lee-Loy A, Barber DL et al. (2002). The T cell protein tyrosine phosphatase is a negative regulator of janus family kinases 1 and 3. *Current biology,* 12, 446-453.

Skinningsrud B, Husebye ES, Gervin K et al. (2008). Mutation screening of PTPN22: association of the 1858T-allele with Addison's disease. *European Journal of Human Genetics,* 16, 977-982.

Skowera A, Ellis RJ, Varela-Calviño R et al. (2008). CTLs are targeted to kill beta cells in patients with type 1 diabetes through recognition of a glucose-regulated preproinsulin epitope. *Journal of Clinical Investigation,* 118, 3390-3402.

Smyth DJ, Plagnol V, Walker NM et al. (2008). Shared and distinct genetic variants in type 1 diabetes and celiac disease. *New England Journal of Medicine,* 359, 2767-2777.

Soranzo N, Spector TD, Mangino M et al. (2009). A genome-wide meta-analysis identifies 22 loci associated with eight hematological parameters in the HaemGen consortium. *Nature Genetics,* 41, 1182-1190.

Suri A, Walters JJ, Gross ML et al. (2005). Natural peptides selected by diabetogenic DQ8 and murine I-A(g7) molecules show common sequence specificity. *Journal of Clinical Investigation,* 115, 2268-2276.

Svoren BM, Volkening LK, Wood JR et al. (2009). Significant vitamin D deficiency in youth with type 1 diabetes mellitus. *Journal of Pediatrics,* 154, 132-134.

Swafford AD, Howson JM, Davison LJ et al. (2011). An allele of IKZF1 (Ikaros) conferring susceptibility to childhood acute lymphoblastic leukemia protects against type 1 diabetes. *Diabetes,* 60, 1041-1044.

Takaki S (2008). Sh2b3/Lnk family adaptor proteins in the regulation of lymphohematopoiesis. *Japanese Journal of Clinical Immunology,* 31, 440-447.

Tobi EW, Lumey LH, Talens RP et al. (2009). DNA methylation differences after exposure to prenatal famine are common and timing- and sex-specific. *Human Molecular Genetics,* 18, 4046-4053.

Todd JA, Walker NM, Cooper JD et al. (2007). Robust associations of four new chromosome regions from genome-wide analyses of type 1 diabetes. *Nature Genetics,* 39, 857-864.

Todd JA (2010). Etiology of type 1 diabetes. *Immunity,* 32, 457-467.

Turley SJ, Lee JW, Dutton-Swain N et al. (2005). Endocrine self and gut non-self intersect in the pancreatic lymph nodes. *Proceedings of the National Academy of Sciences of the U.S.A.,* 102, 17729-17733.

Ueda H, Howson JM, Esposito L et al. (2003). Association of the T-cell regulatory gene CTLA4 with susceptibility to autoimmune disease. *Nature,* 423, 506-511.

Vaarala O, Atkinson MA, Neu J (2008). The "perfect storm" for type 1 diabetes: the complex interplay between intestinal microbiota, gut permeability and mucosal immunity. *Diabetes,* 57, 2555-2562.

Vafiadis P, Bennett ST, Todd JA et al. (1997). Insulin expression in human thymus is modulated by INS VNTR alleles at the IDDM2 locus. *Nature Genetics,* 15, 289-292.

Vandiedonck C, Capdevielle C, Giraud M et al. (2006). Association of the PTPN22*R620W polymorphism with autoimmune myasthenia gravis. *Annals of Neurology,* 59, 404-407.

Vang T, Congia M, Macis MD et al. (2005). Autoimmune-associated lymphoid tyrosine phosphatase is a gain-of-function variant. *Nature Genetics,* 37, 1317-1319.

Vang T, Miletic AV, Arimura Y et al. (2008). Protein tyrosine phosphatases in autoimmunity. *Annual Review of Immunology,* 26, 29-55.

van Ham M, van Lith M, Griekspoor A et al. (2000). What to do with HLA-DO? *Immunogenetics,* 51, 765-770.

van der Auwera BJ, Vandewalle CL, Schuit FC et al. (1997). CTLA-4 gene polymorphism confers susceptibility to insulin-dependent diabetes mellitus (IDDM) independently from age and from other genetic or immune disease markers. The Belgian Diabetes Registry. *Clinical and Experimental Immunology,* 110, 98-103.

Velaga MR, Wilson V, Jennings CE et al. (2004). The codon 620 tryptophan allele of the lymphoid tyrosine phosphatase (LYP) gene is a major determinant of Graves' disease. *Journal of Clinical Endocrinology and Metabolism,* 89, 5862-5865.

Vijayakrishnan L, Slavik JM, Illes Z et al. (2004). An autoimmune disease-associated CTLA-4 splice variant lacking the B7 binding domain signals negatively in T cells. *Immunity,* 20, 563-575.

von Herrath M (2009). Diabetes: A virus-gene collaboration. *Nature,* 459, 518-519.

Wallace C, Smyth DJ, Maisuria-Armer M et al. (2010). The imprinted DLK1-MEG3 gene region on chromosome 14q32.2 alters susceptibility to type 1 diabetes. *Nature Genetics,* 42, 68-71.

Wang Z, Schones DE, Zhao K (2009). Characterization of human epigenomes. *Current Opinion in Genetics & Development,* 19, 127-134.

Waterland RA, Lin JR, Smith CA et al. (2006). Post-weaning diet affects genomic imprinting at the insulin-like growth factor 2 (Igf2) locus. *Human Molecular Genetics,* 15, 705-716.

Wellcome Trust Case Control Consortium (2007). Genome-wide association study of 14,000 cases of seven common diseases and 3,000 shared controls. *Nature,* 447, 661-678.

Wen L, Ley RE, Volchkov PY et al. (2008). Innate immunity and intestinal microbiota in the development of type 1 diabetes. *Nature,* 455, 1109-1113.

Wicker LS, Chamberlain G, Hunter K et al. (2004). Fine mapping, gene content, comparative sequencing, and expression analyses support Ctla4 and Nramp1 as candidates for Idd5.1 and Idd5.2 in the nonobese diabetic mouse. *Journal of Immunology,* 173, 164-173.

Wicker LS, Clark J, Fraser HI et al. (2005). Type 1 diabetes genes and pathways shared by humans and NOD mice. *Journal of Autoimmunity,* 25 (Suppl.), 29-33.

Willcox A, Richardson SJ, Bone AJ et al. (2009). Analysis of islet inflammation in human type 1 diabetes. *Clinical and Experimental Immunology,* 155, 173-181.

Wing K, Onishi Y, Prieto-Martin P et al. (2008). CTLA-4 control over Foxp3+ regulatory T cell function. *Science,* 322, 271-275.

Zhang L, Nakayama M, Eisenbarth GS (2008). Insulin as an autoantigen in NOD/human diabetes. *Current Opinion in Immunology,* 20, 111-118.

27

Genetic Markers, Serological Auto Antibodies and Prediction of Type 1 Diabetes

Raouia Fakhfakh
Immunology Department, Habib Bourguiba Hospital
Sfax,
Tunisia

1. Introduction

The type 1 diabetes mellitus (formerly known as insulin-dependent diabetes mellitus) is a chronic autoimmune disorder that precipitates in genetically susceptible individuals by environmental factors (Atkinson and Eisenbarth 2001). The body's own immune system attacks the beta-cells in the islets of Langerhans of the pancreas, destroying or damaging them sufficiently to reduce and eventually eliminate insulin production.

The increase in understanding of the pathogenesis of type 1 diabetes has made it possible to consider intervention to slow the autoimmune disease process in an attempt to delay or even prevent the onset of hyperglycemia but varying in terms of their genetic, environmental, and amphopometric measures (2003).

Can we really predict type 1 diabetes? This is question has been a major target of diabetes research over the last decade. The aims have been to find a way of identifying individuals at risk and to accurately define their degrees of risk. Subjects who are at high risk for type 1 diabetes (T1D) can be identified using a combination of immune, genetic, and metabolic markers, For example, prediction of T1D among relatives can be quite accurate, by combining screening of relatives by measurement of islet cell autoantibodies with subsequent assessment of insulin autoantibodies (IAAs), first-phase insulin response to intravenous glucose, and oral glucose tolerance, while excluding those relatives with the known protective genetic allele HLA-DQB1-0602 (Pugliese, Gianani et al. 1995).

Using this combination approach and screening approximately 100,000 relatives, it was possible to identify accurately two cohorts of relatives, one (339 individuals) with a projected 5-year risk of greater than 50% and actual 5-year risk of 60%, (2002) and another (372 individuals) with a projected 5-year risk of 25–50% and actual 5-year risk of 35% (Skyler, Krischer et al. 2005).

The seminal research discovery of islet cell cytoplasmic autoantibodies (ICA) in 1974 not only offered clues to the autoimmune basis for type 1 diabetes but in addition, aided in providing some degree of clarity to the aforementioned difficulties associated with disease classification and diagnosis (Bottazzo, Florin-Christensen et al. 1974). The discovery of autoantibodies in T1D also supported the formation of a series of studies defining the natural history of metabolic and immunologic events underling the formation of this disease, the biochemical nature of islet cell autoantigens in the disorder, and trials attempting to predict as well as prevent the formation of T1D.

2. Animal models of type 1 diabetes

The availability of two animal models of type 1 diabetes has made it possible to evaluate plausible therapeutic strategies before starting human trials. Non-obese diabetic (NOD) mice and BioBreeding (BB) rats are in-bred strains that spontaneously develop autoimmune insulitis and diabetes with striking similarities to type 1 diabetes in humans (Mordes, Desemone et al. 1987; Elias and Cohen 1994).

The present landscape of basic and translational research in animal models of T1D is characterized by overuse of the NOD mouse. This scenario has some historic reasons that are understandable, foremost among those being the fact that NOD mice and humans share several susceptibility-related genes, including genes encoding the MHC class II homologs. But it is now also known that there is considerable complexity and heterogeneity in both the disease and in the genetics of the disease, and a singular focus on the NOD model generates too narrow a perspective.

The cumulative incidence of type 1 diabetes in these animals is high, and the onset of insulitis as well as hyperglycemia can be readily detected. Several interventions have been tested in these animals, often at a very early stage in the autoimmune disease process before the onset of insulitis. Examples include subcutaneous and oral insulin, nicotinamide, and the ß-cell antigen glutamic acid decarboxylase. Of note, many interventions have been effective in the murine models when applied before the development of hyperglycemia; however, very few interventions have reversed established diabetes.

3. Natural history of preclinical type 1 diabetes in humans

Type 1 diabetes is usually caused by autoimmune destruction of the insulin-producing ß-cells in the islets of Langerhans (Atkinson and Maclaren 1994). In the new classification of diabetes, immune mediated type 1 diabetes is called type 1A to distinguish it from some rarer cases in which an autoimmune etiology cannot be determined (type 1B); the latter are said to be idiopathic (1997).

Type 1 diabetes (T1D) occurs in genetically susceptible subjects. However many agree that an individual's genetic predisposition to this disease modified by environmental factors likely form a key facet for development (Knip 2003) (figure 1).

Indeed, the genetic predisposition for T1D, like most autoimmune disorders, in large part resides within genes controlling the immune response, principal amongst these being the major histocompatiblity complex (MHC). However, susceptibility and resistance for T1D does not reside in the MHC alone as more than two dozen additional loci outside of the MHC complex have been identified to influence risk for this disease (Melanitou, Fain et al. 2003; Atkinson 2005). Among the many potential candidate genes residing in such loci are BCL2, CD28, CTLA-4, CXCL12, interleukin-2 receptor and INS genes (Atkinson 2005).

The potential influence of environmental factors in T1D development has been suggested through multiple observations, the primary ones being the 500-fold variance in disease incidence based on geographic locale, seasonal variance in disease onset, and somewhat dramatic increases in the frequency of this disease, particularly over the last half-century. While environmental factors influencing T1D development have remained elusive (i.e., none have specifically been isolated), epidemiological studies have associated infant diet, viruses and perhaps increased hygiene as contributing events to this disease (Knip 2003). In terms of how they might contribute to disease, without specific identification, such models remain

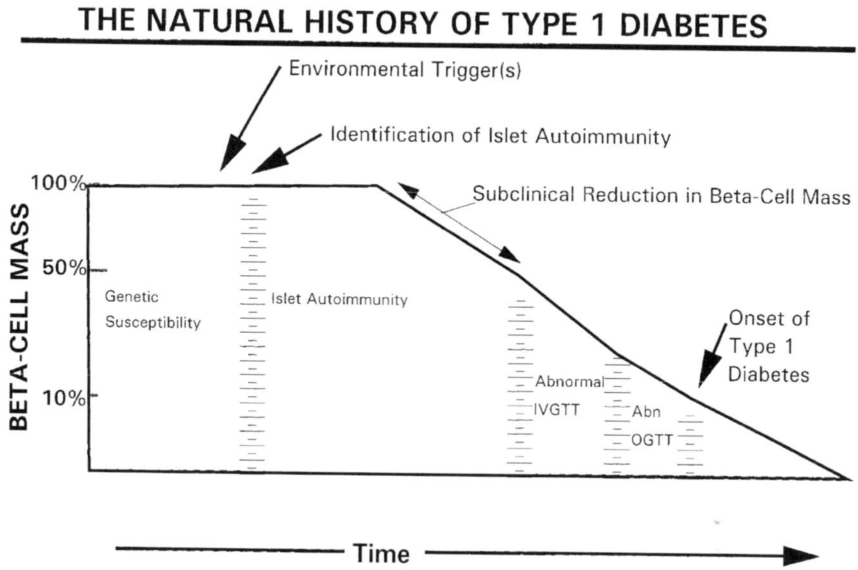

Fig. 1. The natural history of type 1 diabetes is depicted. In individuals with genetic predisposition to beta-cell autoimmunity, exposure to an environmental trigger or triggers is believed to initiate beta-cell autoimmunity, first evidenced in the appearance of islet autoantibodies. If beta-cell necrosis ensues as a consequence of destructive betacell cellular autoimmunity, a subclinical reduction in beta-cell mass ensues. The first clinical evidence of beta-cell dysfunction is an abnormal IVGTT result. With continued damage to the beta-cells, the OGTT will become abnormal. Within 1-2 years, frank symptoms of type 1 diabetes usually evolve (Winter, Harris et al. 2002).

hypothetical, but it is currently speculated that once the pathway to T1D has been initiated, either through as yet unknown triggers or natural physiological processes, various aberrant immune responses begin to play a role. It is important to note that many theories for environmental contributions to T1D development (e.g., viral molecular mimicry, β-cell trophic viruses, cow milk consumption, childhood vaccines, etc.), while popular in terms of their notion, have not proven themselves reproducible across a variety of study populations over time (Litherland, Xie et al. 1999; Atkinson 2005).

Despite genetics and environment forming knowledge voids for T1D pathogenesis, models for T1D development have been proposed that include these factors in combination with other findings (e.g., immunoregulatory defects, rate of metabolic loss, formation of anti-islet antibodies, etc.) which have been subject to better and more detailed description (Litherland, Xie et al. 1999). Under one such natural history model, defects in antigen presentation as well as antigen presenting cell maturation imparts an unnatural arrest in clearance of immune cells from the islets. The additional inability to regulate this response to self-antigens, a facet largely controlled by genetic susceptibility, would ultimately lead to a destructive islet cell inflammation (i.e., insulitis), with death of the insulin secreting β-cells (Brusko, Wasserfall et al. 2005). As the total β-cell mass declines, a critical point is reached where glucose homeostasis is lost and eventually exogenous insulin is an absolute requirement for survival.

Aside from model systems, thoughts continue that T-lymphocytes play the predominant role either directly (cytotoxicity) or indirectly (cytokine mediated β-cell apoptosis) in the destruction of islets. Adoptive transfer experiments in animal models have shown that T-lymphocytes transfer disease and serum does not. At the same time, recent studies have suggested key roles for B-lymphocytes in this process as one mouse model for T1D, the NOD mouse, when rendered deficient in these cells (either through genetic manipulation or through antibody treatment) fail to develop overt disease.

Hence, at one level, it is clear that B-lymphocytes are also involved inasmuch as they do produce autoantibodies (Brusko, Wasserfall et al. 2005) and in reality, it has been hypothesized that antigens presented by B lymphocytes may represent a critical feature to the development of T1D.

However, several aspects of the natural history of preclinical type 1 diabetes remain unclear, including the rate of progression and the changes in and predictive value of genetic and metabolic markers.

4. Biomarkers of susceptibility - tools for disease prediction

4.1 Genetic markers

Genetic markers may be helpful in assessing the risk of type 1 diabetes in close relatives of a patient with type 1 diabetes. The risk is markedly increased in these relatives, averaging about 6 percent in offspring and 5 percent in siblings (versus 0.4 percent in subjects with no family history) (Atkinson and Maclaren 1994).

The major genetic determinants of type 1 diabetes reside in the HLA region within the major histocompatibility complex (MHC) on the short arm of chromosome 6. An association between HLA class I alleles and type 1 diabetes was first described in the early 1970s (Nerup, Platz et al. 1974). More recent observations have indicated that the genes in the HLA-DQ region are even more closely associated with type 1 diabetes than the DR genes (Morel, Dorman et al. 1988). Over 90 percent of patients with type 1 diabetes carry DR4, DQB*0302 and/or DR3, DQB*0201. Thus, if the proband is heterozygous for DR3 and DR4 (the highest risk combination), the incidence of type 1 diabetes in a sibling who shares these two haplotypes rises to 19 percent. On the other hand, the absence of the above alleles makes type 1 diabetes very unlikely, especially if the subject carries a protective allele such as DQB*0301, *0602 (Pugliese, Gianani et al. 1995), DRB*0403, or *0406.

Use of genetic markers plus the family history make it possible to estimate the risk of type 1 diabetes as being as low as one in 5000 (no susceptibility alleles or family history) to as high as one in four (two susceptibility alleles and a positive family history). However, the prevalence of the HLA susceptibility genes is relatively high in whites. As a result, the predictive value of HLA typing is much lower in population screening than it is among families in which one or more members have type 1 diabetes (Bingley, Bonifacio et al. 1993) (Table 1).

In one study, the risk for islet autoimmunity drastically increased in DR3/4-DQ2/DQ8 siblings who shared both HLA hapl9otypes identical by descent with their diabetic proband sibling (63 and 85 percent by ages 7 and 15, respectively) as compared to siblings who did not share both HLA haplotypes with their diabetic proband sibling (Aly, Ide et al. 2006). These data suggest that HLA genotyping at birth may identify individuals at very high risk of developing type 1 diabetes before the occurrence of clear signs of islet autoimmunity and type 1 diabetes onset. Rapid automated assays make it possible to do large-scale population screening for HLA easily, even in newborns (Ilonen, Reijonen et al. 1996; Rewers, Bugawan et al. 1996)

Population	Type 1 Diabetes Risk (%)
Low Risk	
No affected FDR plus HLA protective genes	0.01
No affected FDR	0.4
Affected FDR plus HLA protective genes	0.3
Intermediate Risk	
No affected FDR plus HLA risk genes	4
One affected FDR	5
Mother with T1D	3
Father with T1D	5
Sibling with T1D	8
High Risk	
One affected FDR plus HLA high risk genes	10–20
Multiple affected FDRs	20–25
Very High Risk	
Identical twin affected	30–70
Multiple affected FDRs plus HLA risk genes	50
Sibling affected plus HLA risk genes, identical by descent	30–70

FDR, first-degree relative; HLA risk genes, *HLA DRB1*03,*04;DQB1*0302*; HLA protective genes, *HLA DQB1*0602*.

Table 1. Type 1 Diabetes Risk Stratification by T1D Family History and HLA Genotyping.

In general, the additional measurement of 2 HLA-DQ high-risk haplotypes does not increase the predictive value of combined autoantibody assays. However, in relatives who are seronegative for conventional islet autoantibodies, the presence of two HLA-DQ high-risk haplotypes is associated with an increased risk of progression to type 1 diabetes (Pietropaolo, Becker et al. 2002). This observation suggests that unidentified autoimmune phenomena may be present in seronegative relatives who carry the 2 HLA-DQ high-risk haplotypes.

Furthermore, specific allelic combinations of variants in the insulin gene (INS), the cytotoxic T lymphocyte antigen-4 gene (CTLA4) and the protein tyrosine phosphatase, non-receptor type 22 gene (PTPN22) have been repeatedly associated with type 1 diabetes susceptibility (Undlien, Lie et al. 2001; Pugliese and Miceli 2002; Ueda, Howson et al. 2003) using different approaches and increasing the number of susceptibility loci considered simultaneously generally increases the predictive value for T1D disease. The receiver operating characteristic (ROC) curve analysis confirms that, despite the higher absolute risk for those few with combinations of several risk markers, adding non-HLA genetic markers only marginally increases the utility of the prediction over that of HLA alone.

Despite near-multiplicative effects for most loci, and the fact that groups with very high relative risk of type 1 diabetes can be identified by testing for multiple susceptibility genes, only a small proportion of the population (and cases with type 1 diabetes) simultaneously carry HLA and multiple non-HLA susceptibility genotypes.

4.2 Immunologic markers

4.2.1 Islet autoantibodies:

The most important change in the T1D risk status of a child occurs when islet autoantibodies develop. Several clinically useful serum autoantibodies can be detected during the preclinical period of type 1 diabetes, including islet-cell antibodies (ICA), insulin

autoantibodies (IAA), antibodies to glutamic acid decarboxylase (GAD), and antibodies to tyrosine phosphatase-like proteins such as insulinoma associated protein (IA-2, ICA512).
Furthermore, only 8 to 10% of all cases of type 1 diabetes have a family history, while 90% of cases occur sporadically (Dahlquist, Blom et al. 1985). It was therefore important to examine the prevalence and the prognostic value of autoantibodies in the general population.
ICA is polyclonal autoantibodies that react with all cells of the islet (i.e., α, β, δ, and pancreatic polypeptide cells). The next major discovery in terms of humoral autoimmunity in T1D was that of autoantibodies to insulin or IAA (Williams, Bingley et al. 1999).
The presence of ICA was associated with an increased risk of diabetes, particularly if the ICA titer was high, ICA were persistently detected, or ICA were present in combination with IAA or GAD antibodies (Verge, Stenger et al. 1998).
Similar findings have been reported with IA-2. In one study of first-degree relatives of type 1 diabetic probands, those with IA-2 autoantibodies in the upper three quartiles were at higher risk than relatives with an IA-2 autoantibody titer in the lowest quartile (Achenbach, Bonifacio et al. 2008).
In another study, an autoantibody response directed to the extracellular domain of IA-2 was associated with very high risk of type 1 diabetes progression, suggesting the presence of new antigenic determinants within the extracellular domain of IA-2 (Morran, Casu et al.). This has considerable implications not only for stratifying high type 1 diabetes risk, but also to facilitate the search for pathogenic epitopes to enable the design of peptide-based immunotherapies, which may prevent the progression to overt type 1 diabetes at its preclinical stages.
Unlike NOD mice, an animal model for type 1 diabetes, humans exhibit any combination of ICA, IAA, GAD, and IA-2 antibodies (Kaufman, Clare-Salzler et al. 1993; Tisch, Yang et al. 1993; Greenbaum, Sears et al. 1999). The risk of type 1 diabetes is relatively low with IAA alone, but is higher with the presence of multiple autoantibodies against islet antigens (insulin, GAD, IA-2 and ICA) (Bingley 1996; Pietropaolo and Eisenbarth 2001). Antibodies to GAD are predictive of progression to hyperglycemia even in the absence of ICA or IAA (Verge, Stenger et al. 1998). As with IAA, however, the risk is higher in subjects who are ICA-positive.
Parallel studies have shown the presence of these autoantibodies in the sera of individuals prior to the onset of T1D (Bingley 1996; Bingley, Bonifacio et al. 2001; Achenbach, Warncke et al. 2004). At the onset of disease using GADA, IA-2A and IAA in combination offers N85% sensitivity and 98% specificity (Bingley, Bonifacio et al. 2001). The sensitivity at onset of T1D for ICA is 70–90%, GADA 70–80%, IA-2A 50–70% and IAA 30–50% respectively, with the variances in the ranges reflecting the population differences between studies. In terms of prediction, multiple large intervention trials, while failing to prevent T1D, have validated the predictive value of these autoantibodies for T1D (Gale, Bingley et al. 2004) (Figure 2).
The titter of IAA has been used to predict the time to onset of type 1 diabetes, particularly in children younger than five years of age (Ziegler, Ziegler et al. 1989). In a prospective, cohort study of 1353 offspring of parents with type 1 diabetes, antibodies detected in the first six months were derived by placental transfer from the mother. Autoantibodies began to appear by nine months and frequently persisted. IAA were almost always the first to appear, with other antibodies (ICA, GAD, or IA-2) appearing later. By age five years, nine (1.8 percent) children had developed type 1 diabetes, and all had one or more autoantibodies beforehand. Fifty percent of children who had two or more antibodies

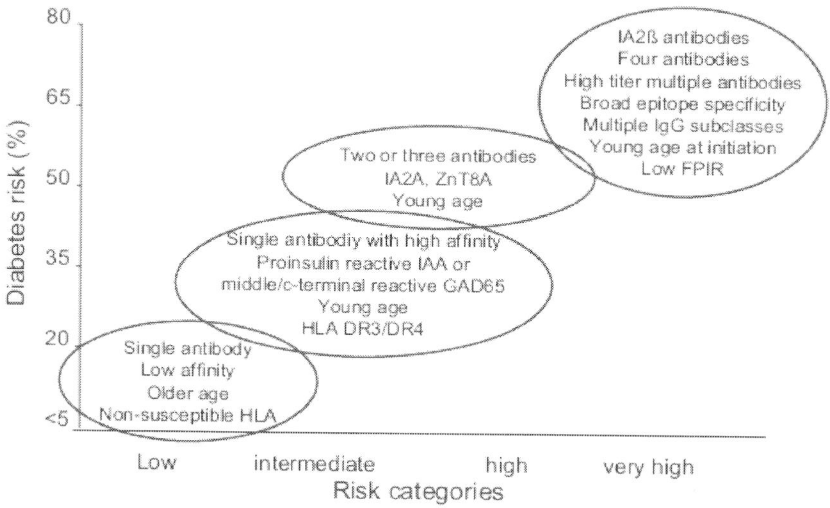

Fig. 2. Type 1 diabetes (T1D) risk stratification by islet autoantibody characteristics. Characteristics associated with low, intermediate, high, and very high risk are grouped from left to right on the abscissa with corresponding T1D risks on the ordinate. Increase in T1D risk is associated with progression of islet autoantibodies from single to multiple autoantibodies. HLA genotype discriminates risk in single antibody-positive children, but multiple antibody-positive children have high risk regardless of HLA genotype.

present by two years had diabetes by age five years (Ziegler, Hummel et al. 1999). In a follow-up report of a slightly larger cohort (1610 offspring), the following results were seen (Hummel, Bonifacio et al. 2004):

- By age five years, the frequencies of islet autoantibodies, multiple autoantibodies, and type 1 diabetes were 5.9, 3.5, and 1.5 percent, respectively.
- The risk of diabetes was highest in those with multiple autoantibodies (40 percent within five years versus 3 percent in those with single autoantibodies).
- Progression to multiple islet autoantibodies was fastest in children who developed their first autoantibody by age two years.
- The risk of progression to diabetes was inversely related to the age of positivity for multiple islet autoantibodies (50 percent of children who had multiple positivity before age 9 months developed diabetes within two years, compared to 7 percent in those who had multiple autoantibodies at age five years).

Thus, children with the earliest evidence of autoimmunity are at greatest risk for and progress more quickly to the development of type 1 diabetes. Periodic testing for islet autoantibodies appears to help assess the risk of diabetes in children of parents with type 1 diabetes.

In another study of 81 Swedish children who later developed type 1 diabetes, 14 (17 percent) had at least one autoantibody present at birth (either GAD, IAA, or ICA512), as compared with 12 of 320 (4 percent) control children (Lindberg, Ivarsson et al. 1999). Four percent had

more than one autoantibody present, compared with none of the control children. This study suggests that the autoimmune process may start in utero, but that this is rare.
In addition to identifying subjects at risk for type 1 diabetes, the presence of ICA and GAD antibodies can also identify late-onset type 1 diabetes in adults thought to have type 2 diabetes. In a study of 97 Swedish diabetic patients who were initially thought to have type 2 or unclassifiable diabetes, 70 became insulin-dependent after six years of follow-up. Among these 70 patients, 60 percent were positive for either ICA or GAD at diagnosis, compared with only 2 percent of the 27 patients who remained responsive to oral therapy.
The presence of these serological markers was closely correlated with histological evidence of insulitis in a study of 29 patients with recently diagnosed type 1 diabetes (Imagawa, Hanafusa et al. 2001). Pancreatic biopsies obtained within these months of diagnosis revealed a T-cell infiltration of pancreatic islets and hyperexpression of HLA class I antigens on islet cells. These features were much more evident among patients with high serum ICA concentration, or the presence of GAD, IAA, or multiple antibodies.
The absence of islet autoantibodies, however, does not exclude type 1 diabetes (House and Winter 1997). The appearance of islet autoantibodies in pancreas transplant recipients predicts recurrence of type 1 diabetes (Bosi, Braghi et al. 2001). Type 1 diabetes can occur after organ donation, and thus living kidney donors from families with histories of type 1 diabetes should be screened for islet autoantibodies (Riley, Maclaren et al. 1990).

4.2.2 Zinc transporter antibodies

In 2007, zinc transporter-8 (ZnT8) was identified as a novel diabetes autoantigen (Wenzlau, Juhl et al. 2007). Autoantibodies against the cation efflux zinc transporter (ZnT8A) have also been identified as a candidate type 1 diabetes autoantigen and proposed as additional markers of rapid disease progression (Wenzlau, Juhl et al. 2007). This study demonstrated that ZnT8 antibodies (ZnTA) were found in 26% of T1D subjects classified as autoantibody-negative on the basis of existing markers (GADA, IA2A, IAA, and ICA). In addition, sixty to 80 percent of patients with newly diagnosed type 1 diabetes have ZnT8 autoantibodies.
The function of this transporter is unknown. But, the combined measurement of ZnT8A, GADA, IA2A, and IAA raised autoimmunity detection rates to 98% at disease onset, a level that approaches that needed to detect prediabetes in a general pediatric population.
A recent study was examined the added value of measuring both IA-2βA and ZnT8A for prediction of impending diabetes in siblings or offspring of type 1 diabetic patients. It confirms the association of IA-2A, IA-2βA and ZnT8A with rapid disease progression and demonstrates that IA-2A and ZnT8A represent the most sensitive combination of two markers to identify relatives with a high progression rate.

4.3 Metabolic markers

Efficacious prevention of T1D will require detection of the earliest events in the process. Autoimmunity is likely the predominant effector mechanism in T1D, but it is possibly not its primary cause. A recent interesting report by Oresic et al. (Oresic, Simell et al. 2008) (see sect. **V***A*) showed that elevated serum concentrations of lysophosphatidyl choline precede the appearance of each islet autoantibody, and thus overt autoimmunity, in T1D. If these results are validated in other well-characterized cohorts, like the German BABYDIAB (Achenbach, Koczwara et al. 2004; Baschal, Aly et al. 2007), the United States-based DAISY (Baschal, Aly et al. 2007) and PANDA (Carmichael, Johnson et al. 2003) studies, and the multinational TEDDY study (Hagopian, Lernmark et al. 2006), metabolome screening could be added to the screening panel to effectively identify pre-diabetic individuals for preventive treatments.

Although glucose tolerance remains normal until close to the onset of hyperglycemia (Atkinson, Maclaren et al. 1990), the acute insulin response to several secretagogues (glucose, arginine, glucagon and isoproterenol) decreases progressively during the preclinical period (Aanstoot, Sigurdsson et al. 1994). The most useful and widely performed test is the acute (or "first phase") insulin response to glucose (FPIR) during an intravenous glucose tolerance test (IVGTT); in this test the rise in serum insulin above baseline is measured during the first 10 minutes after an intravenous glucose challenge; the response correlates with the functioning ß-cell mass (figure 3). The IVGTT has been standardized to allow easier comparison between centers (McCulloch, Bingley et al. 1993). In first-degree relatives of patients with type 1 diabetes, for example, an FPIR below the first percentile of normal is a strong predictor of type 1 diabetes.

In the Diabetes Prevention Trial-Type 1 Diabetes (DPT-1), subjects at high risk for developing diabetes were followed with serial IVGTTs and oral glucose tolerance tests (OGTTs), and in a subsequent study, the metabolic factors associated with progression to diabetes were evaluated (Barker, McFann et al. 2007).

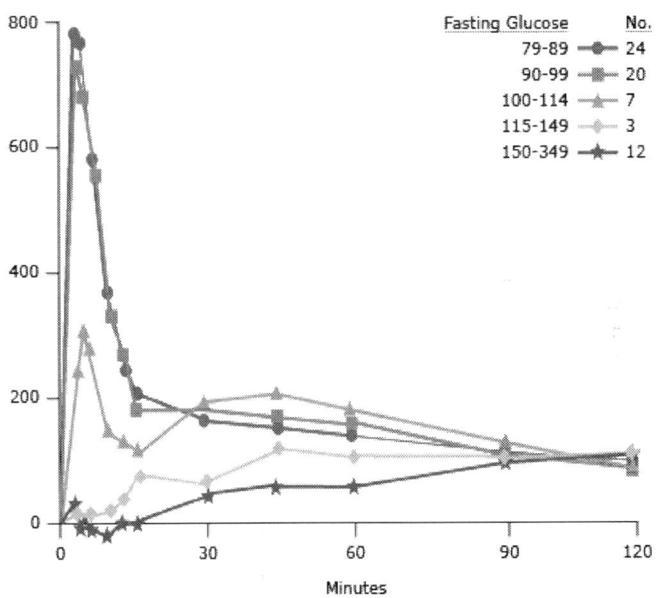

Fig. 3. Relative acute insulin response to IV glucose. Reproduced with permission from Brunzell et al. (Brunzell, Robertson et al. 1976) http://jcem.endojournals.org. Copyright © 1976 The Endocrine Society.

Abnormalities of FPIR and two-hour glucose during OGTT had similar sensitivities for diabetes prediction within six months of diagnosis (76 percent for OGTT [95% CI 60-83%] and 73 percent for FPIR [95% CI 60-83%]). Sensitivity was better when both tests were performed, and the vast majority of these individuals (97 percent) had abnormal IVGTTs and/or OGTTs before the development of the overt diabetes. In contrast, fasting blood glucose levels were a poor predictor of diabetes.
The more important as pathogenetical significance was the finding of increased proinsulin in first degree relatives or descendants from diabetic parents, both with type 1 (Roder, Knip et al. 1994; Truyen, De Pauw et al. 2005). Truyen *et al.* (Truyen, De Pauw et al. 2005) considered that the increased plasma proinsulin levels can be an additional marker for the prediction of type 1 diabetes. A simpler test that may prove useful is to measure the fasting serum concentration of proinsulin, the precursor of insulin. In normal subjects, proinsulin accounts for approximately 15 percent of serum immunoreactive insulin. This proportion rises as ß-cell function declines. One report, as an example, found that serum proinsulin concentrations were three to four times higher among ICA-positive relatives of type 1 diabetes patients as compared with ICA-negative relatives. However, prospective studies are needed to determine whether elevated serum proinsulin values will help in predicting the development of type 1 diabetes.

4.4 Combining risk biomarkers

Since genetic susceptibility is only part of the risk factors for common diseases, genetic markers alone usually do not have adequate specificity. There is growing evidence that combining multiple genetic and clinical markers is the best way to develop a molecular test with clinically useful predictive power.
Various combinations can be used to obtain similar overall risk, and for most combinations the risk can be calculated empirically. Risk can be stratified from less than 0.1% to greater than 70%. Current approaches use a stepwise decision tree (Krischer, Cuthbertson et al. 2003) in which genetic risk is usually the first applied in the form of family history or HLA DR-DQ genotype. Autoantibodies are measured in those individuals who are considered to have sufficient genetic risk to warrant autoantibody testing. Because the risk of developing multiple islet autoantibodies is strongly linked to major histocompatibility complex (MHC) class II genotypes,(Walter, Albert et al. 2003) further typing is unlikely to be helpful in a child who has an armada of islet autoantibodies. Finally, beta cell function is measured in islet autoantibody-positive individuals using either the ability of the beta cell to secrete insulin in response to an intravenous glucose challenge or the ability of the individual to clear glucose after a meal challenge where low insulin secretion (eg, less than the first percentile) or impaired glucose tolerance are indicators of late-stage preclinical T1D.
Although the decision tree approach is logical, it may be expected that once effective preventative therapies become available, the decision tree approach could be replaced by the population-wide application of all the previously mentioned markers in a public health prevention manner. Clinicians may eventually move toward introducing a risk score based on the combination of all markers. This would represent a paradigm shift after years of increasingly complex layers of decisions in screening.
Finally, the T1D risk of an individual is not static throughout life. This is true even for genetically defined risk. Risk in a child who has no family history of T1D at birth increases more than 10-fold if his or her sibling develops T1D, and if the child has an identical twin

who develops T1D, risk immediately increases 100-fold to around 50% (Redondo, Jeffrey et al. 2008). Risk calculated from the autoantibody status usually increases over time as autoantibodies appear and their number rises. Younger age is associated with increased risk than older age. Beta cell function measures are expected to show decrease the closer someone is to disease onset. Over the lifespan of an individual, the calculated T1D risk on the basis of genes, autoantibody, age, and beta cell function change.

5. Conclusions

Type 1 diabetes is an immunemediated disease leading to chronic insulin deficiency due to extensive and selective -cell destruction in subjects with increased genetic disease susceptibility (Atkinson and Eisenbarth 2001). As far as diagnosis of T1D versus other forms of diabetes the autoantibodies and genetic markers are of great value. There remains a subset of patients that are autoantibody negative at onset. This subset may at times present a diagnostic challenge and it is of importance for treatment to know if T1D (absolute requirement for insulin) or type 2 diabetes with a relative insulin resistance is present.

The occurrence of multiple antibodies against islet autoantigens serves as a surrogate marker of disease in primary or secondary intervention strategies aimed at halting the disease process (Pietropaolo and Eisenbarth 2001). Genetic typing for susceptibility or protective HLA alleles can also be performed.

In a research setting, the following approach may be used (McCulloch and Palmer 1991):

- Test individuals at risk for type 1 diabetes progression for GAD65 and IA-2 autoantibodies.
- If they are present and confirmed in a subsequent sample, tests for insulin and islet cell antibodies can be done and the FPIR determined.

Nonetheless, the studies performed to date have given us tremendous insight into the natural history of T1Ds (Eisenbarth 2004; Achenbach, Bonifacio et al. 2005; Sherry, Tsai et al. 2005). As a consequence, at present we can predict the development of T1D. Ideally, we would like to couple such prediction with prevention, but unfortunately we do not yet have a safe and effective preventive therapy.

Successful prevention depends on *1*) a good prediction/ identification of at-risk individuals and 2) a very safe intervention that causes no harm in those individuals who would have never developed T1D. Knowledge of the primary cause of T1D might not be crucial, even at the preventive stage. This statement is based on the fact that immune modulation appears to work in a variety of T1D models and at different stages of the disease. However, many preventive trials are based on data from the NOD mouse model which has improved our understanding of disease pathophysiology. A comprehensive analysis by Shoda et al. (Shoda, Young et al. 2005) concluded that "some popular tenets regarding NOD interventions were not confirmed: all treatments do not prevent disease, treatment dose and timing strongly influence efficacy, and several therapies have successfully treated overtly diabetic mice." So, the good news is that some preventive strategies appear to have a good chance to cure the disease, even during an advanced status of beta-cell destruction. Examples of succesful treatments in NOD mice are ATG, anti-CD3, hsp, and proinsulin DNA vaccine.

Ideally, the balance between therapeutic efficacy and disease stage should be known prior to human trials.

A major problem with preventive trials is that it takes many years before conclusions can be drawn. As can be seen in Table 2, preventive trials divide in two main classes.

Agent	Target/Mechanism	Development Phase, Clinical ID, Organizer
Vitamin D_3	Treg induction	Pilot, NCT00141986*, CDA
Omega-3 fatty acids	Anti-inflammatory	Phase II, NCT00333554*, NIDDK
Hydrolyzed cow's milk	Abnormal handling of intact foreign protein	TRIGR, Phase II, NCT00179777*, CHEO
Oral insulin	Ag-specific tolerance (oral)	Phase II, NCT00419562*, NIDDK
Nasal insulin	Ag-specific tolerance (mucosal)	Phase III, NCT00223613*, University of Turku
		Phase II, NCT00850161*, CPEX Pharma
		Phase II, NCT00336674*, Melbourne Health

* More information is available at http://www.clinicaltrials.gov/.
CDA, Canadian Diabetes Association; CHEO, Children's Hospital of Eastern Ontario; NIDDK, National Institute of Diabetes and Digestive and Kidney Diseases.

Table 2. Prevention trials in T1D.

6. References

(1997). "Report of the Expert Committee on the Diagnosis and Classification of Diabetes Mellitus." Diabetes Care 20(7): 1183-97.

(2002). "Effects of insulin in relatives of patients with type 1 diabetes mellitus." N Engl J Med 346(22): 1685-91.

(2003). "Report of the expert committee on the diagnosis and classification of diabetes mellitus." Diabetes Care 26 Suppl 1: S5-20.

Aanstoot, H. J., E. Sigurdsson, et al. (1994). "Value of antibodies to GAD65 combined with islet cell cytoplasmic antibodies for predicting IDDM in a childhood population." Diabetologia 37(9): 917-24.

Achenbach, P., E. Bonifacio, et al. (2005). "Natural history of type 1 diabetes." Diabetes 54 Suppl 2: S25-31.

Achenbach, P., E. Bonifacio, et al. (2008). "Autoantibodies to IA-2beta improve diabetes risk assessment in high-risk relatives." Diabetologia 51(3): 488-92.

Achenbach, P., K. Koczwara, et al. (2004). "Mature high-affinity immune responses to (pro)insulin anticipate the autoimmune cascade that leads to type 1 diabetes." J Clin Invest 114(4): 589-97.

Achenbach, P., K. Warncke, et al. (2004). "Stratification of type 1 diabetes risk on the basis of islet autoantibody characteristics." Diabetes 53(2): 384-92.

Aly, T. A., A. Ide, et al. (2006). "Extreme genetic risk for type 1A diabetes." Proc Natl Acad Sci U S A 103(38): 14074-9.

Atkinson, M. A. (2005). "ADA Outstanding Scientific Achievement Lecture 2004. Thirty years of investigating the autoimmune basis for type 1 diabetes: why can't we prevent or reverse this disease?" Diabetes 54(5): 1253-63.

Atkinson, M. A. and G. S. Eisenbarth (2001). "Type 1 diabetes: new perspectives on disease pathogenesis and treatment." Lancet 358(9277): 221-9.

Atkinson, M. A. and N. K. Maclaren (1994). "The pathogenesis of insulin-dependent diabetes mellitus." N Engl J Med 331(21): 1428-36.

Atkinson, M. A., N. K. Maclaren, et al. (1990). "The natural history and predictive value of Mr 64,000 autoantibodies for insulin-dependent diabetes mellitus." J Autoimmun 3 Suppl 1: 41-5.

Barker, J. M., K. McFann, et al. (2007). "Pre-type 1 diabetes dysmetabolism: maximal sensitivity achieved with both oral and intravenous glucose tolerance testing." J Pediatr 150(1): 31-36 e6.

Baschal, E. E., T. A. Aly, et al. (2007). "HLA-DPB1*0402 protects against type 1A diabetes autoimmunity in the highest risk DR3-DQB1*0201/DR4-DQB1*0302 DAISY population." Diabetes 56(9): 2405-9.

Bingley, P. J. (1996). "Interactions of age, islet cell antibodies, insulin autoantibodies, and first-phase insulin response in predicting risk of progression to IDDM in ICA+ relatives: the ICARUS data set. Islet Cell Antibody Register Users Study." Diabetes 45(12): 1720-8.

Bingley, P. J., E. Bonifacio, et al. (1993). "Can we really predict IDDM?" Diabetes 42(2): 213-20.

Bingley, P. J., E. Bonifacio, et al. (2001). "Proposed guidelines on screening for risk of type 1 diabetes." Diabetes Care 24(2): 398.

Bosi, E., S. Braghi, et al. (2001). "Autoantibody response to islet transplantation in type 1 diabetes." Diabetes 50(11): 2464-71.

Bottazzo, G. F., A. Florin-Christensen, et al. (1974). "Islet-cell antibodies in diabetes mellitus with autoimmune polyendocrine deficiencies." Lancet 2(7892): 1279-83.

Brunzell, J. D., R. P. Robertson, et al. (1976). "Relationships between fasting plasma glucose levels and insulin secretion during intravenous glucose tolerance tests." J Clin Endocrinol Metab 42(2): 222-9.

Brusko, T. M., C. H. Wasserfall, et al. (2005). "Functional defects and the influence of age on the frequency of CD4+ CD25+ T-cells in type 1 diabetes." Diabetes 54(5): 1407-14.

Carmichael, S. K., S. B. Johnson, et al. (2003). "Prospective assessment in newborns of diabetes autoimmunity (PANDA): maternal understanding of infant diabetes risk." Genet Med 5(2): 77-83.

Dahlquist, G., L. Blom, et al. (1985). "The epidemiology of diabetes in Swedish children 0-14 years--a six-year prospective study." Diabetologia 28(11): 802-8.

Eisenbarth, G. S. (2004). "Prediction of type 1 diabetes: the natural history of the prediabetic period." Adv Exp Med Biol 552: 268-90.

Elias, D. and I. R. Cohen (1994). "Peptide therapy for diabetes in NOD mice." Lancet 343(8899): 704-6.

Gale, E. A., P. J. Bingley, et al. (2004). "European Nicotinamide Diabetes Intervention Trial (ENDIT): a randomised controlled trial of intervention before the onset of type 1 diabetes." Lancet 363(9413): 925-31.

Greenbaum, C. J., K. L. Sears, et al. (1999). "Relationship of beta-cell function and autoantibodies to progression and nonprogression of subclinical type 1 diabetes: follow-up of the Seattle Family Study." Diabetes 48(1): 170-5.

Hagopian, W. A., A. Lernmark, et al. (2006). "TEDDY--The Environmental Determinants of Diabetes in the Young: an observational clinical trial." Ann N Y Acad Sci 1079: 320-6.

House, D. V. and W. E. Winter (1997). "Autoimmune diabetes. The role of autoantibody markers in the prediction and prevention of insulin-dependent diabetes mellitus." Clin Lab Med 17(3): 499-545.

Hummel, M., E. Bonifacio, et al. (2004). "Brief communication: early appearance of islet autoantibodies predicts childhood type 1 diabetes in offspring of diabetic parents." Ann Intern Med 140(11): 882-6.

Ilonen, J., H. Reijonen, et al. (1996). "Rapid HLA-DQB1 genotyping for four alleles in the assessment of risk for IDDM in the Finnish population. The Childhood Diabetes in Finland (DiMe) Study Group." Diabetes Care 19(8): 795-800.

Imagawa, A., T. Hanafusa, et al. (2001). "Pancreatic biopsy as a procedure for detecting in situ autoimmune phenomena in type 1 diabetes: close correlation between serological markers and histological evidence of cellular autoimmunity." Diabetes 50(6): 1269-73.

Kaufman, D. L., M. Clare-Salzler, et al. (1993). "Spontaneous loss of T-cell tolerance to glutamic acid decarboxylase in murine insulin-dependent diabetes." Nature 366(6450): 69-72.

Knip, M. (2003). "Environmental triggers and determinants of beta-cell autoimmunity and type 1 diabetes." Rev Endocr Metab Disord 4(3): 213-23.

Krischer, J. P., D. D. Cuthbertson, et al. (2003). "Screening strategies for the identification of multiple antibody-positive relatives of individuals with type 1 diabetes." J Clin Endocrinol Metab 88(1): 103-8.

Lindberg, B., S. A. Ivarsson, et al. (1999). "Islet autoantibodies in cord blood from children who developed type I (insulin-dependent) diabetes mellitus before 15 years of age." Diabetologia 42(2): 181-7.

Litherland, S. A., X. T. Xie, et al. (1999). "Aberrant prostaglandin synthase 2 expression defines an antigen-presenting cell defect for insulin-dependent diabetes mellitus." J Clin Invest 104(4): 515-23.

McCulloch, D. K., P. J. Bingley, et al. (1993). "Comparison of bolus and infusion protocols for determining acute insulin response to intravenous glucose in normal humans. The ICARUS Group. Islet Cell Antibody Register User's Study." Diabetes Care 16(6): 911-5.

McCulloch, D. K. and J. P. Palmer (1991). "The appropriate use of B-cell function testing in the preclinical period of type 1 diabetes." Diabet Med 8(9): 800-4.

Melanitou, E., P. Fain, et al. (2003). "Genetics of type 1A (immune mediated) diabetes." J Autoimmun 21(2): 93-8.

Mordes, J. P., J. Desemone, et al. (1987). "The BB rat." Diabetes Metab Rev 3(3): 725-50.

Morel, P. A., J. S. Dorman, et al. (1988). "Aspartic acid at position 57 of the HLA-DQ beta chain protects against type I diabetes: a family study." Proc Natl Acad Sci U S A 85(21): 8111-5.

Morran, M. P., A. Casu, et al. "Humoral autoimmunity against the extracellular domain of the neuroendocrine autoantigen IA-2 heightens the risk of type 1 diabetes." Endocrinology 151(6): 2528-37.

Nerup, J., P. Platz, et al. (1974). "HL-A antigens and diabetes mellitus." Lancet 2(7885): 864-6.

Oresic, M., S. Simell, et al. (2008). "Dysregulation of lipid and amino acid metabolism precedes islet autoimmunity in children who later progress to type 1 diabetes." J Exp Med 205(13): 2975-84.

Pietropaolo, M., D. J. Becker, et al. (2002). "Progression to insulin-requiring diabetes in seronegative prediabetic subjects: the role of two HLA-DQ high-risk haplotypes." Diabetologia 45(1): 66-76.

Pietropaolo, M. and G. S. Eisenbarth (2001). "Autoantibodies in human diabetes." Curr Dir Autoimmun 4: 252-82.

Pugliese, A., R. Gianani, et al. (1995). "HLA-DQB1*0602 is associated with dominant protection from diabetes even among islet cell antibody-positive first-degree relatives of patients with IDDM." Diabetes 44(6): 608-13.

Pugliese, A. and D. Miceli (2002). "The insulin gene in diabetes." Diabetes Metab Res Rev 18(1): 13-25.

Redondo, M. J., J. Jeffrey, et al. (2008). "Concordance for islet autoimmunity among monozygotic twins." N Engl J Med 359(26): 2849-50.

Rewers, M., T. L. Bugawan, et al. (1996). "Newborn screening for HLA markers associated with IDDM: diabetes autoimmunity study in the young (DAISY)." Diabetologia 39(7): 807-12.

Riley, W. J., N. K. Maclaren, et al. (1990). "Development of IDDM after donating kidney to diabetic sibling." Diabetes Care 13(8): 883-5.

Roder, M. E., M. Knip, et al. (1994). "Disproportionately elevated proinsulin levels precede the onset of insulin-dependent diabetes mellitus in siblings with low first phase insulin responses. The Childhood Diabetes in Finland Study Group." J Clin Endocrinol Metab 79(6): 1570-5.

Sherry, N. A., E. B. Tsai, et al. (2005). "Natural history of beta-cell function in type 1 diabetes." Diabetes 54 Suppl 2: S32-9.

Shoda, L. K., D. L. Young, et al. (2005). "A comprehensive review of interventions in the NOD mouse and implications for translation." Immunity 23(2): 115-26.

Skyler, J. S., J. P. Krischer, et al. (2005). "Effects of oral insulin in relatives of patients with type 1 diabetes: The Diabetes Prevention Trial--Type 1." Diabetes Care 28(5): 1068-76.

Tisch, R., X. D. Yang, et al. (1993). "Immune response to glutamic acid decarboxylase correlates with insulitis in non-obese diabetic mice." Nature 366(6450): 72-5.

Truyen, I., P. De Pauw, et al. (2005). "Proinsulin levels and the proinsulin:c-peptide ratio complement autoantibody measurement for predicting type 1 diabetes." Diabetologia 48(11): 2322-9.

Ueda, H., J. M. Howson, et al. (2003). "Association of the T-cell regulatory gene CTLA4 with susceptibility to autoimmune disease." Nature 423(6939): 506-11.

Undlien, D. E., B. A. Lie, et al. (2001). "HLA complex genes in type 1 diabetes and other autoimmune diseases. Which genes are involved?" Trends Genet 17(2): 93-100.

Verge, C. F., D. Stenger, et al. (1998). "Combined use of autoantibodies (IA-2 autoantibody, GAD autoantibody, insulin autoantibody, cytoplasmic islet cell antibodies) in type 1 diabetes: Combinatorial Islet Autoantibody Workshop." Diabetes 47(12): 1857-66.

Walter, M., E. Albert, et al. (2003). "IDDM2/insulin VNTR modifies risk conferred by IDDM1/HLA for development of Type 1 diabetes and associated autoimmunity." Diabetologia 46(5): 712-20.

Wenzlau, J. M., K. Juhl, et al. (2007). "The cation efflux transporter ZnT8 (Slc30A8) is a major autoantigen in human type 1 diabetes." Proc Natl Acad Sci U S A 104(43): 17040-5.

Williams, A. J., P. J. Bingley, et al. (1999). "Insulin autoantibodies: more specific than proinsulin autoantibodies for prediction of type 1 diabetes." J Autoimmun 13(3): 357-63.

Winter, W. E., N. Harris, et al. (2002). "Type 1 diabetes islet autoantibody markers." Diabetes Technol Ther 4(6): 817-39.

Ziegler, A. G., M. Hummel, et al. (1999). "Autoantibody appearance and risk for development of childhood diabetes in offspring of parents with type 1 diabetes: the 2-year analysis of the German BABYDIAB Study." Diabetes 48(3): 460-8.

Ziegler, A. G., R. Ziegler, et al. (1989). "Life-table analysis of progression to diabetes of anti-insulin autoantibody-positive relatives of individuals with type I diabetes." Diabetes 38(10): 1320-5.

28

Genetic Determinants of Type 1 Diabetes

Mohamed M. Jahromi
Salmaniya Medical Complex, Ministry of Health, Kingdom of Bahrain

1. Introduction

Type 1 diabetes is (T1D) is an autoimmune disorder characterized by the T-cell-mediated destruction of the insulin-secreting β cells of the pancreatic islet of Langerhans.
T1D is heterogeneous in terms of age at diabetes development with as many adults developing the disorder as children(Barnett et al 1981). Genetic susceptibility is dependent on the degree of genetic identity with the proband, and the risk of diabetes in families has a non-linear correlation with the number of alleles shared with the proband. The highest risk is naturally observed in monozygotic twins (100% sharing) followed by first, second, and third degree relatives (50%, 25%, 12.5% sharing, respectively) (Millward et al 1986).
About 18 regions of the genome have been linked with influencing T1D risk. These regions, each of may contain several genes. Over 40 genes and loci have been associated with T1D (Barett et al 2009) have been labeled *IDDM1* to *IDDM18*.
The most well studied *is IDDM1*, which contains the HLA genes that encode immune response proteins. Variations in HLA genes are an important genetic risk factor, but they alone do not account for the disease and other genes are involved. There is increasing evidence other MHC linked gene or loci with a potential impact on the risk to T1D exist (Renando et al 2001).
There are three other non-MHC genes which have been identified thus far. One of these non-MHC genes is the insulin gene, and the other non-MHC gene maps close to CTLA4, which has a regulatory role in the immune response and the third confirmed non-MHC gene is PTPN22 that is involved in modulating T-cell activation.

2. Global distribution of T1D

T1D is reaching epidemic proportions throughout the world. The incidence of T1D is rapidly increasing in specific regions T1D affects incidence is highly variable among different populations. The overall ratio of incidence of T1D varies from 0.1/100 000 per year in China to more than 36/100 000 per year in Sardinia and in Finland. This drastic variation, a more than 350-fold, among populations is analyzed (Kavvoura &Ionnidis 2005).The polar equatorial gradient (i.e., north-south gradient) described for disease incidence is not as strong as previously thought (e.g. for example Sardinia with extremely high incidence). Most populations with very high incidence rates are Europid. Although it is well established that the incidents rate of T1D is as low as 0.1/100 000 amongst Asians (Kavvoura & Ionnidis 2005) high incidence rates have also been noted in Kuwait(Shaltout et al 2002), Oman

(Abdullah 2005), Bahrain (Jahromi unpublished) and Puerto Rico (Karvonen et al 2000). In fact, a relatively high gradient risk has been reported among some non-Europid ethnicities (i.e., admixed partly African [1/100 000 per year in Mauritius versus 15/100 000 per year in Chicago] and Arab [5/100 000 per year in Sudan vs. 21/100 000 per year in Kuwait] (Shaltout et al 2002).

2.1 Pathogenesis

T1D develops slowly and progressive abnormalities in pancreatic β cell function herald what appears to be a sudden development of hyperglycemia. Rising HbA1c in the normal range(Stene et al 2006), impaired fasting or glucose tolerance, as well as loss of first phase insulin secretion usually precede overt T1D. The exact pancreatic β cell mass remaining at diagnosis is poorly defined and there is almost no studies of insulitis prior to onset of T1D(Gianani et al 2006). For patients with long-term T1D there is evidence of some β cell function remaining (C-peptide secretion) though β cell mass is usually decreased to less than 1% of normal(Meier et al 2005). At present methods to image/quantitate β cell mass and insulitis are only beginning to be developed. However, animal studies have provided the first methods to image islet mass utilizing a labeled amine (dihydrotetrabenazine) (Souza et al 2006) A number of techniques are being evaluated to image insulitis.

An increasing body of evidence indicates that the development of T1D is determined by a balance between pathogenic and regulatory T lymphocytes (Jahromi et al 2010). A fundamental question is whether there is a primary autoantigen for initial T cell autoreactivity with subsequent recognition of multiple islet antigens. A number of investigators have addressed in the NOD mouse (spontaneously develops T1D) the importance of immune reactivity to insulin with the dramatic finding that eliminating immune responses to insulin blocks development of diabetes and insulitis, and importantly immune responses to downstream autoantigens such as the islet specific molecule IGRP(Krishnamurthy et al 2006). Knocking out both insulin genes (mice in contrast to man have two insulin genes) with introduction of a mutated insulin with alanine rather than tyrosine at position 16 of the insulin B chain prevents development of diabetes(Nakayama et al 2005). Recognition of this B-chain peptide of insulin by T lymphocytes depends upon a "non-stringent" T cell receptor with conservation of only the alpha chain sequence (Valpha and Jalpha) and not the N-region of the alpha chain, or the β chain(Homann & Eisenbarth 2006).

Interestingly, a study of pancreatic lymph node from two patients with T1D found a conserved T cell receptor, with T cells reacting with insulin A chain peptide amino acids 1-15.

There are large scale studies such as T1DGC (Barrett et al 2009) (USA), Teddy (International), (Nakayama et al 2005) , DAISY (Liu et al 2005), DIPP BabyDiab(Homann & Eisenbarth 2006) and where tens of thousands of infants have been HLA typed and followed from birth for the development of islet autoantibodies and then progression to diabetes. Although T1D rate is increasing in Arabian countries recently, however, centers with diabetes interest have been found in Kuwait, UAE, Qatar, Bahrain as well as Saudi Arabia that would help in case of international contribution in determining the T1D pathogenesis. Especially since there are likely changing environmental factors contributing to the world-wide increase in the incidence of T1D and the above studies, in addition to providing crucial information for prediction are searching for such factors.

2.2 Genetic of T1D

2.2.1 "Monogenic" inheritance

The immune dysregulation, Polyendocrinopthay, Enteropathy, X-linked (IPEX) syndrome is caused by a mutation of the foxP3 gene, a transcription factor that controls the development of regulatory T cells is a cause of neonatal diabetes(Jahromi & Eisenbarth 2007).

As reflected in the name, children with disorder suffer from overwhelming autoimmunity and usually die as infants. Of note bone marrow transplantation can reverse disease. IPEX syndrome is rare, as is neonatal diabetes. In the differential diagnosis of neonatal diabetes it must be recognized that half of children developing permanent neonatal diabetes have a mutation of the Kir6.2 molecule of the sulfonylurea receptor. These children with their non-autoimmune form of diabetes can be treated with oral sulfonylurea therapy.

Though more common than IPEX syndrome, the APS-1 syndrome (Autoimmune Polyendocrine Syndrome Type 1) is also rare. It results from a mutation of the AIRE gene, another transcription factor(Jahromi & Eisenbarth 2007). Approximately 15% of patients with this syndrome develop autoimmune diabetes. The leading hypothesis as to etiology (e.g. Addison's disease, mucocutaneous candidiasis, and hypoparathyroidism) is that AIRE controls expression of autoantigens and negative selection of autoreactive T lymphocytes within the thymus. A very recent dramatic discovery is the demonstration that essentially 100% of patients with APS-1 have autoantibodies reacting with interferon alpha and other interferons. Such autoantibodies are extremely rare and essentially not found in patients with T1D or Addison's disease outside of the syndrome.

Patients with T1D and their relatives are at risk for development of thyroid autoimmunity, celiac disease, Addison's disease, pernicious anemia and a series of other autoimmune disorders(Aly et al 2006). Approximately 1/20 patients with T1D have celiac disease by biopsy though the majority have no symptoms(Hoffenberg et al 2004). These asymptomatic individuals are usually detected with screening for transglutaminase autoantibodies. The level of transglutaminase autoantibodies relates to the probability of a positive biopsy and it is important for clinicians to know the threshold for likely positive biopsy for the assay they employ(Liu et al 2005). There remains controversy as to whether asymptomatic celiac disease when detected should be treated with a gluten free diet and large clinical trials are needed to address this question.

2.2.2 "Polygenic inheritance"

T1D has become one of the most intensively studied polygenic disorders. There are rare variants of immune mediated diabetes with single gene mutations including the APS-I syndrome (AIRE autoimmune regulator gene) and the IPEX syndrome (Fox P3 mutation) (Jahromi & Eisenbarth 2006). Multiple genetic factors influence both susceptibility and resistance to the common forms of T1D(Barrett et al 2009). Although a significant proportion of patients with T1D lack a family history of the disease, there is significant familial clustering with an average prevalence of 6% in siblings compared to 0.4% in the US Caucasian population. Of note, there is a 3.8 % risk of T1D in Japanese siblings of patients with T1D compared to 0.01~0.02 % prevalence in the general Japanese population (Hoffenberg 2004). The sibling ratio (λs) can be calculated as the ratio of the risk to siblings over the disease prevalence in the general population, and thus λs = 6/0.4= 15 and 3.8/0.01~0.02=>100 for the US and Japan respectively (Hoffenberg 2004).

Genetic susceptibility of different genes and loci have been identified using both association and linkage studies. Using the candidate gene approach, association studies provided evidence for the first two susceptibility loci, the HLA region and the insulin gene (*INS*) locus. These two loci only contribute a portion of the familial clustering (40-50% for *HLA* and 10% for *INS),* suggesting the existence of additional loci (Aly et al 2006, Jahromi & Eisenbarth 2006 & 2007, Barrett et al 2009). The next most potent locus for T1D of man was also discovered using a candidate gene approach, namely the LYP (PTPN22) gene with an odds ratio of approximately 1.7 for a "missense" mutation that contributes to multiple different autoimmune disorders (. Recently, however, Cytotoxic T lymphocyte antigen-4 (CTLA-4) gene and SUMO-4 with weak association were described following genome analysis. For both the associations appear heterogeneous dependent on the population (e.g. stronger association of Sumo-4 in Asian populations and lack of association in multiple European populations) (Nielsen et al 2011) , and nature of the disease (e.g. CTLA-4 associated with diabetes with thyroid autoimmunity) (Meier et al 2005). Undoubtedly, large extensive control case studies will reveal more loci, each providing a piece to the genetic puzzle of T1D, but with difficulty of distinguishing false positive signals with very weak associations.

2.2.2A The Major Histocompatibility Complex (MHC)

The major loci for susceptibility to T1D are located within the HLA (Human Leukocyte Antigen) region on the short arm of chromosome 6 and provide up to 40-50% of the inheritable T1D risk(Jahromi & Eisenbarth 2006, Barrett et al 2009, Jahromi et al 2010, Neilson et al 2011).

2.2.2A1 The HLA classes

Within the MHC region, they are grouped into three classes. **Class I genes:** (HLA - A, HLA - B and HLA-C as major & HLA-D, HLA-E, and HLA-F as minor subclasses) (Marsh et al 2005) encode class I MHC antigens, located on the surface of all nucleated cells (Jahromi & Eisenbarth 2007). The HLA complex was first linked to T1D when associations with several HLA class I antigens (eg HLA-B8, -B18, and -B15) were discovered by serological typing and affected sib-pair analysis showed evidence of linkage(Todd et al 1989, Awata et al 1990). **Class II genes:** (DQ, DR, and DP in that order of risk) were shown to be even more strongly associated with the disease (Todd et al 1989, Mijovic et al 1991). HLA class II antigens are found exclusively on B-lymphocytes, macrophages, epithelial cells of the islets of pancreatic Langerhans and activated T-lymphocytes. Their expression on other cells may be induced by cytokines such as interferon (IFN) and tumor necrosis factor (TNF)-α (Jahromi et al 2000). With the development of typing reagents, HLA class II alleles. However, other loci within or near the HLA complex appear to modulate T1D risk, and add further complexity to the analysis of *IDDM1* -encoded susceptibility. HLA Class III: The TNF (Tumor Necrosis Factor) gene is a strong candidate from class III, Table 1.

Major histocompatibility complex (MHC)/ Human leukocyte antigen (HLA)	**MHC class I**	HLA-A • HLA-B• HLA-C • HLA-E • HLA-F • HLA-G (Bodmer et al 1992)
	MHC class II	HLA-DM (α, β) • HLA-DO (α, β) • HLA-DP (α1, β1) • HLA-DQ (α1, α2, β1, β2, β3) • HLA-DR (α, β1, β3, β4, β5) (Marsh et al 2005)
	MHC class III	

Table 1. Different classes of Major Histocompatibility Complex

The great majority of Caucasian patients have the HLA-DR3(with [DQA1*0501, DQB1*020]DQ2) or -DR4(with [DQA1*0301,DQB1*0302]DQ8) class II alleles and approximately 30% to 50% of patients are DR3/DR4 heterozygotes (Barrett et al 2009). The DR3/DR4 (DQ2, DQ8) genotype confers the highest diabetes risk with a synergistic mode of action, Table 2 (Mitchel et al 2007). However, DR4/DR9 has been reported to be a highly susceptible haplotype in Japanese. The absence of DR3 haplotypes in Japanese population may contribute to lower frequency of the disease in Japan (Fain & Eisenbarth 2002). On the other hand, in Chinese population the DR3/DR9 genotype is highly susceptible (Xiao-mei et al 2009). In fact DQ-DR linkage disequilibrium patterns of HLA haplotypes in different populations may explain part of the world-wide differences in the frequency of incidence of T1D (e.g.DRB1*0405-DQB1*0302 is a high risk haplotype while DRB1*0403-DQB1*0302 is neutral or protective). In Arab population, however, patients with T1D have almost similar HLA genetic susceptibility as Caucasian patients, this may confirms the increase rate of incidents of T1D (Shaltout et al 2002, Al Abbasi et al 2002).

	Relative risk
HLA-DR3	5
HLA allele	6
HLA-DR3/DR4	16

Extracted from Mitchel et al 2007

Table 2. HLA and T1D with increased risk

Furthermore, DRB1*1501-DQB1*0602 is protective in all populations which have been studied to date (shaltout et al 2002, Caillat et al 1997, Escribano-De-Diego et al 1999, Kawasaki et al 2004). Analysis of rare "recombinant" haplotype suggests that DQB1*0602 provides protection and not DRB1*1501.

Specific allelic combination of DR/DQ loci have been shown to determine the haplotypic risk for T1D, protective and susceptible. Table 4 have summarized the most susceptible and the most protective combinations. The comparison of closely related DR-DQ haplotype pairs

DRB1	DQA1	DQB1	Effect on T1D
0405	0301	0302	S1
0401	0301	0302	S2
0301	0501	0201	S3
0402	0301	0302	S4
0404	0301	0302	S5
0701	0201	0503	P1
1401	0101	0503	P2
1501	0102	0602	P3
1104	0501	0301	P4
1303	0501	0301	P5

Haplotype frequency in either proband or control subjects, five most susceptible (S) and five most protective (P) haplotypes are indicated (Erlik et al 2008)

Table 3. Frequency distribution of DRB1-DQB1 haplotype

with different T1D risks allowed identification of specific amino acid positions critical in determining disease susceptibility, only a single change of an amino acid would change degree of genetic susceptibility drastically (Erlick et al 2008).

On the other hand, combined typing of high risk HLA alleles with analysis of HLA haplotype sharing can identify siblings with an extraordinary genetic risk of T1D. This strongly implicates major genes in addition to DR and DQ alleles. The current extensive MHC analysis and multiple studies of conserved haplotypes (eg. A1-B8-DR3-DQ2 common extended haplotype)(Alper et la 1992) conferring increased risk. Increasing studies have confirmed the significant association of HLA-F region in determining the risk for T1D (Al et al 2008, Barett et al 2009, Brorsson et al 2009). Interestingly through out our large affected family based controls (AFBAC) we have found that there is significant signal between patients with T1D and controls in HLA-F region in particular that contributes to T1D risk which seems to go with DRB*0401, but has an independent risk. In other words this signal may have certain link with the possible candidate gene susceptible to T1D other than DQ/DR (Jahromi in process).

2.2.2B Non MHC genes

There are about 40 non MHC genes or loci which are candidates for genetic susceptibility to T1D (Barrett et al 2009). The most well known are discussed in this chapter.

2.2.2B1 Insulin gene

Insulin is composed of two distinct polypeptide chains, chain A and chain B, which are linked by disulfide bonds. Many proteins that contain subunits, such as hemoglobin, are the products of several genes. However, insulin is the product of one gene, INS. The research done by Nakayama and coworkers have strongly shown that insulin is a primary autoantigen in the beginning stages of diabetes (Nakayama et al 2005).

Also, supporting this evidence is the presence of insulin antibodies in the blood of prediabetic and diabetic patients. The insulin gene is the second well established susceptibility locus in T1D on chromosome 11p 15.5 (Jahromi & Eisenbarth 2006).

The 4.1 Kb region containing the insulin gene (*INS)* and its flanking regions contain several polymorphisms in linkage disequilibrium (Stead et al 2000) that have been associated with diabetes risk. All the polymorphisms identified within this region lie outside coding sequences, confirming that diabetes susceptibility must derive from genetic influences on the expression of the insulin gene. Extensive studies involving polymorphisms in the neighboring *HUMTHO1* (tyrosine hydroxylase) and *IGF2* genes provided strong evidence that *INS* is the main susceptibility determinant in this region (Vardi et al 1988,Stead et al 2000). Shortly after its discovery (Vardi et al 1987), the insulin VNTR was found to be associated with T1D (Haskins & Wegman 1996). Susceptibility in the *INS* region, or the *IDDM2* locus, was initially associated to a variable number of tandem repeats (VNTR) located ~0.5 kb upstream of (*INS*) (Vardi et al 1987, Haskins & Wegman 1996, Yu et al 2000). Homozygosity for the short class VNTR I alleles is found in ~75-85% of the patients compared to a frequency of 50-60% in the general population, suggesting that it predisposes to T1D. In contrast, homozygosity for the longer class III VNTR alleles is rarely seen in patients and the class III VNTR is believed to confer a dominant protective effect (Haskins & Wegman 1996, Pugliese et al 2001). The relative risk ratio of the I/I genotype vs. I/III or III/III has been reported to be moderate (in the 3-5 range) and it accounts for about 10% of the familial clustering of T1D (Jahromi & Eisenbarth 2006). However, analyses suggest that it is not possible to discriminate effects of the VNTR from other polymorphisms in this region (Shaltout et al 2002) and that at least two other polymorphisms (-23HphI and +1140A/C) may be important(Heath et al 1998). Moreover, by measuring the *HphI* polymorphism (in tight linkage disequilibrium with the VNTR) (Stead et al 2000), Metcalfe and coworkers showed that homozygosity for the predisposing *INS* genotype increases the likelihood that identical twins will be concordant for T1D (Metcalfe et al 2001).

Insulin associated susceptibility and resistance may derive from quantitative differences in *INS* transcription in the specialized antigen presenting cells found in thymus and peripheral lymphoid tissues, where production of self-antigens such as proinsulin may be crucial for the shaping and maintaining of a self-tolerant T cell repertoire (Vafiadis et al 1997, Alizadeh & Koelman 2008). Such mechanisms may influence the probability of developing autoimmune responses to insulin as a key autoantigen in T1D.

2.2.2B2 LYP gene - PTPN22

LYP gene (encoded by PTPN22 gene belongs to a family of protein tyrosine phosphatases (PTPs) that are involved in modulating T-cell activation. The PTPN22 gene has been associated with development of T1D and other autoimmune diseases (Jahromi & Eisenbarth 2006). Recently, significantly associated of PTPN22 C1858T variant was found to be to lower fasting C-peptide levels, poorer glycemic control in recent onset of T1D subjects and to higher GADA in T1D patients with long disease duration (Mortensen et al 2010).

The gene encodes a lymphoid tyrosine phosphatase (LYP) which by dephosphorylation of Src family kinases negatively regulates T cell receptor (TCR) signaling. The current working hypothesis suggest that the risk carrying allele, T1858, suppresses TCR signaling more efficiently during thymic development resulting in survival of auto reactive T-cells 9(et al 2011). Bottini and co-workers evaluated a functional polymorphism in the lyp gene (no relation to the lymphopenia gene of the BB rat) in two series of patients with T1D, (Bottini et al 2004). They suggested the possible use of PTPN22 SNPs as a prognostic factor for disease severity and variability in autoimmune diseases (Bottini et al 2006).

There are evidence indicating that the diabetes associated allele may result in a "gain of function" (Bottini et al 2006) and thereby contribute to T cell activation. The odds ratio was approximately 1.7, making this polymorphism the most potent after HLA and INS. The polymorphism appears to be a missense mutation that changes an arginine at position 620 to a tryptophan and thereby abrogates the ability of the molecule to bind to the signaling molecule Csk (Bottini et al 2006, Begovich et al 2004). Consistent with a general effect on immune function is the finding that the minor tryptophan encoded allele is associated with a series of autoimmune disorders including T1D, and other autoimmune diseases (Begovich et al 2004, Kyogoku et al 2004). Multiple recent studies have confirmed the association of this missense mutation with T1D including an extensive study from United Kingdom. It is possible that polymorphisms in linkage disequilibrium with R620W determine increased risk of autoimmunity rather than the polymorphism, but this seems unlikely given the rapid confirmation of this polymorphism's association with multiple forms of autoimmune disease in multiple populations and its functional significance.

Recently Nielsen and coworkers have further investigated in the association of PTPN22 C1858T with the disease progression as assessed by liquid meal associated C-peptide and proinsulin, HbA1c, and daily insulin dose, IDAA1C (Petrone et al 2008), production of pancreatic islet antibodies and new onset of T1D(Mortensen et al 2009). They have shown that PTPN22 gene variant may be associated with changes in residual β-cell function and disease pathogenesis during the first year after onset of T1D (Neilsen et al 2011).

2.2.2B3 Cytotoxic T Lymphocyte Antigen-4

CTLA-4 (cytotoxic T lymphocyte-associated antigen 4) is a molecule on T-cells that plays a critical role in regulating natural immune responses.CTLA4 has attracted interest for many years, and multiple studies have established association or linkage between this chromosomal region and autoimmune diseases, particularly T1D(Nistico et al 1996, Ueda et al 2003, , Anjos et al 2004, Concannon et al 2005). Cytotoxic T lymphocyte antigen-4 (CTLA-4) gene is located on chromosome 2q33, is one of the confirmed T1D susceptibility loci. This 300-kilobase region is known to contain at least three genes: CD28, CTLA-4, and the inducible costmulatory molecule (ICOS) gene (Kavvoura & Ioannidid 2005). The LD patterns in this region define two blocks, one comprising the CD28 gene and another including CTLA4 and the 5′ end of ICOS. The first studies limited the signals to the CTLA4-ICOS block and subsequent research determined that the SNPs selected had functional effects on the CTLA- 4 protein while the expression and function of ICOS did not suffer any change. The CTLA4 gene has four exons and three introns. Exon 1 codes for the leader peptide of the protein, exon 2 delivers the ligand-binding domain, exon 3 is the transmembrane domain and exon 4 the cytoplasmic tail. Two of the most studied and replicated polymorphisms in *CTLA4* are rs231775 (+A49G), located in exon 1, and rs3087243 (+6230G>A, also known as CT60) in the 3' region. The A allele of rs231775 codes for a threonine in position 17 of CTLA-4, forming a threonine-X-asparagin glycosilation site. The mutant G allele (alanine) causes an aberrant glycosilation of the derived protein and lower levels of membrane-bound CTLA-4 in *in vitro* experiments(Ueda et al 2003). The change CT60, a transition from a guanine to an adenine in position +6230 of the gene, is correlated to higher levels of a soluble isoform of the CTLA-4 protein.

The CTLA-4 receptor has two variants derived from alternative splicing: the membrane-bound and the soluble form that lacks the transmembrane domain. It is believed that the soluble isoform contributes to downregulate the activation of T cells by binding to CD80-CD86 receptors in antigen presenting cells and preventing the stimulation of *CD28*. Ueda and coworkers found a correlation between high levels of sCTLA-4 in serum and the protective A allele in the CT60 polymorphism(Ueda et al 2003). By mechanisms as yet unknown, the protective allele augments the levels of sCTLA-4 mRNA and patients who carry this allele have higher levels of free sCTLA-4 in serum, that most likely contribute to control the activation of the immune system.

Kavvoura and Ioannidis have a meta analysis on three of them and concluded that the A (49) G gene polymorphism in exon 1 is associated with T1D (Kavvoura & Ioannidis 2005). They have also reported a significant ethnic variation in that polymorphism. On the other hand, the A (CT60) G gene polymorphism have been studied in parallel with A (49) G in different in Caucasian as well as Asian population.

2.2.2B4 Other non-MHC genes and loci

Increasing studies have identified different non-MHC genes apart from insulin gene region, PTPN22, CTLA-4 to be associated in T1D pathogenesis. Other non-MHC genes might also be important in triggering the pathogenesis of T1D. However, further large scale confirmatory association studies might be required. The polygenic nature of T1D pathogenesis functions as a network of genes and loci that exert its effect in the triggering of the disease onset. Our series of human genetic of cytokines work have identified the effect of genetic polymorphisms in cytokines in the pathogenesis of T1D, Figure 1. Given the mediatory role of cytokines in the immune system they might be of a good therapeutic value. However, these findings require large scale confirmatory studies.

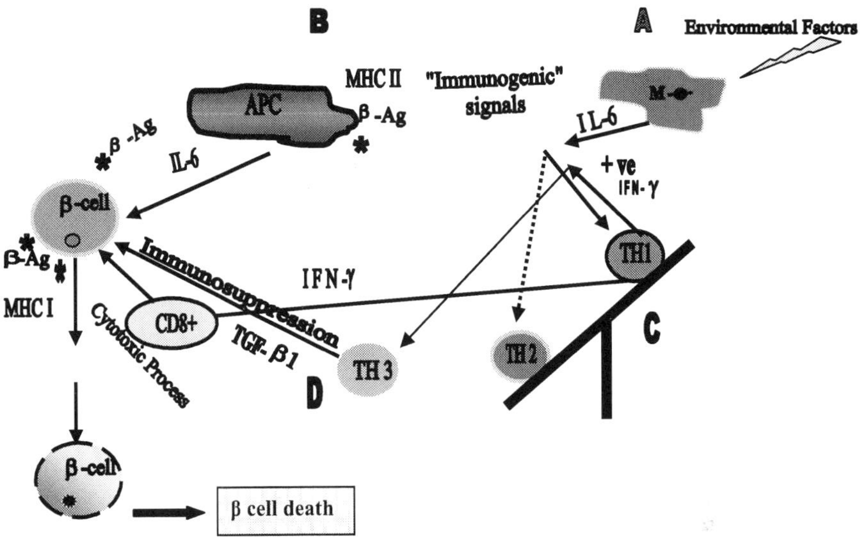

Fig. 1. Diagrammatic presentation of effects of cytokines gene polymorphisms in T1D. This schematic diagram explains the possible effects of cytokines in the initiation triggering of T1D by signals from either environmental factors "A" or immunogenic factors "B" or both. Release of IL-6 would change the counterbalance between TH1/TH2 "C" cytokines level. Increase level of TH1, IFN-γ, cause the cytotoxic process of break down of β-cell by CD8. As a result of deviation of cytokine cross regulation to TH1 dominance TH3 lymphocyte subset produce immunosuppressive cytokines, TGF- β1, however, due to genetic malfunction this cytokines are proved not to be able to bring TH1/TH2 back to normal position, D. Which will lead to the death of pancreatic β cell. This is a simplified schematic descriptions of the impact of cytokines in the pathogenesis of T1D, for detail please refer to Jahromi et al 2000, 2000[a] and 2010.

3. Conclusion

An increasing number of studies indicate that genetic factors influence both susceptibility to and resistance to T1D. Several chromosomal regions have been linked with the disease, suggesting the polygenic nature of disorder in most families. A few rare families have dramatic Mendelian mutations leading to immune mediated diabetes.

Although DR and DQ alleles and their linkage disequilibrium pattern can explain a major portion of disease risk there is evidence for additional genes linked or within the MHC influencing risk. Combination of genes linked to the MHC, have a major effect on risk of T1D in addition to the known potent effects of HLA DR and DQ alleles.

Further, other non-MHC genes such as INS, PTPN22 and CTLA-4 and others with small but significant effects might contribute to pathogenesis of T1D. Differences in disease risk between populations are likely due in part to the distribution within populations of DR and DQ haplotypes. However, the major genetic factors, probably linked to the MHC remain to be defined that will contribute to the remarkable differences in T1D incidence. With the recent biotechnological advancements extensive genetic typing and the formation of cooperative global genetic study groups, international HapMap and Genome Wide Association (GWA) should enhance the speed at which true gene(s) for T1D will be unraveled.

4. References

Abdul Jabbar Al Abbasssy, iman Farid and Dunia Al Hashimi 2002. HLA association with diabetes mellitus type 1 in Bahraini children. Emirates med J; 20: 143-146.

Abdullah , M.A. 2005. Epidemiology of type I diabetes mellitus among Arab children Saudi. Med J. 26: 911-917.

Alizadeh BZ, Koeleman BP 2008. Genetic polymorphisms in susceptibility to Type 1 Diabetes. Clin Chim Acta; 387:9-17.

Alper, C.A., Z.Awdeh & E.J.Yunis 1992. Conserved, extended MHC haplotypes Exp. Clin. Immunogenet. 9: 58-71.

Aly TA, Baschal EE, Jahromi MM, Fernando MS, Babu SR, Fingerlin TE, Kretowski A, Erlich HA, Fain PR, Rewers MJ, Eisenbarth GS 2008. Analysis of single nucleotide polymorphisms identifies major type 1A diabetes locus telomeric of the major histocompatibility complex. Diabetes.;57:770-776.

Aly TA, Ide A, Jahromi MM, Barker J M , Fernando MS, Babu SR, Yu L, Miao D, Erlich HA, Fain PR, Barriga KJ, Norris JM, Rewers MJ, Eisenbarth GS 2006. Extreme Genetic Risk for Type 1A Diabetes. Proc Natl Acad Sci U S A 103: 14074-14079.

Anjos SM, Tessier MC, Polychronakos C 2004. Association of the cytotoxic T lymphocyte-associated antigen 4 gene with type 1 diabetes: Evidence for independent effects of two polymorphisms on the same haplotype block. J Clin Endocrinol Metab;89:6257-6265.

Awata, T., T.Kuzua, A.Matsuda, Y.Iwamoto, Y.Kanzawa, M.Okuyama & T.Juji. 1990. High frequency of aspartic acid at position 57 of HLA-DQ B-chain in Japanese IDDM patients and nondiabetic subjects. Diabetes 39: 266-269.

Barnett, A.H., C.EFF, R.D.Leslie & D.A.Pyke 1981. Diabetes in identical twins. A study of 200 pairs Diabetologia 20: 87-93.

Begovich, A.B., V.E.Carlton, L.A.Honigberg, S.J.Schrodi, A.P.Chokkalingam, H.C.Alexander, K.G.Ardlie, Q.Huang, A.M.Smith, J.M.Spoerke, M.T.Conn, M.Chang, S.Y.Chang, R.K.Saiki, J.J.Catanese, D.U.Leong, V.E.Garcia, L.B.Mcallister, D.A.Jeffery, A.T.Lee, F.Batliwalla, E.Remmers, L.A.Criswell, M.F.Seldin, D.L.Kastner, C.I.Amos, J.J.Sninsky & P.K.Gregersen 2004. A missense single-nucleotide polymorphism in a gene encoding a protein tyrosine phosphatase (PTPN22) is associated with rheumatoid arthritis Am. J. Hum. Genet. 75: 330-337.

Bodmer, JG; Marsh, SG; Albert, ED; Bodmer, WF; Dupont, B; Erlich, HA; Mach, B; Mayr, WR et al. (1992). "Nomenclature for factors of the HLA system, 1991". Human immunology 34 (1): 4–18.

Bottini N, Vang T, Cucca F, Mustelin T 2006: Role of PTPN22 in type 1 diabetes and other autoimmune diseases. Semin Immunol ; 18:207-213.

Bottini, N., MuscumecI L, A.Alonso, S.Rahmouni, K.Nika, M.Rostakhani, J.McMurry, G.Meloni, P.Lucarelli, M.Pellchia, G.Eisenbarth, D.Comings & T.Mustelin 2004. A functional variant of lympoid tyrosine phosphatase is associated with type I diabetes Nature Genet. 36: 337-338.

C. Brorsson, N. T. Hansen, K. Lage, R. Bergholdt, S. Brunak, F. Pociot, and Type 1 Diabetes Genetics Consortium 2009. Identification of T1D susceptibility genes within the MHC region by combining protein interaction networks and SNP genotyping data. Diabetes Obes Metab.;11:60-66.

Caillat-Zucman, S., I.D Jilali-Saiah, J.Timsit, E.Bonifacio, V.Sepe, M.Shattack, G.F.Bottazzo, N.K.McLaren, M.Delamaire, S.Martin, A.-M.Yamamoto, TW.Meade, A.M.Valdes, M.C.Babron, E.Thorsby, F.Clerget-Darpoux, G.Thomson, J.F.Bach & The Participating Centers 1997. Insulin dependent diabetes mellitus (IDDM) joint report. 12th International Histocompatibility Workshop Study. In Genetic diversity of HLA. Functional and medical implications. Charron, D., Ed. 389-398. EDK. Paris.

Concannon P, Erlich HA, Julier C, Morahan G, Nerup J, Pociot F, et al 2005. Type 1 diabetes: evidence for susceptibility loci from four genome-wide linkage scans in 1, 435 multiplex families. Diabetes;54:2995-3001.

Escribano-De-Diego, J., P.Sanchez-Velasco, C.Luzuraga, J.G.Ocego-Vinyals, J.E.Paz-MIiguel & F.Leyva-Cobian 1999. HLA class II immunogenetics and incidence of insulin-dependent diabetes mellitus in the population of Cantabria (Northern Spain) Hum. Immunol. 60: 990-1000.

Fain, P. & G.S.Eisenbarth 2002. Genetics of type 1 diabetes mellitus. In Genetics in Endocrinology. Baxter, J., S.Melmed, M.New & L.Martini, Eds. 37-72. Lippincott Williams & Williams. Philadelphia.

Gianani R, Putnam A, Still T, Yu L, Miao D, Gill RG, Beilke J, Supon P, Valentine A, Iveson A, Dunn S, Eisenbarth GS, Hutton J, Gottlieb P, Wiseman A 2006. Initial results of screening of non - diabetic organ donors for expression of islet autoantibodies. J Clin Endocrinol Metab 91:1855-1861. Meier JJ, Bhushan A, Butler AE, Rizza RA, Butler PC 2005 Sustained beta cell apoptosis in patients with long-standing type 1 diabetes: indirect evidence for islet regeneration? Diabetologia 48:2221-2228.

Haskins, K. & D.Wegmann 1996. Diabetogenic T-cell clones Diabetes 45: 1299-1305.

Heath, V.L., N.C.Moore, S.M.Parnell & D.W.Mason 1998. Intrathymic expression of genes involved in organ specific autoimmune disease J Autoimmun 11: 309-318.

Henry Erlich, Ana Maria Valdes, Janelle Noble, Joyce A. Carlson, Mike Varney, Hoffenberg EJ, Emery LM, Barriga KJ Bao, F, Taylor, J, Eisenbarth GS, Haas JE, Sokol RJ, Taki I, Norris J Cleary P Waberski, B, Greene DA, Stevens MJ, Feldman ELM, Rewers M 2004. Clinical features of children with screening-identified evidence of celiac disease. Peds 113:1254-1259.

Homann D, Eisenbarth GS 2006. An immunologic homunculus for type 1 diabetes. Journal of Clinical Investigation 116: 1212-1215.

Jahromi M, Millward A, Demaine A 2000 . A CA repeat polymorphism of the IFN-gamma gene is associated with susceptibility to type 1 diabetes. J Interferon Cytokine Res.; 20:187-190.

Jahromi MM, Millward BA, Demaine AG 2000[a] . A polymorphism in the promoter region of the gene for interleukin-6 is associated with susceptibility to type 1 diabetes mellitus. Interferon Cytokine Res.;20:885-888.

Jahromi MM, Millward BA, Demaine AG 2010. Significant correlation between association of polymorphism in codon 10 of transforming growth factor-beta1 T (29) C with type 1 diabetes and patients with nephropathy disorder. J Interferon Cytokine Res;30: 59-66.

Jeffrey C. Barrett, David Clayton, Patrick Concannon, Beena Akolkar, Jason D. Jeffrey C. Barrett, David Clayton, Patrick Concannon, Beena Akolkar, Jason D. Cooper, Henry A. Erlich, Cécile Julier, Grant Morahan, Jørn Nerup, Concepcion Nierras, Vincent Plagnol, Flemming Pociot, Helen Schuilenburg, Deborah J. Smyth, Helen Stevens, John A. Todd, Neil M. Walker, Stephen S. Rich, and the Type 1 Diabetes Genetics Consortium 2009. Genome-wide association study and meta-analysis finds over 40 loci affect risk of type 1 diabetes*Nat Genet.* ; 41(6): 703–707.

Karl A Metcalfe, Graham A Hitman, Rachel R Rowe, Mohammed Hawa, Xiaojian Huang, Timothy Stewart, R David G Leslie. Concordance for Type 1 Diabetes in Identical twins is affected by Insulin genotype. Diabetes Care 2001; 24: 838-842.

Karvoen , M., M.Viik-Kajander, E.Moltchanova, I.Libman, R.Laporte & J.TUomilehto 2000. Incidence of childhood type 1 diabetes worldwide. Diabetes Mondiale (DiaMond) Project Group Diabetes Care 23: 1516-1526.

Kavvoura, F.K. & J.P.Ioannidis 2005. CTLA-4 gene polymorphisms and susceptibility to type 1 diabetes mellitus: a HUGE Review and meta-analysis Am. J. Epidemiol. 162: 3-16.

Kawasaki, E. & K.Eguchi 2004. Is Type 1 diabetes in the Japanese population the same as among Caucasians? Ann. N. Y. Acad. Sci. 1037:96-103.: 96-103.

Krishnamurthy B, Dudek NL, McKenzie MD Purcell AW, Brooks AG, Gellert S, Colman PG, Harrison LC, Lew AM, Thomas HE, Kay TW 2006. Responses against islet antigens in NOD mice are prevented by tolerance to proinsulin but not IGRP. J Clin Invest 116:3258-3265.

Kyogoku, C., C.D.Langefeld, W.A.Ortmann, A.Lee, S.Selby, V.E.Carlton, M.Chang, P.Ramos, E.C.Baechler, F.M.Batliwalla, J.Novitzke, A.H.Williams, C.Gillett, P.Rodine, R.R.Graham, K.G.Ardlie, P.M.Gaffney, K.L.Moser, M.Petri, A.B.Begovich, P.K.Gregersen & T.W.Behrens 2004. Genetic Association of the R620W Polymorphism of Protein Tyrosine Phosphatase PTPN22 with Human SLE Am. J Hum. Genet. 75: 504-507.

Liu E, Li M, Bao F Miao D, Rewers MJ, Eisenbarth GS, Hoffenberg EJ 2005. Need for quantitative assessment of transglutaminase autoantibodies for celiac disease in screening-identified children. J Pediatr 146: 494-499.

Lotte B Nielsen, Sven Pörksen, Marie Louise M Andersen, Siri Fredheim, Jannet Svensson, Philip Hougaard, Maurizio Vanelli, Jan Åman, Henrik B Mortensen, Lars Hansen and the Hvidoere Study Group on Childhood Diabetes 2011. The PTPN22 C1858T gene variant is associated with proinsulin in new-onset type 1 diabetes. BMC Med Genetics; 12: 1-6.

Marsh SG, Albert ED, Bodmer WF, Bontrop RE, Dupont B, Erlich HA, Geraghty DE, Hansen JA, Hurley CK, Mach B, Mayr WR, Parham P, Petersdorf EW, Sasazuki T, Schreuder GM, Strominger JL, Svejgaard A, Terasaki PI, and Trowsdale J 2005. "Nomenclature for factors of the HLA System, 2004". Tissue Antigens 65 (4): 301–369.

Meier JJ, Bhushan A, Butler AE, Rizza RA, Butler PC 2005. Sustained beta cell apoptosis in patients with long-standing type 1 diabetes: indirect evidence for islet regeneration? Diabetologia 48:2221-2228.

Mijovic, C.H., A.H.Barnett & J.A.Todd 1991. Genetics of diabetes. Trans-racial gene mapping studies. [Review] Baillieres. Clin. Endocrinol. Metab. 5: 321-340.

Millward, B.A., L.Alviggi, P.J.Hoskins, C.Johnston, D.Heaton, G.F.Bottazzo, D.Vergani , R.D.Leslie & D.A.Pyke 1986. Immune changes associated with insulin dependent diabetes may remit without causing the disease: a study in identical twins BMJ 292: 793-796.

Mitchell, Richard Sheppard; Kumar, Vinay; Abbas, Abul K.; Fausto, Nelson (2007). Robbins Basic Pathology. Philadelphia: Saunders. ISBN 1-4160-2973-7.8th edition.

Mohamed M Jahromi and George S Eisenbarth. Cellular and Molecular Pathology of Type 1 Diabetes. Cell Mol Life Sci 2007; 64: 865-72.

Mohamed M Jahromi and George S Eisenbarth. Genetic Determinants of Type 1 Diabetes Across Populations. Ann NY Acad Sci 2006; 289-299.

Jahromi Mohamed M. Haplotype Specific Alteration of Type 1 Diabetes MHC Risk. (Submitted to Diabetes Care)

Mortensen HB, Hougaard P, Swift P, Hansen L, Holl RW, Hoey H, Bjoerndalen H, de Beaufort C, Chiarelli F, Danne T, Schoenle EJ, Aman J, on behalf of the Hvidoere Study Group on Childhood Diabetes: New Definition for the Partial Remission Period in Children and Adolescents with T1D. Diabetes Care 2009, 32:1384-1390.

Mortensen HB, Swift PG, Holl RW, Hougaard P, Hansen L, Bjoerndalen H, de Beaufort CE, Knip M, Hvidoere Study Group on Childhood Diabetes: Multinational study in children and adolescents with newly diagnosed type 1 diabetes: association of age, ketoacidosis, HLA status, and autoantibodies on residual beta-cell function and glycemic control 12 months after diagnosis. Pediatr Diabetes 2010, 11:218-226.

Nakayama M, Abiru N, Moriyama H Babaya N, Liu E, Miao D, Yu L, Wegmann DR, Hutton JC, Elliott JF, Eisenbarth, GS 2005 Prime role for an insulin epitope in the development of type 1 diabetes in NOD mice. Nature 435:220-223.

Nistico L, Buzzetti R, Pritchard LE, Van der Auwera B, Giovannini C, Bosi E, et al. The CTLA-4 gene region of chromosome 2q33 is linked to, and associated with, type 1 diabetes. Belgian Diabetes

Pat Concannon, Josyf C. Mychaleckyj, John A. Todd, Persia Bonella, Anna Lisa Fear, Eva Lavant, Anthony Louey, and Priscilla Moonsamy for the Type 1 Diabetes Genetics Consortium. HLA DR-DQ Haplotypes and Genotypes and Type 1 Diabetes Risk:Analysis of the Type 1 Diabetes Genetics Consortium Families. Diabetes 2008; 57:1084-1092.

Petrone, A., T.L.Bugawan, C.A.Mesturino, L.Nistco, A.Galgani, G.Giorgi, I.Cascino, H.A.Erlich, U.Di Mario & R.Buzzetti 2001. The distribution of HLA class II susceptible/protective haplotypes could partially explain the low incidence of type 1 diabetes in continental Italy (Lazio region) Tissue Antigens 58: 385-394.

Pugliese, A., D.Brown, Garza D, M.Zeller, M.J.Redondo, G.S.Eisenbarth, D.D.Patel & C.Ricodi 2001. Self-Antigen Presenting Cells Expressing Islet Cell Molecules in Human Thymus and Peripheral Lymphoid Organs: Phenotypic Characterization and Implications for Immunological Tolerance and Type 1 Diabetes J Clin Invest 107: 555-564.

Redondo MJ, Fain PR, Eisenbarth GS. Genetics of type 1A diabetes.Recent Prog Horm Res 2001;56:69-89.

Registry. Hum Mol Genet 1996;5:1075-1080.

Shaltout AA, Moussa MA, Qabazard M, et al 2002 Further evidence for the rising incidence of childhood Type 1 diabetes in Kuwait. Diabet Med; 19:522-525.

Souza F, Simpson N, Raffo A, Saxena C, Maffei A, Hardy M, Kilbourn M, Goland R, Leibel R, Mann JJ, Van Heertum R, Harris PE 2006 Longitudinal noninvasive PET-based beta cell mass estimates in a spontaneous diabetes rat model. J Clin Invest 116:1506-1513.

Stead, J.D., J.Buard, J.A.Todd & A.J.Jefferys 2000. Influence of allele lineage on the role of the insulin minisatellite in susceptibility to type 1 diabetes Hum. Mol. Genet. 9: 2929-2935.

Stene LC, Barriga K, Hoffman M, Kean J , Klingensmith G, Norris JM, Erlich HA, Eisenbarth GS, Rewers M. 2006 Normal but increasing hemoglobin A1c levels predict progression from islet autoimmunity to overt type 1 diabetes: Diabetes Autoimmunity Study in the Young (DAISY). Pediatr Diabetes 7:247-253.

Todd, J.A., C.Mijovic, J.Fletcher, D.Jenkins, A.R.Bradwell & A.H.Barnett 1989. Identification of susceptibility loci for insulin-dependent diabetes mellitus by trans-racial gene mapping Nature 338: 587-589.

Ueda H, Howson JM, Esposito L, Heward J, Snook H, Chamberlain G, et al. Association of the T-cell regulatory gene CTLA4 with susceptibility to autoimmune disease. Nature 2003;423:506-511.

Vafiadis P, Bennett ST, Todd JA, Nadeau J, Grabs R, Goodyer CG, et al. Insulin expression in human thymus is modulated by INS VNTR alleles at the IDDM2 locus. Nat Genet 1997;15:289-292.

Vardi, P., A.G.Ziegler, J.H.Matthews, S.Dib, R.J.Keller, A.T.Ricker, J.I.Wolfsdof, R.D.Herskowitz, A.Rabizadeh, G.S.Eisenbarth & J.S.Soeldner 1988. Concentration of insulin autoantibodies at onset of type I diabetes. Inverse log-linear correlation with age Diabetes Care 11: 736-739.

Vardi, P., S.A.Dib, M.Tuttleman, J.E.Connelly, M.Grinbergs, A.Rabizadeh, W.J.Rilley, N.K.McLaren, G.S.Eisenbarth & J.S.Soeldner 1987. Competitive insulin autoantibody assay. Prospective evaluation of subjects at high risk for development of type I diabetes mellitus Diabetes 36: 1286-1291.

Yu, L., D.T.Robles, N.Abiru, P.Kaur, M.Rewers, K.Kelman & G.S.Eisenbarth 2000. Early expression of antiinsulin autoantibodies of humans and the NOD mouse: evidence for early determination of subsequent diabetes Proc Natl Acad Sci USA 97: 1701-1706.

Zhang Xiao-mei, Wang Hong-yuan, Luo Ying-ying and JI Li-nong. HLA-DQ, DR allele polymorphism of type 1 diabetes in the Chinese population: a meta-analysis. Chin Med J 2009;122(8):980-986.